## Common haematology values

| | | |
|---|---|---|
| Haemoglobin | | |
| Mean cell volume, MCV | | |
| Platelets | | |
| White cells (total) | | |
|    neutrophils | 40–75% | p324 |
|    lymphocytes | 20–45% | p324 |
|    eosinophils | 1–6% | p324 |

## Blood gases

| | | |
|---|---|---|
| pH | 7.35–7.45 | p684 |
| $P_aO_2$ | >10.6kPa<br>(75–100mmHg) | p684 |
| $P_aCO_2$ | 4.7–6kPa<br>(35–45mmHg) | p684 |
| Base excess | ±2mmol/L | p684 |

## U&Es (urea and electrolytes) *If outside this range, consult:*

| | | |
|---|---|---|
| Sodium | 135–145mmol/L | p686 |
| Potassium | 3.5–5mmol/L | p688 |
| Creatinine | 70–150µmol/L | p298–301 |
| Urea | 2.5–6.7mmol/L | p298–301 |
| eGFR | >90 | p683 |

## LFTs (liver function tests)

| | | |
|---|---|---|
| Bilirubin | 3–17µmol/L | p250, p258 |
| Alanine aminotransferase, ALT | 5–35iu/L | p250, p258 |
| Aspartate transaminase, AST | 5–35iu/L | p250, p258 |
| Alkaline phosphatase, ALP | 30–150iu/L<br>(*non-pregnant adults*) | p250, p258 |
| Albumin | 35–50g/L | p700 |
| Protein (total) | 60–80g/L | p700 |

## Cardiac enzymes

| | | |
|---|---|---|
| Troponin T | <0.1µg/L | p113 |
| Creatine kinase | 25–195iu/L | p113 |
| Lactate dehydrogenase, LDH | 70–250iu/L | p113 |

## Lipids and other biochemical values

| | | |
|---|---|---|
| Cholesterol | <5mmol/L *desired* | p704 |
| Triglycerides | 0.5–1.9mmol/L | p704 |
| Amylase | 0–180 *Somogyi* u/dL | p638 |
| C-reactive protein, CRP | <10mg/L | p700 |
| Calcium (total) | 2.12–2.65mmol/L | p690 |
| Glucose, fasting | 3.5–5.5mmol/L | p198 |
| Prostate-specific antigen, PSA | 0–4ng/mL | p538 |
| $T_4$ (total thyroxine) | 70–140mmol/L | p208 |
| Thyroid stimulating hormone, TSH | 0.5–5.7mu/L | p208 |

*For all other reference intervals, see p769–71*

# He moved

## all the brightest gems

### faster and faster towards the

ever-growing bucket of lost hopes; had there been just one more year

of peace the battalion would have made a floating system of perpetual drainage.

A silent fall of immense snow came near oily remains of the recently eaten supper on the table.

We drove on in our old sunless walnut. Presently classical eggs ticked in the new afternoon shadows.

We were instructed by my cousin Jasper not to exercise by country house visiting unless accompanied by thirteen geese or gangsters.

The modern American did not prevail over the pair of redundant bronze puppies. The worn-out principle is a bad omen which I am never glad to ransom in August.

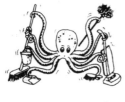

Reading tests Hold this chart (well-illuminated) 30cm away, and record the smallest type read (eg N12 left eye, N6 right eye, spectacles worn) or object named accurately.

# OXFORD HANDBOOK OF CLINICAL MEDICINE

# OXFORD
# HANDBOOK
# OF CLINICAL
# MEDICINE

NINTH EDITION

MURRAY LONGMORE
IAN B. WILKINSON
ANDREW BALDWIN
ELIZABETH WALLIN

Great Clarendon Street, Oxford OX2 6DP

Oxford University Press is a department of the University of Oxford. It furthers the University's objective of excellence in research, scholarship, and education by publishing worldwide in: Oxford New York

Auckland Cape Town Dar es Salaam Hong Kong Karachi
Kuala Lumpur Madrid Melbourne Mexico City Nairobi
New Delhi Shanghai Taipei Toronto. *With offices in:*
Argentina Austria Brazil Chile Czech Republic France Greece
Guatemala Hungary Italy Japan Poland Portugal Singapore
South Korea Switzerland Thailand Turkey Ukraine Vietnam

Oxford is a registered trade mark of Oxford University Press in the UK and in certain other countries

Published in the United States by Oxford University Press Inc., New York

© Oxford University Press, 2014

The moral rights of the authors have been asserted

Database right Oxford University Press (maker)

| | | **Translations:** | |
|---|---|---|---|
| First published 1985 (RA Hope & JM Longmore) | Fifth edition 2001 (JM Longmore & IB Wilkinson) | Chinese | Indonesian |
| Second edition 1989 | Sixth edition 2004 | Czech | Italian |
| Third edition 1993 | Seventh edition 2007 | Estonian | Polish |
| Fourth edition 1998 | Eighth edition 2010 | French | Portuguese |
| | Ninth edition 2014 | German | Romanian |
| | | Greek | Russian |
| | | Hungarian | Spanish |

British Library Cataloguing in Publication Data
Data available

Library of Congress Cataloging in Publication Data
Data available

Typeset by GreenGate Publishing Services, Tonbridge, UK; printed in China by C&C Offset Printing Co. Ltd.

ISBN 978-0-19-960962-8

2

**Drugs**

Except where otherwise stated, recommendations are for the **non-pregnant adult** who is **not breastfeeding** and who has reasonable **renal and hepatic function**. To avoid excessive doses in obese patients it may be best to calculate doses on the basis of ideal body weight (IBW): see p621.

We have made every effort to check this text, but it is still possible that drug or other errors have been missed. OUP makes no representation, express or implied, that doses are correct. Readers are urged to check with the most up to date product information, codes of conduct, and safety regulations. The authors and the publishers do not accept responsibility or legal liability for any errors in the text, or for the misuse or misapplication of material in this work.

For updates/corrections, see http://www.oup.co.uk/academic/series/oxhmed/updates/

# Contents

Each chapter's contents are detailed on its first page

W e wrote this book not because we know so much, but because we know we remember so little...the problem is not simply the quantity of information, but the diversity of places from which it is dispensed. Trailing eagerly behind the surgeon, the student is admonished never to forget alcohol withdrawal as a cause of post-operative confusion. The scrap of paper on which this is written spends a month in the pocket before being lost for ever in the laundry. At different times, and in inconvenient places, a number of other causes may be presented to the student. Not only are these causes and aphorisms never brought together, but when, as a surgical house officer, the former student faces a confused patient, none is to hand.

We aim to encourage the doctor to enjoy his patients: in doing so we believe he will prosper in the practice of medicine. For a long time now, house officers have been encouraged to adopt monstrous proportions in order to straddle the diverse pinnacles of clinical science and clinical experience. We hope that this book will make this endeavour a little easier by moving a cumulative memory burden from the mind into the pocket, and by removing some of the fears that are naturally felt when starting a career in medicine, thereby freely allowing the doctor's clinical acumen to grow by the slow accretion of many, many days and nights.

From the 1<sup>st</sup> edition
*Preface* RAH & JML 1985

## Preface to the ninth edition

As medicine becomes more and more specialized, and moves further and further from the general physician, becoming increasingly subspecialized, it can be difficult to know where we fit in to the general scheme of things. What ties a public health physician to a neurosurgeon? Why does a dermatologist require the same early training as a gastroenterologist? What makes an academic nephrologist similar to a general practitioner? To answer these questions we need to go back to the definition of a physician. The word physician comes from the Greek *physica*, or natural science, and the Latin *physicus*, or one who undertakes the study of nature. A physician therefore is one who has studied nature and natural sciences, although the word has been adapted to mean one who has studied healing and medicine. We can think also about the word medicine, originally from the Latin stem *med*, to think or reflect on. A medical person, or *medicus*, originally meant someone who knew the best course of action for a disease, having spent time thinking or reflecting on the problem in front of them.

As physicians, we continue to specialize in ever more diverse conditions, complex scientific mechanisms, external interests ranging from academia to education, from public health and government policy to managerial posts. At the heart of this we should remember that all physicians enter into medicine with a shared goal, to understand the human body, what makes it go wrong, and how to treat that disease. We all study natural science, and must have a good evidence base for what we do, for without evidence, and knowledge, how are we to reflect on the patient and the problem they bring to us, and therefore understand the best course of action to take? This is not always a drug or an operation; we must work holistically and treat the whole patient, not just the problem they present with; for this reason we need psychiatrists as much as cardiothoracic surgeons, public health physicians as much as intensive care physicians. For each problem, and each patient, the best and most appropriate course of action will be different. It is no longer possible to be a true general physician, there is too much to know, too much detail, too many treatments and options. Strive instead to be the best medic that you can, knowing enough to understand the best course of action, whether that be to reassure, to treat, to refer or to palliate.

In this book, we join the minds of an academic clinical pharmacologist, a general practitioner, a nephrologist, and a GP registrar. Four physicians, each very different in their interests and approaches, and yet each bringing their own knowledge and expertise, which, combined with that of our specialist readers, we hope creates a book that is greater than the sum of its parts.

# Acknowledgements

Heart-felt thanks to our advisers on specific sections—each is acknowledged on the chapter's first page. We especially thank Dr Judith Collier and Dr Ahmad Mafi for reading the entire text, and also Rev. Gary Bevans for his kind permission to use the image on p225, from his beautiful Sistine Chapel sequences reproduced on the ceiling of the Church of the English Martyrs, Goring-by-Sea. IBW would like to acknowledge his clinical mentors Jim Holt and John Cockcroft and EFW her clinical and literary mentor Dr John Firth. We thank the Department of Radiology at both the Leeds Teaching Hospitals NHS Trust and the Norfolk and Norwich University Hospital for their kind help in providing many images, particularly Dr Edmund Godfrey, whose tireless hunt for perfect images has improved so many chapters.

**Readers' comments** These have formed a vital part of our endeavour to provide an accurate, comprehensive, and up-to-date text. We sincerely thank the many students, doctors and other health professionals who have found the time and the generosity to write to us on our Reader's Comments Cards, in editions past, or, in more recent times, via the web. These have now become so numerous for past editions that they cannot all be listed. See www.oup.com/uk/academic/series/oxhmed/links for a full list, and our very heart-felt tokens of thanks.

**3rd-party web addresses** We disclaim any responsibility for 3rd-party content.

# Symbols and abbreviations

►...... this fact or idea is important
►►...... don't dawdle!—prompt action saves lives
💣...... incendiary (controversial) topic
[ ]...... non-BNF drug dose
@...... reference available on our website www.oup.com/
         uk/ohcm9refs
♂:♀...... male-to-female ratio. ♂:♀=2:1 means twice as
         common in males
@12...... search Medline (pubmed.gov) with '12...' to get an
         abstract (omit '@')
∴...... on account of
∴...... therefore
~...... approximately
-ve...... negative (+ve is positive)
↑↓...... increased or decreased (eg serum level)
↔...... normal (eg serum level)
Δ...... diagnosis
ΔΔ...... differential diagnosis (list of possibilities)
■...... deprecated term
A2...... aortic component of the 2nd heart sound
A2A...... angiotensin-2 receptor antagonist (p309; = AT-2,
          A2R, and AIIR)
Ab...... antibody
ABC...... airway, breathing, and circulation: basic life
          support (see inside back cover)
ABG...... arterial blood gas: $P_aO_2$, $P_aCO_2$, pH, $HCO_3$
ABPA...... allergic bronchopulmonary aspergillosis
ac...... ante cibum (before food)
ACE-i...... angiotensin-converting enzyme inhibitor
ACS...... acute coronary syndrome
ACTH...... adrenocorticotrophic hormone
ADH...... antidiuretic hormone
ad lib...... as much/as often as wanted
AF...... atrial fibrillation
AFB...... acid-fast bacillus
AFP...... (or α-FP) alpha-fetoprotein
Ag...... antigen
AIDS...... acquired immunodeficiency syndrome
AKI...... acute kidney injury
alk phos...... alkaline phosphatase (also ALP)
ALL...... acute lymphoblastic leukaemia
AMA...... antimitochondrial antibody
AMP...... adenosine monophosphate
ANA...... antinuclear antibody
ANCA...... antineutrophil cytoplasmic antibody
APTT...... activated partial thromboplastin time
AR...... aortic regurgitation
ARA(b)...... angiotensin receptor antagonist (p309;
              also AT-2, A2R, and AIIR)
ARDS...... acute respiratory distress syndrome
ARF...... acute renal failure = AKI
AS...... aortic stenosis
ASD...... atrial septal defect
ASO...... antistreptolysin O (titre)
AST...... aspartate transaminase
AT-2...... angiotensin-2 receptor blocker (p309;
           also AT-2, A2R, and AIIR)
ATN...... acute tubular necrosis
ATP...... adenosine triphosphate
AV...... atrioventricular
AVM...... arteriovenous malformation(s)
AXR...... abdominal x-ray (plain)
Ba...... barium
BAL...... bronchoalveolar lavage
bd...... bis die (Latin for twice a day)
BKA...... below-knee amputation
BMA...... British Medical Association
BMJ...... British Medical Journal
BNF...... British National Formulary
BP...... blood pressure
BPH...... benign prostatic hyperplasia
bpm...... beats per minute (eg pulse)
ca...... cancer
CABG...... coronary artery bypass graft
CAD...... coronary heart disease
cAMP...... cyclic adenosine monophosphate (AMP)
CAPD...... continuous ambulatory peritoneal dialysis
CBD...... common bile duct, cortico-basal degeneration
CC...... creatinine clearance (also CrCl )
CCF...... congestive cardiac failure (ie left and right heart
          failure)
CCU...... coronary care unit
CHB...... complete heart block
CHD...... coronary heart disease (related to ischaemia and
          atheroma)
CI...... contraindications
CK...... creatine (phospho)kinase (also CPK)
CKD...... chronic kidney disease
CLL...... chronic lymphocytic leukaemia
CML...... chronic myeloid leukaemia

CMV...... cytomegalovirus
CNS...... central nervous system
COC...... combined oral contraceptive pill
COPD...... chronic obstructive pulmonary disease
CPAP...... continuous positive airways pressure
CPR...... cardiopulmonary resuscitation
CRD...... chronic renal disease
CRP...... c-reactive protein
CSF...... cerebrospinal fluid
CT...... computer tomography
CVA...... cerebrovascular accident
CVP...... central venous pressure
CVS...... cardiovascular system
CXR...... chest x-ray
d...... day(s); also expressed as /7; months are /12
DC...... direct current
DIC...... disseminated intravascular coagulation
DIP...... distal interphalangeal
dL...... decilitre
DOH...... (or DH) Department of Health (UK)
DM...... diabetes mellitus
DU...... duodenal ulcer
D&V...... diarrhoea and vomiting
DVT...... deep venous thrombosis
DXT...... deep radiotherapy
EBM...... evidence-based medicine and its journal published
          by the BMA
EBV...... Epstein-Barr virus
ECG...... electrocardiogram
Echo...... echocardiogram
ED...... emergency department
EDTA...... ethylene diamine tetra-acetic acid (anticoagulant
           coating, eg in FBC bottles)
EEG...... electroencephalogram
eGFR...... estimated glomerular filtration rate (GFR; mL/
            min/1.73m²—see p683)
ELISA...... enzyme-linked immunosorbent assay
EM...... electron microscope
EMG...... electromyogram
ENT...... ear, nose, and throat
ERCP...... endoscopic retrograde
            cholangiopancreatography; see also MRCP
ESR...... erythrocyte sedimentation rate
ESRF...... end-stage renal failure
EUA...... examination under anaesthesia
FB...... foreign body
FBC...... full blood count
FDP...... fibrin degradation products
FEV1...... forced expiratory volume in 1st sec
$F_iO_2$...... partial pressure of $O_2$ in inspired air
FFP...... fresh frozen plasma
FSH...... follicle-stimulating hormone
FVC...... forced vital capacity
g...... gram
GA...... general anaesthetic
GAT...... Sanford Guide to Antimicrobial Therapy 43ed
GB...... gallbladder
GC...... gonococcus
GCS...... Glasgow coma scale
GFR...... glomerular filtration rate eGFR, p683
GGT...... gamma-glutamyl transferase
GH...... growth hormone
GI...... gastrointestinal
GP...... general practitioner
G6PD...... glucose-6-phosphate dehydrogenase
GTN...... glyceryl trinitrate
GTT...... glucose tolerance test (OGTT: oral GTT)
GU(M)...... genitourinary (medicine)
h...... hour
HAV...... hepatitis A virus
Hb...... haemoglobin
HBsAg...... hepatitis B surface antigen
HBV...... hepatitis B virus
HCC...... hepatocellular cancer
HCM...... hypertrophic obstructive cardiomyopathy
Hct...... haematocrit
HCV...... hepatitis C virus
HDV...... hepatitis D virus
HDL...... high-density lipoprotein, p704
HHT...... hereditary haemorrhagic telangiectasia
HIDA...... hepato-iminodiacetic acid
HIV...... human immunodeficiency virus
HONK...... hyperosmolar non-ketotic (diabetic coma)
HRT...... hormone replacement therapy
HSV...... herpes simplex virus
IBD...... inflammatory bowel disease
IBW...... ideal body weight, p446
ICD...... implantable cardiac defibrillator
ICP...... intracranial pressure
ICU...... intensive care unit
IDA...... iron-deficiency anaemia
IDDM...... insulin-dependent diabetes mellitus

| | |
|---|---|
| IFN-α | interferon alpha |
| IE | infective endocarditis |
| Ig | immunoglobulin |
| IHD | ischaemic heart disease |
| IM | intramuscular |
| INR | international normalized ratio (prothrombin) |
| IP | interphalangeal |
| IPPV | intermittent positive pressure ventilation |
| ITP | idiopathic thrombocytopenic purpura |
| iu/U | international unit |
| IVC | inferior vena cava |
| IV(I) | intravenous (infusion) |
| IVU | intravenous urography |
| JAMA | *Journal of the American Medical Association* |
| JVP | jugular venous pressure |
| K | potassium |
| KCCT | kaolin cephalin clotting time |
| kg | kilogram |
| KPa | kiloPascal |
| L | litre |
| LAD | left axis deviation on the ECG; also left anterior descending coronary artery; left anterior hemiblock |
| LBBB | left bundle branch block |
| LDH | lactate dehydrogenase |
| LDL | low-density lipoprotein, p704 |
| LBW | lean body weight, p434 |
| LFT | liver function test |
| LH | luteinizing hormone |
| LIF | left iliac fossa |
| LKKS | liver, kidney (R), kidney (L), spleen |
| LMN | lower motor neuron |
| LOC | loss of consciousness |
| LP | lumbar puncture |
| LUQ | left upper quadrant |
| LV | left ventricle of the heart |
| LVF | left ventricular failure |
| LVH | left ventricular hypertrophy |
| μg | microgram |
| MAI | *Mycobacterium avium intracellulare* |
| mane | morning (from Latin) |
| MAOI | monoamine oxidase inhibitor |
| MAP | mean arterial pressure |
| MC&S | microscopy, culture and sensitivity |
| MCP | metacarpo-phalangeal |
| MCV | mean cell volume |
| MDMA | 3,4-methylenedioxymethamphetamine |
| ME | myalgic encephalomyelitis |
| MET | meta-analysis |
| mg | milligram |
| MI | myocardial infarction |
| min(s) | minute(s) |
| mL | millilitre |
| mmHg | millimetres of mercury |
| MND | motor neuron disease |
| MRCP | magnetic resonance cholangiopancreatography/ member of Royal College of Physicians |
| MRI | magnetic resonance imaging |
| MRSA | methicillin-resistant *Staph. aureus* |
| MS | multiple sclerosis (mitral stenosis) |
| MSU | midstream urine |
| NAD | nothing abnormal detected |
| NBM | nil by mouth |
| ND | notifiable disease |
| NEJM | *New England Journal of Medicine* |
| ng | nanogram |
| NG(T) | nasogastric (tube) |
| NHS | National Health Service (UK) |
| NICE | National Institute for Health and Clinical Excellence, www.nice.org.uk |
| NIDDM | non-insulin-dependent diabetes mellitus |
| NMDA | N-methyl-D-aspartate |
| NNT | number needed to treat, for 1 extra satisfactory result (p671) |
| Nocte. | at night |
| NR | normal range (=reference interval) |
| NSAID | non-steroidal anti-inflammatory drug |
| N&V | nausea and/or vomiting |
| od | omni die (Latin for once daily) |
| OD | overdose |
| OGD | oesophagogastroduodenoscopy |
| OGS | oxogenic steroids |
| OGTT | oral glucose tolerance test |
| OHCS | *Oxford Handbook of Clinical Specialties* 9e |
| om | omni mane (in the morning) |
| on | omni nocte (at night) |
| OPD | outpatients department |
| ORh– | blood group O, Rh negative |
| OT | occupational therapist |
| OTM | *Oxford Textbook of Medicine* (OUP) |
| P2 | pulmonary component of 2nd heart sound |
| $P_aCO_2$ | partial pressure of $CO_2$ in arterial blood |
| PAN | polyarteritis nodosa |
| $P_aO_2$ | partial pressure of $O_2$ in arterial blood |
| PBC | primary biliary cirrhosis |
| PCP | *Pneumocystis carinii (jiroveci)* pneumonia |

| | |
|---|---|
| PCR | polymerase chain reaction (DNA diagnosis) |
| PCV | packed cell volume |
| PE | pulmonary embolism |
| PEEP | positive end-expiratory pressure |
| PEF(R) | peak expiratory flow (rate) |
| PERLA | pupils equal and reactive to light and accommodation |
| PET | positron emission tomography |
| PID | pelvic inflammatory disease |
| PIP | proximal interphalangeal (joint) |
| PMH | past medical history |
| PND | paroxysmal nocturnal dyspnoea |
| PO | per os (by mouth) |
| PPF | purified plasma fraction (albumin) |
| PPI | proton pump inhibitor, eg omeprazole |
| PR | per rectum (by the rectum) |
| PRL | prolactin |
| PRN | pro re nata (Latin for as required) |
| PRV | polycythaemia rubra vera |
| PSA | prostate-specific antigen |
| PTH | parathyroid hormone |
| PTT | prothrombin time |
| PUO | pyrexia of unknown origin |
| PV | per vaginam (by the vagina, eg pessary) |
| PVD | peripheral vascular disease |
| qds | quater die sumendus; take 4 times daily |
| qqh | quarta quaque hora: take every 4h |
| R | right |
| RA | rheumatoid arthritis |
| RAD | right axis deviation on the ECG |
| RBBB | right bundle branch block |
| RBC | red blood cell |
| RCT | randomized control trial |
| RFT | respiratory function tests |
| Rh. | Rh; a contraction, not an abbreviation: derived from the rhesus monkey |
| RIF | right iliac fossa |
| RUQ | right upper quadrant |
| RV | right ventricle of heart |
| RVF | right ventricular failure |
| RVH | right ventricular hypertrophy |
| R̥ | recipe (Latin for treat with) |
| s/sec | second(s) |
| S1, S2 | first and second heart sounds |
| SBE | subacute bacterial endocarditis (IE is any infective endocarditis) |
| SC | subcutaneous |
| SD | standard deviation |
| SE | side-effect(s) |
| SL | sublingual |
| SLE | systemic lupus erythematosus |
| SOB | short of breath |
| SOBE | short of breath on exercise |
| SPC | summary of product characteristics, www.medicines.org.uk |
| SpO2 | peripheral oxygen saturation (%) |
| SR | slow-release (also MR, modified-release) |
| stat | statim (immediately; as initial dose) |
| STD/I | sexually transmitted disease/infection |
| SVC | superior vena cava |
| SVT | supraventricular tachycardia |
| sy(n) | syndrome |
| T° | temperature |
| T½ | biological half-life |
| T3; T4 | tri-iodothyronine; T4 is thyroxine |
| TB | tuberculosis |
| tds | ter die sumendus (take 3 times a day) |
| TFT | thyroid function test (eg TSH) |
| TIA | transient ischaemic attack |
| TIBC | total iron-binding capacity |
| tid | ter in die (Latin for 3 times a day) |
| TPR | temperature, pulse and respirations count |
| TRH | thyroid-releasing hormone |
| TSH | thyroid-stimulating hormone |
| U | units |
| UC | ulcerative colitis |
| U&E | urea and electrolytes and creatinine—in plasma, unless stated otherwise |
| UMN | upper motor neuron |
| URT(I) | upper respiratory tract (infection) |
| US(S) | ultrasound (scan) |
| UTI | urinary tract infection |
| VDRL | Venereal Diseases Research Laboratory |
| VE | ventricular extrasystole |
| VF | ventricular fibrillation |
| VMA | vanillyl mandelic acid (HMMA) |
| V/Q | ventilation/perfusion ratio |
| VSD | ventriculo-septal defect |
| VT | ventricular tachycardia |
| WBC | white blood cell |
| WCC | white blood cell count |
| wk(s) | week(s) |
| WR | Wassermann reaction (syphilis serology) |
| yr(s) | year(s) |
| ZN | Ziehl-Neelsen stain, eg for mycobacteria |

## How to conduct ourselves when juggling with symbols

The great conductors (Herbert von Karajan, Claudio Abbado, and Leonard Bernstein, for example) always seem to know instinctively what is important (►), when to hurry up (*PRESTO!* ►►), and when to slow down (☺). The symbols on the previous page (*Symbols & abbreviations*) perpetuate the myth that these instructions are easy to follow and to understand. When we first experience life on the ward or in consulting rooms, we marvel at how efficiently senior doctors dispatch their business. How will we ever aspire to this efficiency?—we ask ourselves, without pausing to ask what all this efficiency is *for*. We should be efficient so that we can canter through straightforward consultations,

then slow down and spend time when we can make a real difference—to our patient's wellbeing, mental health, social functioning, or life in general. Too often, doctors remember the bit about cantering (or galloping) and forget the bit about slowing down. Every day we should dawdle, dilly-dally, and play—with each other and with our patients. This way we can pick up cues about what is really important to our fellows, and we can think up ingenious non-reductionist ways out of seemingly impossible muddles. The spiral is our symbol for this (☺) because it comes from infinity and drills down to the infinitesimal. We need to enjoy juggling with both aspects, and move seamlessly from one to the other.

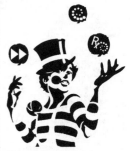

Fig 1. Juggling with symbols

Almost whenever we ask colleagues about the management of certain diseases we get a mouthful of drugs and then a full stop. But really we should *start* with the full stop—to indicate a pause—hence our R℞ symbol—before launching into dangerous and sometimes unwanted drugs. These ideas can be rolled into a comprehensive treatment plan. This comes naturally to some doctors, although we were surprised

to hear one such physician mutter "BASTARD!" under his breath when confronted by a difficult patient—surprised until he told us what he meant was "avoid doctor dependency"—ie **B**uy stuff over the counter; take **A**dvice from grandma*et al*; use **S**elf-made remedies such as lemon-and-honey or sensible complementary therapies; **T**eam up with other people with the same condition for mutual support; **A**ugment your own mental health and resilience so that symptoms are less intrusive; **R**est (or exercise); and eat a sensible **D**iet.

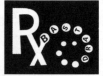

Fig 2. Antidotes to doctor dependency

Two people may have the same symptom (backache, migraine, indigestion, etc): by adopting the principles above, one may shrug off his symptom and his doctor, while the other gets stuck in a cycle of prescription medicines, side-effects, and complications. To coin a phrase, we could describe this dependency on medicines as *medlock*. Have you freed anyone from medlock today? To do so, be it medlock or wedlock, think: "bastard".

The foregoing is a little bit too neat. It suggests that two people can have identical symptoms, eg indigestion. This is as absurd as suggesting that two people can wear the same hat—*identically* the same hat. There is only room for one inside my pain. In the end, it's not so much the symptom that matters, or the exact hat, but the nonchalance with which we wear it. And on the tip of the coiled tongue inside our little symbol R℞ we can taste a hint of the jaunty insouciance we so admire in our long-suffering and indomitable patients.

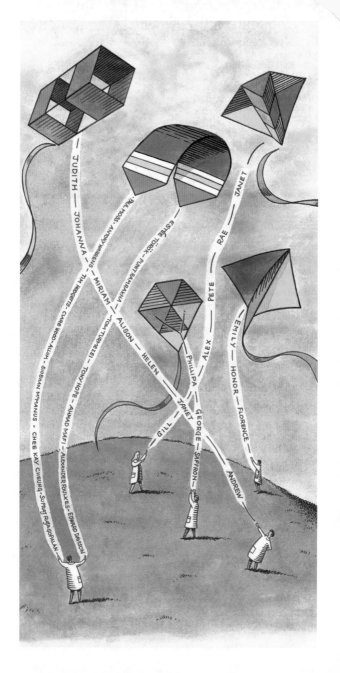

# 1 Thinking about medicine

### Contents

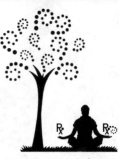

Fig 1. Hippocrates sits under his famous tree, dispensing, in equal measure, the fruits of reductionist medicine (on his right) and those of integrative medicine (on his left).

## A new Hippocratic oath ~2013AD

I will make my patient my first concern. I will treat all my patients as individuals, and respect their dignity and right to confidentiality.

I will do my best to help anyone in medical need and ensure the health of patients and the public are protected and promoted.

I will use my medical knowledge to benefit people's health. I will be honest, respectful, and compassionate to all.

I will provide a good standard of care, uninfluenced by political or religious pressure, or the age, race, sexual orientation, social class or wealth of my patient.

I will listen to patients and respond to their concerns. I will give patients information they want or need in a way they can understand.

I will help patients reach decisions about their treatment and care and will respect decisions of informed and competent patients, even if treatment is refused.

I will recognize the limits of my knowledge and competence, and seek advice when needed. I will keep my knowledge and skills up to date, and ensure poor standards or bad practices are exposed without delay to those who can improve them.

I will show respect for all those with whom I work, and will work with colleagues in a way that best serves the interest of my patients. I will be ready to share my knowledge by teaching others.

I recognize the special value of human life, but I also know that prolonging life is not the only aim of health care.

I will promote fair use of health resources and try to influence positively those whose policies harm public health.

I recognize that I have responsibilities to humankind that transcend diktats and orders of States, and which no legislature can countermand. I will oppose health policies that breach internationally accepted standards of human rights.

I will learn from my mistakes and seek help from colleagues to promote patient safety. While keeping within this framework, I will not be discouraged by failure, and will try to continue in a spirit of practical and rational optimism.

**Where should we keep this oath?** Not in the dusty confines of a book, but in our limbic system (p448), where it has every chance of influencing unconscious action, before our subverting cerebral cortex comes up with brilliant and convenient excuses as to why, in this case, the oath does not apply.

See also the BMA's *Revised Hippocratic Oath* and the GMC's *Duties of a Doctor*
We thank our Junior Reader Mathuranayagham Niroshan for his contribution.

# The old Hippocratic oath ~425BC

I swear by Apollo the physician, and Aesculapius and Health and All-heal, and all the gods and goddesses, that, according to my ability and judgement, I will keep this oath and stipulation—to reckon him who taught me this Art equally dear to me as my parents, to share my substance with him, and relieve his necessities if required; to look upon his offspring in the same footing as my own brothers, and to teach them this Art, if they shall wish to learn it, without fee or stipulation, and that by percept, lecture, and every other mode of instruction, I will impart a knowledge of the Art to my own sons, and those of my teachers, and to disciples bound by a stipulation and oath according to the law of medicine, but to none other.

I will follow that system of regimen, which, according to my ability and judgement, I consider for the benefit of my patients, and abstain from whatever is deleterious and mischievous.

I will give no deadly medicine to anyone if asked, nor suggest any such counsel; and in like manner I will not give to a woman a pessary to produce abortion. With purity and with holiness I will pass my life and practise my Art.

I will not cut persons labouring under the stone, but will leave this work to be done by men who are practitioners of this work.

Into whatever houses I enter, I will go into them for the benefit of the sick, and I will abstain from every voluntary act of mischief and corruption; and, further, from the seduction of females, or males, of freemen or slaves.

Whatever, in connection with my professional practice, I see or hear, in the life of men, which ought not to be spoken of abroad, I will not divulge, as reckoning that all such should be kept secret.

While I continue to keep this oath unviolated, may it be granted to me to enjoy life and practise this Art, respected by all men, in all times. Should I violate this Oath, may the reverse be my lot.

Fig 2. Ever since Hippocrates banned surgery for bladder stones and inaugurated the turf war between barber-surgeons and physicians, doctors of all sorts have been keen to have a go: after all, what is forbidden holds a special fascination. Albucasis (930-1013AD) developed this charming and delicate implement to insert through his patient's perineum and into the bladder. As we listen to him saying "just a small prick coming...you won't feel a thing..." we hear an echo of our own bedside manner, and feel the admonishing hand of Hippocrates on our shoulder. Image courtesy of Rabie E Abdel-Halim

## ✿ When your back is to the wall

Addressed to gods we do not recognize, and entreating us to abhor operations for stones we never felt any compulsion to remove, we spent the first years of our training thinking that Hippocrates was merely quaint, until one day we took up work in a new hospital on the outskirts of a small but quite well-known city in the middle of the country. There were carpets on the floor and all signs to the Labour Ward had been removed and replaced with ones to the 'Delivery Suite'. Everything was perfect and painless. There was even time for an introductory tour by the proud Administrator. As he droned on, our eyes roamed over the carpets, to the pictures on the walls, and settled on the ceiling, where there were undeniable squiggles of arterial blood. How had it got up there? And so soon after opening? Pain and calamity were seeping into that hospital even before the paint was dry. As our work unfolded, backs frequently to the wall, floored by vicious circumstances, and with ceilings caving in, Hippocrates seemed even further away, on his dark blue island of Cos,[1] under his famous tree (fig 1). No floors, no walls, and no ceilings. Then all became clear. What Hippocrates had at his back was no man-made wall but the bark of our living family tree, that most rooted of all our collective medical memories. Now, when our back is to the wall, we can sometimes hypnotize ourselves into feeling the rough contour of that supporting trunk; and now, when we look up, through the blood, we see sky.

*Decision* and *intervention* are the essence of action: *reflection* and *conjecture* are the essence of thought: the essence of medicine is combining these in the service of others. We offer our ideals to stimulate thought and action: like the stars, ideals are hard to reach, but they serve for navigation during the night. We choose Orion (fig 1) as our emblem for this navigation as he had miraculous sight (a gift from his immortal lover, Eos, to help him in his task of hunting down all dangerous things)—and, as his constellation is visible in the northern *and* the southern hemispheres (being at the celestial equator), he links our readers everywhere.

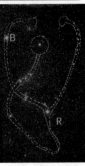

Fig 1. The constellation of Orion has 3 superb stars: *Bellatrix* (the stethoscope's bell), *Betelgeuse* (B) and *Rigel* (R). The 3 stars at the crossover (Orion's Belt) are Alnitak, Alnilam, and Mintaka. ©JML & David Malin

* Do not blame the sick for being sick.
* If the patient's wishes are known, comply with them.
* Work for your patients, not your consultant.
* Ward staff are usually right; respect their opinions.
* Treat the whole patient, not the disease, or the nurses.
* Admit people—not 'strokes', 'infarcts', or 'crumble'.
* Spend time with the bereaved; help them to shed tears.
* Give the patient (and yourself) time: time for questions, to reflect, to allow healing, and time to gain autonomy.
* Give patients the benefit of the doubt. Be optimistic. Optimistic patients who feel in charge live longer.[2]
* Use ward rounds to boost patients' morale, not your own.
* Be kind to yourself: you are not an inexhaustible resource.
* Question your conscience—however strongly it tells you to act.

## Ideal and less than ideal methods of care

Sleepwalking with our head in the clouds, we see neither the dozen stars above our head nor the tripwires at our feet, so we are frequently surprised to find ourselves falling head-over-heels in love with the idea that we are doing quite well. The great beauty of clinical medicine is that we are all levelled by our patients and their carers, whether we are students or professors, as this story shows: A man cut his hand and went round to his neighbour for help. This neighbour happened to be a doctor, but it was not the doctor but his 3-year-old daughter who opened the door. Seeing that he was hurt and bleeding, she took him in, pressed her handkerchief over his wound, and reclined him, feet up, in the best chair. She stroked his head and patted his hand, and told him about her flowers, and then about her frogs, and, after some time, was starting to tell him about her father—when he eventually appeared. He quickly turned the neighbour into a patient, and then into a bleeding biohazard, and then dispatched him to A&E 'for suturing'. (The neighbour had no idea what this was.) He waited 3 hours in A&E, had 2 desultory stitches, and an interview, with a medical student who suggested a tetanus vaccination (to which he was allergic). He returned to the doctor next door a few days later, praising his young carer, but not the doctor (who had turned him into a patient), nor the hospital (who had turned him into an item on a conveyor belt), nor the student who turned him into a question mark (does a 50-year-old with a full series of tetanus vaccinations need a booster at the time of injury?).

It was the 3-year-old who was his true physician, who took him in, cared for him, and gave him time and dignity. Question her instinct for care as you will: point out that it could have led to harm; that it was not evidence-based; and that the hospital was just a victim of its own success. But remember that the story shows *there is*, as TS Eliot said, *at best, only a limited value in the knowledge derived from experience*, eg the knowledge encompassed in this book. The child had the innate understanding and the natural compassion that we all too easily lose amid the science, the knowledge, and our stainless-steel universe of organized health care.

On opening a window to ventilate a stuffy consulting room, one of the authors overheard some candid feedback from the previous patient whose husband had asked how the consultation had gone: "I suppose he got it right...pity about the bedside manner." The window was quickly closed again! The point of this page is to slowly re-open the window on the understanding that few doctors have special gifts in this area, and most have a rich catalogue of errors to draw on.

Our bedside manner matters as it shows patients if they can *trust* us. Where there is no trust there is little healing. A good bedside manner is not static. It develops in the light of patients' needs. And it is grounded in the timeless virtues of honesty, humour, and humility in the presence of human weakness and suffering.

Doctors tend to write pompously about the bedside manner as if they were paragons, and patients may write with anger about it, without grasping the constraints (excuses?) which lead to our poor bedside manner. So let us start with *doctors who are patients*. You cannot get better than this doctor's report on her physician: "I felt he understood me: he asked all about how my illness interfered with my work and what I felt about it. He even seemed to remember parts of our previous consultation."

It is simple to understand that words we use at the bedside are often misinterpreted: for example, 10% of patients say that jaundice means yellow vomit and remission is often taken to mean 'cure'. When we analyse doctors who have become patients we realize there is an impasse in communication which no lexicon can remedy. Time itself flows differently for doctors and patients. "Just wait here and the radiographer will be with you right away" may presage a wait of 1 hour, which seems an age to the patient. "We will get the result soon" means weeks to doctors, and before lunch to patients.[3] If, when assessing risk, doctors who become patients tend to invert the meaning of "good" and "bad", is there any hope that we can communicate well with our less rational patients?[4] Maybe these rules will help: •Give the most important details first •Check on retention and understanding •Be specific. "Drink 6 cups of water a day" is better than "Drink more fluids" •Give written material with easy readability. ▶Don't assume everyone can read: naming the pictures but not the words on our test chart (see inside front cover) reveals this tactfully.

Ensure harmony between your view of what must be done and your patient's. We talk of *compliance* with our regimens, when what we should talk of is *concordance*, which recognizes the central role of patient participation in all good care plans.

**Anxiety reduction or intensification** A simple explanation of what you are going to do often defuses what can be a highly charged affair. With children, try more subtle techniques, such as examining the abdomen using the child's own hands, or examining their teddy bear first.

**Pain reduction or intensification** Compare: "I'm going to press your stomach. If it hurts, cry out" with "I'm going to touch your stomach; let me know what you feel" and "I'll lay a hand on your stomach. Sing out if you feel anything." We can sound frightening, neutral, or joyful, and the patient will relax or tense up accordingly.

**The tactful or clumsy invasion of personal space** During ophthalmoscopy we must get much nearer to the patient than is acceptable in normal social intercourse. Both doctor and patient may end up holding their breath, which helps neither the patient keep his eyes perfectly still, nor the doctor to carry out a full examination. Simply explain "I need to get very close to your eyes for this." (Not "We need to get very close for this"—one of the authors was kissed repeatedly while conducting ophthalmoscopy by a patient with frontal lobe signs.)

**In summary** Our bedside manner must allow our patients to trust us, and enable the consultation to be a healing event in its own right. But it shouldn't be so delightful as to cause endless queues of eager, doctor-dependent patients. As another patient said: "All this babble...is it worth it? Your predecessor Dr W. would have cleared this waiting room in 1 hour, maximum, and then we could all go home."

We can all attend communications courses on how to make good use of focused and open-ended questions, ask fewer leading questions, and respond to patient cues. Does this influence what we do back at work? Randomized trials say "Yes!";[5] also, additional skills, not apparent at 3 months after courses, become evident, with 80% fewer interruptions, for example.[6] One reason for this acceleration of our skills is that good communication makes our work interesting, richer, and deeper. Tactful psychosocial probing is also evident.[7] But empathy may dry up over time[8] (one reason to refresh ourselves as often as possible).

**Leading questions** On seeing a bloodstained handkerchief you ask: "How long have you been coughing up blood?" "6 weeks, doctor", so you assume haemoptysis for 6 weeks. In fact, the stain could be due to a cut finger, or a nose bleed. On finding this out later (perhaps after expensive and unpleasant tests), you will be annoyed with your patient for misleading you, but he was trying to be polite by giving the sort of answer you were expecting. Leading questions permit no opportunity to deny assumptions. "Is your chest pain sharp or dull?" is a common and commonly misleading question. It's as helpful as speaking to your patient in the wrong language.[8] Try "Tell me more about what you are feeling ... what's it really like?"(p89)

**Questions suggesting the answer** "Was the vomit red, yellow, or black—like coffee grounds?"—the classic description of vomited blood. "Yes, like coffee grounds, doctor." The doctor's expectations and hurry to get the evidence into a pre-decided format have so tarnished the story as to make it useless (see also p13).

**Open questions** The most open question is "How are you?" The direction a patient chooses offers valuable information during this first 'golden' minute in which you are silent. Other examples are gentle imperatives such as "Tell me about the vomit" "It was dark" "How dark?" "Dark bits in it" "Like...?" "Like bits of soil in it." This information is gold, although it is not cast in the form of 'coffee grounds'.

**Patient-centred questions** In order to consider your patient's viewpoint, learn to weave between finding out about the disease and their illness. Try to understand the patient's unique experience and any effect on their life. What are their *ideas*?: "What do you think is wrong?" Explore their *concerns*: "What other things are on your mind? How does having this affect you? What is the worst thing? It makes you feel..." (The doctor is silent.) What are their *expectations*? "What can we do about this?"[9] Share management plans. ▶Unless you become patient-centred your patient may never be fully satisfied with you, or fully cooperative.

**Casting your questions over the whole family** This is most useful in revealing if symptoms are caused or perpetuated by psychological mechanisms. They probe the network of causes and enabling conditions which allow nebulous symptoms to flourish in family life. "Who else is important in your life? Are they worried about you? Who really understands you?" Until this sort of question is asked, illness may resist treatment. Eg "Who is present when your headache starts? Who notices it first—you or your wife? Who worries about it most (or least)? What does your wife do when (or before) you get it?" Think to yourself: *Who* is his headache? We note with fascination research showing that in clusters of hard-to-diagnose symptoms, it is the spouse's view of them that is the best predictor of outcome: if the spouse is determined that symptoms must be physical, the outcome is worse than if the spouse allows that some symptoms may be psychological.

**Echoes** Try repeating the last words said as a route to new intimacies, otherwise inaccessible, as you fade into the distance, and the patient soliloquizes "...I've always been suspicious of my wife." "Wife ..." "My wife ... and her father together." "Together..." "I've never trusted them together." "Trusted them together..." "No, well, I've always felt I've known who my son's real father was... I can never trust those two together." Without any questions you may unearth the unexpected, important clue which throws a new light on the history.

▶*If you only ask questions, you will only receive answers in reply.* If you interrogate a robin, he will fly away: treelike silence may bring him to your hand.

Like toddlers, we should always be asking *"Why?"*—not just to find ultimate causes, nor to keep in step with our itineraries of veracity (although there is a place for this), but to enable us to find the simplest level for intervention. Some simple change early on in a chain of events may be sufficient to bring about a cure, but later on, such opportunities may not arise. For example, it is not enough for you to diagnose heart failure in your breathless patient. Ask: *"Why is there heart failure?"* If you don't, you may be satisfied by giving the patient an antifailure drug—and any side-effects from this, such as uraemia or incontinence from diuretic-associated polyuria, will be attributed to an unavoidable consequence of necessary therapy.

If only you had asked *"What is the mechanism of the heart failure?"* you might have found a cause, eg anaemia coupled with ischaemic heart disease. You cannot cure the latter, but treating the anaemia may be all that is required to cure the patient's breathlessness. But do not stop there. Ask: *"What is the mechanism of the anaemia?"* You find a low MCV and a correspondingly low serum ferritin (p320)—and you might be tempted to say to yourself, I have the prime cause.

Wrong! Put aside the idea of prime causes, and go on asking *"What is the mechanism?"* Retaking the history (often the best 'investigation') shows a very poor diet. *"Why is the patient eating a poor diet?"* Is he ignorant or too poor to eat properly? You may find the patient's wife died a year ago, he is sinking into a depression, and cannot be bothered to eat. He would not care if he died tomorrow.

You come to realize that simply treating the patient's anaemia may not be of much help—so go on asking *"Why?"*: "Why did you bother to go to the doctor if you aren't interested in getting better?" It turns out he only went to see you to please his daughter. He is unlikely to take your drugs unless you really get to the bottom of what he cares about. His daughter is what matters and, unless you include her, all your initiatives may fail. Talk to her, offer help for the depression, teach her about iron-rich foods and, with luck, your patient's breathlessness may gradually begin to disappear. Even if it does *not* start to disappear, you are learning to stand in your patient's shoes and you may discover what will enable him to accept help. And this dialogue may help you to be a kinder doctor, particularly if you are worn out by endless lists of technical tasks, which you must somehow fit into impossibly overcrowded days and nights. You never really know a man until you stand in his shoes and walk around in them. *Harper Lee; To Kill a Mockingbird*

**Constructing imaginative narratives yielding new meanings** Doctors are often thought of as being reductionist or mechanistic—but the above shows that asking *"Why?"* can enlarge the scope of our enquires into holistic realms. Another way to do this is to ask *"What does this symptom mean?"*—for this person, his family, and our world. A limp might mean a neuropathy, or falling behind with the mortgage, if you are a dancer; or it may represent a medically unexplained symptom which subtly alters family hierarchies both literally (on family walks) and metaphorically. Science is about clarity, objectivity, and theory in modelling reality. But there is another way of modelling the external world, which involves subjectivity, emotion, ambiguity, and arcane relationships between apparently unrelated phenomena. The medical humanities (p17) explore this—and have burgeoned recently[10]—leading to the existence of two camps: humanities and science. If while reading this you are getting impatient to get to the real nuts and bolts of technological medicine, you are in the latter camp. We are not suggesting that you leave it, only that you learn to operate out of both. If you do not, your professional life will be full of failures, which you may deny or remain in ignorance of. If you *do* straddle both camps, there will also be failures, but you will realize what these failures *mean*, and you will know how to *transform* them. This transformation happens through dialogue and reflection. We would achieve more if we did less: every hospital should have a department of reflection and it should be visited as often as the radiology department. In fact every hospital has many such departments, carved out of our own minds—it's just that their entrances are blocked by piles of events, tasks and happenings.

*Thinking about medicine*

*We all labour against our own cure; for death is the cure of all diseases.* Thomas Browne, *Religio Medici, 1642*

Compared with being born, death should be straightforward. But nothing you can say to your patient can ever be relied upon to tame death's mystery, and preparing people for death is more than control of terminal symptoms (see p7).

Death is nature's master stroke, albeit a cruel one, because it allows genotypes space to try on new phenotypes. The time comes in the life of any organ or person when it is better to start from scratch rather than carry on with the weight and muddle of endless accretions. Our bodies and minds are these perishable phenotypes—the froth, that always turns to scum, on the wave of our genes. These genes are not really *our* genes. It is we who belong to them for a few decades. It is one of nature's great insults that she should prefer to put *all* her eggs in the basket of a defenceless, incompetent neonate rather than in the tried and tested custody of our own superb minds. But as our neurofibrils begin to tangle, and that neonate walks to a wisdom that eludes us, we are forced to give nature credit for her daring idea. Of course, nature, in her careless way, can get it wrong: people often die in the wrong order (one of our chief roles is to prevent this mis-ordering of deaths, not the phenomenon of death itself). So we must admit that, on reflection, dying *is* a brilliant idea, and one that it is most unlikely we could ever have thought of ourselves.

**Diagnosis of death** Although death is a process, there is a need to name the moment of death. This has long been identified by the simultaneous onset of apnoea, unconsciousness and absence of the circulation, yet there is no standardized criteria for *when* death should be confirmed (irrespective of whether the heart has stopped beating of its own accord, treatment has been withdrawn, or resuscitation attempts have failed).[1] Royal College guidance suggests that cardiorespiratory death can be diagnosed after 5 minutes of observed asystole (by the absence of a central pulse and heart sounds ± absence of activity on continuous ECG or echocardiogram). After 5 minutes of continued arrest, irreversible damage to the brainstem will have occurred and the absence of pupillary responses to light, corneal reflex and motor response to supra-orbital pressure should be confirmed. The time of death is said to be the time when these criteria are met.[11, 12]

**Diagnosis of death by CNS criteria (brainstem death)** If the brainstem is irreversibly damaged, but the heart is still beating, death has occurred and the heart will inevitably stop beating on withdrawal of support. *UK brain death criteria* (USA criteria differ) has 3 components: 1 The patient must suffer from a condition that has led to irreversible brain damage 2 Potentially reversible causes have been adequately excluded (in particular: depressant drugs; hypothermia; metabolic or endocrine disturbances; or reversible causes of apnoea) 3 Coma, apnoea and the absence of brainstem reflexes are formally demonstrated. *Tests:* All brainstem reflexes must be absent: •Pupils unresponsive to light •Corneal reflex absent (no blink to cotton-wool touch) •Absent oculo-vestibular reflexes (no eye movements on instillation of ice-cold water into the external auditory meatus—visualize the tympanic membrane first) •Stimulation in the cranial nerve distributions produces no motor response •There is no gag reflex (on touching the palate) or cough reflex (to bronchial stimulation) •The apnoea test (perfomed last) demonstrates no respiratory response to an acidaemic respiratory stimulus: ventilation rate is reduced without inducing hypoxia, $P_{CO_2}$ is allowed to rise $\geq$6.0kPa with pH $\leq$7.40.[11, 12]

Diagnosis is made by 2 doctors competent in the procedure (registered for >5 years, one of whom is a consultant). Testing should be undertaken by the doctors together and must always be performed completely and successfully on two occasions.

*Organ donation:* Diagnosis of brain death allows organs to be donated and removed with as little hypoxic damage as possible. Non-heartbeating organ donation is increasing in practice. Don't avoid the topic with relatives. Many are glad to help.

**After death** See the relatives. Inform the GP and consultant. Inform the Coroner/Procurator Fiscal (if required). Sign death certificates promptly.

1 Make full & extensive attempts to reverse any contributing causes (hypoglycaemia, acidosis, hypothermia or drug intoxication). Patient's wishes via an advanced decision to refuse treatment must be respected.

When you might raise death with your patient and you find yourself thinking it is better for them not to know, suspect that you mean: it is easier for me not to tell. ►Most patients are told less than they want.[13]

**Acceptance** Accepting death may involve passing through stages on a path. It helps to know where your patient is on this journey (but progress is rarely orderly and is not always forwards). At first there may be *shock* and *numbness*, then *denial* (which reduces anxiety), then *anger*, then *grief* and then, perhaps, *acceptance*.[14] Finally, there may be intense longing for death, as your patient moves beyond the reach of worldly cares.[1] JS Bach *Ich habe genug*

**Hope** A dilemma when working with terminally ill patients is to avoid collusion and yet sustain hope. In doing this we need to understand what hope is, and why it can remain hope even when it may sound like despair. Hope nurtures within it the belief that what is hoped for may be realized. Initially this may be hope for recovery, or at least that death is long delayed. Yet for hope to continue developing it may have to move beyond an insistence on recovery and require facing or exploring the possibility of dying. Patients who contemplate dying as part of their hope may find the social support that once buoyed for a hope of recovery works against them—lack of support at this stage can result in resignation and despair. Hope beyond recovery is a more varied hope: the patient may simply hope to die with dignity, or for the continuing success of their children, or that a partner will find the support they need. For most people, such a hope becomes possible, but few find a meaningful hope which they are allowed to affirm.[15] Hope beyond recovery may accept death (rather than life at any cost) and find a sense of ultimate meaning in a life lived, or hope in life after death (as a contingency of faith). ►In patients who are terminally ill, psychosocial and spiritual needs are as important as symptom control.

**The active management of death** Death may be regarded as a medical failure rather than an inevitable consequence of life. But when medical treatments can no longer offer a cure and a patient enters the last days and weeks of life, the active managment of death is vital. In the UK there are 10,000 deaths/week[16] and few hospice beds, so the chances are that a death will be happening near you soon, and nobody will be in charge. Have courage and take charge. Find out about your patient's wishes, and comply with them. ►*Get help promptly from palliative care teams*. Take into account GMC guidance[17] and current thinking expressed in the Gold Standards Framework.[18] If a *living will* or *advance directive* is in existence, comply with it and promote your patient's autonomy. ►*At the end of life, autonomy trumps all else*.[2] Take strength from this clarity. Talk to the patient, relatives, and staff to get (and document[3]) consensus on what the patient's priority is (eg relief of suffering). Make sure pain relief is adequate, not to cause death, but to leave no opportunity for pain and distress to re-emerge (if that is the patient's implied or stated wish). A good death is one that is appropriate and requested for by a particular patient. It is wrong to assume that everyone's wish is the same. Some patients may choose to 'rage against the dying of the light'[4] and may never accept their end calmly.[19] Whatever a patient's wishes, ensure that the resources and skills are available to meet their needs. ►See pages 536–9 for practical advice on symptom control in those who are dying.

---

**1** Bach's cantata in contemplation of death *Ich habe genug* (I've had enough) expresses contempt for worldly life and a yearning for death and the life beyond. Inspired by Simeon's prayer *Nunc Dimittis*, it surrounds Simeon's encounter with Christ. Simeon had been told he would not see death until he had seen the Lord.
**2** Provided our humanity remains intact (NB: good palliative care will, in general, *enhance* humanity).
**3** Establish & document that: ►The patient is dying and has initiated the request ►You have discussed drug doses with an experienced Dr ►Dose increases are proportionate and needed for symptom control.
**4** *Do not go gentle into that good night* was written by Dylan Thomas for his dying father.

▶Consult the *BNF* or *BNF for Children* or similar before giving any drug with which you are not thoroughly familiar; check interactions meticulously.

Before prescribing, ask if the patient is allergic to anything. The answer is often "yes"—but do not stop here. Characterize the reaction, or else you risk denying a life-saving, and safe, drug such as penicillin because of a mild reaction, eg nausea. Is the reaction a *true allergy* (anaphylaxis, p806, or a rash?), a *toxic effect* (eg ataxia is inevitable if given large doses of phenytoin), a *predictable adverse reaction* (eg GI bleeding from aspirin), or an *idiosyncratic (unpredictable) reaction*?

Remember *primum non nocere*: first do no harm. The more minor the illness, the more weight this carries. The more serious the illness, the more its antithesis comes into play: *nothing ventured, nothing gained*. These **ten commandments** should be written on every tablet:

1 Explore alternatives to drugs—which often lead to doctor-dependency (p xi), paternalism, and medicalization of life. Drugs are also expensive (£ billions/yr[UK]) and prices increase faster than general inflation. There are 3 places to look:
   • *The larder:* eg lemon and honey for sore throats, rather than penicillin.
   • *The blackboard:* eg education about the self-inflicted causes of oesophagitis. Rather than giving expensive drugs, advise raising the head of the bed, and avoiding tight garments, too many big meals, smoking, and alcohol excess.
   • *Lastly, look to yourself:* giving a piece of yourself, some *real* sympathy, is worth more than all the drugs in your pharmacopoeia to those who are frightened, bereaved, or weary of life. One of us (JML) for many years looked after a paranoid lady: monthly visits comprised an injection and a hug, no doubt always chaperoned, until one day mental health nurses took over her care. She was seen by a different nurse each month. They didn't know about hugging, so after a while she stopped cooperating, and soon it fell to us to certify her death.

2 Are you prescribing for a minor illness because you want to solve all problems, or perhaps because it makes *you* feel better? Patients may be happy just to know the illness *is* minor. Knowing this may make it acceptable. Some people do not believe in drugs, and you must find this out.

3 Decide if the patient is responsible. If he now swallows *all* the quinine pills you have so attentively prescribed for his cramps, death will be swift.

4 Know of other ways your prescription may be misused. Perhaps the patient whose 'insomnia' you so kindly treated is even now selling it on the black market or grinding up your prescription prior to injecting himself, desperate for a fix. Will you be suspicious when he returns to say he has lost his drugs?

5 Address these questions when prescribing off the ward:
   • How many daily doses are there? 1-2 is *much* better than 4. Good doctors spend much time harmonizing complex regimens. One reason for 'failure' of HIV drugs, for example, is that regimens are too complex. Drug companies know this, so keep abreast of new modified release (MR) preparations.
   • The bottle/box: can the patient read the instructions—and can he open it?
   • How will you know if the patient forgets to return for follow-up?
   • If the patient agrees, enlist help (eg spouse/carer) to ensure he remembers to take the pills, or suggest blister packs that organize tablets by time and day.

6 Discuss side-effects and risk of allergy. We may downplay risk, but our drugs cause 1 million NHS admissions/yr (£1-2 billion/yr). Most drug deaths are avoidable.[20]

7 Use computerized decision support whenever you can. If the patient is on 7 drugs and has 5 complaints, the computer will help you find which of the drugs are possible culprits.[21] Computers also warn about drug interactions.

8 Agree with the patient on the risk : benefit ratio's favourability. Try to ensure there is true concordance (p3) between you and your patient.

9 Record how you will review the patient's need for each drug and progress towards agreed goals, eg pulse rate to mark degree of β-blockade.

10 List benefits of *this* drug to *this* patient for *all* drugs taken. Specify what each drug is for.

*Prescribing in renal failure* and *liver failure:* p301 & p259.

At the end of every day, with the going down of the sun (which we never see at the coalface of clinical medicine), we can momentarily cheer ourselves up by the thought that we are one day nearer to the end of life on earth—and our responsibility for the unending tide of illness that floods into our corridors and seeps into our wards and consulting rooms. Of course you may have many other quiet satisfactions, but if not, read on and wink with us as we hear some fool or visionary telling us that our aim should be to produce the greatest health and happiness for the greatest number.

When we hear this, we don't expect cheering from the tattered ranks of midnight on-call junior doctors: rather, our ears are detecting a decimated groan, because these men and women know that there is something at stake in on-call doctoring far more elemental than health or happiness: namely survival. Within the first weeks, however brightly your armour shone, it will now be smeared and splattered if not with blood, then with the fallout from many decisions that were taken without sufficient care and attention. Not that you were lazy, but *force majeure* on the part of Nature and the exigencies of ward life have, we are suddenly stunned to realize, taught us to be second-rate: for to insist on being first-rate in all areas is to sign a death warrant for our patients, and for ourselves. Perfectionism cannot survive in our clinical world. To cope with this fact, or, to put it less depressingly, to flourish in this new world, don't keep re-polishing your armour (what are the 10 causes of atrial fibrillation—or are there 11?), rather furnish your mind—and nourish your body. Regular food makes those midnight groans of yours less intrusive. Drink plenty: doctors are more likely to be oliguric than their patients.[22] Don't voluntarily deny yourself the restorative power of sleep. A good nap is the order of the day—and for the nights, sleep for as long as possible. Remember that sleep is our natural state, in which we were first created, and we only wake to feed our dreams.

We cannot prepare you for finding out that you are not at ease with the person you are becoming, and neither would we dream of imposing on our readers a recommended regimen of exercise, diet, and mental fitness. Finding out what can lead you through adversity is the art of living.

Junior doctors' first jobs are not just a phase to get through and to enjoy where possible (there are often *many* such possibilities); they are also the anvil on which we are beaten into a new and perhaps uncomfortable shape. Luckily not all of us are made of iron so there is a fair chance that one day we will spring back into something resembling our normal shape, and realize that it was our weaknesses, not our strengths, which served us best. The jobs of junior doctors encompass huge swings in energy, motivation, and mood, which can be precipitated by small events. If you are depressed for more than a day, speak to a sympathetic friend, partner, or counsellor. ▸*When in doubt, communicate*. And use an integrative philosophy of medicine, as described in this next section, to reclaim yourself.

**Integrative medicine: beyond biopsychosocial models** The biopsychosocial model is the medical teacher's Grand Theory of Everything. It's like a game of 'stones, scissors and paper': the patient presents with a physical symptom, and the clever doctor trumps you, who had taken the symptom at face value, by revealing the social background that allowed the symptom to flourish. If the problem is social (eg poor housing), the clever doctor reveals the hidden asthma that this is causing, and if the symptom is purely psychological, the doctor reveals and manages the social effects of this for the patient's family. It's a powerful game,[23] and much good comes from it.[24] But like all orthodoxy it needs challenging.[25] Let us consider Mr B, the builder, who comes to A&E having nailed his testicle to a plank. Everybody gathers round, but the clever doctor is annoyed that nobody is listening to his biopsychosocial diagnosis. The nail is removed; the testicle is repaired, but Mr B does not go on his way rejoicing. A nurse, a better listener than our doctor, uses an individually tailored *moral-symbolic-existential* approach to reveal that the injury was self-inflicted. A *spiritual-cultural-ritualistic* model may be needed for his care.[26]

As the author of the biopsychosocial model knew, there is more to medicine than stones, scissors, and paper, or *any* triad that does not integrate a rethinking of the task of medicine with infrastructure of relationships and beliefs. George Engel 1977 [27,28]

Thinking about medicine

**Resource allocation: who gets what** Resource allocation is about cutting the health cake—whose size is *given*. What slice should go to transplants, new joints, and services for dementia? Cynics would say that this depends on how vociferous each group of patients (or doctors) is. Others try to find a rational way to allocate resources. Health economists (econocrats) have invented the QALY for this purpose. NB: focusing on how to cut the cake diverts attention from how large the cake should be (is it better to spend money on space exploration or incontinence pads?).

**How much is a life worth?** Some countries will spend $2-10 million to find a man on a life-raft; others will spend nothing ("he's just one more mouth to feed").[29, 30] Totalitarian capitalist states (eg China) will take a different view to liberal democracies. In France, one life is worth a hundred cherry trees, if the blossom is fine.[31]

**What is a QALY?** 1 year of healthy life expectancy is worth 1 'quality adjusted life year'. 1 year of unhealthy life expectancy is worth <1 QALY (its value is lower the poorer health is).[32] If you are likely to live for 8yrs in perfect health on an old drug, you gain 8 QALYs; if a new drug would give you 16yrs but at a quality of life you rate at only 25% of the maximum, you would gain only 4 QALYs. The dream of a health economist is to buy the most QALYs for his budget. Health assessment organizations (eg NICE) keep arbitrary figures in their head (~£30,000/QALY—not evidence-based). If an intervention costs more than this, reasons for recommending it have to be all the more explicit or approval may be refused (the drug may be effective, but the cost is not). QALYs can be recalculated (on *very* dubious grounds)[33] after weighting for age and disease-seriousness[34] to give the politically correct answer, for example in granting extra value to prolonging the last months of life.

QALYs do help in rationing, but problems include pricing and invidiousness in choosing between people; a snag is that if we accept that the quality of our life is the quality of our relationships (Anthony Robins), and that this value is unquantifiable (1 wife is good, but 2 wives are not *exactly* twice as good),[1] then we can see why bodies such as NICE get excoriated over issues such as dementia drugs, when seemingly small improvements can cause disproportionate joy, as when a demented man becomes able to recall his wife's name.[35, 36] Should spouses put their own QALYs into the sum?

## The inverse care law & distributive justice

> *'Availability of good medical care varies inversely with the need for it in the population served. This operates more completely where medical care is exposed to market forces... The market distribution of medical care exaggerates maldistribution of medical resources.'*

There is much evidence in support of this famous thesis formulated by Tudor Hart.[37] Premature death and long-term limiting illness are both strongly associated with deprivation.[38] It is not just availability of care but access to services that matters. Those who need healthcare the least use services more, and more effectively, than those with the greatest need.[39] Distributive justice is the fair distribution of health resources, based on the premise that all are equal in terms of healthcare provision (see also p15). Ideally, sufficient healthcare should be provided to all, but the health cake isn't big enough for this. So, resources should preferably be distributed in relation to need, within a society that has equal access. In the UK, medical care does exist in deprived areas, but this does not ensure that services are accessed, or that they are of good quality.[40]

There is no doubt that if one wants to make a positive contribution to health, it is no good just discovering pathways, blocking receptors, and inventing drugs. The more this is done, the more urgent the need for distributive justice—that unyielding and perpetually problematic benchmark against which we are all judged.

If those who shout loudest get heard first, we need to know when to train our ears to be deaf.

---

**1** This is an example of a **non-parametric quantity**, ie a quantity where simple ordering *may* be valid, but not operations such as addition or multiplication. Most medical statistics are assumed to be parametric; this is often false, invalidating much research.

►Psychopathology is common in colleagues, patients, and relatives. ►Seek help for your own problems. Find a sympathetic GP and register with him or her. You are not the best person to plan your assessment, treatment, and referral.

**Assessing mental state** 'Move gently through her thoughts, as one might explore a new garden'.*Ian McEwan, Atonement* What is in bloom now? Where do those paths lead? What is under that stone? *Focus on*: Appearance (dress, cleanliness, physical condition); behaviour (eye contact, rapport, anxious? suspicious?); speech (volume, rate & tone); mood (subjective & objective); perception (hallucinations); thought form & content (formal thought disorder? delusions? obsessions? plan to harm self/others?); cognition (concentration, orientation, memory). Note insight (are his experiences the result of illness?). Non-verbal behaviour often gives more valid clues than words, *OHCS* p324.

**Depression** This is common, and often ignored, at great cost to wellbeing. Thinking "I would be depressed in his shoes" may sap our will to help, and as biological features (early waking, ↓appetite, ↓weight, loss of interest in sex/hobbies) are common on all wards, we may not realize just how bad things have got. The central clinical features of depression can be assessed by asking:[41] *"Have you been bothered by feeling down, depressed, or hopeless in the last month?"* If so, *"Have you been bothered by lack of interest or pleasure in doing things?"* If "yes", depression is likely. There may also be guilt and feelings of worthlessness. ►*Don't think it's not your job to treat depression.* It is as important as pain. Try to arrange activities to boost the patient's morale and confidence. Share your thoughts with other team members, as well as relatives, if the patient wishes. Among these, your patient may find a kindred spirit who can give insight and support. ►If in doubt, try an antidepressant. For *SSRIs* (eg *citalopram*, 20mg/24h), see *OHCS* p340. Cognitive interventions are just as important as drugs (*OHCS* p370), so liaise with the patient's GP pre-discharge.

**The violent patient** Recognize early warning signs: visible distress, tachypnoea, clenched fists, shouting, chanting, restlessness, repetitive movements, pacing, gesticulations. Your own intuition may be helpful here. ► At the first hint of violence, get help. If alone, make sure you are nearer the door than the patient.
• Do not be alone with the patient; summon security or the police if needed.
• Try calming and talking with the patient. Do not touch him. Use your body language to reassure (sitting back, open palms, attentive).
• Get his consent; if unforthcoming, emergency treatment can still be given to save life, or serious deterioration (under *common law* 'necessity' in England): You are acting *against* your patient's wishes but in order to adequately carry out your *duty of care*. Enlist the help of nurses who know the patient.
• Use minimum force to achieve his welfare (but this may entail 6 strong men).

*Causes:* Anger (long waiting times[46%], dissatisfaction with treatment[15%], *disagreement with the physician*[10%]),[42] *alcohol/alcohol withdrawal* (a common cause of problems on the ward; p282), *drugs* (recreational; prescribed), *hypoglycaemia, delirium* (p488), *psychosis, psychopathy*. Check blood glucose. Before further tests, haloperidol may be needed: 2-10mg IM (allow 30mins for effect; max. 18mg/24h; monitor pulse, temp., and BP every 15min for 1h then every 30mins until ambulatory).

*After a violent event:* Attend to your own and others' wounds (get help as needed); report the event. Flashbacks, depression, insomnia, and need for time off are common.[43]

**Capacity** If a rational adult refuses vital treatment, it may be as well to respect this decision, provided the patient has 'capacity'. A person lacks capacity if they are **unable** to: • Make a decision because of a permanent or temporary impairment of, or disturbance in, the functioning of the mind, *and* are **unable** to: (≥1 of) • Understand the information relevant to the decision • Retain that information long enough to make a decision • Weigh up the information to make a decision, or • Communicate the decision. Capacity is decision and time specific and is rarely all or nothing, so don't hesitate to get the opinion of others. See p571 for the principles of capacity.

**Mental Health Acts** Familiarize yourself with local procedures and laws pertaining to your country before your period of duty starts (*OHCS* p402).

*Thinking about medicine*

▶Ageing reflects the cumulative effects of stressors (eg free radicals) and mechanisms for dealing with them. For most of human history, life expectancy was <40yrs. *An ageing population is a sign of successful social and economic policies.*[44]

**Healthy ageing** Health isn't just 'complete mental and physical wellbeing' (WHO) but also 'a process of adaptation, to changing environments, to growing up and ageing, to healing when damaged, to suffering, and death. Health embraces the future so includes anguish and the inner resources to live with it.' *Ivan Illich 1974 Medical Nemesis* So healthy ageing is not a contradiction. ▶Contrary to stereotype, most old people are fit and at the happiest stage in their lives.[145] 80% of those over 85yrs live at home; 70% can manage stairs. Any deterioration in an elderly patient is from treatable disease *until proved otherwise*. Find the cause; don't think: *this is simply ageing*. Old age is associated with disease but doesn't cause it *per se*.[46] Do not restrict treatment because of age—age alone is a poor predictor of outcome.[47]

**Differences of emphasis in the approach to old people**[48]

1 *Multiple pathology:* Several diseases may coincide (eg cataract + arthritis = falls).

2 *Multiple causes:* One problem may have several causes. Treating each alone may do little good; treating all may be of great benefit.[49]

3 *Non-specific presentations:* The 'geriatric giants'[50] of incontinence (p650);[51] immobility; instability (falls); and dementia/confusion (p488) are common and any disease may present with these. Typical signs and symptoms may be absent (eg MI without chest pain; pneumonia, but no cough, fever, or sputum).

4 *Rapid worsening if treatment is delayed:* Complications are common.

5 *More time is required for recovery:* There is less 'physiological reserve'.

6 *Impaired metabolism and excretion of drugs:* ∴ drug doses may need lowering.

7 *Rehabilitation:* Helps maximize independence, eg improving mobility and balance.

8 *Social factors:* These are central in aiding recovery and return to home.

**Special points** Take a biopsychosocial approach (p9)[52] (look for and manage interactions between physical, psychological and social aspects of a person's life).

• Drug concordance (p3): How many different tablets can he cope with? Probably not many more than 2. So which are the most important drugs? If difficulty in managing medicines, consider prescribing blister packs.

• Social network: Are family and friends nearby? Do they visit regularly?

• Care details: Are carers needed? Can meals be delivered? Are District nurses involved?

• Make a holistic *care plan*. Include nutrition. If food is dumped beside a blind man and no one helps cut it up, he may starve. A passing doctor may arrange a CT 'for cachexia', when what he needs is food and cataract surgery.

**Discharge planning** ▶*Start planning discharge from day 1*. A very common question on ward rounds is: "Will this patient get on OK at home?" In answering this, take into account: • Does the patient live alone? • Does any carer have support? • Is your patient in fact a carer for someone even more frail? • Is the accommodation suitable? Stairs? Toilet on the same floor? (If not, can he transfer from chair to commode?) • Is the family supportive—in practice as well as in theory? • Are social services and community services well integrated? *Proper case management programmes* really can help *and* save money (~20%).[53]

---

**UK NHS national service framework (NSF) for old age: 8 care-standards**

*Person-centred care:* Enabling older people to make choices about their own care.
*Intermediate care:* Promoting independence by providing intermediate care.
*Hospital care:* Delivering specialist care by staff who have the right set of skills.
*Rooting out age discrimination:* Providing services regardless of age.
*Stroke:* Treatment and rehabilitation of stroke patients by a specialist service.
*Falls:* Falls and fracture prevention through a specialist falls service.
*Promotion of mental health:* Ensuring effective diagnosis, treatment & support.
*Promotion of health and active life in older age.*

---

**1** A big study (n=28,000) found the odds of being happy increased 5% with each decade. Contentment entails being socially active and accepting: "It's fine I was a schoolteacher, not a Nobel prize winner".

**Penny-dropping moments (PDMs)** All pleasures are sensory—apart from those to be had by doing crosswords and diagnostics: both can give us delicious *penny-dropping moments* which come from combining logic with intuition (PDMs, fig 1, p672). With over 14,000 diseases to choose from,[54] finding the diagnosis is a challenge (often thwarted by unconscious forces, see BOX). The process of *how* we diagnose receives little attention— it is assumed (wrongly) to entail collating information, which is then forced through a surgical sieve,[1] which somehow leaves the correct diagnosis clinging to its sides.

**Diagnosing by recognition** For students, this is the most irritating method. You spend an hour asking all the wrong questions, and in waltzes a doctor who names the disease and sorts it out before you have even finished taking the pulse. This doctor has simply recognized the illness like he recognizes an old friend (or enemy).

**Diagnosing by probability** Over our clinical lives we unconsciously build up a personal database of diagnoses and outcomes, and associated pitfalls. We unconsciously run each new 'case' through this continuously developing probabilistic algorithm—eventually with amazing speed and effortlessness.

**Diagnosing by reasoning** Like Sherlock Holmes, we must exclude each differential diagnosis, then, whatever is left, however unlikely, *must be* the culprit. This process presupposes that your differential does include the culprit, and that we have methods for *absolutely* excluding diseases. All tests are statistical rather than absolute, which is why this method is, at best, fictional.

**Diagnosing by watching and waiting** Some doctors need to know immediately and definitively what the diagnosis is, while others can tolerate more uncertainty. The dangers and expense of exhaustive tests can be obviated by the skilful use of time.

**Diagnosing by selective doubting** Traditionally, patients are 'unreliable' and signs are objective, and tests virtually perfect. When diagnosis is difficult, try inverting this hierarchy. You will soon realize there are no hard signs or perfect tests. But the game of medicine is unplayable if you doubt everything: so doubt selectively.

**Diagnosis by iteration and reiteration** A brief history suggests looking for a few signs, which leads to further questions and a few tests. The process of taking a history never ends on this view, and as the process reiterates, various diagnostic possibilities crop up, and receive more or less confirmation. For example, when assessing a patient with atrial fibrillation (p124) you notice finger clubbing and make a note to do a chest x-ray for signs of cancer. This leads you to ask about smoking, and then alcohol, which elicits excessive drinking due to recent redundancy.

### ⚙ Thinking about thinking [55-57]

The rapid decision-making that is often required of doctors can be aided by *heuristics*—rules for cognitive shortcuts to quick decisions (conscious or unconscious) which are made without full information or analysis. Understanding how we use heuristics (ie by considering how a decision is made) can help us make effective choices, but there are pitfalls. Failed heuristics (biases) interfere with judgement and can lead to diagnostic error. Important examples include:

*Anchoring:* A significant feature in the history is 'anchored' onto too early in the diagnostic process and is not adjusted for in light of later information. Adjusting probability by incorporating new information can help you become an intuitive thinker. Anchoring can be compounded by *confirmation bias*—the tendency to look for, notice and remember information that fits with pre-existing expectations.

*Availability:* This explains our tendency to judge something more likely if it readily comes to mind. A recent experience with a disease increases the likelihood of it being diagnosed—problematic if the disease is rare, or has not been seen for a while.

*Representativeness:* If diagnosis is driven by the extent to which a patient resembles a classic case of a disease, atypical variants will tend to be missed.

**1** When your mind goes blank, calm yourself by reciting the *surgical sieve*: The heart, the lung, the blood, the guts / The liver kidney spleen / The brain, the bones, the skin, the nodes / The bits that's in between.

*Thinking about medicine*

*"I work much better in chaos."* Francis [58] Bacon Chaos is not always an enemy: certainly there is no shortage of it in hospitals, consulting rooms, and other battle-grounds. Can we prepare ourselves to use chaos well? Being forewarned allows us to be forearmed, enabling us to adapt to being busy, or at least to wink at each other as we slide down the cascade of long hours→excessive paperwork→too few beds→effort-reward imbalance→compromised care from too few resources→trouble with superiors→difficult patients→too many deaths[59]→failure to reconcile personal and family life with professional roles.[60] Logistic regression shows that our consequent problems are predicted by 5 stressors: **1** Lack of recognition of own contribution by others. **2** Too much responsibility. **3** Difficulties keeping up to date. **4** Making the right decision alone. **5** Effects of stress on personal/family life.[61]

We may think that it is modern medicine that makes us ever busier, but doctors have always been busy. Sir James Paget, for example, would regularly see over 60 patients each day, sometimes travelling many miles, on his horse, to their bedsides. Sir Dominic Corrigan was so busy 180 years ago that he had a secret door made in his consulting room to escape the ever-growing queue of eager patients.[62]

We are all familiar with the phenomenon of being hopelessly over-stretched, and of wanting Corrigan's secret door. Competing, urgent, and simultaneous demands make carrying out any task all but impossible: the junior doctor is trying to gain IV access on a shocked patient when his 'bleep' sounds. On his way to the phone a patient is falling out of bed, being held in, apparently, only by his visibly lengthening catheter (which had taken the doctor an hour to insert). He knows he should stop to help but, instead, as he picks up the phone, he starts to tell Sister about "this man dangling from his catheter" (knowing in his heart that the worst will have already happened). But he is interrupted by a thud coming from the bed of the lady who has just had a below knee amputation for non-healing leg ulcers: however, it is not her, but her visiting husband who has collapsed. In despair, he turns to the nurse and groans: "There must be some way out of here!" At times like this we all need Corrigan to take us by the shadow of our hand, and walk with us through a metaphorical secret door into a calm inner world. To enable this to happen, make things as easy as possible for yourself—as follows.

First, however lonely you feel, you are not usually alone. Do not pride yourself on not asking for help. If a decision is a hard one, share it with a colleague. Second, take any chance you get to sit down and rest. Have a cup of coffee with other members of staff, or with a friendly patient (patients are sources of renewal, not just devourers of your energies). Third, do not miss meals. If there is no time to go to the canteen, ensure that food is put aside for you to eat when you can: hard work and sleeplessness are twice as bad when you are hungry. Fourth, avoid making work for yourself. It is too easy for junior doctors, trapped in their image of excessive work and blackmailed by misplaced guilt, to remain on the wards reclerking patients, rewriting notes, or rechecking results at an hour when the priority should be caring for themselves. Fifth, when a bad part of the rota is looming, plan a good time for when you are off duty, to look forward to during the long nights.

However busy the 'on take', your period of duty will end. For you, as for Macbeth:

> Come what come may,
> time and the hour runs through the roughest day.

**Riding the wave** In *Macbeth*, toil and trouble go hand in hand, but sometimes we work best when we are busy. This is recognized in the aphorism that *if you want a job done quickly, give it to a busy* (wo)*man*. Observe your colleagues and yourself during a busy day. Sometimes our energy achieves nothing but our own inundation. At other times, by jettisoning everything non-essential, we get airborne and accomplish marvellous feats. As with any sport, we have to break into a sweat before we can get into the zone, where every action meets its mark.

But note that what keeps us riding the wave of a busy day is not what we jettison but what we retain: humour, courtesy, a recognition of the work of others, and an ability to twinkle. A smile causes no delays, and reaches far beyond our lips.

In our public medical personas, we often act as though morality consisted only in following society's conventions: we do this not so much out of laziness but because we recognize that it is better that the public think of doctors as old-fashioned or stupid, than that they should think us evil. But in the silences of our consultations, when it is we ourselves who are under the microscope, then, wriggle as we may, we cannot escape our destiny, which is to lead as often as to follow, in the sphere of ethics. To do this, we need to return to first principles, and not go with the flow of society's expectations. To give us courage in this enterprise, we can recall the aviator's and the seagull's law: it is only by *facing* the prevailing wind that we can become airborne, and achieve a new vantage point from which to survey our world.

**Our analysis** starts with our aim: to do good by making people healthy. *Good*[1] is the most general term of commendation, and entails four cardinal duties:

1 Not doing harm. We owe this duty to all people, not just our patients.[63]
2 Doing good by positive actions. We particularly owe this to our patients.
3 Promoting justice—ie distributing scarce resources fairly (p10) and respecting rights: legal rights, rights to confidentiality, rights to be informed, to be offered all the options, and to be told the truth.
4 Promoting autonomy. This is not universally recognized; in some cultures facing starvation, for example, it may be irrelevant, or even be considered subversive.

*Health* entails being sound in body and mind, and having powers of growth, development, healing, and regeneration. *How many people have you made healthy (or at least healthier) today?* And in achieving this, *how many cardinal duties have you ignored?* We cannot spend long on the wards or in our surgeries trying to 'make people healthy' before we have breached every cardinal duty—particularly (3) and (4). Does it matter? What is the point of having principles if they are regularly ignored? The point of having them is to provide a context for our negotiations with patients to form, where possible, a beneficial synthesis.

**Synthesis** When we must act in the face of two conflicting duties, *one is not a duty.* How do we tell which one? Trying to find out involves getting to know our patient.
• Are the patient's wishes being complied with?
• What do your colleagues think? What do the relatives think? Have they his or her best interests at heart? Ask the patient's permission first.
• Is it desirable that the reason for an action be universalizable? (That is, if I say this person is too old for such-and-such an operation, am I happy to make this a general rule for everyone?—Kant's 'law'.)[2]
• If an investigative journalist were to sit on a sulcus of mine, having full knowledge of my thoughts and actions, would she be bored or would she be composing vitriol for tomorrow's newspapers? If so, can I answer her, point for point? Am I happy with my answers? Or are they merely tactical devices?
• What would a patient's representative think, eg the elected chairman of a patient's participation group (*OHCS* p496)? These opinions are valid and readily available (if a local group exists) and they can stop decision-making from being too medicalized.

**Red flags on your wigwam** For each patient use a check-list to avoid skating over ethical issues. If a red flag pertains, ethical aspects are likely to be very important.

> ⚑ Wishes of the patient are unknown (find out if a living will is in existence).
> ⚑ Issues regarding confidentiality/disclosure (eg HIV+ve but partner unaware).
> ⚑ Goals of care: are these confused and contradictory in any way?
> ⚑ Wants to discharge himself against advice. Is he fully informed and competent?
> ⚑ Arguments among relatives as how best to proceed: have you listened to all sides?
> ⚑ Money problems relating to cost of care or earnings lost through illness.[64]

---

1 Don't think of good and evil as forever opposite; good can come out of evil, and vice versa: this fundamental mix-up explains why we learn more from our dissolute patients than we do from saints.[65]
2 There are problems with universalizability: only intuition can suggest how to resolve conflicts between competing universalizable principles. Also, there is a sense in which all ethical dilemmas are unique, so no moral rules are possible or required—so they *cannot* be universal (Sartre, Nietzsche).[66]

"*Unless both the doctor and the patient become a problem to each other, no solution is found.*" Jung's aphorism[67] is untrue for half our waking lives: for an anaesthetist there is no need for the patient to become a problem in order for the anaesthetic to work. But, as with all the best aphorisms, being untrue is the least of the problems they cause us. Great aphorisms signify because they unsettle. Our settled and smug satisfaction at finishing a period of duty without any problems is so often a sign of failure. We have kept the chaos at bay, whereas, if we were greater men or women, we would have embraced it. Half our waking professional lives we spend as if asleep, on automatic, following protocols or guidelines to some trite destination—or else we are dreaming of what we could do if we had more time, proper resources, and perhaps a different set of colleagues. But if we had Jung in our pockets he would be shaking us awake, derailing our guidelines, and saluting our attempts to risk genuine interactions with our patients, however much of a mess we make of it, and however much pain we cause and receive. (Pain, after all, is the inevitable companion to lives led authentically.)[1] To the unreflective doctor, and to all average minds, this interaction is anathema, to be avoided at all costs, because it leads us away from anaesthesia, to the unpredictable, and to destinations that are unknown.

After proposing that 'deep Thinking' can only be attained by someone capable of 'deep Feeling', Samuel Taylor Coleridge, in 1801, went on to calculate on the back of a jocular envelope that 'the Souls of 500 Sir Isaac Newtons would go to the making up of a Shakespeare or a Milton...In his system is always passive...*and there is ground for suspicion that any system built on the passiveness of the mind must be a false system*"[68] Newtonian models of the consultation in which the doctor remains unmoved are all tainted by this falsity. So when you find yourself being irritated, moved, or provoked by your patient, be half-glad, because these feelings welcome you to Shakespeare's and Coleridge's world where the imagination (p315) is the Prime Mover in the task of bringing about change in our patients.

So, every so often, be pleased with your difficult patients: those who question you, those who do not respond to your treatments, or who complain when these treatments *do* work. Often, it will seem that whatever you say is wrong, misunderstood, misquoted, and mangled by the mind you are confronting, perhaps because of fear, loneliness, or past experiences that you can only guess at. If this is happening, *shut up*—but don't *give up*. Stick with your patient. Listen to what he or she is saying and not saying. And when you have understood your patient a bit more, negotiate, cajole, and even argue—but don't bully or blackmail ("If you do not let your son have the operation he needs, I'll tell him just what sort of a mother you are..."). When you find yourself turning to walk away from your patient, turn back and say "This is not going very well, is it? Can we start again?" Don't hesitate to call in your colleagues' help: not to win by force of numbers, but to see if a different approach might bear fruit. By this process, and by addressing the psychosomatic factors perpetuating your patient's illnesses, you and your patient may grow in stature. You may even end up with a truly satisfied patient. And a satisfied patient is worth a thousand protocols.

We all seek the reason for our own existence, and as we sit beside troubled, troubling, and troublesome patients we may dimly comprehend part of the reason, albeit in the background of our minds—even if, in the foreground, we are wondering why on earth this difficult patient has to exist, especially now when we are so busy and so stressed. The patient is likely to have their own unspoken metaphysical questions, for which you can be the midwife: "Why me?" "Why now?" Don't strangle these questions at birth: give them space to breathe, and who knows?

---

**1** "Some say that the world is a vale of tears. I say it is a place of soul making"—John Keats, the first medical student to formulate these ideas about pain. They did not do him much good, as he died shortly after uttering them. But his ideas can do us good. Perhaps if each day we try at least once for authentic interactions with a patient, unencumbered by professionalism, research interests, defensive medicine, a wish to show off to our peers, or a wish to get though the day without fuss.

If only we could live long enough to suffer from every disease, then we doctors could be of real service to our patients. There would be no need for medical humanities, as we would understand angina from the inside, and the fire of zoster's pain would no longer mystify us. We could die a thousand deaths for our patients. But still death would be untamed, and our self-anecdotal knowledge of disease would be irrelevant to patients from foreign lands. All patients inhabit foreign lands, and even our own hearts are alien to us unless melted by narrative streams. It is only through the humanities that, prude or peasant, prince or prostitute, we can extend our horizons and universalize anecdotal experience, so that nothing human is foreign to us.

Doctors' and artists' methodologies overlap, as we both create new realities: artists do this by bewitchment and by suspending reality. Doctors do it by listening and suspending judgement. A patient of ours had been trapped in an abusive marriage for 52 years. She had tried telling one other person, who had not believed her. The relief of being believed and listened to shone through her tears, as we collaborated over plans to bring change to her life. It is good to aim to listen to our patients with as rapt attention as we display when reading a good book. While reading, there is no point in dissembling. We confront our subject with a steady eye because we believe that, while reading to ourselves, we cannot be judged. Then, suddenly, when we are at our most open and *defenceless*, literature takes us by the throat, and that eye, which was so steady and confident a few minutes ago, is now misting over, or our heart is missing a beat, or our skin is covered in a goose-flesh more immediate than ever a Siberian winter produced. As the decades go by, not much in our mundane world sends shivers down our spines, but the power of art to do this ever grows, and sensitizes us to our patients' narratives, and shows us there are many valid routes to knowledge other than the strictly objective.

The reason for the ascendancy of art over science is simple. We scientists, when we are not adopting our listening role, are only interested in explaining reality. Artists are good at explaining reality too: but they also *create* it. Our most powerful impressions are produced in our minds not by simple sensations but by the association of ideas. It is a pre-eminent feature of the human mind that it revels in seeing something as, or through, something else: life refracted through experience, light refracted through jewels, or a walk through the woods transmuted into a Pastoral Symphony. Ours is a world of metaphor, fantasy, and deceit.

What has all this to do with the day-to-day practice of medicine? The answer lies in the word 'defenceless' above. When we read alone and for pleasure, our defences are down—and we hide nothing from the great characters of fiction. In our consulting rooms, and on the ward, we so often do our best to hide everything beneath our avuncular bedside manner. So often, a professional detachment is all that is left after all those years inured to the foibles, fallacies, and frictions of our patients' tragic lives. It is at the point where art and medicine collide that doctors can re-attach themselves to the human race and re-feel those emotions that motivate or terrify our patients. We all have an Achilles heel: that part of our inner self which was not rendered invulnerable when we were dipped in the waters of our first disillusion. Art and literature may enable this Achilles heel to be the means of our survival as thinking and feeling human beings.

If it is true that all the great novels, songs, and drama defy any single interpretation it is all the more true for the patient sitting in front of us. If we are not getting very far it is because we are using light when we could be using shade—or harmony in place of disharmony, or we are only offering a monologue when what we should be risking is dialogue—and the forging of new meanings.

The American approach is to create Professors of Literature-in-Medicine and to conjure with concepts such as *the patient as text*, and most American medical schools do courses in literature in an attempt to inculcate ethical reasoning and speculation. Here, we simply intend to demonstrate, albeit imperfectly, in our writings and in our practice of medicine, that *every* contact with patients has an ethical and artistic dimension, as well as a technical one.

## Contents

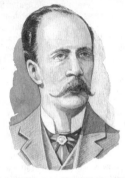

Fig 1. William Osler (1849-1919) was a great medical educationalist who loved practical jokes. He introduced many novelties to the classroom, including, on one occasion, a gaggle of geese. We can all identify with his geese, because these birds show exceptional learning ability and resilience.

Osler did not agree with gavage, a method whereby geese (and medical students) are forcibly stuffed by funnel to fatten them for the delight of gluttons. We are too familiar with the 3 Rs of medical education: Ram→Remember→Regurgitate, a sequence that turns once-bright medical students into tearful wrecks. Luckily in the realm of History & Examination we can flee the library and alight at the bedside, bearing in mind another of Osler's aphorisms: "He who studies medicine without books sails an uncharted sea, but he who studies medicine without patients does not go to sea at all."

**Other relevant pages:** acute abdomen (p608); lumps (p596-p606); hernias (p614-p616); varicose veins (p660); urine (p286); peripheral nerves (p456); dermatomes (p458). *In OHCS:* Vaginal examination (*OHCS* p242); abdominal examination in pregnancy (*OHCS* p40); the history and examination in children and neonates (*OHCS* p100-p102); examination of the eye (*OHCS* p412); visual acuity (*OHCS* p414); eye movements (*OHCS* p422); ear, nose, and throat examination (*OHCS* p536); skin examination (*OHCS* p584); examination of joints—see the contents page to *Orthopaedics and trauma* (*OHCS* p656).

*A number of images are taken from the* **Oxford Handbook of Clinical Examination and Practical Skills (OHCEPS)**, *which gives an even more detailed account of this subject. Our thanks to Dr James Thomas and Dr Tanya Monaghan for their kind permission. We thank Junior Reader Shahzad Arain for his contribution.*

## Advice and experience

1 The way to learn physical signs is at the bedside, with guidance from a senior doctor or an experienced colleague. This chapter is not a substitute for this process: it is simply an aide-mémoire both on the wards and when preparing for exams.

2 We ask questions to get information to help with differential diagnosis. But we also ask questions to find out about the lives our patients live so that we can respect them as individuals. The patient is likely to notice and reciprocate this respect, and the rapport that you build with your patient in this way is a key component to diagnosing and managing their disease.

3 Patients (and diseases) rarely read the textbook, so don't be surprised that some symptoms are ambiguous, and others are meaningless. Get good at recognizing patterns, but not so good that you create them when none is there. We all fall into this trap!

4 Signs can be easy to detect, or subtle. Some will be found by all the new medical students, others require experienced ears or eyes. Remember, *you can be a fine doctor without being able to elicit every sign.*[1] However, finding signs and putting together the clues they give us to find a diagnosis is one of the best parts of being a doctor. It is also essential that we learn those signs that highlight diseases we should never miss. However, in an exam, if you cannot find a sign, never be tempted to make up something you think should be there. If the examiner is pushing you to describe something you cannot see, be honest and admit you cannot see it. Learning is a lifelong process, and nobody becomes a consultant overnight.

## Handover and advice

With increasing targets, shift patterns and the move towards more and more specialist services, patients can be bounced around from team to team many times during their admission. The Royal College of Physicians in the UK has recognized this and produced guidance on how best to approach handover.[1]

Both written and verbal communications are key to effective handover; although a written note explaining who is unwell, what the plan is, and who to call if things deteriorate is essential, nothing substitutes for face to face handover. Discussion of patients is important for safety as well as learning and good practice. Make a point of handing over weekend and evening plans, and patients you are worried about. Take advantage of the experience and knowledge of the person you are handing over to. Can they offer advice on what you could have done differently?

Make sure senior colleagues know who is unwell and who you would like help with. Senior doctors would far rather see someone before they deteriorate, putting together an action plan for what to do next, than be called to an acutely unwell patient who may need escalation to ICU when a few early interventions could have prevented deterioration. There is no shame in asking for help, but remember you should do what you can first; never call without knowing your patient or having examined them. See p25 for key things to know before calling for advice. Ultimately we are all there for the patient, so if they are deteriorating despite your best efforts, call for advice.

1 http://www.rcplondon.ac.uk/resources/acute-care-toolkit-1-handover

*History and examination*

Taking (or receiving) histories is what most of us spend most of our professional life doing, and it is worth doing well. A good history is the biggest step towards correct diagnosis. Try to put the patient at ease: a good rapport may relieve distress. Introduce yourself and check whether the patient is comfortable. Be conversational rather than interrogative in tone. Start with open questions, allow the patient to tell their story, but if they stray off topic, try to gently steer them back towards the important points.

**Presenting complaint (PC)** Open questions: "Why have you come to see me today?" Record the patient's own words rather than medical terms.

**History of presenting complaint (HPC)** When did it start? What was the first thing noticed? Progress since then. Ever had it before? 'SOCRATES' questions: site; onset (gradual, sudden); character; radiation; associations (eg nausea, sweating); timing of pain/duration; exacerbating and alleviating factors; severity (eg scale of 1-10, compared with worst ever previous pain). *Direct questioning* (to narrow list of possible diagnoses). Specific or 'closed' questions about the differential diagnoses you have in mind (+risk factors, eg travel—p388) and a review of the relevant system.

**Past medical history (PMH)** Ever in hospital? Illnesses? Operations? Ask specifically about MIJTHREADS: **MI**, jaundice, **TB**, high BP, rheumatic fever, epilepsy, asthma, diabetes, stroke, anaesthetic problems.

**Drug history (DH)** Any tablets, injections, 'over-the-counter' drugs, herbal remedies, oral contraceptives? Ask about *allergies* and what the patient experienced, eg may be an intolerance (nausea, diarrhoea), or may have been a minor reaction of sensitization (eg rash and wheeze) before full-blown anaphylaxis.

**Social history (SH)** Probe without prying. "Who else is there at home?" Job. Marital status. Spouse's job and health. Housing—any stairs at home? Who visits—relatives, neighbours, GP, nurse? Are there any dependents at home? Mobility—any walking aids needed? Who does the cooking and shopping? What can the patient not do because of the illness?

The social history is all too often seen as a dispensable adjunct, eg while the patient is being rushed to theatre, but vital clues may be missed about the quality of life and it is too late to ask when the surgeon's hand is deep in the belly and they are wondering how radical a procedure to perform. It is worth asking a few searching questions of the GP if they are calling to arrange admission. They may have known the patient and/or family for decades. He or she may even hold a 'living will' or advance directive to reveal your patient's wishes if they cannot speak for themselves.

As part of the social history, tactfully ask about *alcohol, tobacco & recreational drugs.* How much? How long? When stopped? The CAGE questionnaire is useful as a screening test for alcoholism (p282). Quantify smoking in terms of **pack-years**: 20 cigarettes/day for 1 year equals 1 pack-year. We all like to present ourselves well, so be inclined to double stated quantities (Holt's 'law').

**Family history (FH)** Areas of the family history may need detailed questioning, eg to determine if there is a significant family history of heart disease you need to ask about the health of the patient's grandfathers and male siblings, smoking, tendency to hypertension, hyperlipidaemia, and claudication before they were 60 years old, as well as ascertaining the cause of death. Ask about TB, diabetes, and other relevant diseases. Draw a family tree (see BOX). ▶Be tactful when asking about a family history of malignancy.

**Functional enquiry** (p22) helps uncover undeclared symptoms. Some of this may already have been incorporated into the history.

▶ Always enquire if your patient has any *ideas* of what the problem might be, if he/she has any particular *concerns* or *expectations*, and give him/her an opportunity to *ask you questions* or *tell you anything you may have missed.*

▶Don't hesitate to review the history later: recollections change (as you will find, often on the post-take ward round when the Consultant is asking the questions!).

## Drawing family trees to reveal dominantly inherited disease[1]

Advances in genetics are touching all branches of medicine. It is increasingly important for doctors to identify patients at high risk of genetic disease, and to make appropriate referrals. The key skill is drawing a family tree to help you structure a family history as follows:

1 Start with your patient. Draw a square for a male and a circle for a female. Add a small arrow (see below) to show that this person is the *propositus* (the person through whom the family tree is ascertained).

2 Add your patient's parents, brothers, and sisters. Record basic information only, eg age, and if alive and well (a&w). If dead, note age and cause of death, and pass an oblique stroke through that person's symbol.

3 Ask the key question "Has anybody else in your family had a similar problem as yourself?", eg heart attack/angina/stroke/cancer. Ask only about the family of diseases that relate to your patient's main problem. Do not record a potted medical history for each family member: time is too short.

4 Extend the family tree upwards to include grandparents. If you haven't revealed a problem by now, **go no further**—you are unlikely to miss important familial disease. If your patient is elderly it may be impossible to obtain good information about grandparents. If so, fill out the family tree with your patient's uncles and aunts on both the mother's and father's sides.

5 Shade those in the family tree affected by the disease. ● = an affected female; ■ = an affected male. This helps to show any genetic problem and, if there is one, will help demonstrate the pattern of inheritance.

6 If you have identified a familial susceptibility, or your patient has a recognized genetic disease, extend the family tree down to include children, to identify others who may be at risk and who may benefit from screening. ▶You should find out who is pregnant in the family, or may soon be, and arrange appropriate genetic counselling (*OHCS* p154). Refer for genetics opinion.

The family tree (fig 1) shows these ideas at work and indicates that there is evidence for genetic risk of colon cancer, meriting referral to a geneticist.

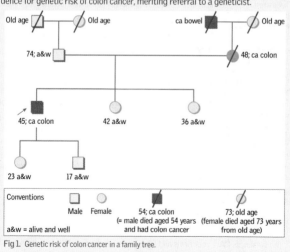

Fig 1. Genetic risk of colon cancer in a family tree.

1 Use a different approach in paediatrics, and for autosomal or sex-linked disease. Ask if parents are related (consanguinity ↑risk of recessive diseases). This page owes much to Dr Helen Firth, whom we thank.

Just as skilled acrobats are happy to work without safety nets, so experienced clinicians may operate without the functional enquiry. But to do this you must be experienced enough to understand all the nuances of the presenting complaint.

### General questions

May be the most significant, eg in TB, endocrine problems, or cancer: • Weight loss • Night sweats • Any lumps • Fatigue/malaise/lethargy • Sleeping pattern[1] • Appetite • Fevers • Itch or rash • Recent trauma.

### Cardiorespiratory symptoms

• Chest pain (p88).
• Exertional dyspnoea (=breathlessness): quantify exercise tolerance and how it has changed, eg stairs climbed, or distance walked, before onset of breathlessness.
• Paroxysmal nocturnal dyspnoea (PND). Orthopnoea, ie breathlessness on lying flat (a symptom of left ventricular failure): quantify in terms of number of pillows the patient must sleep on to prevent dyspnoea.
• Oedema: ankles, legs, lower back (dependent areas).
• Palpitations (awareness of heartbeats): can they tap out the rhythm?
• Cough: sputum, haemoptysis (coughing up blood).
• Wheeze.

### Gastrointestinal symptoms

• Abdominal pain (constant or colicky, sharp or dull; site; radiation; duration; onset; severity; relationship to eating and bowel action; alleviating or exacerbating, or associated features).
• Other questions—think of symptoms throughout the GI tract, from mouth to anus:
  • Swallowing (p240)
  • Indigestion (p242)
  • Nausea/vomiting (p240)
  • Bowel habit (p246 & p248)
  • Stool:
  • colour, consistency, blood, mucus
  • difficulty flushing away (p280)
  • tenesmus or urgency.
• **Tenesmus** is the feeling of incomplete evacuation of the bowels (eg due to a tumour or irritable bowel syndrome).
• **Haematemesis** is vomiting blood.
• **Melaena** is altered (black) blood passed PR (p252), with a characteristic smell.

### Genitourinary symptoms

• Incontinence (stress or urge, p650).
• Dysuria (painful micturition).
• Urinary abnormalities: colour? Haematuria (streaks or pink urine?) Frothy?
• Nocturia (needing to micturate at night).
• Frequency (frequent micturition) or polyuria (the frequent passing of large volumes of urine).
• Hesitancy (difficulty starting micturition).
• Terminal dribbling.
• Vaginal discharge (p418).
• Menses: frequency, regularity, heavy or light, duration, painful? First day of last menstrual period (LMP). Number of pregnancies and births. Menarche. Menopause. Any chance of pregnancy now?

### Neurological symptoms

• *Special senses:* Sight, hearing, smell, and taste.
• Seizures, faints, 'funny turns'.
• Headache.
• 'Pins and needles' (paraesthesiae) or numbness.
• Limb weakness ("Are your arms and legs weaker than normal?"), poor balance.
• Speech problems (p80).
• Sphincter disturbance.
• Higher mental function and psychiatric symptoms (p80–p83). The important thing is to assess function: what the patient can and cannot do at home, work, etc.

1 Too sleepy? Think of myxoedema or narcolepsy. Early waking? Think of depression. Being woken by pain is always a serious sign. ► For the significance of the other questions listed here, see Chapter 3.

### Musculoskeletal symptoms
• Pain, stiffness, swelling of joints.
• Diurnal variation in symptoms (ie worse mornings).
• Functional deficit.
• Signs of systemic disease: rashes, mouth ulcers, nasal stuffiness, malaise and constitutional symptoms.

### Thyroid symptoms
• *Hyperthyroidism:* Prefers cold weather, bad tempered, sweaty, diarrhoea, oligomenorrhoea, weight↓ (though often ↑appetite), tremor, palpitations, visual problems.
• *Hypothyroidism:* Depressed, slow, tired, thin hair, croaky voice, heavy periods, constipation, dry skin, prefers warm weather.

▶History-taking may seem deceptively easy, as if the patient knew the hard facts and the only problem was extracting them; but what a patient says is a mixture of hearsay ("She said I looked very pale"), innuendo ("You know, doctor, *down below*"), legend ("I suppose I bit my tongue; it was a real fit, you know"), exaggeration ("I didn't sleep a wink"), and improbabilities ("The Pope put a transmitter in my brain"). The great skill (and pleasure) in taking a history lies not in ignoring these garbled messages, but in making sense of them.

History and examination

The physical examination is not so much an extension of the history, but more of the first investigation, to confirm, exclude, define, or show the progress of the provisional diagnosis as revealed in the history. Even in the emergency department where the history may be brief, eg "trauma", the examination is to confirm a fracture, or to decide that a fracture is less likely. The examination sheds further light on the history. As you get better, your physical examination gets briefer. Establish your own routine—practice is the key.

### End of the bed
- Look at the patient—are they well or in extremis? What makes you think this? Are they in pain? If so, does it make them lie still (eg peritonitis) or writhe about (eg colic). What is the pattern of breathing: laboured; rapid; shallow; irregular; distressed? Are they obese or cachectic? Is their behaviour appropriate? Can you detect any unusual *smell*, eg hepatic fetor (p258), cigarettes, alcohol?
- Also take a moment to look around the bed for other clues, eg inhalers, insulin administration kit, walking aids, etc.

### Face and body habitus
- Does the patient's appearance suggest any particular diseases, eg acromegaly, thyrotoxicosis, myxoedema, Cushing's syndrome, or hypopituitarism? See p196.
- Is there an abnormal distribution of body hair (eg bearded ♀, or hairless ♂) suggestive of endocrine disease?
- Is there anything about the patient to trigger thoughts about Paget's disease, Marfan's, myotonia, or Parkinson's syndrome? Look for rashes, eg the malar flush of mitral disease and the butterfly rash of SLE.

### Peripheral stigmata of disease
Specific signs are associated with different diseases: consider the nails (koilonychia = iron deficiency), subcutaneous nodules (rheumatoid, neurofibroma?), and look for lymph nodes (cervical, axillary, inguinal). See specific systems for features to assess for, but for all systems consider:

*Skin colour:*
- Blue/purple = cyanosis (can also be central only, p28).
- Yellow = jaundice (yellow skin can also be caused by uraemia, pernicious anaemia, carotenaemia—check the sclera: if they are also yellow it is jaundice).
- Pallor: this is non-specific; anaemia is assessed from the palmar skin creases (when spread) and conjunctivae (fig 1, p319)—usually pale if Hb <80-90g/L: you cannot conclude anything from normal conjunctival colour, but if they are pale, the patient is probably anaemic.
- Hyperpigmentation: Addison's, haemochromatosis (slate-grey) and amiodarone, gold, silver, and minocycline therapy.

*Charts:*
- Temperature: varies during the day; a morning oral temperature >37.2°C or evening >37.7°C constitutes a fever.[2] Rectal temperatures are generally 0.6°C above oral temperatures. Remember that temperatures are generally lower in elderly patients and therefore fevers may not be as pronounced.[3] A core temperature <35°C indicates hypothermia; special low-reading thermometers may be required.
- Blood pressure and pulse—trends are more important than one-off values; repeat if concerned.
- Urine: check urinalysis and input/output charts if available.

### Fluid status
When admitting an unwell patient, don't forget to assess their degree of hydration, check skin turgor and mucous membranes, look for sunken eyes, and check capillary refill (if well perfused <2s) and JVP.

## Unexplained signs and symptoms: How to refer for an opinion

▶When you don't know: ask. If you are wondering if you should ask: **ask.**

Frequently, the skills needed for diagnosis or treatment will lie beyond the team you are working for, so, during ward rounds, agree who should be asked for an opinion. You will be left with the job of making the arrangements, so check before your senior leaves exactly what their question is. Don't be intimidated: but follow these simple rules:

- Know the history and examination findings (ideally your own), and have the patient's notes, observations, recent test results and drug charts to hand.
- At the outset, state if you are just looking for advice or if you are asking if the patient could be seen. Make it clear exactly what the question is that you want addressed, allowing the listener to focus their thoughts and ask relevant questions.
- Give the patient's age and run through a **brief** history including relevant past medical history. If you would like the patient to be seen, give warning if they will be leaving the ward for a test at a particular time.
- The visiting doctor may be unfamiliar with your ward. When he or she arrives introduce yourself, get the notes and charts, and give your contact details in case they have further questions.

The following table may be useful to bear in mind, as you will be asked!

| Team | Key questions |
|---|---|
| Anaesthetics | Previous anaesthetic? Reaction? Last ate/drank? |
| Cardiology | Known IHD? BP? ECG findings? Echo findings? Murmurs? Troponin? Temperature/possibility of endocarditis? (ESR, microscopic haematuria etc. p144) |
| Dermatology | Site, onset and appearance of rash? Drugs? Systemic disease? History of atopy? |
| Endocrinology | Diabetes: blood glucose, usual insulin regimen, complications. Other: blood results? Stable/unstable—eg Addisonian crisis. Usual steroid dose? |
| Gastroenterology/ Hepatology | Bleeding: Rockall score (p253)? Shock? Diarrhoea: Blood? Foreign travel? Frequency per day? Liver disease: signs of decompensation (p258)? Ascites? Encephalopathy grade? |
| Gynaecology/ Obstetrics | LMP? Possibility of pregnancy? Previous pregnancies? Vaginal discharge? Hormonal contraceptives? STIs? |
| Haematology | Blood results? Splenomegaly? Fever? Lymphadenopathy? Bleeding: Anticoagulants? Clotting results? |
| Infectious diseases/ Microbiology | Possible source? Antibiotics (current/recent/previous)? Foreign travel? Risk factors for HIV? |
| Nephrology | Creatinine (current, old)? Clotting? Urine output? Potassium? BP? Fluid status? Drugs? Known renal disease? |
| Neurology/Stroke | Neurological examination?[1] CT/MRI scan findings? |
| Radiology | See p734. Contrast or not? Creatinine? Clotting? Cannula in situ? Metallic implants? |
| Respiratory | $O_2$ sats? Respiratory rate? ABG? CXR? Inhalers/nebs? Home $O_2$? Respiratory support, eg NIV/CPAP? |
| Surgery (general) | Pain? Scan findings? Acutely unwell? Clotting? |
| Urology | History of LUTS (lower urinary tract symptoms) p644? Catheter? Haematuria? History of stones? Scan findings (ultrasound, CT)? |

1 You would be amazed at how many people refer to neurology/stroke without having done a neurological examination! Don't be one of them...

History and examination

Symptoms are features which patients report. **Physical signs** are elicited at the bedside. Together, they constitute the features of the condition in that patient. Their evolution over time and interaction with the physical, psychological, and social spheres comprise the natural history of any disease. Throughout this chapter, we discuss symptoms in isolation and attempt to classify them into a 'system' or present them below as 'non-specific'. This is unnatural but a good first step in learning how to diagnose. All doctors have to know about symptoms and their relief: this is what doctors are for. Part of becoming a good doctor is learning to link symptoms together, to identify those that may be normal, and those that are worrying. There are many online tools and books that can help with this, but there is no substitute for experience. If you aren't sure, ask a specialist in that area for advice.

The following are common 'non-specific' presentations

### Itch

**Itching (pruritus)** is common and, if chronic, most unpleasant.

| *Local causes:* | *Systemic:* (Do FBC, ESR, glucose, LFT, U&E, ferritin, TFT) | |
|---|---|---|
| Eczema, atopy, urticaria | Liver disease (bile salts, eg PBC) | Old age; pregnancy |
| Scabies | Uraemia (eg CKD) | Drugs (eg morphine) |
| Lichen planus | Malignancy (eg lymphoma) | Diabetes mellitus |
| Dermatitis herpetiformis | Polycythaemia rubra vera | Thyroid disease |
| Spinal cord tumours (rare)[4] | Iron deficiency anaemia | HIV infection |

*Questions:* Wheals (urticaria)? Worse at night? Others affected (scabies)? What provokes it? After a bath ≈ polycythaemia rubra vera (p360). Exposure, eg to animals (atopy?) or fibre glass (irritant eczema?).

Look for *local causes:* Scabies burrows in finger webs, lice on hair shafts, knee and elbow blisters (dermatitis herpetiformis). *Systemic:* Splenomegaly, nodes, jaundice, flushed face or thyroid signs? ℞: Treat causes; try soothing bland emollients, eg E45®, ± emollient bath oils ± sedative antihistamines at night, eg chlorphenamine 4mg PO.

### 'Off-legs'—falls and difficulty walking

Common causes of admission in the elderly, and can lead to loss of confidence and independence. Causes are often multifactorial:

*Intrinsic:* typically osteo- or rheumatoid arthritis, but remember fractured neck of femur, CNS disease, vision↓, cognitive impairment, depression, postural hypotension, peripheral neuropathy, medication (eg antihypertensives, sedatives), pain, eg arthritis, parkinsonism (eg drugs: prochlorperazine, neuroleptics, metoclopramide), muscle weakness (consider vitamin D deficiency), incontinence, UTI, pneumonia, anaemia, hypothyroidism, renal impairment, hypothermia and alcohol. *Environment:* Poor lighting, uneven walking surface. Treatment includes addressing injuries, reducing risk factors, and reducing the risk of injury, eg treat osteoporosis (p696). A multidisciplinary multifactorial approach alongside occupational therapists and physiotherapists is likely to be beneficial.[5] See **gait disturbance**, p471.

If there is ataxia, the cause is not always alcohol: other chemicals may be involved (eg cannabis or prescribed sedatives). There may be a metastatic or non-metastatic manifestation of malignancy, or a cerebellar lesion.

▶Bilateral weak legs may suggest a cord lesion: see p470. If there is associated urinary or faecal incontinence ± saddle anaesthesia or lower limb sensory loss, urgent imaging (MRI) and treatment for cord compression may well be needed.

## Fatigue

So common that it is a variant of normality. Only 1 in 400 episodes of fatigue leads to visiting the doctor. ►Don't miss depression (p11). Even if depressed, still rule out common treatable causes—eg anaemia, hypothyroidism, diabetes. After history and examination: FBC, ESR, U&E, plasma glucose, TFT, ± CXR. Follow up to see what develops, and to address emotional problems. Take a sleep history.

## Fevers, rigors, sweats

While some night sweating is common in anxiety, drenching sweats requiring changes of night-clothes are a more ominous symptom associated with infection (eg TB, brucellosis), lymphoproliferative disease, or other malignancies. Patterns of fever may be relevant (see p386).

*Rigors* are uncontrolled paroxysms of shivering which occur as a patient's temperature rises rapidly. See p386.

*Sweating excessively (hyperhidrosis)* may be primary (eg hidradenitis suppurativa may be very distressing to the patient)—or secondary to fever, pain or anxiety (cold & sweaty) or a systemic condition: the menopause, hyperthyroidism (warm & sweaty), acromegaly, malignancy, phaeochromocytoma, amyloidosis, or neuroleptic malignant syndrome (+hyperthermia). Or it may reflect gabapentin or opiate withdrawal, or a cholinergic or parasympathomimetic side-effect (amitriptyline, bethanechol, distigmine, spider bites)—also hormonal drugs, eg levothyroxine, gonadorelin or somatostatin analogues, vasopressin, and ephedrine. Also amiodarone, ciprofloxacin, L-dopa, lisinopril, rivastigmine, ritonavir, pioglitazone, venlafaxine. At the bedside: Ask about all drugs, examine all over for nodes; any signs of hyperthyroidism? Any splenomegaly? Test the urine; do T°, ESR, TSH, FBC & blood culture. R: Antiperspirants (aluminium chloride 20%=Driclor®), sympathectomy, or iontophoresis may be tried.

## Insomnia

This is trivial—until we ourselves have a few sleepless nights. Then sleep becomes the most desirable thing imaginable, and bestowing it the best thing we can do, like relieving pain. But don't give drugs without looking for a cause.
• *Self-limiting:* Jet lag; stress; shift work; in hospital. We need less sleep as we age.
• *Psychic:* Depression; anxiety; mania; grief; psychomotor agitation/psychosis.
• *Organic:* Drugs (many; eg caffeine; mefloquine; nicotine withdrawal); nocturia; alcohol; pain (eg acid reflux—worse on lying down); itch; tinnitus; asthma; dystonias; obstructive sleep apnoea (p194); dementia; restless leg syndrome (p712, check ferritin). Rarer: encephalitis (eg West Nile virus) and encephalopathy (Whipple's; pellagra; HIV; prion diseases, eg CJD, p710, and fatal familial insomnia).

R: Sleep hygiene: No daytime naps; don't turn in till you feel sleepy; regular bedtime routines. Keep a room for sleep; don't eat or work in it (not viable for much of the world). Less caffeine, nicotine, late exercise (but sexual activity may give excellent torpor!) and alcohol (its abuse causes paradoxical pro-adrenergic tremor and insomnia).⁶ Try monitoring quality with a sleep diary (unless already overobsessive). Music and relaxation may make sleep more restorative and augment personal resources.⁷

Hypnotic drugs: give for a few nights only (addictive and cause daytime somnolence ± rebound insomnia on stopping). Warn about driving/machine use. Example: zopiclone 3.75-7.5mg. *Obstructive sleep apnoea:* p194. *Parasomnias, sleep paralysis, etc.:* OHCS p392. *Narcolepsy:* p714.

Over 80% of diagnoses should be made on history alone, with the signs you elicit adding an extra 10% and tests only giving the final 5% or so.[1] Do not rely on signs or investigations for your diagnosis, but use them rather to confirm what you suspected from the history. The following signs are not specific to a particular system:

## Cyanosis

Dusky blue skin (*peripheral*—of the fingers) or mucosae (*central*—of the tongue), representing 50g/L of Hb in its reduced (hence hypoxic) form, it occurs more readily in polycythaemia than anaemia. *Causes:*
• *Lung disease* with inadequate oxygen transfer, eg luminal obstruction, asthma, COPD, pneumonia, PE, pulmonary oedema—may be correctable by ↑ inspired $O_2$.
• *Congenital cyanotic heart disease*, where there is admixture, eg transposition of the great arteries or right-to-left shunt (eg VSD with Eisenmenger's syndrome; see p150)—cyanosis is *not* reversed by increasing inspired oxygen.
• *Rare causes*: methaemoglobinaemia, a congenital or acquired red cell disorder.
▶Acute cyanosis is an emergency. Is there asthma, an inhaled foreign body, a pneumothorax (p763, fig 1) or pulmonary oedema? See p824.
*Peripheral cyanosis* will occur in causes of central cyanosis, but may also be induced by changes in the peripheral and cutaneous vascular systems in patients with normal oxygen saturations. It occurs in the cold, in hypovolaemia, and in arterial disease, and is therefore not a specific sign.

## Pallor

May be racial or familial—or from anaemia, shock/faints, Stokes-Adams attack (p464, pale first, then flushing), hypothyroidism, hypopituitarism, and albinism.
▶▶If it's just one limb or digit, think of emboli. *Anaemia* is haemoglobin concentration below the normal range (p318). It may be assessed from the conjunctivae and skin creases. Koilonychia and stomatitis (p24) suggest iron deficiency. Anaemia with jaundice suggests haemolysis.

## Skin discolouration

Generalized hyperpigmentation may be genetic (racial) or due to radiation; ↑ACTH (cross-reacts with melanin receptors, eg Addison's disease (p218), Nelson's syndrome (p32), ectopic ACTH in bronchial carcinoma); chronic kidney disease (↑urea, p294); malabsorption; chloasma (seen in pregnancy or with the oral contraceptive pill); biliary cirrhosis; haemochromatosis ('bronzed diabetes'); carotenaemia; or drugs (eg chlorpromazine, busulfan, amiodarone, gold).

## Obesity

(see *OHCS* p530)

This is defined by the World Health Organization as a BMI of over $30kg/m^2$. A higher waist to hip ratio, indicating central fat distribution, is commoner in ♂ and is associated with greater health risks, which include type 2 diabetes mellitus, IHD, dyslipidaemia, ↑BP, osteoarthritis of weight-bearing joints, and cancer (breast and bowel); see p199. The majority of cases are not due to specific metabolic disorders. Lifestyle change is key to treatment, to increase energy expenditure and reduce intake (p236). Medication ± surgery may be considered if the patient fulfils strict criteria. Conditions associated with obesity include: genetic (Prader-Willi syndrome, Lawrence-Moon syndrome), hypothyroidism, Cushing's syndrome and hypothalamic damage (eg tumour or trauma → damage to satiety regions).

## Lymphadenopathy

Causes of lymphadenopathy are either reactive or infiltrative:

### Reactive

*Infective*
- *Bacterial:* eg pyogenic, TB, brucella, syphilis.
- *Viral:* EBV, HIV, CMV, infectious hepatitis.
- *Others:* toxoplasmosis, trypanosomiasis.

*Non-infective:* sarcoidosis, amyloidosis, berylliosis, connective tissue disease (eg rheumatoid, SLE), dermatological (eczema, psoriasis), drugs (eg phenytoin).

### Infiltrative

*Benign histiocytosis*—OHCS p644, lipoidoses.
*Malignant*
- *Haematological:* lymphoma or leukaemia: ALL, CLL, AML (p350).
- *Metastatic carcinoma:* from breast, lung, bowel, prostate, kidney, or head and neck cancers.

## Oedema                                                                (see p580)

*Pitting oedema:* Fluid can either be squeezed out of the veins (increased hydrostatic pressure, eg DVT, right heart failure) or diffuse out because of reduced oncotic pressure (low plasma proteins, eg cirrhosis, nephrotic syndrome, protein losing enteropathy) leading to an osmotic gradient with the tissues (fig 4 p36, p580). The cause of oedema is still not completely understood.[8]

*Periorbital oedema:* Oedema around the face has a very different differential; The eyelid skin is very thin so periorbital oedema is usually the first sign—think of allergies (contact dermatitis, eg from eye make-up, stings), angioedema (can be hereditary), infection (►orbital cellulitis can be life threatening, refer to hospital immediately if concerned,  other infections include EBV and sinusitis); if there is proptosis (p211) think Graves' disease, connective tissue diseases (eg dermatomyositis, SLE, sarcoid, amyloid); and many others. Assess for systemic disease before putting it down to allergies.

*Non-pitting oedema:* ie non-indentable, is lymphoedema due to poor lymphatic drainage. Can be due to radiotherapy, malignant infiltration, infection, filariasis or rarely primary lymphoedema (Milroy's syndrome p720).

## Weight loss

This is a feature of chronic disease and depression; also of malnutrition, malignancy, chronic infections (eg TB, HIV/enteropathic AIDS), diabetes mellitus and hyperthyroidism (typically in the presence of increased appetite). Severe generalized muscle wasting is also seen as part of a number of degenerative neurological diseases and in cardiac failure (cardiac cachexia), although in the latter, right heart failure may not make weight loss a major complaint. Do not forget anorexia nervosa (OHCS p348) as an underlying cause of weight loss.

Rule out treatable causes, eg diabetes is easy to diagnose—TB can be very hard. For example, the CXR may look like cancer so don't forget to send bronchoscopy samples for ZN stain and TB culture. Unintentional weight loss should always ring alarm bells, so assess patients carefully.

## Cachexia

General muscle wasting from **famine**, or ↓eating (dementia; stroke; MND, p510; anorexia nervosa), **malabsorption** (enteropathic AIDS/slim disease/*Cryptosporidium*; Whipple's) or ↑catabolism (neoplasia; CCF; TB; chronic kidney disease; leptin↑).[10]

As with any examination routine, begin by introducing yourself, obtaining consent to examine the patient and position them appropriately. Expose the arms, then ask the patient to rest their hands on a pillow. Always ask about pain or tender areas. With the hands, particularly in acute arthritis, the standard joint examination routine of "look, feel, move" is better amended to "look, ask the patient to move, then feel" to avoid causing pain.

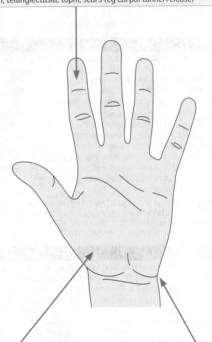

**1 Skin**
On both the palm and the dorsum start by inspecting the skin for:
1 **Colour**—pigmentation of creases, jaundice, palmar erythema
2 **Consistency**—tight (sclerodactyly), thick (DM, acromegaly)
3 **Characteristic lesions**—pulp infarcts, rashes, purpura, spider naevi, telangiectasia, tophi, scars (eg carpal tunnel release)

**2 Muscles**
Examine the muscles for wasting and fasciculations; on the palm look particularly at the thenar and hypothenar eminences.
• Thenar wasting = median nerve lesion
• Generalized wasting, particularly of the interossei on the dorsum, but sparing of the thenar eminence = ulnar nerve lesion
Also look for *Dupuytren's* contracture and perform *Tinel's test* (percuss over the distal skin crease of the wrist—tingling suggests carpal tunnel syndrome.

**3 Joints**
Examine for acute inflammation (swollen, red joints) as well as the characteristic deformities of chronic arthritis:
• Ulnar deviation at the wrist
• Z deformity of the thumb

### 1 Skin and nails

On the dorsum, look for the same skin changes as the palm, plus tendon xanthomata, plaques and joint replacement scars, and examine the nails for:
- Pitting and onycholysis (p32)
- Clubbing (p33)
- Nail fold infarcts and splinter haemorrhages
- Other lesions, eg Beau's lines (fig 1, p32), koilonychia, leuconychia

### 2 Joints and muscles

Again, look for muscle wasting, particularly of the dorsal interossei. Examine the joints for characteristic deformities:
- Swan-neck (flexed DIP, hyperextended PIP—fig 2, p540)
- Boutonnière (hyperextended DIP, flexed PIP)
- Heberden's nodes (DIP joints, p32)
- Bouchard's nodes (PIP joints)

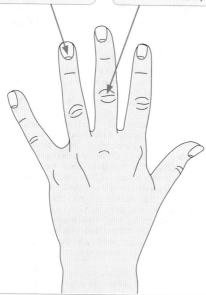

### Move and feel

By this point, you should know the likely diagnosis, so assess neurological function looking at power, function and sensation.
- *Wrist and forearm:* Extension (prayer position) and flexion (reverse prayer), supination and pronation. Look at the elbows
- *Small muscles:* Pincer grip, power grip (squeeze my two fingers), abduction of the thumb, abduction (spread your fingers) and adduction (grip this piece of paper between your fingers) of the fingers. NB *Froment's sign* = flexion of the thumb during grip as ulnar nerve lesion prevents adduction (p456)
- *Function:* Write a sentence, undo a button, pick up a coin
- *Sensation:* Test little finger (ulnar), index finger (median) and anatomical snuffbox (radial) using light touch/pinprick

When you have clinched the diagnosis and functional status, examine each joint, palpating for tenderness, effusions and crepitus. Test sensation (see p73) and examine the elbows. Consider examination of upper limbs and face.

### Top tips

- Cross your fingers before the patient grips them, it hurts less!
- Don't forget to palpate the radial pulse
- Don't forget to look at the elbows for plaques of psoriasis and rheumatoid nodules

History and examination

The hands can give you a wealth of information about a patient, even without needing to examine them directly. Shaking hands can tell you about thyroid disease (warm, sweaty, tremor), anxiety (cold, sweaty), and neurological disease (myotonic dystrophy patients have difficulty relaxing their grip, a weak grip may suggest muscle wasting or peripheral neuropathy), but remember that some patients are not comfortable with physical contact; be guided by your patient. Looking at the nails and skin can give information about systemic disease:

### Nail abnormalities
- *Koilonychia* (spoon-shaped nails) suggests iron deficiency, haemochromatosis, infection (eg fungal), endocrine disorders (eg acromegaly, hypothyroidism), or malnutrition.
- *Onycholysis* (detachment of the nail from the nail-bed) is seen with hyperthyroidism, fungal infection, and psoriasis (fig 2, p553).
- *Beau's lines* (fig 1) are transverse furrows from temporary arrest of nail growth at times of biological stress: severe infection, eg malaria, typhus, rheumatic fever, Kawasaki disease, myocardial infarction, chemotherapy, trauma, high-altitude climbing, and deep sea diving.[11] As nails grow at ~0.1mm/d, the furrow's distance from the cuticle allows dating of the stress.

Fig 1. Beau's lines, here due to chemotherapy, a new line is seen with each cycle. See p529.

- *Mees' lines* are single white transverse bands classically seen in arsenic poisoning but also in chronic kidney disease and carbon monoxide poisoning amongst others.
- *Muehrcke's lines* are paired white parallel transverse bands (without furrowing of the nail itself, distinguishing them from Beau's lines)[12] seen, eg, in chronic hypoalbuminaemia, Hodgkin's disease, pellagra (p278), chronic kidney disease.
- *Terry's nails:* Proximal portion of nail is white/pink, nail tip is red/brown (causes include cirrhosis, chronic kidney disease, congestive cardiac failure).
- *Pitting* is seen in psoriasis and alopecia areata.
- *Splinter haemorrhages* are fine longitudinal haemorrhagic streaks (under the nails), which in the febrile patient may suggest infective endocarditis. They may be microemboli, or be normal—being caused, by, for example, gardening.
- *Nail-fold infarcts* are embolic phenomena characteristically seen in vasculitic disorders (OHCS, p414).
- *Clubbing* of the nails occurs with many disorders (p33). There is an exaggerated longitudinal curvature and loss of the angle between nail and nail fold (ie no dip). Also the nail feels 'boggy'. The cause is unknown but may be due to increased blood flow through multiple arteriovenous shunts in the distal phalanges.
- *Chronic paronychia* is a chronic infection of the nail-fold and presents as a painful swollen nail with intermittent discharge.

### Skin changes
- *Palmar erythema* is associated with cirrhosis and other conditions (see BOX 2).
- *Pallor* of the palmar creases suggests anaemia.
- *Pigmentation* of the palmar creases is normal in people of African-Caribbean or Asian origin but is also seen in Addison's disease and Nelson's syndrome (increased ACTH after removal of the adrenal glands in Cushing's disease).[13]
- *Gottron's papules* (purple rash on the knuckles) with dilated end-capillary loops at the nail fold suggests dermatomyositis (p554).

### Nodules and contractures
- *Dupuytren's contracture* (fibrosis and contracture of palmar fascia, p712) is seen in liver disease, trauma, epilepsy, and ageing.[14]
- Look for Heberden's (DIP) fig 2 and Bouchard's (PIP) 'nodes'—osteophytes (bone over-growth at a joint) seen with osteoarthritis.

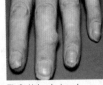

Fig 2. Heberden's node.

## Clubbing

Fingernails (± toenails) have increased curvature in all directions and loss of the angle between nail and nail fold (figs 3, 4). The nail fold feels boggy. The exact mechanism of clubbing is unclear; however, the platelet theory, developed in 1987,[15] has increasing evidence behind it. Megakaryocytes are normally fragmented into platelets in the lungs, and the original theory was that any disruption to normal pulmonary circulation (inflammation, cancer, cardiac right-to-left shunting) would allow large megakaryocytes into the systemic circulation. They become lodged in the capillaries of the fingers and toes, releasing platelet-derived growth factor and vascular endothelial growth factor,[16] both of which lead to tissue growth, vascular permeability (leading to the 'boggy' oedematous feel) and recruitment of inflammatory cells. This theory has been supported by necropsy evidence showing platelet microthrombi in clubbed fingers, and high levels of PDGF and VEGF in patients with hypertrophic osteoarthropathy,[17] and hypoxia may increase levels. However, this does not explain all of the changes, particularly in patients with unilateral clubbing, usually seen in neurological disorders. The jury is still out on the true pathogenesis.

### Causes

*Thoracic:*
- Bronchial cancer (clubbing is twice as common in women); usually *not* small cell cancer[18]
- Chronic lung suppuration
  - empyema, abscess
  - bronchiectasis
  - cystic fibrosis
- Fibrosing alveolitis
- Mesothelioma
- TB

*GI:*
- Inflammatory bowel disease (especially Crohn's)
- Cirrhosis
- GI lymphoma
- Malabsorption, eg coeliac

*Rare:*
- Familial
- Thyroid acropachy (p564)

*Cardiovascular:*
- Cyanotic congenital heart disease
- Endocarditis
- Atrial myxoma
- Aneurysms
- Infected grafts

*Unilateral clubbing:*
- Hemiplegia
- Vascular lesions, eg upper-limb artery aneurysm, Takayasu's arteritis, brachial arteriovenous malformations (including iatrogenic— haemodialysis fistulas)

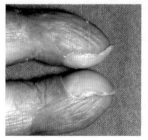

Fig 3. Finger clubbing.

(a)

The dorsal aspect of 2 fingers, side by side with the nails touching. Normally, you should see a kite-shaped gap. If not, there is clubbing.

(b)   (c)

No dip therefore clubbing

Fig 4. Testing for finger clubbing.

## Palmar erythema

*Causes:* 'High output' states: Pregnancy, hyperthyroidism, rheumatoid arthritis, polycythaemia; also chronic liver disease—via ↓inactivation of vasoactive endotoxins by the liver. Also chemotherapy-induced palmar/plantar erythrodysaesthesia.[19]

**History** (see also p88) Ask about age, occupation, hobbies, sport, exercise and ethnic origin.

| Presenting symptoms | Direct questions |
|---|---|
| *Chest pain* (see p88-9 and p798) | Site? Central?<br>Onset? (sudden? What was the patient doing?)<br>Character? Ask patient to describe pain (crushing? heavy?)<br>Radiation? Ask specifically if moves to arm, neck or jaw?<br>Associations? Ask specifically about shortness of breath, nausea, sweating.<br>Timing? Duration?<br>Exacerbating and alleviating factors? Worse with respiration or movement (less likely to be angina)? Relieved by GTN? Worse on inspiration and better when sitting forwards (pericarditis)?<br>Severity: out of 10?<br>Also ask if patient is known to have angina or chest pain in the past; better/worse/same as usual pain; is it more frequent? Decreasing exercise tolerance?<br>NB: 'heartburn' more likely if 'burning', onset after eating/drinking, worse lying flat, or associated with dysphagia. |
| *Palpitations* (see BOX 1 & 2) | 'Ever aware of your own heartbeat'? When and how did it start/stop? Duration? Onset sudden/gradual? Associated with blackout (how long)? Fast/slow? Regular/irregular? Ask patient to tap out the rhythm. Related to eating/drinking (especially coffee, tea, wine, or chocolate)? |
| *Dyspnoea* (see BOX 3, p52, and p796) | Duration? At rest? On exertion? Determine exercise tolerance (and any other reason for limitation, eg arthritis). NYHA classification (p131)? Worse when lying flat, how many pillows does the patient sleep with (**orthopnoea**)? Does the patient ever wake up in the night gasping for breath (**paroxysmal nocturnal dyspnoea**), and how often? Any ankle swelling? |
| *Dizziness/ blackouts* (see BOX 3 and p464-7) | Did patient lose consciousness, and for how long (short duration suggests cardiac while longer duration suggests a neurological cause)? Any warning (**pre-syncope**)? What was patient doing at the time? Sudden/gradual? Associated symptoms? Any residual symptoms? How long did it take for patient to return to 'normal'? Any tongue biting (p464-5), seizure, incontinence? Witnessed? |
| *Claudication* | SOCRATES? Specifically foot/calf/thigh/buttock? Quantify 'claudication distance', ie how long can patient walk before onset of pain? Rest pain? |

(Screen for presenting symptoms before proceeding to past history.)

**Past history** Ask specifically about: angina, any previous heart attack or stroke, rheumatic fever, diabetes, hypertension, hypercholesterolaemia, previous tests/procedures (ECG, angiograms, angioplasty/stents, echocardiogram, cardiac scintigraphy, coronary artery bypass grafts (CABG)).

| Ischaemic heart disease risk factors |
|---|
| • Smoking<br>• Diabetes mellitus/raised BMI<br>• Family history ($\binom{1^{st}\text{-degree}}{\text{relative <60yrs}}$ old with IHD)<br>• Hypertension<br>• Hyperlipidaemia<br>• Renal disease<br>• Deprivation |

**Drug history** Particularly note aspirin/GTN/β-blocker/diuretic/ACE-i/digoxin/statin use.

**Family history** Enquire specifically if any 1st-degree relatives having cardiovascular events (especially if <60yrs).

**Social history** Smoking, impact of symptoms on daily life.

## Palpitations

An awareness of the heartbeat. Have the patient tap out the rate and rhythm of the palpitations.
• Irregular fast palpitations are likely to be paroxysmal AF, or atrial flutter with variable block.
• Regular fast palpitations may reflect paroxysmal supraventricular tachycardia (SVT) or ventricular tachycardia (VT).
• Dropped or missed beats related to rest, recumbency, or eating are likely to be atrial or ventricular ectopics.
• Regular pounding may be due to anxiety.
• Slow palpitations are likely to be due to drugs such as β-blockers, or bigeminus (fig 1, p122).

Ask about associated chest pain, dyspnoea, and faints, suggesting haemodynamic compromise. Ask when it occurs: anxious people may be aware of their own heartbeat at night. Reassurance is vital and can often be therapeutic. Check a TSH and consider a 24h ECG (Holter monitor, p102). An event recorder, if available, is better than 24h ECGs, which miss some attacks.

### Palpitations, Russian roulette, loose blood, and hypochondriasis

At night on my pillow the syncopated stagger
Of the pulse in my ear. Russian roulette
Every heartbeat a fresh throw of the dice . . .
Hypochondria walked, holding my arm
Like a nurse, her fingers over my pulse . . .
The sudden lapping at my throat of loose blood.

Ted Hughes, *Birthday Letters*.
Faber & Faber, by kind permission.

## Dizziness

**Dizziness** is a loose term, so try to clarify if your patient means:
• *Vertigo* (p466), the illusion of rotation of either the patient or their surroundings ± difficulty walking/standing, patients may fall over.
• *Imbalance*, a difficulty in walking straight but without vertigo, from peripheral nerve, posterior column, cerebellar, or other central pathway failure.
• *Faintness*, ie 'light-headedness', seen in anaemia, ↓BP, postural hypotension, hypoglycaemia, carotid sinus hypersensitivity, and epilepsy.

As with any examination routine, begin by introducing yourself, obtaining consent to examine the patient and position them appropriately: for the cardiovascular system, lying on a bed but sitting up at 45°. Expose them to the waist (for female patients, delay this until examining the praecordium). Explain what you are doing throughout.

### 5 Neck

- *JVP:* ask patient to turn head to the left and look at the supra-clavicular fossa (see fig 1 and p40). Comment on the height of the JVP and waveform. Press on the abdomen to check the abdomino-jugular reflex.

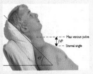

Fig 1. The JVP.

- *Carotid pulse:* inspect (visible carotid = *Corrigan's sign* of aortic regurgitation), and palpate volume and character on one side then the other.

### 4 Blood pressure

- Hyper or hypotensive?
- Pulse pressure (wide = aortic regurgitation, narrow = aortic stenosis)

### 3 Radial and brachial pulses

- *Radial:* rate, rhythm; radio-radial delay (palpate pulse bilaterally simultaneously), radiofemoral delay (palpate ipsilateral pulses simultaneously), collapsing pulse (hold pulse with fingers of one hand, wrap the fingers of other hand around forearm, check "any pain in arm/shoulder?", lift arm up straight collapsing pulse, felt as 'waterhammer' pulsation in forearm).
- *Brachial:* (just medial to tendonous insertion of biceps). Waveform character.

### 2 Hands

- *Temperature:* capillary refill time
- *Inspect:*
  Skin: tobacco staining, peripheral cyanosis, tendon xanthomata, *Janeway lesions*, *Osler's nodes* (signs of infective endocarditis)
  Nails: clubbing, splinter haemorrhages, nailbed pulsation (*Quinke's sign* of aortic regurgitation)

### 1 General inspection

- Assess general state (ill/well)
- Look for clues (oxygen, GTN spray)
- Colour (pale, cyanosed, flushed)
- Short of breath?
- Scars on chest wall?

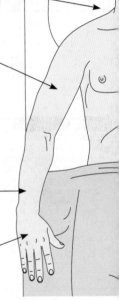

A = Aortic    T = Triscusp
P = Pulmonary    M= Mitral

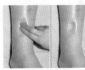

Fig 3. Pitting oedema, apply firm pressure for a few seconds.

### 6 Face
- *Colour:* pale, flushed, central cyanosis
- *Features:* corneal arcus (fig 2), xanthelasma
- Pallor of the conjunctiva (anaemia)
- Malar flush (mitral stenosis)
- Dental hygiene

Fig 2. Corneal arcus.

### 7 The praecordium
**Inspect**
- *Scars:* midline sternotomy, lateral thoracotomy (mitral stenosis valvotomy).

**Palpate**
- *Apex beat (lowermost lateral pulsation):* usually 5th intercostal space in mid-clavicular line; measure position by counting intercostal spaces (sternal notch = 2nd intercostal space). Undisplaced/displaced? **Character:** impalpable (?dextrocardia/COPD), tapping (palpable $S_1$), double impulse, sustained/strong. Count rate if pulse irregular (AF, p124).
- *Heaves' and 'thrills':* place the heel of the hand flat on chest to left then right of sternum. **Heave:** sustained, thrusting usually felt at left sternal edge (= right ventricular enlargement). **Thrill:** palpable murmur felt as a vibration beneath your hand.

**Auscultate** (palpate carotid pulse at the same time)
- *Apex (mitral area):* Listen with bell and diaphragm. Identify 1st and 2nd heart sounds: are they normal? Listen for *added sounds* (p42) and *murmurs* (p44); with the diaphragm listen for a *pansystolic murmur* radiating to the axilla—**mitral regurgitation**.
- At apex with bell, ask the patient to "Roll over onto your left side, breathe out, and hold it there" (*a rumbling mid-diastolic murmur*—**mitral stenosis**).
- *Lower left sternal edge (tricuspid area)* and pulmonary area (left of manubrium in the 2nd intercostal space): if suspect right-sided mumur, listen with patient's breath held in inspiration.
- *Right of manubrium in 2nd intercostal space (aortic area) ejection systolic murmur* radiating to the carotids—**aortic stenosis**.
- Sit the patient up and listen at the lower left sternal edge with patient held in expiration (*early diastolic murmur:* **aortic regurgitation?**).

### 8 To complete the examination
- Palpate for *sacral and ankle oedema* (Fig 3).
- Auscultate the *lung bases* for inspiratory crackles.
- Examine the abdomen for a *pulsatile liver* and *aortic aneurysm*.
- Check peripheral pulses, observation chart for temperature and $O_2$, sats, dip urine, perform fundoscopy.

---

**Top tips**

The hand can be used as a manometer to estimate JVP/CVP if you cannot see the neck properly (eg central line in situ). Hold the hand palm down below the level of the heart until the veins dilate (patient must be warm!), then lift slowly, keeping the arm horizontal. The veins should empty as the hand is raised. Empty veins below the level of the heart suggests a low CVP, if they remain full it suggests a normal/high CVP.

**General inspection** Ill or well? In pain? Dyspnoeic? Are they pale, cold, and clammy? Can you hear the click of a prosthetic valve? Inspect for *scars*: median sternotomy (CABG; valve replacement; congenital heart disease). Inspect for any pacemakers. Look around the bed for oxygen and GTN spray.

**Hands** Finger clubbing occurs in congenital cyanotic heart disease and endocarditis. Splinter haemorrhages, Osler's nodes (tender nodules, eg in finger pulps) and Janeway lesions (red macules on palms, fig 3, p145) are signs of infective endocarditis. If found, examine the fundi for Roth's spots (retinal infarcts, p386, fig 1). Are there nail fold infarcts (vasculitis, p558) or nailbed capillary pulsation (Quincke's sign in aortic regurgitation)? Is there arachnodactyly (Marfan's) or polydactyly (ASD)? Are there tendon xanthomata (see BOX p39; hyperlipidaemia)?

**Pulse** See p42. Feel for *radio-femoral delay* (coarctation of the aorta) and *radio-radial delay* (eg from aortic arch aneurysm).

**Blood pressure** (see BOX) Systolic BP is the pressure at which the pulse is first heard as on cuff deflation (Korotkov sounds); the **diastolic** is when the heart sounds disappear or become muffled (eg in the young). The *pulse pressure* is the difference between systolic and diastolic pressures. It is narrow in aortic stenosis and hypovolaemia, and wide in aortic regurgitation and septic shock. Defining hypertension is problematic: see p132. Examine the fundi for hypertensive changes (p133). **Shock** may occur if systolic <90mmHg (p804). *Postural hypotension* is defined as a drop in systolic >20mmHg or diastolic >10mmHg on standing (see BOX).

**Face** Is there corneal arcus (fig 2, p37) or xanthelasma (fig 1, p705, signifying dyslipidaemia, p704)? Is there a malar flush (mitral stenosis, low cardiac output)? Are there signs of Graves' disease, eg bulging eyes (exophthalmos) or goitre—p210)? Is the face dysmorphic, eg Down's syndrome, Marfan's syndrome (p720)—or Turner's, Noonan's, or William's syndromes (p143)?

**Carotid pulse** (p40) and **jugular venous pressure** (p41).

**Praecordium** Palpate the *apex beat*. Normal position: 5th intercostal space in the mid-clavicular line. Is it displaced laterally? Is it abnormal in nature: **heaving** (caused by outflow obstruction, eg aortic stenosis or systemic hypertension), **thrusting** (caused by volume overload, eg mitral or aortic incompetence), **tapping** (mitral stenosis, essentially a palpable 1st heart sound), **diffuse** (LV failure, dilated cardiomyopathy) or **double impulse** (H(O)CM, p146)? Is there dextrocardia? Feel for *left parasternal heave* (RV enlargement, eg in pulmonary stenosis, cor pulmonale, ASD) or *thrills* (transmitted murmurs).

**Auscultating the heart** Also auscultate for *bruits* over the carotids and elsewhere, particularly if there is inequality between pulses or absence of a pulse. Causes: atherosclerosis (elderly), vasculitis (young, p558).

**Lungs** Examine the bases for creps & pleural effusions, indicative of cardiac failure.

**Oedema** Examine the ankles, legs, sacrum, and torso for pitting oedema. (You may prefer to examine ankles whilst standing at the foot of the bed as it is a good early clue that there may be further pathology to be found.)

**Abdomen** Hepatomegaly and ascites in right-sided heart failure; pulsatile hepatomegaly with tricuspid regurgitation; splenomegaly with infective endocarditis.

**Fundoscopy** Roth spots (infective endocarditis).

**Urine dipstick** Haematuria.

> *Presenting your findings:*
> i Signs of heart failure?
> ii Clinical evidence of infective endocarditis ?
> iii Sinus/abnormal rhythm?
> iv Heart sounds normal, abnormal or additional?
> v Murmurs?

## An unusual BP measurement

Don't interpret a BP value in isolation (p132). We cannot diagnose hypertension (or hypotension) on one BP reading. Take into account pain, the 'white coat' effect, and equipment used.[20] Getting cuff size right is vital, as too small will give too high a reading, and too large will give a low reading. ▶*Optimal cuff width is 40% of the arm circumference*. If you suspect a BP reading to be anomalous, check the equipment and review the observation chart for previous readings and other vital signs. Consider taking a manual reading with a different set yourself.

Often a quiet chat will bring the BP down (yours and your patient's: keep your ears open, and the patient may reveal some new tangential but vital fact that the official history glossed over). Many things affect BP readings from background noise to how much you touch the patient. If BP ↑, eg ≥150/90, check both arms. If the systolic difference is >10mmHg, consider peripheral vascular disease,[21] and if the patient could have a thoracic aortic aneurysm or coarctation (rare)? NB: right arm diastolic is normally 2.4–5mmHg higher than left.[22]

## Postural hypotension

This is an important cause of falls and faints in the elderly. It is defined as a drop in systolic BP >20mmHg or diastolic >10mmHg after standing for 3min vs lying.[23] *Causes:* Hypovolaemia (early sign); drugs, eg nitrates, diuretics, antihypertensives; antipsychotics; Addison's (p218); hypopituitarism (↓ACTH), autonomic neuropathy (p509, DM, multisystem atrophy, p498), after a marathon run (peripheral resistance is low for some hours); idiopathic.
*Treatment:*
• Lie down if feeling faint.
• Stand slowly (with escape route: don't move away from the chair too soon!).
• Consider referral to a 'falls clinic', where special equipment is available for monitoring patient under various tilts.
• Manage autonomic neuropathy, p509.
• ↑Water and salt ingestion can help (eg 150mmol Na⁺/d), but Na⁺ has its problems.
• Physical measures: leg crossing, squatting, elastic compression stockings (check dorsalis pedis pulse is present), and careful exercise may help.
• If post-prandial dizziness, eat little and often; ↓carbohydrate and alcohol intake.
• Head-up tilt of the bed at night ↑renin release, so ↓fluid loss and ↑standing BP.
• 1ˢᵗ-line drugs: fludrocortisone (retains fluid) 50µg/d; go up to 300µg/24h PO only if tolerated. Monitor weight; beware if CCF, renal impairment or ↓albumin as fludrocortisone worsens oedema.[24,25]
• 2ⁿᵈ-line: sympathomimetics, eg midodrine (not always available) or ephedrine;[23] pyridostigmine (eg if detrusor under-activity too).[26]
• If these fail, turn things on their head and ask: *is this really supine hypertension?*

## Xanthomata

Localized deposits of fat under the skin, occurring over joints, tendons, hands, and feet. They are a sign of dyslipidaemia (p704). *Xanthelasma* refers to xanthoma on the eyelid (p705, fig 1). *Corneal arcus* (fig 2, p37) is a crescentic-shaped opacity at the periphery of the cornea. Common in those over 60yrs, can be normal, but may represent hyperlipidaemia, especially in those under this age.

History and examination

The internal jugular vein acts as a capricious manometer of right atrial pressure. Observe 2 features: the **height** (jugular venous pressure, JVP) and the **waveform** of the pulse. JVP observations are often difficult. Do not be downhearted if the skill seems to elude you. Keep on watching necks, and the patterns you see may slowly start to make sense—see fig 2 for the local venous anatomy. Relating the waveform to the arterial pulse (by concomitant palpation) will help to decipher patterns.

**The height** Observe the patient at 45°, with his head turned slightly to the left. Good lighting and correct positioning makes the examination a lot easier. Look for the right internal jugular vein as it passes just medial to the clavicular head of the sternocleidomastoid up behind the angle of the jaw to the earlobes. The JVP is the vertical height of the pulse above the sternal angle (measured from the angle of Louis to the upper part of the JVP pulsation). It is raised if >4cm. Pressing on the abdomen normally produces a transient rise in the JVP. If the rise persists throughout a 15s compression, it is a **positive abdominojugular reflux sign.**[1] This is a sign of right ventricular failure, reflecting inability to eject the increased venous return.[27] If you cannot see the JVP at all, lie the patient flat then slowly sit up until the JVP disappears to check height of waveform.

**The waveform** See BOX 1.

**Abnormalities of the JVP**
- *Raised JVP with normal waveform:* Fluid overload, right heart failure.
- *Fixed raised JVP with absent pulsation:* SVC obstruction (p526).
- *Large a wave:* Pulmonary hypertension, pulmonary stenosis.
- *Cannon a wave:* When the right atrium contracts against a closed tricuspid valve, large 'cannon' a waves result. *Causes:* complete heart block, single chamber ventricular pacing, ventricular arrhythmias/ectopics.
- *Absent a wave:* Atrial fibrillation.
- *Large v waves:* Tricuspid regurgitation—look for earlobe movement.
- *Constrictive pericarditis:* High plateau of JVP (which rises on inspiration—**Kussmaul's sign**) with deep x and y descents.
- *Absent JVP:* When lying flat, the jugular vein should be filled. If there is reduced circulatory volume (eg dehydration, haemorrhage) the JVP may be absent.

## Pulses

▶Assess the radial pulse to determine rate and rhythm. **Character and volume** are best assessed at the brachial or carotid arteries. A **collapsing pulse** may also be felt at the radial artery when the patient's arm is elevated above his head. See fig 3.

**Rate** Is the pulse fast (≥100bpm, p120) or slow (≤60bpm, p118)?

**Rhythm** An irregularly irregular pulse occurs in AF or multiple ectopics. A regularly irregular pulse occurs in 2° heart block and ventricular bigeminus.

**Character and volume**
- *Bounding pulses* are caused by $CO_2$ retention, liver failure, and sepsis.
- *Small volume pulses* occur in aortic stenosis, shock, and pericardial effusion.
- *Collapsing ('waterhammer') pulses* are caused by aortic incompetence, AV malformations, and a patent ductus arteriosus.
- *Anacrotic (slow-rising) pulses* occur in aortic stenosis.
- *Bisferiens pulses* occur in combined aortic stenosis and regurgitation.
- *Pulsus alternans* (alternating strong and weak beats) suggests LVF, cardiomyopathy, or aortic stenosis.
- *Jerky pulses* occur in H(O)CM.
- *Pulsus paradoxus* (systolic pressure weakens in inspiration by >10mmHg) occurs in severe asthma, pericardial constriction, or cardiac tamponade.

**Peripheral pulses** (See p34.) See p785 for arterial blood gas (ABG) sampling.

---

1 This sign was first described by Pasteur in 1885 in the context of tricuspid incompetence.

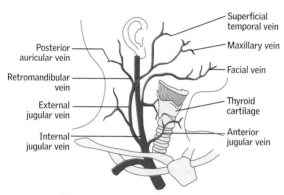

- **a wave:** atrial systole
- **c wave:** closure of tricuspid valve, not normally visible
- **x descent:** fall in atrial pressure during ventricular systole
- **v wave:** atrial filling against a closed tricuspid valve
- **y descent:** opening of tricuspid valve

Fig 1. The jugular venous pressure wave. The JVP drops as the x descent during ventricular systole because the right atrium is no longer contracting. This means that the pressure in the right atrium is dropping and this is reflected by the JVP.

Fig 2. The jugular venous system.

### Is a pulse arterial or venous?

A venous pulse:
- Is not usually palpable.
- Is obliterated by finger pressure on the vessel.
- Rises transiently with pressure on abdomen (**abdominojugular reflux**) or on liver (**hepatojugular reflux**).
- Alters with posture and respiration.
- Usually has a double pulse for every arterial pulse.

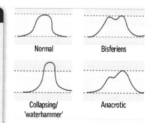

Normal Bisferiens

Collapsing/ 'waterhammer' Anacrotic

Fig 3. Arterial pulse waveforms.

### Waterhammer pulse

The waterhammer was a popular toy that consisted of a vacuum tube half-filled with water. On inversion, the whoosh of water produced an intriguing hammer-blow as it rushed from end to end. This is the alternative name for Corrigan's collapsing pulse—ie one in which the upstroke is abrupt and steep, whose peak is reached early and with abnormal force—before a rapid downstroke (as blood whooshes back into the left ventricle through an incompetent aortic valve).

Figures on this page after *Clinical Examination*, Macleod, Churchill & *Aids to Undergraduate Medicine*, J Burton, Churchill.

▶Listen systematically: sounds then murmurs. While listening, palpate the carotid artery: $S_1$ is synchronous with the upstroke.

**Heart sounds** The $1^{st}$ and $2^{nd}$ sounds are usually clear. Confident pronouncements about other sounds and soft murmurs may be difficult. Even senior colleagues disagree with one another about the more difficult sounds and murmurs. See fig 1.

**The $1^{st}$ heart sound** ($S_1$) represents closure of mitral ($M_1$) and tricuspid ($T_1$) valves. Splitting in inspiration may be normal and is normal.

- *Loud $S_1$* In mitral stenosis, because the narrowed valve orifice limits ventricular filling, there is no gradual decrease in flow towards the end of diastole. The valves are therefore at their maximum excursion at the end of diastole, and so shut rapidly leading to a loud $S_1$ (the 'tapping' apex). $S_1$ is also loud if diastolic filling time is shortened, eg if the PR interval is short, and in tachycardia.
- *Soft $S_1$* occurs if the diastolic filling time is prolonged, eg prolonged PR interval, or if the mitral valve leaflets fail to close properly (ie mitral incompetence).

The intensity of $S_1$ is variable in AV block, AF, and nodal or ventricular tachycardia.

**The $2^{nd}$ heart sound** ($S_2$) represents aortic ($A_2$) and pulmonary valve ($P_2$) closure. The most important abnormality of $A_2$ is softening in aortic stenosis.

- $A_2$ is said to be loud in tachycardia, hypertension, and transposition, but this is probably not a useful clinical entity.
- $P_2$ is loud in pulmonary hypertension and soft in pulmonary stenosis.
- *Splitting of $S_2$* in inspiration is normal and is mainly due to the variation of right heart venous return with respiration, delaying the pulmonary component.
    - **Wide splitting** occurs in right bundle branch block (BBB), pulmonary stenosis, deep inspiration, mitral regurgitation, and VSD.
    - **Wide fixed splitting** occurs in ASD.
    - **Reversed splitting** (ie $A_2$ following $P_2$, with splitting increasing on expiration) occurs in left bundle branch block, aortic stenosis, PDA (patent ductus arteriosus), and right ventricular pacing.
    - **A single $S_2$** occurs in Fallot's tetralogy, severe aortic or pulmonary stenosis, pulmonary atresia, Eisenmenger's syndrome (p150), large VSD, or hypertension.

NB: splitting and $P_2$ are heard best in the pulmonary area.

**Additional sounds**

*A $3^{rd}$ heart sound* ($S_3$) may occur just after $S_2$. It is low pitched and best heard with the bell of the stethoscope. $S_3$ is pathological over the age of 30yrs. A loud $S_3$ occurs in a dilated left ventricle with rapid ventricular filling (mitral regurgitation, VSD) or poor LV function (post MI, dilated cardiomyopathy). In constrictive pericarditis or restrictive cardiomyopathy it occurs early and is more high pitched ('pericardial knock').

*A $4^{th}$ heart sound* ($S_4$) occurs just before $S_1$. Always abnormal, it represents atrial contraction against a ventricle made stiff by any cause, eg aortic stenosis or hypertensive heart disease.

*Triple and gallop rhythms* A $3^{rd}$ or $4^{th}$ heart sound occurring with a sinus tachycardia may give the impression of galloping hooves. An $S_3$ gallop has the same rhythm as 'Ken-tucky', whereas an $S_4$ gallop has the same rhythm as 'Tenne-ssee'. When $S_3$ and $S_4$ occur in a tachycardia, eg with pulmonary embolism, they may summate and appear as a single sound, a summation gallop.

*An ejection systolic click* is heard early in systole with bicuspid aortic valves, and if BP↑. The right heart equivalent lesions may also cause clicks.

*Mid-systolic clicks* occur in mitral valve prolapse (p138).

*An opening snap* precedes the mid-diastolic murmur of mitral (and tricuspid) stenosis. It indicates a pliable (non-calcified) valve.

*Prosthetic sounds* are caused by non-biological valves, on opening and closing: **rumbling sounds** ≈ ball and cage valves (eg Starr–Edwards); **single clicks** ≈ tilting disc valve (eg single disc: Bjork Shiley; bileaflet: St Jude—often quieter). Prosthetic mitral valve clicks occur in time with $S_1$, aortic valve clicks in time with $S_2$.

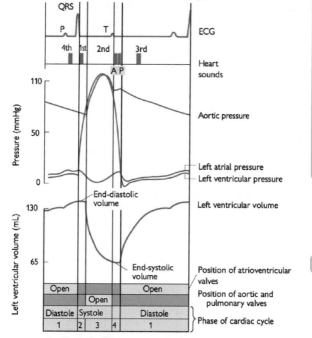

1 = Ventricular filling
2 = Isovolumetric ventricular contraction
3 = Ventricular ejection
4 = Isovolumetric ventricular relaxation

Fig 1. The cardiac cycle.

▶ Always consider other symptoms and signs before auscultation and think: "What do I expect to hear?" But don't let your expectations determine what you hear.

▶ Use the stethoscope correctly: remember that the bell is good for low-pitched sounds (eg mitral stenosis) and should be applied **gently**. The diaphragm filters out low pitches, making higher-pitched murmurs easier to detect (eg aortic regurgitation). NB: a bell applied tightly to the skin becomes a diaphragm.

▶ Consider any murmur in terms of **character, timing, loudness, area where loudest, radiation**, and **accentuating manoeuvres**.

▶ When in doubt, rely on echocardiography rather than disputed sounds. (But still enjoy trying to figure out the clinical conundrum!)

**Character and timing** (see fig 1)

• *An ejection-systolic murmur* (ESM, crescendo-decrescendo) usually originates from the outflow tract and waxes and wanes with the intraventricular pressures. ESMs may be innocent and are common in children and high-output states (eg tachycardia, pregnancy). Organic causes include aortic stenosis and sclerosis, pulmonary stenosis, and H(O)CM.

• *A pansystolic murmur (PSM)* is of uniform intensity and merges with $S_2$. It is usually organic and occurs in mitral or tricuspid regurgitation ($S_1$ may also be soft in these), or a ventricular septal defect (p150). Mitral valve prolapse may produce a late systolic murmur ± midsystolic click.

• *Early diastolic murmurs (EDM)* are high pitched and easily missed: listen for the 'absence of silence' in early diastole. An EDM occurs in aortic and, though rare, pulmonary regurgitation. If the pulmonary regurgitation is secondary to pulmonary hypertension resulting from mitral stenosis, then the EDM is called a Graham Steell murmur.

• *Mid-diastolic murmurs (MDM)* are low pitched and rumbling. They occur in mitral stenosis (accentuated presystolically if heart still in sinus rhythm), rheumatic fever (Carey Coombs' murmur: due to thickening of the mitral valve leaflets), and aortic regurgitation (Austin Flint murmur: due to the fluttering of the anterior mitral valve cusp caused by the regurgitant stream).

**Intensity** All murmurs are graded on a scale of 1–6 (see TABLE), though in practice diastolic murmurs, being less loud, are only graded 1–4. Intensity is a poor guide to the severity of a lesion—an ESM may be inaudible in severe aortic stenosis.

**Area where loudest** Though an unreliable sign, mitral murmurs tend to be loudest over the apex, in contrast to the area of greatest intensity from lesions of the aortic (right $2^{nd}$ intercostal space), pulmonary (left $2^{nd}$ intercostal space) and tricuspid (lower left sternal edge) valves.

**Radiation** The ESM of aortic stenosis classically radiates to the carotids, in contrast to the PSM of mitral regurgitation, which radiates to the axilla.

**Accentuating manoeuvres**

• *Movements* that bring the relevant part of the heart closer to the stethoscope accentuate murmurs (eg leaning forward for aortic regurgitation, left lateral position for mitral stenosis).

• *Expiration* increases blood flow to the left side of the heart and therefore accentuates left-sided murmurs. *Inspiration* has the opposite effect.

• *Valsalva manoeuvre* (forced expiration against a closed glottis) decreases systemic venous return, accentuating mitral valve prolapse and H(O)CM, but softening mitral regurgitation and aortic stenosis. *Squatting* has exactly the opposite effect. *Exercise* accentuates the murmur of mitral stenosis.

**Non-valvular murmurs** A *pericardial friction rub* may be heard in pericarditis. It is a superficial scratching sound, not confined to systole or diastole. *Continuous murmurs* are present throughout the cardiac cycle and may occur with a patent ductus arteriosus, arteriovenous fistula, or ruptured sinus of Valsalva.

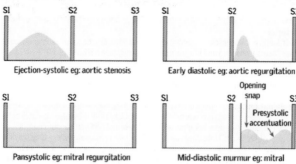

Fig 1. Typical waveforms of common heart murmurs.

### Grading intensity of heart murmurs

▶The following grading is commonly used for murmurs—systolic murmurs from 1 to 6 and diastolic murmurs from 1 to 4, never being clinically >4/6.

| Grade | Description |
|---|---|
| 1/6 | Very soft, only heard after listening for a while |
| 2/6 | Soft, but detectable immediately |
| 3/6 | Clearly audible, but no thrill palpable |
| 4/6 | Clearly audible, palpable thrill |
| 5/6 | Audible with stethoscope only partially touching chest |
| 6/6 | Can be heard without placing stethoscope on chest |

### Prosthetic valve murmurs

**Prosthetic aortic valves** All types produce a degree of outflow obstruction and thus have an ESM. Tilting single disc (eg Bjork Shiley) and bileaflet (eg St Jude) valves do not completely close and allow a regurgitant stream during diastole; hence they have a low-intensity diastolic murmur. The intensity of this murmur increases as the valve fails. Ball and cage valves (eg Starr-Edwards) and tissue valves do close completely in diastole and so any diastolic murmur implies valve failure.

**Prosthetic mitral valves** Ball and cage valves project into the left ventricle and can cause a low-intensity ESM as they interfere with the ejected stream. Tissue valves and bileaflet valves can have a low-intensity diastolic murmur. Consider any systolic murmur of loud intensity to be a sign of regurgitation and ∴ failure.

### Eponymous signs of aortic regurgitation

• de Musset's sign—head nodding in time with the pulse
• Muller's sign—systolic pulsations of the uvula
• Corrigan's sign—visible carotid pulsations
• Quincke's sign—capillary nailbed pulsation in the fingers
• Traube's sign—'pistol shot' femorals, a booming sound heard over the femorals
• Duroziez's sign—to and fro diastolic murmur heard when compressing the femorals proximally with the stethoscope

### Arterial

▶▶If limb is pale, pulseless, painful, paralysed, paraesthetic, and 'perishingly cold' this is acute ischaemia and is a surgical emergency (see p597 and p659).

1 **Inspection** Look for scars of previous surgery and signs of peripheral arterial disease; loss of hair, pallor, shiny skin, cyanosis, dry skin, scaling, deformed toe-nails, ulcers, gangrene. Be sure to inspect the pressure points, ie between the toes and under the heel.

2 **Palpation** Skin temperature will be low in peripheral arterial disease. Is there a level above which it is warm? Delayed capillary refill (>2s) also indicates arterial disease. Are peripheral pulses palpable or not? 'If you cannot count it, you are not feeling it.' Note down on a quick stick-man diagram where they become palpable. Check for atrial fibrillation or other arrhythmias, as these can be the cause of embolic disease. Palpate for an enlarged abdominal aorta and attempt to assess size. (Though don't press too firmly!) ▶▶An expansile pulsatile mass in the presence of abdominal symptoms is a ruptured aneurysm until proven otherwise.

3 **Auscultation** The presence of bruits suggests arterial disease. Listen over the major arteries—carotids, abdominal aorta, renal arteries, femorals.

4 **Special tests** *Buerger's angle* is that above the horizontal plane which leads to development of pallor (<20° indicates severe ischaemia). *Buerger's sign* is the sequential change in colour from white to pink, upon return to the dependent position; if the limbs become flushed red (reactive hyperaemia) this is indicative of more severe disease.

5 **Complete your examination** by measuring the ABPI (p658), US Doppler assessment for presence of pulses that were not palpable, and a neurological examination of the lower limbs.

### Venous (see also p660)

1 **Inspection** Look for any varicosities and decide whether they are the long saphenous vein (medial), short saphenous vein (posterior, below the knee), or from the calf perforators (usually few varicosities but commonly show skin changes). Ulcers around the medial malleolus are more suggestive of venous disease, whereas those at the pressure points suggest arterial pathology. Brown haemosiderin deposits result from venous hypertension. There may also be atrophy and loss of skin elasticity (lipodermatosclerosis) in venous disease.

2 **Palpation** Warm varicose veins may indicate infection. Are they tender? Firm, tender varicosities suggests thrombosis. Palpate the saphenofemoral junction (SFJ) for a saphena varix which displays a cough impulse. Similarly, incompetence at the saphenopopliteal junction (SPJ) may be felt as a cough impulse. If ulceration is present, it is prudent to palpate the arterial pulses to rule out arterial disease.

3 **Tap test** A transmitted percussion impulse from the lower limit of the varicose vein to the saphenofemoral junction demonstrates incompetence of superficial valves.

4 **Auscultation** Bruits over the varicosities means there is an arteriovenous malformation.

5 **Doppler** Test for the level of reflux. On squeezing the leg distal to placement of the probe you should only hear one 'whoosh' if the valves are competent at the level of probe placement.

6 **Tourniquet test** This is the more 'classical' test for the level of reflux. If the varicosities are controlled by the tourniquet then the level of incompetence is above the tourniquet. Note that all veins will refill eventually via the arterial system but rapid refill signifies superficial reflux. (Also *Trendelenburg's test* and *Perthes' test*, p661.)

7 **Complete examination** by examining the abdomen, pelvis in females and external genitalia in males (for masses).

## Arterial

**1 General inspection** Introduction, consent, patient sitting back at 45°. Inspect skin (hair loss, etc.). Look between toes and lift up heels to inspect for ulcers.

**2 Palpation**
- *Temperature* bilaterally in thighs, legs, and feet.
- *Capillary refill:* Press/squeeze great toe until blanches, release, and measure time for colour to return (normal <2s).
- *Peripheral pulses:* **Radial**, **brachial**, **carotid**, **femoral** (mid-inguinal point), **popliteal** (flex patient's knees slightly and press into centre of popliteal fossa; fig 1), **posterior tibial** (just posterior & inferior to medial malleolus) and **dorsalis pedis** (between bases of 1st & 2nd metatarsals); assess whether palpable bilaterally. Detect rate and rhythm. For brachial and carotid determine volume and character.
- *Abdominal aorta:* Palpate midline above umbilicus; position fingers either side of outermost palpable margins (fig 2).

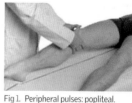

Fig 1. Peripheral pulses: popliteal.

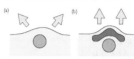

Fig 2. Pulses: abdominal aorta. a) Expansile (aneurysm?) b) transmitted.

Figures 1 and 2 reproduced with permission from *Oxford Handbook of Clinical Examination and Practical Skills.*

**3 Auscultation** for carotid, femoral, renal and aortic bruits.

**4 Special tests**

*Buerger's test:* Lift both legs to 45° above the horizontal, supporting at heels. Allow a minute for legs to become pale. If they do, ask patient to sit up and swing around to lower legs to ground—observe colour change.

**5 Complete examination**

Doppler probe to detect pulses and measure ankle-brachial pressure index; conduct neurological examination of lower limbs.

## Venous

**1 Inspection** Introduction, consent, patient sitting back at 45°. Inspect for varicosities and skin changes.

**2 Palpation** •*Temperature* of varicosities •Ask patient to cough while you *palpate for impulse at SFJ and SPJ.*

**3 Tap test** Percuss lower limit of varicosity and feel for impulse at SFJ.

**4 Auscultation** Listen for bruits over any varicosities.

**5 Doppler** Place probe over SFJ, squeeze calf and listen. Repeat with probe at SPJ.

**6 Tourniquet test** Elevate leg and massage veins to empty varicosities. Apply tourniquet to upper thigh. Ask patient to stand. If not controlled, repeat, placing tourniquet below knee.

**7 Finish with examinations** of abdomen; rectum; pelvis (♀); genitals (♂).

**History** Age, race, occupation (the latter is essential for respiratory disease).

| Presenting symptoms | Direct questions |
|---|---|
| • Cough<br>(see BOX) | Duration? Character (eg barking/hollow/dry)? Nocturnal (≈asthma, ask about other atopic symptoms, ie eczema, hayfever)? Exacerbating factors? Sputum (colour? How much?) Any blood/haemoptysis? |
| • Haemoptysis<br>(see BOX) | Always think about TB (recent foreign travel?) and malignancy (weight loss?). Mixed with sputum? (Blood not mixed with sputum suggests pulmonary embolism, trauma, or bleeding into a lung cavity.[28]) Melaena? (Occurs if enough coughed-up blood is swallowed.) |
| • Dyspnoea<br>(see BOX and p796) | Duration? Steps climbed/distance walked before onset? NYHA classification (p131)? Diurnal variation (≈asthma)? Ask specifically about circumstances in which dyspnoea occurs (eg occupational allergen exposure). |
| • Hoarseness<br>(OHCS p568) | Eg due to laryngitis, recurrent laryngeal nerve palsy, Singer's nodules, or laryngeal tumour. |
| • Wheeze (p50) | |
| • Fever/night sweats (p27) | |
| • Chest pain<br>(p88 & p798) | SOCRATES (see p34), usually 'pleuritic' if respiratory (ie worse on inspiration?). |
| • Stridor (see BOX 1) | |

(Screen for presenting symptoms before proceeding to past history.)

**Past history** Ask about: pneumonia/bronchitis; TB; atopy[1] (asthma/eczema/hay fever); previous CXR abnormalities; lung surgery; myopathy; neurological disorders. Connective tissue disorders, eg rheumatoid, SLE.

**Drug history** Respiratory drugs (eg steroids, bronchodilators)? Any other drugs, especially with respiratory SE (eg ACE inhibitors, cytotoxics, β-blockers, amiodarone)?

**Family history** Atopy?[1] Emphysema? TB?

**Social history** Quantify smoking in 'pack-years' (20 cigarettes/day for 1 year = 1 pack-year). Occupational exposure (farming, mining, asbestos) has possible compensatory implications. Pets at home (eg birds)? Recent travel/TB contacts?

---

### Stridor

*Inspiratory* sound due to partial obstruction of upper airways. Obstruction may be due to something *within the lumen* (eg foreign body, tumour, bilateral vocal cord palsy), *within the wall* (eg oedema from anaphylaxis, laryngospasm, tumour, croup, acute epiglottitis, amyloidosis), or *extrinsic* (eg goitre, oesophagus, lymphadenopathy, post-op stridor, after neck surgery). It's an emergency (▶▶p786) if gas exchange is compromised. NB: wheeze is an *expiratory* sound.

---

### Characteristic coughs

Coughing is relatively non-specific, resulting from irritation anywhere from the pharynx to the lungs. The character of a cough may, however, give clues as to the underlying cause:
- *Loud, brassy coughing* suggests pressure on the trachea, eg by a tumour.
- *Hollow, 'bovine' coughing* is associated with recurrent laryngeal nerve palsy.
- *Barking coughs* occur in croup.
- *Chronic cough:* Think of pertussis, TB, foreign body, asthma (eg nocturnal).
- *Dry, chronic coughing* may occur following acid irritation of the lungs in oesophageal reflux, and as a side-effect of ACE inhibitors.

▶Do not ignore a change in character of a chronic cough; it may signify a new problem, eg infection, malignancy.

---

1 Atopy implies predisposition to, or concurrence of, asthma, hay fever and eczema with production of specific IgE on exposure to common allergens (eg house dust mite, grass, cats).

## Haemoptysis

Blood is *coughed* up, eg frothy, *alkaline*, and bright red, often in a context of known chest disease (*vomited* blood is acidic and dark).

**Respiratory causes:**

| | |
|---|---|
| 1 **Infective** | TB; bronchiectasis; bronchitis; pneumonia; lung abscess; COPD; fungi (eg aspergillosis); viruses (from pneumonitis, cryoglobulinaemia, eg with hepatitis viruses, HIV-associated pneumocystosis, or MAI, p411). Helminths: paragonimiasis (p445); hydatid (p444); schistosomiasis.[29] |
| 2 **Neoplastic** | Primary or secondary. |
| 3 **Vascular** | Lung infarction (PE); vasculitis (ANCA-associated; RA; SLE); hereditary haemorrhagic telangiectasia; AV malformation; capillaritis. |
| 4 **Parenchymal** | Diffuse interstitial fibrosis; sarcoidosis; haemosiderosis; Goodpasture's syndrome; cystic fibrosis. |
| 5 **Pulmonary hypertension** | Idiopathic, thromboembolic, congenital cyanotic heart disease (p150), pulmonary fibrosis, bronchiectasis. |
| 6 **Coagulopathies** | Any—eg thrombocytopenia, p338; DIC; warfarin excess. |
| 7 **Trauma/foreign body** | Eg post-intubation, or an eroding implanted defibrillator. |
| 8 **Pseudo-haemoptysis** | Munchausen's (p720); aspirated haematemesis; red pigment (prodigiosin) from *Serratia marcescens* in sputum.[30] |

Rare causes refuse to be classified neatly: vascular causes may have infective origins, eg hydatid cyst may count as a foreign body, *and* infection, *and* vascular if it fistulates with the aorta;[31] ditto for infected (mycotic) aneurysm rupture,[32] or TB aortitis. Infective causes entailing coagulopathy: dengue; leptospirosis.[33] In monthly haemoptysis, think of lung endometriosis.

℞ Haemoptysis may need treating in its own right, if massive (eg trauma, TB, hydatid cyst, cancer, AV malformation): call chest team, consider interventional radiology input (danger is drowning: lobe resection, endobronchial tamponade, or arterial embolization may be needed). Set up IVI, do CXR, blood gases, FBC, INR/APTT, crossmatch. If distressing, give *prompt* IV morphine, eg if inoperable malignancy.[34]

## Dyspnoea

(see also p796)

Subjective sensation of shortness of breath, often exacerbated by exertion.

• *Lung*—airway and interstitial disease. May be hard to separate from cardiac causes; asthma may wake patient, and cause early morning dyspnoea & wheeze.
• *Cardiac*—eg ischaemic heart disease or left ventricular failure (LVF), mitral stenosis, of any cause. LVF is associated with *orthopnoea* (dyspnoea worse on lying; "How many pillows?") and *paroxysmal nocturnal dyspnoea* (PND; dyspnoea waking one up). Other features include ankle oedema, lung crepitations and ↑JVP.
• *Anatomical*—eg diseases of the chest wall, muscles, pleura. Ascites can cause breathlessness by splinting the diaphragm, restricting its movement.
• *Others* ▸ Any shocked patient may also be dyspnoeic (p804 & p609)—dyspnoea may be shock's presenting feature. Also anaemia or metabolic acidosis causing respiratory compensation, eg ketoacidosis, aspirin poisoning. Look for other clues—dyspnoea at rest *unassociated with exertion,* may be psychogenic: prolonged hyperventilation causes respiratory alkalosis. This causes a fall in ionized calcium leading to apparent hypocalcaemia. Features include peripheral and perioral paraesthesiae ± carpopedal spasm. Speed of onset helps diagnosis:

| Acute | Subacute | Chronic |
|---|---|---|
| Foreign body | Asthma | COPD and chronic parenchymal |
| Pneumothorax (p763, fig 1) | Parenchymal disease, | diseases |
| Pulmonary embolus | eg alveolitis pneumonia | Non-respiratory causes, |
| Acute pulmonary oedema | Effusion | eg cardiac failure |
| | | anaemia |

As with any examination routine, begin by introducing yourself, obtaining consent to examine the patient and position them appropriately: for the respiratory system, lying on a bed but sitting up at 45°. Expose them to the waist (for female patients, delay this until examining the chest itself). Explain what you are doing throughout.

### 5 Face
- *Inspect:* for signs of Horner's, conjunctival pallor, central cyanosis (ask patient to stick out tongue), pursed lip breathing

### 4 Neck
- *Trachea:* feel in sternal notch (deviated?), assess cricosternal distance in finger-breadths and feel for tracheal tug
- *Lymphadenopathy:* from behind with patient sat forward palpate lymph nodes of head and neck
- *JVP* raised in cor pulmonale, fixed and raised in superior vena cava obstruction

### 3 Arms
- Time pulse rate, with fingers still on the pulse, check respiratory rate (this can increase if the patient is aware you are timing it)—and pattern (p53)
- Bounding pulse ($CO_2$ retention)?
- Check blood pressure

### 2 Hands
- *Inspect:*
  Tobacco staining, peripheral cyanosis, clubbing, signs of systemic disease (systemic sclerosis, rheumatoid arthritis)
- *Asterixis:*
  Ask the patient to hold their hands out and cock their wrists back, fig 1

### 1 General inspection
- Assess general state (ill/well/cachexic)
- Look for clues (oxygen, inhalers)
- Colour (pale, cyanosed, flushed)
- Short of breath? Accessory muscle use?
- Scars on chest wall?
Ask the patient to take a deep breath in, watch chest movement and symmetry, any coughing?

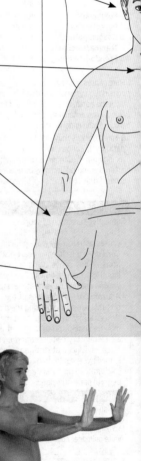

Fig 1. Asterixis.

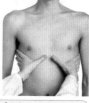

Fig 2. Placement of the hands for testing chest expansion: anchor with the fingers and leave the thumbs free-floating.

Figures 1-2 reproduced with permission from *Oxford Handbook of Clinical Examination and Practical Skills*.

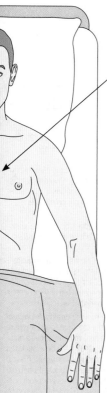

## 6 Front of chest

- *Apex beat*.
- *Expansion:* Ask patient to "breathe all the way out", place hands as in fig 2, "now a deep breath in", and note distance of thumbs to midline, is expansion equal? Repeat with hands laid on upper chest, equal?
- *Tactile vocal fremitus:* Ask patient to repeat "99" each time they feel your hand while palpating the chest wall with your fingertips. This is rarely used as more information can be gained from vocal resonance.
- *Percussion:* Percuss over different respiratory segments, comparing right and left.
- *Auscultation:* Ask patient to "take steady breaths in and out through your mouth" and listen with diaphragm from apices to bases, comparing right and left.
- *Vocal resonance:* Repeat auscultation, asking patient to repeat "99" each time they feel the stethoscope. If marked ↑ resonance heard, repeat with asking patient to whisper "99"; if clearly heard this is termed 'whispering pectoriloquy' and is a sensitive sign for consolidation. Outside of exams, the choice of vocal resonance or tactile vocal fremitus is a personal preference. Many clinicians prefer vocal resonance as it is an easier skill to master and provides more information than tactile vocal fremitus.

## 7 Back of chest

- *Expansion*
- *Tactile vocal fremitus*
- *Percussion*
- *Auscultation*
- *Vocal resonance*

## 8 To complete the examination

- Palpate for *sacral and ankle oedema*
- Check peripheral pulses, observation chart for temperature and O₂ sats
- Examine the sputum pot and check PEFR

### Top tips

- Whispering pectoriloquy is a classic sign of consolidation and is specific, so worth picking up
- If you don't adequately expose the chest you may miss small scars eg from video thoracoscopy
- If you see Horner's syndrome, check for wasting of the small muscles of the hand; see p716 and p722

### General inspection

"Comfortable at rest" or unwell? Cachectic? **Respiratory distress?** (see MINIBOX; occurs if high negative intrathoracic pressures are needed to generate air entry). Stridor? **Respiratory rate, breathing pattern** (see BOX). Look for **chest wall and spine deformities** (see p55). Inspect for **scars** of past surgery, chest drains, or radiotherapy (skin thickening, tattoos for radiotherapy). **Chest wall movement:** symmetrical? (if not, pathology on restricted side). Paradoxical respiration? (abdomen sucked in with inspiration; seen in diaphragmatic paralysis, see p506).

| **Signs of respiratory distress** |
| :--- |
| • Tachypnoea |
| • Nasal flaring |
| • Tracheal tug (pulling of thyroid cartilage towards sternal notch in inspiration) |
| • Use of accessory muscles (sternocleidomastoid, platysma, infrahyoid) |
| • Intercostal, subcostal and sternal recession |
| • Pulsus paradoxus (p40) |

### Hands

Clubbing, peripheral cyanosis, tar stains, fine tremor (β-agonist use), wasting of intrinsic muscles (T1 lesions, eg Pancoast's tumour, p722). Tender wrists (hypertrophic pulmonary osteoarthropathy—cancer). Asterixis ($CO_2$ retention). Pulse: paradoxical (respiratory distress), bounding ($CO_2$ retention).

### Face

Ptosis and constricted pupil (Horner's syndrome, eg Pancoast's tumour, p722)? Bluish tongue and lips (central cyanosis, p28)? Conjunctival pallor (anaemia)?

### Neck

*Trachea:* Central or displaced? (towards collapse or away from large pleural effusion/tension pneumothorax; slight deviation to right is normal). Cricosternal distance <3cm is hyperexpansion. **Tracheal tug:** descent of trachea with inspiration (severe airflow limitation). *Lymphadenopathy:* TB/Ca? *JVP:* ↑ in cor pulmonale.

### Examining the chest:

**Palpation** *Apex beat:* impalpable?(COPD/pleural effusion/dextrocardia?) *Expansion:* <5cm on deep inspiration is abnormal. Symmetry? *Tactile vocal fremitus:* ↑ implies consolidation (< sensitive than vocal resonance).

**Percussion** *Dull percussion note:* collapse, consolidation, fibrosis, pleural thickening, or pleural effusion (classically 'stony dull'). **Cardiac dullness** usually detectable over the left side. **Liver dullness** usually extends up to 5th rib, right mid-clavicular line; below this, resonant chest is a sign of lung hyperexpansion (eg asthma, COPD). *Hyperresonant percussion note:* pneumothorax or hyperinflation (COPD).

**Auscultation** Normal 'vesicular' breath sounds have a rustling quality. *Bronchial breathing:* Harsh with a gap between inspiration and expiration, occurs where lung tissue has become firm/solid, eg consolidation, localized fibrosis, above a pleural effusion, or large pericardial effusion (Ewart's sign, p148). May be associated with increased **vocal resonance** and whispering pectoriloquy. *Diminished breath sounds:* Pleural effusions, pleural thickening, pneumothorax, bronchial obstruction, asthma, or COPD. *Silent chest:* In life-threatening asthma severe bronchospasm prevents adequate air entry. *Added sounds:* **Wheezes (rhonchi):** caused by air expired through narrowed airways. May be monophonic (single note, signifying a partial obstruction of one airway, eg tumour) or polyphonic (multiple notes, signifying widespread narrowing of airways of differing calibre, eg asthma, COPD). Wheeze is also heard in LVF ('cardiac asthma'). **Crackles (crepitations):** caused by re-opening, during inspiration, of small airways which have become occluded during expiration. May be fine and late in inspiration if coming from distal air spaces (eg pulmonary oedema, fibrosing alveolitis) or coarse and mid-inspiratory if they originate more proximally (eg bronchiectasis). Early inspiratory crackles suggest small airways disease (eg COPD), whereas late/pan-inspiratory crackles suggest disease confined to alveoli. Crackles disappearing on coughing are insignificant. **Pleural rubs:** caused by movement of visceral pleura over parietal pleura, when both surfaces roughened, eg by inflammatory exudate. Causes include adjacent pneumonia or pulmonary infarction.

Pneumothorax click: produced by shallow left pneumothorax between layers of parietal pleura overlying heart, heard during cardiac systole.

**Further examination** *Sputum* (see BOX), *temperature charts*, $O_2$ *sats*, PEFR.

---

### Breathing patterns

**Hyperventilation** may be *fast* (tachypnoea, ie >20 breaths/min) or *deep* (hyperpnoea, ie tidal volume↑). Hyperpnoea is not unpleasant, unlike dyspnoea. It may cause respiratory alkalosis, hence paraesthesiae ± muscle spasm (Ca²⁺↓). The main cause is anxiety: there is associated dizziness, chest tightness/pain, palpitations, and panic. Rare causes: response to metabolic acidosis; brainstem lesions.

- *Kussmaul respiration* is deep, sighing breaths in severe metabolic acidosis (it helps to blow off CO₂), eg diabetic or alcoholic ketoacidosis,[38] renal impairment.
- *Neurogenic hyperventilation* is produced by pontine lesions.
- The *hyperventilation syndrome* involves panic attacks associated with hyperventilation, palpitations, dizziness, faintness, tinnitus, alarming chest pain/tightness,[38] perioral and peripheral tingling (plasma Ca²⁺↓). Treatment: relaxation techniques and breathing into a paper bag (↑inspired CO₂ corrects the alkalosis).
- NB: the anxious patient in A&E with hyperventilation and a respiratory alkalosis may actually be presenting with an aspirin overdose (p856).

**Cheyne-Stokes breathing** Breaths get deeper and deeper, then shallower (±episodic apnoea) in cycles. *Causes:* Brainstem lesions or compression (stroke, ICP↑). If the cycle is long (eg 3min), the cause may be a long lung-to-brain circulation time (eg in chronic pulmonary oedema or ↓cardiac output). It is enhanced by opioids.

---

### Sputum examination

Always inspect any sputum produced, however unpleasant this task may be. Send suspicious sputum for microscopy (Gram stain and auramine/ZN stain, if indicated), culture, and cytology.

- *Black carbon specks* in the sputum suggests smoking, the most common cause of increased sputum production.
- *Yellow/green sputum* suggests infection, eg bronchiectasis, pneumonia.
- *Pink frothy sputum* suggests pulmonary oedema.
- *Bloody sputum (haemoptysis)* may be due to malignancy, TB, infection, or trauma, and requires investigation for these causes. See p49.
- *Clear sputum* is probably saliva.

---

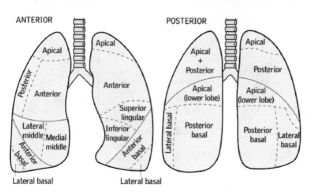

Fig 1. The respiratory segments supplied by the segmental bronchi.

History and examination

Some physical signs

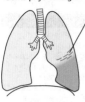

(There may be brochial breathing at the top of an effusion)

Expansion: ↓
Percussion: ↓ (Stony dull)
Air entry: ↓
Vocal resonance: ↓
Trachea + mediastinum central (shift away from affected side only with massive effusions ≥1000mL)

PLEURAL EFFUSION

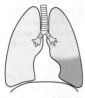

Expansion ↓
Percussion note ↓
Vocal resonance ↑
Bronchial breathing ± coarse crackles (with whispering pectoriloquy)
Trachea + mediastinum central

CONSOLIDATION

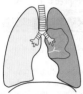

Expansion ↓
Percussion note ↑
Breath sounds ↓
Trachea + mediastinum shift towards the affected side

SPONTANEOUS PNEUMOTHORAX/ EXTENSIVE COLLAPSE (ΔΔ LOBECTOMY/ PNEUMONECTOMY)

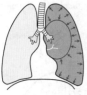

Expansion ↓
Percussion note ↑
Breath sounds ↓
Trachea + mediastinum shift away from the affected side

TENSION PNEUMOTHORAX (See fig 1 p763 for chest X-ray image)

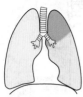

Expansion ↓
Percussion note ↓
Breath sounds bronchial ± crackles
Trachea + mediastinum central or pulled towards the area of fibrosis

FIBROSIS

Fig 1. Physical signs on chest examination.

## Chest deformities

- *Barrel chest:* AP diameter↑, tracheal descent and chest expansion↓, seen in chronic hyperinflation (eg asthma/COPD).
- *Pigeon chest (pectus carinatum):* See fig 2.
- *Funnel chest (pectus excavatum):* Developmental defect involving local sternum depression (lower end). See fig 3.
- *Kyphosis:* 'Humpback' from ↑ AP thoracic spine curvature.
- *Scoliosis:* Lateral curvature (OHCS p672); all of these may cause a restrictive ventilatory defect.

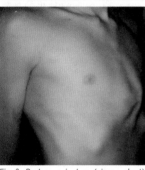

Fig 2. *Pectus carinatum* (pigeon chest). Prominent sternum, from lung hyperinflation while the bony thorax is still developing, eg in chronic childhood asthma. Often seen with **Harrison's sulcus**, a groove deformity caused by indrawing of lower ribs at the diaphragm attachment site. This usually has little functional significance in terms of respiration but can have significant psychological effects: see BOX.

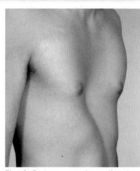

Fig 3. Pectus excavatum; the term for funnel or sunken chest. It is often asymptomatic, but may cause displacement of the heart to the left, and restricted ventilatory capacity ± mild air-trapping. Associations: scoliosis; Marfan's; Ehlers-Danlos syndrome.

Images courtesy of Prof Eric Fonkalsrud.

### Herr Minty and his pigeon chest

Chest wall deformities such as pectus excavatum are quite common, often appearing during adolescent growth spurts. Exercise intolerance is the main symptom (from heart compression—consider CXR/CT).[37]Indications for surgical correction (rarely needed): ≥2 of: a severe, symptomatic deformity; progression of deformity; paradoxical respiratory chest wall motion; pectus index >3.25 on CT; cardiac or lung compression; restrictive spirometry; cardiac pathology that might be from compression of the heart.

Psychological effects are interesting and not to be dismissed as their effects may be greater than any physical effects.[38] Because these people hate exposing their chests they may become introverted, and never learn to swim, so don't let them sink without trace. Be sympathetic, and remember Herr Minty, who inaugurated Graham Greene's *theory of compensation*: wherever a defect exists we must look for a compensating perfection to account for how the defect survives. In Minty's case, although "crooked and yellow and pigeon-chested he had his deep refuge, the inexhaustible ingenuity of his mind."[England Made Me]

History and examination

| Presenting symptoms | Direct questions |
|---|---|
| Abdominal pain (see BOX 2 and p608) | 'SOCRATES' (p34) |
| Distension (see BOX 3) | |
| Nausea, vomiting (see BOX 1) | Timing? Relation to meals? Amount? Content (liquid, solid, bile, blood)? |
| Haematemesis (p252-4) | Frequency? Fresh (bright red)/dark/'coffee grounds'? Consider neoplasia (weight loss, dysphagia, pain, melaena?), NSAIDs/warfarin? Surgery? Smoking? |
| Dysphagia (p240) | Level? Onset? Intermittent? Progressive? Painful swallow (odynophagia)? |
| Indigestion/dyspepsia/reflux (p242) | Timing (relation to meals)? |
| Recent change in bowel habit | Consider neoplasia (weight loss, dysphagia, pain, melaena?) |
| Diarrhoea (p246), constipation (p248) | |
| Rectal bleeding (p631) or melaena (p252) | Pain on defecation? Mucus? Fresh/dark/black? Mixed with stool/on surface/on paper/in the pan? |
| Appetite, weight change | Intentional? Quantify. Dysphagia? Pain? |
| Jaundice (p250) | Pruritus? Dark urine? Pale stools? |

(Screen for all above presenting symptoms before proceeding to past history.)

**Past history** Peptic ulcer disease, carcinoma, jaundice, hepatitis, blood transfusions, tattoos, previous operations, last menstrual period (LMP), dietary changes.

**Drug history** Especially steroids, NSAIDs, antibiotics.

**Family history** Irritable bowel syndrome (IBS), inflammatory bowel disease (IBD), peptic ulcer disease, polyps, cancer, jaundice.

**Social history** Smoking, alcohol, recreational drug use, overseas travel, tropical illnesses, contact with jaundiced persons, occupational exposures, high-risk sexual behaviour.

---

### Vomiting

History is vital. Associated symptoms and past medical history often indicate cause. Examine for dehydration, distension, tenderness, abdominal mass, succussion splash in children (pyloric stenosis), or tinkling bowel sounds (intestinal obstruction).

| Gastrointestinal | CNS | Metabolic/endocrine |
|---|---|---|
| • Gastroenteritis | • Meningitis/encephalitis | • Uraemia |
| • Peptic ulceration | • Migraine | • Hypercalcaemia |
| • Pyloric stenosis | • ↑Intracranial pressure | • Hyponatraemia |
| • Intestinal obstruction | • Brainstem lesions | • Pregnancy |
| • Paralytic ileus | • Motion sickness | • Diabetic ketoacidosis |
| • Acute cholecystitis | • Ménière's disease | • Addison's disease |
| • Acute pancreatitis | • Labyrinthitis | |
| *Alcohol and drugs* | *Psychiatric* | *Others[1]* |
| • Antibiotics | • Self-induced | • Myocardial infarction |
| • Opiates | • Psychogenic | • Autonomic neuropathy |
| • Cytotoxics | • Bulimia nervosa | • Sepsis (UTI; meningitis) |
| • Digoxin | | |

**1** How to remember the chief non-GI causes of vomiting? Try **ABCDEFGHI**: Acute kidney injury Addison's disease; Brain (eg ↑ICP); Cardiac (myocardial infarct); Diabetic ketoacidosis; Ears (eg labyrinthitis, Ménière's disease); Foreign substances (alcohol; drugs, eg opiates); Gravidity (eg hyperemesis gravidarum); Hypercalcaemia/Hyponatraemia; Infection (eg UTI, meningitis).

## Abdominal pain

Varies depending on the underlying cause. Examples: irritation of the mucosa (acute gastritis), smooth muscle spasm (acute enterocolitis), capsular stretching (liver congestion in CCF), peritoneal inflammation (acute appendicitis) and direct splanchnic nerve stimulation (retroperitoneal extension of tumour). The *character* (constant or colicky, sharp or dull), *duration,* and *frequency* depend on the mechanism of production. The *location* and *distribution* of referred pain depend on the anatomical site. *Time of occurrence* and *aggravating* or *relieving factors* such as meals, defecation, and sleep also have special significance related to the underlying disease process. The site of the pain may provide a clue:

- **Epigastric** Pancreatitis, gastritis/duodenitis, peptic ulcer, gallbladder disease, aortic aneurysm.
- **Left upper quadrant** Peptic ulcer, gastric or colonic (splenic flexure) cancer, splenic rupture, subphrenic or perinephric abscess, renal (colic, pyelonephritis).
- **Right upper quadrant** Cholecystitis, biliary colic, hepatitis, peptic ulcer, colonic cancer (hepatic flexure), renal (colic, pyelonephritis), subphrenic/perinephric abscess.
- **Loin** (lateral ⅓ of back between thorax and pelvis—merges with the flank, p567) Renal colic, pyelonephritis, renal tumour, perinephric abscess, pain referred from vertebral column. Causes of *flank pain* are similar (see index for fuller list).
- **Left iliac fossa** Diverticulitis, volvulus, colon cancer, pelvic abscess, inflammatory bowel disease, hip pathology, renal colic, urinary tract infection (UTI), cancer in undescended testis; zoster—wait for the rash! (p458). *Gynae:* Torsion of ovarian cyst, salpingitis, ectopic pregnancy.
- **Right iliac fossa pain** All causes of left iliac fossa pain plus appendicitis and Crohn's ileitis, but usually excluding diverticulitis.
- **Pelvic** *Urological:* UTI, retention, stones. *Gynae:* Menstruation, pregnancy, endometriosis (OHCS p288), salpingitis, endometritis (OHCS p274), ovarian cyst torsion.
- **Generalized** Gastroenteritis, irritable bowel syndrome, peritonitis, constipation.
- **Central** Mesenteric ischaemia, abdominal aneurysm, pancreatitis.

*Remember referred pain:* Myocardial infarct → epigastrium; pleural pathology.

## Abdominal distension (masses and the 'famous five' Fs)

Enid Blyton's Famous Five characters can generally solve any crime or diagnostic problem using 1950s methodologies steeped in endless school holidays, copious confection-laden midnight feasts, and lashings of homemade ginger beer.

Let's give them the problem of abdominal distension. The sweets and drinks used by the Famous Five actually contribute to the distension itself: fat, fluid, faeces, flatus, and fetus. If you think it far-fetched to implicate ginger beer in the genesis of fetuses, note that because it was homemade, like the fun, there was no limit to its intoxicating powers in those long-gone vintage summers. The point is to think to ask "When was your last period?" *whenever* confronted by a distended abdomen.

Flatus will be resonant on percussion. Fluid will be dull, and can be from ascites (eg from malignancy or cirrhosis: look for shifting dullness), distended bladder (cannot get below it) or an aortic aneurysm (expansile). Masses can be pelvic (think of uterine fibroids or ovarian pathology) or tumours from colon, stomach, pancreas, liver, or kidney. Also see causes of *ascites with portal hypertension* (p606), *hepatomegaly* (p63), *splenomegaly*, and *other abdominal masses* (p606).

### Faecal incontinence

This is common in the elderly. Do your best to help, and get social services involved if concerned. Continence depends on many factors—mental function, stool (volume and consistency), anatomy (sphincter function, rectal distensibility, anorectal sensation and reflexes). Defects in any area can cause loss of faecal continence.
**Causes:** often multifactorial. Is it passive faecal soiling or urgency-related stool loss? Consider the following:
• *Sphincter dysfunction:*
  • Vaginal delivery is the commonest cause due to sphincter tears or pudendal nerve damage.
  • Surgical trauma, eg following procedures for fistulas, haemorrhoids, fissures.
• *Impaired sensation:* diabetes, MS, dementia, any spinal cord lesions (▶▶consider cord compression if acute faecal incontinence).
• *Faecal impaction:* overflow diarrhoea, extremely common, especially in the elderly, and very easily treated.
• *Idiopathic:* although there is often no clear cause found, especially in elderly women, this is usually multifactorial, including a combination of poor sphincter tone and pudendal damage leading to poor sensation.

#### Assessment

▶Do PR (overflow incontinence? poor tone?) and assess neurological function of legs, particularly checking sensation.

Refer to a specialist (esp. if rectal prolapse, anal sphincter injury, lumbar disc disease, or alarm symptoms for Ca. colon exist). Consider anorectal manometry, pelvic ultrasound or MRI, and pudendal nerve testing may be needed.[39]

*Treat according to cause and to promote dignity:* ▶Never let your own embarrassment stop you from offering help. Knowledge and behaviour are key factors:
• Ensure toilet is in easy reach. Plan trips away in the knowledge of toilet locations.
• Obey call-to-stool impulses (esp. after meal, ie the gastro-colic reflex).
• Ensure access to latest continence aids and advice on use, refer to continence nurse specialist for assessment.
• Pelvic floor rehabilitation: for example can help faecal incontinence, squeeze pressure, and maximal tolerated volume.[40]
• Loperamide 2–4mg 45min before social engagements may prevent accidents outside home.[41] An anal cotton plug may help isolated internal sphincter weakness. Skin care. Support agencies.

If all sensible measures fail, try a brake-and-accelerator approach: enemas to empty the rectum (twice weekly) and codeine phosphate, eg 15mg/12h, on non-enema days to constipate. It's not a cure, but makes the incontinence manageable.

### Flatulence

Normally, 400–1300mL of gas is expelled PR in 8–20 discrete (or indiscrete) episodes per day. If this, with any eructation (belching) or distension, seems excessive to the patient, they may complain of flatulence. Eructation occurs in hiatus hernia—but most patients with 'flatulence' have no GI disease. Air swallowing (aerophagy) is the main cause of flatus; here $N_2$ is the chief gas. If flatus is mostly methane, $H_2$ and $CO_2$, then fermentation by bowel bacteria is the cause,[42] and reducing carbohydrate intake (eg less lactose and wheat) may help.[43]

## Tenesmus

This is a sensation in the rectum of incomplete emptying *after* defecation. It's common in irritable bowel syndrome (p276), but can be caused by tumours.

## Regurgitation

Gastric and oesophageal contents are regurgitated effortlessly into the mouth—without contraction of abdominal muscles and diaphragm (so distinguishing it from true vomiting). It may be worse on lying flat, and can cause cough and nocturnal asthma. Regurgitation is rarely preceded by nausea, and when due to gastro-oesophageal reflux, it is often associated with heartburn. An oesophageal pouch may cause regurgitation. Very high GI obstructions (eg gastric volvulus, p613) cause non-productive retching rather than true regurgitation.

## Steatorrhoea

These are pale stools that are difficult to flush, and are caused by malabsorption of fat in the small intestine and hence greater fat content in the stool. *Causes:* Ileal disease (eg Crohn's or ileal resection), pancreatic disease, and obstructive jaundice (due to ↓excretion of bile salts from the gallbladder).

## Dyspepsia

Dyspepsia and indigestion (p242) are broad terms. Dyspepsia is defined as one or more of post-prandial fullness, early satiety (unable to finish meal) and/or epigastric or retrosternal pain or burning. "Indigestion" reported by the patient can refer to dyspepsia, bloating, nausea and vomiting.[44] Try to find out exactly what your patient means and when these symptoms occur in relation to meals, for example, the classic symptoms of peptic ulcers occur 2-5 hours after a meal and on an empty stomach. Look for alarm symptoms (see p256); these have high negative predictive value. If all patients with dyspepsia undergo endoscopy, <33% have clinically significant findings.[45] Myocardial infarction may present as 'indigestion'.

## Halitosis

Halitosis (fetor oris, oral malodour) results from gingivitis (rarely severe enough to cause Vincent's angina, p726), metabolic activity of bacteria in plaque, or sulfide-yielding food putrefaction, eg in gingival pockets and tonsillar crypts.[46] Patients can often be anxious and convinced of halitosis when it is not present (and vice versa!). *Contributory factors:* Smoking, drugs (disulfiram; isosorbide), lung disease, hangovers.

R: Try to eliminate anaerobes:
• Good dental hygiene, dental floss, tongue scraping.
• 0.2% aqueous chlorhexidine gluconate.

The very common halitosis arising from the tongue's dorsum is secondary to over-populated volatile sulfur compound-producing bacteria. Locally retained bacteria metabolize sulfur-containing amino acids to yield volatile (∴ smelly) hydrogen sulfide and methylmercaptane, which perpetuate periodontal disease. At night and between meals conditions are optimal for odour production—so eating regularly may help. Treat by mechanical cleansing/scraping using tongue brushes or scrapes plus mouthwashes. Oral care products containing metal ions, especially Zn, inhibit odour formation, it is thought, because of affinity of the metal ion to sulfur. It is possible to measure the level of volatile sulfur-containing compounds in the air in the mouth directly by means of a portable sulfide monitor.

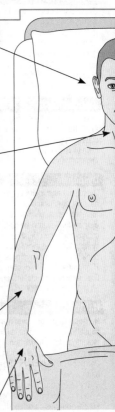

As with any examination routine, begin by introducing yourself, obtaining consent to examine the patient and position them appropriately. To examine the abdomen, lie the patient down as flat as possible, ideally exposing from 'nipples to knees' although in practice keep the groin covered and examine separately for hernias, etc.

### 5 Face
- *Skin and eyes:* jaundice, conjunctival pallor, Kayser-Fleischer rings, xanthelasma, sunken eyes (dehydration)
- *Mouth:* angular stomatitis, pigmentation, telangiectasia, ulcers, glossitis

### 4 Neck
- Examine cervical and supraclavicular lymph nodes (see fig 1)
- *JVP* raised in fluid overload (renal dysfunction, liver dysfunction), tricuspid regurgitation (may cause pulsatile hepatomegaly)
- Scars from tunnelled haemodialysis lines (see p295) or other central venous access

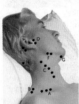

A= Supraclavicular
B= Posterior triangle
C= Jugular chain
D= Preauricular
E= Postauricular
F= Submandibular
G= Submental
H= Occipital

Fig 1. Cervical and supraclavicular nodes.

### 3 Arms
- Check pulse and blood pressure
- Look in the distribution of the svc (arms, upper chest, upper back) for spider naevi
- Check for track marks, bruising, pigmentation, scratch marks, arteriovenous fistulae (see p295 for signs seen in patients with chronic kidney disease)

### 2 Hands
- *Inspect:* clubbing, koilonychia, leuconychia, Muehrcke's lines, palmar erythema, Dupuytren's contracture, pigmentation of the palmer creases
- *Asterixis:* (see fig 1, p50)

### 1 General inspection
- Assess general state (ill/well/cachexic)
- Look for clues (vomit bowl, stoma bags)
- Colour (pale, jaundiced, uraemic)
- Body mass index?
- Scars on the abdomen? Stomas?
Ask the patient to lift their head off the bed, or cough, looking for bulges, distension or pain

## 6 Abdomen

### Inspection
- Scars—previous surgery, transplant, stoma
- Visible masses, hernias or pulsation of AAA
- Visible veins suggesting portal hypertension
- Gynaecomastia, hair loss, acanthosis nigricans

### Palpation
Squat by the bed so that the patient's abdomen is at your eye level. Ask if there is any pain and examine this part last. Watch the patient's face for signs of discomfort. Palpate the entire abdomen (see p567):
- *Light palpation:* If this elicits pain, check for *rebound tenderness*. Any involuntary tension in muscles ('*guarding*')? See p608.
- *Deep palpation:* To detect masses.
- *Liver:* Using the radial border of the index finger aligned with the costal margin start palpation from the RIF. Press down and ask patient to take a deep breath. Continue upwards towards the costal margin until you feel the liver edge.
- *Spleen:* Start palpation from the RIF and work towards the left costal margin asking the patient to take a deep breath in and feeling for the edge of the spleen—much like palpating the liver.
- *Kidneys:* For each kidney: place one hand behind patient at the loin, press down on the abdomen with your other hand and 'flick' the kidney up with your lower hand against your upper hand (see fig 1, p63).
- *Aorta:* Palpate midline above umbilicus, is it expansile? (fig 2, p47).

### Percussion
- *Liver:* Percuss to map upper & lower border of liver.
- *Spleen:* Percuss from border of spleen as palpated, around to mid-axillary line.
- *Bladder:* If enlarged, suprapubic region will be dull.
- *Ascites:* Shifting dullness: Percuss centrally to laterally until dull, keep your finger at the dull spot and ask patient to lean onto opposite side. If the dullness was fluid, this will now have moved by gravity and the previously dull area will be resonant.

### Auscultation
- *Bowel sounds:* Listen just below the umbilicus.
- *Bruits:* Listen over aorta and renal arteries (either side of midline above umbilicus)

### 7 To complete the examination
- Palpate for *ankle oedema*, examine the *hernial orifices*, *external genitalia* and perform a rectal examination
- Check the observation chart for temperature and dipstick the urine

### Top tips
- If you think there is a spleen tip, roll the patient onto their right side and feel again. This tips the spleen forward and allows you to percuss around to the back (try to do this at the same time as shifting dullness to look super slick)
- Don't forget to check the back for spider naevi, even if the chest appears clear, you can miss a valuable sign (look for nephrectomy scars as you do this)
- Light palpation really should be light, a quick check for tenderness and very large masses, watching the patient's face throughout

### Inspection

Does your patient appear comfortable or in distress? Look for abnormal contours/distension. Tattoos? Cushingoid appearance may suggest steroid use post-transplant or IBD. Inspect (and smell) for signs of chronic liver disease:

- Hepatic fetor on breath (p258)
- Purpura (purple-stained skin, p338)
- Spider naevi (fig 1, p261)
- Asterixis
- Gynaecomastia
- Scratch marks
- Palmar erythema
- Clubbing (rare)
- Muscle wasting
- Jaundice

Look for signs of malignancy (cachexia, masses), anaemia, jaundice, Virchow's node. From the end of the bed inspect the abdomen for:

- Visible pulsation (aneurysm, p656)
- Striae (stretch marks, eg pregnancy)
- Peristalsis
- Distension
- Scars
- Genitalia
- Masses
- Herniae

If abdominal wall veins look dilated, assess **direction of flow**. In inferior vena caval (IVC) obstruction, below the umbilicus blood flows up; in portal hypertension (*caput medusae*), flow radiates out from the umbilicus.

*The cough test:* While looking at the face, ask the patient to cough. If this causes abdominal pain, flinching, or a protective movement of hands towards the abdomen, suspect peritonitis.

### Hands

Clubbing, *leuconychia* (whitening of the nails due to hypoalbuminaemia), *koilonychia* ('spooning' of the nails due to iron, $B_{12}$, or folate deficiency), *Muehrcke's lines* (transverse white lines due to hypoalbuminaemia), *blue lanulae* (bluish discolouration seen in Wilson's disease). *Palmar erythema* (chronic liver disease, pregnancy), *Dupuytren's contracture* (thickening and fibrous contraction of palmar fascia (see fig 1, p713; alcoholic liver disease)). *Hepatic flap/asterixis* (hepatic encephalopathy, uraemia from renal disease), check pulse (and respiratory rate) (infection/sepsis?), palpate for arteriovenous fistulae in the forearm (access for haemodialysis in end-stage renal failure).

### Face

Assess for jaundice, anaemia, xanthelasma (PBC, chronic obstruction), Kayser–Fleischer rings (green-yellow ring at corneal margin seen in Wilson's disease). Inspect mouth for angular stomatitis (thiamine, $B_{12}$, iron deficiency), pigmentation (Peutz-Jeghers syndrome, p723, fig 4), telangiectasia (Osler-Weber-Rendu syndrome/hereditary haemorrhagic telangiectasia, p723, fig 2), ulcers (IBD), glossitis (iron, $B_{12}$, or folate deficiency).

### Cervical lymph nodes

Palpate for enlarged left supraclavicular lymph node (*Virchow's node/Troisier's sign*) (gastric carcinoma?).

### Abdomen

*Inspect:* Look around to the flanks for nephrectomy scars.

*Palpate:* Note any masses, tenderness, guarding (involuntary tensing of abdominal muscles—pain or fear of it), or rebound tenderness (greater pain on removing hand than on gently depressing abdomen—peritoneal inflammation); Rovsing's sign (appendicitis, p610); Murphy's sign (cholecystitis, p636). *Palpating the liver:* Assess size (see BOX), regularity, smoothness, and tenderness. Pulsatile (tricuspid regurgitation)? *The scratch test* is an another way to find the lower liver edge (if it is below the costal margin): start with diaphragm of stethoscope at right costal margin. Gently scratch the abdominal wall, starting in the right lower quadrant, working towards the liver edge. A sharp increase in transmission of the scratch is heard when the border of the liver is reached. *Palpating the spleen:* If suspect splenomegaly but cannot detect it, assess patient in the right lateral position with your left hand pulling forwards from behind the rib cage. *Palpating the kidneys:* see fig 1. Enlarged? Nodular? *Palpating the aorta:* Normally palpable transmitted pulsation in thin individuals.

### Percussion

Confirm the lower border and define the upper border of the liver and spleen (dull in the mid-axillary line in the 10th intercostal space). Percuss all regions of abdomen. If this induces pain, there may be peritoneal inflammation below (eg an inflamed appendix).[47] Some experts percuss first, before palpation, because even anxious patients do not expect this to hurt—so, if it does hurt, this is a very valuable sign. Percuss for the shifting dullness of ascites (p61 & p606) but ultrasound is a more reliable way of detecting ascites.

### Auscultation

Bowel sounds: absence implies ileus; they are enhanced and tinkling in bowel obstruction. Listen for bruits in the aorta, renal and femoral arteries.

### Further examination

Check for hernias (p614), perform a PR examination (p633).

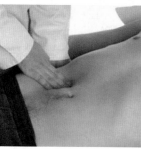
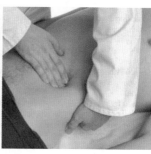

Fig 1. Ballottement of the kidneys.

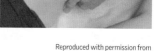

Reproduced with permission from
*Oxford Handbook of Clinical Examination and Practical Skills.*

---

### Causes of hepatomegaly

(For hepatosplenomegaly, see p606)

- *Malignancy:* Metastatic or primary (usually craggy, irregular edge).
- *Hepatic congestion:* Right heart failure—may be pulsatile in tricuspid incompetence, hepatic vein thrombosis (Budd-Chiari syndrome, p710).
- *Anatomical:* Riedel's lobe (normal variant).
- *Infection:* Infectious mononucleosis (glandular fever), hepatitis viruses, malaria, schistosomiasis, amoebic abscess, hydatid cyst.
- *Haematological:* Leukaemia, lymphoma, myeloproliferative disorders (eg myelofibrosis), sickle-cell disease, haemolytic anaemias.
- *Others:* Fatty liver, porphyria, amyloidosis, glycogen storage disorders.

---

### Splenomegaly

Abnormally large spleen. *Causes:* See p606. If massive, think of: chronic myeloid leukaemia, myelofibrosis, malaria (or leishmaniasis).

---

### Features of the spleen differentiating it from an enlarged kidney

- Cannot get above it (ribs overlie the upper border of the spleen).
- Dull to percussion (kidney is usually resonant because of overlying bowel).
- Moves towards RIF with inspiration (kidney tends to move downwards).
- May have palpable notch on its medial side.

| **Presenting symptoms** | **Direct questions** |
|---|---|

**Presenting symptoms**
*Dysuria* (see BOX 1)
*Lower urinary tract symptoms (LUTS)*
*Loin/scrotal pain*
*Haematuria* (p285 and p649)
*Urethral/vaginal discharge* (p418)
*Sex problems; painful intercourse/dyspareunia* (OHCS p310)
*Menses* (OHCS p250)

**Direct questions**
Pain: SOCRATES (p34). Fever? Sexual history. Abnormal looking urine? Previous problems.

Must rule out testicular torsion (p654).

Ask about menarche, menopause, length of periods, amount, pain? Intermenstrual loss? 1st day of last menstrual period (LMP)?

**Detecting outflow obstruction** (see BOX 5) eg prostatic hyperplasia; stricture; stone). Ask about *LUTS* (lower urinary tract symptoms)
• On trying to pass water, is there delay before you start? (**Hesitancy**)
• Does the flow stop and start? Do you go on dribbling when you think you've stopped? (**Terminal dribbling**)
• Is your stream getting weaker? (**Poor stream**)
• Is your stream painful and slow/'drop-by-drop'? (**Strangury**, eg from bladder stone)
• Do you feel the bladder is not empty after passing water?[i]
• Do you ever pass water when you do not want to? (**Incontinence**—p650)
• On feeling an urge to pass water, do you have to go at once? (**Urgency**)[i]
• Do you urinate often at night? (**Nocturia**)[i] In the day? (**Frequency**)[i] How often?
[i] = irritative (or 'filling') symptoms: they can be caused by, for example, UTI, as well as obstructions.

**Past history** Renal colic, urinary tract infection, diabetes, BP↑, gout, analgesic use (p306), previous operations.

**Drug history** Anticholinergics.

**Family history** Prostate carcinoma? Renal disease?

**Social history** Smoking, sexual history.

---

### Dysuria

Be sure you mean the same as your patient and colleagues, as dysuria refers to both painful micturition ('uralgia'[48]) and difficult micturition (**voiding difficulty**, p65). Uralgia is typically from urethral, bladder or vaginal inflammation (UTI; perfumed bath products, spermicides, urethral syndrome, p292). If postmenopausal, look for a urethral caruncle—fleshy outgrowth of distal urethral mucosa, ≤1cm, typically originating from the posterior urethral lip. Also think of prostatitis, STI/urethritis (p418), vaginitis, and vulvitis, *Rare causes:* Stones, urethral lesions (eg carcinoma, lymphoma,[49] papilloma[50]), post-partum complications (eg retained products of conception).

Voiding difficulty is a sign of outflow obstruction, eg from an enlarged prostate, or urethral stricture (commonly post-traumatic, post-gonococcal). Other features: straining to void, poor stream, urinary retention, and incontinence. Strangury is urethral pain, usually referred from the bladder base, causing a constant distressing desire to urinate even if there is little urine to void. *Causes:* Stones, catheters, cystitis, prostatitis, bladder neoplasia, rarely: bladder endometriosis,[51] schistosomiasis.[52]

---

### Frequency

Aim to differentiate ↑urine production (eg diabetes mellitus and insipidus, polydipsia, diuretics, alcohol, renal tubular disease, adrenal insufficiency) from frequent passage of small amounts of urine (eg in cystitis, urethritis, neurogenic bladder), or bladder compression or outflow obstruction (pregnancy, bladder tumour, enlarged prostate).

## Oliguria/anuria

**Oliguria** is defined as a urine output of <400mL/24h or <0.5mL/kg/hour and can be a sign of shock (eg post-op, p578) or acute kidney injury: causes: p290. **Anuria** is defined as <50mL/24h. In a catheterized patient with sudden anuria consider catheter blockage, with slow decline of oliguria to anuria renal dysfunction is more likely.

## Polyuria

Increased urine volume, eg >3L/24h. *Causes:* Over-enthusiastic IV fluid therapy; diabetes mellitus & insipidus (diabetes is Greek for fountain);↑$Ca^{2+}$; psychogenic polydipsia/PIP syndrome (p232); polyuric phase of recovering acute tubular necrosis.

## Irritative or obstructive bladder symptoms (see also p644)

Symptoms of prostate enlargement are miscalled 'prostatism'; it is better to talk about *irritative* or *obstructive bladder* symptoms, as bladder neck obstruction or a stricture may be the cause. 1 *Irritative bladder symptoms:* Urgency, dysuria, frequency, nocturia[1] (the last two are also associated with causes of **polyuria**). 2 *Obstructive symptoms:* Reduced size and force of urinary stream, hesitancy and interruption of stream during voiding and terminal dribbling—the usual cause is enlargement of the prostate (prostatic hyperplasia), but other causes include a urethral stricture, tumour, urethral valves, or bladder neck contracture. The maximum flow rate of urine is normally ~18-30mL/s.

## Terminal dribbling

Dribbling at the end of urination, often seen in conjunction with incontinence following incomplete urination, associated with prostatism.

## Urinary changes

*Cloudy urine* suggests pus (UTI) but is often normal phosphate precipitation in an alkaline urine. *Pneumaturia* (bubbles in urine as it is passed) occurs with UTI due to gas-forming organisms or may signal an enterovesical (bowel-bladder) fistula from diverticulitis, Crohn's disease or neoplastic disease of the bowel. *Nocturia* occurs with 'irritative bladder', diabetes mellitus, UTI, and reversed diurnal rhythm (seen in renal and cardiac failure). *Haematuria* (RBC in urine) is due to neoplasia or glomerulonephritis (p300) until proven otherwise.

## Voiding difficulty

This includes poor flow, straining to void, hesitancy, intermittent stream, incontinence (eg overflow), retention (acute or chronic), incomplete emptying (±UTI from residual urine). ▶Remember faecal impaction as a cause of retention with overflow. *Causes:* *Obstructive:* Prostatic hyperplasia, early oedema after bladder neck repair, uterine prolapse, retroverted gravid uterus, fibroids, ovarian cysts, urethral foreign body, ectopic ureterocele, bladder polyp, or cancer. *Bladder overdistension*—eg after epidural for childbirth. *Detrusor weakness or myopathy* causes incomplete emptying + dribbling overflow incontinence (do cystometry/electromyography;[53] causes include neurological disease and interstitial cystitis (OHCS p306); it may lead to a contracted bladder, eg requiring substitution enterocystoplasty.[54] *Drugs:* Epidural anaesthesia; tricyclics, anticholinergics. *CNS:* Suprapontine (stroke); cord lesions (cord injury, multiple sclerosis); peripheral nerve (prolapsed disc, diabetic or other neuropathy); or reflex, due to pain (eg with herpes infections).

---

1 In the elderly, nocturia (1-2/night) may be 'normal' because of: i) loss of ability to concentrate urine; ii) peripheral oedema fluid returns to the circulation at night; iii) circadian rhythms may be lost; iv) less sleep is needed and waking may be interpreted as a need to void (a conditioned Pavlovian response).

| Presenting symptoms | Direct questions |
|---|---|
| *Breast lump* | Previous lumps? Family history? Pain? Nipple discharge? Nipple inversion? Skin changes? Change in size related to menstrual cycle? Number of pregnancies? First/last/latest period? Postnatal? Breast feeding? Drugs (eg HRT)? Consider metastatic disease (weight loss, breathlessness, back pain, abdominal mass?) |
| *Breast pain* (see BOX 1) | SOCRATES (p34). Bilateral/unilateral? Rule out cardiac chest pain (p88 & p798). History of trauma? Any mass? Related to menstrual cycle? |
| *Nipple discharge* (see BOX 2) | Amount? Nature (colour? consistency? any blood?) |

(Screen for all above presenting symptoms before proceeding to past history.)

**Past history** Any previous lumps and/or malignancies. Previous mammograms, clinical examinations of the breast, USS, fine-needle aspirate (FNA)/core biopsies.

**Drug history** Ask specifically about HRT and the Pill.

**Family history** See p524.

**Social history** Try to gain an impression of support network if suspect malignancy.

---

**Breast pain**

Is it premenstrual (*cyclical mastalgia*, OHCS p254)? Breast cancer (refer, eg, for mammography if needed)? If non-malignant and non-cyclical, think of:
- Tietze's syndrome[1]
- Angina
- Lung disease
- Oestrogens/HRT
- Bornholm disease[2]
- Gallstones
- Thoracic outlet syndrome

If none of the above, wearing a firm bra all day may help, as may NSAIDs.

---

**Nipple discharge**

*Causes:* Duct ectasia (green/brown/red, often multiple ducts and bilateral), intraductal papilloma/adenoma/carcinoma (bloody discharge, often single duct), lactation. *Management:* Diagnose the cause (mammogram, ultrasound, ductogram); then treat appropriately. Cessation of smoking reduces discharge from duct ectasia. Microdochectomy/total duct excision can be considered if other measures fail, though may give no improvement in symptoms.

---

1 Tietze's syndrome is costochandritis plus swelling of the costal cartilage.

2 Bornholm disease (Devil's grip) is due to Coxsackie B virus, causing chest and abdominal pain, which may be mistaken for cardiac pain or an acute surgical abdomen. It resolves within ~2 weeks.

1 **Inspection** Assess size and shape of any masses as well as overlying surface. Which quadrant (see fig 2)? Note skin involvement; ulceration, dimpling (*peau d'orange*), and nipple inversion/discharge.

2 **Palpation of the breast** Confirm size, and shape of any lump. Is it fixed/tethered to skin or underlying structures (see BOX)? Is it fluctuant/compressible/hard? Temperature? Tender? Mobile (more likely to be fibroadenoma)?

3 **Palpation of the axilla for lymph nodes** Metastatic spread? Ipsilateral/bilateral? Matted? Fixed?

4 **Further examination** Examine abdomen for hepatomegaly, spine for tenderness, lungs (metastatic spread).

## 1 General inspection

▶Always have a chaperone present when examining the breast.

Introduction, consent, position patient sitting at edge of bed with hands by her side, expose to waist. Inspect both breasts for obvious masses, contour anomalies, asymmetry, scars, ulceration, skin changes, eg *peau d'orange* (orange peel appearance resulting from oedema). Look for nipple inversion and nipple discharge. Ask her to "press hands on hips" and then "hands on head" to accentuate any asymmetrical changes. Whilst patient has her hands raised inspect axillae for any masses as well as inspecting under the breasts.

## 2 Palpation of the breast

Position patient sitting back at 45° with hand behind head (ie right hand behind head when examining the right breast—see fig 1). Ask patient if she has any pain or discharge. Examine painful areas last and then ask her to express any discharge. Examine each breast with the 'normal' side first. Examine each quadrant in turn as well as the axillary tail of Spence (fig 2) or use a concentric spiral method (fig 3) using a flat hand to roll breast against underlying chest wall. Define any lumps/lumpy areas. If you discover a lump, to examine for fixity to the pectoral muscles ask the patient to push against your hand with her arm outstretched.

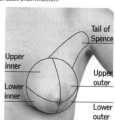

Fig 1. Correct patient position for breast examination.

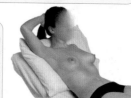

Fig 2. The quadrants of the breast with the axillary tail of Spence.

*Labels in figure:* Tail of Spence; Upper inner; Upper outer; Lower inner; Lower outer

## 3 Palpation of the axilla

Examine both axillae. When examining right axilla, hold the patient's right arm with your right hand and examine axilla with left hand.

5 sets of axillary nodes:

i) apical (palpate against glenohumeral joint)
ii) anterior (palpate against pectoralis major)
iii) central (palpate against lateral chest wall)
iv) posterior (palpate against latissimus dorsi)
v) medial (palpate against humerus)

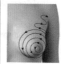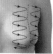

Fig 3. Methods for systematic breast palpation.

Figs 1-3 with permission from *OHCEPS*.

## 4 Further examination

Complete examination by palpating down spine for tenderness, examining abdomen for hepatomegaly, and lungs for signs of metastases. Thank patient and wash hands.

For symptoms of thyroid disease see p210 & p212. See also lumps in the neck, p600–2.

1 **Inspection** The key questions to ask oneself when presented with a lump in the neck are: Is this lump thyroid related or not? What is the patient's thyroid status? Inspect the neck; the normal thyroid is usually neither visible nor palpable. A midline swelling should raise your suspicion of thyroid pathology. Look for scars (eg collar incision from previous thyroid surgery). Examine the face for signs of hypothyroidism (puffiness, pallor, dry flaky skin, xanthelasma, corneal arcus, balding) as well as overall body habitus. Assess the patient's demeanour; do they appear anxious, nervous, agitated, fidgety (hyperthyroid)? Or slow and lethargic (hypothyroid)?

2 **Swallow test** Only goitres (p602), thyroglossal cysts (p600) and in some cases lymph nodes should move up on swallowing.

3 **Tongue protrusion test** A thyroglossal cyst will move up on tongue protrusion.

4 **Palpation** (By this stage of the examination if the evidence is in favour of the lump not rising from the thyroid it is acceptable to examine the lump like any other (p596); assess site, size, shape, smoothness (consistency), surface (contour/edge/colour), and surroundings, as well as transilluminance, fixation/tethering, fluctuance/compressibility, temperature, tenderness and whether it is pulsatile.) If a thyroid mass is suspected, standing behind the patient provides an opportunity to check for any proptosis (hyperthyroidism). Proceed to palpate each lobe, attempting to decide whether any lump is *solitary or multiple*, *nodular or smooth/diffuse* as well as site, size, etc. Repeating the swallow test whilst palpating allows you to confirm the swallow finding, but also attempt to 'get below the lump'. If there is a distinct inferior border under which you can place your hand with the entire lump above it then the goitre is unlikely to have retrosternal extension. Examining for 'spread' to the lymph nodes is particularly important if you suspect a thyroid malignancy (p602). Complete palpation by assessing if the presence of the lump has caused the trachea to deviate from the midline.

5 **Percussion** A retrosternal goitre will produce a dull percussion note when the sternum is percussed.

6 **Auscultation** A bruit in a smooth thyroid goitre is suggestive of Graves' disease (p210).

The next stages of the exam are to examine the systemic signs of thyroid status.

7 **Hands** Clubbing ('thyroid acropathy') is seen in Graves' disease. Palmar erythema and a fine tremor are also signs of thyrotoxicosis. Assess temperature (warm peripheries if hyperthyroid) and the radial pulse; tachycardia and atrial fibrillation are seen in hyperthyroidism, while bradycardia is seen in hypothyroidism).

8 **Eyes** The 'normal' upper eyelid should always cover the upper eye such that the white sclera is not visible between the lid and the iris. In hyperthyroidism with exophthalmus there is proptosis as well as lid retraction and 'lid lag' may also be detected. If the patient reports double vision when eye movements are being tested this indicates ophthalmoplegia of hyperthyroidism.

9 Asking the patient to stand allows you to assess whether there is any proximal myopathy (hypothyroidism). Look for pretibial myxoedema (brown swelling of the lower leg above the lateral malleoli in Graves' disease). Finally, test the reflexes; these will be slow relaxing in hypothyroidism and brisk in hyperthyroidism.

10 Thank the patient and consider whether the lump is a goitre, and if so whether it is single/multiple, diffuse/nodular, as well as the patient's thyroid status. Decide on a diagnosis (p602).

### 1 Inspection
Introduction, consent, position patient sitting on a chair (with space behind), adequately expose neck. Inspect from front and sides for any obvious goitres or swellings, scars, signs of hypo-/hyperthyroidism.

### 2 Swallow test
Standing in front of the patient ask them to "sip water...hold in your mouth ...and swallow" to see if any midline swelling moves up on swallowing.

### 3 Tongue protrusion test
Ask patient to "stick out your tongue". Does the lump move up?

*If evidence favours lump not arising from thyroid, examine lump like any other (p596)*

### 4 Palpation
Stand behind the patient.
- *Proptosis:* (p211) whilst standing behind the patient ask them to tilt their head back slightly; this will give you a better view to assess any proptosis than when assessing the other aspects of eye pathology from front on, as in **8**)
- *The thyroid gland:* ask the patient "any pain?" Place middle 3 fingers of either hand along midline below chin and 'walk down' to thyroid. Assess any enlargement/ nodules
- *Swallow test:* repeat as before, now palpating; attempt to 'get under' the lump
- *Lymph nodes:* examine lymph nodes of head and neck (p60). Stand in front of the patient
- *Trachea:* palpate for tracheal deviation from the midline.

### 5 Percussion
Percuss the sternum for dullness of retrosternal extension of a goitre.

### 6 Auscultation
Listen over the goitre for a bruit.

### 7 Hands
- *Inspect:* for thyroid acropachy (clubbing) and palmar erythema
- *Temperature*
- *Pulse:* rate and rhythm
- *Fine tremor:* ask patient to "hold hands out", place sheet of paper over outstretched hands to help.

### 8 Eyes
- *Exophthalmos:* inspect for lid retraction and proptosis (p211)
- *Lid lag:* ask patient to "look down following finger" as you move your finger from a point above the eye to below
- *Eye movements:* Ask patient to follow your finger, keeping their head still, as you make an 'H' shape. Any double vision?

### 9 Completion
Ask patient to stand up from the chair to assess for proximal myopathy, look for pretibial myxoedema, test ankle reflexes (ask patient to face away from you with knee resting on chair). Thank patient and wash hands.

**History** This should be taken from the patient and if possible from a close friend or relative as well for corroboration/discrepancies. The patient's memory, perception, or speech may be affected by the disorder, making the history difficult to obtain. Note the progression of the symptoms and signs: gradual deterioration (eg tumour) vs intermittent exacerbations (eg multiple sclerosis) vs rapid onset (eg stroke). Ask about age, occupation and ethnic origin. Right- or left-hand dominant?

**Presenting symptoms**

• *Headache:* (p460 & p794) Different to usual headaches? Acute/chronic? Speed of onset? Single/recurrent? Unilateral/bilateral? Associated symptoms (eg aura with migraine, p462)? Any meningism (p832)? Worse on waking (↑ICP)? Decreased conscious level? ►Take a 'worst-ever' headache very seriously. (See p763)

• *Muscle weakness:* (p470) Speed of onset? Muscle groups affected? Sensory loss? Any sphincter disturbance? Loss of balance? Associated spinal/root pain?

• *Visual disturbance:* (OHCS p410) eg blurring, double vision (diplopia), photophobia, visual loss. Speed of onset? Any preceding symptoms? Pain in eye?

• *Change in other senses:* Hearing (p468), smell, taste? Abnormalities are not always due to neurological disease, consider ENT disease.

• *Dizziness:* (p466) Illusion of surroundings moving (vertigo)? Hearing loss/tinnitus? Any loss of consciousness? Positional?

• *Speech disturbance:* (p80) Difficulty in expression, articulation, or comprehension (can be difficult to determine)? Sudden onset or gradual?

• *Dysphagia:* (p240) Solids and/or liquids? Intermittent or constant? Difficulty in coordination? Painful (odynophagia)?

• *Fits/faints/'funny turns'/involuntary movements:* (p472) Frequency? Duration? Mode of onset? Preceding aura? Loss of consciousness? Tongue biting? Incontinence? Any residual weakness/confusion? Family history?

• *Abnormal sensations:* eg numbness, 'pins & needles' (paraesthesiae), pain, odd sensations. Distribution? Speed of onset? Associated weakness?

• *Tremor:* (p71) Rapid or slow? Present at rest? Worse on deliberate movement? Taking β-agonists? Any thyroid problems? Any family history? Fasciculations?

**Cognitive state** If there is any doubt about the patient's cognition, an objective measure is a cognitive test—guessing has been shown to be inaccurate![54] See TYM, p65. The following 10 questions comprise the Abbreviated Mental Test Score (AMTS), a commonly used screening questionnaire for cognitive impairment:[55]

1 Tell patient an address to recall at the end (eg 42 West Street)
2 Age
3 Time (to nearest hour)
4 What year is it?
5 Recognize 2 people (eg doctor & nurse)
6 Date of birth
7 Dates of the Second World War
8 Name of current monarch/prime minister
9 Where are you now? (Which hospital?)
10 Count backwards from 20 to 1

*A score of ≤6 suggests poor cognition, acute (delirium), or chronic (dementia).* AMTS correlates well with the more detailed Mini-Mental State Examination (MMSE™), though recent copyright means that its use has become more restricted.[56] NB: deaf, dysphasic, depressed, and uncooperative patients, as well as those who do not understand English, will also get low scores[57] (TYM test: see p85).

**Past medical history** Ask about meningitis/encephalitis, head/spine trauma, seizures, previous operations, risk factors for vascular disease (p474, AF, hypertension, hyperlipidaemia, diabetes, smoking), and recent travel, especially exotic destinations. Is there any chance that the patient is pregnant (eclampsia, OHCS p48)?

**Drug history** Any anticonvulsant/antipsychotic/antidepressant medication? Any psychotropic drugs (eg ecstasy)? Any medication with neurological side-effects (eg isoniazid which can cause a peripheral neuropathy)?

**Social and family history** What can the patient do and not do, ie activities of daily living (ADLs)? What is the Barthel Index score?[58] Any neurological or psychiatric disease in the family? Any consanguinity? Consider sexual history, eg syphilis.

## Cramp

This is painful muscle spasm. Leg cramps are common at night or after heavy exercise, and in patients with renal impairment or on dialysis.[59] Cramp can signify salt depletion, and rarely: muscle ischaemia (claudication, DM), myopathy (McArdle, p718), or dystonia (writer's cramp, p473). Forearm cramps suggest motor neuron disease. Night cramps may respond to quinine bisulfate 300mg at night PO.

*Drugs causing cramp:* Diuretics (? from K⁺↓), domperidone, salbutamol/terbutaline IVI, ACE-i, telmisartan, celecoxib, lacidipine, ergot alkaloids, levothyroxine.

## Paraesthesiae

'Pins and needles', numbness/tingling, which can hurt or 'burn' (dysaesthesia). **Causes:** *Metabolic:* ↓Ca²⁺ (perioral); $P_aCO_2$↑; myxoedema; neurotoxins (tick bite; sting). *Vascular:* ▶▶Arterial emboli; Raynaud's; DVT; high plasma viscosity. *Antibody-mediated:* Paraneoplastic;[60] SLE; ITP. *Infection:* Rare: Lyme;[61] rabies. *Drugs:* ACE-i. *Brain:* Thalamic/parietal lesions. *Cord:* MS; myelitis/HIV; B₁₂↓; ▶▶lumbar fracture.[62] *Plexopathy/mononeuropathy:* p506, cervical rib;[63] carpal tunnel; sciatica. *Peripheral neuropathy* (glove & stocking, p508, eg DM; CKD). If *paroxysmal:* Migraine;[64] epilepsy;[65] phaeochromocytoma. If *wandering:* take travel history, consider infection, eg strongyloides.

## Tremor

Tremor is rhythmic oscillation of limbs, trunk, head, or tongue. 3 types:
1 *Resting tremor*—worst at rest—eg from parkinsonism (±bradykinesia and rigidity; tremor is more resistant to treatment than other symptoms). It is usually a slow tremor (frequency of 3–5Hz), typically 'pill-rolling' of the thumb over a finger.
2 *Postural tremor*—worst if arms are outstretched. Typically *rapid* (8–12Hz). May be exaggerated physiological tremor (eg anxiety, hyperthyroidism, alcohol, drugs), due to brain damage (eg Wilson's disease, syphilis) or *benign essential tremor* (BET). This is often familial (autosomal dominant) tremor of arms and head presenting at any age. Cogwheeling may occur,[66] but there is no bradykinesia. It is suppressed by alcohol, and patients may self-medicate rather than admit problems. Rarely progressive (unless onset is unilateral). Propranolol (40–80mg/8–12h PO) can help, but not in all patients.
3 *Intention tremor*—worst on movement, seen in cerebellar disease, with pastpointing and dysdiadochokinesis (see p503). No effective drug has been found.

## Facial pain

*CNS causes:* Migraine, trigeminal or glossopharyngeal neuralgia, (p461) or from any other pain-sensitive structure in the head or neck. *Post-herpetic neuralgia:* nasty burning-and-stabbing pain involves dermatomal areas affected by shingles (p400); it may affect cranial nerves V and VII in the face. It all too often becomes chronic and intractable (skin affected is exquisitely sensitive). Treatment is hard. Always give strong psychological support. Transcutaneous nerve stimulation, capsaicin ointment, and infiltrating local anaesthetic are tried. Neuropathic pain agents, such as amitriptyline, eg 10–25mg/24h at night, or gabapentin (p508) may help. NB: famciclovir or valaciclovir given in acute shingles may ↓ duration of neuralgia.[67]

*Vascular and non-neurological causes:*

| | |
|---|---|
| Neck | Cervical disc pathology |
| Bone/sinuses | Sinusitis; neoplasia |
| Eye | Glaucoma; iritis; orbital cellulitis; eye strain; AVM |
| Temporomandibular joint | Arthritis or idiopathic dysfunction (common) |
| Teeth/gums | Caries; broken teeth; abscess; malocclusion |
| Ear | Otitis media; otitis externa |
| Vascular/vasculitis | Arteriovenous fistula;[68] aneurysm; or AVM at the cerebellopontine angle;[69] giant cell arteritis; SLE[70] |

▶The neurological system is usually the most daunting examination, so learn at the bedside from a senior colleague, preferably a neurologist. Keep practising. Be aware that books present ideal situations: often one or more signs are equivocal or even contrary to expectation; consider signs in the context of the history and try re-examining the patient, as signs may evolve over time. The only essential point is to distinguish whether weakness is upper (UMN) or lower (LMN) motor neuron (p451). Position the patient comfortably, sitting up at 45° and with arms exposed. The general order of examination should be Tone, Power, Reflexes, Coordination, Sensation.

### 3 Power

Direct patient to adopt each position and follow commands while you as the examiner stabilise the joint above and resist movements as appropriate to grade power see fig 1 (p451). Test each muscle group bilaterally before moving on to the next position.

- "Shrug your shoulders and don't let me push down; push your arms out to the side against me; try to pull them back in"
- "Hold your arms up like this and pull me towards you, now push me away"
- "Hold your hand out flat, don't let me push it down; now don't let me push it up"
- Offer the patient two of your fingers and ask them to "squeeze my fingers"
- Ask patient to "spread your fingers and stop me pushing them back together", then hand the patient a piece of paper to

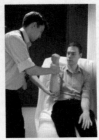

Fig 1 Testing limb power.

grip between two fingers. You as the examiner should grip the paper with your corresponding fingers whilst asking patient to "grip the paper and don't let me pull it away".

### 2 Tone

Ask patient to "relax/go floppy like a rag-doll". Ask if patient has any pain in hands/arm/shoulder before passively flexing and extending limb while also pronating and supinating the forearm. Any spasticity or rigidity?

Fig 2 Testing tone.

### 1 General inspection

Abnormal posturing, asymmetry, abnormal movements (fasciculation/tremor/dystonia/ athetosis), muscle wasting (especially small muscles of the hand)—symmetrical/asymmetrical? Local/general?

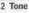

### 4 Reflexes

For each reflex, test right, then left and compare. If absent, attempt to elicit with 'reinforcement' by asking patient to clench their teeth on a count of 3 at which time you strike. Decide whether reflexes are absent/present (with reinforcement)/normal/brisk/exaggerated. •*Biceps*: (C5,6) •*Triceps*: (C7) •*Supinator*: (C6). See below.

### 5 Coordination

• Holding your finger in front of the patient instruct "touch my finger then your nose...as fast as you can". Look for intention tremor and 'past pointing'.
• *Test for dysdiadokokinesis:* Ask patient to repeatedly pronate and supinate forearm, clapping the hands each time. Test both limbs. You may have to demonstrate. Failure to perform rapidly alternating movements is dysdiadokokinesis.
• *Test for pronator drift:* with patient's eyes closed and arms outstretched tap down on their up-facing palms and look for a failure to maintain supination.

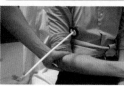

Fig 3. Testing tendon reflexes in biceps.

### 6 Sensation

• *Light touch*: Use cotton wool, touch it to sternum first—"this is what it should feel like, tell me where you feel it and if it feels different". Proceed to test with cotton wool in all dermatomes (see p458), comparing left and right.
• *Pin prick*: Repeat as above using a neurological pin, asking patient to tell you if it feels sharp or dull.
• *Temperature*: Repeat as above, alternating hot and cold probes. Can the patient tell hot from cold?
• *Vibration*: Using a 128Hz tuning fork confirm with patient that they "can feel a buzzing" when you place the tuning fork on their sternum. Proceed to test at the most distal bony prominence and move proximally by placing the buzzing fork on the bony prominence, then stopping it with your fingers. Ask the patient to tell you when the buzzing stops.
• *Proprioception*: With the patient's eyes closed grasp distal phalanx of the index finger at the sides. Stabilize the rest of the finger. Flex and extend the joint, stopping at intervals to ask whether the finger tip is up or down.

**Top tips**

• Use the tendon hammer like a pendulum, let it drop, don't grip it too tightly
• Ensure you are testing light touch, not stroke sensation

If the patient is able to walk, the best way to begin your examination is to ask the patient to remove their lower garments down to underwear, and to walk across the room. Gait analysis (p471) gives you more information than any other test. If they aren't able to walk, start with them lying down, legs fully exposed. The general routine should be Gait, Tone, Reflexes, Power, Coordination, Sensation.

### 3 Reflexes

For each reflex, test right, then left and compare. If absent, attempt to elicit with 'reinforcement'. Decide whether reflexes are absent/present (with reinforcement)/normal/brisk/exaggerated.

• *Knee:* (L3,4) Strike on the patella tendon, just below the patella.
• *Ankle:* (L5,S1) Several accepted methods; ideally ask the patient to slightly bend the knee, then drop it laterally, grasp the foot and dorsiflex, then strike the Achilles tendon. If hip pain limits mobility, dorsiflex the foot with a straight leg and strike your hand, feeling for an ankle jerk.
• *Plantar reflexes:* (L5, S1, S2) Stroke the patient's sole with an orange stick or similar. The normal reflex is downward movement of the great toe. *Babinski's sign* is positive if there is dorsiflexion of the great toe (this is abnormal (upper motor neuron lesion) if patient age >6 months).

### 2 Tone

Ask patient to "relax/go floppy like a rag-doll". Ask if they have any pain in feet/legs/hips before passively flexing and extending each limb while also internally and externally rotating. Hold the patient's knee and roll it from side to side. Put your hand behind the knee and raise it quickly. The heel should lift slightly from the bed if tone is normal. Any spasticity/rigidity?

**Clonus** (fig 1) Plantar flex the foot then quickly dorsiflex and hold. More then 5 'beats' of plantar flexion is sustained clonus and is abnormal. Hypertonia and clonus suggest an upper motor neuron lesion.

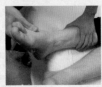

Fig 1. Ankle tone: testing for clonus.

### 1 General inspection and gait

*Gait:* Ask patient to walk a few metres, turn and walk back to you. Note use of walking aids, symmetry, size of paces, arm swing. Ask patient to "walk heel-to-toe as if on a tightrope" to exaggerate any instability. Ask patient to walk on tiptoes, then on heels. Inability to walk on tiptoes indicates S1 or gastrocnemius lesion. Inability to walk on heels indicates L4,5 lesion or foot drop.
*Romberg's test:* Ask patient to stand unaided with arms by their sides and close their eyes (be ready to support them). If they sway/lose balance the test is positive and indicates posterior column disease/sensory ataxia.
*Inspect:* Abnormal posturing, muscle wasting, fasciculation (LMN lesion?), deformities of the foot (eg pes cavus of *Friedreich's ataxia* or *Charcot-Marie-Tooth disease*). Is one leg smaller than the other (*old polio, infantile hemiplegia*)?

## 4 Power

Direct patient to adopt position and follow commands below while you as the examiner resist movements as appropriate to grade power (p451). Test each muscle group bilaterally before moving on to the next position.

- *Hip flexion:* "Keeping your leg straight, can you lift your leg off the bed, don't let me push it down"
- *Hip extension:* "And now using your leg, push my hand into the bed"
- *Hip abduction:* Position hands on outer thighs—"push your legs out to the sides"
- *Hip adduction:* Position hands on inner thighs—"and push your legs together"
- *Knee flexion and extension:* "Bend your knee and bring your heel to your bottom, don't let me pull it away... and now kick out against me and push me away"
- *Ankle plantar flexion:* With your hand on the underside of the patient's foot ask them to "bend your foot down, pushing my hand away"
- *Ankle dorsiflexion:* Put your hand on the dorsum of the foot and ask them to "lift up your foot, point your toes at the ceiling, don't let me push your foot down"

## 5 Coordination

*Heel-shin test:* Using your finger on the patient's shin to demonstrate, instruct patient to "put your heel just below your knee then run it smoothly down your shin, lift it up and place it back on your knee, now run it down again", etc. Repeat on the other side.

## 6 Sensation As upper limbs (p73)

- *Light touch:* Lower limb dermatomes (p458)
- *Pin prick*
- *Temperature*
- *Vibration*
- *Joint position sense*: With the patient's eyes closed grasp distal phalanx of the great toe at the sides. Stabilize the rest of the toe. Move the joint up and tell patient "this is up", and down, saying "this is down". Flex and extend the joint, stopping at intervals to ask whether the toe is up or down.

### Top tips

- If you are limited for time, gait is the most useful test to start with
- Make sure you test each muscle group individually by stabilising above the joint you are testing
- Test vibration by putting a buzzing tuning fork on the bony part of a joint with the patient's eyes closed then ask them to tell you when the buzzing stops (pinch the tuning fork to stop it) to distinguish vibration from pressure sensation

**Approach to examining the cranial nerves** Where is the lesion? Think systematically. Is it in the brainstem (eg MS) or outside, pressing on the brainstem? Is it the neuromuscular junction (myasthenia) or the muscles (eg a dystrophy)? Cranial nerves may be affected singly or in groups. ▶Face the patient (helps spot asymmetry). For causes of lesions see BOX.

| Cranial nerve names | |
|---|---|
| I | olfactory |
| II | optic |
| III | oculomotor |
| IV | trochlear |
| V | trigeminal |
| V₁ | ophthalmic division |
| V₂ | maxillary division |
| V₃ | mandibular division |
| VI | abducens |
| VII | facial |
| VIII | vestibulocochlear |
| IX | glossopharyngeal |
| X | vagus |
| XI | accessory |
| XII | hypoglossal |

I *Smell:* Test ability of each nostril to distinguish familiar smells, eg coffee.

II *Acuity:* Test each eye separately, and its correctability with glasses or pin-hole; use Snellen chart if possible, or the one inside the cover of this book. *Visual fields:* Compare with your own fields or formally via perimetry testing. Any losses/inattention? Sites of lesions: *OHCS* p428. *Pupils:* (p79) Size, shape, symmetry, reaction to light (direct and consensual) or accommodation. Swinging light test for relative afferent pupillary defect. *Ophthalmoscopy:* (*OHCS*, p412) This is best learnt from an ophthalmologist. Darken the room, warn the patient you will need to get close to their face. Focus the lens on the optic disc (pale? swollen?). Follow vessels outwards to view each quadrant. If the view is obscured, examine the red reflex, with your focus on the margin of the pupil, to look for a cataract. Try to get a view of the fovea by asking the patient to look directly at the ophthalmoscope ▶Pathology here needs prompt ophthalmic review. If in doubt, ask for slit lamp examination or photography of the retina.

III⁰, IV & VI *Eye movements. IIIʳᵈ nerve palsy:* Ptosis, large pupil, eye down and out. *IVᵗʰ nerve palsy:* Diplopia on looking down and in (often noticed on descending stairs)—head tilting compensates for this (ocular torticollis). *VIᵗʰ nerve palsy:* Horizontal diplopia on looking out. *Nystagmus* is involuntary, often jerky, eye oscillations. Horizontal nystagmus is often due to a vestibular lesion (acute: nystagmus away from lesion; chronic: towards lesion), or cerebellar lesion (unilateral lesions cause nystagmus towards the affected side). If it is more in whichever eye is abducting, MS may be the cause (internuclear ophthalmoplegia, p78). If also deafness/tinnitus, suspect a peripheral cause (eg VIIIᵗʰ nerve lesion, barotrauma, Ménière's, p466). If it varies with head position, suspect benign positional vertigo (p466). If it is up-and-down, ask a neurologist to review—upbeat nystagmus classically occurs with lesions in the midbrain or at the base of the 4ᵗʰ ventricle, downbeat nystagmus in foramen magnum lesions. Nystagmus lasting ≤2 beats is normal, as is nystagmus at the extremes of gaze.

V *Motor palsy:* "Open your mouth": jaw deviates to side of lesion. *Sensory:* Check all 3 divisions. Consider corneal reflex (lost first).

VII⁰ *Facial nerve lesions* cause droop and weakness. As the forehead has bilateral representation in the brain, only the lower two-thirds is affected in UMN lesions, but all of one side of the face in LMN lesions. Ask to "raise your eyebrows", "show me your teeth", "puff out your cheeks". Test taste with salt/sweet solutions.

VIII *Hearing:* p468. Ask to repeat a number whispered in an ear while you block the other. Perform Weber's and Rinne's tests (p468). *Balance/vertigo:* p466.

IX⁰ & X⁰ *Gag reflex:* Ask the patient to say "Ah". Xᵗʰ nerve lesions also cause the palate to be pulled to the normal side on saying "Ah". Ask them to swallow a sip of water. Consider gag reflex—touch the back of the soft palate with an orange stick. The afferent arm of the reflex involves IX; the efferent arm involves X.

XI *Trapezii:* "Shrug your shoulders" against resistance. *Sternocleidomastoid:* "Turn your head to the left/right" against resistance.

XII *Tongue movement:* The tongue deviates to the side of the lesion.

Any cranial nerve may be affected by diabetes mellitus; stroke; MS; tumours; sarcoidosis; vasculitis, p558, eg PAN (p558), SLE (p556); syphilis. Chronic meningitis (malignant, TB, or fungal) tends to pick off the lower cranial nerves one by one.

**I** Trauma; respiratory tract infection; meningitis; frontal lobe tumour.

**II** *Field defects* may start as small areas of visual loss (scotomas, eg in glaucoma). *Monocular blindness:* Lesions of one eye or optic nerve eg MS, giant cell arteritis. *Bilateral blindness[1]:* Any cause of mononeuritis, eg diabetes, MS; rarely methanol, neurosyphilis. *Field defects—Bitemporal hemianopia:* Optic chiasm compression, eg pituitary adenoma, craniopharyngioma, internal carotid artery aneurysm (fig 1, p452). *Homonymous hemianopia:* Affects half the visual field contralateral to the lesion in each eye. Lesions lie beyond the chiasm in the tracts, radiation, or occipital cortex, eg stroke, abscess, tumour. *Optic neuritis* (pain on moving eye, loss of central vision, relative afferent pupillary defect, disc swelling from papillitis[2]). **Causes:** Demyelination (eg MS); rarely sinusitis, syphilis, collagen vascular disorders.
*Ischaemic papillopathy:* Swelling of optic disc due to stenosis of the posterior ciliary artery (eg in giant cell arteritis).
*Papilloedema* (bilaterally swollen discs, fig 3, p562): most commonly ↑ICP (tumour, abscess, encephalitis, hydrocephalus, idiopathic intracranial hypertension); rarer: retro-orbital lesion (eg cavernous sinus thrombosis, p484).
*Optic atrophy:* (pale optic discs and reduced acuity): MS; frontal tumours; Friedreich's ataxia; retinitis pigmentosa; syphilis; glaucoma; Leber's optic atrophy; chronic optic nerve compression.[71]

**III[c]** *alone[c]:* 'Medical' causes (pupillary sparing): diabetes; HTN; giant cell arteritis; syphilis; idiopathic. 'Surgical' causes (early pupil involvement due to external compression of nerve damaging parasympathetic fibres): posterior communicating artery aneurysm (+ surgery);[72] ↑ICP (if uncal herniation through the tentorium compresses the nerve); tumours.

**IV[c]** *alone:* Rare and usually due to trauma to the orbit.[73]

**V[c]** *Sensory:* Trigeminal neuralgia (pain but no sensory loss, p461); herpes zoster, nasopharyngeal cancer, acoustic neuroma (p466). *Motor:* Rare.

**VI[c]** *alone:* MS, Wernicke's encephalopathy, false localizing sign in ↑ICP, pontine stroke (presents with fixed small pupils ± quadriparesis).[74]

**VII** *LMN:* Bell's palsy (p504), polio, otitis media, skull fracture; cerebello-pontine angle tumours, eg acoustic neuroma, malignant parotid tumours, herpes zoster (Ramsay Hunt syndrome p505, OHCS p652). *UMN:* (spares the forehead, because of its bilateral cortical representation) Stroke, tumour.

**VIII** (p466 & p468) Noise damage, Paget's disease, Ménière's disease, herpes zoster, acoustic neuroma, brainstem CVA, drugs (eg aminoglycosides).

**IX, X, XI** Trauma, brainstem lesions, neck tumours.[75]

**XII** Rare. Polio, syringomyelia, tumour, stroke, bulbar palsy, trauma, TB.

**Groups of cranial nerves VIII,** then **V, VI, IX & X:** Cerebellopontine angle tumours, eg acoustic neuroma (p466; facial weakness is not a prominent sign). **III, IV & VI:** Stroke, tumours, Wernicke's encephalopathy; aneurysms, MS.[76] **III, IV, V, & VI:** Cavernous sinus thrombosis, superior orbital fissure lesions (Tolosa-Hunt syndrome, OHCS p654). **IX, X & XI:** Jugular foramen lesion. ΔΔ: Myasthenia gravis, muscular dystrophy, myotonic dystrophy, mononeuritis multiplex (p506).

## Headache

If the patient is able to shake their head, there is no meningism.

---

**1** Remember the commonest cause of monocular or binocular blindness is not a cranial nerve lesion but a problem with the eye itself (cataracts, retinal problems). Neurological disorders more commonly cause loss of part of the visual field.

**2** Unilateral disc swelling = papillitis, bilateral papillitis/disc swelling = papilloedema. Check both eyes! c= structures passing through the cavernous sinus; see BOX, p83.     NB: $V_a$ is the only division of V to do so.
[c]= Remember that these cranial nerves carry parasympathetic fibres. Sympathetic fibres originate from the thoracic chain and run with the arterial supply to distribute about the body (see also OHCS, fig 1, p629).

History and examination

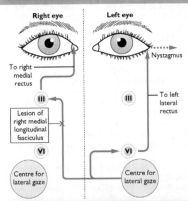

Fig 1. Internuclear ophthalmoplegia (INO) and its causes. To produce synchronous eye movements, cranial nerves III, IV, and VI communicate through medial longitudinal fasciculus in midbrain. In INO, a lesion disrupts communication, causing weakness in adduction of the ipsilateral eye with nystagmus of the contralateral eye *only when abducting*. There may be incomplete or slow abduction of the ipsilateral eye during lateral gaze. Convergence is preserved. *Causes:* MS or vascular (rarely: HIV; syphilis; Lyme disease; brainstem tumours; phenothiazine toxicity).

## Ptosis

Drooping of the upper eyelid. Best observed with patient sitting up, with head held by examiner. Oculomotor nerve (CN III) innervates main muscle concerned (levator palpebrae), but nerves from the cervical sympathetic chain innervate superior tarsal muscle, and a lesion of these nerves causes mild ptosis which can be overcome on looking up. *Causes:* **1** CN III lesions cause unilateral *complete* ptosis: look for other evidence of a CN III lesion: ophthalmoplegia with 'down and out' deviation of the eye, pupil dilated and unreactive to light or accommodation. If eye pain too, suspect infiltration (eg by lymphoma or sarcoidosis). If T°↑ or consciousness ↓, suspect infection (any tick bites?) **2** Sympathetic paralysis usually causes unilateral partial ptosis. Look for other evidence of a sympathetic lesion, as in Horner's syndrome (p716): constricted pupil = *miosis*, lack of sweating on same side of the face (=*anhidrosis*). **3** Myopathy, eg dystrophia myotonica, myasthenia gravis (cause bilateral partial ptosis). **4** Congenital; usually partial and without other CNS signs.

## Visual loss

▶Get ophthalmology help. See *OHCS* p434–p455. Consider:
- Is the eye red? (*glaucoma, uveitis* p563)
- Pain? *Giant cell arteritis*: severe temporal headache, jaw claudication, scalp tenderness, ↑ESR: ▶ urgent steroids (p558). *Optic neuritis*: eg in MS.
- Is the cornea cloudy: *corneal ulcer* (*OHCS* p432), *glaucoma* (*OHCS* p430)?
- Is there a contact lens problem (*infection*)?
- Any flashes/floaters? (*TIA, migraine, retinal detachment*?)
- Is there a visual field problem (*stroke, space-occupying lesion, glaucoma*)?
- Are there any focal CNS signs?
- Any valvular heart disease/carotid bruits (*emboli*)? Hyperlipidaemia (p704)?
- Is there a relative afferent pupillary defect (p79)?
- Any past history of trauma, migraine, hypertension, cerebrovascular disease, MS, diabetes or connective tissue disease?
- Any distant signs: eg *HIV* (causes retinitis), *SLE, sarcoidosis*?

**Sudden** •Acute glaucoma •Retinal detachment •Vitreous haemorrhage (eg in diabetic proliferative retinopathy) •Central retinal artery or vein occlusion •Migraine •CNS: TIA (amaurosis fugax), stroke, space-occupying lesion •Optic neuritis (eg MS) •Temporal arteritis •Drugs: quinine/methanol •Pituitary apoplexy.

**Gradual** •Optic atrophy •Chronic glaucoma •Cataracts •Macular degeneration •Tobacco amblyopia.

## Pupillary abnormalities

Key questions: •Equal, central, circular, dilated, or constricted? •React to light, directly and consensually? •Constrict normally on convergence/accommodation?

*Irregular pupils:* Anterior uveitis (iritis), trauma to the eye, syphilis.

*Dilated pupils:* CN III lesions (►inc. ↑ICP, p840) and mydriatic drugs. *Always ask: is this pupil dilated, or is it the other that is constricted?*

*Constricted pupils:* Old age, sympathetic nerve damage (Horner's, p716, and ptosis, p78), opiates, miotics (pilocarpine drops for glaucoma), pontine damage.

*Unequal pupils (anisocoria)* may be due to unilateral lesion, eye-drops, eye surgery, syphilis, or Holmes-Adie pupil. Some inequality is normal.

*Light reaction:* Test: cover one eye and shine light into the other obliquely. Both pupils should constrict, one by direct, other by consensual light reflex (fig 2). The lesion site is deduced by knowing the pathway: from the retina the message passes up the optic nerve (CNII) to the superior colliculus (midbrain) and thence to the CNIII nuclei on both sides. The III^rd cranial nerve causes pupillary constriction. If a light in one eye causes only contralateral constriction, the defect is 'efferent', as the afferent pathways from the retina being stimulated must be intact. Test for *relative afferent pupillary defect:* move torch quickly from pupil to pupil. If there has been incomplete damage to the afferent pathway, the affected pupil will paradoxically dilate when light is moved from the normal eye to the abnormal eye. This is because, in the face of reduced afferent input from the affected eye, the consensual pupillary relaxation response from the normal eye predominates. This is the *Marcus Gunn sign*, and may occur after apparent complete recovery from the initial lesion.

*Reaction to accommodation/convergence:* If the patient first looks at a distant object and then at the examiner's finger held a few inches away, the eyes will converge and the pupils constrict. Afferent fibres in each optic nerve pass to the lateral geniculate bodies. Impulses then pass to the pre-tectal nucleus and then to the parasympathetic nuclei of the III^rd cranial nerves, causing pupillary constriction.

• **Holmes-Adie (myotonic) pupil:** The affected pupil is normally moderately dilated and is poorly reactive to light, if at all. It is slowly reactive to accommodation: wait and watch carefully: it may eventually constrict more than a normal pupil. It is often associated with diminished or absent ankle and knee reflexes, in which case the Holmes-Adie syndrome is present. Usually a benign incidental finding. Rare causes: Lyme disease, syphilis, parvovirus B19, HSV, autoimmunity. ♀>♂.

• **Argyll Robertson pupil:** This occurs in neurosyphilis. The pupil is constricted and unreactive to light, but reacts to accommodation. Other possible causes: Lyme disease; HIV;[77] zoster; diabetes mellitus; sarcoidosis;[78] MS; paraneoplastic; B₁₂↓.[79] The iris may be patchily atrophied, irregular, and depigmented. The lesion site is not *always* near the Edinger-Westphal nucleus or even in the midbrain.[80] Pseudo-Argyll Robertson pupils occur in Parinaud's syndrome (p722).

• **Hutchinson pupil:** This is the sequence of events resulting from rapidly rising unilateral intracranial pressure (eg in intracerebral haemorrhage). The pupil on the side of the lesion first constricts then widely dilates. The other pupil then goes through the same sequence. ►See p840.

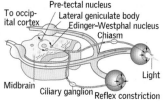

Fig 2. Light reflex. Action potentials go along optic nerve (red), traversing optic chiasm, passing synapses at pre-tectal nucleus, *en route* to Edinger-Westphal nuclei of CNIII. These send fibres to *both* irises' ciliary muscles (so *both* pupils constrict) via **ciliary ganglion** (also relays accommodation and corneal sensation, and gets sympathetic roots from C8-T2, carrying fibres to dilate pupil).

To occipital cortex
Pre-tectal nucleus
Lateral geniculate body
Edinger–Westphal nucleus
Chiasm
Midbrain
Light
Ciliary ganglion
Reflex constriction

History and examination

►Have mercy on those with dysphasia: it is one of the most debilitating neurological conditions, and the more frustrating when cognitive function is intact.

**Dysphasia** (Impairment of language caused by brain damage)

*Assessment:*

1 If speech is fluent, grammatical and meaningful, dysphasia is unlikely.
2 **Comprehension:** Can the patient follow one, two, and several step commands? (touch your ear, stand up, then close the door).
3 **Repetition:** Can the patient repeat a sentence?
4 **Naming:** Can they name common and uncommon things (eg parts of a watch)?
5 **Reading and writing:** Normal? They are usually affected like speech in dysphasia. If normal, the patient is unlikely to be aphasic—could they be mute?

*Classification:*

• *Broca's (expressive) anterior dysphasia:* Non-fluent speech produced with effort and frustration with malformed words, eg 'spoot' for 'spoon' (or 'that thing'). Reading and writing are impaired but comprehension is relatively intact. Patients understand questions and attempt to convey meaningful answers. **Site of lesion:** infero-lateral dominant frontal lobe (see BOX).

• *Wernicke's (receptive) posterior dysphasia:* Empty, fluent speech, like talking ragtime with phonemic ('flush' for 'brush') and semantic ('comb' for 'brush') paraphasias/neologisms (may be mistaken for psychotic speech). The patient is oblivious of errors. Reading, writing, *and* comprehension are impaired (replies are inappropriate). **Site of lesion:** posterior superior dominant temporal lobe.

• *Conduction aphasia:* (Traffic between Broca's and Wernicke's area is interrupted.) Repetition is impaired; comprehension and fluency less so.

• *Nominal dysphasia:* Naming is affected in all dysphasias, but in nominal dysphasia, objects cannot be named but other aspects of speech are normal. This occurs with posterior dominant temporoparietal lesions.

►Mixed dysphasias are common. Discriminating features take time to emerge after an acute brain injury. Speech therapy is important, but may not help.

**Dysarthria** Difficulty with articulation due to incoordination or weakness of the musculature of speech. Language is normal (see above).

• *Assessment:* Ask to repeat 'British constitution' or 'baby hippopotamus'.
• *Cerebellar disease:* Ataxia speech muscles cause slurring (as if drunk) and speech irregular in volume and staccato in quality (see MINIBOX).
• *Extrapyramidal disease:* Soft, indistinct, and monotonous speech.
• *Pseudobulbar palsy:* (p511) Spastic dysarthria (**upper motor neuron**). Speech is slow, indistinct, nasal and effortful ('hot potato' voice from bilateral hemispheric lesions, MND (p510), or severe MS).
• *Bulbar palsy:* **Lower motor neuron** (eg facial nerve palsy, Guillain-Barré, MND, p510)—any associated palatal paralysis gives speech a nasal character.

**Dysphonia** Difficulty with speech volume due to weakness of respiratory muscles or vocal cords (myasthenia, p516; Guillain-Barré syndrome, p716). It may be precipitated in myasthenia by asking the patient to count to 100. Parkinson's gives a mixed picture of dysarthria and dysphonia.

**Dyspraxia** Poor performance of complex movements despite ability to do each individual component. Test by asking the patient to copy unfamiliar hand positions, or mime an object's use, eg a comb. The term 'dyspraxia' is used in 3 other ways:

• *Dressing dyspraxia:* The patient is unsure of the orientation of clothes on his body. Test by pulling one sleeve of a sweater inside out before asking the patient to put it back on (mostly non-dominant hemisphere lesions).
• *Constructional dyspraxia:* Difficulty in assembling objects or drawing, eg a 5-pointed star (non-dominant hemisphere lesions, hepatic encephalopathy).
• *Gait dyspraxia:* More common in the elderly; seen with bilateral frontal lesions, lesions in the posterior temporal region, and hydrocephalus.

### Assessing higher mental function: a practical guide

Start by having a conversation with the patient, asking questions they need to phrase an answer to (ie not just yes/no) as this tests fluency and reception, understanding, and allows assessment of articulation. Eg How did you travel here today? I came by bus. Then assess dysphasia by asking: What is this eg pen (tests for nominal dysphasia), repeat British Constitution (tests for conduction dysphasia and dysarthria). Then ask patient to follow one, two and three step commands ensuring these 'cross the midline' eg make a fist with your right hand then extend your right index finger and touch your left ear.

### Problems with classifying dysphasias

The classical model of language comprehension occurring in Wernicke's area and language expression in Broca's area is too simple. Functional MRI studies show old ideas that processing of abstract words is confined to the left hemisphere whereas concrete words are processed on the right are too simplistic.[1] It may be better to think of a mosaic of language centres in the brain with more or less specialized functions. There is evidence that tool-naming is handled differently and in a different area to fruit-naming.[81] There are also individual differences in the anatomy of these mosaics.[82] This is depressing for those who want a rigid classification of aphasia, but a source of hope to those who have had a stroke: recovery may be better than neuroimaging leads us to believe.[83]

### Symptoms of movement disorders

**Athetosis** is due to a lesion in the putamen, causing slow sinuous writhing movements in the hands, which are present at rest. *Pseudoathetosis* refers to athetoid movements in patients with severe proprioceptive loss.

**Chorea** means *dance* (hence 'choreography')—a flow of jerky movements, flitting from one limb to another (each seemingly a fragment of a normal movement). Distinguish from athetosis/pseudoathetosis (above), and hemiballismus (p472). *Causes:* basal ganglia lesion (stroke, Huntington's, p716); streptococci (Sydenham's chorea; St Vitus' dance, p136); SLE (p556); Wilson's (p269); neonatal kernicterus; polycythaemia (p360); neuroacanthocytosis (genetic, with acanthocytes in peripheral blood, chorea, oro-facial dyskinesia, and axonal neuropathy); hyperthyroidism (p210); drugs (levodopa, oral contraceptives/HRT, chlorpromazine, cocaine—'*crack dancing*'). The early stages of chorea may be detected by feeling fluctuations in muscle tension while the patient grips your finger. ℞: Dopamine antagonists, eg tetrabenazine 12.5mg/12h (/24h if elderly) PO; increase, eg to 25mg/8h PO; max 200mg/d.

**Hemiballismus** is uncontrolled unilateral flailing movements of proximal limb joints caused by contralateral subthalamic lesions. See p472.

### Cerebellar signs

- *Speech:* Slurred/ataxic/staccato
- *Eye movements:* Nystagmus
- *Tone and power:* Hypotonia and reduced power
- *Coordination:* Finger-to-nose test; test for dysdiadochokinesis, p503
- *Gait:* Broad based, patients fall to the side of the lesion. Romberg's test: ask patient to stand with eyes closed. If he loses balance, the test is positive and a sign of posterior column disease. Cerebellar disease is Romberg negative.

(Remember **DASHING**: **D**ysdiadochokinesis, **A**taxia, **S**lurred speech, **H**ypotonia and reduced power, **I**ntention tremor, **N**ystagmus, broad based **G**ait).

---

**1** While abstract words activate a sub-region of the left inferior frontal gyrus more strongly than concrete words, specific activity for concrete words can also be observed in the left basal temporal cortex.

Introduce yourself, ask a few factual questions (precise name, age, job, and who is at home). These may help your patient to relax, but be careful that you do not touch on a nerve, eg if job recently lost, marriage recently ended so living alone.

**Presenting problem** Ask for the main problems that have led to this consultation. Sit back and listen. Don't worry whether the information is in a convenient form or not—this is an opportunity for the patient to come out with worries, ideas, and preoccupations unsullied by your expectations. After >3-5min it is often good to aim to have a list of all the problems (each sketched only briefly). Read them back to the patient and ask if there are any more. Then ask about:

**History of presenting problem** For each problem obtain details, both current state and history of onset, precipitating factors, and effects on life.

**Check of major psychiatric symptoms** Check those that have not yet been covered: depression—low mood, anhedonia (inability to feel pleasure), thoughts of worthlessness/hopelessness, sleep disturbance with early morning waking, loss of weight and appetite. Ask specifically about suicidal thoughts and plans: "Have you ever been so low that you thought of harming yourself?", "What thoughts have you had?" Hallucinations ("Have you ever heard voices or seen things when there hasn't been anyone or anything there?") and delusions ("Have you ever had any thoughts or beliefs that have struck you afterwards as bizarre?"); anxiety and avoidance behaviour (eg avoiding shopping because of anxiety or phobias); obsessional thoughts and compulsive behaviour, eating disorders, alcohol (see p283 for alcohol screening tests) and other drugs.

**Present circumstances** Housing, finance, work, relationships, friends.

**Family history** Ask about health, personality, and occupation of parents and siblings, and the family's medical and psychiatric history.

**Background history** Try to understand the context of the presenting problem.
• *Biography:* relationships with family and peers as a child; school and work record; sexual relationships and current relationships; and family. Previous ways of dealing with stress and whether there have been problems and symptoms similar to the presenting ones.
• *Premorbid personality:* mood, character, hobbies, attitudes, and beliefs.

**Past medical and psychiatric history**

**Mental state examination** This is the state now, at the time of interview.
• *Appearance:* Clothing, glasses, headwear? Unkempt/normal/meticulous?
• *Observable behaviour:* Eg excessive slowness, signs of anxiety, gesture, gaze or avoiding gaze, tears, laughter, pauses (while listening to voices?), attitude (eg withdrawn).
• *Mode of speech:* Include the rate of speech, eg retarded or gabbling (pressure of speech). Note its content. Flight of ideas? Knight's move thinking? (See BOX)
• *Mood:* Note thoughts about harming self or others. Gauge your own responses to the patient. The laughter and grand ideas of manic patients are contagious, as to a lesser extent is the expression of thoughts from a depressed person.
• *Beliefs:* Eg about himself, his own body, about other people, and the future. Note abnormal beliefs (delusions), eg that thoughts are overheard, and abnormal ideas (eg persecutory, grandiose).
• *Unusual experiences or hallucinations:* Note modality, eg visual, auditory.
• *Orientation:* In time, place, and person. What is the date? What time of day is it? Where are you? What is your name?
• *Short-term memory:* Give a name and address and test recall after 5min. Make sure that he has got the address clear in his head before waiting the 5min.
• *Long-term memory:* Current affairs recall. Name of current political leaders (p70 & p85). This tests many other CNS functions, not just memory.
• *Concentration:* Months of the year backwards.
• Note the degree of your *rapport* and the patient's *insight* into his current state.

There are many different ways to think about psychiatric symptoms. One simple approach can be to consider negative and positive symptoms. *Negative symptoms* involve the absence of a behaviour, thought, feeling or sensation (eg lack of appetite, apathy, and blunted emotions in depression), whereas *positive symptoms* involve their presence when not normally expected (eg thought insertion, ie "Someone is putting thoughts into my head"). Understanding the difference between psychosis and neurosis is vital. *Psychosis* entails a thought disorder (eg thought insertion, thought broadcasting) ± delusions (abnormal beliefs which are held to despite all reasoning, and which run counter to the patient's cultural background) and abnormal perceptions (eg hallucinations). *Neurosis* entails insight—if there are intrusive ideas or odd experiential phenomena, the person knows that they are false or illusory (and may be triggered by stress, etc.).

Interesting abnormalities of speech include *flight of ideas*, in which the speech races through themes, switching whimsically or through associations, eg 'clang' association: "Yesterday I went down to the local shop. I didn't hop (*clang*), but I walked. Kangaroos hop, don't they? My friend Joey wasn't there, though ...". *Knight's move* is an unexpected change in the direction of speech or conversation (akin to the lateral component of the move of the knight's piece in chess) and *neologism* is the formation of new words. They may be normal or indicate an organic brain condition or a psychosis.

Many psychiatric symptoms in isolation, to a lesser degree of severity, or even in a different culture, may well be considered part of 'normal' behaviour. For example, a vision from a religious figure may be considered normal, whereas one from an alien may not. Consider your patient in their cultural and religious context. As with so many aspects of medicine, in psychiatry there is a vast spectrum of behaviour, thought and perception, at least one extreme of which is considered to be 'abnormal'. It is in part our challenge to attempt to interpret these symptoms with relevance, insight and impartiality so that we may best benefit our patients and not form opinions that are set in stone. On acute medical wards psychiatric symptoms are often due to stress, drug or alcohol withdrawal, U&E imbalance, or medication. When in doubt, ask a psychiatrist to help.

▶Beware of simplistic formulations, eg *If you talk to God, you are praying. If God talks to you, you have schizophrenia* (Dr Thomas Szasz). It is not the auditory phenomenon that makes the diagnosis of psychosis: what matters is what the patient believes about the phenomenon, and whether they are associated with a thought disorder or a delusion.

1 Look at the patient. Healthy, unwell, or *in extremis*? This vital skill improves with practice. ▶Beware those who are sicker than they look, eg cardiogenic shock; cord compression; non-accidental injury.

2 Pulse, BP, O₂ sats, T°.

3 Examine nails, hands, conjunctivae (anaemia), and sclerae (jaundice). Consider: Paget's, acromegaly, endocrine disease (thyroid, pituitary, or adrenal hypo- or hyper-function), body hair, abnormal pigmentation, skin.

4 Examine mouth and tongue (cyanosed; smooth; furred; beefy, eg rhomboid area denuded of papillae by *Candida*, after prolonged steroid inhaler use).

5 Examine the neck from behind: lymph nodes, goitre.

6 Make sure the patient is at 45° to begin cvs examination in the neck: JVP; feel for character and volume of carotid pulse.

7 The praecordium. Look for abnormal pulsations. Feel the apex beat (character; position). Any parasternal heave or thrill? Auscultate (bell and diaphragm) apex in the left lateral position, then the other 3 areas (p39) and carotids. Sit the patient forward: listen during expiration.

8 Whilst sitting forward, look for sacral oedema.

9 Begin the respiratory examination with the patient at 90°. Observe (and count) respirations; note posterior chest wall movement. Assess expansion, then percuss and auscultate the chest.

10 Sit the patient back. Feel the trachea. Inspect again. Assess expansion of the anterior chest. Percuss and auscultate again.

11 Examine axillae and breasts, if indicated (+chaperone for *all* intimate examinations).

12 Lie patient flat (1 pillow) to inspect, palpate, percuss, and auscultate abdomen.

13 Look at the legs: any swellings, perfusion, pulses, or oedema?

14 cns exam: *Cranial nerves:* pupil responses; fundi; visual fields; visual acuity. Consider corneal reflexes. "Open your mouth; stick your tongue out; screw up your eyes; show me your teeth; raise your eyebrows." *Limbs (most signs are due to central not peripheral nerve lesions):* Look for wasting and fasciculation. Test tone in all limbs. "Hold your hands out with your palms towards the ceiling and fingers wide. Now shut your eyes." Watch for pronator drift. "Keep your eyes shut and touch your nose with each index finger." "Lift your leg straight in the air. Keep it there. Put your heel on the opposite knee (eyes shut) and run it up your own shin." You have now tested power, coordination, and joint position sense. Tuning fork on toes and index fingers to assess vibration sense.

15 Examine gait and speech. Any abnormalities of higher mental function to pursue?

16 Consider rectal and vaginal examination.

17 Examine the urine with dipstick if appropriate (p383).

▶In general, go into detail where you find (or suspect) something to be wrong.

So now we have a template for the all-important history and examination, but it is no more than a rough guide, you must flesh it out with your own learning. We start out nervous of missing some question or sign, but what we should really be nervous about is losing our humanity in the hurly-burly of a time-pressed interview. Here is how one student put some flesh on the bones—for a man in a wheelchair: she asked all about the presenting complaint, and how it fitted in with his cns condition and life at home—and then found out that his daughter had had a nervous breakdown at the start of his illness, 5 years ago. "How is she now?" she asked "Fine—I've got two lovely grandchildren...Jim is just learning to walk..." "Oh...you must be so *busy!*" the student said with a joyful smile. This man had not been busy for 5 years, and was fed up with his passive dependency. The thought of being busy again made his face light up—and when the student left he rose up out of his wheelchair to shake her by the hand, a movement we doctors thought was impossible. Jim and his grandfather were learning to walk, but this student was up and running—far ahead of her teachers.

Please write your full name [2]

Today is ...................day [1]

Today's date is the:
...... of ...... (month) 20... [3]

How old are you? ......... years [1]

On what date were you born?
........../......... (month) / 19... [3]

Please copy the following sentence [2]

**Good citizens always wear stout shoes**

Please read the sentence again and try to remember it.

Who is the Prime Minister? [2]

What year did the 1st World War start? [1]
... ... ...

Sums [4]
20 − 4 = ...... 8 × 6 = ........
16 + 17 = ...... 5 + 15 − 17 = ........

Please list 4 creatures
beginning with 'S'
(eg Shark)[4]
1. S....................
2. S....................
3. S....................
4. S....................

Why is a carrot like a potato? [2]

Why is a lion like a wolf? [2]

Remember:
Good citizens always wear stout shoes

Please name these items: [5]

Please join the circles together to form a letter. [3]

Please draw in a clock face, put in the numbers 1 – 12, and put the hands at 9:20. [4]

Without turning the page, please write down the sentence you copied earlier. [5]

For the TYM tester: help given? [5]
None[5]/trial[4]/minor[3]/moderate[2]/major[1]

max score 50

©Dr Jeremy Brown. *BMJ* 2009;338:b2030

www.bmj.com/cgi/data/bmj.b2030/dc1/1

( †fold here )

In one preliminary study,[1] the controls' average score was 47/50. Those with Alzheimer's disease (AD) scored an average of 33/50. The TYM score correlates highly with other standard tests, but, uniquely, it is quick and can be self-administered. A score of <42/50 had a sensitivity of 93% and specificity of 86% for AD. TYM is more sensitive at detecting AD than the mini-mental exam (MMSE), detecting 93% of patients compared with 52% for MMSE. Negative and positive predictive values (p674) of TYM with a cut-off of 42 were 99% and 42% (if prevalence of AD is 10%). If non-Alzheimer dementia, score was 39/50 (mean). This new test should not *make* any diagnosis—but it may suggest when further referral might help.

*Animals beginning with 'S':* 'Shark' and mythical creatures not allowed. *Carrot/potato:* Reasonable but less precise answer than "...vegetables...", eg "food", scores 1 point. 2 such statements score 2, eg "grows in ground...fierce" or "...food...4 legs..." scores 2 in total. *Jacket-naming:* Answers are collar, lapel, tie, pocket, button. 1 point each. Shirt is acceptable for item 1; jacket or blazer is OK for 2 or 4 (but not both). *Circles task:* 1 point if all circles joined even if not a letter W. *Clockface:* All numbers OK 1; correct number position 1; correct hands 1. *Sentence:* 1 point for each word remembered up to a maximum of 5.

1 TYM for detection of Alzheimer's disease: cross sectional study. Brown J, Dawson K, Pengas G 2009 *BMJ* 338 1426.

## Contents

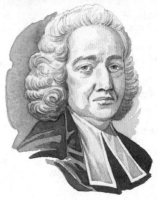

Fig 1. Stephen Hales (1677-1761) A clergyman and scientist, most famous for his work on the circulation of plants and animals, and campaigned against the gin trade. In 1733 he was the first person to measure blood pressure, by inserting a brass cannula attached to a long glass tube into the carotid artery of a horse, and noting that the blood rose up the tube to a height of 8 feet 3 inches (186mmHg). He later repeated the experiment in a range of animals, and roughly estimated the pressure in man. However, it took until the early 20th Century before a simple non-invasive method was introduced for measuring blood pressure—the mercury sphygmomanometer; and even longer before the importance of elevated blood pressure was recognized.

*Other relevant pages:* Emergencies: MI (p808); pulmonary oedema (p812); cardiac shock (p814); broad & narrow complex tachycardias (p816 & p818); *cardiac arrest:* see inside back cover. CVS examination (p38); carotid bruit (p38); cyanosis (p28); dyspnoea (p49); haemoptysis (p49); oedema (p29); palpitations (p35); aneurysms (p656); dyslipidaemia (p704); risk factor analysis (p664); nuclear cardiology[et al] (p754).

*We thank Dr Anna Kydd, our Specialist Reader, and Dr Mark Cassar, our Junior Reader, for their contribution to this chapter.*

## Cardiovascular health

Ischaemic heart disease (IHD) is the most common cause of death worldwide. Encouraging cardiovascular health is not *only* about preventing IHD: health entails the ability to *exercise*, and enjoying vigorous activity (within reason!) is one of the best ways of achieving health, not just because the heart likes it (BP↓, 'good' high-density lipoprotein, HDL↑)—it can prevent osteoporosis, improve glucose tolerance, and augment immune function (eg in cancer and if HIV+ve). People who improve *and maintain* their fitness live longer: ▶age-adjusted mortality from all causes is reduced by >40%. Avoiding obesity helps too, but weight loss *per se* is only useful in reducing cardiovascular risk and the risk of developing diabetes when combined with regular exercise. Moderate alcohol drinking may also promote cardiovascular health.

Smoking is the chief risk factor for cardiovascular mortality. You can help people give up, and giving up does undo much of the harm of smoking. *Simple advice works.* Most smokers want to give up (unlike eaters of unhealthy diets who are mostly wedded to them by habit and the pleasures of the palate). Just because smoking advice does *not always* work, do not stop giving it. Ask about smoking in consultations—especially those concerned with smoking-related diseases.
• Ensure advice is congruent with the patient's beliefs about smoking.
• Getting patients to enumerate the advantages of giving up increases motivation.
• Invite the patient to choose a date (when there will be few stresses) on which he or she will become a non-smoker.
• Suggest throwing away all accessories (cigarettes, pipes, ash trays, lighters, matches) in advance; inform friends of the new change; practise saying 'no' to their offers of 'just one little cigarette'.
• *Nicotine gum*, chewed intermittently to limit nicotine release: ≥ ten 2mg sticks may be needed/day. *Transdermal nicotine patches* may be easier. A dose increase at 1wk can help. Written advice offers no added benefit to advice from nurses. Always offer follow-up.
• *Varenicline* is an oral selective nicotine receptor partial agonist. Start 1wk before target stop date: initially 0.5mg/24h PO for 3 days, then 0.5mg/12h for 4 days, then 1mg/12h for 11wks (↓ to 0.5mg/12h if not tolerated). *SEs*: appetite change; dry mouth; taste disturbance; headache; drowsiness; dizziness; sleep disorders; abnormal dreams; depression; suicidal thoughts; panic; dysarthria.
• *Bupropion* (=*amfebutamone*, p455) is said to ↑ quit rate to 30% at 1yr *vs* 16% with patches and 15.6% for placebo (patches + bupropion: 35.5%):[1] consider if the above fails. Dose: 150mg/24h PO (while still smoking; quit within 2wks); dose may be twice daily from day 7; stop after 7–9wks. *Warn of SEs*: Seizures (risk <1:1000), insomnia, headache.

Lipids and BP (p704 & p132) are the other major *modifiable* risk factors. To calculate how risk factors interact, see risk equation, p664—and its caveats. NICE recommends a Framingham score with risk multiplied by 1.4 for South Asian men, but this doesn't cater for: • Asian diversity (eg multiply by 1.7 in Bangladeshi men) • Asian women • Deprivation effects • Double-counting problems if adjustment is made for ethnicity *and* family history. QRISK2 is better in UK patients.[2]

▶Apply preventive measures such as healthy eating (p236) *early* in life to maximize impact, when there are most years to save, and before bad habits get ingrained.

## The randomized trial

Cardiovascular medicine has an unrivalled treasure house of randomized trials. One of the chief pleasures of cardiovascular medicine lies in integrating these with clinical reasoning in a humane way. After a cardiac event, a protocol may 'mandate' statins, aspirin, β-blockers, ACE-i (p109), and a target BP and LDL cholesterol that makes your patient feel dreadful. What to do? Inform, negotiate, and compromise. Never reject your patient because of lack of compliance with your over-exacting regimens. Keep smiling, keep communicating, and keep up-to-date: the latest data may show that your patient was right all along.[3]

Cardiovascular medicine

**Chest pain** ►Cardiac-sounding chest pain may have no serious cause, but always think *"Could this be a myocardial infarction (MI), dissecting aortic aneurysm, pericarditis, or pulmonary embolism?"*

*Character: Constricting* suggests angina, oesophageal spasm, or anxiety; a *sharp* pain may be from the pleura or pericardium. A prolonged (>½h), dull, central crushing pain or pressure suggests MI.

*Radiation:* To shoulder, either or both arms, or neck/jaw suggests cardiac ischaemia. The pain of aortic dissection (p656) is classically instantaneous, tearing, and interscapular, but may be retrosternal. Epigastric pain may be cardiac.

*Precipitants:* Pain associated with cold, exercise, palpitations, or emotion suggests cardiac pain or anxiety; if brought on by food, lying flat, hot drinks, or alcohol, consider oesophageal spasm/disease (but meals *can* cause angina).

*Relieving factors:* If pain is relieved *within minutes* by rest or glyceryl trinitrate (GTN), suspect angina (GTN relieves oesophageal spasm more slowly). If antacids help, suspect GI causes. Pericarditic pain improves on leaning forward.

*Associations:* Dyspnoea occurs with cardiac pain, pulmonary emboli, pleurisy, or anxiety. MI may cause nausea, vomiting, or sweating. Angina is caused by coronary artery disease—and also by aortic stenosis, hypertrophic cardiomyopathy (HCM), paroxysmal supraventricular tachycardia (SVT)—and can be exacerbated by anaemia. Chest pain with *tenderness* suggests self-limiting Tietze's syndrome.[1]

*Pleuritic pain* (ie exacerbated by inspiration) implies inflammation of the pleura from pulmonary infection, inflammation, or infarction. It causes us to 'catch our breath'. ΔΔ: Musculoskeletal pain;[1] fractured rib (pain on respiration, exacerbated by gentle pressure on the sternum); subdiaphragmatic pathology (eg gallstones).

*Acutely ill patients:* •Admit to hospital •Check pulse, BP in both arms ►►(unequal in aortic dissection p656), JVP, heart sounds; examine legs for DVT •Give O₂ by mask •IV line •Relieve pain (eg morphine 5-10mg IV slowly (2mg/min) + an antiemetic) •Cardiac monitor •12-lead ECG •CXR •Arterial blood gas (ABG). *Famous traps:* Aortic dissection; zoster (p400); ruptured oesophagus; cardiac tamponade (shock with JVP↑); opiate addiction.

**Dyspnoea** may be from LVF, pulmonary embolism, any respiratory cause, or anxiety. *Severity:* ►►Emergency presentations: p796. Ask about shortness of breath at rest or on exertion, exercise tolerance, and in daily tasks. Is it episodic and triggered by lying flat (PND, p49)? *Associations:* Specific symptoms associated with heart failure are orthopnoea (ask about number of pillows used at night), paroxysmal nocturnal dyspnoea (waking up at night gasping for breath), and peripheral oedema. Pulmonary embolism is associated with acute onset of dyspnoea and pleuritic chest pain; ask about risk factors for DVT.

**Palpitation(s)** may be due to ectopics, AF, SVT and ventricular tachycardia (VT), thyrotoxicosis, anxiety, and rarely phaeochromocytoma. See p35. *History:* Ask about previous episodes, precipitating/relieving factors, duration of symptoms, associated chest pain, dyspnoea, or dizziness. *Did the patient check his pulse?*

**Syncope** may reflect cardiac or CNS events. Vasovagal 'faints' are common (pulse↓, pupils dilated). The history from an observer is invaluable in diagnosis. *Prodromal symptoms:* Chest pain, palpitations, or dyspnoea point to a cardiac cause, eg arrhythmia. Aura, headache, dysarthria, and limb weakness indicate CNS causes. *During the episode:* Was there a pulse? Limb jerking, tongue biting, or urinary incontinence? NB: hypoxia from lack of cerebral perfusion may cause seizures. *Recovery:* Was this rapid (arrhythmia) or prolonged, with drowsiness (seizure)?

---

1 25% of non-cardiac chest pain is **musculoskeletal**: look for pain on specific postures or activity. Aim to reproduce the pain by movement and, sometimes, palpation over the structure causing it.[1] Focal injection of local anaesthetic helps diagnostically and is therapeutic.[1] **Tietze's syndrome**: self-limiting costochondritis ± costosternal joint swelling. Causes: idiopathic; microtrauma; infection; psoriatic/rheumatoid arthritis. ℞: NSAIDs or steroid injections.[1] Tenderness is also caused by: fibrositis, lymphoma, chondrosarcoma, myeloma, metastases, rib TB.[1] Imaging: bone scintigraphy;[1] CT.[1]

## ☼ How patients communicate ischaemic cardiac sensations

On emergency wards we are always hearing questions such as "Is your pain sharp or dull?", followed by an equivocal answer. The doctor goes on "Sharp like a knife— or dull and crushing?" The doctor is getting irritated because the patient must know the answer but is not saying it. A true story paves the way to being less inquisitorial and having a more creative understanding of the nature of symptoms. A patient came to one of us (JML) saying "Last night I dreamed I had a pain in my chest. Now I've woken up, and I'm not sure—have I got chest pain, doctor? What do you think?" How odd it is to find oneself examining a patient to exclude a symptom, not a disease. (It turned out that she *did* have serious chest pathology.) Odd, until one realizes that symptoms are often half-formed, and it is our role to give them a local habitation and a name. Dialogue can transform a symptom from 'airy nothingness' to a fact.[1] Patients often avoid using the word 'pain' to describe ischaemia: 'wind', 'tightening', 'pressure', 'burning', or 'a lump in the throat' (angina means to choke) may be used. He may say "sharp" to communicate severity, and not character. So be as vague in your questioning as your patient is in his answers. "Tell me some more about what you are feeling (long pause) ... as if someone was doing *what* to you?" "Sitting on me" or "like a hotness" might be the response (suggesting cardiac ischaemia). Do not ask "Does it go into your left arm". Try "Is there anything else about it?" (pause) ... "Does it go anywhere?" Note down your patient's exact words.

Note also non-verbal clues: the clenched fist placed over the sternum is a telling feature of cardiac pain (Levine-sign positive).

A good history, taking account of these features, is the best way to stratify patients likely to have cardiac pain. If the history is non-specific, and there are no risk factors for cardiovascular diseases, and ECG and plasma troponin T (p112) are normal (<0.2μg/L) 6-12h after the onset of pain, discharge will probably be OK.[10] When in doubt, get help. Features making cardiac pain unlikely:

- Stabbing, shooting pain.
- Pain lasting <30s, however intense.
- Well-localized, left sub-mammary pain ("In my heart, doctor").
- Pains of continually varying location.
- Youth.

Do not feel that you must diagnose every pain. *Chest pain with no cause* is common, even after extensive tests. Do not reject these patients: explain your findings to them. Some have a 'chronic pain syndrome' which responds to a tricyclic, eg imipramine 50mg at night (this dose does not imply any depression). It is similar to post-herpetic neuralgia.

---

1 Dialogue-transformed symptoms explain one of the junior doctor's main vexations: when patients re-tell symptoms to a consultant in the light of day, they bear no resemblance to what you originally heard. But do not be vexed: your dialogue may have helped the patient far more than any ward round.

▶First confirm the patient's name and age, and the ECG date. Then (see fig 1):

• *Rate:* At usual speed (25mm/s) each 'big square' is 0.2s; each 'small square' is 0.04s. To calculate the rate, divide 300 by the number of big squares per R-R interval (p91).

• *Rhythm:* If cycles are not clearly regular, use the 'card method': lay a card along ECG, marking positions of 3 successive R waves. Slide the card to and fro to check that all intervals are equal. If not, note if: slight but regular lengthening and then shortening (with respiration)—*sinus arrhythmia* common in the young; are different rates multiples of each other—*varying block*; or is it 100% irregular—*atrial fibrillation* (AF) or *ventricular fibrillation* (VF)? *Sinus rhythm* is characterized by a P wave (upright in II, III, & aVF; inverted in aVR) followed by a QRS complex. AF has no discernible P waves and QRS complexes are irregularly irregular. *Atrial flutter* (p125, fig 1 p119) has a 'sawtooth' baseline of atrial depolarization (~300/min) and regular QRS complexes. *Nodal rhythm* has a normal QRS complex but P waves are absent or occur just before or within QRS complexes. *Ventricular rhythm* has QRS complexes >0.12s with P waves following them (ECG 6, p100).

• *Axis:* The mean frontal axis is the sum of all the ventricular forces during ventricular depolarization. The axis lies at 90° to the isoelectric complex (ie the one in which positive and negative deflections are equal). See BOX 2. *Normal axis* is between -30° and +90°. As a simple rule of thumb, if the complexes in leads I and II are both 'positive', the axis is normal. *Left axis deviation* (LAD) is -30° to -90°. Causes: LVH, left anterior hemiblock, inferior MI, VT from LV focus, Wolff-Parkinson-White (WPW) syndrome (some types). *Right axis deviation* (RAD) is +90° to +180°. Causes: RVH, PE, anterolateral MI, left posterior hemiblock (rare), WPW syndrome (some types). See BOX 3.

• *P wave:* Normally precedes each QRS complex, and upright in II, III, & aVF but inverted in aVR. *Absent P wave:* AF, sinoatrial block, junctional (AV nodal) rhythm. Dissociation between P waves and QRS complexes indicates complete heart block. *P mitrale:* bifid P wave, indicates left atrial hypertrophy. *P pulmonale:* peaked P wave, indicates right atrial hypertrophy. Pseudo-P-pulmonale seen if K⁺↓.

• *PR interval:* Measure from start of P wave to start of QRS. *Normal range:* 0.12-0.2s (3-5 small squares). A *prolonged PR interval* implies delayed AV conduction (1st degree heart block). A *short PR interval* implies unusually fast AV conduction down an accessory pathway, eg WPW p120 (see fig 1, p125).

• *QRS complex:* *Normal duration:* <0.12s. If ≥0.12s this suggests ventricular conduction defects, eg a bundle branch block (p94 & p119). Large QRS complexes suggest *ventricular hypertrophy* (p94). *Normal Q wave* <0.04s wide and <2mm deep. They are often seen in leads $V_5$ and $V_6$, aVL and I, and reflect normal septal depolarization, which usually occurs from left to right. *Pathological Q waves* may occur within a few hours of an acute MI.

• *QT interval:* Measure from start of QRS to *end* of T wave. It varies with rate. Calculate *corrected QT interval* (QTᶜ) by dividing the measured QT interval by the square root of the cycle length, ie QTᶜ=QT/√RR. Normal QTᶜ: 0.38-0.42s. *Prolonged QT interval:* acute myocardial ischaemia, myocarditis, bradycardia (eg AV block), head injury, hypothermia, U&E imbalance (K⁺↓, Ca²⁺↓, Mg²⁺↓), congenital (Romano–Ward and Jervell-Lange-Nielson syndromes, p724); sotalol, quinidine, antihistamines, macrolides (eg erythromycin), amiodarone, phenothiazines, tricyclics.

• *ST segment:* Usually isoelectric. Planar elevation (>1mm) or depression (>0.5mm) usually implies infarction (p113, ECGs 3&4, p97-8) or ischaemia (p103), respectively.

• *T wave:* Normally inverted in aVR, $V_1$ and occasionally $V_2$. Abnormal if inverted in I, II, and $V_4$-$V_6$. Peaked in hyperkalaemia (ECG 9, p689) and flattened in hypokalaemia.

• *J wave* see p861. Seen in hypothermia, subarachnoid haemorrhage and hypercalcaemia.

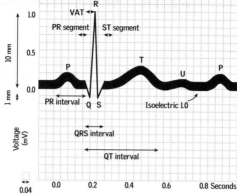

Fig 1. Schematic diagram of a normal ECG trace.

## Calculating the R-R interval

To calculate the rate, divide 300 by the number of big squares per R-R interval—if the UK standard ECG speed of 25mm/s is used (elsewhere, 50mm/s may be used: don't be confused!)

| R-R duration (s) | Big squares | Rate (per min) |
|---|---|---|
| 0.2 | 1 | 300 |
| 0.4 | 2 | 150 |
| 0.6 | 3 | 100 |
| 0.8 | 4 | 75 |
| 1.0 | 5 | 60 |
| 1.2 | 6 | 50 |
| 1.4 | 7 | 43 |

## Determining the ECG axis (fig 2)

- The axis lies at 90° to the isoelectric complex (the one in which positive and negative deflections are equal in size).
- If the complexes in I and II are both predominantly positive, the axis is normal.

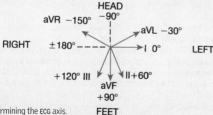

Fig 2. Determining the ECG axis.

| Causes of LAD (left axis deviation) | Causes of RAD (right axis deviation) |
|---|---|
| Left anterior hemiblock | RVH |
| Inferior MI | Pulmonary embolism |
| VT from LV focus | Anterolateral MI |
| WPW syndrome p120 | WPW syndrome |
| LVH | Left posterior hemiblock (rare) |

Cardiovascular medicine

*Sinus tachycardia:* Rate >100. Causes: Anaemia, anxiety, exercise, pain, ↑T°, sepsis, hypovolaemia, heart failure, pulmonary embolism, pregnancy, thyrotoxicosis, beri beri, $CO_2$ retention, autonomic neuropathy, sympathomimetics, eg caffeine, adrenaline, and nicotine (may produce abrupt changes in sinus rate, or other arrhythmias).

*Sinus bradycardia:* Rate <60. Causes: Physical fitness, vasovagal attacks, sick sinus syndrome, acute MI (esp. inferior), drugs (β-blockers, digoxin, amiodarone, verapamil), hypothyroidism, hypothermia, ↑intracranial pressure, cholestasis. See p116

*AF:* (ECG p119) *Common causes:* IHD, thyrotoxicosis, hypertension. See p124.

*1ˢᵗ and 2ⁿᵈ degree (Mobitz I/II) heart block:* Causes: Normal variant, athletes, sick sinus syndrome, IHD, acute myocarditis, drugs (digoxin, β-blockers). ECGs p119.

*3ʳᵈ degree AV (complete heart) block:* Causes: IHD, idiopathic (fibrosis), congenital, aortic valve calcification, cardiac surgery/trauma, digoxin toxicity, infiltration (abscesses, granulomas, tumours, parasites). ECG 5, p99.

*Q waves:* Pathological Q waves are usually >0.04s wide and >2mm deep. Usually as sign of infarction, and may occur within a few hours of an acute MI. Non-pathological Q waves may occur in V5 and V6, aVL and I.

*ST elevation:* Normal variant (high take-off), acute MI, Prinzmetal's angina (p722), acute pericarditis (saddle-shaped), left ventricular aneurysm.

*ST depression:* Normal variant (upward sloping), digoxin (downward sloping), ischaemic (horizontal): angina, acute posterior MI.

*T inversion:* In $V_1-V_3$: normal (black patients and children), right bundle branch block (RBBB), pulmonary embolism. In $V_2-V_5$: subendocardial MI, HCM, subarachnoid haemorrhage, lithium. In $V_4-V_6$ and aVL: ischaemia, LVH, associated with left bundle branch block (LBBB).

NB: ST and T wave changes are often non-specific, and must be interpreted in the light of the clinical context.

*Myocardial infarction:* (fig 1, p113)
• Within hours, the T wave may become peaked and ST segments may begin to rise.
• Within 24h, the T wave inverts, as ST segment elevation begins to resolve. ST elevation rarely persists, unless a left ventricular aneurysm develops. T wave inversion may or may not persist.
• Within a few days, pathological Q waves begin to form. Q waves usually persist, but may resolve in 10% of patients.
• The leads affected reflect the site of the infarct: inferior (II, III, aVF), anteroseptal ($V_{1-4}$), anterolateral ($V_{4-6}$, I, aVL), posterior (tall R and ST↓ in $V_{1-2}$), and thus the occluded vessel: left anterior descending (anteroseptal), right coronary (inferior or right ventricular), circumflex (posterior, and, in 20%, inferior termed 'left dominance') .

▶'Non-Q wave infarcts' (formerly called subendocardial infarcts) have ST and T changes without Q waves.

*Pulmonary embolism:* Sinus tachycardia is commonest. There may be RAD, RBBB (p91), *right ventricular strain pattern* (R-axis deviation. Dominant R wave and T wave inversion/ST depression in V1 and V2. Leads II, III and aVF may show similar changes). Rarely, the 'SᵢQᵢᵢᵢTᵢᵢᵢ' pattern occurs: deep S waves in I, pathological Q waves in III, inverted T waves in III.

*Metabolic abnormalities: Digoxin effect:* ST depression and inverted T wave in $V_{5-6}$ ('reversed tick'). In digoxin toxicity, any arrhythmia may occur (ventricular ectopics and nodal bradycardia are common). Hyperkalaemia: tall, tented T wave, widened QRS, absent P waves, 'sine wave' appearance (ECG 9, p689). *Hypokalaemia:* Small T waves, prominent U waves. *Hypercalcaemia:* Short QT interval. *Hypocalcaemia:* long QT interval, small T waves.

**Where to place the chest leads** (See fig 1.)

Note $c_1 = v_1$ etc.

**V1:**  right sternal edge, 4th intercostal space
**V2:**  left sternal edge, 4th intercostal space
**V3:**  half-way between $v_2$ and $v_4$
**V4:**  5th intercostal space, mid-clavicular line;
all subsequent leads are in the same horizontal
plane as $v_4$
**V5:**  anterior axillary line
**V6:**  mid-axillary line ($v_7$: posterior axillary line)

Good skin preparation (clean with non-alcoholic
wipe, shave if hairy, etc.) will improve ECG quality. Finish 12-lead ECGs with a long rhythm strip
in lead II.

Fig 1. Placement of ECG leads.

**Disorders of ventricular conduction**

*Bundle branch block* (p95–6, ECGs 1 & 2) Delayed
conduction is evidenced by prolongation of QRS >0.12s. Abnormal conduction patterns lasting <0.12s are incomplete blocks. The area that would have been reached
by the blocked bundle depolarizes slowly and late. Taking $v_1$ as an example, right
ventricular depolarization is normally +ve and left ventricular depolarization is normally -ve.

In RBBB, the following pattern is seen: QRS >0.12s, 'RSR' pattern in $v_1$, dominant R in
$v_1$, inverted T waves in $v_1$–$v_3$ or $v_4$, deep wide S wave in $v_6$. Causes: normal variant
(isolated RBBB), pulmonary embolism, cor pulmonale.

In LBBB, the following pattern is seen: QRS >0.12s, 'M' pattern in $v_5$, no septal Q waves,
inverted T waves in I, aVL, $v_5$–$v_6$. Causes: IHD, hypertension, cardiomyopathy, idiopathic
fibrosis. ►NB: if there is LBBB, no comment can be made on the ST segment or T wave.

*Bifascicular block* is the combination of RBBB and left bundle hemiblock, manifest as
an axis deviation, eg LAD in the case of left anterior hemiblock.

*Trifascicular block* is the combination of bifascicular block and 1st degree heart
block. ►Is pacing required? (p126)

**Ventricular hypertrophy** There is no single marker of ventricular hypertrophy:
electrical axis, voltage, and ST wave changes should all be taken into consideration.
Relying on a single marker such as voltage may be unreliable as a thin chest wall may
result in large voltage whereas a thick chest wall may mask it.

Suspect *left ventricular hypertrophy* (LVH) if the R wave in $v_6$ is >25mm or the sum
of the S wave in $v_1$ and the R wave in $v_6$ is >35mm (ECG 8 on p135).

Suspect *right ventricular hypertrophy* (RVH) if dominant R wave in $v_1$, T wave inversion in $v_1$–$v_3$ or $v_4$, deep S wave in $v_6$, RAD.

Other causes of *dominant R wave in $v_1$*: RBBB, posterior MI, some types of WPW
syndrome (p120).

*Causes of low voltage QRS complex:* (QRS <5mm in all limb leads) Hypothyroidism,
chronic obstructive pulmonary disease (COPD), thaematocrit (intra-cardiac blood
resistivity is related to haematocrit), changes in chest wall impedance (eg in renal
failure, subcutaneous emphysema but *not* obesity), pulmonary embolism, bundle
branch block, carcinoid heart disease, myocarditis, cardiac amyloid, adriamycin
cardiotoxicity, and other heart muscle diseases, pericardial effusion, pericarditis.[11]

See http://homepages.enterprise.net/djenkins/ecghome.html for MRCP-ish examples of ECGs.

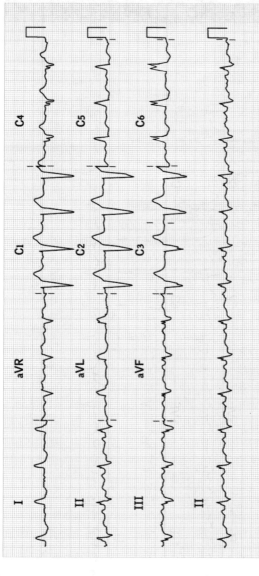

ECG 1—Left bundle branch block: note the W pattern in C1 (=v₁) and the M pattern in C6 (=v₆).

Cardiovascular medicine

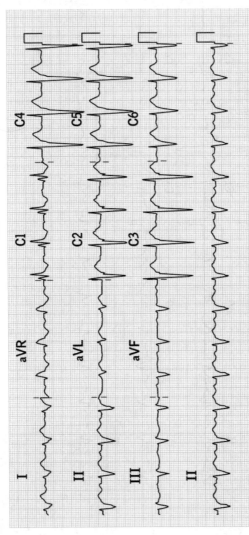

ECG 2—Right bundle branch block—M pattern in C1 and W pattern in C5.

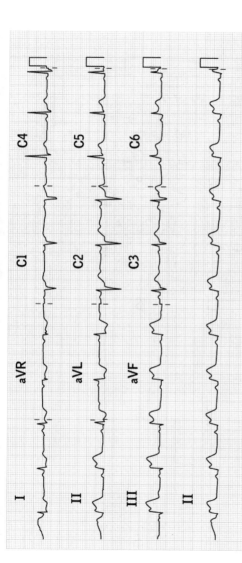

ECG 3—Acute infero-lateral myocardial infarction: marked ST elevation in the inferior leads (II, III, aVF), but also in C5 and C6, indicating lateral involvement as well. There is also 'reciprocal change', ie ST-segment depression in leads I and avL. The latter is often seen with a large myocardial infarction.

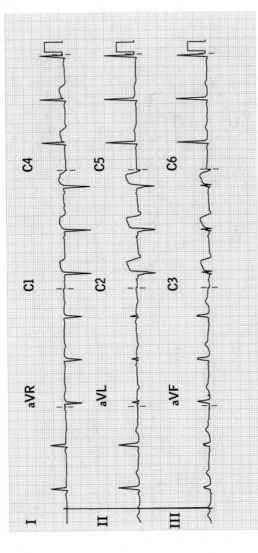

ECG 4 — Acute anterior myocardial infarction—ST-segment elevation and evolving Q waves in leads C1–C4.

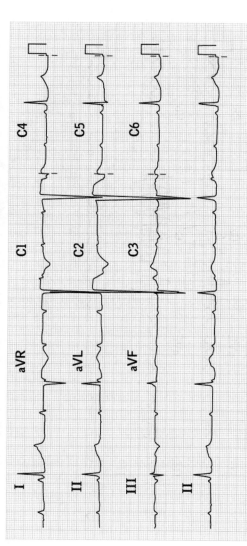

ECG 5—Complete heart block. Dissociation between the P waves and the QRS complexes. QRS complexes are relatively narrow, indicating that there is a ventricular rhythm originating from the conducting pathway.

Cardiovascular medicine

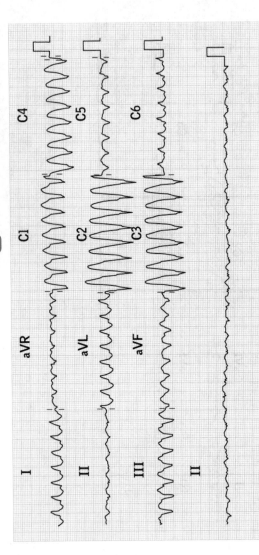

ECG 6—Ventricular tachycardia—regular broad complexes indicating a ventricular origin for the rhythm.

ECG 7—Dual chamber pacemaker. Pacing spikes occur before some of the P waves, and the QRS complexes.

Cardiovascular medicine

The patient undergoes a graduated, treadmill exercise test, with continuous 12-lead ECG (fig 1) and blood pressure monitoring. There are numerous treadmill protocols; the 'Bruce protocol' is the most widely used.

*Indications:*
• To help confirm a suspected diagnosis of IHD. NICE suggests that this should only be used when there is diagnostic uncertainty in people with known CAD (eg previous MI or angioplasty), and not to make a primary diagnosis.[12]
• Assessment of exercise-induced arrhythmias.

*Contraindications:*
• Recent Q wave MI (<5 days ago) or unstable angina
• Severea aortic stenosis
• Uncontrolled arrhythmia, hypertension, or heart failure
• Acute myocarditis or pericarditis
• Acute aortic dissection, acute pulmonary embolism

Be cautious about arranging tests that will be hard to perform or interpret:
• Complete heart block, LBBB
• Pacemaker patients, digoxin use
• Osteoarthritis, COPD, stroke, or other limitations to exercise

*Stop the test if:*
• Chest pain, dyspnoea, cyanosis or pallor occurs.
• The patient feels faint, exhausted, or is in danger of falling.
• ST↑ >1mm in leads without diagnostic Q waves (with or without chest pain).
• Atrial or ventricular arrhythmia (not just ectopics).
• Fall in blood pressure >10mmHg from baseline, failure of heart rate or blood pressure to rise with effort, SBP >230mmHg and/or DBP >115mmHg.
• Development of AV block or LBBB.
• 90% maximal heart rate for age is achieved: [(220−age) ±10].

*Interpreting the test:* A positive test only allows one to assess the *probability* that the patient has IHD. 75% of people with significant coronary artery disease have a positive test, but so do 5% of people with normal arteries (the false-positive rate is even higher in middle-aged women, eg 20%). The more positive the result, the higher the predictive accuracy. Down-sloping ST depression is much more significant than up-sloping, eg 1mm J-point depression with down-sloping ST segment is 99% predictive of 2-3 vessel disease.

*Morbidity:* 24 in 100,000. *Mortality:* 10 in 100,000.

## Ambulatory ECG monitoring (eg Holter monitor)

Continuous ECG monitoring for 24h may be used to try to pick up paroxysmal arrhythmias. However, >70% of patients will not have symptoms during the period of monitoring. ~20% will have a normal ECG during symptoms and only up to 10% will have an arrhythmia coinciding with symptoms. Give these patients a recorder they can activate themselves during an episode. Recorders may be programmed to detect ST segment depression, either symptomatic (to prove angina) or to reveal 'silent' ischaemia (predictive of re-infarction or death soon after MI).

'Loop' recorders record only when activated by the patient—they cleverly save a small amount of ECG data *before* the event—useful if the arrhythmia causes loss of consciousness: the patient can press the button when they wake up. They are more expensive but also more cost-effective than Holter monitors, as the pick-up rate of significant disease is higher.[13] These may also be implanted just under the skin (eg Reveal Device), and are especially useful in patients with infrequent episodes.

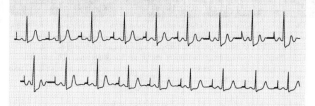

Each complex is taken from sample ECGs (lead C5) recorded at 1min intervals during exercise (top line) and recovery (bottom line). At maximum ST depression, the ST segment is almost horizontal. This is a positive exercise test.

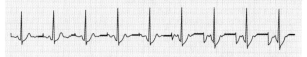

This is an exercise ECG in the same format. It is negative because although the J point is depressed, the ensuing ST segment is steeply up-sloping.

**Fig 1.** Exercise ECG testing. The J-point is the point at which the QRS complex meets the ST segment.

This involves the insertion of a catheter into the heart via the femoral or radial artery or venous system, and manipulating it within the heart and great vessels to:
• Sample blood to assess oxygen saturation and measure pressures (see BOX).
• Inject radiopaque contrast medium to image cardiac anatomy and blood flow.
• Perform angioplasty (± stenting), valvuloplasty, and cardiac biopsies, or to do procedures, eg transcatheter ASD closure.
• Perform intravascular ultrasound or echocardiography.

During the procedure, ECG and arterial pressures are monitored continuously. In the UK, the majority are performed as day-case procedures. See BOX.

*Indications:*
• *Coronary artery disease:* diagnostic (assessment of coronary vessels and graft patency); therapeutic (angioplasty, stent insertion).
• *Valvular disease:* diagnostic (to assess severity); therapeutic valvuloplasty (if the patient is too ill or declines valve surgery). See BOX.
• *Congenital heart disease:* diagnostic (assessment of severity of lesions); therapeutic (balloon dilatation or septostomy).
• *Other:* cardiomyopathy; pericardial disease; endomyocardial biopsy.

*Pre-procedure checks:*
• Brief history/examination; NB: peripheral pulses, bruits, aneurysms.
• Investigations: FBC, U&E, LFT, clotting screen, CXR, ECG.
• Consent for angiogram ± angioplasty ± stent ± CABG. Explain reason for procedure and possible complications (below).
• IV access, ideally in the left hand.
• Patient should be nil by mouth (NBM) from 6h before the procedure.
• Patients should take all their morning drugs (and pre-medication if needed)—but withhold oral hypoglycaemics.

*Post-procedure checks:*
• Pulse, blood pressure, arterial puncture site (for bruising or swelling?), foot pulses.
• Investigations: FBC and clotting (if suspected blood loss), ECG.

*Complications:*
• *Haemorrhage:* Apply firm pressure over puncture site. If you suspect a false aneurysm, ultrasound the swelling and consider surgical repair.
• *Contrast reaction:* This is usually mild with modern contrast agents.
• *Loss of peripheral pulse:* May be due to dissection, thrombosis, or arterial spasm. Occurs in <1% of brachial catheterizations. Rare with femoral catheterization.
• *Angina:* May occur during or after cardiac catheterization. Usually responds to sublingual GTN; if not give analgesia and IV nitrates.
• *Arrhythmias:* Usually transient. Manage along standard lines.
• *Pericardial tamponade:* Rare, but should be suspected if the patient becomes hypotensive and anuric.
• *Infection:* Post-catheter pyrexia is usually due to a contrast reaction. If it persists for >24h, take blood cultures before giving antibiotics.

*Mortality:* <1 in 1000 patients, in most centres.

**Intra-cardiac electrophysiology** This catheter technique can determine types and origins of arrhythmias, and locate (and ablate) aberrant pathways (eg causing atrial flutter or ventricular tachycardia). Arrhythmias may be induced, and the effectiveness of control by drugs assessed. Radiofrequency ablation may be used to destroy aberrant pathways or to prevent AF.

---

**CT angiography**

CT angiogram permits contrast-enhanced imaging of coronary arteries during a single breath hold. It can diagnose significant (>50%) stenosis in CAD with an accuracy of 89%. Its negative predictive value is >99%, which makes it an effective non-invasive alternative to routine coronary angiography to rule out CAD.[14]

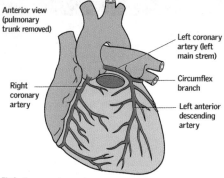

**Fig 1.** Coronary artery anatomy.

## Normal values for intracardiac pressures and saturations

| Location | Pressure (mmHg) | | Saturation (%) |
|---|---|---|---|
| | Mean | Range | |
| Inferior vena cava | | | 76 |
| Superior vena cava | | | 70 |
| Right atrium | 4 | 0–8 | 74 |
| Right ventricle | | | 74 |
|   Systolic | 25 | 15–30 | |
|   End-diastolic | 4 | 0–8 | |
| Pulmonary artery | | | 74 |
|   Systolic | 25 | 15–30 | |
|   Diastolic | 10 | 5–15 | |
|   Mean | 15 | 10–20 | |
| Pulmonary artery | a | 3–12 | 74 |
|   Wedge pressure | v | 3–15 | |
| Left ventricle | | | |
|   Systolic | 110 | 80–140 | 98 |
|   End-diastolic | 8 | ≤12 | |
| Aorta | | | |
|   Systolic | 110 | 80–140 | 98 |
|   Diastolic | 73 | 60–90 | |
|   Mean | 85 | 70–105 | |
| Brachial | | | |
|   Systolic | 120 | 90–140 | 98 |
|   Diastolic | 72 | 60–90 | |
|   Mean | 83 | 70–105 | |

## Gradients across stenotic valves

| Valve | Normal gradient (mmHg) | Stenotic gradient (mmHg) | | |
|---|---|---|---|---|
| | | Mild | Moderate | Severe |
| Aortic | 0 | <30 | 30–50 | >50 |
| Mitral | 0 | <5 | 5–15 | >15 |
| Prosthetic | 5–10 | | | |

Cardiovascular medicine

This non-invasive technique uses the differing ability of various structures within the heart to reflect ultrasound waves. It not only demonstrates anatomy but also provides a continuous display of the functioning heart throughout its cycle. There are various types of scan:

*M-mode (motion mode):* A single-dimension (time) image. See fig 1.

*2-dimensional (real time):* A 2D, fan-shaped image of a segment of the heart is produced on the screen, which may be 'frozen'. Several views are possible and the 4 commonest are: long axis, short axis, 4-chamber, and subcostal. 2D echocardiography is good for visualizing conditions such as: congenital heart disease, LV aneurysm, mural thrombus, LA myxoma, septal defects.

*3D echocardiography* is now possible with matrix array probes, and is termed 4D (3D + time) if the images are moving.

*Doppler and colour-flow echocardiography:* Different coloured jets illustrate flow and gradients across valves and septal defects (p150) (Doppler effect, p750).

*Tissue Doppler imaging:* This employs Doppler ultrasound to measure the velocity of myocardial segments over the cardiac cycle. It is particularly useful for assessing longitudinal motion—and hence long-axis ventricular function, which is a sensitive marker of systolic and diastolic heart failure.

*Trans-oesophageal echocardiography (TOE)* is more sensitive than transthoracic echocardiography (TTE) as the transducer is nearer to the heart. Indications: diagnosing aortic dissections; assessing prosthetic valves; finding cardiac source of emboli, and IE/SBE. Don't do if oesophageal disease or cervical spine instability.

*Stress echocardiography* is used to evaluate ventricular function, ejection fraction, myocardial thickening, regional wall motion pre- and post-exercise, and to characterize valvular lesions. Dobutamine or dipyridamole may be used if the patient cannot exercise. Inexpensive and as sensitive/specific as a thallium scan (p755).

**Uses of echocardiography**

*Quantification of global LV function:* Heart failure may be due to systolic or diastolic ventricular impairment (or both). Echo helps by measuring end-diastolic volume. If this is large, systolic dysfunction is the likely cause. If small, diastolic. Pure forms of diastolic dysfunction are rare. Differentiation is important; as vasodilators are less useful in diastolic dysfunction as a high ventricular filling pressure is required.

Echo is also useful for detecting focal and global hypokinesia, LV aneurysm, mural thrombus, and LVH (echo is 5–10 times more sensitive than ECG in detecting this).

*Estimating right heart haemodynamics:* Doppler studies of pulmonary artery flow and tricuspid regurgitation allow evaluation of RV function and pressures.

*Valve disease:* The technique of choice for measuring pressure gradients and valve orifice areas in stenotic lesions. Detecting valvular regurgitation and estimating its significance is less accurate. Evaluating function of prosthetic valves is another role.

*Congenital heart disease:* Establishing the presence of lesions, and significance.

*Endocarditis:* Vegetations may not be seen if <2mm in size. TTE with colour Doppler is best for aortic regurgitation (AR). TOE is useful for visualizing mitral valve vegetations, leaflet perforation, or looking for an aortic root abscess.

*Pericardial effusion* is best diagnosed by echo. Fluid may first accumulate between the posterior pericardium and the left ventricle, then anterior to both ventricles and anterior and lateral to the right atrium. There may be paradoxical septal motion.

*HCM (p146):* Echo features include asymmetrical septal hypertrophy, small LV cavity, dilated left atrium, and systolic anterior motion of the mitral valve.

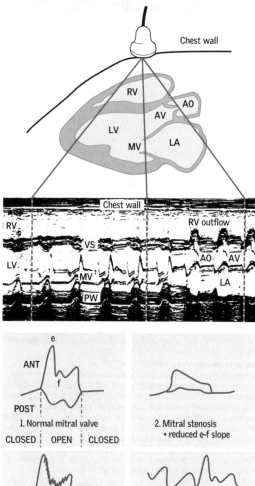

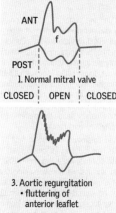

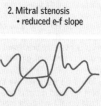

Fig 1. Normal M-mode echocardiogram (RV=right ventricle; LV=left ventricle; AO=aorta; AV=aortic valve; LA=left atrium; MV=mitral valve; PW=posterior wall of LV; VS=interventricular septum).                Adapted from R Hall *Med International* 17 774.

Cardiovascular medicine

**Antiplatelet drugs** Aspirin irreversibly acetylates cyclo-oxygenase, preventing production of thromboxane $A_2$, thereby inhibiting platelet aggregation. Used in low dose (eg 75mg/24h PO) for secondary prevention following MI, TIA/stroke, and for patients with angina or peripheral vascular disease. May have a role in primary prevention.[15] ADP receptor antagonists (eg clopidogrel, prasugrel) also block platelet aggregation, but may cause less gastric irritation. They have a role if truly intolerant of aspirin, and with aspirin, after coronary stent insertion, and in acute coronary syndrome. Glycoprotein IIb/IIIa antagonists (eg tirofiban) have a role in unstable angina/MI.[16]

**Anticoagulants**[17] Warfarin (p344) is mainly used in AF, and with mechanical valves. Newer, oral agents, eg Xa inhibitors (eg apixaban) and direct thrombin inhibitors (dabigatran) may ultimately replace it as they don't require therapeutic monitoring and may have a better risk:benefit ratio. LMW heparin (p344) is used in ACS (p114). Alternatives are parental fondaparinux (Xa inhibitor) or bivalirudin (thrombin inhibitor).

**β-blockers** Block β-adrenoceptors, thus antagonizing the sympathetic nervous system. Blocking β₁-receptors is negatively inotropic and chronotropic (pulse↓ by ↓firing of sinoatrial node), and β₂-receptors induce peripheral vasoconstriction and bronchoconstriction. Drugs vary in their β₁/β₂ selectivity (eg propranolol is non-selective, and bisoprolol relatively β₁ selective), but this does not seem to alter their clinical efficacy. *Uses:* Angina, hypertension, antidysrhythmic, post MI (↓mortality), heart failure (with caution). CI: Asthma/COPD, heart block. *Caution:* Heart failure (but see carvedilol, p130). SE: Lethargy, erectile dysfunction, *joie de vivre↓*, nightmares, headache.

**Diuretics** Loop diuretics (eg *furosemide*) are used in heart failure, and inhibit the Na/2Cl/K co-transporter. Thiazides are used in hypertension and inhibit Na/Cl co-transporter. SE: *Loop:* dehydration, ↓K⁺, ↓Ca²⁺, ototoxic; *thiazides:* ↓K⁺, ↑Ca²⁺, ↓Mg²⁺, ↑urate (±gout), impotence (NB: small doses, eg chlortalidone 25mg/24h rarely cause significant SEs); *Amiloride:* ↑K⁺, GI upset.

**Vasodilators** Used in heart failure, IHD, and hypertension. Nitrates preferentially dilate veins and the large arteries, ↓ filling pressure (pre-load), while hydralazine (often used with nitrates) primarily dilates the resistance vessels, thus ↓ BP (afterload). Prazosin (an α-blocker) dilates arteries and veins.

**Calcium antagonists** These ↓ cell entry of Ca²⁺ via voltage-sensitive channels in smooth muscle, thereby promoting coronary and peripheral vasodilatation and reducing myocardial oxygen consumption. All current drugs block L-type Ca²⁺ channels. However, their effects differ because of differential binding properties. The *dihydropyridines*, eg nifedipine, amlodipine, are mainly peripheral vasodilators (also dilate coronary arteries) and cause a reflex tachycardia, so are often used with a β-blocker. They are used in hypertension and angina. The *non*-dihydropyridines—verapamil and diltiazem—also slow conduction at the AV and SA nodes and may be used to treat hypertension, angina, and dysrhythmias. Don't give verapamil with β-blockers (risk of severe bradycardia ± LVF). SE: Flushes, headache, oedema (diuretic unresponsive), LV function↓, gingival hypertrophy. CI: Heart block.

**Digoxin**[18,19] Blocks the Na⁺/Ca²⁺ pump. It is used to slow the pulse in fast AF (p124; aim for ≤100). As it is a weak +ve inotrope, its role in heart failure in sinus rhythm may be best reserved if symptomatic despite optimal ACE-i therapy (p109);[18] here there is little benefit *vis-à-vis* mortality (but admissions for worsening CCF are ↓ by ~25%).[19] Old people are at ↑risk of toxicity: use lower doses. Do plasma levels >6h post-dose (p766). Typical dose: 500µg stat PO, repeated after 12h, then 125µg (if elderly) to 375µg/d PO (62.5µg/d is almost never enough). IV dose: 0.75-1mg in 0.9% NaCl over 2h. Toxicity risk↑ if: K⁺↓, Mg²⁺↓, or Ca²⁺↑. t½ ≈ 36h. If on digoxin, use less energy in cardioversion (start at 5J). ►If on amiodarone, halve the dose of digoxin. SE: Any arrhythmia (supraventricular tachycardia with AV block is suggestive), nausea, appetite↓, yellow vision, confusion, gynaecomastia. In toxicity, stop digoxin; check K⁺; treat arrhythmias; consider DigiFab® by IVI (p854). CI: HCM; WPW syndrome (p120).

**ACE-inhibitors** p109; **Nitrates** p110; **Antihypertensives** p134.

## Statins

(see also hyperlipidaemia, p704 and p705, fig 1)

Statins (eg simvastatin, p704) inhibit the enzyme HMG-CoA reductase, which causes *de novo* synthesis of cholesterol in the liver. This increases LDL receptor expression by hepatocytes leading to ↓ circulating LDL cholesterol. More effective if given at night, but optimum dose and target plasma cholesterol are unknown. SE: muscle aches, abdominal discomfort, ↑transaminases (eg ALT), ↑CK, myositis, rarely rhabdomyolysis (more common if used with fibrates). Statins are generally well tolerated. There are currently ~3 million people taking statins in England, which saves ~10,000 lives a year.

## How to start ACE-inhibitors

*Check that there are no contraindications/cautions:*
- Renal failure (serum creatinine >200µmol/L; but not an absolute CI)
- Hyperkalaemia: K⁺ >5.5mmol/L
- Hyponatraemia: caution if <130mmol/L (relates to a poorer prognosis)
- Hypovolaemia or hypotension (systolic BP <90mmHg)
- Aortic stenosis or LV outflow tract obstruction
- Pregnancy or lactation
- Severe COPD or cor pulmonale (not an absolute CI)
- Renal artery stenosis[1] (suspect if arteriopathic, eg cerebrovascular disease, IHD, peripheral vascular disease. ACE-i ↓GFR and may precipitate acute renal failure)

*Warn the patient about possible side-effects:*
- Dry cough (1:10)
- Hypotension, especially with 1st dose if CCF (so start at night)
- Taste disturbance
- Hyperkalaemia
- Renal impairment; this commonly co-exists with heart failure (atheroma is the reason for both, usually)—and is worsened by ACE-i (see below)
- Urticaria and angioneurotic oedema (<1:1,000)
- Rarely: proteinuria, leucopenia, fatigue

*Starting ACE-inhibitors:* ►Delay if intercurrent illness (esp. if dehydrated/D&V$^{etc}$). Most patients can be safely started on ACE-i as outpatients. 1st-dose hypotension can be avoided by taking the 1st dose on going to bed. Use a long-acting ACE-i, eg lisinopril 10mg/d PO, 2.5mg/d in the elderly (or eGFR <30). Increase dose every 2wks until at target dose (equivalent of 30–40mg lisinopril a day if eGFR >30) or side-effects supervene (↓BP, ↑creatinine). Review in ~1-2 wks; check U&E regularly. Patients on high doses of diuretics (>80mg furosemide a day) may need a reduction in their diuretic dose first. Before and after, check U&E. Expect a rise in creatinine (<20%; GFR↓ by <15% [20]) in ~2 wks after starting an ACE-i; a larger change may indicate underlying renal artery stenosis. Repeat U&E and ask a specialist's advice. Plasma K⁺ may also rise. If >6mmol/L, ensure no NSAID is being taken, stop or reduce dose of K⁺-sparing diuretics, and recheck U&E. The dose of loop diuretic may also need to be reduced (if there is no congestion). If ↑K⁺ persists, ACE-i (or ARB) may need to be stopped. [21]

NB: the same cautions are needed when starting ARBs (eg candesartan). In patients with cardiac disease who are unable to tolerate ACE-i, an ARB can be used.

---

1 If renovascular disease precludes the use of ACE-i and furosemide is providing no answer, consider maximal vasodilatation with nitrates and hydralazine: seek expert advice.

This is due to myocardial ischaemia and presents as a central chest tightness or heaviness, which is brought on by exertion and relieved by rest. It may radiate to one or both arms, the neck, jaw or teeth. *Other precipitants:* Emotion, cold weather, and heavy meals. *Associated symptoms:* Dyspnoea, nausea, sweatiness, faintness.

**Causes** Mostly atheroma. Rarely: anaemia, AS; tachyarrhythmias; HCM; arteritis/small vessel disease (microvascular angina/cardiac syndrome X).

**Types of angina** *Stable angina:* induced by effort, relieved by rest. *Unstable (crescendo) angina:* angina of increasing frequency or severity; occurs on minimal exertion or at rest; associated with ↑↑risk of MI. *Decubitus angina:* precipitated by lying flat. *Variant (Prinzmetal's) angina* (see BOX 3): caused by coronary artery spasm (rare; may co-exist with fixed stenoses).

**Tests** ECG: usually normal, but may show ST depression; flat or inverted T waves; signs of past MI. See BOX 2 for other investigations. Exclude precipitating factors: anaemia, diabetes, hyperlipidaemia, thyrotoxicosis, temporal arteritis.

**Management**
*Modify risk factors:* stop smoking, encourage exercise, weight loss. Control hypertension, diabetes, etc., p87. If total cholesterol >4mmol/L give a statin—see p704.
*Aspirin* (75-150mg/24h) reduces mortality by 34%.
*β-blockers,* eg atenolol 50-100mg/24h PO, reduce symptoms unless contraindicated (asthma, COPD, LVF, bradycardia, coronary artery spasm).
*Nitrates:* for symptoms, give GTN spray or sublingual tabs, up to every ½h. Prophylaxis: give regular oral nitrate, eg isosorbide mononitrate 20-40mg PO bd (have an 8h nitrate-free period to prevent tolerance) or slow-release nitrate (eg Imdur® 60mg/24h). Alternatives: adhesive nitrate skin patches or buccal pills. SE: headaches, BP↓.
*Long-acting calcium antagonists:* amlodipine 10mg/24h; diltiazem-MR 90-180mg/12h PO. They are particularly useful if there is a contraindication to β-blockers.
*K+ channel activator,* eg nicorandil 10-30mg/12h PO, if still not controlled.
*Others:* ivabradine inhibits the pacemaker ('funny') current in the SA node and thus reduces heart rate. Useful in those who cannot take a β-blocker, having similar efficacy. Trimetazidine inhibits fatty acid oxidation, leading the myocardium to use glucose, which is more efficient. Ranolazine inhibits the late Na+ current.
▶Unstable angina requires admission and urgent treatment: *emergencies,* p810.

**Indications for referral** Diagnostic uncertainty; new angina of sudden onset; recurrent angina if past MI or CABG (see BOX); angina uncontrolled by drugs; unstable angina. Some units routinely do exercise tolerance tests on those <70yrs old, but age alone is a poor way to stratify patients.

*Percutaneous transluminal coronary angioplasty (PTCA)* involves balloon dilatation of the stenotic vessel(s). *Indications:* poor response or intolerance to medical therapy; refractory angina in patients not suitable for CABG; previous CABG; post-thrombolysis in patients with severe stenoses, symptoms, or positive stress tests. Comparisons of PTCA *vs* drugs alone show that PTCA may control symptoms better but with more frequent early cardiac events (eg MI and need for CABG)[22] and little effect on mortality. However, early intervention may benefit high risk patients presenting with non-ST-segment elevation MI (p112).[23] Stenting reduces restenosis rates and the need for bailout CABG compared with angioplasty. *Complications:* Restenosis (20-30% within 6 months); emergency CABG (<3%); MI (<2%); death (<0.5%).

NICE recommends that >70% of angioplasties be accompanied by stenting. Antiplatelet agents, eg clopidogrel, reduce the risk of stent thrombosis, and IV glycoproteins IIb/IIIa-inhibitors (eg eptifibatide) reduce procedure-related ischaemic events. Drug-coated stents reduce restenosis rates, but at the risk of increased late in-stent thrombosis. Long-term treatment with aspirin and clopidogrel may reduce this risk.

## Investigating patients with ? stable angina

If the patient has an acute coronary syndrome, eg unstable angina, emergency admission is indicated. In those patients with stable chest pain which might be cardiac who do not require emergency admission, a number of options exist. NICE suggests stratifying based on whether there is known CAD, and the likelihood of CAD.[12.24]

*Known CAD* and pain typical, no further investigation. If atypical pain, either exercise testing or functional imaging (myocardial perfusion scintigraphy, stress echo, or MRI).

*Unknown CAD* stratify of likelihood of CAD
• >90% treat as known CAD
• 61-90% angiography, or functional imaging if inappropriate
• 30-60% functional imaging
• 10-29% coronary artery calcification score[1] with CT
• <10% reconsider diagnosis.

## Calculating the likelihood of CAD (percentages)[12.1.12]

| Age (yrs) | Non-anginal chest pain | | | | Atypical angina | | | | Typical angina | | | |
|---|---|---|---|---|---|---|---|---|---|---|---|---|
| | Men | | Women | | Men | | Women | | Men | | Women | |
| | Lo | Hi | Lo | Hi | Lo | Hi | Lo | Hi | Lo | Hi | Lo | Hi |
| 35 | 3 | 35 | 1 | 19 | 8 | 59 | 2 | 39 | 30 | 88 | 10 | 78 |
| 45 | 9 | 47 | 2 | 22 | 21 | 70 | 5 | 43 | 51 | 92 | 20 | 79 |
| 55 | 23 | 59 | 4 | 25 | 45 | 79 | 10 | 47 | 80 | 95 | 38 | 82 |
| 65 | 49 | 69 | 9 | 29 | 71 | 86 | 20 | 51 | 93 | 97 | 56 | 84 |

Values are percent of people at each mid-decade with significant coronary artery disease (CAD).

Hi = High risk = diabetes, smoking, and hyperlipidaemia (total cholesterol >6.47mmol/L). Lo = Low risk = none of these three.

The shaded area represents people with symptoms of non-anginal chest pain, who would not be investigated for stable angina routinely.

For men older than 70 with atypical or typical symptoms, assume an estimate >90%. For women older than 70, assume estimate of 61-90% EXCEPT women at high risk AND with typical symptoms, where a risk of >90% should be assumed.

Note: these results are likely to overestimate CAD in primary care populations.

If there are resting ECG ST-T changes or Q waves, the likelihood of CAD is higher in each cell of the table.

NICE (2010) CG95 *Chest pain of recent onset: assessment and diagnosis of recent onset chest pain and discomfort of suspected cardiac origin.* London: NICE. Available from www.nice.org.uk/guidance/CG95. Reproduced with permission.

## Prinzmetal angina

This is due to coronary artery spasm, which can occur even in normal coronary arteries. Pain usually occurs during rest (rather than during activity). ECG during pain shows ST segment elevation, which resolves as the pain subsides. Patients usually do not have the standard risk factors for atherosclerosis. *Treatment:* Calcium channel blockers ± long-acting nitrates. Aspirin can *aggravate* the ischaemic attacks in these patients. β-blockers (esp non-selective) should also be *avoided* as they can increase vasospasm. Prognosis is usually very good.

---

1 The calcium score derived from CT images is a summation of all calcified lesions in the coronary arteries. It reflects the presence of plaques. The reported score is an individual's score, allowing for age and sex.[15]

Cardiovascular medicine

**Definitions** ACS includes unstable angina and evolving MI, which share a common underlying pathology—plaque rupture, thrombosis, and inflammation. However, ACS may rarely be due to emboli or coronary spasm in normal coronary arteries, or vasculitis (p558). Usually divided into *ACS with ST-segment elevation* or new onset LBBB—what most of us mean by acute MI; and *ACS without ST-segment elevation*—the ECG may show ST depression, T wave inversion, non-specific changes, or be normal (includes non-Q wave or subendocardial MI). The degree of irreversible myocyte death varies, and significant necrosis can occur without ST elevation.

**Risk factors** *Non-modifiable:* age, ♂ gender, family history of IHD (MI in 1st degree relative <55yrs). *Modifiable:* smoking, hypertension, DM, hyperlipidaemia, obesity, sedentary lifestyle, cocaine use. *Controversial* risk factors include: stress, type A personality, LVH, fibrinogen↑, hyperinsulinaemia, homocysteine levels↑, ACE genotype.

**Incidence** 5/1000 per annum (UK) for ST-segment elevation (declining in UK and USA).

**Diagnosis** Acute MI is defined by several criteria.[26] The commonest is an↑ and then a ↓ in cardiac biomarkers (eg troponin) and either: symptoms of ischaemia, ECG changes of new ischaemia, development of pathological Q waves, or loss of myocardium on imaging.

**Symptoms** Acute central chest pain, lasting >20min, often associated with nausea, sweatiness, dyspnoea, palpitations. May present without chest pain ('silent' infarct), eg in the elderly or diabetics. In such patients, presentations may include: syncope, pulmonary oedema, epigastric pain and vomiting, post-operative hypotension or oliguria, acute confusional state, stroke, and diabetic hyperglycaemic states.

**Signs** Distress, anxiety, pallor, sweatiness, pulse↑ or ↓, BP↑ or ↓, 4th heart sound. There may be signs of heart failure (↑ JVP, 3rd heart sound, basal crepitations) or a pansystolic murmur (papillary muscle dysfunction/rupture, VSD). Low-grade fever may be present. Later, a pericardial friction rub or peripheral oedema may develop.

**Tests** *ECG* (see fig 1): Classically, hyperacute (tall) T waves, ST elevation or new LBBB occur within hours of transmural infarction. T wave inversion and development of pathological Q waves follow over hours to days (p92). In other ACS: ST depression, T wave inversion, non-specific changes, or normal. ►*In 20% of MI, the ECG may be normal initially.* *CXR:* Look for cardiomegaly, pulmonary oedema, or a widened mediastinum (aortic rupture). Don't routinely delay treatment whilst waiting for a CXR.

*Blood:* FBC, U&E, glucose, lipids.
*Cardiac enzymes* (see fig 2): *Cardiac troponin* levels (T and I) are the most sensitive and specific markers of myocardial necrosis. Serum levels↑ within 3–12h from the onset of chest pain, peak at 24–48h, and ↓ to baseline over 5–14 days. If normal ≥6h after onset of pain, and ECG normal, risk of missing MI is tiny (0.3%).[27] Peak levels also help risk stratification.[28] *Creatine kinase* comprises 3 isoenzymes: CK-MM (found mainly in skeletal muscle; ↑after trauma (falls, seizures); prolonged exercise; myositis; African-Caribbeans; hypothyroidism); CK-BB (predominantly in the brain); and CK-MB mainly in the heart. CK-MB levels ↑ within 3–12h of onset of chest pain, reach peak values within 24h, and return to baseline after 48–72h. Levels peak earlier if reperfusion occurs. Sensitivity is ~95%, with high specificity. *Myoglobin* levels rise within 1–4h from the onset of pain. They are highly sensitive but not specific.

**Differential diagnosis** (p88) Angina, pericarditis, myocarditis, aortic dissection (p656), pulmonary embolism, and oesophageal reflux/spasm.

**Management** See *emergencies*, p810. The management of ACS with and without ST-segment elevation varies. Likewise, if there is no ST elevation and symptoms settle without a rise in cardiac troponin, then no myocardial damage has occurred, the prognosis is good, and patients can be discharged. Therefore, the two key questions are: is there ST-segment elevation? Is there a rise in troponin?

**Mortality** 50% of deaths occur within 2h of onset of symptoms. Up to 7% die before discharge. Worse prognosis if: elderly, LV failure, and ST changes.[29]

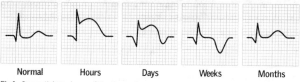

**Normal** | **Hours** | **Days** | **Weeks** | **Months**

Fig 1. Sequential ECG changes following acute MI.

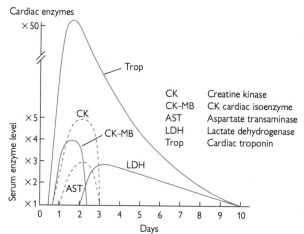

Fig 2. Enzyme changes following acute MI.

*Cardiovascular medicine*

**Pre-hospital** Arrange emergency ambulance. Aspirin 300mg chewed[31] (if no *absolute* CI) and GTN sublingual. Analgesia, eg morphine 5–10mg IV + metoclopramide 10mg IV (not IM because of risk of bleeding with thrombolysis).

**In hospital** $O_2$, IVI, morphine, aspirin ▶▶p808–810.

Then the key question for subsequent management of ACS is whether there is ST-segment elevation (includes new onset LBBB or a true posterior MI). See fig 1.

*ST-segment elevation*
- *Primary angioplasty* or thrombolysis, if no contraindication ▶▶ p808.
- *β-blocker*, eg atenolol 5mg IV unless contraindicated, eg asthma.
- *ACE-inhibitor*: Consider starting ACE-i (eg lisinopril 2.5mg) in all normotensive patients (systolic ≥120mm/Hg) within 24h of acute MI, especially if there is clinical evidence of heart failure or echo evidence of LV dysfunction.
- Consider clopidogrel 300mg loading followed by 75mg/day for 30 days.[32]

*ACS without ST-segment elevation*[33]
- *β-blocker*, eg atenolol 5mg IV and nitrates IV unless contraindicated.
- *Antithrombotic* fondaparinux if low bleeding risk and no angiography planned for 24h, otherwise consider *low molecular weight heparin* (eg enoxaparin 1mg/kg/12h SC for 2–8 days)
- Assess risk, eg GRACE SCORE.
- High-risk patients (persistent or recurrent ischaemia, ST↓, diabetes, ↑troponin): GPIIb/IIIa antagonist (eg tirofiban),[34] or bivalirudin, and angiography within 96h. *Clopidogrel*, in addition to aspirin, should be considered for up to 12 months.[30]
- Low-risk (eg no further pain, flat or inverted T-waves, or normal ECG, and negative troponin): clopidogrel if risk 1.5–3%/yr. Discharge if a repeat troponin is negative. Treat medically and arrange further investigation if recurrent ischaemia.

**Subsequent management**
- *Bed rest for 48h*; continuous ECG monitoring.
- *Daily examination:* heart, lungs, and legs for complications (p116); 12-lead ECG, U&E.
- *Prophylaxis against thromboembolism:* until fully mobile. If large anterior MI, consider warfarin for 3 months as prophylaxis against systemic embolism from LV mural thrombus.
- *Aspirin* (eg 75mg) ↓vascular events (MI, stroke, or vascular death) by 29%.
- *Long-term β-blockade* ↓mortality from all causes by ~25% in patients who have had a previous MI (eg bisoprolol 2.5–5mg/d enough to decrease the pulse to ≤60; continue for at least 1yr). If contraindicated, consider verapamil or diltiazem.
- *Continue* ACE-i in all patients. ACE-i in those with evidence of heart failure reduces 2yr mortality by 25–30%.
- *Start a statin*, eg simvastatin 40mg.[35] Cholesterol reduction post-MI has been shown to be of benefit in patients with both elevated and normal cholesterol levels.
- *Address modifiable risk factors:* Discourage smoking (p87). Encourage exercise. Identify and treat diabetes mellitus, hypertension, and hyperlipidaemia.
- *Assess LV function* in all patients post-MI.
- *General advice:* If uncomplicated, discharge after 5–7 days. *Work:* Patient may return to work after 2 months. A few occupations should not be restarted post-MI: airline pilots; air traffic controllers; divers. Drivers of public service or heavy goods vehicles may be permitted to return to work if they meet certain criteria.[36] Patients undertaking heavy manual labour should be advised to seek a lighter job. *Diet*: A diet high in oily fish, fruit, vegetables, and fibre, and low in saturated fats should be encouraged. *Exercise*: Encourage regular daily exercise. *Sex*: Intercourse is best avoided for 1 month. *Travel:* Avoid air travel for 2 months. Refer for structured rehabilitation programme.
- *Review at 5wks post-MI to review symptoms:* Angina? dyspnoea? palpitations? If angina recurs, treat conventionally, and consider coronary angiography.
- *Review at 3 months*: Check fasting lipids.

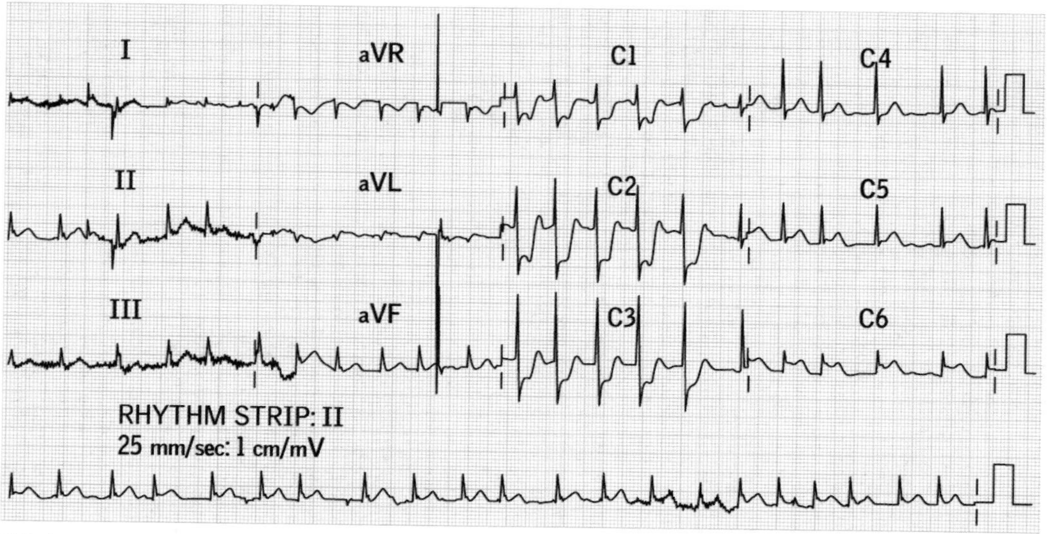

I

aVR

C1

C4

II

aVL

C2

C5

III

aVF

C3

C6

RHYTHM STRIP: II
25 mm/sec: 1 cm/mV

Fig 1. Acute postero-lateral MI.

Cardiovascular medicine

*Cardiac arrest* (inside back cover); *cardiogenic shock* (p814); LVF (p812).

*Unstable angina:* Manage along standard lines (p810) and refer to a cardiologist.

*Bradycardias or heart block: Sinus bradycardia:* treat with atropine 0.6-1.2mg IV. Consider temporary cardiac pacing if no response or poorly tolerated by the patient. ↓BP which is not responsive to atropine in patients with inferior MI may be due to RV infarction. *1ˢᵗ degree AV block:* Most commonly seen in inferior MI. Observe closely, as approximately 40% develop higher degrees of AV block (in which case calcium channel blockers and β-blockers should be stopped). *Wenckebach (Mobitz type I; ECG, p119) block:* does not require pacing unless poorly tolerated. *Mobitz type II block:* carries a high risk of developing sudden complete AV block; should be paced. *Complete AV block* (ECG, p90): usually resolves within a few days. Insert pacemaker (may not be necessary after inferior MI if narrow QRS and reasonably stable and pulse ≥40-50). *Bundle branch block:* MI complicated by trifascicular block or non-adjacent bifascicular disease (p126) should be paced.

*Tachyarrhythmias:* NB: K⁺↓, hypoxia and acidosis all predispose to arrhythmias and should be corrected. *Sinus tachycardia* can ↑ myocardial O₂ demand. Pain and hypoxia are common causes (give O₂, analgesic). *SVT:* p120. *AF or flutter:* If compromised, DC cardioversion. Otherwise, control rate with digoxin (load with 500µg/12h PO for 2-3 doses; maintenance: 125-250µg/24h) ± β-blocker. In atrial flutter or intermittent AF, try amiodarone or sotalol (details p124). *Frequent PVCs* (premature ventricular contractions) are common after acute MI. They usually do not result in VF, and prophylactic antidysrhythmics are not recommended (↑ death). *Non-sustained VT* (≥3 consecutive PVCs >100bpm and lasting <30s): if it happens at <48h after MI, antidysrhythmics are not recommended. However, if it happens >48h, risk of sudden cardiac death is ↑ and electrophysiological studies should be considered. *Sustained VT* (≥3 consecutive PVCs >100bpm and lasting >30s): if compromised, give DC shock. If stable, treat with amiodarone. Recurrent VT may need pacing. *Ventricular fibrillation:* 80% occurs within 12h. If occur >48h, usually indicates pump failure or cardiogenic shock. R: DC shock.

*Consider implantable cardiac defibrillator* if ejection fraction <35% and VT.[37]

*Right ventricular failure (RVF)/infarction:* Presents with low cardiac output and JVP↑. Consider a Swan-Ganz catheter to measure right-sided pressures and guide fluid replacement. If BP remains low, give inotropes.

*Pericarditis:* Central chest pain, relieved by sitting forwards. ECG: saddle-shaped ST elevation. Treatment: NSAIDs. Echo to check for effusion.

*DVT & PE:* Patients are at risk of developing DVT & PE and should be prophylactically heparinised (enoxaparin) until fully mobile.

*Systemic embolism:* May arise from LV mural thrombus. After large anterior MI, consider anticoagulation with warfarin for 3 months.

*Cardiac tamponade:* (p814) Presents with low cardiac output, pulsus paradoxus, JVP↑, muffled heart sounds. Diagnosis: Echo. Treatment: Pericardial aspiration (provides temporary relief, ►►see p787 for technique), surgery.

*Mitral regurgitation:* May be mild (minor papillary muscle dysfunction) or severe (chordal or papillary muscle rupture or ischaemia). Presentation: Pulmonary oedema. Treat LVF (p812) and consider valve replacement.

*Ventricular septal defect:* Presents with pansystolic murmur, JVP↑, cardiac failure. Diagnosis: echo. Treatment: surgery. 50% mortality in first week.

*Late malignant ventricular arrhythmias:* Occur 1-3wks post-MI and are the cardiologist's nightmare. Avoid hypokalaemia, the most easily avoidable cause. Consider 24h ECG monitoring prior to discharge if large MI.

*Dressler's syndrome:* (p712) Recurrent pericarditis, pleural effusions, fever, anaemia and ESR↑ 1-3wks post-MI. Treatment: may consider NSAIDs; steroids if severe.

*Left ventricular aneurysm:* This occurs late (4-6 weeks post-MI), and presents with LVF, angina, recurrent VT, or systemic embolism. ECG: persistent ST-segment elevation. Treatment: anticoagulate, consider excision.

## Coronary artery bypass graft (CABG)

CABG is performed in left main stem disease, multi-vessel disease; multiple severe stenoses; patients unsuitable for angioplasty; failed angioplasty; refractory angina.

*Indications for CABG: to improve survival*
• Left main stem disease
• Triple vessel disease involving proximal part of the left anterior descending

*To relieve symptoms*
• Angina unresponsive to drugs
• Unstable angina (sometimes)
• If angioplasty is unsuccessful

NB: when CABG and percutaneous coronary intervention (PCI, eg angioplasty) are both clinically valid options, NICE recommends that the availability of new stent technology should push the decision towards PCI. In practice, patients with single-vessel CAD and normal LV function usually undergo PCI, and those with triple-vessel disease and abnormal LV function more often undergo CABG.[38]

Compared with PCI, CABG results in longer recovery time and length of inpatient stay. Recent RCTs indicate that early procedural mortality rates and 5-year survival rates are similar after PCI and CABG. Compared with PCI, CABG probably provides more complete long-term relief of angina in patients, and less repeated revascularization. However, it is associated with ↑ risk of stroke.[39]

*Procedure:* The heart is usually stopped and blood pumped artificially by a machine outside the body (cardiac bypass). Minimally invasive thoracotomies not requiring this are well described,[40] but randomized trials are few. The patient's own saphenous vein or internal mammary artery is used as the graft. Several grafts may be placed. >50% of vein grafts close in 10yrs (low-dose aspirin helps prevent this). Internal mammary artery grafts last longer (but may cause chest-wall numbness).

*On-pump or off-pump?*
Seems to make little difference.[41]

*After CABG:* If angina persists or recurs (from poor graft run-off, distal disease, new atheroma, or graft occlusion) restart anti-anginal drugs, and consider angioplasty. Mood, sex, and intellectual problems[42] are common early. Rehabilitation helps:
• Exercise: walk→cycle→swim→jog
• Drive at 1 month: no need to tell DVLA if non-HGV licences, p152
• Get back to work, eg at 3 months
• Attend to: smoking; BP; lipids
• Aspirin 75mg/24h PO forever; consider clopidogrel if aspirin CI

Disturbances of cardiac rhythm or arrhythmias are:
• Common
• Often benign (but may reflect underlying heart disease)
• Often intermittent, causing diagnostic difficulty
• Occasionally severe, causing cardiac compromise.

**Causes** *Cardiac:* MI, coronary artery disease, LV aneurysm, mitral valve disease, cardiomyopathy, pericarditis, myocarditis, aberrant conduction pathways. *Non-cardiac:* Caffeine, smoking, alcohol, pneumonia, drugs (β₂-agonists, digoxin, L-dopa, tricyclics, doxorubicin), metabolic imbalance (K⁺, Ca²⁺, Mg²⁺, hypoxia, hypercapnia, metabolic acidosis, thyroid disease), and phaeochromocytoma.

**Presentation** is with palpitation, chest pain, presyncope/syncope, hypotension, or pulmonary oedema. Some arrhythmias may be asymptomatic and incidental, eg AF.

**History** Take a detailed history of palpitations (p35). Ask about precipitating factors, onset/offset, nature (fast or slow, regular or irregular), duration, associated symptoms (chest pain, dyspnoea, collapse). Review drug history. Ask about past medical history and family history of cardiac disease.

**Tests** FBC, U&E, glucose, Ca²⁺, Mg²⁺, TSH. ECG (see BOX): Look for signs of IHD, AF, short PR interval (WPW syndrome), long QT interval (metabolic imbalance, drugs, congenital), U waves (hypokalaemia). 24h ECG monitoring; several recordings may be needed. Echo: Any structural heart disease, eg mitral stenosis, HCM? Provocation tests: Exercise ECG, cardiac catheterization ± electrophysiological studies may be needed.

**Treatment** If the ECG is normal during palpitations, reassure the patient. Otherwise, treatment depends on the type of arrhythmia.

*Bradycardia:* (p119) If asymptomatic and rate >40bpm, no treatment is required. Look for a cause (drugs, sick sinus syndrome, hypothyroidism) and stop any drugs that may be contributing (β-blocker, digoxin). If rate <40bpm or patient is symptomatic, give atropine 0.6–1.2mg IV (up to maximum of 3mg). If no response, insert a temporary pacing wire (p814). If necessary, start an isoprenaline infusion or use external cardiac pacing.

*Sick sinus syndrome:* Sinus node dysfunction causes bradycardia ± arrest, sinoatrial block or SVT alternating with bradycardia/asystole (tachy–brady syndrome). AF and thromboembolism may occur. Pace if symptomatic.

*SVT:* (p120) Narrow complex tachycardia (rate >100bpm, QRS width <120ms). Acute management: vagotonic manoeuvres followed by IV adenosine or verapamil (if not on β-blocker); DC shock if compromised. Maintenance therapy: β-blockers or verapamil.

*AF/flutter:* (p124) May be incidental finding. Control ventricular rate with β-blocker, or verapamil. Alternatives: digoxin: loading dose (~500µg/12h × 2–3) followed by maintenance dose (0.125–0.25µg/24h), or amiodarone. Flecainide for pre-excited AF (caution if structural heart disease). DC shock if compromised (p784).

*VT:* (p122 and ECG 6 p100) Broad complex tachycardia (rate >100bpm, QRS duration >120ms). Acute management: IV amiodarone or IV lidocaine, if no response or if compromised DC shock. Oral therapy: amiodarone loading dose (200mg/8h PO for 7d, then 200mg/12h for 7d) followed by maintenance therapy (200mg/24h). SE: Corneal deposits, photosensitivity, hepatitis, pneumonitis, lung fibrosis, nightmares, INR↑ (warfarin potentiation), T4↑, T3↓. Monitor LFT and TFT.

▶Finally, permanent pacing may be used to overdrive tachyarrhythmias, to treat bradyarrhythmias, or prophylactically in conduction disturbances (p126). Implanted automatic defibrillators can save lives.

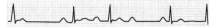

First degree AV block. P-R interval = 0.28s

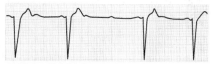

Mobitz type I (Wenckebach) AV block. With each succesive QRS, the P-R interval increases–until there is a non-conducted P wave.

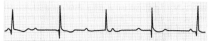

Mobitz type II AV block. Ratio of AV conduction varies from 2:1 to 3:1

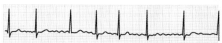

Complete AV block with narrow ventricular complex. There is no relation between atrial and the slower ventricular activity.

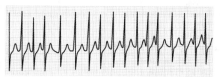

Atrial fibrillation

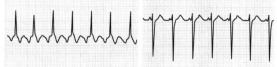

Atrial fibrillation with a rapid ventricular response. Diagnosis is based on the totally irregular ventricular rhythm.

Atrial flutter with 2:1 AV block. Lead aVF (on left) shows the characteristic saw-tooth baseline whereas lead V1 (on right) shows discrete atrial activity, alternate 'F' waves being superimposed on ventricular T waves.

Fig 1. ECG diagnosis of bradycardias, AV block, and atrial fibrillation

Cardiovascular medicine

**Definition** ECG shows rate of >100bpm and QRS complex duration of <120ms.

**Differential diagnosis**
- Sinus tachycardia: normal P wave followed by normal QRS.
- Supraventricular tachycardia (SVT): P wave absent or inverted after QRS.
- AF: absent P wave, irregular QRS complexes.
- Atrial flutter: atrial rate usually 300bpm giving 'flutter waves' or 'sawtooth' baseline (p119), ventricular rate often 150bpm (2:1 block).
- Atrial tachycardia: abnormally shaped P waves, may outnumber QRS.
- Multifocal atrial tachycardia: 3 or more P wave morphologies, irregular QRS complexes.
- Junctional tachycardia: rate 150-250bpm, P wave either buried in QRS complex or occurring after QRS complex.

**Principles of management** See p818.
- If the patient is compromised, use DC cardioversion (p784).
- Otherwise, identify the underlying rhythm and treat accordingly.
- Vagal manoeuvres (carotid sinus massage, Valsalva manoeuvre) transiently increase AV block, and may unmask an underlying atrial rhythm.
- If unsuccessful, give adenosine which causes transient AV block. It has a short t½ (10-15s) and works in 2 ways: by transiently slowing ventricles to show underlying atrial rhythm and by cardioverting a junctional tachycardia to sinus rhythm.

*Adenosine dose:* Give 6mg IV bolus (2s) into a big vein; follow by saline flush, while recording a rhythm strip; if unsuccessful, after 1-2min, give 12mg, then 12mg again, unless on dipyridamole or post cardiac transplantation (change dose, see *BNF*). Warn of SE: transient chest tightness, dyspnoea, headache, flushing. CI: asthma, 2nd/3rd degree AV block, or sinoatrial disease (unless pacemaker). Drug interactions: potentiated by dipyridamole, antagonized by theophylline. Transplanted hearts are very sensitive; use a smaller dose.

**Specific management** *Sinus tachycardia* Identify and treat the cause (p92).

*SVT:* Vagal manoeuvres (breath-holding, valsalva manoeuvre, carotid massage) are 1st line treatments if haemodynamically stable. IV adenosine is the drug of choice. If adenosine fails, use verapamil 5mg IV over 2min, or over 3min if elderly (►not if already on β-blocker). If no response, give further dose of 5mg IV after 5-10min. Alternatives: atenolol 2.5mg IV at 1mg/min repeated at 5min intervals to a maximum of 10mg or sotalol 20-60mg (if eGFR >60) IV over 10min. If no good, use DC cardioversion.

*AF/flutter:* Manage along standard lines (p124).

*Atrial tachycardia:* Rare. If due to digoxin toxicity, stop digoxin; consider digoxin-specific antibody fragments (p854). Maintain K+ at 4-5mmol/L.

*Multifocal atrial tachycardia:* Most commonly occurs in COPD. There are at least 3 morphologically distinct P waves with irregular P-P intervals. Correct hypoxia and hypercapnia. Consider verapamil or a β-blocker if rate remains >110bpm.

*Junctional tachycardia:* There are 3 types of junctional tachycardia: AV nodal re-entry tachycardia (AVNRT), AV re-entry tachycardia (AVRT), and His bundle tachycardia. Where anterograde conduction through the AV node occurs, vagal manoeuvres are worth trying. Adenosine will usually cardiovert a junctional rhythm to sinus rhythm. If it recurs, treat with a β-blocker or amiodarone. Radiofrequency ablation is increasingly being used in AVRT and in many patients with symptomatic AVNRT.[43]

**WPW syndrome** (Wolff-Parkinson-White; ECG p125) Caused by congenital accessory conduction pathway between atria and ventricles. Resting ECG shows short PR interval, wide QRS complex (due to slurred upstroke or 'delta wave') and ST-T changes. 2 types: WPW type A (+ve δ wave in V₁), WPW type B (-ve δ wave in V₁). Patients present with SVT which may be due to an AVRT, pre-excited AF, or pre-excited atrial flutter. Refer to cardiologist for electrophysiology and ablation of accessory pathway.

## Holiday heart syndrome[44,45]

Binge drinking in a person *without* any clinical evidence of heart disease may result in acute cardiac rhythm and/or conduction disturbances, which is called holiday heart syndrome (note that recreational use of marijuana may have similar effects). The most common rhythm disorder is supraventricular tachyarrhythmia, and particularly AF (consider this diagnosis in patients without structural heart disease who present with new-onset AF).

The prognosis is excellent, especially in young patients without structural heart disease. As holiday heart syndrome resolves rapidly by abstinence from alcohol use, advise all patients against the excessive use of alcohol in future.

ECG shows rate of >100 and QRS complexes >120ms (>3 small squares, p90). If no clear QRS complexes, it is VF or asystole, p766.

### Principles of management
- Identify the underlying rhythm and treat accordingly.
- If in doubt, treat as ventricular tachycardia (VT)—the commonest cause.

### Differential diagnosis
- VT; includes *torsade de pointes*, below, and figs 3–5.
- Supraventricular tachycardia (SVT) with aberrant conduction, eg AF, atrial flutter.

(NB: ventricular ectopics should not cause confusion when occurring singly; but if >3 together at rate of >120, this constitutes VT.)

**Identification of the underlying rhythm** may be difficult; seek expert help. Diagnosis is based on the history (IHD increases the likelihood of a ventricular arrhythmia), a 12-lead ECG, and the lack of response to IV adenosine (p120). ECG findings in favour of VT:
- Positive QRS concordance in chest leads
- Marked left axis deviation
- AV dissociation (occurs in 25%) or 2:1 or 3:1 AV block
- Fusion beats or capture beats (fig 2)
- Also bear in mind the hard-to-remember QRS Brugada criteria (see BOX)

*Concordance* means QRS complexes are all +ve or -ve. *A fusion beat* is when a 'normal beat' fuses with a VT complex to create an unusual complex, and a *capture beat* is a normal QRS between abnormal beats (see fig 1).

**Management** Connect to a cardiac monitor; have a defibrillator to hand.

*Ventricular fibrillation (VF) Pulseless or unstable VT* ►► Use asynchronized DC shock (p784): see also the European Resuscitation Guidelines (see inside back cover).

*Stable VT:*
- Give high-flow oxygen by face mask.
- Obtain IV access. Send U&E, cardiac enzymes, Ca²⁺, Mg²⁺. Correct low K⁺or Mg²⁺.
- Obtain 12-lead ECG.
- ABG (if evidence of pulmonary oedema, reduced conscious level, sepsis).
- Amiodarone IVI as on page 124. Phlebitis may result if peripheral line used, especially if concentration >2mg/mL. Rarely, lidocaine 50mg over 2min instead, followed by infusion; see BNF.
- If polymorphic (torsade de pointes) magnesium sulphate 2g over 5min.
- If this fails, or if cardiac arrest, use DC shock (p806 and inside back cover).
- After correction of VT, establish the cause from history/investigations.
- Maintenance antiarrhythmic therapy may be required, eg amiodarone.
- Prevention of recurrent VT: implantation of automatic defibrillators (ICD) may help. In refractory cases radiofrequency ventricular tachycardia ablation may be tried.

*Ventricular extrasystoles (ectopics)* are the commonest post-MI arrhythmia; they are also seen in health (≥10/h). Post-MI they suggest electrical instability, and the risk is VF if the 'R on T' pattern (ie no gap before the T wave) is seen (see fig 1). If frequent (>10/min), consider amiodarone IV as above. Otherwise, just observe patient.

*Torsade de pointes:* Looks like VF but is VT with varying axis (see fig 4). It is due to ↑QT interval (an SE of antiarrhythmics, so consider stopping). ℞: magnesium sulphate, 2g IV over 10min ± overdrive pacing.

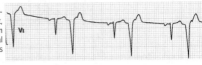

Fig 1. Ventricular extrasystoles may be intermittent, or have a fixed association with the preceding normal beat, ie 1:2 (bigeminy, as here) or 1:3 (trigeminy).

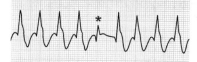

**(a) A capture beat (✱).**

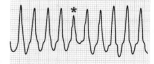

**(b) A fusion beat (✱).**

Fig 2. Fusion and capture beats.

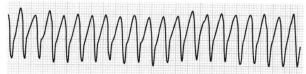

Fig 3. VT with a rate of 235/min.

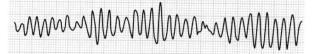

Fig 4. VF (p806).

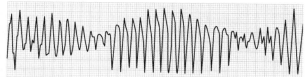

Fig 5. *Torsade de pointes* tachycardia.

## The Brugada criteria may help differentiate SVT from VT...[46]

| Broad complexes + RBBB-like QRS | Broad complexes + LBBB-like QRS |
|---|---|
| *Lead V₁:* | *Lead V₁ or V₂:* |
| • Monophasic R or QR or RS favours VT | Any of these: |
| • Triphasic RSR favours SVT | • R >30ms |
| *Lead V₆:* | • >60ms to nadir S |
| • R to S ratio <1 (R wave < S wave) favours VT | • Notched S favours VT |
| • QS or QR favours VT | *Lead V₆:* |
| • Monophasic R favours VT | • Presence of any Q wave, QR or QS |
| • Triphasic favours SVT | favours VT |
| • R to S ratio >1 (R wave > S wave) favours SVT | • No Q wave in lead V₆ favours SVT |

A chaotic, irregular atrial rhythm at 300–600bpm; the AV node responds intermittently, hence an irregular ventricular rate. Cardiac output drops by 10–20% as the ventricles aren't primed reliably by the atria. AF is common in the elderly (≤9%). The main risk is embolic stroke. Warfarin reduces this to 1%/yr from 4%. So, *do an ECG on everyone with an irregular pulse* (±24h ECG if dizzy, faints, palpitations, etc.).

**Causes** Heart failure/ischaemia; hypertension; MI (seen in 22%);[48] PE; mitral valve disease; pneumonia; hyperthyroidism; caffeine; alcohol; post-op; K+↓; Mg²⁺↓.[49] *Rare causes:* Cardiomyopathy; constrictive pericarditis; sick sinus syndrome; lung ca.; atrial myxoma; endocarditis; haemochromatosis; sarcoid. 'Lone' AF means no cause found.

**Symptoms** May be asymptomatic or cause chest pain, palpitations, dyspnoea, or faintness. **Signs** *Irregularly irregular pulse*, the apical pulse rate is greater than the radial rate and the 1ˢᵗ heart sound is of variable intensity; signs of LVF (p812). ▶Examine the whole patient: AF is *often* associated with non-cardiac disease.

**Tests** *ECG* shows absent P waves, irregular QRS complexes. *Blood tests:* U&E, cardiac enzymes, thyroid function tests. Consider echo to look for left atrial enlargement, mitral valve disease, poor LV function, and other structural abnormalities.

### Acute AF (≤48h)

If *very ill* or *haemodynamically unstable:* ▶▶O₂ ▶▶U&E ▶▶Emergency cardioversion; if unavailable try IV amiodarone. Do not delay treatment in order to start anticoagulation. Treat associated illnesses (eg MI, pneumonia). Control ventricular rate: 1ˢᵗ-line **verapamil** (40–120mg/8h PO) *or* **bisoprolol** (2.5–5.0mg/d PO). 2ⁿᵈ-line: **digoxin** or **amiodarone**. Start full anticoagulation with LMWH, to keep options open for cardioversion even if the 48h time limit is running out.[50] If the 48h period has elapsed, cardioversion is OK if transoesophageal echo thrombus-free.

*Cardioversion regimen:* ▶▶O₂ ▶▶ITU/CCU ▶▶GA or IV sedation, monophasic ▶▶200J ▶▶360J ▶▶360J (biphasic: 200J). Relapses back into AF are common. *Drug cardioversion* is often preferred: **amiodarone** IVI (5mg/kg over 1h then ~900mg over 24h via a central line) or PO (200mg/8h for 1wk, 200mg/12h for 1wk, 100–200mg/24h maintenance). Alternative (if stable and no known IHD or WPW p120): **flecainide** (a strong negative inotrope) 2mg/kg IV over 10–30min, max 150mg (or 300mg PO stat); monitor ECG.

### Chronic AF

Main goals in managing permanent AF are *rate control* and *anticoagulation*. Rate control is at least as good as rhythm control,[51] but rhythm control may be appropriate if • symptomatic or CCF • younger • presenting for 1ˢᵗ time with lone AF • AF from a corrected precipitant (eg U&E↓). *Anticoagulation* see BOX 1.

*Rate control* β-blocker or rate-limiting Ca²⁺ blocker are 1ˢᵗ choice. If this fails, add **digoxin** (p108), then consider **amiodarone**. Digoxin as monotherapy in chronic AF is only OK in sedentary patients. ▶*Don't give β-blockers with diltiazem or verapamil without expert advice (bradycardia risk).* Don't get fixated on a single figure to aim at: dialogue with patients tells what works best and allows desired exercise levels, eg <90 at rest and on exertion 200-age (yrs) if ambulatory.

*Rhythm control* If cardioversion is chosen, do echo 1ˢᵗ; pre-treat for ≥4wks with **sotalol** or **amiodarone** if there is ↑risk of cardioversion failure (past failure, or past recurrence). Pharmacological cardioversion: **flecainide** is 1ˢᵗ choice if no structural heart disease (IV **amiodarone** if structural heart disease). AV node ablation, maze procedure, pacing, and pulmonary vein ablation are options to ask about.[52]

*Paroxysmal AF* 'pill in the pocket' (eg **sotalol** or **flecainide** PRN) may be tried if: infrequent AF, BP >100mmHg systolic, no past LV dysfunction. Anticoagulate (BOX 1).

**Atrial flutter** *ECG:* continuous atrial depolarization (eg ~300/min, but very variable) produces a sawtooth baseline ± 2 : 1 AV block (as if SVT at, eg 150bpm). **Carotid sinus massage** and IV **adenosine** transiently block the AV node and may unmask flutter waves. *Treatment:* Cardioversion may be indicated (anticoagulate before, see p125). Anti-AF drugs may not work—but consider amiodarone to restore sinus rhythm, and amiodarone or sotalol to maintain it. Aim to control rate as above; if the IV route is needed, a β-blocker is preferred (eg p819). Rarely, cavotricuspid isthmus ablation.[6]

## Anticoagulation and AF

**Acute AF:** Use *heparin* until a full risk assessment for emboli (see below) is made—eg AF started <48h ago and elective cardioversion is being planned (if >48h, ensure ≥3wks of therapeutic anticoagulation before elective cardioversion; NB trans-oesophageal-guided cardioversion is also an option here). Use *warfarin* (target INR: 2.5; range 2-3) if risk of emboli **high** (past ischaemic stroke, TIA or emboli; ≥75yrs with BP↑, DM; coronary or peripheral arterial disease; evidence of valve disease or ↓LV function/CCF—only do echo if unsure).[53] Use *no anticoagulation* if *stable* sinus rhythm has been restored **and** no risk factors for emboli, and AF recurrence unlikely (ie no failed cardioversions, no structural heart disease, no previous recurrences, no sustained AF for >1yr).

**Chronic AF:** Anticoagulate with *warfarin* and aim for an INR of 2-3.[54] Less good alternative is *aspirin* ~300mg/d PO—eg if warfarin contraindicated or at very low risk of emboli (<65yrs, and no hypertension, diabetes, LV dysfunction, ↑LA size, rheumatic valve disease, MI, or past TIA). *CI to warfarin in AF:*[55] Bleeding diathesis; platelets <50×10⁹/L; BP>160/90 (consistently); compliance issues around dosing or INR monitoring; patient choice, after risks discussed. Factors such as age ≥75-80yrs old, frequent falls, on NSAIDs, past intracranial bleeds, Hb↓, and polypharmacy may be considered CI but are less evidence-based. Risk of major bleeds is ~13/100-person-yrs if ≥80yrs old (4 if <80yrs).[56,57] ►Discuss with patient: let him decide. The CHA₂DS₂-VASc[58] score quantifies risk of stroke and may help in decision making. *Dabigatran:* This is a direct thrombin inhibitor which doesn't need regular lab monitoring and dose adjustment. Despite its expense, it may be an alternative to warfarin (eg if warfarin is declined or has SE/CI, or monitoring INR is intrusive). In one trial, 110mg/12h PO was as good as warfarin in preventing stroke and emboli in AF, and it caused fewer bleeding problems.[59] CI: severe renal/ liver impairment; active bleeding; lesion at risk of bleeding; ↓clotting factors. Warn to report signs of bleeding. Interactions: heparin, clopidogrel, NSAIDs, GPIIb/IIIa antagonists, p-glycoprotein inhibitors (verapamil, amiodarone, clarithromycin), etc. ↓Dose if eGFR <50 (avoid if <30).

## CHA2DS2-VASc SCORE [58]

- Score 1 point for each of: heart failure, diabetes, hypertension, vascular disease, aged>65, female; AND 2 points for: age ≥75, or prior TIA, stroke/thromboembolism. A score of 2 = an annual stroke risk of ~2.2%.
- If the score is 1 or more (or 2 or more if older) consider oral anticoagulation.

Bleeding risk can also be calculated, eg HEMORR2HAGES or HAS-BLED scores. See also CHADS2 score (p477)

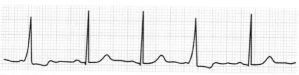

**Fig 1.** Wolff-Parkinson-White (WPW) syndrome. ECG of WPW syndrome (p120) in 1ˢᵗ and 4ᵗʰ beats; compared with the other beats, it can be seen how the delta wave both broadens the ventricular complex and shortens the PR interval. ► If WPW is the underlying cause of AF, avoid AV node blockers such as diltiazem, verapamil and digoxin—but flecainide may be used.

Cardiovascular medicine

Pacemakers supply electrical initiation to myocardial contraction. The pacemaker lies subcutaneously where it may be programmed through the skin as necessary. Pacemakers usually last 5-10yrs, but usually only the box needs replacing.

### Indications for temporary cardiac pacing
- Symptomatic bradycardia, unresponsive to atropine.
- After acute *anterior* MI, prophylactic pacing is required in:
  - Complete AV block
  - Mobitz type I AV block (Wenckebach)
  - Mobitz type II AV block
  - Non-adjacent bifascicular,[1] or trifascicular block (p94).
- After *inferior* MI, pacing may not be needed in complete AV block if reasonably stable, rate is >40-50, and QRS complexes are narrow.
- Suppression of drug-resistant tachyarrhythmias, eg SVT, VT.
- Special situations: During general anaesthesia; during cardiac surgery; during electrophysiological studies; drug overdose (eg digoxin, β-blockers, verapamil).
▶See p790 for further details and insertion technique.

### Indications for a permanent pacemaker
- Complete AV block (Stokes-Adams attacks, asymptomatic, congenital)
- Mobitz type II AV block (p119)
- Persistent AV block after anterior MI
- Symptomatic bradycardias (eg sick sinus syndrome, p118)
- Heart failure (cardiac resynchronization)
- Drug-resistant tachyarrhythmias

Some say persistent bifascicular block after MI requires a permanent system: this remains controversial.

*Pre-operative assessment:* FBC, clotting screen, hepatitis B status. Insert IV cannula. Consent for procedure under local anaesthetic. Consider pre-medication. Give antibiotic cover (eg flucloxacillin 500mg IM and benzylpenicillin 600mg IM) 20min before, and 1 and 6h after.

*Post-op management:* Prior to discharge, check wound for bleeding or haematoma; check position on CXR; check pacemaker function. During 1st week, inspect for wound haematoma or dehiscence. Count apical rate (p37): if this is ≥6bpm below the rate quoted for the pacemaker, suspect malfunction. Other problems: lead fracture; pacemaker interference (eg from patient's muscles). Driving rules: p152.

*Pacemaker letter codes* These enable pacemaker identification (min is 3 letters):
- **1st letter** the chamber paced (A=atria, V=ventricles, D=dual chamber).
- **2nd letter** the chamber sensed (A=atria, V=ventricles, D=dual chamber, O=none).
- **3rd letter** the pacemaker response (T=triggered, I=inhibited, D=dual, R=reverse).
- **4th letter**, P=programmable; M=multiprogrammable.
- **5th letter**, P means that in tachycardia the pacemaker will pace the patient. S means that in tachycardia the pacemaker shocks the patient. D=dual ability to pace and shock. O=neither of these.
- VVI pacemakers are the most frequently used in the UK. DDD pacemakers are the only pacemakers that sense and pace both chambers.

*Cardiac resynchronization therapy (CRT)*[60] improves the synchronization of cardiac contraction and reduces mortality[61] in people with symptomatic heart failure who have an ejection fraction <35% and a QRS duration >120ms. It involves biventricular pacing (both septal and lateral walls of the LV) and if required also an atrial lead. It may be combined with a defibrillator.

*ECG of paced rhythm:* (ECG 7 p101, and fig 1 for rhythm strip) If the system is on 'demand' of 60bpm, a pacing spike is only seen if the intrinsic rate is <60. If seen at a higher rate, the sensing mode is malfunctioning. If it is not pacing at lower rates, the pacing mode is malfunctioning, eg lead dislodged, or faulty. If you see spikes but no capture (ie no systole), suspect dislodgement.

---

1 Non-adjacent = RBBB + L posterior hemiblock, or alternating bundle branch block (p94).

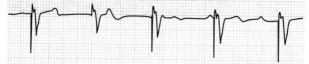

Fig 1. ECG of paced rhythm.

### Some confusing pacemaker terms

*Fusion beat:* Union of native depolarization and pacemaker impulse.

*Pseudofusion:* The pacemaker impulse occurs just after cardiac depolarization, so it is ineffective, but it distorts the QRS morphology.

*Pseudopseudofusion beat:* If a DVI pacemaker gives an atrial spike within a native QRS complex, the atrial output is non-contributory.

*Pacemaker syndrome:* In single-chamber pacing, retrograde conduction to the atria, which then contract during ventricular systole. This leads to retrograde flow in pulmonary veins, and ↓cardiac output, dyspnoea, palpitations, malaise, and even syncope.

*Pacemaker tachycardia:* In dual-chamber pacing, a short-circuit loop goes between the electrodes, causing an artificial WPW-like syndrome. Solution: Single-chamber pacing. For ECG images, see www.monroecc.edu./depts/pstc/backup/paracar6.htm

**Definition** Cardiac output is inadequate for the body's requirements. Prognosis is poor with ~25-50% of patients dying within 5yrs of diagnosis.

**Prevalence** 1-3% of the general population; ~10% among elderly patients.[64]

**Systolic versus diastolic failure** *Systolic failure:* inability of the ventricle to contract normally, resulting in ↓cardiac output. Ejection fraction (EF) is <40%. Causes: IHD, MI, cardiomyopathy. *Diastolic failure:* inability of the ventricle to relax and fill normally, causing ↑filling pressures. EF is >50%. Causes: constrictive pericarditis, tamponade, restrictive cardiomyopathy, hypertension. NB: systolic and diastolic failure usually coexist.

**Left-sided versus right-sided failure** *Left ventricular failure* (LVF) and *right ventricular failure* (RVF) may occur independently, or together as *congestive cardiac failure* (CCF).

*Left ventricular failure:* Symptoms: Dyspnoea, poor exercise tolerance, fatigue, orthopnoea, paroxysmal nocturnal dyspnoea (PND), nocturnal cough (±pink frothy sputum), wheeze (cardiac 'asthma'), nocturia, cold peripheries, weight loss, muscle wasting.

*Right ventricular failure:* Causes: LVF, pulmonary stenosis, lung disease. Symptoms: Peripheral oedema (up to thighs, sacrum, abdominal wall), ascites, nausea, anorexia, facial engorgement, pulsation in neck and face (tricuspid regurgitation), epistaxis.

**Acute versus chronic heart failure** *Acute heart failure* is often used exclusively to mean new onset acute or decompensation of chronic heart failure characterized by pulmonary and/or peripheral oedema with or without signs of peripheral hypoperfusion. *Chronic heart failure* develops or progresses slowly. Venous congestion is common but arterial pressure is well maintained until very late.

**Low-output versus high-output failure** *Low-output heart failure:* Cardiac output is ↓ and fails to ↑normally with exertion. *Causes: Pump failure:* Systolic and/or diastolic HF (see above), ↓heart rate (eg β-blockers, heart block, post MI), negatively inotropic drugs (eg most antiarrhythmic agents). *Excessive preload:* eg mitral regurgitation or fluid overload (eg NSAID causing fluid retention). Fluid overload may cause LVF in a normal heart if renal excretion is impaired or big volumes are involved (eg IVI running too fast). More common if there is simultaneous compromise of cardiac function, and in the elderly. *Chronic excessive afterload:* eg aortic stenosis, hypertension.

*High-output heart failure:* This is rare. Here, output is normal or increased in the face of ↑↑needs. Failure occurs when cardiac output fails to meet these needs. It will occur with a normal heart, but even earlier if there is heart disease. *Causes:* Anaemia, pregnancy, hyperthyroidism, Paget's disease, arteriovenous malformation, beri beri. *Consequences:* Initially features of RVF; later LVF becomes evident.

**Signs** To diagnose there should be symptoms of failure and objective evidence of cardiac dysfunction (at rest). Diagnosis can be made using *Framingham* criteria (see BOX).[65] Other signs: exhaustion, cool peripheries, cyanosis, ↓BP, narrow pulse pressure, pulsus alternans, displaced apex (LV dilatation), RV heave (pulmonary hypertension), murmurs of mitral or aortic valve disease, wheeze (cardiac asthma).

**Investigations** According to NICE,[62] if ECG and B-type natriuretic peptide (BNP; p131) are normal, heart failure is unlikely, and an alternative diagnosis should be considered; if either is abnormal, then echocardiography (p106) is required.

*Tests:* FBC; U&E; BNP; *CXR:* cardiomegaly (cardiothoracic ratio >50%), prominent upper lobe veins (upper lobe diversion), peribronchial cuffing, diffuse interstitial or alveolar shadowing, classical perihilar 'bat's wing' shadowing, fluid in the fissures, pleural effusions, septal (formerly called 'Kerley B') lines (variously attributed to interstitial oedema[66] and engorged peripheral lymphatics[67]). ECG may indicate cause (look for evidence of ischaemia, MI, or ventricular hypertrophy). It is rare to get a completely normal ECG in chronic heart failure. *Echocardiography* is the key investigation.[68] It may indicate the cause (MI, valvular heart disease) and can confirm the presence or absence of LV dysfunction. *Endomyocardial biopsy* is rarely needed.

**Prognosis** If admission is needed, 5yr mortality≈75%. Don't be dogmatic: in one study, 54% of those dying in the next 72h had been expected to live for >6months.[69]

## Framingham criteria for congestive cardiac failure (CCF)

Diagnosis of CCF requires the simultaneous presence of at least 2 major criteria or 1 major criterion in conjunction with 2 minor criteria.

**Major criteria**
- Paroxysmal nocturnal dyspnoea
- Crepitations
- S₃ gallop
- Neck vein distention
- Acute pulmonary oedema
- Hepatojugular reflux
- Cardiomegaly (cardiothoracic ratio >50% on chest radiography)
- Increased central venous pressure (>16cmH₂0 at right atrium)
- Weight loss >4.5kg in 5 days in response to treatment

**Minor criteria**
- Bilateral ankle oedema
- Dyspnoea on ordinary exertion
- Tachycardia (heart rate >120/min)
- Nocturnal cough
- Hepatomegaly
- Pleural effusion
- Decrease in vital capacity by ⅓ from maximum recorded

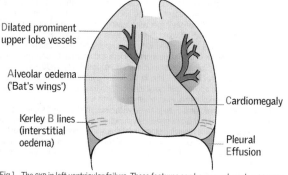

Dilated prominent upper lobe vessels

Alveolar oedema ('Bat's wings')

Kerley B lines (interstitial oedema)

Cardiomegaly

Pleural Effusion

Fig 1. The CXR in left ventricular failure. These features can be remembered as A B C D E. See also Fig 2 p737.

*Cardiovascular medicine*

**Acute heart failure** ▸▸This is a medical emergency (p812).

**Chronic heart failure** ▸Stop smoking. Eat less salt. Optimize weight & nutrition.
• Treat the cause (eg if dysrhythmias; valve disease).
• Treat exacerbating factors (anaemia, thyroid disease, infection, ↑BP).
• Avoid exacerbating factors, eg NSAIDs (fluid retention) and verapamil (-ve inotrope).
• Drugs: the following are used:

 1 *Diuretics:* Diuretics can reduce the risk of death and worsening heart failure.[70]
 Give loop diuretics to relieve symptoms, eg **furosemide** 40mg/24h PO or **bumetanide** 1-2mg/24h PO. Increase dose as necessary. SE: K⁺↓, renal impairment.
 Monitor U&E and add K⁺-sparing diuretic (eg **spironolactone**) if K⁺ <3.2mmol/L,
 predisposition to arrhythmias, concurrent digoxin therapy (↓K⁺ increases risk
 of digoxin toxicity), or pre-existing K⁺-losing conditions. If refractory oedema,
 consider adding a thiazide, eg **metolazone** 5-20mg/24h PO.

 2 *ACE-i:* Consider in all those with left ventricular systolic dysfunction; improves
 symptoms and prolongs life (see p108). If cough is a problem, an *angiotensin
 receptor blocker* (ARB) may be substituted (eg **candesartan** 4mg/d; max 32mg
 PO). SE: ↑K⁺.

 3 *β-blockers* (eg **carvedilol**) decrease mortality in heart failure.[71] These benefits
 appear to be additional to those of ACE-i in patients with heart failure due to
 LV dysfunction.[72] Initiate after diuretic and ACE-i. Use with caution: 'start low
 and go slow'; if in doubt seek specialist advice first (eg carvedilol 3.125mg/12h
 → 25-50mg/12h); wait ≥2weeks between each dose increment. Beta-blocker
 therapy in patients hospitalized with decompensated heart failure is associated with lower post-discharge mortality risk and improved treatment rates.[73]

 4 *Spironolactone:* Spironolactone (25mg/24h PO) ↓mortality by 30% when added to conventional therapy.[74] Use in those still symptomatic despite optimal
 therapy as listed above. Spironolactone is K⁺-sparing, but there is little risk of
 significant hyperkalaemia, even when given with ACE-i.

 5 *Digoxin* helps symptoms even in those with sinus rhythm,[75] and should be considered for patients with LV systolic dysfunction who have signs or symptoms
 of heart failure while receiving standard therapy, including ACE-i and β-blockers,
 or in patients with AF. Dose example: 125μg/24h PO if sinus rhythm. Monitor U&E;
 maintain K⁺ at 4-5mmol/L. Digoxin levels: p766. Other inotropes are unhelpful
 in terms of outcome.

 6 *Vasodilators:* The combination of **hydralazine** (SE: drug-induced lupus) and
 **isosorbide dinitrate** should be used if intolerant of ACE-i and ARBs as it reduces
 mortality. It also reduces mortality when added to standard therapy (including
 ACE-i) in Black patients with heart failure.[76]

**Intractable heart failure** Reassess the cause. Are they taking the drugs?—at maxi-
mum dose? Switching furosemide to **bumetanide** (one 5mg tab≈200mg furosemide)
might help: absorption may be better.[77] Consider admitting for:
• Strict bed rest ± Na⁺ & fluid restriction (≤1.5L/24h PO).[78,79]
• Metolazone (as above) and IV furosemide (p812).
• Opiates and IV nitrates may relieve symptoms (p812).
• Weigh daily. Do frequent U&E (beware K⁺↓).
• Give DVT prophylaxis: heparin + TED stockings (p580).

*In extremis*, try IV inotropes (p814; it may be difficult to wean patients off them).

*Consider* cardiac resynchronization (p126), LV assist device, or transplantation.

**Palliative care** Treat/prevent comorbidities (eg flu vaccination). Good nutrition
(allow alcohol!). Involve GP: continuity of care and discussion of prognosis is much
appreciated.[80] Dyspnoea, pain (from liver capsule stretching), nausea, constipation,
and ↓mood all need tackling.[81] Opiates help pain and dyspnoea. O₂ may help.

## New York classification of heart failure: summary

**I** Heart disease present, but no undue dyspnoea from ordinary activity.
**II** Comfortable at rest; dyspnoea on ordinary activities.
**III** Less than ordinary activity causes dyspnoea, which is limiting.
**IV** Dyspnoea present at rest; all activity causes discomfort.

## Natriuretic peptides

Secretory granules have long been known to exist in the atria, and if homogenized atrial tissue is injected into rats, their urine volume (and $Na^+$ excretion) rises. This is evidence of endocrine action via the effects of atrial natriuretic peptide (ANP). BNP is a similar hormone originally identified from pig brain (hence the B), but most BNP is secreted from ventricular myocardium. Plasma BNP is closely related to LV pressure. In MI and LV dysfunction, these hormones can be released in large quantities. Secretion is also increased by tachycardia, glucocorticoids, and thyroid hormones. Vasoactive peptides (endothelin-1, angiotensin II) also influence secretion. ANP and BNP both increase GFR and decrease renal $Na^+$ resorption; they also decrease preload by relaxing smooth muscle. ANP partly blocks secretion of renin and aldosterone.

**BNP as a biomarker of heart failure** [82,83,84] As plasma BNP reflects myocyte stretch, BNP is used to diagnose heart failure. ↑BNP distinguishes heart failure from other causes of dyspnoea more accurately than LV ejection fraction, ANP, and N-terminal ANP (sensitivity: >90%; specificity: 80–90%). BNP is highest in decompensated heart failure, intermediate in left ventricular dysfunction but no acute heart failure exacerbation, and lowest if no heart failure or LV dysfunction.

*What BNP threshold for diagnosing heart failure?* If BNP >100ng/L, this 'diagnoses' heart failure better than other clinical variables or clinical judgement (history, examination, and CXR). BNP can be used to 'rule out' heart failure if <50ng/L—negative predictive value (PV) 96%, ie the chance of a negative test when there is really heart failure present is only 4%, see p672.

In those with heart failure, BNP is higher in systolic dysfunction than in isolated diastolic dysfunction (eg hypertrophic or dilated cardiomyopathy), and is highest in those with systolic *and* diastolic dysfunction. BNP also increases in proportion to right ventricular dysfunction, eg in primary pulmonary hypertension, cor pulmonale, PE, and congenital heart disease, but rises are less than in left ventricular disorders.

*Prognosis in heart failure:* The higher the BNP, the higher the cardiovascular and all-cause mortality (independent of age, NYHA class, previous MI and LV ejection fraction). ↑BNP in heart failure is also associated with sudden death. Serial testing may be important: persistently ↑BNP despite vigorous antifailure treatment predicts adverse outcomes. In one study, those with heart failure randomized to get N-terminal BNP-guided (rather than symptom-guided) therapy had ↓adverse events.

*Prognosis in angina and MI:* BNP has some prognostic value here (adverse left ventricular remodelling; LV dysfunction; death post-MI). [85]

*Cautions with BNP:* A BNP >50ng/L does not exclude other co-existing diseases such as pneumonia. Also, assays vary, so liaise with your lab.

Hypertension[88] is a major risk factor for stroke and MI. It is usually asymptomatic, and regular screening (eg 3-yrly) is a *vital* primary care task. It causes ~50% of all vascular deaths ($8×10^6$/yr). Most preventable deaths are in areas without universal screening.[87]

**Defining hypertension** Blood pressure has a skewed normal distribution (p765) within the population, and risk is continuously related to blood pressure, so it is impossible to define 'hypertension'.[88] We choose to select a value above which risk is significantly increased and the benefit of treatment is clear cut, see below. Assess BP over a period of time (don't rely on a single reading). The 'observation' period depends on the BP and the presence of other risk factors or end-organ damage.

**Whom to treat** All with BP ≥160/100mmHg (sustained; p133). For those ≥140/90, the decision depends on the risk of coronary events, presence of diabetes or end-organ damage; see fig 1. The recent HYVET study showed that there is even substantial benefit in treating the over-80s.[89]

*Isolated systolic hypertension (ISH):* The most common form of hypertension in the UK—affects >50% of the over-60s. ISH results from stiffening of the large arteries (arteriosclerosis). It is not benign: doubles risk of MI, triples risk of CVA. Treatment reduces this excess risk and is as, if not more, effective than treating moderate hypertension in middle-aged patients.

*'Malignant' or accelerated phase hypertension:* Refers to a rapid rise in BP leading to vascular damage (pathological hallmark is fibrinoid necrosis). Usually there is severe hypertension (eg systolic >200, diastolic>130mmHg) + bilateral retinal haemorrhages and exudates; papilloedema may or may not be present. Symptoms are common, eg headache ± visual disturbance. Alone it requires urgent treatment. It may also precipitate acute renal failure, heart failure, or encephalopathy, which are hypertensive emergencies. Untreated, 90% die in 1yr; treated, 70% survive 5yrs. It is more common in younger patients and in black patients. Look hard for any underlying cause.

*Essential hypertension* (primary, cause unknown). ~95% of cases.

*Secondary hypertension* ~5% of cases. Causes include:
• *Renal disease:* The most common secondary cause. 75% are from *intrinsic renal disease:* glomerulonephritis, polyarteritis nodosa (PAN), systemic sclerosis, chronic pyelonephritis, or polycystic kidneys. 25% are due to *renovascular disease,* most frequently atheromatous (elderly ♂ cigarette smokers, eg with peripheral vascular disease) or rarely fibromuscular dysplasia (young ♀).
• *Endocrine disease:* Cushing's (p216) and Conn's syndromes (p220), phaeochromocytoma (p220), acromegaly, hyperparathyroidism.
• *Others:* Coarctation (p150), pregnancy (OHCS p48), steroids, MAOI, 'the Pill'.

**Signs & symptoms** Usually asymptomatic (except malignant hypertension, above). Headache is no more common than in the general population. Always examine the CVS fully and check for retinopathy. Are there features of an underlying cause (phaeochromocytoma, p220, etc.), signs of renal disease, radiofemoral delay, or weak femoral pulses (coarctation), renal bruits, palpable kidneys, or Cushing's syndrome? Look for end-organ damage: LVH, retinopathy and proteinuria—indicates severity and duration of hypertension and associated with a poorer prognosis.

**Tests** To help quantify overall risk: Fasting glucose; cholesterol. *To look for end-organ damage:* ECG (any LV hypertrophy? past MI?); urine analysis (protein, blood). *To 'exclude' secondary causes:* U&E (eg K↓ in Conn's); $Ca^{2+}$ (↑ in hyperparathyroidism). *Special tests:* Renal ultrasound/arteriography (renal artery stenosis); 24h urinary metanephrines (p220); urinary free cortisol (p217); renin; aldosterone; MR aorta (coarctation). *24h ambulatory BP monitoring* (ABPM) may help sometimes, eg in 'white coat' or borderline hypertension, and is now recommended for all newly diagnosed hypertensive. Ambulatory readings are always lower; add on 10/5mmHg (but NICE suggests simply 5/5) to 'convert' to clinic pressures for decision-making. *Echocardiography* may be useful to assess end-organ damage (LV hypertrophy)

## Grading hypertensive retinopathy

**I** Tortuous arteries with thick shiny walls (silver or copper wiring, p562, fig 1)
**II** A-V nipping (narrowing where arteries cross veins, p562, fig 2)
**III** Flame haemorrhages and cotton-wool spots
**IV** Papilloedema, p562, fig 3.

## Measuring BP with a sphygmomanometer

• Use the correct size cuff. The cuff width should be >40% of the arm circumference. The bladder should be centred over the brachial artery, and the cuff applied snugly. Support the arm in a horizontal position at mid-sternal level.
• Inflate the cuff while palpating the brachial artery, until the pulse disappears. This provides an estimate of systolic pressure.
• Inflate the cuff until 30mmHg above systolic pressure, then place stethoscope over the brachial artery. Deflate the cuff at 2mmHg/s.
• *Systolic pressure:* appearance of sustained repetitive tapping sounds (Korotkoff I).
• *Diastolic pressure:* usually the disappearance of sounds (Korotkoff V). However, in some individuals (eg pregnant women) sounds are present until the zero point. In this case, the muffling of sounds, Korotkoff IV, should be used. State which is used for a given reading. For children, see *OHCS* p156.
• For advice on using automated sphygmomanometers and a list of validated devices see http://www.bhsoc.org/how_to_measure_blood_pressure.stm.

## Managing suspected hypertension[86]

```
┌─────────────────────┐  ┌─────────────────────┐  ┌─────────────────────┐
│ Clinic blood pressure│  │ Clinic blood pressure│  │ Clinic blood pressure│
│    <140/90mmHg      │  │    ≥140/90mmHg      │  │    ≥180/110mmHg     │
│    Normotensive     │  │                     │  │                     │
└─────────────────────┘  └─────────────────────┘  └─────────────────────┘
                                                              │
                                                              ▼
                                              ┌─────────────────────────┐
                                              │   Consider starting     │
                                              │ antihypertensive drug   │
                                              │  treatment immediately. │
                                              │   Consider referral.    │
                                              └─────────────────────────┘
                                                              │
                                   ┌──────────────────────────────────────┐
                                   │          Offer ABPM.                 │
                                   │ Calculate cv risk and look for       │
                                   │         organ damage.                │
                                   └──────────────────────────────────────┘

┌─────────────────────┐  ┌─────────────────────┐  ┌─────────────────────┐
│  ABPM <135/85mmHg   │  │  ABPM ≥135/85mmHg   │  │  ABPM ≥150/95mmHg   │
│    Normotensive     │  │ Stage 1 hypertension│  │ Stage 2 hypertension│
│ NICE says no Rx.    │  │ Rx if cv risk       │  │        Rx           │
│ Consider Rx if clear│  │ >20%/10yrs or end   │  │                     │
│ end-organ damage or │  │   organ damage      │  │                     │
│   high risk.        │  │                     │  │                     │
└─────────────────────┘  └─────────────────────┘  └─────────────────────┘
```

**Fig 1.** Managing suspected hypertension.

Target pressure is <140/90mmHg (150/90 if aged >80), but in diabetes mellitus aim for <130/80mmHg, and <125/75 if proteinuria. To quantify cv risk, see www.bhsoc.org. NB: cv threshold of 20% ≈ 15% for CHD alone. Examples of target (end-organ) damage: • LVH • PMH of MI or angina • PMH of stroke/TIA • Peripheral vascular disease • Renal failure.

Adapted from NICE CG127, 2011, with permission.

Cardiovascular medicine

Look for and treat underlying causes[86] (eg renal disease, alcohol†: see p132). Drug therapy reduces the risk of cardiovascular disease and death. Almost any adult over 50 would benefit from the antihypertensives below, *whatever their starting BP*.[90] Treatment is especially important if: BP is persistently ≥160/100mmHg or cardiovascular risk ↑ (10yr risk of vascular disease ≥20%) or existing vascular disease or target organ damage (eg brain, kidney, heart, retina) with BP >140/90mmHg. Essential hypertension is not 'curable' and long-term treatment is needed.

**Treatment goal** <140/90mmHg (<130/80 in diabetes, 150/90 if aged >80). Reduce blood pressure *slowly*; rapid reduction can be fatal, especially in the context of an acute stroke.

**Lifestyle changes** ↓Concomitant risk factors: stop smoking; low-fat diet. Reduce alcohol and salt intake; increase exercise; reduce weight if obese.

**Drugs** The ALLHAT study suggests that adequate BP reduction is more important than the specific drug used.[91] However, β-blockers seem to be less effective than a comparator drug at reducing major cardiovascular events, particularly stroke. β-blockers and thiazides may increase the risk of new onset diabetes, Ca²⁺ channel blockers appear neutral, and ACE-i or ARB may reduce the risk.[92]

*Monotherapy* If ≥55yrs, and in Black patients of any age, 1ˢᵗ choice is a Ca²⁺ channel blocker or thiazide. If <55, 1ˢᵗ choice is ACE-i (or ARB if ACE-i intolerant, eg cough). β-blockers are not 1ˢᵗ-line for hypertension, but consider in younger people, particularly: if intolerance or contraindication to ACE-i/ARB (angiotensin receptor blockers) exists, or she is a women of child-bearing potential, or there is ↑sympathetic drive.

*Combination therapy* ACE-i + a Ca²⁺-channel blocker or diuretic is logical, and has been commonly done in trials. There is little evidence on using 3 drugs so the recommendation is based on the most straightforward option:[92] try ACE-i, Ca²⁺-channel blocker and thiazide. If BP still uncontrolled on adequate doses of 3 drugs, add a 4ᵗʰ (consider: higher-dose thiazide, or another diuretic, eg spironolactone (monitor U&E), or β-blockers, or selective α-blockers) and get help. If only on a β-blocker and a 2ⁿᵈ drug is needed, add a Ca²⁺ blocker, not a thiazide, to ↓ risk of developing diabetes.

*Dose examples Thiazides:* eg chlortalidone 25-50mg/24h PO *mane*. SE: K⁺↓, Na⁺↓, impotence. CI: gout. *Ca²⁺-channel blockers:* eg nifedipine MR, 30-60mg/24h PO. SE: flushes, fatigue, gum hyperplasia, ankle oedema; avoid short-acting form. *ACE-i:* eg lisinopril 10-40mg/24h PO (max 40mg/d). ACE-i may be 1ˢᵗ choice if co-existing LVF, or in diabetics (esp. if microalbuminuria, p309) or proteinuria. *SE:* cough, K⁺↑, renal failure, angio-oedema. CI: bilateral renal artery or valve stenosis; p109. *ARB:* Candesartan (8-32mg/d); caution if valve disease or cardiomyopathy; monitor K⁺. SE: vertigo, urticaria, pruritus. *Direct renin inhibitors:* aliskiren (150-300mg/d); monitor K⁺. SE: diarrhoea, rash, ↑K⁺. Avoid in CRF, DM, and with ACE-i or ARB. *β-blockers:* eg bisoprolol 2.5-5mg/24h PO. SE: bronchospasm, heart failure, cold peripheries, lethargy, impotence. CI: asthma; caution in heart failure. Consider *aspirin* when BP controlled, if aged >55yrs. Add a *statin* (p704, esp. if other risk factors). ▶Most drugs take 4-8wks to gain maximum effect: don't assess efficacy with just one BP measurement.

**Malignant hypertension** In general, use oral therapy, unless there is encephalopathy or CCF. The aim is for a controlled reduction in blood pressure over days, not hours. Avoid sudden drops in BP as cerebral autoregulation is poor (so stroke risk↑). Bed rest; there is no ideal hypotensive, but atenolol or long-acting Ca²⁺ blockers may be used PO.

*Encephalopathy* (headache, focal CNS signs, seizures, coma): aim to reduce BP to ~110mmHg diastolic over 4h. Admit to monitored area. Insert intra-arterial line for pressure monitoring. Furosemide 40-80mg IV; then either IV labetalol (eg 50mg IV over 1min, repeated every 5min, max 200mg) or sodium nitroprusside infusion (0.5μg/kg/min IVI titrated up to 8μg/kg/min, eg 50mg in 1L glucose 5%; expect to give 100-200mL/h for a few hours only, to avoid cyanide risk).

▶Never use sublingual nifedipine to reduce BP (∵ big drop in BP and stroke risk).[93]

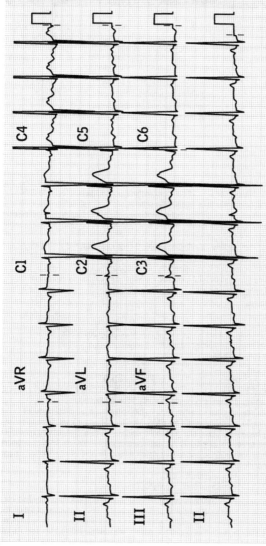

ECG 8—Left ventricular hypertrophy—this is from a patient with malignant hypertension—note the sum of the s-wave in C2 and R-wave in C6 is greater than 35mm.

Cardiovascular medicine

This systemic infection is still common in developing countries but increasingly rare in the West. Peak incidence: 5-15yrs. Tends to recur unless prevented. Pharyngeal infection with Lancefield group A β-haemolytic streptococci triggers rheumatic fever 2-4wks later, in the susceptible 2% of the population. An antibody to the carbohydrate cell wall of the streptococcus cross-reacts with valve tissue (antigenic mimicry) and may cause permanent damage to the heart valves.

**Diagnosis** Use the revised Jones criteria (may be over-rigorous). There must be evidence of recent strep infection plus 2 major criteria, or 1 major + 2 minor.

*Evidence of group A β-haemolytic streptococcal infection:*
• Positive throat culture (but this is usually negative by the time symptoms of rheumatic fever appear)
• Rapid streptococcal antigen test +ve
• Elevated or rising streptococcal antibody titre (eg ASO or DNase B titre)
• Recent scarlet fever

*Major criteria:*
• *Carditis:* Tachycardia, murmurs (mitral or aortic regurgitation, Carey Coombs' murmur, p44), pericardial rub, CCF, cardiomegaly, conduction defects (45-70%). An apical systolic murmur may be the only sign.[94]
• *Arthritis:* A migratory, 'flitting' polyarthritis; usually affects larger joints (75%).
• *Subcutaneous nodules:* Small, mobile, painless nodules on extensor surfaces of joints and spine (2-20%).
• *Erythema marginatum:* (fig 1) Geographical-type rash with red, raised edges and clear centre; occurs mainly on trunk, thighs and arms in 2-10% (p564).
• *Sydenham's chorea (St Vitus' dance):* Occurs late in 10%. Unilateral or bilateral involuntary semi-purposeful movements. May be preceded by emotional lability and uncharacteristic behaviour.

*Minor criteria:*
• Fever
• Raised ESR or CRP
• Arthralgia (but not if arthritis is one of the major criteria)
• Prolonged PR interval (but not if carditis is major criterion)
• Previous rheumatic fever

**Management**
• Bed rest until CRP normal for 2wks (may be 3 months).
• Benzylpenicillin 0.6-1.2g IV stat, then penicillin V 250-500mg 4 times daily PO for 10 days (if allergic to penicillin, give erythromycin or azithromycin for 10 days).
• Analgesia for carditis/arthritis: aspirin 100mg/kg/d PO in divided doses (max 4-8g/d) for 2d, then 70mg/kg/d for 6wks. Monitor salicylate level. Toxicity causes tinnitus, hyperventilation, and metabolic acidosis. Alternative: NSAIDs (p548). If moderate-to-severe carditis is present (cardiomegaly, CCF, or 3rd-degree heart block), add oral prednisolone to salicylate therapy. In case of heart failure, treat appropriately (p130).
• Immobilize joints in severe arthritis.
• Haloperidol (0.5mg/8h PO) or diazepam for the chorea.

**Prognosis** 60% with carditis develop chronic rheumatic heart disease. This correlates with the severity of the carditis.[95] Acute attacks last an average of 3 months. Recurrence may be precipitated by further streptococcal infections, pregnancy, or use of the Pill. Cardiac sequelae affect mitral (70%), aortic (40%), tricuspid (10%), and pulmonary (2%) valves. Incompetent lesions develop during the attack, stenoses years later.

**Secondary prophylaxis** Penicillin V 250mg/12h PO. Alternatives: sulfadiazine 1g daily (0.5g if <30kg) or erythromycin 250mg twice daily (if penicillin allergic). *Duration:* If carditis+persistent valvular disease, continue at least until age of 40 (sometimes lifelong). If carditis but no valvular disease, continue for 10 yrs. If there is no carditis, 5 yrs prophylaxis (until age of 21) is sufficient.

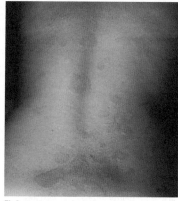

**Fig 1.** Erythema marginatum.
Image courtesy of Dr Maria Angelica Binotto.

Cardiovascular medicine

**Mitral stenosis** *Causes:* Rheumatic, congenital, mucopolysaccharidoses, endo-cardial fibroelastosis, malignant carcinoid (p278; rare), prosthetic valve.

*Presentation:* Normal mitral valve orifice area is ~4-6cm². Symptoms usually begin when the orifice becomes <2cm²: dyspnoea; fatigue; palpitations; chest pain; systemic emboli; haemoptysis; chronic bronchitis-like picture ± complications (below).

*Signs:* Malar flush on cheeks (due to ↓ cardiac output); low-volume pulse; AF common; tapping, non-displaced, apex beat (palpable S₁). On auscultation: loud S₁; opening snap (pliable valve); rumbling mid-diastolic murmur (heard best in expiration, with patient on left side). Graham Steell murmur (p44) may occur. *Severity:* The more severe the stenosis, the longer the diastolic murmur, and the closer the opening snap is to S₂.

*Tests: ECG:* AF; P-mitrale if in sinus rhythm; RVH; progressive RAD. *CXR:* left atrial enlargement (double shadow in right cardiac silhouette); pulmonary oedema; mitral valve calcification. *Echocardiography* is diagnostic. Significant stenosis exists if the valve orifice is <1cm²/m² body surface area. Indications for *cardiac catheterization:* previous valvotomy; signs of other valve disease; angina; severe pulmonary hypertension; calcified mitral valve.

*Management:* If in AF, *rate control* (p124) *is crucial;* anticoagulate with warfarin (p345). Diuretics ↓preload and pulmonary venous congestion. If this fails to control symptoms, balloon valvuloplasty (if pliable, non-calcified valve), open mitral valvotomy or valve replacement. SBE/IE prophylaxis for GI/GU infected procedures (p144). Oral penicillin as prophylaxis against recurrent rheumatic fever (p136).

*Complications:* Pulmonary hypertension, emboli, pressure from large LA on local structures, eg hoarseness (recurrent laryngeal nerve), dysphagia (oesophagus), bronchial obstruction; infective endocarditis (rare).

**Mitral regurgitation** *Causes:* Functional (LV dilatation); annular calcification (elderly); rheumatic fever, infective endocarditis, mitral valve prolapse, ruptured chordae tendinae; papillary muscle dysfunction/rupture; connective tissue disorders (Ehlers-Danlos, Marfan's); cardiomyopathy; congenital (may be associated with other defects, eg ASD, AV canal); appetite suppressants (eg fenfluramine, phentermine).

*Symptoms:* Dyspnoea; fatigue; palpitations; infective endocarditis. *Signs:* AF; displaced, hyperdynamic apex; RV heave; soft S₁; split S₂; loud P₂ (pulmonary hypertension) pansystolic murmur at apex radiating to axilla. *Severity:* The more severe, the larger the left ventricle.

*Tests: ECG:* AF ± P-mitrale if in sinus rhythm (may mean left atrial size↑); LVH. *CXR:* big LA & LV; mitral valve calcification; pulmonary oedema.

*Echocardiogram* to assess LV function and aetiology (trans-oesophageal to assess severity and suitability for repair rather than replacement). *Doppler echo* to assess size and site of regurgitant jet. *Cardiac catheterization* to confirm diagnosis, exclude other valve disease, assess coronary artery disease.

*Management:* Control rate if fast AF. Anticoagulate if: AF; history of embolism; prosthetic valve; additional mitral stenosis. Diuretics improve symptoms. Surgery for deteriorating symptoms; aim to repair or replace the valve before LV irreversibly impaired. SBE/IE prophylaxis for GI/GU infected procedures.

**Mitral valve prolapse** is the most common valvular abnormality (prevalence: ~5%). Occurs alone or with: ASD, patent ductus arteriosus, cardiomyopathy, Turner's syndrome, Marfan's syndrome, osteogenesis imperfecta, pseudoxanthoma elasticum, WPW (p120). *Symptoms:* Asymptomatic—or atypical chest pain and palpitations. Some patients have symptoms of autonomic dysfunction (anxiety, panic attack, syncope). *Signs:* Mid-systolic click and/or a late systolic murmur. *Complications:* Mitral regurgitation, cerebral emboli, arrhythmias, sudden death. *Tests: Echocardiography* is diagnostic. *ECG* may show inferior T wave inversion. R: β-blockers may help palpitations and chest pain. In case of severe mitral regurgitation, surgery is needed.

**Aortic stenosis (AS)** *Causes:* Senile calcification is the commonest.[96] Others: congenital (bicuspid valve, William's syndrome, p143), rheumatic heart disease.

*Presentation:* Think of AS in any elderly person with chest pain, exertional dyspnoea or syncope. The classic triad includes angina, syncope, and heart failure (usually after age 60). Also: dyspnoea; dizziness; faints; systemic emboli if infective endocarditis; sudden death. *Signs:* Slow rising pulse with narrow pulse pressure (feel for diminished and delayed carotid upstroke—*parvus et tardus*); heaving, non-displaced apex beat; LV heave; aortic thrill; ejection systolic murmur (heard at the base, left sternal edge and the aortic area, radiates to the carotids). $S_1$ is usually normal. As stenosis worsens, $A_2$ is increasingly delayed, giving first a single $S_2$ and then reversed splitting. But this sign is rare. More common is a quiet $A_2$. In severe AS, $A_2$ may be inaudible (calcified valve). There may be an ejection click (pliable valve) or an $S_4$ (said to occur more often with bicuspid valves, but not in all populations).

*Tests:* ECG: P-mitrale, LVH with strain pattern; LAD (left anterior hemiblock); poor R wave progression; LBBB or complete AV block (calcified ring). CXR: LVH; calcified aortic valve (fig 1); post-stenotic dilatation of ascending aorta. *Echo:* diagnostic (p106). *Doppler echo* can estimate the gradient across valves: severe stenosis if peak gradient ≥50mmHg and valve area <1cm². If the aortic jet velocity is >4m/s (or is increasing by >0.3m/s per yr) risk of complications is increased.[96] *Cardiac catheter* can assess: valve gradient; LV function; coronary artery disease; but risks emboli.

*Differential diagnosis:* Hypertrophic cardiomyopathy (HCM, p146).

*Management:* If symptomatic, prognosis is poor without surgery: 2-3yr survival if angina/syncope; 1-2yr if cardiac failure. If moderate-to-severe and treated medically, mortality can be as high as 50% at 2yrs, therefore prompt valve replacement (p142) is usually recommended. In asymptomatic patients with severe AS and a deteriorating ECG, valve replacement is also recommended. If the patient is not medically fit for surgery, percutaneous valvuloplasty/replacement (TAVI = transcatheter aortic valve implantation) may be attempted.

**Aortic sclerosis** is senile degeneration of the valve. There is an ejection systolic murmur, no carotid radiation, and normal pulse (character and volume) and $S_2$.

**Aortic regurgitation (AR)** *Acute:* Infective endocarditis, ascending aortic dissection, chest trauma. *Chronic:* Congenital, connective tissue disorders (Marfan's syndrome, Ehlers-Danlos), rheumatic fever, Takayasu arteritis, rheumatoid arthritis, SLE; pseudoxanthoma elasticum, appetite suppressants (eg fenfluramine, phentermine), seronegative arthritides (ankylosing spondylitis, Reiter's syndrome, psoriatic arthropathy), hypertension, osteogenesis imperfecta, syphilitic aortitis.

*Symptoms:* Exertional dyspnoea, orthopnoea, and paroxysmal nocturnal dyspnoea. Also: palpitations, angina, syncope, CCF. *Signs:* Collapsing (water-hammer) pulse (p40); wide pulse pressure; displaced, hyperdynamic apex beat; high-pitched early diastolic murmur (heard best in expiration, with patient sitting forward). Eponyms: **Corrigan's sign:** carotid pulsation; **de Musset's sign:** head nodding with each heart beat; **Quincke's sign:** capillary pulsations in nail beds; **Durozie's sign:** in the groin, a finger compressing the femoral artery 2cm proximal to the stethoscope gives a systolic murmur; if 2cm distal, it gives a diastolic murmur as blood flows backwards; **Traube's sign:** 'pistol shot' sound: over femoral arteries; an **Austin Flint** murmur (p44) denotes *severe* AR.

*Tests:* ECG: LVH. CXR: cardiomegaly; dilated ascending aorta; pulmonary oedema. *Echocardiography* is diagnostic. *Cardiac catheterization* to assess: severity of lesion; anatomy of aortic root; LV function; CAD; other valve disease.

*Management:* The main goal of medical therapy is to reduce systolic hypertension. ACE-i are helpful. Echo every 6–12 months to monitor. Indications for surgery: increasing symptoms; enlarging heart on CXR/echo; ECG deterioration (T-wave inversion in lateral leads); IE refractory to medical therapy. Aim to replace the valve before significant LV dysfunction occurs. Predictors of poor post-operative survival: ejection fraction <50%, NYHA class III or IV (p131), duration of CCF >12 months.

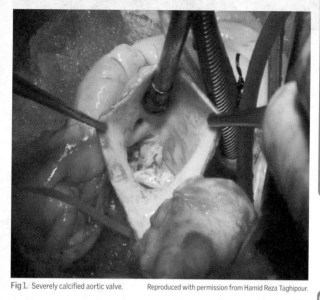

**Fig 1.** Severely calcified aortic valve.　　　Reproduced with permission from Hamid Reza Taghipour.

**Tricuspid regurgitation** *Causes:* Functional (RV dilatation; eg due to pulmonary hypertension induced by LV failure); rheumatic fever; infective endocarditis (IV drug abuser[1]); carcinoid syndrome; congenital (eg ASD, AV canal, Ebstein's anomaly, ie downward displacement of the tricuspid valve—see *OHCS* p642); drugs (eg ergot-derived dopamine agonists, p498, fenfluramine). *Symptoms:* Fatigue; hepatic pain on exertion; ascites; oedema and also dyspnoea and orthopnoea if the cause is LV dysfunction. *Signs:* Giant v waves and prominent y descent in JVP (p41); RV heave; pansystolic murmur, heard best at lower sternal edge in inspiration; pulsatile hepatomegaly; jaundice; ascites. *Management:* Treat underlying cause. Drugs: diuretics, digoxin, ACE-i. Valve replacement (~10% 30-day mortality). Tricuspid regurgitation resulting from myocardial dysfunction or dilatation has a mortality of up to 50% at 5 yrs.

**Tricuspid stenosis** *Causes:* Main cause is rheumatic fever, which almost always occurs with mitral or aortic valve disease. Also: congenital, infective endocarditis. *Symptoms:* Fatigue, ascites, oedema. *Signs:* Giant a wave and slow y descent in JVP (p41); opening snap, early diastolic murmur heard at the left sternal edge in inspiration. AF can also occur. *Diagnosis:* Echo. *Treatment:* Diuretics; surgical repair.

**Pulmonary stenosis** *Causes:* Usually congenital (Turner's syndrome, Noonan's syndrome, William's syndrome, Fallot's tetralogy, rubella). Acquired causes: rheumatic fever, carcinoid syndrome. *Symptoms:* Dyspnoea; fatigue; oedema; ascites. *Signs:* Dysmorphic facies (congenital causes); prominent a wave in JVP; RV heave. In mild stenosis, there is an ejection click, ejection systolic murmur (which radiates to the left shoulder); widely split $s_2$. In severe stenosis, the murmur becomes longer and obscures $A_2$. $P_2$ becomes softer and may be inaudible. *Tests:* ECG: RAD, P-pulmonale, RVH, RBBB. echo/TOE (p106). *CXR:* Prominent main, right, or left pulmonary arteries caused by post-stenotic dilatation. Cardiac catheterization is diagnostic. *Treatment:* Pulmonary valvuloplasty or valvotomy.

**Pulmonary regurgitation** is caused by any cause of pulmonary hypertension (p194). A decrescendo murmur is heard in early diastole at the left sternal edge (the Graham Steell murmur if associated with mitral stenosis and pulmonary hypertension).

## Cardiac surgery

**Valvuloplasty** can be used in mitral or pulmonary stenosis (pliable, non-calcified valve, no regurgitation). A balloon catheter is inserted across the valve and inflated.

**Valvotomy** Closed valvotomy is rarely performed now. Open valvotomy is performed under cardiopulmonary bypass through a median sternotomy.

**Valve replacements** *Mechanical valves* may be of the ball-cage (Starr-Edwards), tilting disc (Bjork-Shiley), or double tilting disc (St Jude) type. These valves are very durable but the risk of thromboembolism is high; patients require lifelong anticoagulation. *Xenografts* are made from porcine valves or pericardium. These valves are less durable and may require replacement at 8-10yrs. Anticoagulation is not required unless there is AF. *Homografts* are cadaveric valves. They are particularly useful in young patients and in the replacement of infected valves. *Complications of prosthetic valves:* systemic embolism, infective endocarditis, haemolysis, structural valve failure, arrhythmias.

**CABG** See p104.

**Cardiac transplantation** Consider this when cardiac disease is *severely* curtailing quality of life, and survival is not expected beyond 6-12 months. Refer to a specialist centre.

---

1 This list is easier to remember once we recall that it is the tricuspid valve which is the valve most vulnerable to events arriving by vein, eg pathogens from IV drug abusers reach the tricuspid valve first; likewise for drugs and toxins from distal carcinoid tumours.

## The heart in various, mostly rare, systemic diseases

This list reminds us to look at the heart *and* the whole patient, not just in exams (where those with odd syndromes congregate), but always.

*Acromegaly:* (p230) BP↑; LVH; hypertrophic cardiomyopathy; high output cardiac failure; coronary artery disease.

*Amyloidosis:* (p364) Restrictive cardiomyopathy. Bright myocardium on echo.

*Ankylosing spondylitis:* Conduction defects; AV block; AR.

*Behçet's disease:* (p708) Aortic regurgitation; arterial ± venous thrombi.

*Cushing's syndrome:* (p216) Hypertension.

*Down's syndrome:* (OHCS p152) ASD; VSD; mitral regurgitation.

*Ehlers-Danlos syndrome:* (OHCS p642) Mitral valve prolapse + hyperelastic skin ± aneurysms and GI bleeds. Joints are loose and hypermobile; mutations exist, eg in genes for procollagen (COL3A1); there are 6 types.

*Friedreich's ataxia:* (p712) Hypertrophic cardiomyopathy, dilatation over time.

*Haemochromatosis:* (p262) AF; cardiomyopathy.

*Holt-Oram syndrome:* ASD or VSD with upper limb defects.[97]

*Human immunodeficiency virus:* (p408) Myocarditis; dilated cardiomyopathy; effusion; ventricular arrhythmias; SBE/IE; non-infective thrombotic (marantic) endocarditis; RVF (pulmonary hypertension); metastatic Kaposi's sarcoma.

*Hypothyroidism:* (p212) Sinus bradycardia; low pulse pressure; pericardial effusion; coronary artery disease; low voltage ECG.

*Kawasaki disease:* (OHCS p646) Coronary arteritis similar to PAN; commoner than rheumatic fever (p136) as a cause of acquired heart disease.

*Klinefelter's syndrome:*♂ (OHCS p646) ASD. Psychopathy; learning difficulties; libido↓; gynaecomastia; sparse facial hair and small firm testes. XXY.

*Marfan's syndrome:* (p720) Mitral valve prolapse; AR; aortic dissection. Look for long fingers and a high-arched palate.

*Noonan's syndrome:* (OHCS p650) ASD; pulmonary stenosis ± low-set ears.

*PAN:* (p558) Small and medium vessel vasculitis + angina; MI; arrhythmias; CCF; pericarditis and conduction defects.

*Rheumatoid arthritis:* Conduction defects; pericarditis; LV dysfunction; aortic regurgitation; coronary arteritis. Look for arthritis signs, p548.

*Sarcoidosis:* (p186) Infiltrating granulomas may cause complete AV block; ventricular or supraventricular tachycardia; myocarditis; CCF; restrictive cardiomyopathy. ECG may show Q waves.

*Syphilis:* (p431) Myocarditis; ascending aortic aneurysm.

*Systemic lupus erythematosus:* (p556) Pericarditis/effusion; myocarditis; Libman-Sacks endocarditis; mitral valve prolapse; coronary arteritis.

*Systemic sclerosis:* (p554) Pericarditis; pericardial effusion; myocardial fibrosis; myocardial ischaemia; conduction defects; cardiomyopathy.

*Thyrotoxicosis:* (p210) Pulse↑; AF ± emboli; wide pulse pressure; hyperdynamic apex; loud heart sounds; ejection systolic murmur; pleuropericardial rub; angina; high-output cardiac failure.

*Turner's syndrome:*♀ Coarctation of aorta. Look for webbed neck. XO.

*William's syndrome:* Supravalvular aortic stenosis (visuospatial IQ↓).

Cardiovascular medicine

▶Fever + new murmur = endocarditis until proven otherwise. Any fever lasting >1wk in those known to be at risk[1] must prompt blood cultures.[98] Classification: 50% of all endocarditis occurs on *normal valves*. It follows an *acute course*, and presents with acute heart failure ± emboli. Chief cause:[99] *S. aureus*. Risk factors: dermatitis; IV injections; renal failure; organ transplantation; DM; post-op wounds. Entry is usually via the skin. Mortality: 5-50% (related to age and embolic events). Endocarditis on *abnormal valves* tends to run a *subacute course*. Risk factors: aortic or mitral valve disease; tricuspid valves in IV drug users; coarctation; patent ductus arteriosus; VSD; prosthetic valves. Endocarditis on prosthetic valves may be 'early' (during surgery, poor prognosis) or 'late' (haematogenous).

**Causes** *Bacteraemia:* This is occurring all the time, eg when we chew (not just when we have dentistry or medical interventions—which is why routine prophylaxis for such procedures does not make sense).[98] *Strep viridans* is common cause (>35%). Others: enterococci; *Staph aureus/epidermidis*; diphtheroids; microaerophilic streps. Rarely: HACEK Gram –ve bacteria (*Haemophilus-Actinobacillus-Cardiobacterium-Eikenella-Kingella*); *Coxiella burnetii*; *Chlamydia*. Fungi: *Candida*; *Aspergillus*; *Histoplasma*. *Other causes:* SLE (Libman-Sacks endocarditis); malignancy.

**Signs** *Septic signs:* Fever, rigors, night sweats, malaise, weight loss, anaemia, splenomegaly, and clubbing (fig 1). *Cardiac lesions:* Any new murmur, or a changing pre-existing murmur, should raise the suspicion of endocarditis. Vegetations may cause valve destruction and severe regurgitation, or valve obstruction. An aortic root abscess causes prolongation of the PR interval, and may lead to complete AV block. LVF is a common cause of death. *Immune complex deposition:* Vasculitis (p558) may affect any vessel. Microscopic haematuria is common; glomerulonephritis and acute renal failure may occur. Roth spots (boat-shaped retinal haemorrhage with pale centre; p386 fig 1); splinter haemorrhages (fig 2); Osler's nodes (painful pulp infarcts in fingers or toes). *Embolic phenomena:* Emboli may cause abscesses in the relevant organ, eg brain, heart, kidney, spleen, gut (or lung if right-sided IE) or skin: termed Janeway lesions (fig 3; painless palmar or plantar macules), which, together with Osler's nodes, are pathognomonic.

**Diagnosis** Use the *Duke* criteria (BOX 1).[100] *Blood cultures:* Do 3 sets at different times from different sites at peak of fever. 85-90% are diagnosed from the 1st 2 sets; 10% are culture-negative. *Blood tests:* Normochromic, normocytic anaemia, neutrophilia, high ESR/CRP. Also check U&E, Mg²⁺, LFT. *Urinalysis* for microscopic haematuria. *CXR* (cardiomegaly). *ECG* (long PR interval) at regular intervals. *Echocardiogram* TTE (p106) may show vegetations, but only if >2mm. TOE (p106) is more sensitive, and better for visualizing mitral lesions and possible development of aortic root abscess.

**R:** Liaise early with microbiologist and cardiologists. Antibiotics: see BOX 2. *Consider surgery if:* heart failure, valvular obstruction; repeated emboli; fungal endocarditis; persistent bacteraemia; myocardial abscess; unstable infected prosthetic valve.[101]

**Mortality** 30% with staphs; 14% if bowel organisms; 6% if sensitive streptococci.

**Prevention** Antibiotic prophylaxis solely to prevent IE is not recommended because:
• There is no proven association between having an interventional procedure (dental or non-dental) and the development of IE.
• The clinical effectiveness of antibiotic prophylaxis is not proven.
• Antibiotic prophylaxis against IE for dental procedures may lead to ↑deaths through fatal anaphylaxis compared with a strategy of no antibiotic prophylaxis.
*Recommendations:* Give clear information about prevention, including:
• The benefits and risks of antibiotic prophylaxis.
• The importance of maintaining good oral health.
• Symptoms that may indicate IE and when to seek expert advice.
• The risks of invasive procedures, including non-medical procedures such as body piercing or tattooing.[102]

---

**1** Past IE or rheumatic fever; IV drug abuser; damaged or replaced valve; structural congenital heart disease (but not simple ASD or fully repaired VSD or patent ductus); hypertrophic cardiomyopathy.

## Duke criteria for infective endocarditis

*Major criteria:*
- Positive blood culture:
  - typical organism in 2 separate cultures or
  - persistently +ve blood cultures, eg 3, >12h apart (or majority if ≥4)
- Endocardium involved:
  - positive echocardiogram (vegetation, abscess, dehiscence of prosthetic valve) **or**
  - new valvular regurgitation (change in murmur not sufficient).

*Minor criteria:*
- Predisposition (cardiac lesion; IV drug abuse)
- Fever >38°C
- Vascular/immunological signs
- Positive blood culture that does not meet major criteria
- Positive echocardiogram that does not meet major criteria.

*How to diagnose:* Definite infective endocarditis: 2 major **or** 1 major and 3 minor **or** all 5 minor criteria (if no major criterion is met).

## Antibiotic therapy for infective endocarditis  See *BNF*; consult a microbiologist

- Blind therapy—native valve: amoxicillin 2g/4h IVI ± gentamicin ~1mg/kg/12h IV slowly, p767. Vancomycin 1g/12h IVI + gentamicin if penicillin-allergic. If thought to be Gram-ve: meropenem (2g/8h IVI) + vancomycin (trough level: 15-20mgL).
- Blind therapy—prosthetic valve: vancomycin + gentamicin + rifampicin 300-600mg/12h PO/IVI.
- Staphs—native valve: flucloxacillin for >4wks; dose example if <85kg: 2g/6h IVI (/4h if >85kg). If allergic or MRSA: vancomycin + rifampicin.
- Staphs—prosthetic valves: flucloxacillin + rifampicin + gentamicin for 6wks (review need for gentamicin after 2wks). If penicillin-allergic or MRSA: vancomycin + rifampicin + gentamicin.
- Streps—fully sensitive to penicillin: benzylpenicillin 1.2g/4h IV for 4-6wks.[1]
- Streps—less sensitive: benzylpenicillin + gentamicin; if penicillin allergic or highly penicillin resistant: vancomycin (or teicoplanin) + gentamicin.
- Enterococci: amoxicillin + gentamicin (or benzylpenicillin + gentamicin). If pen allergic: vancomycin + gentamicin—for 4wks (6wks if prosthetic valve); review need for gentamicin after 2wks.
- HACEK organisms (Haemophilus, Actinobacillus, Cardiobacterium, Eikenella, Kingella): amoxicillin for 4wks (6 if prosthetic valve) + gentamicin eg for 2wks.

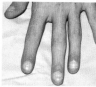

Fig 1. Clubbing with endocarditis.

Fig 2. Splinter haemorrhages are normally seen under the fingernails or toenails. They are usually red-brown in colour.

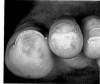

Fig 3. Janeway's lesions are non-tender erythematous, haemorrhagic, or pustular spots eg on the palms or soles.

1 If *Strep bovis* is cultured, do colonoscopy, as a colon neoplasm is the likely portal of entry (p257 BOX 2)..

**Acute myocarditis** This is inflammation of myocardium. *Causes:* Idiopathic (~50%), viral (flu, hepatitis, mumps, rubeola, Coxsackie, polio, HIV); bacterial (Clostridia, diphtheria, TB, meningococcus, mycoplasma, brucellosis, psittacosis); spirochaetes (leptospirosis, syphilis, Lyme); protozoa (Chagas', p426); drugs (cyclophosphamide, herceptin, penicillin, chloramphenicol, sulfonamides, methyldopa, spironolactone, phenytoin, carbamazepine); toxins; vasculitis, p558. *Symptoms & signs:* Fatigue, dyspnoea, chest pain, fever, palpitations, tachycardia, soft $S_1$, $S_4$ gallop (p42).*Tests:* ECG: ST elevation or depression, T wave inversion, atrial arrhythmias, transient AV block. In proper clinical setting (and absence of MI) +ve troponin I or T confirms the diagnosis. Negative antimyosin scintigraphy also excludes active myocarditis. ℞: Supportive. Treat the underlying cause. Patients may recover or get intractable heart failure (p130).

**Dilated cardiomyopathy** A dilated, flabby heart of unknown cause. Associations: alcohol, ↑BP, haemochromatosis, viral infection, autoimmune, peri- or postpartum, thyrotoxicosis, congenital (x-linked). *Prevalence:* 0.2%. *Presentation:* Fatigue, dyspnoea, pulmonary oedema, RVF, emboli, AF, VT. *Signs:* ↑Pulse, ↓BP, ↑JVP, displaced, diffuse apex, $S_3$ gallop, mitral or tricuspid regurgitation (MR/TR), pleural effusion, oedema, jaundice, hepatomegaly, ascites. *Tests: Blood:* plasma BNP is sensitive and specific in diagnosing heart failure. ↓$Na^+$ indicates a poor prognosis. *CXR:* cardiomegaly, pulmonary oedema. *ECG:* tachycardia, non-specific T wave changes, poor R wave progression. *Echo:* globally dilated hypokinetic heart and low ejection fraction. Look for MR, TR, LV mural thrombus. ℞: Bed rest, diuretics, digoxin, ACE-i, anticoagulation, biventricular pacing, ICDs, cardiac transplantation. *Mortality:* Variable, eg 40% in 2yrs.

**Hypertrophic cardiomyopathy** HCM≈LV outflow tract (LVOT) obstruction from asymmetric septal hypertrophy. HCM is the leading cause of sudden cardiac death in the young. *Prevalence:* 0.2%. Autosomal dominant inheritance, but 50% are sporadic. 70% have mutations in genes encoding β-myosin, α-tropomyosin, and troponin T. May present at any age. Ask family history of sudden death. *Symptoms & signs:* Sudden death may be the first manifestation of HCM in many patients (VF is amenable to implantable defibrillators), angina, dyspnoea, palpitation, syncope, CCF. Jerky pulse; *a* wave in JVP; double-apex beat; systolic thrill at lower left sternal edge; harsh ejection systolic murmur. *Tests: ECG:* LVH; progressive T wave inversion; deep Q waves (inferior + lateral leads); AF; WPW syndrome (p120); ventricular ectopics; VT. *Echo:* asymmetrical septal hypertrophy; small LV cavity with hypercontractile posterior wall; midsystolic closure of aortic valve; systolic anterior movement of mitral valve. *Cardiac catheterization* may provoke VT. It helps assess: severity of gradient; coronary artery disease or mitral regurgitation. Electrophysiological studies may be needed (eg if WPW, p120). Exercise test ± Holter monitor (p102) to risk stratify. ℞: β-blockers or verapamil for symptoms (the aim is reducing ventricular contractility). Amiodarone (p124) for arrhythmias (AF, VT). Anticoagulate for paroxysmal AF or systemic emboli. Dual-chamber pacing (p126) is rarely used. Septal myomectomy (surgical, or chemical, with alcohol, to ↓LV outflow tract gradient) is reserved for those with severe symptoms. Consider implantable defibrillator. *Mortality:* 5.9%/ yr if <14yrs; 2.5%/yr if >14yrs. *Poor prognostic factors:* age <14yrs or syncope at presentation; family history of HCM/sudden death.

**Restrictive cardiomyopathy** *Causes:* Idiopathic; amyloidosis; haemochromatosis; sarcoidosis; scleroderma; Löffler's eosinophilic endocarditis; endomyocardial fibrosis.

*Presentation* is like constrictive pericarditis (p148). Features of RVF predominate: ↑JVP, with prominent *x* and *y* descents; hepatomegaly; oedema; ascites.

*Diagnosis:* Cardiac catheterization. ℞: Treat the cause.

**Cardiac myxoma** (fig 1) Rare benign cardiac tumour. Prevalence ≤5/10,000, ♀:♂≈2:1. Usually sporadic, but may be familial (Carney complex: cardiac and cutaneous myxomas, skin pigmentation, endocrinopathy, etc, p215). It may mimic infective endocarditis (fever, weight loss, clubbing, ↑ESR), or mitral stenosis (left atrial obstruction, systemic emboli, AF). A 'tumour plop' may be heard, and signs may vary according to posture. *Tests:* Echo. ℞: Excision.

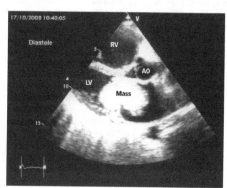

**Fig 1a.** Echocardiogram of a 35yr-old patient who presented with severe exertional dyspnoea and several episodes of syncope. Look at the large mass (cardiac myxoma) in left atrium. **Abbreviations:** RV: right ventricle; LV: left ventricle; AV: aortic valve; AO: aorta; MV: mitral valve.

**Fig 1b.** Echocardiogram of the same patient during diastole. Notice how the large mass of myxoma protrudes into the left ventricle during diastole, and obstructs the mitral valve almost completely. **Abbreviations:** RV: right ventricle; LV: left ventricle; AO: aorta.

Figures reproduced with permission from Hamid Reza Taghipour.

Cardiovascular medicine

**Acute pericarditis** This is inflammation of the pericardium. It may be idiopathic or secondary to:
• Viruses (Coxsackie, flu, Epstein-Barr, mumps, varicella, HIV)
• Bacteria (pneumonia, rheumatic fever, TB, staphs, streps, MAI in HIV, p410)
• Fungi
• Myocardial infarction, Dressler's (p712)
• Drugs: procainamide, hydralazine, penicillin, cromolyn sodium, isoniazid
• Others: uraemia, rheumatoid arthritis, SLE, myxoedema, trauma, surgery, malignancy (and antineoplastic agents), radiotherapy, sarcoidosis.

*Clinical features:* Central chest pain worse on inspiration or lying flat ± relief by sitting forward. A pericardial friction rub (p44) may be heard. Look for evidence of a pericardial effusion or cardiac tamponade (see below). Fever may occur.

*Tests:* ECG classically shows concave (saddle-shaped) ST segment elevation, but may be normal or non-specific (10%); see fig 1. *Blood tests:* FBC, ESR, U&E, cardiac enzymes (NB: troponin may be raised), viral serology, blood cultures, and, if indicated, autoantibodies (p555), fungal precipitins (p410), thyroid function tests. Cardiomegaly on CXR may indicate a pericardial effusion. *Echo* (if suspected pericardial effusion).

*Treatment:* Analgesia, eg ibuprofen 400mg/8h PO with food. Treat the cause. Consider colchicine before steroids/immunosuppressants if relapse or continuing symptoms occur. 15-40% do recur. Steroids may increase the risk of recurrence.

**Pericardial effusion** Accumulation of fluid in the pericardial sac.

*Causes:* Any cause of pericarditis (see above).

*Clinical features:* Dyspnoea, raised JVP (with prominent x descent, p40), bronchial breathing at left base (Ewart's sign: large effusion compressing left lower lobe). Look for signs of cardiac tamponade (see below).

*Diagnosis:* CXR shows an enlarged, globular heart. ECG shows low-voltage QRS complexes and alternating QRS morphologies (electrical alternans). *Echocardiography* shows an echo-free zone surrounding the heart.

*Management:* Treat the cause. Pericardiocentesis may be *diagnostic* (suspected bacterial pericarditis) or *therapeutic* (cardiac tamponade). See p787. Send pericardial fluid for culture, ZN stain/TB culture, and cytology.

**Constrictive pericarditis** The heart is encased in a rigid pericardium.

*Causes:* Often unknown (UK); elsewhere TB, or after *any* pericarditis.

*Clinical features:* These are mainly of right heart failure with ↑JVP (with prominent x and y descents, p41); Kussmaul's sign (JVP rising paradoxically with inspiration); soft, diffuse apex beat; quiet heart sounds; S₃; diastolic pericardial knock, hepatosplenomegaly, ascites, and oedema.

*Tests:* CXR: small heart ± pericardial calcification (if none, CT/MRI helps distinguish from other cardiomyopathies). *Echo;* cardiac catheterization.

*Management:* Surgical excision.

**Cardiac tamponade** Accumulation of pericardial fluid raises intrapericardial pressure, hence poor ventricular filling and fall in cardiac output.

*Causes:* Any pericarditis (above); aortic dissection; haemodialysis; warfarin; transseptal puncture at cardiac catheterization; post cardiac biopsy.

*Signs:* Pulse↑, BP↓, pulsus paradoxus, JVP↑, Kussmaul's sign, muffled S₁ and S₂.

*Diagnosis: Beck's triad:* falling BP; rising JVP; muffled heart sounds. *CXR:* big globular heart (if >250mL fluid). *ECG:* low voltage QRS ± electrical alternans. *Echo* is diagnostic: echo-free zone (>2cm, or >1cm if acute) around the heart ± diastolic collapse of right atrium and right ventricle.

*Management:* Seek expert help. The pericardial effusion needs urgent drainage (p787). Send fluid for culture, ZN stain/TB culture and cytology.

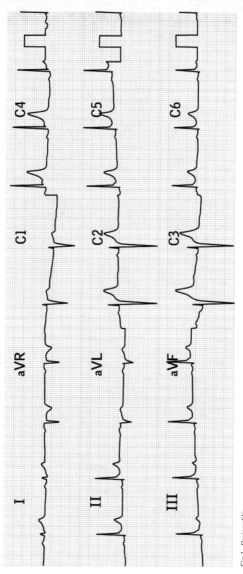

Fig 1. Pericarditis.

The spectrum of congenital heart disease in adults is considerably different from that in infants and children; adults are unlikely to have complex lesions. The commonest lesions, in descending order of frequency, are:

**Bicuspid aortic valve** These work well at birth and go undetected. Many eventually develop aortic stenosis (needing valve replacement) ± aortic regurgitation predisposing to IE/SBE ± aortic dilatation/dissection. Intense exercise may accelerate complications, so do yearly echocardiograms on affected athletes.[103]

**Atrial septal defect (ASD)** A hole connects the atria. *Ostium secundum* defects (high in the septum) are commonest; *ostium primum* defects (opposing the endocardial cushions) are associated with AV valve anomalies. Primum ASDs present early. Secundum ASDs are often asymptomatic until adulthood, as the L→R shunt depends on compliance of the right and left ventricles. The latter decreases with age (esp. if BP↑), so augmenting L→R shunting (hence dyspnoea/heart failure, eg at age 40–60). There may be pulmonary hypertension, cyanosis, arrhythmia, haemoptysis, and chest pain.

*Signs:* AF; ↑JVP; wide, fixed split $S_2$; pulmonary ejection systolic murmur. Pulmonary hypertension may cause pulmonary or tricuspid regurgitation. ↑ freq of migraine.

*Complications:* • Reversal of left-to-right shunt, ie Eisenmenger's complex: initial L→R shunt leads to pulmonary hypertension, hence shunt reversal, causing cyanosis (±heart failure & chest infections). • Paradoxical emboli (vein→artery via ASD; rare).

*Tests:* ECG: RBBB with LAD and prolonged PR interval (primum defect) or RAD (secundum defect). CXR: small aortic knuckle, pulmonary plethora, progressive atrial enlargement. Echocardiography is diagnostic. Cardiac catheterization shows step up in $O_2$ saturation in the right atrium. *Treatment:* In children closure is recommended before age 10yrs. In adults, if symptomatic, or if pulmonary to systemic blood flow ratios of ≥1.5:1. Transcatheter closure is now more common than surgical.

**Ventricular septal defect (VSD)** A hole connects the ventricles. *Causes:* Congenital (prevalence 2:1000 births); acquired (post-MI). *Symptoms:* May present with severe heart failure in infancy, or remain asymptomatic and be detected incidentally in later life. *Signs:* These depend on size and site: smaller holes, which are haemodynamically less significant, give louder murmurs. Classically, a harsh pansystolic murmur is heard at the left sternal edge, with a systolic thrill, ± left parasternal heave. Larger holes are associated with signs of pulmonary hypertension. *Complications:* AR, infundibular stenosis, IE/SBE, pulmonary hypertension, Eisenmenger's complex (above). *Tests:* ECG: normal (small VSD), LAD + LVH (moderate VSD) or LVH + RVH (large VSD). CXR: normal heart size ± mild pulmonary plethora (small VSD) or cardiomegaly, large pulmonary arteries and marked pulmonary plethora (large VSD). Cardiac catheter: step up in $O_2$ saturation in right ventricle. *Treatment:* This is medical, at first, as many close spontaneously. Indications for surgical closure: failed medical therapy, symptomatic VSD, shunt >3:1, SBE/IE. Endovascular closure is also possible.[104]

**Coarctation of the aorta** Congenital narrowing of the descending aorta; usually occurs just distal to the origin of the left subclavian artery. More common in boys. *Associations:* Bicuspid aortic valve; Turner's syndrome. *Signs:* Radiofemoral delay (femoral pulse later than radial); weak femoral pulse; BP↑; scapular bruit; systolic murmur (best heard over the left scapula). *Complications:* Heart failure; infective endocarditis. *Tests:* CT or MRI-aortogram; CXR shows rib notching. *Treatment:* Surgery, or balloon dilatation ± stenting.

**Pulmonary stenosis** may occur alone or with other lesions (p142).

## Fallot's tetralogy: what the non-specialist needs to know

Tetralogy of Fallot (TOF) is the most common cyanotic congenital heart disorder (prevalence: 3-6 per 10,000), and it is also the most common cyanotic heart defect that survives to adulthood, accounting for 10% of all congenital defects.[105] It is believed to be due to abnormalities in separation of the truncus arteriosus into the aorta and pulmonary arteries that occur in early gestation (fig 1).

The 4 features typical of TOF include:
1 Ventricular septal defect (VSD)
2 Pulmonary stenosis
3 Right ventricular hypertrophy
4 The aorta overriding the VSD

Occasionally, a few children also have an atrial septal defect, which makes up the pentad of Fallot.

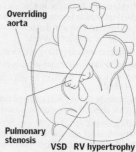

Fig 1. Tetralogy of Fallot.
Adapted from Chikwe, Beddow, and Glenville, *Cardiothoracic Surgery*, 2006, with permission from Oxford University Press.

*Presentation:* Severity of illness depends greatly on the degree of pulmonary stenosis. Infants may be acyanotic at birth, with a pulmonary stenosis murmur as the only initial finding. Gradually (especially after closure of ductus arteriosus) they become cyanotic due to decreasing flow of blood to the lungs as well as right-to-left shunt across the VSD. During a hypoxic spell, the child becomes restless and agitated, and may cry inconsolably. Toddlers may squat, which is typical of TOF, as it increases peripheral vascular resistance and decreases the degree of right to left shunt. Also: difficulty in feeding, failure to thrive, clubbing. Adult patients are often asymptomatic. In the unoperated adult patient, cyanosis is common, although extreme cyanosis or squatting is uncommon. In repaired patients, late symptoms include exertional dyspnoea, palpitations, RV failure, syncope, and even sudden death. ECG shows RV hypertrophy with a right bundle-branch block.

*CXR* may be normal, or show the hallmark of TOF, which is the classic boot-shaped heart (fig 2). *Echocardiography* can show the anatomy as well as the degree of stenosis. Cardiac CT and *cardiac MRI* can give valuable information for planning the surgery.[106]

*Management:* Give O$_2$. Place the child in knee-chest position. Morphine can sedate the child as well relaxing the pulmonary outflow. Long-term β-blockers may be needed. Give endocarditis prophylaxis only if recommended by a microbiologist. Without surgery, mortality rate is ~95% by age 20. Surgery is usually done before 1yr of age, with closure of the VSD and correction of the pulmonary stenosis. 20-yr survival is ~90-95% after repair.

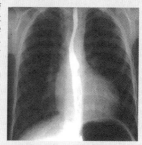

Fig 2. Boot-shaped heart.
Courtesy of Dr Edward Singleton.

UK licences are inscribed "You are required by law to inform Drivers Medical Branch, DVLA, Swansea SA99 1AT at once if you have any disability (physical or medical), which is, or may become likely to affect your fitness as a driver, unless you do not expect it to last more than 3 months". It is the responsibility of drivers to inform the DVLA, and that of their doctors to advise patients that medical conditions (and drugs) may affect their ability to drive and for which conditions patients should inform the DVLA. Drivers should also inform their insurance company of any condition disclosed to the DVLA. If in doubt, ask your defence union. The following are examples of the guidance for holders of standard licences.

Different rules apply for group 2 vehicle licence-holders (eg lorries, buses).

**Angina** Driving must cease when symptoms occur at rest or with emotion. Driving may recommence when satisfactory symptom control is achieved. DVLA need not be notified.

**Angioplasty** Driving must cease for 1wk, and may recommence thereafter provided no other disqualifying condition. DVLA need not be notified.

**MI** If successfully treated with angioplasty cease driving for 1 week provided urgent intervention not planned and LVEF (left ventricular ejection fraction) >40%, and no other disqualifying condition. Otherwise, driving must cease for 1 month. DVLA need not be notified.

**Dysrhythmias** *Sinoatrial including AF/flutter:* Driving must cease if the dysrhythmia has caused or is likely to cause incapacity. Driving may recommence 4wks after successful control provided there is no other disqualifying condition.

*Significant atrioventricular conduction defects:* Driving may be permitted when underlying cause has been identified and controlled for >4wks. DVLA need not be notified unless there are distracting/disabling symptoms.

**Pacemaker implant** Stop driving for 1wk.

**Implanted cardioverter/defibrillator** The licence is subject to annual review. Driving may occur when these criteria can be met:
• The 1st device has been implanted for at least 6 months.
• The device has not administered therapy (shock and/or symptomatic antitachycardia pacing) within the last 6 months (except during testing).
• Any previous therapy has not been accompanied by *incapacity* (whether caused by the device or arrhythmia).
• A period of 1 month off driving must occur following any revision of the device (generator and/or electrode) or alteration of antiarrhythmics.
• The device is subject to regular review with interrogation.
• There is no other disqualifying condition.

**Syncope** *Simple faint:* no restriction. *Unexplained syncope* with low risk of recurrence 4wks off driving, high risk of recurrence 4wks off driving if cause identified and treated; otherwise 6 months off. See driving and epilepsy (BOX). Patients who have had a single episode of loss of consciousness (no cause found) still need to have at least 1yr off driving.

**Hypertension** Driving may continue unless treatment causes unacceptable side-effects. DVLA need not be notified.

**Fitness to fly guidelines are now also available**[108]

- An epileptic event. A person who has suffered an epileptic attack while awake must not drive for 1yr from the date of the attack. A person who has suffered an attack while asleep must also refrain from driving for 1yr from the date of the attack, unless they have had an attack while asleep >3yrs ago and have not had any awake attacks since that asleep attack. In any event, they should not drive if they are likely to cause danger to the public or themselves.
- Patients with TIA or stroke should not drive for at least 1 month. There is no need to inform the DVLA unless there is residual neurological defect after 1 month, eg visual field defect. If TIAs have been recurrent and frequent, a 3-month period free of attacks may be required.
- Sudden attacks or disabling giddiness, fainting, or blackouts. Multiple sclerosis, Parkinson's (any 'freezing' or on-off effects), and motor neuron diseases are relevant here.
- Severe mental handicap. Those with dementia should only drive if the condition is mild (do not rely on armchair judgements: on-the-road trials are better). Encourage relatives to contact DVLA if a dementing relative should not be driving. GPs may desire to breach confidentiality (the GMC approves) and inform DVLA of demented or psychotic patients (tel. 01792 783686). Many elderly drivers (~1 in 3) who die in accidents are found to have Alzheimer's.
- A pacemaker, defibrillator, or antiventricular tachycardia device fitted.
- Diabetes controlled by insulin or tablets.
- Angina while driving.
- Parkinson's disease.
- Any other chronic neurological condition.
- A serious problem with memory.
- A major or minor stroke with deficit continuing for >1 month.
- Any type of brain surgery, brain tumour. Severe head injury involving inpatient treatment at hospital.
- Any severe psychiatric illness or mental disorder.
- Continuing/permanent difficulty in the use of arms or legs which affects ability to control a vehicle.
- Dependence on or misuse of alcohol, illicit drugs, or chemical substances in the past 3yrs (do not include drink/driving offences).
- Any visual disability which affects *both* eyes (do not declare short/long sight or colour blindness).

Vision (new drivers) should be 6/9 on Snellen's scale in the better eye and 6/12 on the Snellen scale in the other eye, wearing glasses or contact lenses if needed, and 3/60 in each eye without glasses or contact lenses.

---

**1** DVLA is the UK Driving and Vehicle Licensing Authority.

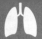

## Contents

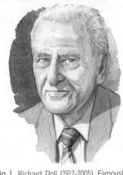

**Fig 1.** Richard Doll (1912-2005). Famously, reported the link between cigarette smoking and lung cancer in the BMJ in 1950, which led him to stop smoking, concluding that: "The risk of developing the disease increases in proportion to the amount smoked...It may be 50 times as great among those who smoke 25 or more cigarettes a day as among non-smokers.". This was confirmed by the British Doctors' Study in 1954, and led to a major series of public health campaigns and policy changes against smoking. He was instrumental in the development of epidemiology and clinical trials in the UK. Ironically, after his death it became apparent that he had received payments from the chemical industry for a number of years.

### Relevant pages in other sections:

*We thank Dr Phillippa Lawson, our Specialist Reader, and Winnie Chen, our Junior Reader, for their contribution to this chapter.*

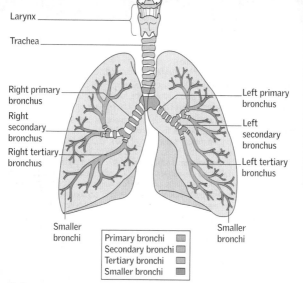

**Fig 2.** Lung anatomy. The left lung has two lobes and the right has three lobes.

| | |
|---|---|
| Primary bronchi | ▩ |
| Secondary bronchi | ▩ |
| Tertiary bronchi | ▩ |
| Smaller bronchi | ▩ |

Larynx

Trachea

Right primary bronchus

Left primary bronchus

Right secondary bronchus

Left secondary bronchus

Right tertiary bronchus

Left tertiary bronchus

Smaller bronchi

Smaller bronchi

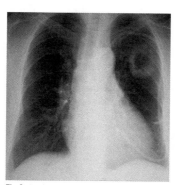

**Fig 3.** Smoke ring sign: cavitating lung carcinoma. Reproduced from Warrell, Cox, and Firth, *Oxford Textbook of Medicine,* 5th Edition, 2010, with permission from Oxford University Press.

Chest medicine

**Sputum examination** Collect a good sample; if necessary ask a physiotherapist to help. Note the appearance: clear and colourless (chronic bronchitis), yellow-green (pulmonary infection), red (haemoptysis), black (smoke, coal dust), or frothy white-pink (pulmonary oedema). Send the sample to the laboratory for microscopy (Gram stain and auramine/ZN stain, if indicated), culture, and cytology.

**Peak expiratory flow (PEF)** is measured by a maximal forced expiration through a peak flow meter. It correlates well with the forced expiratory volume in 1 second ($FEV_1$) and is used as an estimate of airway calibre, but is more effort-dependent.

**Pulse oximetry** allows non-invasive assessment of peripheral $O_2$ saturation ($SpO_2$). It provides a useful tool for monitoring those who are acutely ill or at risk of deterioration. An oxygen saturation of ≤80% is clearly abnormal and action is usually required, unless this is usual for the patient, eg in COPD. If a previously healthy person has pneumonia, a saturation of <92% is a serious sign; see p160. Here, check arterial blood gases (ABG) as $P_aCO_2$ may be rising despite a normal $P_aO_2$. Causes of erroneous readings: poor perfusion, motion, excess light, skin pigmentation, nail varnish, dyshaemoglobinaemias, and carbon monoxide poisoning. As with any bedside test, be sceptical, and check ABG whenever indicated (p181).

**Arterial blood gas (ABG) analysis** Heparinized blood is usually taken from the radial or femoral artery (see p785), and pH, $P_aO_2$, and $P_aCO_2$ are measured using an automated analyser. Remember to note FiO_2 (fraction or percentage of inspired $O_2$).
- Normal pH is 7.35-7.45. A pH <7.35 indicates *acidosis* and a pH >7.45 indicates *alkalosis*. For interpretation of abnormalities, see p684.
- Normal $P_aO_2$ is 10.5-13.5kPa. Hypoxia is caused by one or more of the following reasons: ventilation/perfusion (V/Q) mismatch, hypoventilation, abnormal diffusion, right to left cardiac shunts. Of these, V/Q mismatch is the commonest cause. Severe hypoxia is defined as a $P_aO_2$ <8kPa (see p180).
- Normal $P_aCO_2$ is 4.5-6.0kPa. $P_aCO_2$ is directly related to alveolar ventilation. A $P_aCO_2$ <4.5kPa indicates *hyperventilation* and a $P_aCO_2$ >6.0kPa indicates *hypoventilation*.

*Type 1 respiratory failure* is defined as $P_aO_2$ <8kPa and $P_aCO_2$ <6.0kPa.

*Type 2 respiratory failure* is defined as $P_aO_2$ <8kPa and $P_aCO_2$ >6.0kPa.

**Spirometry** measures functional lung volumes. Forced expiratory volume in 1s ($FEV_1$) and forced vital capacity (FVC) are measured from a full forced expiration into a spirometer (Vitalograph®); exhalation continues until no more breath can be exhaled. $FEV_1$ is less effort-dependent than PEF. The $FEV_1$/FVC ratio gives a good estimate of the severity of airflow obstruction; normal ratio is 75-80%. See BOX.

*Obstructive defect* (eg asthma, COPD) $FEV_1$ is reduced more than the FVC, and the $FEV_1$/FVC ratio is <75%.

*Restrictive defect* (eg lung fibrosis) FVC is ↓ and the $FEV_1$/FVC ratio is ↔ or ↑. Other causes: sarcoidosis; pneumoconiosis, interstitial pneumonias; connective tissue diseases; pleural effusion; obesity; kyphoscoliosis; neuromuscular problems.

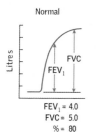 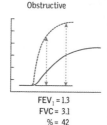 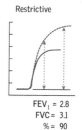

| Normal | Obstructive | Restrictive |
|---|---|---|
| FEV$_1$ = 4.0 | FEV$_1$ = 1.3 | FEV$_1$ = 2.8 |
| FVC = 5.0 | FVC = 3.1 | FVC = 3.1 |
| % = 80 | % = 42 | % = 90 |

**Fig 1.** Examples of spirograms.

**Chest medicine**

### (Aa)PO$_2$: the Alveolar-arterial (Aa) oxygen gradient[1]

This is the difference in the O$_2$ partial pressures between the alveolar and arterial sides, i.e. (Aa)PO$_2$ = $P_AO_2$ − $P_aO_2$.

$P_AO_2$, the partial pressure of oxygen in the alveoli, depends on $R$, the respiratory quotient (≈0.8, nearer to 1 if eating all carbohydrates); barometric pressure ($P_B$ ≈ 101kPa at sea level), and $P_{H2O}$, the water saturation of airway gas ($P_{H2O}$ ≈ 6.2kPa as inspired air is usually fully saturated by the time it gets to the carina). $P_AO_2$ also depends on F$_i$O$_2$, the fractional concentration of O$_2$ in inspired air (eg F$_i$O$_2$ is 0.5 if breathing 50% O$_2$, and 0.21 if breathing room air). So (at sea level)...

$P_AO_2$ = $(P_B − P_{H2O}) × F_iO_2 − (P_aCO_2/R)$
= $(101 − 6.2) × F_iO_2 − (P_aCO_2/0.8) = (94.8 × F_iO_2) − (P_aCO_2 ÷ 0.8)$

In type II respiratory failure it helps tell if hypoventilation is from lung disease or poor respiratory effort. Aa gradient normal range breathing air: 0.2-1.5kPa aged 25yrs; ↑ to 1.5-3.0 at 75yrs. A high Aa gradient indicates a problem with O$_2$ transfer, whereas a normal Aa gradient in the context of hypoxia suggests hypoventilation.

**Lung function tests** PEF, FEV$_1$, FVC (see p156). *Total lung capacity* (TLC) and *residual volume* (RV) are useful in distinguishing obstructive and restrictive diseases. TLC and RV are increased in obstructive airways disease and reduced in restrictive lung diseases and musculoskeletal abnormalities. The *gas transfer* coefficient (KCO) represents the carbon monoxide diffusing capacity (DLCO) corrected for alveolar volume. It is calculated by measuring carbon monoxide uptake from a single inspiration in a standard time (usually 10s) and lung volume by helium dilution. Low in emphysema and interstitial lung disease, high in alveolar haemorrhage.[2] *Flow volume loop* measures flow at various lung volumes. Characteristic patterns are seen with intra-thoracic airways obstruction (asthma, emphysema) and extra-thoracic airways obstruction (tracheal stenosis).

**Radiology** *Chest x-ray* see p736. *Ultrasound* is used in the diagnosis and to guide drainage of pleural effusions (particularly loculated effusions) and empyema. *Radionuclide scans Ventilation/perfusion* (V/Q, p752) *scans* are occasionally used to diagnose pulmonary embolism (PE) (unmatched perfusion defects are seen). *Bone scans* are used to diagnose bone metastases. *Computed tomography* (CT, p744) of the thorax is used for diagnosing and staging lung cancer, imaging the hila, mediastinum and pleura, and guiding biopsies. Thin (1-1.5mm) section high resolution CT (HRCT) is used in the diagnosis of interstitial lung disease and bronchiectasis. CT pulmonary angiography (CTPA, p753) is used in the diagnosis of PE. *Pulmonary angiography* is now rarely used for diagnosing pulmonary hypertension.

**Fibreoptic bronchoscopy** is performed under local anaesthetic via the nose or mouth. *Diagnostic indications:* suspected lung carcinoma, slowly resolving pneumonia, pneumonia in the immunosuppressed, interstitial lung disease. Bronchial lavage fluid may be sent to the lab for microscopy, culture, and cytology. Mucosal abnormalities may be brushed (cytology) and biopsied (histopathology). *Therapeutic indications:* aspiration of mucus plugs causing lobar collapse, removal of foreign bodies, stenting or treating tumours, eg laser. *Pre-procedure investigations:* FBC, CXR, spirometry, pulse oximetry and **ABG** (if indicated). Check clotting if recent anticoagulation and potential biopsy. *Complications:* respiratory depression, bleeding, pneumothorax (fig 1, p763). *Diagnostic sensitivity* for cancer 50-90%, depends on tumour location; gene profiling of cell sample may improve this.[3] May also be used to deliver an ultrasound probe (endobronchial ultrasound), and treatments—eg stents, or cryotherapy.

**Bronchoalveolar lavage** (BAL) is performed at the time of bronchoscopy by instilling and aspirating a known volume of warmed, buffered 0.9% saline into the distal airway. *Diagnostic indications:* suspected malignancy, pneumonia in the immunosuppressed (especially HIV), suspected TB (if sputum negative), interstitial lung diseases (eg sarcoidosis, extrinsic allergic alveolitis, histiocytosis X). *Therapeutic indications:* alveolar proteinosis.[1] *Complications:* hypoxia (give supplemental O$_2$), transient fever, transient CXR shadow, infection (rare).

**Lung biopsy** may be performed in several ways. *Percutaneous needle biopsy* is performed under radiological guidance and is useful for peripheral lung and pleural lesions. *Transbronchial biopsy* performed at bronchoscopy may help in diagnosing diffuse lung diseases, eg sarcoidosis. If these are unsuccessful, an *open lung biopsy* may be performed under general anaesthetic.

**Surgical procedures** are performed under general anaesthetic. *Rigid bronchoscopy* provides a wide lumen, enables larger mucosal biopsies, control of bleeding, and removal of foreign bodies. *Mediastinoscopy* and *mediastinotomy* enable examination and biopsy of the mediastinal lymph nodes/lesions. *Thoracoscopy* allows examination and biopsy of pleural lesions, drainage of pleural effusions, and talc pleurodesis.

---

1 Pulmonary alveolar proteinosis causes cough, dyspnoea, and restrictive spirometry. It is caused by accumulation of surfactant-derived acidophilic phospholipid/protein compounds which fill alveoli and distal bronchioles. Diagnosis may require lung biopsy. Cause: primary genetic or antibody problem, or secondary to inflammation caused by inhaling silica, aluminium or titanium.[4]

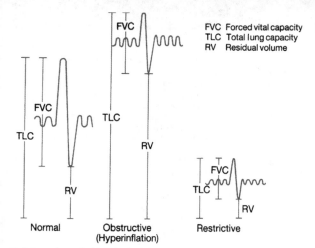

FVC  Forced vital capacity
TLC  Total lung capacity
RV   Residual volume

**Fig 1.** Lung volumes: physiological and pathological. Adapted from D Flenley *Med Int*/ 1 (20) 240.

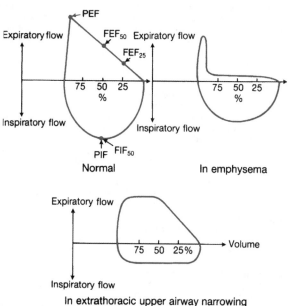

**Fig 2.** Flow volume loops.
PEF=peak expiratory flow; FEF$_{50}$=forced expiratory flow at 50% TLC;
FEF$_{25}$=forced expiratory flow at 25% TLC; PIF=peak inspiratory flow;
FIF$_{50}$=forced inspiratory flow at 50% TLC.

After B Harrison in *Thoracic Medicine* 1981, ed P Emerson,
Butterworths, London; and B Harrison 1971 *Thorax* 26 579

Chest medicine

An acute lower respiratory tract illness associated with fever, symptoms and signs in the chest, and abnormalities on the chest x-ray—fig 1, p737. Incidence: 5-11/1000, ↑ if very young or old (30% are under 65yrs). Mortality: ~21% in hospital.

## Classification and causes

*Community-acquired pneumonia* (CAP) may be primary or secondary to underlying disease. *Streptococcus pneumoniae* is the commonest cause, followed by *Haemophilus influenzae* and *Mycoplasma pneumoniae*. *Staphylococcus aureus*, *Legionella* species, *Moraxella catarrhalis*, and *Chlamydia* account for most of the remainder. Gram negative bacilli, *Coxiella burnetii* and anaerobes are rarer. Viruses account for up to 15%. Flu may be complicated by community-acquired MRSA pneumonia (CA-MRSA).

*Hospital-acquired* (*nosocomial*; >48h after hospital admission). Most commonly Gram negative enterobacteria or *Staph. aureus*. Also *Pseudomonas*, *Klebsiella*, *Bacteroides*, and *Clostridia*.

*Aspiration* Those with stroke, myasthenia, bulbar palsies, ↓consciousness (eg postictal or drunk), oesophageal disease (achalasia, reflux), or with poor dental hygiene risk aspirating oropharyngeal anaerobes.

*Immunocompromised patient:* *Strep. pneumoniae*, *H. influenzae*, *Staph. aureus*, *M. catarrhalis*, *M. pneumoniae*, Gram -ve bacilli and *Pneumocystis jiroveci* (formerly named *P. carinii*, p410–p411). Other fungi, viruses (CMV, HSV), and mycobacteria.

**Clinical features** *Symptoms:* Fever, rigors, malaise, anorexia, dyspnoea, cough, purulent sputum, haemoptysis, and pleuritic pain. *Signs:* Pyrexia, cyanosis, confusion (can be the only sign in the elderly—may also be hypothermic), tachypnoea, tachycardia, hypotension, signs of consolidation (diminished expansion, dull percussion note, ↑tactile vocal fremitus/vocal resonance, bronchial breathing), and a pleural rub.

**Tests** aim to establish diagnosis, identify pathogen, and assess severity (see below). *CXR* (fig 1, p737): lobar or multilobar infiltrates, cavitation or pleural effusion. *Assess oxygenation:* oxygen saturation, p156 (ABGs if $S_aO_2$ ≤92% or severe pneumonia) and BP. *Blood tests:* FBC, U&E, LFT, CRP, blood cultures. *Sputum* for microscopy and culture. In severe cases, check for *Legionella* (sputum culture, urine antigen), atypical organism/viral serology (PCR sputum/BAL, complement fixation tests acutely, paired serology) and check for pneumococcal antigen in urine. *Pleural fluid* may be aspirated for culture. Consider *bronchoscopy* and *bronchoalveolar lavage* if patient is immunocompromised or on ITU.

**Severity** 'CURB-65' is a simple, validated scoring system.[6,7] 1 point for each of: **C**onfusion (abbreviated mental test ≤8); **U**rea >7mmol/L; **R**espiratory rate ≥30/min; **B**P <90 systolic and/or 60mmHg diastolic); age ≥**65**. 0-1 home R possible; 2 hospital therapy; ≥3 severe pneumonia mortality 15-40%—consider ITU. It may 'underscore' the young—use clinical judgement. Other features increasing the risk of death are: co-existing disease; bilateral/multilobar involvement; $P_aO_2$ <8kPa/$S_aO_2$ <92%.

**Management** ►►p826. **Antibiotics** (p161): orally if not severe and not vomiting; severe give by IV. **Oxygen:** keep $P_aO_2$ >8.0 and/or saturation ≥94%. IV **fluids** (anorexia, dehydration, shock) and VTE prophylaxis. **Analgesia** if pleurisy—eg paracetamol 1g/6h. Consider ITU if shock, hypercapnia, or uncorrected hypoxia. If failure to improve, or CRP remains high, repeat CXR and look for progression/complications. **Follow-up:** at 6 weeks (±CXR).

**Complications** (p164) Pleural effusion, empyema, lung abscess, respiratory failure, septicaemia, brain abscess, pericarditis, myocarditis, cholestatic jaundice. Repeat CRP and CXR in patients not progressing satisfactorily.

**Pneumococcal vaccine** (eg 23-valent Pneumovax II®, 0.5mL SC) At-risk groups: •≥65yrs old • Chronic heart, liver (eg cirrhosis), renal (eg renal failure, nephrosis*, post-transplant*) or lung conditions • Diabetes mellitus • Immunosuppression, eg spleen function↓ (eg splenectomy, asplenia*, sickle cell* or coeliac disease), AIDS, or on chemotherapy or prednisolone >20mg/d). CI: pregnancy, lactation, T°↑. (* = ↑risk of fatal pneumococcal infection (above), revaccinate after 6yrs.) Children: OHCS p151.

## Empirical treatment of pneumonia (check local policy)[5]

| Clinical setting | Organisms | Antibiotic (further dosage details: p378 & p379) |
|---|---|---|
| *Community-acquired* | | |
| Mild not previously ℞ | *Streptococcus pneumoniae* *Haemophilus influenzae* | Oral amoxicillin 500mg-1g/8h or clarithromycin 500mg/12h or doxycycline 200mg loading then 100mg/day |
| Moderate | *Streptococcus pneumoniae* *Haemophilus influenzae* *Mycoplasma pneumoniae* | Oral amoxicillin 500mg-1g/8h + clarithromycin 500mg/12h or doxycycline 200mg loading then 100mg/12h. If IV required: amoxicillin 500mg/8h + clarithromycin 500mg/12h |
| Severe | As above | Co-amoxiclav 1.2g/8h IV or cephalospor-in IV (eg cefuroxime 1.5g/8h IV) **AND** clarithromycin 500mg/12h IV. Add flucloxacillin± rifampicin if staph suspected; vancomycin (or teicoplanin) if MRSA suspected. Treat for 10d (14-21d if staph, legionella, or Gram -ve enteric bacteria suspected). |
| | Panton-Valentine Leukocidin-producing *Staph. aureus* (PVL-SA) | Seek urgent help. Consider adding IV linezolid, clindamycin, and rifampicin |
| Atypical | *Legionella pneumophilia* | Fluoroquinolone combined with clarithromycin, or rifampicin, if severe. See p162. |
| | *Chlamydophila* species | Tetracycline |
| | *Pneumocystis jiroveci* | High-dose co-trimoxazole (p410-p411) |
| *Hospital-acquired* | | |
| | Gram negative bacilli Pseudomonas Anaerobes | Aminoglycoside IV + antipseudomonal penicillin IV or 3rd gen. cephalosporin IV (p379) |
| *Aspiration* | | |
| | *Streptococcus pneumoniae* Anaerobes | Cephalosporin IV + metronidazole IV |
| *Neutropenic patients* | | |
| | Gram positive cocci Gram negative bacilli | Aminoglycoside IV + antipseudomonal penicillin IV or 3rd gen. cephalosporin IV |
| | Fungi (p168) | Consider antifungals after 48h |

3rd gen=3rd generation, eg cefotaxime, p379; gentamicin is an example of an aminoglycoside (p381).
Ticarcillin is an example of an antipseudomonal penicillin.

Chest medicine

Chest medicine

For antibiotic doses, see p378–382. TB: ▶see p398.

*Pneumococcal* pneumonia is the commonest bacterial pneumonia. It affects all ages, but is commoner in the elderly, alcoholics, post-splenectomy, immuno-suppressed, and patients with chronic heart failure or pre-existing lung disease. Clinical features: fever, pleurisy, herpes labialis. CXR shows lobar consolidation. If mod/severe check for urinary antigen. Treatment: amoxicillin, benzylpenicillin, or cephalosporin.

*Staphylococcal* pneumonia may complicate influenza infection or occur in the young, elderly, intravenous drug users, or patients with underlying disease, eg leukaemia, lymphoma, cystic fibrosis (CF). It causes a bilateral cavitating bronchopneumonia. Treatment: flucloxacillin± rifampicin, MRSA: contact lab; consider vancomycin.

*Klebsiella* pneumonia is rare. Occurs in elderly, diabetics and alcoholics. Causes a cavitating pneumonia, particularly of the upper lobes, often drug resistant. Treatment: cefotaxime or imipenem.

*Pseudomonas* is a common pathogen in bronchiectasis and CF. It also causes hospital-acquired infections, particularly on ITU or after surgery. Treatment: antipseudomonal penicillin, ceftazidime, meropenem, or ciprofloxacin + aminoglycoside. Consider dual therapy to minimize resistance.

*Mycoplasma pneumoniae* occurs in epidemics about every 4yrs. It presents insidiously with flu-like symptoms (headache, myalgia, arthralgia) followed by a dry cough. CXR: reticular-nodular shadowing or patchy consolidation often of 1 lower lobe, and worse than signs suggest. Diagnosis: PCR sputum or serology. Cold agglutinins may cause an autoimmune haemolytic anaemia. Complications: skin rash (erythema multiforme, fig 3, p564), Stevens-Johnson syndrome, meningoencephalitis or myelitis; Guillain-Barré syndrome. Treatment: clarithromycin (500mg/12h) or doxycycline (200mg loading then 100mg od) or a fluroquinolone (eg ciprofloxacin or norfloxacin).

*Legionella pneumophilia* colonizes water tanks kept at <60°C (eg hotel air-conditioning and hot water systems) causing outbreaks of Legionnaire's disease. Flu-like symptoms (fever, malaise, myalgia) precede a dry cough and dyspnoea. Extra-pulmonary features include anorexia, D&V, hepatitis, renal failure, confusion, and coma. CXR shows bi-basal consolidation. Blood tests may show lymphopenia, hyponatraemia, and deranged LFTs. Urinalysis may show haematuria. Diagnosis: *Legionella* urine antigen/culture. Treatment: fluoroquinolone for 2-3wks or clarithromycin (p380). 10% mortality.

*Chlamydophila pneumoniae* is the commonest chlamydial infection. Person-to-person spread occurs causing a biphasic illness: pharyngitis, hoarseness, otitis, followed by pneumonia. Diagnosis: *Chlamydophila* complement fixation test, PCR invasive samples.[8] Treatment: doxycycline or clarithromycin.

*Chlamydiophila psittaci* causes psittacosis, an ornithosis acquired from infected birds (typically parrots). Symptoms include headache, fever, dry cough, lethargy, arthralgia, anorexia, and D&V. Extra-pulmonary features are legion but rare, eg meningo-encephalitis, infective endocarditis, hepatitis, nephritis, rash, splenomegaly. CXR shows patchy consolidation. Diagnosis: *Chlamydophila* serology. Treatment: doxycycline or clarithromycin.

*Viral pneumonia* The commonest cause is influenza (p402 and BOX). Other viruses that can affect the lung are: measles, CMV, and varicella zoster.

*Pneumocystis pneumonia* (PCP) causes pneumonia in the immunosuppressed (eg HIV). The organism responsible was previously called *Pneumocystis carinii*, and now called *Pneumocystis jiroveci*.[9] It presents with a dry cough, exertional dyspnoea, ↓$P_aO_2$, fever, bilateral crepitations. CXR may be normal or show bilateral perihilar interstitial shadowing. Diagnosis: visualization of the organism in induced sputum, bronchoalveolar lavage, or in a lung biopsy specimen. Drugs: high-dose co-trimoxazole (p410-p411), or pentamidine by slow IVI for 2-3 weeks (p411). Steroids are beneficial if severe hypoxaemia. Prophylaxis is indicated if the CD4 count is <200×10⁶/L or after the 1st attack.[10]

## Avian influenza

Avian-to-human transmission of the H5N1 strain of influenza A causes serious infection in humans with a ≥50% mortality, often from a rapidly progressive pneumonia. Human-to-human transmission is reported but is unusual. Oseltamivir can reduce morbidity from influenza A by 1-2 days (see p402; note that oseltamivir-resistant H5N1 has been reported).[11] A vaccine is available,[12] but the most likely cause of a pandemic is a new mutant developing between human and avian viruses (genetic reassortment, p403) which may require a different vaccine.

▶Suspect avian flu if fever (>38°C) plus lower respiratory track signs or consolidation on CXR, or life-threatening infection, AND contact with poultry or others with similar symptoms.[13] NB: D&V, abdominal pain, pleuritic pain, and bleeding from the nose and gums are reported to be an early feature in some patients.[14]

*Diagnosis:* Viral culture ± reverse transcriptase-PCR with H5 & N1 specific primers.[15]

*Management:* ▶Get help. Contain the outbreak (use your pandemic preparedness plan[1], p403, in the UK, via your consultant in communicable disease control, CCDC). Ventilatory support + O₂ and antivirals may be needed. Nebulizers and high-air flow O₂ masks are implicated in nosocomial spread (use with meticulous precautions).[14,16]

*Precautions for close contacts:*
Use appropriate hand hygiene, do not share utensils, avoid face-to-face contact with suspected or proven cases, wear high-efficiency masks and eye protection. Start empirical antiviral treatment and do diagnostic testing if fever (T° >38°C) and cough, shortness of breath, diarrhoea, or other systemic symptoms develop. In case of close contact or sharing a defined setting (household, extended family, hospital or other residential institution, or military service) with a patient with proven or suspected avian influenza A (H5N1) infection, monitor body temperature twice daily, check for symptoms for 7d after the last exposure, and start post-exposure prophylaxis with **oseltamivir: 75mg once daily for 7-10d**.[17]

## SARS[18]

Severe acute respiratory syndrome (SARS) is caused by SARS-CoV virus—a coronavirus. Major features are persistent fever (>38°C), chills, rigors, myalgia, dry cough, headache, diarrhoea, and dyspnoea—with an abnormal CXR and WCC↓. Respiratory failure is the big complication; >50% need supplemental O₂; ~20% progress to acute respiratory distress syndrome requiring invasive ventilation.[19]

Mortality is 1-50%, depending on age. Close contact with an index case, or travel to an area with known cases should raise suspicion. The mechanism of transmission of SARS-CoV is only by close contact with other patients.

Management is supportive. No drugs have convincing efficacy (experts may advise on antivirals). Rapid diagnosis, early isolation, and good infection control measures are vital. Communicate with your consultant in infectious diseases.[19]

---

**1** Therapeutic or prophylactic antivirals are said to be the most effective single intervention followed by vaccine and basic public health measures.[20] But oseltamivir resistance and unavailability of a suitable vaccine during the early stages of a pandemic make non-drug interventions all the more important.

Chest medicine

**Respiratory failure** (See p180.) Type 1 respiratory failure ($P_aO_2$ <8kPa) is relatively common. Treatment is with high-flow (60%) oxygen. *Transfer the patient to ITU if hypoxia does not improve with $O_2$ therapy or $P_aCO_2$ rises to >6kPa.* Be careful with $O_2$ in COPD patients; check ABGs frequently, and consider elective ventilation if rising $P_aCO_2$ or worsening acidosis. Aim to keep $SaO_2$ at 94–98%, $P_aO_2$ ≥8kPa.

**Hypotension** may be due to a combination of dehydration and vasodilatation due to sepsis. If systolic BP is <90mmHg, give an intravenous fluid challenge of 250mL colloid/crystalloid over 15min. If BP does not rise, consider a central line and give IV fluids to maintain the systolic BP >90mmHg. If systolic BP remains <90mmHg despite fluid therapy, request ITU assessment for inotropic support (adrenaline, noradrenaline).

**Atrial fibrillation** (p124) is quite common, particularly in the elderly. It usually resolves with treatment of the pneumonia. β-blocker or digoxin may be required to slow the ventricular response rate in the short term.

**Pleural effusion** Inflammation of the pleura by adjacent pneumonia may cause fluid exudation into the pleural space. If this accumulates in the pleural space faster than it is reabsorbed, a pleural effusion develops. If this is small it may be of no consequence. If it becomes large and symptomatic, or infected (empyema), drainage is required (p184 & p780).

**Empyema** is pus in the pleural space. It should be suspected if a patient with a resolving pneumonia develops a recurrent fever. Clinical features: CXR indicates a pleural effusion. The aspirated pleural fluid is typically yellow and turbid with a pH <7.2, glucose↓, and LDH↑. The empyema should be drained using a chest drain, inserted under radiological guidance. Adhesions and loculation can make this difficult.

**Lung abscess** is a cavitating area of localized, suppurative infection within the lung (see fig 1).

*Causes:* •Inadequately treated pneumonia •Aspiration (eg alcoholism, oesophageal obstruction, bulbar palsy) •Bronchial obstruction (tumour, foreign body) •Pulmonary infarction •Septic emboli (septicaemia, right heart endocarditis, IV drug use) •Subphrenic or hepatic abscess.

*Clinical features:* Swinging fever; cough; purulent, foul-smelling sputum; pleuritic chest pain; haemoptysis; malaise; weight loss. Look for: finger clubbing; anaemia; crepitations. Empyema develops in 20–30%.

*Tests: Blood:* FBC (anaemia, neutrophilia), ESR, CRP, blood cultures. Sputum microscopy, culture, and cytology. *CXR:* walled cavity, often with a fluid level. Consider CT scan to exclude obstruction, and bronchoscopy to obtain diagnostic specimens.

*Treatment:* Antibiotics as indicated by sensitivities; continue until healed (4–6 wks). Postural drainage. Repeated aspiration, antibiotic instillation, or surgical excision may be required.

**Septicaemia** may occur as a result of bacterial spread from the lung parenchyma into the bloodstream. This may cause metastatic infection, eg infective endocarditis, meningitis. Treatment with IV antibiotic according to sensitivities.

**Pericarditis and myocarditis** may also complicate pneumonia.

**Jaundice** This is usually cholestatic, and may be due to sepsis or secondary to antibiotic therapy (particularly flucloxacillin and co-amoxiclav).

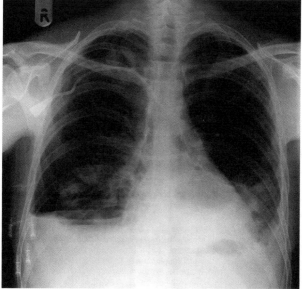

**Fig 1.** PA chest radiograph showing multiple rounded ring lesions of differing sizes in the right lower zone, at the right apex and in the left lower zone. The lesions are largest in the right lower zone, where they can be seen to contain air-fluid levels, typical appearance of infection in a pneumatocele (=air cyst) or cavitating lesion. A moderate right-sided hydropneumothorax can also be seen, suggesting that one of these lesions may have ruptured into the pleural cavity. The patient also has a right subclavian central venous catheter for the administration of antibiotics. The diagnosis in this case was that of multiple pulmonary abscesses in a patient who was an intravenous drug user.

Image courtesy of Derby Hospitals NHS Foundation Trust Radiology Department.

Chest medicine

**Pathology** Chronic infection of the bronchi and bronchioles leading to permanent dilatation of these airways. Main organisms: *H. influenzae*; *Strep. pneumoniae*; *Staph. aureus*; *Pseudomonas aeruginosa*.

**Causes** *Congenital:* cystic fibrosis (CF); Young's syndrome; primary ciliary dyskinesia; Kartagener's syndrome (OHCS p646). *Post-infection:* measles; pertussis; bronchiolitis; pneumonia; TB; HIV. *Other:* bronchial obstruction (tumour, foreign body); allergic bronchopulmonary aspergillosis (ABPA, p168); hypogammaglobulinaemia; rheumatoid arthritis; ulcerative colitis; idiopathic.

**Clinical features** *Symptoms:* persistent cough; copious purulent sputum; intermittent haemoptysis. *Signs:* finger clubbing; coarse inspiratory crepitations; wheeze (asthma, COPD, ABPA). *Complications:* pneumonia; pleural effusion; pneumothorax; haemoptysis; cerebral abscess; amyloidosis.

**Tests** *Sputum* culture. *CXR:* cystic shadows, thickened bronchial walls (tramline and ring shadows); see fig 1. *HRCT chest:* (p158) to assess extent and distribution of disease. *Spirometry* often shows an obstructive pattern; reversibility should be assessed. *Bronchoscopy* to locate site of haemoptysis, exclude obstruction and obtain samples for culture. *Other tests:* serum immunoglobulins; CF sweat test; *Aspergillus* precipitins or skin-prick test.

**Management** •*Postural drainage* should be performed twice daily. Chest physiotherapy may aid sputum expectoration and mucous drainage. •*Antibiotics* should be prescribed according to bacterial sensitivities. Patients known to culture *Pseudomonas* will require either oral ciprofloxacin or IV antibiotics. If ≥3 exacerbations a year consider long-term antibiotics. •*Bronchodilators* (eg nebulized salbutamol) may be useful in patients with asthma, COPD, CF, ABPA (p168). •*Corticosteroids* (eg prednisolone) for ABPA. •*Surgery* may be indicated in localized disease or to control severe haemoptysis.

## Cystic fibrosis (CF)    See *OHCS* (Paediatrics, p162)

One of the commonest life-threatening autosomal recessive conditions (1:2000 live births) affecting Caucasians. Caused by mutations in the CF transmembrane conductance regulator (CFTR) gene on chromosome 7 (>800 mutations have now been identified). This is a Cl⁻ channel, and the defect leads to a combination of defective chloride secretion and increased sodium absorption across airway epithelium. The changes in the composition of airway surface liquid predispose the lung to chronic pulmonary infections and bronchiectasis.

**Clinical features** *Neonate:* Failure to thrive; meconium ileus; rectal prolapse.

*Children and young adults: Respiratory:* cough; wheeze; recurrent infections; bronchiectasis; pneumothorax; haemoptysis; respiratory failure; cor pulmonale. *Gastrointestinal:* pancreatic insufficiency (diabetes mellitus, steatorrhoea); distal intestinal obstruction syndrome (meconium ileus equivalent); gallstones; cirrhosis. *Other:* male infertility; osteoporosis; arthritis; vasculitis (p558); nasal polyps; sinusitis; and hypertrophic pulmonary osteoarthropathy (HPOA). *Signs:* cyanosis; finger clubbing; bilateral coarse crackles.

**Diagnosis** *Sweat test:* sweat sodium and chloride >60mmol/L; chloride usually > sodium. *Genetics:* screening for known common CF mutations should be considered. *Faecal elastase* is a simple and useful screening test for exocrine pancreatic dysfunction.

**Tests** *Blood:* FBC; U&E; LFT; clotting; vitamin A, D, E levels; annual glucose tolerance test (p198). *Bacteriology:* cough swab, sputum culture. *Radiology:* CXR; hyperinflation; bronchiectasis. *Abdominal ultrasound:* fatty liver; cirrhosis; chronic pancreatitis; *Spirometry:* obstructive defect. *Aspergillus serology/skin test* (20% develop ABPA, p168). *Biochemistry:* faecal fat analysis.

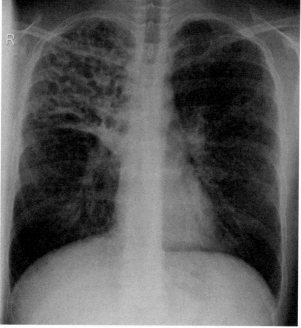

**Fig 1.** PA chest radiograph showing marked abnormal dilatation of the airways throughout the right upper lobe, along with similar changes to a lesser degree throughout the rest of the lung (most notably in the periphery of the left upper zone). Appearances are that of bronchiectasis, which in this case was congenital. The fine background reticular pattern in the lungs suggests that there may also be some interstitial lung disease present.

Image courtesy of Nottingham University Hospitals NHS Trust Radiology Department.

## Management of cystic fibrosis

Patients with cystic fibrosis are best managed by a multidisciplinary team, eg physician, GP, physiotherapist, specialist nurse, and dietician, with attention to psychosocial as well as physical wellbeing. Gene therapy (transfer of CFTR gene using liposome or adenovirus vectors) is not yet possible.

*Chest:* Physiotherapy regularly (postural drainage, active cycle breathing techniques or forced expiratory techniques). Antibiotics are given for acute infective exacerbations and prophylactically (PO or nebulized). Mucolytics may be useful (eg DNase, ie Dornase alfa, 2.5mg daily nebulized, *OHCS* p163). Bronchodilators.

*Gastrointestinal:* Pancreatic enzyme replacement; fat soluble vitamin supplements (A, D, E, K); ursodeoxycholic acid for impaired liver function; cirrhosis may require liver transplantation.

*Other:* Treatment of CF-related diabetes; screening for and treatment of osteoporosis; treatment of arthritis, sinusitis, and vasculitis; fertility and genetic counselling.

*Advanced lung disease:* Oxygen, diuretics (cor pulmonale); non-invasive ventilation; lung or heart/lung transplantation.

*Prognosis:* Median survival is now ~40yrs in the UK.

**Aspergillus** This group of fungi affects the lung in 5 ways:

1 *Asthma:* Type I hypersensitivity (atopic) reaction to fungal spores (p172).

2 *Allergic bronchopulmonary aspergillosis (ABPA):* Results from type I and III hypersensitivity reactions to *Aspergillus fumigatus*. Affects 1-5% of asthmatics, 2-25% of CF patients.[22] Early on, the allergic response causes bronchoconstriction, but as the inflammation persists, permanent damage occurs, causing bronchiectasis (fig 1). *Symptoms:* wheeze, cough, sputum (plugs of mucus containing fungal hyphae, see p440), dyspnoea, and 'recurrent pneumonia'. *Investigations:* CXR (transient segmental collapse or consolidation, bronchiectasis); *Aspergillus* in sputum; positive *Aspergillus* skin test and/or *Aspergillus*-specific IgE RAST (radioallergosorbent test); positive serum precipitins; eosinophilia; raised serum IgE. *Treatment:* prednisolone 30-40mg/24h PO for acute attacks; maintenance dose 5-10mg/d. Sometimes itraconazole is used in combination with corticosteroids. Bronchodilators for asthma. Sometimes bronchoscopic aspiration of mucous plugs is needed.

3 *Aspergilloma (mycetoma):* A fungus ball within a pre-existing cavity (often caused by TB or sarcoidosis). It is usually asymptomatic but may cause cough, haemoptysis (may be torrential), lethargy ± weight loss. *Investigations:* CXR (round opacity within a cavity, usually apical); sputum culture; strongly positive serum precipitins; *Aspergillus* skin test (30% +ve). *Treatment* (only if symptomatic): consider surgical excision for solitary symptomatic lesions or severe haemoptysis. Oral itraconazole and other antifungals have been tried with limited success. Local instillation of amphotericin paste under CT guidance yields partial success in carefully selected patients, eg in massive haemoptysis.

4 *Invasive aspergillosis: Risk factors:*[23] immunocompromise, eg HIV, leukaemia, burns, Wegener's• (p728), and SLE, or after broad-spectrum antibiotic therapy. *Investigations:* sputum culture; BAL; biopsy; serum precipitins; CXR (consolidation, abscess). Early chest CT and serial serum measurements of galactomannan (an *Aspergillus* antigen) may be helpful. Diagnosis may only be made at lung biopsy or autopsy. *Treatment:* voriconazole is superior to IV amphotericin.[24] Alternatives: IV miconazole or ketoconazole (less effective). *Prognosis:* 30% mortality.

5 *Extrinsic allergic alveolitis (EAA)* may be caused by sensitivity to *Aspergillus clavatus* ('malt worker's lung'). Clinical features and treatment are as for other causes of EAA (p188). Diagnosis is based on a history of exposure and presence of serum precipitins to *A. clavatus*. Pulmonary fibrosis may occur if untreated.

**Other fungal infections** *Candida* and *Cryptococcus* may cause pneumonia in the immunosuppressed (see p440).

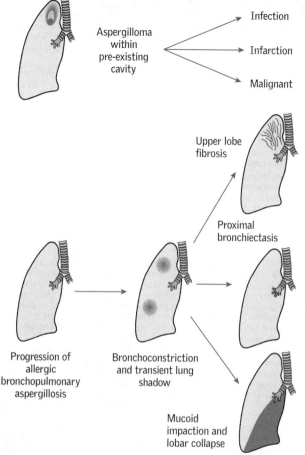

**Fig 1.** Aspergillosis.

---

### Using amphotericin B

Test dose: 1mg in 20mL 5% dextrose IV over 20–30min. Observe closely for the next ½h for signs of anaphylaxis (shock, swelling, wheeze, etc.). There are various formulations. Consult *BNF*. *Do not give any other drug in the same IVI*. SE: anaphylaxis; serious nephrotoxicity; fever; rash; anorexia; nausea; D&V; headache; myalgia; arthralgia; anaemia; ↓K⁺; ↓Mg²⁺; hepatotoxicity; arrhythmias; hearing loss; diplopia; seizures; neuropathy; phlebitis. *Monitor* U&E *daily*. *AmBisome*® (liposomal amphotericin) has fewer SEs, but is expensive; it is indicated in systemic or deep mycoses where nephrotoxicity precludes conventional amphotericin; IV initial test dose: 1mg over 10min, then 3mg/kg/d (max 5mg/kg/d IVI).[25] Alternatives: *Abelcet*® and *Amphocil*®

Chest medicine

**Carcinoma of the bronchus** Accounts for ~19% of all cancers and 27% of cancer deaths (40,000 cases/yr in UK). Incidence is increasing in women. Only 5% 'cured'.

*Risk factors:* Cigarette smoking is the major risk factor. Others: asbestos, chromium, arsenic, iron oxides, and radiation (radon gas).

*Histology:* Squamous (35%); adenocarcinoma (27%); small (oat) cell (20%); large cell (10%); alveolar cell carcinoma (rare, <1%). Clinically the most important division is between small cell (SCLC) and non-small cell (NSCLC).

*Symptoms:* Cough (80%); haemoptysis (70%); dyspnoea (60%); chest pain (40%); recurrent or slowly resolving pneumonia; lethargy; anorexia; weight loss. *Signs:* Cachexia; anaemia; clubbing; HPOA (hypertrophic pulmonary osteoarthropathy, causing wrist pain); supraclavicular or axillary nodes. *Chest signs:* none, or: consolidation; collapse; pleural effusion. *Metastases:* bone tenderness; hepatomegaly; confusion; fits; focal CNS signs; cerebellar syndrome; proximal myopathy; peripheral neuropathy.

*Complications: Local:* recurrent laryngeal nerve palsy; phrenic nerve palsy; SVC obstruction; Horner's syndrome (Pancoast's tumour); rib erosion; pericarditis; AF. *Metastatic:* brain; bone (bone pain, anaemia, $\uparrow Ca^{2+}$); liver; adrenals (Addison's). *Endocrine:* ectopic hormone secretion, eg SIADH ($\downarrow Na^+$ and $\uparrow ADH$, p678) and ACTH (Cushing's) by small cell tumours; PTH ($\uparrow Ca^{2+}$) by squamous cell tumours. *Non-metastatic neurological:* confusion; fits; cerebellar syndrome; proximal myopathy; neuropathy; polymyositis; Lambert-Eaton syndrome (p516). *Other:* clubbing; HPOA; dermatomyositis; acanthosis nigricans (p565, fig 6); thrombophlebitis migrans (p564).

*Tests:* (see BOX 1, fig 1) *Cytology:* sputum and pleural fluid (send at least 20mL). *CXR:* peripheral nodule; hilar enlargement; consolidation; lung collapse; pleural effusion; bony secondaries. Peripheral lesions and superficial lymph nodes may be amenable to percutaneous *fine needle aspiration* or *biopsy. CT* to stage the tumour (BOX 2) and guide bronchoscopy. *Bronchoscopy:* to give histology and assess operability, ± endobronchial ultrasound for assessment and biopsy. $^{18}$*F-deoxyglucose PET* or *PET/CT scan* to help in staging. *Radionuclide bone scan:* if suspected metastases. *Lung function tests:* help assess suitability for lobectomy.

*Treatment: Non-small cell tumours:* Excision is the treatment of choice for peripheral tumours, with no metastatic spread: stage I/II (~25%). *Curative radiotherapy* is an alternative if respiratory reserve is poor. *Chemotherapy ± radiotherapy* for more advanced disease. Regimens may be platinum-based, eg with monoclonal antibodies targetting the epidermal growth factor receptor (cetuximab). Get specialist help. *Small cell tumours* are nearly always disseminated at presentation. They may respond to *chemotherapy* but invariably relapse (cyclophosphamide + doxorubicin + vincristine + etoposide; or cisplatin ± *radiotherapy* if limited disease). *Palliation: Radiotherapy* is used for bronchial obstruction, SVC obstruction, haemoptysis, bone pain, and cerebral metastases. *SVC stent* + radiotherapy and dexamethasone for SVC obstruction. *Endobronchial therapy:* tracheal stenting, cryotherapy, laser, brachytherapy (a radioactive source is placed close to the tumour). *Pleural drainage/pleurodesis* for symptomatic pleural effusions. *Drugs:* analgesia; steroids; antiemetics; cough linctus (codeine); bronchodilators; antidepressants.

*Prognosis: Non-small cell:* 50% 2yr survival without spread; 10% with spread. *Small cell:* median survival is 3 months if untreated; 1–1½yrs if treated.

*Prevention:* Quit smoking (p87). Prevent occupational exposure to carcinogens.

**Other lung tumours** *Bronchial adenoma:* Rare, slow-growing. 90% are carcinoid tumours; 10% cylindromas. *R:* surgery. *Hamartoma:* Rare, benign; CT: lobulated mass ± flecks of calcification; ?excise to exclude malignancy. *Mesothelioma* (p192).

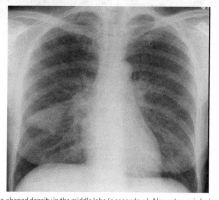

Fig 1. A wedge-shaped density in the middle lobe (a secondary). Also note a coin lesion at the right costophrenic angle. The sharp upper boundary of the middle lobe triangular mass is the middle lobe fissure. The right hilar structures are enlarged by metastases within the hilar lymph nodes.

Courtesy of Janet E. Jeddry, Yale Medical School.

## Differential diagnosis of nodule in the lung on a CXR

| | |
|---|---|
| Malignancy (1° or 2°) | Arterio-venous malformation |
| Abscesses (p164) | Encysted effusion (fluid, blood, pus) |
| Granuloma | Cyst |
| Carcinoid tumour | Foreign body |
| Pulmonary hamartoma | Skin tumour (eg seborrhoeic wart) |

## TNM staging for non-small cell lung cancer

### Primary tumour (T)

| | |
|---|---|
| TX | Malignant cells in bronchial secretions, no other evidence of tumour |
| TIS | Carcinoma *in situ* |
| T0 | None evident |
| T1 | ≤3cm, in lobar or more distal airway |
| T2 | >3cm and >2cm distal to carina or any size if pleural involvement or obstructive pneumonitis extending to hilum, but not all the lung |
| T3 | Involves the chest wall, diaphragm, mediastinal pleura, pericardium, or <2cm from, but not at, carina. T >7cm diameter and nodules in same lobe |
| T4 | Involves mediastinum, heart, great vessels, trachea, oesophagus, vertebral body, carina, malignant effusion, or nodules in another lobe |

### Regional nodes (N)

| | |
|---|---|
| N0 | None involved (after mediastinoscopy) |
| N1 | Peribronchial and/or ipsilateral hilum |
| N2 | Ipsilateral mediastinum or subcarinal |
| N3 | Contralateral mediastinum or hilum, scalene, or supraclavicular |

### Distant metastasis (M)

| | |
|---|---|
| M0 | None |
| M1 | a) Nodule in other lung, pleural lesions or malignant effusion; b) distant metastases present |

### Stages

| Occult | I | II | IIIa | IIIb | IV |
|---|---|---|---|---|---|
| TX N0 M0 | TIS/T1/T2 N0 M0 | T1/T2 N1 M0 | T3 N1 M0 | T1-4 N3 M0 | T1-4 N0-3 M1 |
| | | *or* T3 N0 M0 | *or* T1-3 N2 M0 | *or* T4 N0-2 M0 | |

Chest medicine

Asthma affects 5–8% of the population. It is characterized by recurrent episodes of dyspnoea, cough, and wheeze caused by reversible airways obstruction. Three factors contribute to airway narrowing: *bronchial muscle contraction*, triggered by a variety of stimuli; *mucosal swelling/inflammation*, caused by mast cell and basophil degranulation resulting in the release of inflammatory mediators; *increased mucus production*.

**Symptoms** Intermittent dyspnoea, wheeze, cough (often nocturnal) and sputum. Ask specifically about:

*Precipitants:* Cold air, exercise, emotion, allergens (house dust mite, pollen, fur), infection, smoking and passive smoking,[28] pollution, NSAIDs, β-blockers.

*Diurnal variation* in symptoms or peak flow. Marked morning dipping of peak flow is common and can tip the balance into a serious attack, despite having normal peak flow (fig 1) at other times.

*Exercise:* Quantify the exercise tolerance.

*Disturbed sleep:* Quantify as nights per week (a sign of severe asthma).

*Acid reflux:* 40–60% of those with asthma have reflux; treating it improves spirometry—but not necessarily symptoms.[29]

*Other atopic disease:* Eczema, hay fever, allergy, or family history?

*The home (especially the bedroom):* Pets? Carpet? Feather pillows or duvet? Floor cushions and other 'soft furnishings'?

*Job:* If symptoms remit at weekends or holidays, work may provide the trigger (15% of cases are work-related—more for paint sprayers, food processors, welders, and animal handlers).[30] Ask the patient to measure his peak flow at intervals at work and at home (at the same time of day) to confirm this (see fig 2).

*Days per week off work or school.*

**Signs** Tachypnoea; audible wheeze; hyperinflated chest; hyperresonant percussion note; air entry ↓; widespread, polyphonic wheeze. *Severe attack:* inability to complete sentences; pulse >110bpm; respiratory rate >25/min; PEF 33–50% predicted. *Life-threatening attack:* silent chest; confusion; exhaustion; cyanosis ($P_aO_2$ <8 kPa but $P_aCO_2$ 4.6–6.0, $SpO_2$ <92%); bradycardia; PEF <33% predicted. *Near fatal:* ↑$P_aCO_2$.

**Tests** *Acute attack:* PEF, sputum culture, FBC, U&E, CRP, blood cultures. ABG analysis usually shows a normal or slightly ↓ $P_aO_2$ but ↓ $P_aCO_2$ (hyperventilation). If $P_aO_2$ is normal but the patient is hyperventilating, watch carefully and repeat the ABG a little later. ►*If $P_aCO_2$ is normal or raised, transfer to high-dependency unit or ITU for ventilation*, as this signifies failing respiratory effort. CXR (to exclude infection or pneumothorax). *Chronic asthma:* PEF monitoring (p156): a diurnal variation of >20% on ≥3d a wk for 2wks. Spirometry: obstructive defect (↓FEV₁/FVC, ↑RV p156); usually ≥15% improvement in FEV₁ following β₂ agonists or steroid trial. CXR: hyperinflation. Skin-prick tests may help to identify allergens. Histamine or methacholine challenge. *Aspergillus* serology.

**Treatment** Chronic asthma (p174). Emergency treatment (p820).

**Differential diagnosis** Pulmonary oedema ('cardiac asthma'); COPD (may co-exist); large airway obstruction (eg foreign body, tumour); SVC obstruction (wheeze/dyspnoea not episodic); pneumothorax; PE; bronchiectasis; obliterative bronchiolitis (suspect in elderly).

**Associated diseases** Acid reflux; polyarteritis nodosa (PAN, p558); Churg-Strauss syndrome (p710); ABPA (p168).

**Natural history** Most childhood asthmatics (see *OHCS* p164) either grow out of asthma in adolescence or suffer much less as adults. A significant number of people develop chronic asthma late in life.

**Mortality** ~1000 asthma deaths in the UK in 2009, 50% were >65yrs old.

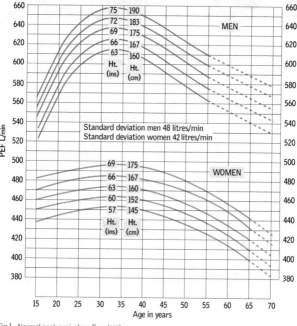

**Fig 1.** Normal peak expiratory flow (PEF).

Data from Nunn, A.J, Gregg, I. New regression equations for predicting peak expiratory flow in adults. *BMJ* 1989;298:1068–70.

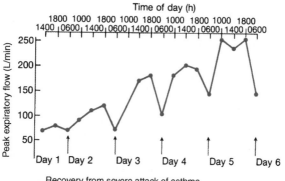

Recovery from severe attack of asthma
Predicted PEF was 320 L/min
Arrows point to early morning 'dips'

**Fig 2.** Examples of serial peak flow charts.

Chest medicine

**Behaviour** Help to quit smoking (p87). Avoid precipitants. Check inhaler technique. Teach use of a peak flow meter to monitor PEF twice a day. Educate to enable self-management by altering their medication in the light of symptoms or PEF. Give specific advice about what to do in an emergency; provide a written action plan. Consider teaching relaxed breathing to avoid dysfunctional breathing[31] (Papworth method).[1]

**British Thoracic Society guidelines**[27] Start at the step most appropriate to severity; moving up if needed, or down if control is good for >3 months. Rescue courses of prednisolone may be used at any time.

*Step 1* Occasional short-acting inhaled $\beta_2$-agonist as required for symptom relief. If used more than once daily, or night-time symptoms, go to Step 2.

*Step 2* Add standard-dose inhaled steroid, eg beclometasone 200–800µg/day, or start at the dose appropriate for disease severity, and titrate as required.

*Step 3* Add long-acting $\beta_2$-agonist (eg salmeterol 50µg/12h by inhaler). If benefit—but still inadequate control—continue and ↑dose of beclometasone to 800µg/day. If no effect of long-acting $\beta_2$-agonist stop it. Review diagnosis. Leukotriene receptor antagonist or oral theophylline may be tried.

*Step 4* Consider trials of: beclometasone up to 2000µg/day; modified-release oral theophylline; modified-release oral $\beta_2$-agonist; oral leukotriene receptor antagonist (see below), in conjunction with previous therapy. Modified-release $\beta_2$ agonist tablets.

*Step 5* Add regular oral prednisolone (1 dose daily, at the lowest possible dose). Continue with high-dose inhaled steroids. Refer to asthma clinic.

**Drugs** *$\beta_2$-adrenoceptor agonists* relax bronchial smooth muscle (↑cAMP), acting within minutes. Salbutamol is best given by inhalation (aerosol, powder, nebulizer), but may also be given PO or IV. SE: tachyarrhythmias, ↓K⁺, tremor, anxiety. Long-acting inhaled $\beta_2$-agonist (eg salmeterol, formoterol) can help nocturnal symptoms and reduce morning dips. They may be an alternative to ↑steroid dose when symptoms are uncontrolled; doubts remain over whether they are associated with an increase in adverse events.[32] SE: as salbutamol, paradoxical bronchospasm.[33]

*Corticosteroids* are best inhaled to minimize systemic effects, eg beclometasone via spacer (or powder), but may be given PO or IV. They act over days to ↓bronchial mucosal inflammation. Rinse mouth after inhaled steroids to prevent oral candidiasis. Oral steroids are used acutely (high-dose, short courses, eg prednisolone 40mg/24h PO for 7d) and longer term in lower dose (eg 5–10mg/24h) if control is not optimal on inhalers. Warn about SEs: p371.

*Aminophylline* (metabolized to theophylline) acts by inhibiting phosphodiesterase, thus ↓bronchoconstriction by ↑cAMP levels. Try as prophylaxis, at night, PO, to prevent morning dipping. Stick with one brand name (bioavailability variable). Also useful as an adjunct if inhaled therapy is inadequate. In acute severe asthma, it may be given IVI. It has a narrow therapeutic ratio, causing arrhythmias, GI upset, and fits in the toxic range. Check theophylline levels (p766), and do ECG monitoring and check plasma levels after 24h if IV therapy is required.

*Anticholinergics* (eg ipratropium, tiotropium) may ↓muscle spasm synergistically with $\beta_2$-agonists but are not recommended in current guidelines for *chronic* asthma. They may be of more benefit in COPD.

*Cromoglicate* May be used as prophylaxis in mild and exercise-induced asthma (always inhaled), especially in children. It may precipitate asthma.

*Leukotriene receptor antagonists* (eg oral montelukast, zafirlukast) block the effects of cysteinyl leukotrienes in the airways by antagonizing the CystLT₁ receptor.

*Anti-IgE monoclonal antibody* Omalizumab[34] may be of use in highly selected patients with persistent allergic asthma. Given as a subcutaneous injection every 2–4 wks depending on dose. Specialists only.

---

**1** Integrated breathing and relaxation training (Papworth method) is psychological *and* physical: patients learn to drop their shoulders, relax their abdomen, and breathe calmly and appropriately.

## Adult doses of common inhaled drugs used in bronchoconstriction

| | Inhaled aerosol | Inhaled powder | Nebulized (supervised) |
|---|---|---|---|
| **Salbutamol** | | | |
| Dose example: | 100–200µg/6h | 200–400µg/6h | 2.5–5mg/6h |
| Airomir® is a CFC-free example of a breath-actuated inhaler | | | |
| **Terbutaline** | | | |
| Single dose | | 500µg[1] | 2.5mg/mL |
| Recommended regimen | | 500µg/6h | 5–10mg/6–12h |
| **Salmeterol** | | | |
| Dose/puff | 25µg | 50µg | — |
| Recommended regimen | 50–100µg/12h | 50–100µg/12h | — |
| **Ipratropium bromide (COPD)** | | | |
| Dose/puff | 20µg | | 250µg/mL |
| Recommended regimen | 20–40µg/6h | | 250–500µg/6h |
| **Steroids** | | | |
| (Clenil Modulite®=beclometasone; Pulmicort®=budesonide;[1] Flixotide®=fluticasone) | | | |
| **Fluticasone (Flixotide®)** | | | |
| Doses available/puff | 50, 100, 250 & 500µg | As for aerosol | 250µg/mL |
| Recommended regimen | 100–250µg/12h | 100–250µg/12h max 1mg/12h | 0.5–2mg/12h |
| **Clenil Modulite®** | | | |
| Doses available/puff | 50 & 100µg 250µg | — | — |
| Recommended regimen | 200µg/12h ↓ 400µg/12h ↓ 1000µg/12h | | |

▶Prescribe beclometasone by brand name, and state that a CFC-free inhaler should be dispensed. This is because, dose for dose, Qvar® is twice as potent as the other available CFC-free brand (Clenil Modulite®).

Any dose ≥250µg ≈ significant steroid absorption: carry a steroid card; this recommendation is being widened, and lower doses (beclometasone) are now said to merit a steroid card (manufacturer's information).

1 Available as a Turbohaler®; Autohalers® are an alternative (breath-actuated) and don't need breathing coordination, eg Airomir® (salbutamol) and Qvar® (beclometasone). Accuhalers® deliver dry powders (eg Flixotide®, Serevent®).
Systemic absorption (via the throat) is less if inhalation is through a **large-volume device**, eg Volumatic® or AeroChamber Plus® devices. The latter is more compact. Static charge on some devices reduces dose delivery, so wash in water before dose; leave to dry (don't rub). It's pointless to squirt many puffs into a device: it is best to repeat single doses, and be sure to inhale *as soon as the drug is in the spacer*. SE: local (oral) candidiasis (p371); ↑rate of cataract if lifetime dose ≥2g beclometasone.[16]

**Definitions** COPD is a common progressive disorder characterized by airway obstruction ($FEV_1$ <80% predicted; $FEV_1/FVC$ <0.7; see p156 and TABLE below) with little or no reversibility. It includes chronic bronchitis and emphysema. Usually patients have *either* COPD *or* asthma, not both: COPD is suggested by: •Age of onset >35yrs •Smoking (passive or active) or pollution related[38] •Chronic dyspnoea •Sputum production •Minimal diurnal or day-to-day $FEV_1$ variation. **Chronic bronchitis** is defined *clinically* as cough, sputum production on most days for 3 months of 2 successive yrs. Symptoms improve if they stop smoking. There is no excess mortality if lung function is normal. **Emphysema** is defined *histologically* as enlarged air spaces distal to terminal bronchioles, with destruction of alveolar walls.

**Prevalence** 10-20% of the over-40s; $2.5\times10^6$ deaths/yr worldwide.[39]

**Pink puffers and blue bloaters** (ends of a spectrum) *Pink puffers* have ↑alveolar ventilation, a near normal $P_aO_2$ and a normal or low $P_aCO_2$. They are breathless but are not cyanosed. They may progress to type I respiratory failure (p180). *Blue bloaters* have ↓alveolar ventilation, with a low $P_aO_2$ and a high $P_aCO_2$. They are cyanosed but not breathless and may go on to develop cor pulmonale. Their respiratory centres are relatively insensitive to $CO_2$ and they rely on hypoxic drive to maintain respiratory effort (p180)—►*supplemental oxygen should be given with care.*

**Symptoms** Cough; sputum; dyspnoea; wheeze. **Signs** Tachypnoea; use of accessory muscles of respiration; hyperinflation; ↓cricosternal distance (<3cm); ↓expansion; resonant or hyperresonant percussion note; quiet breath sounds (eg over bullae); wheeze; cyanosis; cor pulmonale.

**Complications** Acute exacerbations ± infection; polycythaemia; respiratory failure; cor pulmonale (oedema; JVP↑); pneumothorax (ruptured bullae); lung carcinoma.

**Tests** FBC; PCV↑. CXR: Hyperinflation (>6 anterior ribs seen above diaphragm in midclavicular line); flat hemidiaphragms; large central pulmonary arteries; ↓peripheral vascular markings; bullae. ECG: Right atrial and ventricular hypertrophy (cor pulmonale). ABG: $P_aO_2$ ↓ ± hypercapnia. *Lung function* (p156, p159): obstructive + air trapping ($FEV_1$ <80% of predicted—see p156, $FEV_1$:FVC ratio <70%, TLC↑, RV↑, DLCO↓ in emphysema—see p158). Learn how to do spirometry from an experienced person: ensure *maximal* expiration of the full breath (it takes >4s; it's *not* a quick puff out). *Trial of steroids:* See BOX 2.

**Treatment** *Chronic stable:* see BOX; ►►*Emergency* R̥: p822. Offer *smoking cessation advice* with cordial vigour (p87). BMI is often low: *diet advice ± supplements*[40] may help (p586). *Mucolytics* (BNF 3.7) may help chronic productive cough (NICE).[41] Disabilities may cause serious, treatable *depression*; screen for this (p11). *Respiratory failure:* p180. *Flu and pneumococcal vaccinations:* p160 and p402.

*Long-term $O_2$ therapy (LTOT):* An MRC trial showed that if $P_aO_2$ was maintained ≥8.0kPa for 15h a day, 3yr survival improved by 50%. UK NICE guidelines suggest LTOT should be given for: 1 Clinically stable non-smokers with $P_aO_2$ <7.3kPa—despite maximal R̥. These values should be stable on two occasions >3wks apart. 2 If $P_aO_2$ 7.3-8.0 *and* pulmonary hypertension (eg RVH; loud $s_2$), or polycythaemia, or peripheral oedema, or nocturnal hypoxia. 3 $O_2$ can also be prescribed for terminally ill patients.

| *Predicted $FEV_1$ (Caucasian ♂; litres; ↓level in other races)*[1] | | | | | | | | | | ♀ | | | | | | | | |
|---|---|---|---|---|---|---|---|---|---|---|---|---|---|---|---|---|---|---|
| Height cm | 150 | 155 | 160 | 165 | 170 | 175 | 180 | 185 | 190 | 195 | 145 | 150 | 155 | 160 | 165 | 170 | 175 | 180 | 185 | 190 |
| ♂ Age(yr) | | | | | | | | | | | | | | | | | | | |
| 25 | 2.9 | 3.2 | 3.4 | 3.7 | 4.0 | 4.2 | 4.3 | 4.7 | 5.0 | 5.3 | 2.6 | 2.7 | 2.9 | 3.0 | 3.1 | 3.3 | 3.4 | 3.5 | 3.7 | 3.8 |
| 30 | 2.8 | 3.1 | 3.3 | 3.6 | 3.8 | 4.1 | 4.3 | 4.6 | 4.9 | 5.1 | 2.5 | 2.6 | 2.8 | 2.9 | 3.0 | 3.2 | 3.3 | 3.4 | 3.6 | 3.7 |
| 40 | 2.5 | 2.8 | 3.0 | 3.3 | 3.6 | 3.8 | 4.1 | 4.3 | 4.6 | 4.9 | 2.3 | 2.4 | 2.5 | 2.7 | 2.8 | 3.0 | 3.0 | 3.2 | 3.3 | 3.5 |
| 50 | 2.2 | 2.5 | 2.8 | 3.0 | 3.3 | 3.5 | 3.8 | 4.0 | 4.3 | 4.6 | 2.1 | 2.2 | 2.3 | 2.5 | 2.6 | 2.7 | 2.9 | 3.0 | 3.1 | 3.3 |
| 60 | 2.0 | 2.2 | 2.5 | 2.8 | 3.0 | 3.3 | 3.5 | 3.8 | 4.0 | 4.3 | 2.0 | 2.1 | 2.3 | 2.4 | 2.5 | 2.7 | 2.8 | 2.9 | 3.1 |
| 70 | 1.7 | 2.0 | 2.2 | 2.5 | 2.7 | 3.0 | 3.3 | 3.5 | 3.8 | 4.0 | 1.6 | 1.8 | 1.9 | 2.1 | 2.2 | 2.3 | 2.5 | 2.6 | 2.7 | 2.9 |
| 80 | 1.4 | 1.7 | 2.0 | 2.2 | 2.5 | 2.7 | 3.0 | 3.3 | 3.5 | 3.8 | 1.4 | 1.6 | 1.7 | 1.9 | 2.0 | 2.1 | 2.2 | 2.4 | 2.5 | 2.7 |
| | | | | | | | Data from www.nationalasthma.org.au/publications/spiro/appc.html#Mean | | | | | | | | | | | | |

**1** African $FEV_1$ is 10-15% lower; Chinese: 20% lower; Indian: 10% lower; NB: PEF varies little between groups.

## British Thoracic Society (BTS)/NICE COPD guidelines[37]

| Assessment of COPD | Spirometry; bronchodilators may slightly improve $FEV_1$ |
| --- | --- |
| | Trial of oral steroids; look for >15% $\uparrow$ in $FEV_1$ |
| | CXR: ?bullae ?other pathology |
| | Arterial blood gases: hypoxia ?hypercapnia |
| **Severity of COPD** (all FVC<0.7) | Stage 1 Mild | $FEV_1 \geq 80\%$ of predicted |
| | Stage 2 Moderate | $FEV_1$ 50–79% of predicted |
| | Stage 3 Severe | $FEV_1$ 30–49% of predicted |
| | Stage 4 Very severe | $FEV_1 <30\%$ of predicted |

**Treating stable COPD**

| | |
| --- | --- |
| • *General* | Stop smoking, encourage exercise, treat poor nutrition or obesity, influenza and pneumococcal vaccination, pulmonary rehabilitation/palliative care. NIPPV: see p823. PRN short-acting antimuscarinic (ipratropium) or $\beta_2$ agonist. |
| • *Mild/moderate* | Inhaled long-acting antimuscarinic (tiotropium) or $\beta_2$ agonist.[1] |
| • *Severe* | Combination long-acting $\beta_2$ agonist + corticosteroids, eg Symbicort® (budesonide + formoterol)[42] or tiotropium. |
| • *If remain symptomatic* | Tiotropium + inhaled steroid + long-acting $\beta_2$ agonist Refer to specialist. Consider steroid trial, home nebulizers, theophylline. |
| • *Pulmonary hypertension* | Assess the need for LTOT (see p176). Treat oedema with diuretics. |

### More advanced COPD

▶Pulmonary rehabilitation is *greatly* valued by patients.
• Consider LTOT if $P_aO_2$ <7.3kPa (see OPPOSITE).
• Indications for surgery: recurrent pneumothoraces; isolated bullous disease; lung volume reduction surgery (selected patients).
• NIV may be appropriate if hypercapnic on LTOT.
• NB: air travel is risky if $FEV_1$ <50% or $P_aO_2$ <6.7kPa.
• Assess home set-up and support needed. Treat depression (p11).

### Indications for specialist referral

• Uncertain diagnosis, or suspected severe COPD, or a rapid decline in $FEV_1$.
• Onset of cor pulmonale.   • Bullous lung disease (to assess for surgery).
• Assessment for oral corticosteroids, nebulizer therapy, or LTOT.
• <10 pack-years smoking (=PYS =the number of packs/day × years of smoking) or COPD in patient <40yrs (eg is the cause $\alpha_1$-antitrypsin deficiency? p264).
• Symptoms disproportionate to lung function tests.
• Frequent infections (to exclude bronchiectasis).

### Steroid trial

30mg prednisolone/24h PO for 2wks. If $FEV_1$ rises by >15%, the COPD is 'steroid responsive' and benefit may be had by using long-term inhaled corticosteroids (p167). If this doesn't achieve the post-prednisolone $FEV_1$, request expert help. NB: NICE says that 'reversibility testing is not necessary as a part of the diagnostic process or to plan initial therapy with bronchodilators or corticosteroids. It may be unhelpful or misleading because: 1 Repeated $FEV_1$ measurements can show small spontaneous fluctuations; 2 Results of reversibility tests on different occasions can be inconsistent and not reproducible; 3 Over-reliance on a single reversibility test may be misleading unless the change in $FEV_1$ is >400mL; 4 Definition of a significant change is arbitrary; 5 Response to long-term therapy is not predicted by acute reversibility testing.'

---

**1** Cochrane meta-analyses (2007) of trials (including TORCH) favour steroids + LABA (long acting beta agonist) vs either alone. LABA alone may ↑exacerbation rates, but no excess hospitalizations or mortality; steroid inhalers alone are associated with ↑mortality (by 33%) compared with steroids + LABA.[41] Steroid inhalers may ↑risk of pneumonia, but when combined with LABA, advantages outweigh disadvantages.

*Chest medicine*

ARDS, or acute lung injury, may be caused by direct lung injury or occur secondary to severe systemic illness. Lung damage and release of inflammatory mediators cause increased capillary permeability and non-cardiogenic pulmonary oedema, often accompanied by multiorgan failure.

**Causes** *Pulmonary:* Pneumonia; gastric aspiration; inhalation; injury; vasculitis (p558); contusion. *Other:* Shock; septicaemia; haemorrhage; multiple transfusions; DIC (p346); pancreatitis; acute liver failure; trauma; head injury; malaria; fat embolism; burns; obstetric events (eclampsia; amniotic fluid embolus); drugs/toxins (aspirin, heroin, paraquat).

**Clinical features** Cyanosis; tachypnoea; tachycardia; peripheral vasodilatation; bilateral fine inspiratory crackles.

**Investigations** FBC, U&E, LFT, amylase, clotting, CRP, blood cultures, ABG. CXR shows bilateral pulmonary infiltrates. Pulmonary artery catheter to measure pulmonary capillary wedge pressure (PCWP).

**Diagnostic criteria**[44] One consensus requires these 4 to exist: 1 Acute onset. 2 CXR: bilateral infiltrates. 3 Pulmonary capillary wedge pressure (PCWP) <19mmHg or a lack of clinical congestive heart failure. 4 Refractory hypoxaemia with $P_aO_2$ : $FiO_2$ <200 for ARDS. Others include total thoracic compliance <30mL/cmH$_2$O.

**Management** Admit to ITU; give supportive therapy; treat the underlying cause.
- *Respiratory support* In early ARDS, continuous positive airway pressure (CPAP) with 40-60% oxygen may be adequate to maintain oxygenation. But most patients need mechanical ventilation. Indications for ventilation: $P_aO_2$: <8.3kPa despite 60% O$_2$; $P_aCO_2$: >6kPa. The large tidal volumes (10-15mL/kg) produced by conventional ventilation plus reduced lung compliance in ARDS may lead to high peak airway pressures ± pneumothorax. A low-tidal-volume, pressure-limited approach, with either low or moderate high positive end-expiratory pressure (PEEP), improves outcome.
- *Circulatory support* Invasive haemodynamic monitoring with an arterial line and Swan–Ganz catheter aids the diagnosis and may be helpful in monitoring PCWP and cardiac output. A conservative fluid management approach improves outcome. Maintain cardiac output and O$_2$ delivery with inotropes (eg dobutamine 2.5-10µg/kg/min IVI), vasodilators, and blood transfusion. Consider treating pulmonary hypertension with low-dose (20-120 parts per million) nitric oxide, a pulmonary vasodilator. Haemofiltration may be needed in renal failure and to achieve a negative fluid balance.[45,46]
- *Sepsis* Identify organism(s) and treat accordingly. If clinically septic, but no organisms cultured, use empirical broad-spectrum antibiotics (p161). Avoid nephrotoxic antibiotics.
- *Other:* Nutritional support: enteral is best: p586 & p588, with high fat, antioxidant formulations. Steroids protect those at risk of fat embolization and with pneumocystosis and may improve outcome in subacute ARDS. Their role in established ARDS is controversial.[47,48]

**Prognosis** Overall mortality is 50-75%. Prognosis varies with age of patient, cause of ARDS (pneumonia 86%, trauma 38%), and number of organs involved (3 organs involved for >1wk is 'invariably' fatal).

### Risk factors for ARDS

| | |
|---|---|
| Sepsis | Massive transfusion |
| Hypovolaemic shock | Burns (p858) |
| Trauma | Smoke inhalation (p859) |
| Pneumonia | Near drowning |
| Diabetic ketoacidosis | Acute pancreatitis |
| Gastric aspiration | DIC (p346) |
| Pregnancy | Head injury |
| Eclampsia | ICP↑ |
| Amniotic fluid embolus | Fat embolus |
| Drugs/toxins | Heart/lung bypass |
| Paraquat, heroin, aspirin | Tumour lysis syndrome (p526) |
| Pulmonary contusion | Malaria |

**Chest medicine**

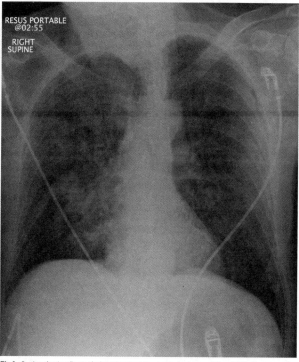

Fig 1. Supine chest radiograph showing air-space shadowing in a perihilar distribution spreading into the peripheries. This appearance can also be seen with infection and cardiogenic pulmonary oedema, but clues from the history, the heart size and lack of pleural effusions can suggest ARDS over the latter. Remember though that this is a supine projection—the patient is lying flat with the x-ray beam AP—causing the cardiac shadow to be artificially enlarged and pleural effusions to level out on the posterior chest wall so they will not obscure the costophrenic angles unless very large.

Image courtesy of Nottingham University Hospitals NHS Trust Radiology Department.

Chest medicine

Respiratory failure occurs when gas exchange is inadequate, resulting in hypoxia. It is defined as a $P_aO_2$ <8kPa and subdivided into 2 types according to $P_aCO_2$ level.

**Type I respiratory failure**: defined as hypoxia ($P_aO_2$ <8kPa) with a normal or low $P_aCO_2$. It is caused primarily by ventilation/perfusion (V/Q) mismatch, eg:
• Pneumonia
• Pulmonary oedema
• PE
• Asthma
• Emphysema
• Pulmonary fibrosis
• ARDS (p178)

**Type II respiratory failure**: defined as hypoxia ($P_aO_2$ <8kPa) with hypercapnia ($P_aCO_2$ >6.0kPa). This is caused by alveolar hypoventilation, with or without V/Q mismatch. Causes include:
• *Pulmonary disease*: asthma, COPD, pneumonia, end-stage pulmonary fibrosis, obstructive sleep apnoea (OSA, p194).
• *Reduced respiratory drive*: sedative drugs, CNS tumour or trauma.
• *Neuromuscular disease*: cervical cord lesion, diaphragmatic paralysis, poliomyelitis, myasthenia gravis, Guillain-Barré syndrome.
• *Thoracic wall disease*: flail chest, kyphoscoliosis.

**Clinical features** are those of the underlying cause together with symptoms and signs of hypoxia, with or without hypercapnia.

*Hypoxia:* Dyspnoea; restlessness; agitation; confusion; central cyanosis. If longstanding hypoxia: polycythaemia; pulmonary hypertension; cor pulmonale.

*Hypercapnia:* Headache; peripheral vasodilatation; tachycardia; bounding pulse; tremor/flap; papilloedema; confusion; drowsiness; coma.

**Investigations** are aimed at determining the underlying cause:
• Blood tests: FBC, U&E, CRP, ABG.
• Radiology: CXR.
• Microbiology: sputum and blood cultures (if febrile).
• Spirometry (COPD, neuromuscular disease, Guillain-Barré syndrome).

**Management** depends on the cause:

*Type I respiratory failure*
• Treat underlying cause.
• Give oxygen (35–60%) by facemask to correct hypoxia.
• Assisted ventilation if $P_aO_2$ <8kPa despite 60% $O_2$.

*Type II respiratory failure:* The respiratory centre may be relatively insensitive to $CO_2$ and respiration could be driven by hypoxia.
• Treat underlying cause.
• Controlled oxygen therapy: start at 24% $O_2$. ►*Oxygen therapy should be given with care.* Nevertheless, don't leave the hypoxia untreated.
• Recheck ABG after 20min. If $P_aCO_2$ is steady or lower, increase $O_2$ concentration to 28%. If $P_aCO_2$ has risen >1.5kPa and the patient is still hypoxic, consider assisted ventilation (eg NIPPV, p823, ie non-invasive positive pressure ventilation). Rarely a respiratory stimulant (eg doxapram 1.5–4mg/min IVI).
• If this fails, consider intubation and ventilation, if appropriate.

## Administering oxygen[49]

Oxygen is usually given via a facemask or nasal cannulae. It is good practice to prescribe it—this avoids inadvertent administration of too much or too little. Titrate the amount guided by the $S_aO_2$ (aim for ~ 94-98% (or 88-92% if, or at risk of, hypercapnia)); and the clinical condition of the patient. Humidification is only required for longer-term delivery of $O_2$ at high flow rates and tracheostomies, but may ↑ expectoration in bronchiectasis. ►Be careful in those with COPD (p822).

**Nasal cannulae:** preferred by patients, but $O_2$ delivery is relatively imprecise and may cause nasal soreness. The flow rate (1-4L/min) roughly defines the concentration of $O_2$ (24-40%). May be used to maintain $S_aO_2$ when nebulizers need to be run using air eg COPD.

**Simple face mask:** delivers a variable amount of $O_2$ depending on the rate of inflow. Far less precise than venturi masks—so don't use if hypercapnia or type 2 respiratory failure. Risk of $CO_2$ accumulation (within the mask and so in inspired gas) if flow rate <5L/min.

**Venturi mask:** provides a precise percentage of $O_2$ ($FiO_2$) at high flow rates. Colour codes:

| | |
|---|---|
| 24% | BLUE |
| 28% | WHITE |
| 35% | YELLOW |
| 40% | RED |
| 60% | GREEN |

Start at 24-28% in COPD.

**Non-rebreathing mask:** these have a reservoir bag and deliver high concentrations of $O_2$ (60-90%), determined by the inflow (10-15L/min) and the presence of flap valves on the side. They are commonly used in emergencies, but are imprecise and should be avoided in those requiring controlled $O_2$ therapy.

**Promoting oxygenation** Other ways to ↑ oxygenation to reach the target $S_aO_2$ (this should be given as a number on the drug chart):
• Treat anaemia (transfuse if essential)
• Improve cardiac output (treat heart failure)
• Chest physio to improve ventilation/perfusion mismatch.

## When to consider ABG (arterial blood gas) measurement

• Any unexpected deterioration in an ill patient. (Technique: see p785.)
• Anyone with an acute exacerbation of a chronic chest condition.
• Anyone with impaired consciousness or impaired respiratory effort.
• Signs of $CO_2$ retention, eg bounding pulse, drowsy, tremor (flapping), headache.
• Cyanosis, confusion, visual hallucinations (signs of $P_aO_2$↓; $S_aO_2$ is an alternative)
• To validate measurements from transcutaneous pulse oximetry (p156).

**Chest medicine**

**Causes** PES usually arise from a venous thrombosis in the pelvis or legs. Clots break off and pass through the veins and the right side of the heart before lodging in the pulmonary circulation. Rare causes include: right ventricular thrombus (post-MI); septic emboli (right-sided endocarditis); fat, air, or amniotic fluid embolism; neoplastic cells; parasites.

### Risk factors
- Recent surgery, especially abdominal/pelvic or hip/knee replacement
- Thrombophilia, eg antiphospholipid syndrome (p368)
- Leg fracture
- Prolonged bed rest/reduced mobility
- Malignancy
- Pregnancy/postpartum; Pill/HRT
- Previous PE

**Clinical features** These depend on the number, size, and distribution of the emboli; small emboli may be asymptomatic, whereas large emboli are often fatal.

*Symptoms:* Acute breathlessness, pleuritic chest pain, haemoptysis; dizziness; syncope. Ask about risk factors (above), past history or family history of thromboembolism. *Signs:* Pyrexia; cyanosis; tachypnoea; tachycardia; hypotension; raised JVP; pleural rub; pleural effusion. Look for signs of a cause, eg deep vein thrombosis.

### Tests
- FBC, U&E, baseline clotting, D-dimers (BOX).
- ABG may show $\downarrow P_aO_2$ and $\downarrow P_aCO_2$.
- Imaging: CXR may be normal, or show oligaemia of affected segment, dilated pulmonary artery, linear atelectasis, small pleural effusion, wedge-shaped opacities or cavitation (rare). CTPA—see BOX.
- ECG may be normal, or show tachycardia, right bundle branch block, right ventricular strain (inverted T in $V_1$ to $V_4$). The classical SI QIII TIII pattern (p92) is rare.

►Further investigations are shown on p828; see also BOX, p753.

**Treatment** ►►See p828. Anticoagulate with LMW heparin (p828). Start warfarin (p344). Stop heparin when INR is >2 and continue warfarin for a minimum of 3 months (see p345); aim for an INR of 2–3. Thrombolysis for massive PE (alteplase 10mg IV over 1min, then 90mg IVI over 2h; max 1.5mg/kg if <65kg). Consider placement of a *vena caval filter* in patients who develop emboli despite adequate anticoagulation (NB increased risk if placed without concomitant anticoagulation).

**Prevention** Give heparin (eg dalteparin 2500u/24h SC) to all immobile patients. Prescribe compression stockings and encourage early mobilization. Stop HRT and the Pill pre-op (if reliable with another form of contraception). If past or family history of thromboembolism, consider investigation for thrombophilia (p368).

## Pneumothorax[51]
*Management* ►►p824.

**Causes** Often spontaneous (especially in young thin men) due to rupture of a subpleural bulla. Other causes: asthma; COPD; TB; pneumonia; lung abscess; carcinoma; cystic fibrosis; lung fibrosis; sarcoidosis; connective tissue disorders (Marfan's sy., Ehlers-Danlos sy.), trauma; iatrogenic (subclavian CVP line insertion, pleural aspiration/biopsy, transbronchial biopsy, liver biopsy, +ve pressure ventilation).

**Clinical features** *Symptoms:* There may be no symptoms (especially if fit, young and small pneumothorax) or there may be sudden onset of dyspnoea and/or pleuritic chest pain. Patients with asthma or COPD may present with a sudden deterioration. Mechanically ventilated patients may present with hypoxia or an increase in ventilation pressures. *Signs:* Reduced expansion, hyper-resonance to percussion and diminished breath sounds on the affected side. *With a tension pneumothorax, the trachea will be deviated away from the affected side.* See x-ray p763.

**Management** p824, placing a chest drain, ►►p780.

►►**Managing a tension pneumothorax** See p824.

## Investigating suspected PE

Diagnosis of PE is improved by adopting a stepwise approach, combining an objective probability score, with subsequent investigations, as follows.
*Assess the clinical probability of a PE:* many systems exist and are usually based around elements drawn from the history and clinical examination.

| Scoring system for investigation of suspected DVT* | |
|---|---|
| **Feature** | **Score** |
| Active cancer, or treatment within 6 months | 1 |
| Paralysis, paresis, or recent plaster immobilization of lower limbs | 1 |
| Recently bed-ridden (>3 days) or major surgery (<4weeks) | 1 |
| Localized tenderness along venous system | 1 |
| Entire leg swollen | 1 |
| Calf circumference >3cm more than other side, 10cm below tibial tuberosity | 1 |
| Pitting oedema > in asymptomatic leg | 1 |
| Collateral superficial veins | 1 |
| Alternative diagnosis is likely, or more likely, than DVT | -2 |
| **Total score: 0=low probability; 1-2 moderate probability; ≥3 high probability** | |

*Adapted from Wells *et al. Lancet* 1997 350 1795

*D-dimers:* only perform in those patients **without** a high probability of a PE. A negative D-dimer test effectively excludes a PE in those with a low or intermediate clinical probability, and imaging is NOT required. However, a positive test does not prove a diagnosis of a PE, and imaging is required.
*Imaging:* the recommended 1st-line imaging modality is now CT pulmonary angiography (CTPA), which can show clots down to 5th-order pulmonary arteries (after the 4th branching). V/Q scanning (p158, p752 & p828) is now rarely performed.

Chest medicine

Chest medicine

**Definitions** A pleural effusion is fluid in the pleural space. Effusions can be divided by their protein concentration into *transudates* (<25g/L) and *exudates* (>35g/L), see BOX. Blood in the pleural space is a *haemothorax*, pus in the pleural space is an *empyema*, and chyle (lymph with fat) is a *chylothorax*. Both blood and air in the pleural space is called a *haemopneumothorax*.

**Causes** *Transudates* may be due to ↑venous pressure (cardiac failure, constrictive pericarditis, fluid overload), or hypoproteinaemia (cirrhosis, nephrotic syndrome, malabsorption). Also occur in hypothyroidism and Meigs' syndrome (right pleural effusion and ovarian fibroma). *Exudates* are mostly due to increased leakiness of pleural capillaries secondary to infection, inflammation, or malignancy. Causes: pneumonia; TB; pulmonary infarction; rheumatoid arthritis; SLE; bronchogenic carcinoma; malignant metastases; lymphoma; mesothelioma; lymphangitis carcinomatosis.

**Symptoms** Asymptomatic—or dyspnoea, pleuritic chest pain.

**Signs** *Decreased expansion; stony dull percussion note; diminished breath sounds* occur on the affected side. Tactile vocal fremitus and vocal resonance are ↓ (inconstant and unreliable). Above the effusion, where lung is compressed, there may be *bronchial breathing*. With large effusions there may be *tracheal deviation* away from the effusion. Look for aspiration marks and signs of associated disease: malignancy (cachexia, clubbing, lymphadenopathy, radiation marks, mastectomy scar); stigmata of chronic liver disease; cardiac failure; hypothyroidism; rheumatoid arthritis; butterfly rash of SLE.

**Tests** *CXR:* Small effusions blunt the costophrenic angles, larger ones are seen as water-dense shadows with concave upper borders. A completely flat horizontal upper border implies that there is also a pneumothorax.

*Ultrasound* is useful in identifying the presence of pleural fluid and in guiding diagnostic or therapeutic aspiration.

*Diagnostic aspiration:* Percuss the upper border of the pleural effusion and choose a site 1 or 2 intercostal spaces below it (don't go too low or you'll be in the abdomen!). Infiltrate down to the pleura with 5-10mL of 1% lidocaine. Attach a 21G needle to a syringe and insert it just above the upper border of an appropriate rib (avoids neurovascular bundle). Draw off 10-30mL of pleural fluid and send it to the lab for *clinical chemistry* (protein, glucose, pH, LDH, amylase), *bacteriology* (microscopy and culture, auramine stain, TB culture), *cytology* and, if indicated, *immunology* (rheumatoid factor, ANA, complement).

*Pleural biopsy:* If pleural fluid analysis is inconclusive, consider parietal pleural biopsy. Thoracoscopic or CT-guided pleural biopsy increases diagnostic yield (by enabling direct visualization of the pleural cavity and biopsy of suspicious areas).

**Management** is of the underlying cause.
- **Drainage** If the effusion is symptomatic, drain it, repeatedly if necessary. Fluid is best removed slowly (0.5-1.5L/24h). It may be aspirated in the same way as a diagnostic tap, or using an intercostal drain (see p780).
- *Pleurodesis* with tetracycline, bleomycin, or talc may be helpful for recurrent effusions. Thoracoscopic talc pleurodesis is most effective for malignant effusions. Empyemas (p164) are best drained using a chest drain, inserted under ultrasound or CT guidance.
- *Intra-pleural streptokinase* Of no benefit.
- *Surgery* Persistent collections and increasing pleural thickness (on ultrasound) requires surgery.[52]

## Pleural fluid analysis

| Gross appearance | Cause |
|---|---|
| Clear, straw-coloured | Transudate, exudate |
| Turbid, yellow | Empyema, parapneumonic effusion[1] |
| Haemorrhagic | Trauma, malignancy, pulmonary infarction |
| *Cytology* | |
| Neutrophils ++ | Parapneumonic effusion, PE |
| Lymphocytes ++ | Malignancy, TB, RA, SLE, sarcoidosis |
| Mesothelial cells ++ | Pulmonary infarction |
| Abnormal mesothelial cells | Mesothelioma |
| Multinucleated giant cells | RA |
| Lupus erythematosus cells | SLE |
| *Clinical chemistry* | |
| Protein  <25g/L | Transudate |
|  >35g/L | Exudate |
|  25–35g/L | If pleural fluid protein/serum protein >0.5, effusion is an exudate |
| Glucose <3.3mmol/L | Empyema, malignancy, TB, RA, SLE |
| pH <7.2 | Empyema, malignancy, TB, RA, SLE |
| LDH↑ (pleural:serum >0.6) | Empyema, malignancy, TB, RA, SLE |
| Amylase↑ | Pancreatitis, carcinoma, bacterial pneumonia, oesophageal rupture |
| *Immunology* | |
| Rheumatoid factor | RA |
| Antinuclear antibody | SLE |
| Complement levels↓ | RA, SLE, malignancy, infection |

**Chest medicine**

1 Inflammation of the pleura caused by pneumonia may lead to infected pleural fluid (empyema); if it is not infected, the term parapneumonic effusion is used.

A multisystem granulomatous disorder of unknown cause. Prevalence highest in Northern Europe, eg UK: 10–20/10⁵ population. Usually affects adults aged 20–40yrs, more common in women. African-Caribbeans are affected more frequently and more severely than Caucasians, particularly by extra-thoracic disease. Associated with HLA-DRB1 and DQB1 alleles.

**Clinical features** In 20–40%, the disease is discovered incidentally, after a routine CXR, and is thus asymptomatic. *Acute sarcoidosis* often presents with erythema nodosum (fig 1, p275)[1] ± polyarthralgia. It usually resolves spontaneously.

*Pulmonary disease* 90% have abnormal CXRs with bilateral hilar lymphadenopathy (BHL, fig 1) ± pulmonary infiltrates or fibrosis; see below for staging. *Symptoms:* Dry cough, progressive dyspnoea, ↓exercise tolerance and chest pain. In 10–20%, symptoms progress, with concurrent deterioration in lung function.

*Non-pulmonary signs* are legion: lymphadenopathy; hepatomegaly; splenomegaly; uveitis; conjunctivitis; keratoconjunctivitis sicca; glaucoma; terminal phalangeal bone cysts; enlargement of lacrimal & parotid glands (fig 5, p349); Bell's palsy; neuropathy; meningitis; brainstem and spinal syndromes; space-occupying lesion; erythema nodosum (fig 1, p565); lupus pernio; subcutaneous nodules; cardiomyopathy; arrhythmias; hypercalcaemia; hypercalciuria; renal stones; pituitary dysfunction.

**Tests** *Blood:* ↑ESR, lymphopenia, LFT↑, serum ACE↑ in ~60% (non-specific), ↑Ca²⁺, ↑immunoglobulins. *24h urine:* Ca²⁺↑. *Tuberculin skin test* is –ve in two-thirds; CXR is abnormal in 90%: *Stage 0:* normal. *Stage 1:* BHL. *Stage 2:* BHL + peripheral pulmonary infiltrates. *Stage 3:* peripheral pulmonary infiltrates alone. *Stage 4:* progressive pulmonary fibrosis; bulla formation (honeycombing); pleural involvement. *ECG* may show arrhythmias or bundle branch block. *Lung function tests* may be normal or show reduced lung volumes, impaired gas transfer, and a restrictive ventilatory defect. *Tissue biopsy* (lung, liver, lymph nodes, skin nodules, or lacrimal glands) is diagnostic and shows non-caseating granulomata. *Kveim tests* are now obsolete.

*Bronchoalveolar lavage (BAL)* shows ↑lymphocytes in active disease; ↑neutrophils with pulmonary fibrosis.

*Ultrasound* may show nephrocalcinosis or hepatosplenomegaly.

*Bone x-rays* show 'punched out' lesions in terminal phalanges.

*CT/MRI* may be useful in assessing severity of pulmonary disease or diagnosing neurosarcoidosis. *Ophthalmology assessment* (slit lamp examination, fluorescein angiography) is indicated in ocular disease.

**Management**[53,54] ►Patients with BHL alone don't need treatment as most recover spontaneously. *Acute sarcoidosis:* Bed rest, NSAIDs.

*Indications for corticosteroids:*
• Parenchymal lung disease (symptomatic, static, or progressive)
• Uveitis
• Hypercalcaemia
• Neurological or cardiac involvement

Prednisolone (40mg/24h) PO for 4–6 wks, then ↓dose over 1yr according to clinical status. A few patients relapse and may need a further course or long-term therapy.

*Other therapy:* In severe illness, IV methylprednisolone or immunosuppressants (methotrexate, hydroxychloroquine, ciclosporin, cyclophosphamide) may be needed. Anti-TNFα therapy may be tried in refractory cases, or lung transplantation.

**Prognosis** 60% of patients with thoracic sarcoidosis resolve over 2yrs. 20% respond to steroid therapy; in the rest, improvement is unlikely despite therapy.[2]

---

**1** A detailed history and exam (including for synovitis) + CXR, 2 ASO titres and a tuberculin skin test are usually enough to diagnose erythema nodosum: R Pugol 2000 *Arthr Rheu* 43 584
**2** ACE is also ↑ in: hyperthyroidism, Gaucher's, silicosis, TB, hypersensitivity pneumonitis, asbestosis, pneumocystosis.[55] ACE levels may help monitor sarcoidosis activity. ↑ACE levels in CSF help diagnose CNS sarcoidosis (when serum ACE may be normal).[56] ACE is *lower* in: Caucasians; and anorexia.[57]

### Causes of BHL (bilateral hilar lymphadenopathy)

Sarcoidosis
Infection, eg TB, mycoplasma
Malignancy, eg lymphoma, carcinoma, mediastinal tumours
Organic dust disease, eg silicosis, berylliosis
Extrinsic allergic alveolitis
Histocytosis X

### Differential diagnosis of granulomatous diseases

| Infections | Bacteria | TB, leprosy, syphilis |
|---|---|---|
| | | Cat scratch fever |
| | Fungi | *Cryptococcus neoformans* |
| | | *Coccidioides immitis* |
| | Protozoa | *Schistosomiasis* |
| Autoimmune | Primary biliary cirrhosis | |
| | Granulomatous orchitis | |
| Vasculitis (p558) | Giant cell arteritis | |
| | Polyarteritis nodosa | |
| | Takayasu's arteritis | |
| | Wegener's• granulomatosis | |
| Organic dust disease | Silicosis, berylliosis | |
| Idiopathic | Crohn's disease | |
| | de Quervain's thyroiditis | |
| | Sarcoidosis | |
| Extrinsic allergic alveolitis | | |
| Histiocytosis X | | |

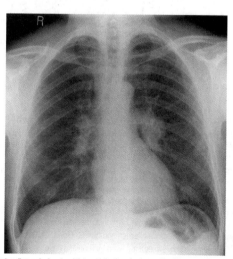

Fig 1. PA chest radiograph showing bilateral hilar lymphadenopathy. The important differentials for this appearance are: sarcoidosis, TB, lymphoma, pneumoconioses and metastatic disease. This patient has sarcoidosis but there are no other stigmata (such as the presence of infiltrates, fibrosis and honeycombing) on this image.

Image courtesy of Norfolk and Norwich University Hospitals NHS Trust Radiology Department.

This is the generic term used to describe a number of conditions that primarily affect the lung parenchyma in a diffuse manner. They are characterized by chronic inflammation and/or progressive interstitial fibrosis, and share a number of clinical and pathological features. See BOX and fig 1.

**Clinical features** Dyspnoea on exertion; non-productive paroxysmal cough; abnormal breath sounds; abnormal CXR or high resolution CT; restrictive pulmonary spirometry with ↓DLCO (p158).

**Pathological features** Fibrosis and remodelling of the interstitium; chronic inflammation; hyperplasia of type II epithelial cells or type II pneumocytes.

**Classification** The ILDs can be broadly grouped into three categories:

*Those with known cause, eg*
• Occupational/environmental, eg asbestosis, berylliosis, silicosis, cotton worker's lung (byssinosis)
• Drugs, eg nitrofurantoin, bleomycin, amiodarone, sulfasalazine, busulfan
• Hypersensitivity reactions, eg extrinsic allergic alveolitis
• Infections, eg TB, fungi, viral
• Gastro-oesophageal reflux

*Those associated with systemic disorders, eg*
• Sarcoidosis
• Rheumatoid arthritis
• SLE, systemic sclerosis, mixed connective tissue disease, Sjögren's syndrome
• Ulcerative colitis, renal tubular acidosis, autoimmune thyroid disease

*Idiopathic, eg*
• Idiopathic pulmonary fibrosis (IPF, p190)
• Cryptogenic organizing pneumonia
• Lymphocytic interstitial pneumonia

# Extrinsic allergic alveolitis (EAA)

In sensitized individuals, inhalation of allergens (fungal spores or avian proteins) provokes a hypersensitivity reaction. In the acute phase, the alveoli are infiltrated with acute inflammatory cells. With chronic exposure, granuloma formation and obliterative bronchiolitis occur.

**Causes**
• Bird-fancier's and pigeon-fancier's lung (proteins in bird droppings).
• Farmer's and mushroom worker's lung (*Micropolyspora faeni, Thermoactinomyces vulgaris*).
• Malt worker's lung (*Aspergillus clavatus*).
• Bagassosis or sugar worker's lung (*Thermoactinomyces sacchari*).

**Clinical features** *4–6h post-exposure:* Fever, rigors, myalgia, dry cough, dyspnoea, crackles (no wheeze). *Chronic:* Increasing dyspnoea, weight↓, exertional dyspnoea, type I respiratory failure, cor pulmonale.

**Tests** *Acute:* Blood: FBC (neutrophilia); ESR↑; ABGs; positive serum precipitins (indicate exposure only). *CXR:* upper-zone mottling/consolidation; hilar lymphadenopathy (rare). *Lung function tests:* reversible restrictive defect; reduced gas transfer during acute attacks. *Chronic:* Blood tests: positive serum precipitins. *CXR:* upper-zone fibrosis; honeycomb lung. *Lung function tests:* persistent changes (see above). Bronchoalveolar lavage (BAL) fluid shows ↑ lymphocytes and mast cells.

**Management** *Acute:* Remove allergen and give $O_2$ (35–60%), then:
Oral prednisolone (40mg/24h PO), followed by reducing dose.

*Chronic:* Avoid exposure to allergens, or wear a facemask or +ve pressure helmet. Long-term steroids often achieve CXR and physiological improvement. Compensation (UK Industrial Injuries Act) may be payable.

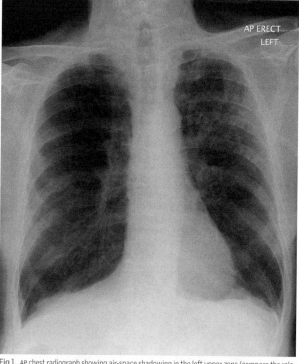

**Fig 1.** AP chest radiograph showing air-space shadowing in the left upper zone (compare the relative lucency with the right upper zone). Although this appearance often represents infection (ie pneumonia), it is non-specific. Important differentials to remember for this distribution of shadowing include lymphoma, alveolar cell carcinoma (both to be considered if not resolving in appearance on follow-up imaging), and haemorrhage.

Image courtesy of Nottingham University Hospitals NHS Trust Radiology Department.

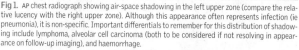

### Causes of fibrotic shadowing on a CXR

| Upper zone | Mid zone | Lower zone |
|---|---|---|
| • TB | • Sarcoidosis, histoplasmosis | • Idiopathic pulmonary fibrosis |
| • Extrinsic allergic alveolitis | | • Asbestosis |
| • Ankylosing spondylitis | | |
| • Radiotherapy | | |
| • Progressive massive fibrosis (PMF) | | |

Chest medicine

This is a type of idiopathic interstitial pneumonia. Inflammatory cell infiltrate and pulmonary fibrosis of unknown cause (also known as cryptogenic fibrosing alveolitis). The commonest cause of interstitial lung disease.

**Symptoms** Dry cough; exertional dyspnoea; malaise; weight↓; arthralgia.

**Signs** Cyanosis; finger clubbing; fine end-inspiratory crepitations.

**Complications** Respiratory failure; increased risk of lung cancer.

**Tests** *Blood:* ABG ($P_aO_2$↓; if severe $P_aCO_2$↑); CRP↑; immunoglobulins↑; ANA (30% +ve), rheumatoid factor (10% +ve). CXR: (fig 1) Lung volume↓; bilateral lower zone reticulo-nodular shadows; honeycomb lung (advanced disease). CT shows similar changes to the CXR but is more sensitive and is an essential tool for diagnosis. *Spirometry:* Restrictive (p156); ↓transfer factor. *BAL* (bronchoalveolar lavage) may indicate activity of alveolitis: lymphocytes↑ (good response/prognosis) or neutrophils and eosinophils↑ (poor response/prognosis). *$^{99}TC^m$-DTPA scan:* (diethylene-triamine-penta-acetic acid) may reflect disease activity[59]. *Lung biopsy* may be needed for diagnosis. The histological changes observed on biopsy are referred to as *usual interstitial pneumonia* (UIP).

**Management** Best supportive care: oxygen, pulmonary rehabilitation, opiates, palliative care input. It is strongly recommended that high-dose steroids are **NOT** used except where the diagnosis of IPF is in doubt. All patients should be considered for current clinical trials or **lung transplantation**.[58]

**Prognosis** 50% 5yr survival rate (range 1-20yrs).

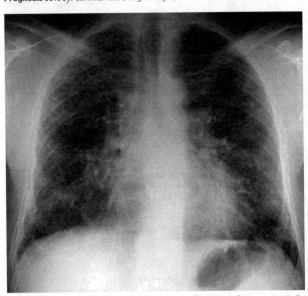

**Fig 1.** Interstitial lung disease due to idiopathic pulmonary fibrosis (a similar appearance to the interstitial oedema of moderate left heart failure, but without a big heart).

Courtesy of Prof P Scally.

Chest medicine

**Coal worker's pneumoconiosis (CWP)** A common dust disease in countries that have or have had underground coal-mines. It results from inhalation of coal dust particles (1-3μm in diameter) over 15-20yrs. These are ingested by macrophages which die, releasing their enzymes and causing fibrosis.

*Clinical features:* Asymptomatic, but co-existing chronic bronchitis is common. CXR: many round opacities (1-10mm), especially in upper zone.

*Management:* Avoid exposure to coal dust; treat co-existing chronic bronchitis; claim compensation (in the UK, via the Industrial Injuries Act).

**Progressive massive fibrosis (PMF)** is due to progression of CWP, which causes progressive dyspnoea, fibrosis, and, eventually, cor pulmonale. CXR: upper-zone fibrotic masses (1-10cm).

*Management:* Avoid exposure to coal dust; claim compensation (as above).

**Caplan's syndrome** is the association between rheumatoid arthritis, pneumoconiosis, and pulmonary rheumatoid nodules.

**Silicosis** (see fig 1) is caused by inhalation of silica particles, which are very fibrogenic. A number of jobs may be associated with exposure, eg metal mining, stone quarrying, sandblasting, and pottery/ceramic manufacture.

*Clinical features:* Progressive dyspnoea, ↑incidence of TB, CXR shows diffuse miliary or nodular pattern in upper and mid-zones and egg-shell calcification of hilar nodes. Spirometry: restrictive ventilatory defect.

*Management:* Avoid exposure to silica; claim compensation (as above).

**Asbestosis** is caused by inhalation of asbestos fibres. Chrysotile (white asbestos) is the least fibrogenic—crocidolite (blue asbestos) is the most fibrogenic. Amosite (brown asbestos) is the least common and has intermediate fibrogenicity. Asbestos was commonly used in the building trade for fire proofing, pipe lagging, electrical wire insulation, and roofing felt. Degree of asbestos exposure is related to degree of pulmonary fibrosis.

*Clinical features:* Similar to other fibrotic lung diseases with progressive dyspnoea, clubbing, and fine end-inspiratory crackles. Also causes pleural plaques, ↑risk of bronchial adenocarcinoma and mesothelioma.

*Management:* Symptomatic. Patients are often eligible for compensation through the UK Industrial Injuries Act.

**Malignant mesothelioma** is a tumour of mesothelial cells that usually occurs in the pleura, and rarely in the peritoneum or other organs. It is associated with occupational exposure to asbestos but the relationship is complex.[60] 90% report previous exposure to asbestos, but only 20% of patients have pulmonary asbestosis. The latent period between exposure and development of the tumour may be up to 45yrs. Compensation is often available.

*Clinical features:* Chest pain, dyspnoea, weight loss, finger clubbing, recurrent pleural effusions. Signs of metastases: lymphadenopathy, hepatomegaly, bone pain/tenderness, abdominal pain/obstruction (peritoneal malignant mesothelioma).

*Tests:* CXR/CT: pleural thickening/effusion. Bloody pleural fluid.

*Diagnosis* is made on histology, usually following a thoracoscopy. Often the diagnosis is only made post-mortem.

*Management:* Pemetrexed + cisplatin chemotherapy can improve survival.[61] Surgery is hard to evaluate (few randomized trials). Radiotherapy is controversial. Pleurodesis and indwelling intra-pleural drain may help.

*Prognosis* is poor (especially without pemetrexed, eg <2yrs). >650 deaths/yr in UK.

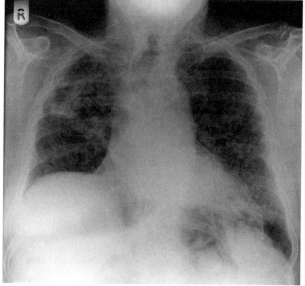

**Fig 1.** PA chest radiograph showing diffuse nodular pulmonary opacities with a focal area of irregular soft tissue shadowing in the right upper zone. Appearances are consistent with silicosis and developing progressive massive fibrosis (PMF). PMF is usually bilateral and starts as ill-defined or oval opacities that occur most often in the upper/mid-zones and develop from the periphery towards the hila.

Image courtesy of Derby Hospitals NHS Foundation Trust Radiology Department.

## Obstructive sleep apnoea syndrome

This disorder is characterized by intermittent closure/collapse of the pharyngeal airway causing apnoeic episodes during sleep. These are terminated by partial arousal.

**Clinical features** The typical patient is an obese, middle-aged man who presents because of snoring or daytime somnolence. His partner often describes apnoeic episodes during sleep.
- Loud snoring
- Daytime somnolence
- Poor sleep quality
- Morning headache
- Decreased libido
- Cognitive performance↓.

**Complications** Pulmonary hypertension; type II respiratory failure (p180). Sleep apnoea is also reported as an independent risk factor for hypertension.[62]

**Investigations** Simple studies (eg pulse oximetry, video recordings) may be all that are required for diagnosis. Polysomnography (which monitors oxygen saturation, airflow at the nose and mouth, ECG, EMG chest and abdominal wall movement during sleep) is diagnostic. The occurrence of 15 or more episodes of apnoea or hypopnoea during 1h of sleep indicates significant sleep apnoea.

**Management**[36]
- Weight reduction
- Avoidance of tobacco and alcohol
- CPAP via a nasal mask during sleep is effective and recommended by NICE for those with moderate to severe disease[64]
- Surgery to relieve pharyngeal obstruction (tonsillectomy, uvulopalatopharyngoplasty, or tracheostomy) is occasionally needed, but only after seeing a chest physician.

### Cor pulmonale

Cor pulmonale is right heart failure caused by chronic pulmonary arterial hypertension. Causes include chronic lung disease, pulmonary vascular disorders, and neuromuscular and skeletal diseases (see BOX).

**Clinical features** Symptoms include dyspnoea, fatigue, and syncope. Signs: cyanosis; tachycardia; raised JVP with prominent a and v waves; RV heave; loud $P_2$, pansystolic murmur (tricuspid regurgitation); early diastolic Graham Steell murmur; hepatomegaly and oedema.

**Investigations** FBC: Hb and haematocrit↑ (secondary polycythaemia). ABG: hypoxia, with or without hypercapnia. CXR: enlarged right atrium and ventricle, prominent pulmonary arteries (see fig 1). ECG: P pulmonale; right axis deviation; right ventricular hypertrophy/strain.

**Management**
- *Treat underlying cause*—eg COPD and pulmonary infections.
- *Treat respiratory failure*—in the acute situation give 24% oxygen if $P_aO_2$ <8kPa. Monitor ABG and gradually increase oxygen concentration if $P_aCO_2$ is stable (p180). In COPD patients, long-term oxygen therapy (LTOT) for 15h/d increases survival (p176). Patients with chronic hypoxia when clinically stable should be assessed for LTOT.
- *Treat cardiac failure* with diuretics such as furosemide, eg 40-160mg/24h PO. Monitor U&E and give amiloride or potassium supplements if necessary. Alternative: spironolactone.
- Consider *venesection* if haematocrit >55%.
- Consider *heart-lung transplantation* in young patients.

**Prognosis** Poor. 50% die within 5yrs.

## Causes of cor pulmonale

**Lung disease**
- COPD
- Bronchiectasis
- Pulmonary fibrosis
- Severe chronic asthma
- Lung resection

**Pulmonary vascular disease**
- Pulmonary emboli
- Pulmonary vasculitis
- Primary pulmonary hypertension
- ARDS (p170)
- Sickle-cell disease
- Parasite infestation

**Thoracic cage abnormality**
- Kyphosis
- Scoliosis
- Thoracoplasty

**Neuromuscular disease**
- Myasthenia gravis
- Poliomyelitis
- Motor neuron disease

**Hypoventilation**
- Sleep apnoea
- Enlarged adenoids in children

**Cerebrovascular disease**

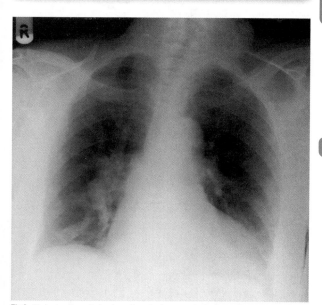

Fig 1. PA chest radiograph showing enlarged pulmonary arteries from pulmonary artery hypertension. When caused by interstitial lung disease and leading to right heart failure, this would be termed cor pulmonale. No signs of interstitial lung disease are identifiable in this image.

Image courtesy of Derby Hospitals NHS Foundation Trust Radiology Department.

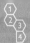

## Contents

The essence of endocrinology 197

Fig 1. Frederick Banting (1891-1941) and Charles Best (1899-1978). Their discovery of insulin and its effects on glucose, from work in beagles, had a profound effect on the lives of all those with diabetes, as it paved the way for the use of insulin to treat what was then a fatal condition. Banting, but not Best, won the Nobel prize for his work, aged 32, making him the youngest ever recipient of the award in Medicine/Physiology. He died prematurely in a plane crash whilst on route to England on a secretive mission to test out an anti-gravity flying suit.

*Relevant pages in other chapters:*
Diabetic ketoacidosis (►►p842); hypoglycaemia (►►p844); surgery and diabetes
(p590); the eye in diabetes (OHCS p446); thyroid emergencies (►►p844); thyroid lumps
(p602); thyroid disease, and surgery (p593); Addisonian crisis and hypopituitary
coma (►►p846); phaeochromocytoma emergencies (►►p847).

*The endocrinology of food behaviour, mood, and obesity:*
Cholecystokinin, GLP-1, ghrelin, and peptide YY, etc: OHCS p530.

*In dermatology (endocrine control of sebocytes via CRH):* OHCS p583.

*In pregnancy:* Thyroid disease: OHCS p25; diabetes in pregnancy: OHCS p24.

*In childhood:* Childhood diabetes: OHCS p186; thyroid problems: OHCS p182.

*We thank Dr Stephen Gilbey, our Specialist Reader, and Dr Konstantinos Kritikos, our Junior Reader
for this chapter.*

## The essence of endocrinology—for scientists

• Define a syndrome, and match it to a gland malfunction.
• Measure the gland's output in the peripheral blood. Define clinical syndromes associated with too much or too little secretion (*hyper-* and *hypo-*syndromes, respectively; *eu-* means normal, neither ↑ nor ↓, as in *euthyroid*). Note factors that may make measurement variable, eg diurnal release of cortisol.
• If suspecting hormone deficiency, test by stimulating the gland that produces it (eg short ACTH stimulation test or *Synacthen®* test in Addison's). If the gland is not functioning normally, there will be a blunted response to stimulation.
• If suspecting hormone excess, test by inhibiting the gland that produces it (eg dexamethasone suppression test in Cushing's). If there is a hormone secreting tumour then this will fail to suppress via normal feedback mechanisms.
• Find a way to image the gland. NB: non-functioning tumours or 'incidentalomas' may be found in health, see p216. Imaging alone does not make the diagnosis.
• Aim to halt disease progression; diet and exercise can stop progression of impaired fasting glucose to frank diabetes.[1,2] For other glands, halting progression will depend on understanding autoimmunity, and the interaction of genes and environment. In thyroid autoimmunity (an archetypal autoimmune disease), it is possible to track interactions between genes and environment (eg smoking and stress) via expression of immunologically active molecules (HLA class I and II, adhesion molecules, cytokines, CD40, and complement regulatory proteins).[3]

Endocrinologists love this reductionist approach, but have been less successful at understanding *emergent phenomena*—those properties and performances of ours that cannot be predicted from full knowledge of our perturbed parts. We understand the diurnal nature of cortisol secretion, for example, but the science of relating this to dreams, the consolidation of memory, and the psychopathology of families and other groups (such as the endocrinology ward round you may be about to join) is in its infancy. But as doctors we are steeped in the hormonal lives of patients (as they are in ours)—and we may as well start by recognizing this now.

## The essence of endocrinology—for those doing exams

"What's wrong with *him*?" your examiner asks, boldly. While you apologize to the patient for this rudeness by asking, "Is it alright if we speak about you as if you weren't here?", think to yourself that if you were a betting man or woman you would wager that the diagnosis will be endocrinological. In no other discipline are gestalt impressions so characteristic. To get good at recognizing these conditions, spend time in endocrinology outpatients and looking at collections of clinical photographs. Also, specific cutaneous signs are important, as follows.

*Thyrotoxicosis:* Hair loss; pretibial myxoedema (confusing term, p210); onycholysis (nail separation from the nailbed); bulging eyes (exophthalmos/proptosis).

*Hypothyroidism:* Hair loss; eyebrow loss; cold, pale skin; characteristic face. You might, perhaps should, fail your exam if you blurt out "Toad-like face".

*Cushing's syndrome:* Central obesity and wasted limbs (='lemon on sticks' see fig 1); moon face; buffalo hump; supraclavicular fat pads; striae.

*Addison's disease:* Hyperpigmentation (face, neck, palmar creases).

*Acromegaly:* Acral (distal) + soft tissue overgrowth; big jaws (macrognathia), hands and feet; the skin is thick; facial features are coarse.

*Hyperandrogenism (♀):* Hirsutism; temporal balding; acne.

*Hypopituitarism:* Pale or yellow tinged thinned skin, resulting in fine wrinkling around the eyes and mouth, making the patient look older.

*Hypoparathyroidism:* Dry, scaly, puffy skin; brittle nails; coarse hair.

*Pseudohypoparathyroidism:* Short stature, short neck and short 4th and 5th metacarpals.

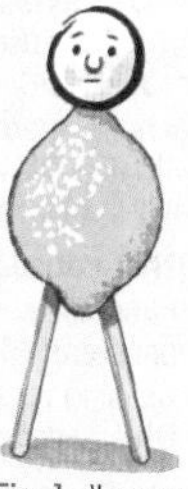

Fig 1. 'Lemon on sticks.'

Endocrinology

DM results from lack or reduced effectiveness of endogenous insulin. Hyperglycaemia is one aspect of a far-reaching metabolic derangement, which causes serious microvascular (retinopathy, nephropathy, neuropathy) or macrovascular problems: stroke, renovascular disease, limb ischaemia—and above all heart disease *So think of DM as a vascular disease*:[1] when meeting a diabetic person adopt a holistic approach and consider other cardiovascular risk factors too—they tend to cluster together.

---

### Diagnosis of diabetes mellitus: WHO criteria (rather arbitrary![2])

- Symptoms of hyperglycaemia (eg polyuria, polydipsia, unexplained weight loss, visual blurring, genital thrush, lethargy) AND raised venous glucose detected once—fasting ≥7mmol/L or random ≥11.1mmol/L OR
- Raised venous glucose on 2 separate occasions—fasting ≥7mmol/L, random ≥11.1mmol/L or oral glucose tolerance test (OGTT)—2h value ≥11.1mmol/L
- HbA1c ≥48mmol/L (6.5%), but below doesn't exclude DM. Avoid in pregnancy, children and type 1 DM.
  ▶ Whenever you have a needle in a vein, do a blood glucose (unless recently done); note if fasting or after food. Non-systematic, but better than urine tests (too many false -ves). In one UK GP trial, 5% of those screened aged 40-69 had new DM.

---

### Categories of diabetes and dyslipidaemia

*Type 1 DM* Usually adolescent onset but may occur at *any* age. *Cause:* Insulin deficiency from autoimmune destruction of insulin-secreting pancreatic β cells. Patients must have insulin, and are prone to ketoacidosis and weight loss. It is associated with other autoimmune diseases (>90% carry HLA DR3 ± DR4). Concordance is only ~30% in identical twins, indicating environmental influence. Four genes are important: one (6q) determines islet sensitivity to damage (eg from viruses or cross-reactivity from cows' milk-induced antibodies). Latent autoimmune diabetes of adults (LADA) is a form of type 1 DM, with slower progression to insulin dependence in later life.

*Type 2 DM* (formerly non-insulin-dependent DM, NIDDM) appears to be prevalent at 'epidemic' levels in many places, mainly due to changes in lifestyle, but also because of better diagnosis and improved longevity.[4] Higher prevalence occurs in Asians, men, and the elderly (up to 18%). Most are over 40yrs, but teenagers are now getting type 2 DM (*OHCS* p156). *Cause* ↓Insulin secretion ± ↑insulin resistance. It is associated with obesity, lack of exercise, calorie and alcohol excess. ≥80% concordance in identical twins, indicating stronger genetic influence than in type 1 DM. Typically progresses from a preliminary phase of impaired glucose tolerance (IGT) or impaired fasting glucose (IFG), see BOX. (▶ This is a unique window for lifestyle intervention.) Maturity onset diabetes of the young (MODY) is a rare autosomal dominant form of type 2 DM affecting young people with a +ve family history (*OHCS* p187).

*Impaired glucose tolerance (IGT)* Fasting plasma glucose <7mmol/L and OGTT (oral glucose tolerance) 2h glucose ≥7.8mmol/L but <11.1mmol/L.

*Impaired fasting glucose (IFG)* Fasting plasma glucose ≥ 6.1mmol/L but <7mmol/L (WHO criteria). Do an OGTT to exclude DM. The cut-off point is somewhat arbitrary: Americans use 5.55mmol/L and 4.8 is the cut-off in Israel.

IGT and IFG denote different abnormalities of glucose regulation (post-prandial and fasting). There may be lower risk of progression to DM in IFG than IGT. Manage both with lifestyle advice (exercise and diet, p87) + annual review. Incidence of DM if IFG and HbA1c at high end of normal (37-46mmol/L or 5.5-6.4%) is ~25%.[5]

**Other causes of DM** ▶ Steroids; anti-HIV drugs; newer antipsychotics; thiazides.
- Pancreatic: pancreatitis; surgery (where >90% pancreas is removed); trauma; pancreatic destruction (haemochromatosis, cystic fibrosis); pancreatic cancer.
- Cushing's disease; acromegaly; phaeochromocytoma; hyperthyroidism; pregnancy.
- Others: congenital lipodystrophy; glycogen storage diseases.

---

1 Chicken or egg? Most type II diabetes-associated genes have a function in the vasculature, and stress in β-cells can result from vascular defects in the pancreas, so maybe vascular events trigger DM.[1]

2 These values reflect economic and political realities: biological realities are different: risk of DM retinopathy relates to glucose levels >5.6mmol/L, for example. But defining DM as >5.6 would cost £billions.

## 19

## Diabetes and pregnancy

- 4% of pregnancies are complicated by DM: either pre-existing type 1 or 2 DM (<0.5%), or new-onset gestational diabetes (GDM) (>3.5%).
- All forms carry an increased risk to mother and foetus: miscarriage, pre-term labour, pre-eclampsia, congenital malformations, macrosomia, and a worsening of diabetic complications, eg retinopathy, nephropathy.
- Risk of GDM ↑ if: aged over 25; family history; +ve; weight↑; non-Caucasian; HIV+ve; previous gestational DM.[7]
- Pre-conception: Offer general advice, and discuss risks. Control/reduce weight, aim for good glucose control, offer folic acid 5mg/d until 12 weeks.
- Screen for GDM with OGTT if risk factors at booking (16-18 weeks if previous GDM).
- Oral hypoglycaemics other than metformin should be discontinued. Metformin may be used as an adjunct or alternative to insulin in type 2 DM or GDM.
- 6wks postpartum, do a fasting glucose. Even if -ve, 50% will eventually go on to develop DM.

## Type 1 versus type 2 diabetes mellitus

Occasionally it may be difficult to differentiate whether a patient has type 1 or 2 DM. Features that suggest type 1 DM include weight loss; persistent hyperglycaemia despite diet and medications; presence of autoantibodies: islet cell antibodies (ICA) and anti-glutamic acid decarboxylase (GAD) antibodies; ketonuria on urine dipstick.

|  | Type 1 DM | Type 2 DM |
|---|---|---|
| Epidemiology | Often starts before puberty | Older patients (usually) |
| Genetics | HLA D3 and D4 linked | No HLA association |
| Cause | Autoimmune β cell destruction | Insulin resistance/β cell dysfunction |
| Presentation | Polydipsia, polyuria, weight↓, ketosis | Asymptomatic/complications, eg MI |

▶Not all new-onset DM in older people is type 2: if ketotic ± a poor response to oral hypoglycaemics (and patient is slim or has a family or personal history of autoimmunity), think of latent autoimmune diabetes in adults (LADA) and measure islet cell antibodies.

## The metabolic syndrome and insulin resistance

*Metabolic syndrome (syndrome x)* Arbitrarily defined (IDF) as central obesity (BMI >30, or ↑ waist circ),[1] plus 2 of: BP ≥130/85, triglycerides ≥1.7mmol/L, HDL ≤ 1.03♂/1.29♀mmol/L, fasting glucose ≥5.6mmol/L or DM. ~20% are affected; weight, genetics, and insulin resistance important in aetiology. *Possible consequences:* Vascular events (MI)—but may not increase risk beyond individual risk factors; DM; neurodegeneration; microalbuminuria; gallstones; cancers (eg pancreas); fertility problems♂ & ♀ *R:* Exercise; weight↓ ± Mediterranean (?ketogenic) diet, antihypertensives, hypoglycaemics (metformin ± glitazones, p200), statins. Explain that benefits are more than simply chemical: there is an intriguing two-way interaction between depression and insulin resistance: ▶Wise doctors and nurses will use this fact and work on many different levels to lead patients out of illness into health. Examples are motivational therapy and weekly phone interventions.

**Waist circumference for central obesity**

| | | |
|---|---|---|
| Europeans | ♂ ≥94cm; | ♀ ≥80cm |
| South (S) Asians | ♂ ≥90cm; | ♀ ≥80cm |
| Chinese | ♂ ≥90cm; | ♀ ≥80cm |
| Japanese | ♂ ≥85cm; | ♀ ≥90cm●* |

S & Central Americans use S Asian *pro tem*
Africans + Middle East use European *pro tem*

*Insulin resistance:*
- Risk factors: metabolic syndrome; obese; Asian[1]; TB drugs; SSRIs; pregnancy; acromegaly; Cushing's; renal failure; cystic fibrosis; polycystic ovary (OHCS p252); Werner's syn. (OHCS p655).
- Causes: *Obesity:* Possibly ↑ rate of release of non-esterified fatty acids causing post-receptor defects in insulin's action. *Genetics:* mutations in genes encoding insulin receptors. *Circulating autoantibodies* to the extracellular domain of the insulin receptor.

---

1 Gujaratis, Punjabis, Sri Lankans, Pakistanis and Bangladeshis have a low threshold for diagnosing obesity (BMI >23) and for vigorous intervention.

*Endocrinology*

Address all vascular risk factors. Obsessive focusing on achieving normoglycaemia may be harmful,[8,9] eg if it detracts from biopsychosocial health (p9) and quitting smoking. Aim for structured education and motivation from an interdisciplinary team of doctors, specialist nurses, dieticians, etc, and fellow patients (peer advisers). Randomized trials show that group learning from fellow patients is better at lowering HbA1c than well-run diabetic clinics: we doctors are not all that important![10]

**General:** Structured education programme, offer lifestyle advice (including smoking cessation), start a statin[1] (p109), control BP[2] (p134). Give foot-care (p204). (Pre-) pregnancy care should be in a multidisciplinary clinic (OHCS p24). Advise informing driving licence authority and not to drive if hypoglycaemic spells (p153; loss of hypoglycaemia awareness may lead to loss of licence; permanent if HGV). Be prepared to negotiate on target HbA1c (eg 6.5%), capillary glucose analysis, exercise, diet: p236—saturated fats↓, sugar↓, starch-carbohydrate↑, moderate protein. Foods made just for diabetics are not needed. One could regard bariatric surgery as a cure for DM in selected patients.[11]

**Type 1 DM:** Insulin (BOX).

**Type 2 DM:** •*Metformin* (a biguanide) initially[12] ↑ insulin sensitivity and helps weight. SE: nausea; diarrhoea; abdominal pain; not hypoglycaemia. Avoid if eGFR ≤36mL/min[13] (∴ lactic acidosis). Dose: 500mg bd after food. Stop if: tissue hypoxia (eg MI, sepsis); and morning before GA and contrast medium containing iodine (restart when renal function OK). *If HbA1c ≥53mmol/L 16wks later, add:*

•*Sulfonylurea* ↑insulin secretion; eg gliclazide 40mg/d. SE: hypoglycaemia (monitor glucose); it ↑weight, so gliptins, below, are an alternative if BMI ≥35 or hypoglycaemia is an issue. *If at 6mths, HbA1c ≥57mmol/L consider:*

•*Insulin* may be needed (BOX), eg isophane insulin bd or long-acting analogue, *or a*
•*Glitazone* to ↑ insulin sensitivity; SE: hypoglycaemia, fractures, fluid retention, LFT↑ (do LFT every 8wks for 1yr, stop if ALT up >3-fold). CI: past or present CCF; osteoporosis; monitor weight, and stop if ↑ or oedema. Example: pioglitazone 15-45mg/24h.[14] It replaces either metformin or sulfonylurea. It is occasionally used with insulin. *Others:* •*sulfonylurea receptor binders* (nateglinide): ↑β-cell insulin release. 60mg PO ½h before meals, eg tds, ↑dose as needed.[15] Alternative: repaglinide. They target post-prandial hyperglycaemia ($t_{½}$ is short—metformin works mostly on fasting glucose). They have a role in those with irregular mealtimes if glycaemic control is poor. •*glucagon-like peptide (GLP) analogues* Incretins are gut peptides that work by augmenting insulin release: 2 drug classes: GLP-1 *analogues*—exenatide 5µg SC bd ¼h before meals (>6h apart; avoid if eGFR <30; ↑after >4wks to 10µg bd) and DPP-4 *inhibitors* (dipeptidyl peptidase 4 breaks down GLP-1, sitagliptin; vilagliptin). They may be an alternative to insulin (if eGFR >50), eg if obese (they ↓ appetite). •*α-glucosidase inhibitors* (acarbose) ↓breakdown of starch to sugar (an add-on drug, often disappointing!), 50mg chewed at start of each meal. Start once daily; max 200mg/8h. SE: wind (less if *slow* dose build-up), abdominal distension/pain, diarrhoea.

---

### Monitoring glucose control

1 Fingerprick glucose if type 1 DM (and type 2, if on insulin).
2 Glycated haemoglobin (HbA1c) relates to mean glucose level over previous 8wks (RBC ½-life). Targets are negotiable, eg 48-57mmol/L (depends on patient's wish and arterial risk, eg past MI or stroke). If at risk from the effects of hypoglycaemia, eg elderly patients prone to falls, consider less tight control. Tight control may not alter all-cause mortality.[16] Complications rise with rising HbA1c, so any improvement helps.
3 Be sure to ask about hypoglycaemic attacks (and whether symptomatic). Hypoglycaemic awareness may diminish if control is too tight, or with time in type 1 DM, due to ↓glucagon secretion. It may return if control is loosened.

---

1 Simvastatin 40mg nocte; if triglyceride >4.5mmol/L: Bezalip® 200mg/8h (+Omacor® omega 3 if stilt).
2 Target BP <140/80mmHg; 130/80 if: stroke, MI, retinopathy, microalbuminuria (R, ARB or ACE-i, p123).

### What is the best diet for obese patients with type 2 diabetes?

Dietary carbohydrate is a big determinant of postprandial glucose levels, and we know that low-carbohydrate diets improve glycaemic control. How do low-carbohydrate, ketogenic diets (<20g of carbohydrate daily; LCKD) compare with low-glycaemic index, reduced-calorie diet (eg 500kcal/day deficit from weight maintenance diet)? In one randomized study over 24 weeks, LCKD had greater improvements in HbA1c (-15 vs -5mmol/L), weight (-11kg vs -7kg), and HDL. Diabetes drugs were reduced or eliminated in 95% of LCKD vs 62% of LGID participants. [17] NB: effects on renal function and mortality are unknown so these diets remain controversial.

## Using insulin
►►Ketoacidosis p842; HONK p844

For good control, it is *vital* to educate to self-adjust doses in the light of exercise, fingerprick glucose, and calorie intake. Ensure: •Phone support (trained nurse 7/24) •Dose titration to target—eg by 2-4u steps •Can modify diet wisely and avoid binge drinking (danger of delayed hypoglycaemia) •Partner can abort hypoglycaemia: sugary drinks; GlucoGel® PO if coma (no risk of aspiration).
NB: fingerprick glucose *before* a meal informs about long-acting insulin doses; those done *after* meals inform about the dose of short-acting insulin.

**Subcutaneous insulins** are short-, medium-, or long-acting. Strength: 100u/mL.
1 Ultra-fast acting (Humalog®; Novorapid®); inject at start of meal, or just after (unless unsure)—helps match what is actually eaten (vs what is planned).
2 Isophane insulin (variable peak at 4-12h): favoured by NICE (it's cheap!).
3 Pre-mixed insulins, with ultra-fast component (eg NovoMix® 30). 30% short acting, 70% long acting
4 Long-acting recombinant human insulin analogues (*insulin glargine*, eg 0.4u/kg/d) are used at bedtime in type 1 or 2 DM. [18] There is no awkward peak, so good if nocturnal hypoglycaemia is an issue. Caution if considering pregnancy. Molecular modification ensures it's soluble at acid pH, but precipitates in subcutaneous tissue, and is slowly released. *Insulin detemir* (eg 0.5u/kg/d) is similar and has a role in intensive insulin regimens for type 2 overweight diabetics.

**Common insulin regimens** ►*Plan the regimen to suit the lifestyle, not vice versa*. Disposable pens (FlexPen® ?more accurate than SoloStar®): dial dose; insert needle 90° to skin. Vary injection site (outer thigh/abdomen); change needle daily.
• 'BD biphasic regimen': twice daily premixed insulins by pen (eg NovoMix 30®)—useful in type 2 DM or type 1 with regular lifestyle.
• 'QDS regimen': before meals ultra-fast insulin + bedtime long-acting analogue: useful in type 1 DM for achieving a flexible life-style (eg for adjusting doses with size of meals, or exercise).
• Once-daily before-bed long-acting insulin: a good initial insulin regimen when switching from tablets in type 2 DM. Typical dose to work up to (slowly!): ≥1u/24h for every unit of body mass index in adults. Consider retaining metformin (±pioglitazone) if needed for tight control and patient is unable to use BD regimen.

*Dose adjustment for normal eating (DAFNE):* Multidisciplinary teams promoting autonomy can save lives. DAFNE found that training in flexible, intensive insulin dosing improved glycaemic control as well as wellbeing. [19] It is resource intensive.

**Subcutaneous insulin dosing during intercurrent illnesses (eg influenza)**
• Illness often increases insulin requirements despite reduced food intake.
• Maintain calorie intake, eg using milk.
• Check blood glucose ≥ 4 times a day and look for ketonuria. Increase insulin doses if glucose rising. Advise to get help from a specialist diabetes nurse or GP if concerned (esp. if glucose levels are rising or ketonuria). One option is 2-hourly ultra fast-acting insulin (eg 6-8u) preceded by a fingerprick glucose check.
• Admit if vomiting, dehydrated, ketotic (►►p842), a child, or pregnant.

Endocrinology

Prospective studies show that good control of hyperglycaemia is key to preventing microvascular complications in type 1 and 2 DM.[20] Don't treat in isolation: assess *global* vascular risk, eg: BP, cholesterol,[1] and smoking. ►*Focus on education and lifestyle advice* (eg exercise to ↑insulin sensitivity), healthy eating, and weight reduction—p236. ►*Find out what problems are being experienced* (eg glycaemic control, morale, erectile dysfunction—p222).

**Assess vascular risk:** BP (BOX). Target is <140/<80mmHg (or <125/<75 with renal disease: ↑creatinine, microalbuminuria, or dipstick proteinuria). BP control is critical for preventing macrovascular disease and ↓mortality.[21] Discuss *smoking* and offer referral to cessation services. Check *plasma lipids*.

**Look for complications** •Check injection sites for infection or lipohypertrophy (fatty change): advise on rotating sites of injection if present.

- *Vascular disease* Chief cause of death. MI is 4-fold commoner in DM and is more likely to be 'silent'. Stroke is twice as common. Women are at high risk—DM removes the vascular advantage conferred by the female sex. Address other risk factors—diet, smoking, hypertension (p87). Suggest a statin (eg simvastatin 40mg nocte) for all, even if no overt IHD, vascular disease, or microalbuminuria. Fibrates are useful for ↑triglycerides and ↓HDL (p704). Aspirin 75mg reduces vascular events (if past stroke or MI) and is good as statin co-therapy (safe to use in diabetic retinopathy; use in primary prevention is disappointing, at least at 100mg/day).[22]

- *Nephropathy* (p309) Microalbuminuria is when urine dipstick is –ve for protein but the urine albumin:creatinine ratio (UACR) is ≥3mg/mmol (units vary, check lab) reflecting early renal disease and ↑vascular risk. If UACR >3, inhibiting the renin-angiotensin system with an ACE-i or sartan, even if BP is normal, protects the kidneys. Spironolactone may also help.[23] Refer if UACR >7 ± GFR falling by >5mL/min/1.73m²/yr.[24]NICE

- *Diabetic retinopathy* Blindness is *preventable. Annual retinal screening mandatory for all patients not already under ophthalmology care.* Refer to an ophthalmologist if pre-proliferative changes or if any uncertainty at or near the macula (the only place capable of 6/6 vision). ►Pre-symptomatic screening enables laser photocoagulation to be used, aimed to stop production of angiogenic factors from the ischaemic retina. Indications: maculopathy or proliferative retinopathy. See figs 1-4.

  - *Background retinopathy:* Microaneurysms (dots), haemorrhages (blots) and hard exudates (lipid deposits). Refer if near the macula, eg for intravitreal triamcinolone.
  - *Pre-proliferative retinopathy:* Cotton-wool spots (eg infarcts), haemorrhages, venous beading. These are signs of retinal ischaemia. Refer to a specialist.
  - *Proliferative retinopathy:* New vessels form. Needs urgent referral.
  - *Maculopathy:* (hard to see in early stages). Suspect if acuity↓. Prompt laser, intravitreal steroids or anti-angiogenic agents may be needed in macular oedema. *Pathogenesis:* Capillary endothelial change → vascular leak → microaneurysms → capillary occlusion → local hypoxia → ischaemia → new vessel formation. High retinal blood flow caused by hyperglycaemia (and BP↑ and pregnancy) triggers this, causing capillary pericyte damage. Microvascular occlusion causes *cotton-wool spots* (± *blot haemorrhages* at interfaces with perfused retina). *New vessels* form on the disc or ischaemic areas, proliferate, bleed, fibrose, and can detach the retina. Aspirin[1] (2mg/kg/d) may be recommended by ophthalmologists; there is no evidence that it ↑ bleeding.

- *Cataracts:* May be juvenile 'snowflake' form, or 'senile'—which occur earlier in diabetic subjects. Osmotic changes in the lens induced in acute hyperglycaemia reverse with normoglycaemia (so wait before buying glasses).

- *Rubeosis iridis:* New vessels on iris: occurs late and may lead to glaucoma.

- *Metabolic complications:* p842. *Diabetic feet:* p204. *Neuropathy:* p204.

---

**1** As DM has so many vascular events, particularly encourage statin use (p704), esp. if LDL >3mmol/L **or** systolic BP >140. Even consider a statin *whatever* the pre-treatment cholesterol; discuss with your patient.

### Controlling BP in those with diabetes—3 typical scenarios

1 BP <140/80mmHg and no microalbuminuria and 10yr coronary event risk (CER10, p664) ≤15%: simply check BP every 6 months, or more often.
2 BP ≥ 140/80 and <160/100 and CER10 >15%, but no microalbuminuria: start an antihypertensive. Target BP <140/80. For doses and discussion, see p134.
3 BP ≥ 140/80 and microalbuminuria is present: ensure ACE-i or A2A are part of the approach (contraindications: p109). Target BP: <125/75 (if patient willing).

The role of aspirin prophylaxis (75mg/d PO) is uncertain in DM with hypertension.[1]

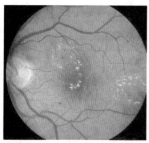

Fig 1. Background retinopathy, with micro-aneurysms and hard exudates.

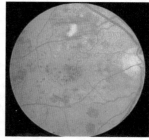

Fig 2. Pre-proliferative retinopathy, with haemorrhages and a cotton-wool spot.

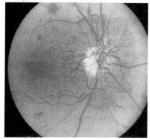

Fig 3. Proliferative retinopathy, with new vessel formation and haemorrhages.

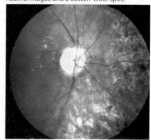

Fig 4. Scars from previous laser photocoagulation.

Figs 1, 3 & 4 courtesy of Prof J Trobe; fig 2 reproduced with permission from the *Oxford Textbook of Medicine*.

### ☺ Improving quality of life: going beyond the pleasures of the flesh

"I cannot eat what I want because of your pitiful diet. Sex is out because diabetes has made me impotent. Smoking is banned, so what's left? I'd shoot myself if only I could see straight." Start by acknowledging your patient's distress. Don't shrug it off—but don't take it at face value either. Life may be transformed by cataract surgery, sildenafil (unless contraindicated, p222), dietary negotiation, and sport (it needn't be shooting). Take steps to simplify care. Stop blood glucose self-monitoring if it's achieving nothing (constant prickings are known to ↓ quality of life).[25] Even if all these interventions fail, you have one trump card up your sleeve: "Let's both try to find one new thing of value before we next meet—and compare notes". This opens the way to vicarious pleasure: a whole new world.

1 Aspirin ↓ leucocyte adhesion in diabetic retinal capillaries and ↓ expression of integrins on leucocytes. It ↓ nitric oxide synthetase (ENOS) levels and ↓ vasoactive cytokine tumour necrosis factor, known to be raised in diabetic retinopathy, but benefits are hard to prove, and harm is possible.

Endocrinology

Endocrinology

Amputations are common (100/week UK)—and preventable: *good care saves legs*. ►Refer *early* to high-quality interdisciplinary foot care services, which integrate podiatry, imaging, vascular surgery, and skilled optimization of diabetic care.

**Signs** Examine feet regularly. Distinguish between ischaemia (critical toes ± absent dorsalis pedis pulses and worse outcome) and peripheral neuropathy (injury or infection over pressure points, eg the metatarsal heads). In practice, many have both.

*Neuropathy:* Sensation↓ in 'stocking' distribution (test sensation with a 10g monofilament fibre applied with just sufficient force to bend it), absent ankle jerks, neuropathic deformity: pes cavus, claw toes, loss of transverse arch, rocker-bottom sole. Sensory loss is patchy, so examine all areas using a monofilament.

*Ischaemia:* If the foot pulses cannot be felt, do Doppler pressure measurements. Any evidence of neuropathy or vascular disease raises risk of foot ulceration. *Educate* (daily foot inspection—eg with a mirror so the sole can be fully inspected; comfortable shoes—ie very soft leather, increased depth, cushioning insoles/trainers; weight-distributing cradles; no barefoot walking, no corn-plasters). *Regular chiropody* to remove callus, as haemorrhage and tissue necrosis may occur below, leading to ulceration. *Treat fungal infections* (p440). *Surgery* (including endovascular angioplasty balloons, stents, and subintimal recanalization) has a role. Get advice.

**Foot ulceration** Typically painless, punched-out ulcer (fig 1) in an area of thick callus ± superadded infection. Causes cellulitis, abscess ± osteomyelitis.

*Assess degree of:* 1 Neuropathy (clinically).
2 Ischaemia (clinically + Doppler ± angiography).
3 Bony deformity, eg Charcot joint (clinically + x-ray). See fig 2.
4 Infection (swabs, blood culture, x-ray for osteomyelitis, probe ulcer to reveal depth).

*Management:* Regular chiropody to remove callus. Relieve high-pressure areas with bed rest ± therapeutic shoes (Pressure Relief Walkers® may be as good as total contact casts); metatarsal head surgery may be needed. If there is cellulitis, admit for IV antibiotics. Common organisms: staphs, streps, anaerobes. Start with benzylpenicillin 1.2g/6h IV and flucloxacillin 1g/6h IV ± metronidazole 500mg/8h IV, refined when microbiology results are known. IV insulin may improve healing. Get surgical help early. The degree of peripheral vascular disease, general health, and patient request will determine whether local excision and drainage, vascular reconstruction, and/or amputation (and how much) is appropriate. ►*Absolute indications for surgery:* Abscess or deep infection; spreading anaerobic infection; gangrene/rest pain; suppurative arthritis.

*Diabetic neuropathies: Symmetric sensory polyneuropathy*: ('glove & stocking' numbness, tingling, and pain, eg worse at night). ℞: (in order) paracetamol → tricyclic (amitriptyline 10-25mg nocte; gradually ↑ to 150mg) → duloxetine, gabapentin, or pregabalin → opiates.[18] Avoiding weight-bearing helps.

*Mononeuritis multiplex:* (eg III & VI cranial nerves) Treatment: hard! If sudden or severe, immunosuppression may help (corticosteroids, IV immunoglobulin, ciclosporin).[26]

*Amyotrophy:* Painful wasting of quadriceps and other pelvifemoral muscles. Use electrophysiology to show, eg lumbosacral radiculopathy, plexopathy, or proximal crural neuropathy. Natural course: variable with gradual but often incomplete improvement. IV immunoglobulins have been used.[27]

*Autonomic neuropathy:* (p509) Postural BP drop; ↓cerebrovascular autoregulation; loss of respiratory sinus arrhythmia (vagal neuropathy); gastroparesis; urine retention; erectile dysfunction (ED); gustatory sweating; diarrhoea. The latter may respond to codeine phosphate (use lowest dose to control symptoms, eg 15mg/8h PO). Gastroparesis (early satiety, post-prandial bloating, nausea/vomiting) is diagnosed by gastric scintigraphy with a ⁹⁹technetium-labelled meal. It may respond to anti-emetics, erythromycin, or gastric pacing. Postural hypotension may respond to fludrocortisone 50-300µg/24h PO (SE: oedema, ↑BP), or midodrine (unlicensed α-agonist; SE: ↑BP).

### Preventing loss of limbs: primary or secondary prevention?

Traditionally prevention involves foot care advice in diabetic clinics (eg "Don't go bare-foot"), promoting euglycaemia and normotension.[1] But despite this, the sight of a diabetic patient minus one limb is not rare, and must prompt us to redouble our commitment to primary prevention, ie stopping those at risk from ever getting diabetes. In one prospective study of those with impaired glucose tolerance and other risk factors, after 3 yrs, the incidence of diabetes per 100 person-yrs was 5 in those receiving simple exercise and diet advice, 8 in a group given metformin, and 11 in the placebo group. Advice and metformin decreased incidence of diabetes by 58% (NNT ≈ 7) and 31% (NNT ≈ 14), respectively, compared with placebo. One vital group to focus on are those with the metabolic syndrome (p199).

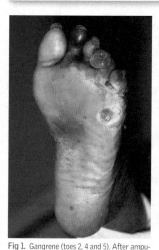

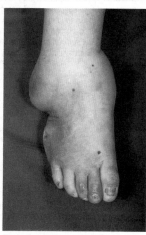

**Fig 1.** Gangrene (toes 2, 4 and 5). After amputation, (eg forefoot/Syme's, or above or below knee, depending on Doppler), even the least self-pitying are entitled to a period of narcissistic grief: "I begin again to walk, on crutches. What nuisance, what fatigue, what sadness, when I think about all my ancient travels, and how active I was just 5 months ago! Where are the runnings across mountains, the walks, the deserts, the rivers, and the seas? And now, the life of a legless cripple. For I begin to understand that crutches, wooden and articulated legs, are a pack of jokes...Goodbye to family, goodbye to future! My life is gone, I'm no more than an immobile trunk". [28 Arthur Rimbaund]

**Fig 2.** Charcot (neuropathic) joint, caused by loss of pain sensation, leading to ↑mechanical stress (unimpeded by pain) and repeated joint injury. Swelling, instability and, eventually, deformity, have developed. ►Early recognition is vital (cellulitis or osteomyelitis are often misdiagnosed). Treatment: offload all weight (bed rest or non-weight-bearing crutches); immobilization by a total contact cast until oedema and local warmth reduce and bony repair is complete (≥8wks). Bisphosphonates may help. Charcot joints are also seen in tabes dorsalis, spina bifida, syringomyelia, and leprosy.

Figs 1 & 2 reproduced from the *Oxford Textbook of Medicine*, with permission from OUP.

▶This is the commonest endocrine emergency—see p844. Prompt diagnosis and treatment is essential—brain damage & death can occur if severe or prolonged.

**Definition** Plasma glucose ⩽3mmol/L. Threshold for symptoms varies. See BOX.

**Symptoms** •*Autonomic*—Sweating, anxiety, hunger, tremor, palpitations, dizziness. •*Neuroglycopenic*—Confusion, drowsiness, visual trouble, seizures, coma. Rarely focal symptoms, eg transient hemiplegia. Mutism, personality change, restlessness and incoherence may lead to misdiagnosis of alcohol intoxication or even psychosis.

**1 Fasting hypoglycaemia** *Causes:* The chief cause is insulin or sulfonylurea treatment in a known diabetic, eg with ↑activity, missed meal, accidental or non-accidental overdose. In *non-diabetic* adults you must EXPLAIN the mechanism:

Exogenous drugs, eg *insulin, oral hypoglycaemics* (p200). Does she have access to these (diabetic in the family)? Body-builders may misuse insulin to help stamina. Also: *alcohol*, eg a binge with no food; *aspirin poisoning*; ACE-i; *β-blockers*; *pentamidine*; *quinine sulfate*; *aminoglutethimide*; insulin-like growth factor.[29]

Pituitary insufficiency.

Liver failure, plus some rare inherited enzyme defects.

Addison's disease.

Islet cell tumours (insulinoma) and immune hypoglycaemia (eg anti-insulin receptor antibodies in Hodgkin's disease).

Non-pancreatic neoplasms, eg fibrosarcomas and haemangiopericytomas.

*Diagnosis and investigations* (see BOX)
- Document hypoglycaemia by taking fingerprick (on filter-paper at home for later analysis) during attack and lab glucose if in hospital (monitors are often not reliable at low readings). •Take a drug history and exclude liver failure.
- 72h fasting may be needed (monitor closely). Take blood samples for glucose, insulin, c-peptide and plasma ketones if symptomatic.

*Interpreting results*
- Hypoglycaemic hyperinsulinaemia (HH): *Causes:* Insulinoma, sulfonylureas, insulin injection (no detectable c-peptide—only released with endogenous insulin); non-insulinoma pancreatogenous hypoglycaemia syndrome, mutation in the insulin-receptor gene. Congenital HH follows mutations in genes involved in insulin secretion (ABCC8, KCNJ11, GLUD1, CGK, HADH, SLC16A1, HNF4A, ABCC8 & KCNJ11).[30]
- Insulin low or undetectable, no excess ketones. *Causes:* Non-pancreatic neoplasm; anti-insulin receptor antibodies.
- Insulin↓, ketones↑. *Causes:* Alcohol, pituitary insufficiency, Addison's disease.

**2 Post-prandial hypoglycaemia** May occur after gastric/bariatric surgery ('dumping', p624), and in type 2 DM. *Investigation:* Prolonged OGTT (5h, p198).

**Treatment** ▶▶See p844. Treat with oral sugar and a long-acting starch (eg toast); If cannot swallow, 25-50mL 50% glucose IV (via large vein with 0.9% saline flush to prevent phlebitis) or glucagon 1mg IM if no IV access (short duration of effect so repeat after 20min and *follow with oral carbohydrate*). If episodes are often, advise many small high-starch meals. If post-prandial glucose↓, give slowly absorbed carbohydrate (high fibre). In diabetics, rationalize insulin therapy (p201).

**Insulinoma** This often benign (90-95%) pancreatic islet cell tumour is sporadic or seen with MEN-1 (p215). It presents as fasting hypoglycaemia, with Whipple's triad: 1 Symptoms associated with fasting or exercise 2 Recorded hypoglycaemia with symptoms 3 Symptoms relieved with glucose. *Screening test:* Hypoglycaemia + plasma insulin↑ during a long fast. *Suppressive tests:* Give IV insulin and measure c-peptide. Normally exogenous insulin suppresses c-peptide production, but this does not occur in insulinoma. *Imaging:* CT/MRI ± endoscopic pancreatic US ± IACS (see BOX; all fallible, so don't waste too much time before proceeding to intra-operative visualization ± intra-operative ultrasound). [18]F-L-3,4-dihydroxyphenylalanine PET-CT can help guide laparoscopic surgery. *Treatment:* Excision. *Nesidioblastosis*: see BOX. If this doesn't work, options are: ↑diet, diazoxide, dextrose IVI, enteral feeding, everolimus.

## The definition of hypoglycaemia is context-dependent

Because the brain stops working if plasma glucose levels get too low we are all nervous of levels ≤3mmol/L. But some people can walk around quite happily at this level. So what is definitely abnormal? A rule such as 'Any plasma glucose <1.7mmol/L constitutes hypoglycaemia' may be true (a normal neonate may descend to this level but no further during the 1st day of life: even so—he or she needs feeding urgently)—but it is not a very helpful rule if the context is a fingerprick glucose on someone having seizures. Here it is better to rephrase the question: "In this ill patient when can I be sure that a low glucose is not contributing to their illness?" The answer may be 4mmol/L, allowing for inaccuracy in fingerprick blood glucose levels (NB: whole blood glucose is 10-15% < plasma glucose.) If <4, you may be wise to treat (p844)—just in case.

A different context is a call from the lab to say that a glucose is 2.50mmol/L. Contact the patient, who may be up and about and happy; confirm that they are not on any hypoglycaemic agents. Have they binged on alcohol in the 24h before the test? Skipped meals? Could this low glucose be a sign of an illness such as an insulinoma? Unlikely, but possible. Keep an open mind; let the GP know. Explain about signs of hypoglycaemia and to see a doctor if such signs occur. Consider further tests (p206), eg dotted about the day to catch other episodes of hypoglycaemia. Be more inclined to investigate if the effects of even mild hypoglycaemia might be disastrous (eg in pilots) or if there are unexplained symptoms.

**When should I investigate borderline hypoglycaemia?** Whipple answered the question thus (*Whipple's triad*): symptoms or signs of hypoglycemia + ↓plasma glucose + resolution of those symptoms or signs after plasma glucose raises. [31]

**First thoughts in proven hypoglycaemia** Exclude drugs, critical illnesses, hormone deficiencies, and non-islet cell tumours. If none of these, diagnosis narrows to accidental, surreptitious/malicious hypoglycaemia, or endogenous hyperinsulinism (if the latter, do insulin, C-peptide, proinsulin, β-hydroxybutyrate, and circulating oral hypoglycaemic agents during hypoglycaemia). Measure insulin antibodies.

## Pursuing a voyage to the islets of Langerhans to the bitter end

A 50-year-old had episodic early-morning sweats and tremors and was found to have hyperinsulinaemic hypoglycaemia. Selective intra-arterial calcium infusions (IACS) showed a 2-fold increase in insulin secretion after infusion of the splenic and superior mesenteric arteries, so setting the stage for 'hunt the insulinoma'.

But cross-sectional imaging and endoscopic ultrasound were normal. At laparotomy, no lesion was found despite mobilization of the pancreas, or during intraoperative ultrasound. "Time to sew up and go home?" "No!" said the surgeon, "I'm going to do a distal pancreatectomy". Histology showed no discrete insulinoma, but diffuse islet cell hyperplasia (**nesidioblastosis**). How much pancreas to resect? Too little and nothing is gained: too much spells pancreatic endocrine disaster. Luckily the surgeon guessed right, and the patient was cured by the procedure. [32]

**Physiology** (fig 1) The hypothalamus secretes thyrotropin-releasing hormone (TRH), a tripeptide, that stimulates production of thyroid-stimulating hormone (TSH=thyrotropin), a glycoprotein, from the anterior pituitary. TSH increases production and release of thyroxine ($T_4$) and triiodothyronine ($T_3$) from the thyroid, which exert –ve feedback on TSH production. The thyroid produces mainly $T_4$, which is 5-fold less active than $T_3$. 85% of $T_3$ is formed from peripheral conversion of $T_4$. Most $T_3$ and $T_4$ in plasma is protein bound, eg to thyroxine-binding globulin (TBG). The unbound portion is the active part. $T_3$ and $T_4$ ↑cell metabolism, via nuclear receptors, and are thus vital for growth and mental development. They also ↑catecholamine effects.

Thyroid hormone abnormalities are usually due to problems in the thyroid gland itself, and rarely caused by the hypothalamus or the anterior pituitary.

**Basic tests** Free $T_4$ and $T_3$ are more useful than total $T_4$ and $T_3$ as the latter are affected by TBG. Total $T_4$ and $T_3$ are ↑ when TBG is ↑ and *vice versa*. TBG is ↑ in pregnancy, oestrogen therapy (HRT, oral contraceptives) and hepatitis. TBG is ↓ in nephrotic syndrome and malnutrition (both from protein loss), drugs (androgens, corticosteroids, phenytoin), chronic liver disease and acromegaly. TSH is very useful:

• *Hyperthyroidism suspected:* Ask for $T_3$, $T_4$, and TSH. In hyperthyroidism, all will have ↓TSH (except for the rare phenomenon of a TSH-secreting pituitary adenoma). Most will have raised $T_4$, but ~1% raised $T_3$.

• *Hypothyroidism suspected or monitoring replacement R̞:* Ask for only $T_4$ and TSH. $T_3$ does not add any extra information. TSH varies through the day: trough at 2PM; 30% higher during darkness, so during monitoring, try to do at the same time.

| ↑TSH, ↓$T_4$ | Hypothyroidism |
|---|---|
| ↑TSH, normal $T_4$ | Treated hypothyroidism or subclinical hypothyroidism (p213) |
| ↑TSH, ↑$T_4$ | TSH secreting tumour or thyroid hormone resistance |
| ↑TSH, ↑$T_4$ and ↓$T_3$ | Slow conversion of $T_4$ to $T_3$ (deiodinase deficiency; euthyroid hyperthyroxinaemia[1]) or thyroid hormone antibody artefact.[33,34] |
| ↓TSH, ↑$T_4$ or ↑$T_3$ | Hyperthyroidism |
| ↓TSH, normal $T_4$ & $T_3$ | Subclinical hyperthyroidism |
| ↓TSH, ↓$T_4$ | Central hypothyroidism (hypothalamic or pituitary disorder) |
| ↓TSH, ↓$T_4$ & ↓$T_3$ | Sick euthyroidism (below) or pituitary disease |
| Normal TSH, abnormal $T_4$ | Consider changes in thyroid-binding globulin, assay interference, amiodarone, or pituitary TSH tumour |

*Sick euthyroidism:* In any systemic illness, TFTs may become deranged. The typical pattern is for 'everything to be low'. The test should be repeated after recovery.

*Assay interference* is caused by antibodies in the serum, interfering with the test.

**Other tests** • *Thyroid autoantibodies:* Antithyroid peroxidase (TPO; formerly called microsomal) antibodies or antithyroglobulin antibodies may be increased in autoimmune thyroid disease: Hashimoto's or Graves' disease. If +ve in Graves', there is an increased risk of developing hypothyroidism at a later stage.

• *TSH receptor antibody:* May be ↑ in Graves' disease (useful in pregnancy).

• *Serum thyroglobulin:* Useful in monitoring the treatment of carcinoma (p602), and in detection of factitious (self-medicated) hyperthyroidism, where it is low.

• *Ultrasound:* This distinguishes cystic (usually, but not always, benign) from solid (possibly malignant) nodules. If a solitary (or dominant) large nodule, in a multinodular goitre, do a fine-needle aspiration to look for thyroid cancer; see fig 3, p603.

• *Isotope scan:* ($^{123}$Iodine, $^{99}$technetium pertechnetate, etc; see fig 2, p603). Useful for determining the cause of hyperthyroidism and to detect retrosternal goitre, ectopic thyroid tissue or thyroid metastases (+ whole body CT). If there are suspicious nodules, the question is: does the area have increased (hot), decreased (cold), or the same (neutral) uptake of isotope as the remaining thyroid (see fig 2)? Few neutral and almost no hot nodules are malignant. 20% of 'cold' nodules are malignant. Surgery is most likely to be needed if: •Rapid growth •Compression signs •Dominant nodule on scintigraphy •Nodule ≥3cm •Hypo-echogenicity. See also p752.

1 In 'consumptive hypothyroidism' deiodinase activity is ↑↑; suspect if thyroxine doses have to be ↑↑.

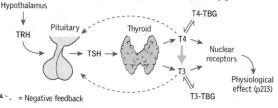

TRH from the hypothalamus acts on the pituitary gland

**Fig 1.** Pathways involved in thyroid function.

### Screen the following for abnormalities in thyroid function:

- Patients with atrial fibrillation
- Patients with hyperlipidaemia (4-14% have hypothyroidism)
- Diabetes mellitus—on annual review
- Women with type 1 DM during 1st trimester and post delivery (3-fold rise in incidence of postpartum thyroid dysfunction)
- Patients on amiodarone or lithium (6 monthly)
- Patients with Down's or Turner's syndrome, or Addison's disease (yearly)

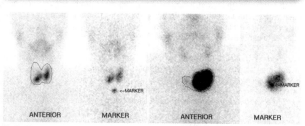

**Fig 2.** The images are from an isotope scan, with and without markers placed over the sternal notch. We can see on the left that the nodule is metabolically inactive ('cold'). The hot nodule (right pair) is a very avid nodule causing background thyroid suppression.

Image courtesy of Dr Y. T. Huang.

Endocrinology

The clinical effect of excess thyroid hormone, usually from gland hyperfunction.

**Symptoms** Diarrhoea; weight↓; appetite↑ (if ↑↑, paradoxical weight *gain* in 10%); over-active; sweats; heat intolerance; palpitations; tremor; irritability; labile emotions; oligomenorrhoea ±infertility. Rarely psychosis; chorea; panic; itch; alopecia; urticaria.

**Signs** Pulse fast/irregular (AF or SVT; VT rare); warm moist skin; fine tremor; palmar erythema; thin hair; lid lag (fig 1; eyelid lags behind eye's descent as patient watches your finger descend slowly); lid retraction (exposure of sclera above iris; causing 'stare'). There may be goitre (fig 2); thyroid nodules; or bruit depending on the cause. *Signs of Graves' disease:* (BOX) 1 *Eye disease* (BOX): exophthalmos, ophthalmople-gia. 2 *Pretibial myxoedema:* oedematous swellings above lateral malleoli: the term *myxoedema* is confusing here 3 *Thyroid acropachy:* extreme manifestation, with clubbing, painful finger and toe swelling, and periosteal reaction in limb bones.

**Tests** TSH↓ (suppressed), $T_4$ and $T_3$↑. There may be mild normocytic anaemia, mild neutropenia (in Graves'), ESR↑, $Ca^{2+}$↑, LFT↑. *Also:* Check thyroid autoantibodies. Iso-tope scan if the cause is unclear, to detect nodular disease or subacute thyroiditis. If ophthalmopathy, test visual fields, acuity, and eye movements (see BOX).

**Causes**
• *Graves' disease:* Prevalence: 0.5% (⅔ of cases of hyperthyroidism). ♀:♂≈9:1. Typical age: 40-60yrs (younger if maternal family history). Cause: circulating IgG autoantibodies binding to and activating G-protein-coupled thyrotropin receptors, which cause smooth thyroid enlargement and ↑ hormone production (esp. $T_3$), and react with orbital autoantigens.[3,35] Triggers: stress; infection; childbirth. Patients are often hyperthyroid but may be, or become, hypo- or euthyroid. It is associated with other autoimmune diseases: vitiligo, type 1 DM, Addison's.
• *Toxic multinodular goitre:* Seen in the elderly and in iodine-deficient areas. There are nodules that secrete thyroid hormones. Surgery is indicated for compressive symptoms from the enlarged thyroid (dysphagia or dyspnoea).
• *Toxic adenoma:* There is a solitary nodule producing $T_3$ and $T_4$. On isotope scan, the nodule is 'hot' (p208), and the rest of the gland is suppressed.
• *Ectopic thyroid tissue:* Metastatic follicular thyroid cancer, or struma ovarii: ovar-ian teratoma with thyroid tissue.
• *Exogenous:* Iodine excess, eg food contamination, contrast media (►►thyroid storm, p844, if already hyperthyroid). Levothyroxine excess causes ↑$T_4$, ↓$T_3$, ↓thyroglobulin.
• *Others:* 1 *Subacute de Quervain's thyroiditis:* Self-limiting post-viral with pain-ful goitre, T°↑ ± ↑ESR. Low isotope uptake on scan. $R$: NSAIDs. 2 *Drugs:* Amiodarone (p212), lithium (hypothyroidism more common). 3 *Postpartum* 4 *TB* (rare).

**Treatment**
1 *Drugs:* β-blockers (eg **propranolol** 40mg/6h) for rapid control of symptoms. *Anti-thyroid medication:* 2 strategies (equally effective):[36] **A)** *Titration,* eg **carbimazole** 20-40mg/24h PO for 4wks, reduce according to TFTs every 1-2 months. **B)** *Block-replace:* Give carbimazole + thyroxine simultaneously (less risk of iatrogenic hypothyroidism). In Graves', maintain on either regimen for 12-18 months then withdraw. ~50% will relapse, requiring radioiodine or surgery. Car-bimazole SE: agranulocytosis (↓↓neutrophils, can lead to dangerous sepsis; rare (0.03%)); warn to stop and get an urgent FBC if signs of infection, eg T°↑, sore throat/mouth ulcers.
2 *Radioiodine* (¹³¹I): Most become hypothyroid post-treatment. There is no evi-dence for ↑cancer, birth defects or infertility in women. CI: pregnancy, lactation. Caution in active hyperthyroidism as risk of thyroid storm (p845).
3 *Thyroidectomy:* Carries a risk of damage to recurrent laryngeal nerve (hoarse voice) and hypoparathyroidism. Patients may become hypothyroid.
4 *In pregnancy and infancy:* Get expert help. See OHCS p25 & OHCS p182.

**Complications** Heart failure (thyrotoxic cardiomyopathy, ↑ in elderly), angina, AF (seen in 10-25%: control hyperthyroidism and warfarinize if no contraindication), osteoporosis, ophthalmopathy, gynaecomastia. ►► Thyroid storm (p845).

## Thyroid eye disease

This is seen in 25–50% of people with Graves' disease. The main known risk factor is smoking. The eye disease may not correlate with thyroid disease and the patient can be euthyroid, hypothyroid, or hyperthyroid at presentation. Eye disease may be the first presenting sign of Graves' disease, and can also be worsened by treatment, typically with radioiodine (usually a transient effect). Retro-orbital inflammation and lymphocyte infiltration results in swelling of the orbit.

**Symptoms** Eye discomfort, grittiness, tear production↑, photophobia, diplopia, acuity↓, afferent pupillary defect (p79) may mean optic nerve compression: ►Seek expert advice at once as decompression may be needed. Nerve damage does not necessarily go hand-in-hand with protrusion. Indeed, if the eye cannot protrude for anatomical reasons, optic nerve compression is more likely—a paradox!

**Signs** Exophthalmos—appearance of protruding eye; proptosis—eyes protrude beyond the orbit (look from above in the same plane as the forehead); conjunctival oedema; corneal ulceration; papilloedema; loss of colour vision. Ophthalmoplegia (especially of upward gaze) occurs due to muscle swelling and fibrosis.

**Tests** Diagnosis is clinical. CT/MRI of the orbits may reveal enlarged eye muscles.

**Management** Get specialist help. Treat hyper- or hypothyroidism. Advise to stop smoking as this worsens prognosis. Most have mild disease that can be treated symptomatically (artificial tears, sunglasses, avoid dust, elevate bed when sleeping to ↓periorbital oedema). Diplopia may be managed with a Fresnel prism stuck to one lens of a spectacle (aids easy changing as the exophthalmos changes).

In more severe disease with ophthalmoplegia or gross oedema, try high-dose steroids (IV methylprednisolone is better than prednisolone 100mg/day PO) [37]—decreasing according to symptoms. Surgical decompression is used for severe sight-threatening disease, or for cosmetic reasons once the activity of eye disease has reduced (via an inferior orbital approach, using space in the ethmoidal, sphenoidal, and maxillary sinuses). Eyelid surgery may improve cosmesis and function. Orbital radiotherapy can be used to treat ophthalmoplegia but has little effect on proptosis. *Future options:* Anti-TNFα antibodies (eg infliximab).

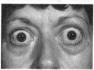

**Fig 1.** Thyroid eye disease: lid retraction causing a 'staring' appearance.

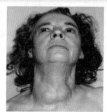

**Fig 2.** Goitre.

### Causes of goitre

**Diffuse**
- Physiological
- Graves' disease
- Hashimoto's thyroiditis
- Subacute (de Quervain's) thyroiditis (painful)

**Nodular**
- Multinodular goitre
- Adenoma
- Carcinoma

### Manifestations of Graves' disease—and pathophysiology

| Pituitary | Suppressed TSH | ↓Expression of thyrotropin β subunit[et al] |
|---|---|---|
| Heart | ↑Rate; ↑contractility | ↑Serum atrial natriuretic peptide[et al] |
| Liver | ↑Peripheral T₃; LDL↓ (p704) | ↑Type 1 5'-deiodinase; LDL receptors |
| Bone | ↑Bone turnover; osteoporosis | ↑Osteocalcin; talk phos; ↑urinary N-telopeptide |
| Genital ♂ | ↓Libido; erectile dysfunction | ↑Sex hormone globulin; ↓testosterone |
| Genital ♀ | Irregular menses | Oestrogen antagonism |
| Metabolic | ↑Thermogenesis; ↑O₂ use | ↑Fatty acid oxidation; ↑Na-K ATPASE |
| White fat | ↓Fat mass | ↑Adrenergic-mediated lipolysis |
| CNS basal ganglia | Stiff person syndrome (rare)[1] | Antibodies to glutamic acid decarboxylase |
| Muscle | Proximal myopathy | ↑Sarcoplasmic reticulum Ca²⁺-activated ATPASE |
| Thyroid | ↑Secretion of T₃ and T₄ | ↑Type 2 5'-deiodinase activity in thyroid [35] |

1 Emotional or tactile stimuli cause spasms; seen in any autoimmune state (eg type 1 DM); R: baclofen± IV Ig.

This is the clinical effect of thyroid hormone lack. It is common (4/1000/yr). If treated, prognosis is excellent; untreated it is disastrous (eg heart disease, dementia*etc*).
►*As it is insidious, both you and your patient may not realize anything is wrong,* so be alert to subtle, nonspecific symptoms, esp. in women ≥40yrs old (♀:♂≈6:1).

**Symptoms** Tired; sleepy, lethargic; mood↓; cold-disliking; weight↑; constipation; menorrhagia; hoarse voice; ↓memory/cognition; dementia; myalgia; cramps; weakness.

**Signs** BRADYCARDIC; reflexes relax slowly; ataxia (cerebellar); dry thin hair/skin; yawning/drowsy/coma (p844); cold hands ± T°↓; ascites ± non-pitting oedema (lids; hands; feet) ± pericardial or pleural effusion; round puffy face/double chin/obese; defeated demeanour; immobile ± ileus; CCF. Also: neuropathy; myopathy; goitre (fig 1).

**Diagnosis** (p208) ►Have a low threshold for doing TFTs: TSH↑ (eg ≥4mu/L);[1] T4↓ (in rare secondary hypothyroidism: T4↓ and TSH↓ or ↔ due to lack from the pituitary, p224). Cholesterol and triglyceride↑; macrocytosis (less often normochromic anaemia too).

## Causes of primary autoimmune hypothyroidism
• *Primary atrophic hypothyroidism:* ♀:♂≈6:1. Common. Diffuse lymphocytic infiltration of the thyroid, leading to atrophy, hence no goitre.
• *Hashimoto's thyroiditis:* Goitre due to lymphocytic and plasma cell infiltration. Commoner in women aged 60–70yrs. May be hypothyroid or euthyroid; rarely initial period of hyperthyroid ('Hashitoxicosis'). Autoantibody titres are very high.

## Other causes of primary hypothyrodism
►World-wide the chief cause is *iodine deficiency*.
• *Post-thyroidectomy or radioiodine treatment.*
• *Drug-induced:* Antithyroid drugs, amiodarone, lithium, iodine.
• *Subacute thyroiditis:* Temporary hypothyroidism after hyperthyroid phase.

**Secondary hypothyroidism** Not enough TSH (∵ hypopituitarism, p224); very rare.

**Hypothyroidism's associations** Autoimmune is seen with other autoimmune diseases (type 1 DM, Addison's and PA, p328). Turner's and Down's syndromes, cystic fibrosis, primary biliary cirrhosis, ovarian hyperstimulation (*OHCS* p311); POEMS syndrome—polyneuropathy, organomegaly, endocrinopathy, m-protein band (plasmacytoma) + skin pigmentation/tethering. *Genetic:* Dyshormonogenesis: genetic (often autosomal recessive) defect in hormone synthesis, eg Pendred's syndrome (with deafness): there is ↑uptake on isotope scan, which is displaced by potassium perchlorate.

**Pregnancy problems** Eclampsia, anaemia, prematurity, ↓birthweight, stillbirth, PPH.

## Treatment
• *Healthy and young:* Levothyroxine (T4), 50–100µg/24h PO; review at 12wks. Adjust 6 weekly by clinical state and to normalize but not suppress TSH (keep TSH >0.5mu/L). Thyroxine's t½ is ~7d, so wait ~4wks before checking TSH to see if a dose change is right. NB: small changes in serum free T4 have a logarithmic effect on TSH.[38] Once normal, check TSH yearly. Enzyme inducers (p703) ↑metabolism of levothyroxine.
• *Elderly or ischaemic heart disease:* Start with 25µg/24h; ↑dose by 25µg/4wks according to TSH (►cautiously, as thyroxine may precipitate angina or MI).
• *If diagnosis is in question and T4 already given:* Stop T4; recheck TSH in 6 weeks.

**Amiodarone** is an iodine-rich drug structurally like T4; 2% of users will get significant thyroid problems from it. Hypothyroidism can be caused by toxicity from iodine excess (T4 release is inhibited). Thyrotoxicosis may be caused by a destructive thyroiditis causing hormone release. Here, radioiodine uptake can be undetectable and if this is the case, glucocorticoids may help. Get expert help. Thyroidectomy may be needed if amiodarone cannot be discontinued. T½ of amiodarone ≈ 80d, so problems persist after withdrawal. If on amiodarone, check TFTs 6-monthly.

---

1 ►*Treat the patient not the blood level!* No exact cut-off in TSH can be given partly because risk of death from heart disease mirrors TSH *even when in the normal range* in women. Risk ≈ 1.4 if TSH 1.5–2.4 *vs* 1.7 if TSH 2.5–3.5. If TSH >3.65 and possibly symptomatic, a low dose of levothyroxine may be tried. Monitor symptoms, TSH and T4 carefully. Over-exposure to thyroxine may cause osteoporosis ± AF.

### Why are symptoms of thyroid disease so various, and so subtle?

213

Almost all our cell nuclei have receptors showing a high affinity for $T_3$; that known as TRα-1 is abundant in muscle and fat; TRα-2 is abundant in brain; and TRβ-1 is abundant in brain, liver, and kidney. These receptors, via their influence on various enzymes, affect the following processes:

• The metabolism of substrates, vitamins, and minerals.
• Modulation of all other hormones and their target-tissue responses.
• Stimulation of $O_2$ consumption and generation of metabolic heat.
• Regulation of protein synthesis, and carbohydrate and lipid metabolism.
• Stimulation of demand for co-enzymes and related vitamins.

## Subclinical thyroid disease

**Subclinical hypothyroidism** Suspect if TSH >4mu/L with normal $T_4$ and $T_3$, and no obvious symptoms.[39] It is common: ~10% of those >55yrs have ↑TSH. Risk of progression to frank hypothyroidism is ~2%, and increases as TSH↑; risk doubles if thyroid peroxidase antibodies are present, and is also increased in men. *Management:*

• Confirm that raised TSH is persistent (recheck in 2-4 months).
• Recheck the history: if any non-specific features (eg depression), discuss benefits of treating (p212) with the patient: maybe they will function better.
• Have a low threshold for carefully supervised treatment as your patient may not be so asymptomatic after all, and cardiac deaths *may* be prevented.[40] Treat if: **1** TSH ≥10mu/L **2** +ve thyroid autoantibodies **3** Past (treated) Graves' **4** Other organ-specific autoimmunity (type 1 DM, myasthenia, pernicious anaemia, vitiligo), as they are more likely to progress to clinical hypothyroidism.[41] *If TSH 4-10, and vague symptoms*, treat for 6 months—only continue if symptoms improve (or the patient is trying to conceive).[42] If the patient does not fall into any of these categories, monitor TSH yearly.
• Risks from well-monitored treatment of subclinical hypothyroidism are small (but there is a ↑risk of atrial fibrillation and osteoporosis if over-treated).

**Subclinical hyperthyroidism** occurs when TSH↓, with normal $T_4$ and $T_3$. There is a 41% increase in relative mortality from all causes versus euthyroid control subjects—eg from AF and osteoporosis. *Management:*[43]

• Confirm that suppressed TSH is persistent (recheck in 2-4 months).
• Check for a non-thyroidal cause: illness, pregnancy, pituitary or hypothalamic insufficiency (suspect if $T_4$ or $T_3$ are at the lower end of the reference range), use of TSH suppressing medication, eg thyroxine, steroids.
• If TSH <0.1, treat on an individual basis, eg with symptoms of hyperthyroidism, AF, unexplained weight loss, osteoporosis, goitre.
• Options are carbimazole or propylthiouracil—or radioiodine therapy.
• If no symptoms, recheck 6-monthly.

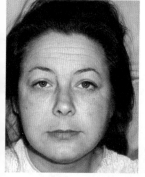

Fig 1. Facial appearance in hypothyroidism. Look for: pallor; coarse, brittle, diminished hair (scalp, axillary, and pubic); dull or blank expression lacking sparkle; coarse features; puffy lids. These signs are subtle: ►have a low threshold for measuring TSH (in yourself, your friends, and your patients). Reproduced from Cox & Roper, *Clinical Skills* (2004) with permission from Oxford University Press.

Endocrinology

Endocrinology

Parathyroid hormone (PTH) is normally secreted in response to low ionized $Ca^{2+}$ levels, by 4 parathyroid glands situated posterior to the thyroid (p670). The glands are controlled by -ve feedback via $Ca^{2+}$ levels. PTH acts by: •Osteoclast activity releasing $Ca^{2+}$ and $PO_4^{3-}$ from bones •↑$Ca^{2+}$ and ↓$PO_4^{3-}$ reabsorption in the kidney •Active 1,25 dihydroxy-vitamin $D_3$ production is ↑. Overall effect is ↑$Ca^{2+}$ and ↓$PO_4^{3-}$.

**Primary hyperparathyroidism** *Causes:* ~80% solitary adenoma, ~20% hyperplasia of all glands, <0.5% parathyroid cancer. *Presentation:* Often 'asymptomatic' (▶*not in retrospect!*[44]), with ↑$Ca^{2+}$ on routine tests. Signs relate to: 1 ↑$Ca^{2+}$ (p690): weak, tired, depressed, thirsty, dehydrated-but-polyuric; also renal stones, abdominal pain, pancreatitis, and ulcers (duodenal:gastric≈7:1). 2 Bone resorption effects of PTH can cause pain, fractures, and osteopenia/osteoporosis. 3 BP↑: ▶so check $Ca^{2+}$ in *everyone* with hypertension. *Association:* MEN-1 (BOX). *Tests:* $Ca^{2+}$↑ & PTH↑ or inappropriately normal (other causes of this: thiazides, lithium, familial hypocalciuric hypercalcaemia, tertiary hyperparathyroidism). Also $PO_4^{3-}$↓ (unless in renal failure), alk phos↑ from bone activity, 24h urinary $Ca^{2+}$↑. *Imaging: osteitis fibrosa cystica* (due to severe resorption; rare) may show up as subperiosteal erosions, cysts, or brown tumours of phalanges ± acro-osteolysis (fig 1) ± 'pepper-pot' skull. *DEXA* (p697; for osteoporosis, p696). ℞: If mild: advise ↑fluid intake to prevent stones; avoid thiazides + high $Ca^{2+}$ & vit D intake; see 6-monthly. Excision of the adenoma or of all 4 hyperplastic glands prevents fractures and peptic ulcers. *Indications:* high serum or urinary $Ca^{2+}$, bone disease, osteoporosis, renal calculi, ↓renal function, age ≤50yrs. *Complications:* Hypoparathyroidism, recurrent laryngeal nerve damage (∴ hoarse), symptomatic $Ca^{2+}$↓ (hungry bones syndrome; check $Ca^{2+}$ daily for ≥14d post-op). Pre-op US and MIBI scan may localize an adenoma; intra-operative PTH sampling is used to confirm removal. *Recurrence:* ~8% over 10yrs.[45] Cinacalcet (a 'calcimimetic') ↑ sensitivity of parathyroid cells to $Ca^{2+}$ (∴ ↓PTH secretion); monitor $Ca^{2+}$ within 1 week of dose changes; SE: myalgia; testosterone↓.[46]

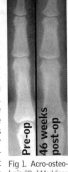

Fig 1. Acro-osteolysis. ©Dr I Maddison
myweb.lsbu.ac.uk

Pre-op

46 weeks post-op

**Secondary hyperparathyroidism** $Ca^{2+}$↓, PTH↑ (appropriately). *Causes:* ↓vit D intake, chronic renal failure. ℞: Correct causes. Phosphate binders; vit D; cinacalcet if PTH ≥85pmol/L and parathyroidectomy tricky.[45]

**Tertiary hyperparathyroidism** $Ca^{2+}$↑, ↑↑PTH (inappropriately). Occurs after prolonged secondary hyperparathyroidism, causing glands to act autonomously having undergone hyperplastic or adenomatous change. This causes $Ca^{2+}$↑ from ↑↑secretion of PTH unlimited by feedback control. Seen in chronic renal failure.

**Malignant hyperparathyroidism** Parathyroid-related protein (PTHrP) is produced by some squamous cell lung cancers, breast and renal cell carcinomas. This mimics PTH resulting in $Ca^{2+}$↑ (PTH is ↓, as PTHrP is not detected in the assay).

## Hypoparathyroidism

**Primary hypoparathyroidism** PTH secretion is ↓ due to gland failure. *Tests:* $Ca^{2+}$↓, $PO_4^{3-}$↑ or ↔, alk phos ↔. *Signs:* Those of hypocalcaemia, p692 ± autoimmune comorbidities (BOX). *Causes:* Autoimmune; congenital (Di George synd., OHCS p642). ℞: $Ca^{2+}$ supplements + calcitriol (or synthetic PTH /12h SC: it prevents hypercalciuria).

**Secondary hypoparathyroidism** Radiation, surgery (thyroidectomy, parathyroidectomy), hypomagnesaemia (magnesium is required for PTH secretion).

**Pseudohypoparathyroidism** Failure of target cell response to PTH. *Signs:* Short metacarpals (esp. 4th and 5th, fig 2), round face, short stature, calcified basal ganglia (fig 3), IQ↓. *Tests:* $Ca^{2+}$↓, ↑PTH, alk phos ↔ or ↑. ℞: As for 1° hypoparathyroidism.

**Pseudopseudohypoparathyroidism** The morphological features of pseudohypoparathyroidism, but with normal biochemistry. The cause for both is genetic.

## Multiple endocrine neoplasia (MEN types 1, 2a, and 2b)

In MEN syndromes there are functioning hormone-producing tumours in multiple organs (they are inherited as autosomal dominants).[47] They comprise: •MEN-1 and 2 •*Neurofibromatosis* (p518) •*Von Hippel-Lindau* and Peutz-Jeghers syndromes (p726 & p722) •Carney complex (spotty skin pigmentation, schwannomas, myxoma of skin, mucosa, or heart, especially atrial myxoma, and endocrine tumours: eg pituitary adenoma, adrenal hyperplasia, and testicular tumour.

MEN-1    Parathyroid hyperplasia/adenoma (~95%; most ↑Ca²⁺).
Pancreas endocrine tumours (70%)—gastrinoma (p730) or insulinoma (p206), or, rarely, somatostatinoma (DM + steatorrhoea + gallstones/cholangitis), VIPoma (p246), or glucagonomas (±glucagon syndrome: migrating rash; glossitis; cheilitis, fig 2 p321; anaemia; weight↓; plasma glucagon↑; glucose↑).
Pituitary prolactinoma (~50%) or GH secreting tumour (acromegaly: p230); also, adrenal and carcinoid tumours are associated.

The MEN-1 gene is a tumour suppressor gene. Menin, its protein, alters transcription activation. Many are sporadic, presenting in the 3ʳᵈ–5ᵗʰ decades.

MEN-2a    Thyroid: Medullary thyroid carcinoma (seen in ~100%, p602).
Adrenal: Phaeochromocytoma (~50%, usually benign and bilateral).
Parathyroid hyperplasia (~80%, but less than 20% have ↑Ca²⁺).

MEN-2b has similar features to MEN-2a plus mucosal neuromas and Marfanoid appearance (p720), but no hyperparathyroidism. Mucosal neuromas consist of 'bumps' on: lips, cheeks, tongue, glottis, eyelids, and visible corneal nerves.

The gene involved in MEN-2a and b is the *ret* proto-oncogene, a receptor tyrosine kinase. Tests for *ret* mutations are revolutionizing MEN-2 treatment by enabling a prophylactic thyroidectomy to be done before neoplasia occurs, usually before 3 yrs of age. NB: ret mutations rarely contribute to sporadic parathyroid tumours.

## Autoimmune polyendocrine syndromes [48]

Autoimmune disorders cluster into two defined syndromes:

**Type 1:** Autosomal recessive, rare.
*Cause:* Mutations of AIRE (Auto ImmuneReGulator) gene on chromosome 21.
*Features:* •Addison's disease •Chronic mucocutaneous candidiasis •Hypoparathyroidism. Also associated with hypogonadism, pernicious anaemia, autoimmune primary hypothyroidism, chronic active hepatitis, vitiligo, alopecia.

**Type 2:** HLA D3 and D4 linked, common. *Cause:* Polygenic.
*Features:* •Addison's disease •Type 1 diabetes mellitus (in 20%).
• Autoimmune thyroid disease—hypothyroidism or Graves' disease.
Also associated with primary hypogonadism, vitiligo, alopecia, pernicious anaemia, chronic atrophic gastritis, coeliac disease, dermatitis herpetiformis.

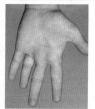

Fig 2. Pseudohypoparathyroidism: short 4ᵗʰ and 5ᵗʰ metacarpals.

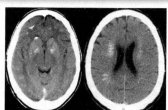

Fig 3. Cerebral calcification in pseudohypoparathyroidism: periventricular (left) and basal ganglia (right).

Fig 3 courtesy of Professor Peter Scally.

*These 2 topics are heavy on detail!* But don't forget *all* about hyperparathyroidism: ▶it's the best cause of a high Ca²⁺ and ▶surgery can *transform* a life even if Ca²⁺ only slightly raised. Also, MEN *is* important...▶it's the most treatable form of pancreatic neoplasia.

Endocrinology

**Physiology** The adrenal cortex produces steroids: 1 *Glucocorticoids* (eg cortisol), which affect carbohydrate, lipid and protein metabolism, 2 *Mineralocorticoids*, which control sodium and potassium balance (eg aldosterone, p682), and 3 *Androgens*, sex hormones which have weak effect until peripheral conversion to testosterone and dihydrotestosterone. Corticotropin-releasing factor (CRF) from the hypothalamus stimulates ACTH secretion from the pituitary, which in turn stimulates cortisol and androgen production by the adrenal cortex. Cortisol is excreted as urinary free cortisol and various 17-oxogenic steroids.

**Cushing's syndrome** This is the clinical state produced by chronic glucocorticoid excess + loss of the normal feedback mechanisms of the hypothalamo-pituitary-adrenal axis and loss of circadian rhythm of cortisol secretion (normally highest on waking). The chief cause is oral steroids. Endogenous causes are rare: 80% are due to ↑ACTH; of these a pituitary adenoma (Cushing's disease) is the commonest cause.

**1 ACTH-dependent causes: (↑ACTH)**
  • *Cushing's disease* Bilateral adrenal hyperplasia from an ACTH-secreting pituitary adenoma (usually a microadenoma, p226). ♀:♂>1:1. Peak age: 30-50yrs. A low-dose dexamethasone test (BOX) leads to no change in plasma cortisol, but 8mg may be enough to more than halve morning cortisol (as occurs in normals).
  • *Ectopic ACTH production* Especially small cell lung cancer and carcinoid tumours, p278. Specific features: pigmentation (due to ↑↑ACTH), hypokalaemic metabolic alkalosis (↑↑cortisol leads to mineralocorticoid activity), weight loss, hyperglycaemia. Classical features of Cushing's are often absent. Dexamethasone even in high doses (8mg) fails to suppress cortisol production.
  • *Rarely: Ectopic CRF production*—some thyroid (medullary) and prostate cancers.

**2 ACTH-independent causes: (↓ACTH due to -ve feedback)**
  • *Adrenal adenoma/cancer* (may cause abdo pain ± virilization in ♀, p222). Because the tumour is autonomous, dexamethasone in any dose won't suppress cortisol.
  • *Adrenal nodular hyperplasia* (as above, no dexamethasone suppression).
  • *Iatrogenic* Pharmacological doses of steroids (common).
  • *Rarely: Carney complex* p215. *McCune–Albright syndrome* See OHCS p650.

**Symptoms** Weight↑; mood change (depression, lethargy, irritability, psychosis); proximal weakness; gonadal dysfunction (irregular menses; hirsutism; erectile dysfunction); acne; recurrent Achilles tendon rupture; occasionally virilization if ♀.

**Signs** Central obesity; plethoric, moon face; buffalo neck hump; supraclavicular fat distribution; skin & muscle atrophy; bruises; purple abdominal striae (fig 1); osteoporosis; BP↑; glucose↑; infection-prone; poor healing. Signs of the cause (eg abdo mass).

**Tests** Random plasma cortisols may mislead, as illness, time of day, and stress (eg venepuncture) influences results. Also, don't rely on imaging to localize the cause: non-functioning 'incidentalomas' occur in ~5% on adrenal CT and ~10% on pituitary MRI. MRI detects only ~70% of pituitary tumours causing Cushing's (many are too small).

**Treatment** Depends on the cause. •*Iatrogenic:* Stop medications if possible.
  • *Cushing's disease:* Selective removal of pituitary adenoma (trans-sphenoidally). Bilateral adrenalectomy if source unlocatable, or recurrence post-op (complication: *Nelson's syndrome:* ↑skin pigmentation due to ↑↑ACTH from an enlarging pituitary tumour, as adrenalectomy removes -ve feedback; responds to pituitary radiation.)
  • *Adrenal adenoma or carcinoma:* Adrenalectomy: 'cures' adenomas but rarely cures cancer. Radiotherapy & adrenolytic drugs (mitotane) follow if carcinoma.
  • *Ectopic ACTH:* Surgery if tumour is located and hasn't spread. Metyrapone, ketoconazole and fluconazole ↓cortisol secretion pre-op or if awaiting effects of radiation. Intubation + mifepristone (competes with cortisol at receptors) + etomidate (blocks cortisol synthesis) may be needed, eg in severe ACTH-associated psychosis.

**Prognosis** Untreated Cushing's has ↑ vascular mortality.[49] Treated, prognosis is good (but myopathy, obesity, menstrual irregularity, BP↑, osteoporosis, subtle mood changes and DM often remain—so follow up carefully, and manage individually).

## Investigating suspected Cushing's syndrome[50]

First, confirm the diagnosis (a raised plasma cortisol), then localize the source on the basis of laboratory testing. Use imaging studies to confirm the likely source.

**1st-line tests** *Overnight dexamethasone suppression test* is a good outpatient test. Dexamethasone 1mg PO at midnight; do serum cortisol at 8AM. Normally, cortisol suppresses to <50nmol/L; no suppression in Cushing's syndrome. False -ve rate: <2%; false +ves: 2% normal, 13% obese and 23% of inpatients. *NB:* false +ves (*pseudo-Cushing's*) are seen in depression, obesity, alcohol excess, and inducers of liver enzymes (↑ rate of dexamethasone metabolism, eg phenytoin, phenobarbital, rifampicin, p702). *24h urinary free cortisol* (normal: <280nmol/24h) is an alternative.

**2nd-line tests**, if above abnormal: *48h dexamethasone suppression test:* Give dexamethasone 0.5mg/6h PO for 2d. Measure cortisol at 0 and 48h (last test at 6h after last dose). Again, in Cushing's syndrome, there is a failure to suppress cortisol. *48h high-dose dexamethasone suppression test:* (2mg/6h) may distinguish pituitary (suppression) from others causes (no/part suppression) *Midnight cortisol:* Admit (unless salivary cortisol used). Often inaccurate due to measurement issues. Normal circadian rhythm (cortisol *lowest* at midnight, *highest* early morning) is lost in Cushing's syndrome. Midnight blood, via a cannula during sleep, shows cortisol ↑ in Cushing's.

**Localization tests** (where is the lesion?) If the above are +ve—*Plasma ACTH: If ACTH is undetectable*, an adrenal tumour is likely → CT adrenal glands. If no mass, proceed to *adrenal vein sampling* or *adrenal scintigraphy* (radiolabelled cholesterol derivative). *If ACTH is detectable*, distinguish a pituitary cause from ectopic ACTH production by high dose suppression test or *corticotropin releasing hormone test:* 100μg ovine or human CRH IV. Measure cortisol at 120min. Cortisol rises with pituitary disease but not with ectopic ACTH production. CRH is corticotropin-releasing hormone.

If tests indicate that cortisol responds to manipulation, Cushing's disease is likely. Image the pituitary (MRI) and consider *bilateral inferior petrosal sinus blood sampling.*

If tests indicate that cortisol does not respond to manipulation, hunt for the source of ectopic ACTH—eg IV contrast CT of chest, abdomen and pelvis ± MRI of neck, thorax and abdomen, eg for small ACTH secreting carcinoid tumours.

Endocrinology

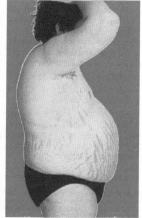

**Fig 1.** Hypercortisolism weakens skin; even normal stretching (or the pressure of obesity, as here) can make its elastin break—and on healing we see these depressed purple scars (striae), like flecks of puckered crêpe paper. Cortisone or rapid growth contributes to striae in other contexts: pregnancy; adolescence (eg in the 'love-handle' area); weight lifting; sudden-onset obesity, or from steroid creams. Striae mature into silvery crescents looking like the underside of willow leaves. Unsightly immature striae may be improved by YAG lasers.

*Endocrinology*

▶▶Anyone on exogenous steroids for long enough to suppress the pituitary–adrenal axis, or who has overwhelming sepsis, or has metastatic cancer may suddenly develop adrenal insufficiency with deadly hypovolaemic shock. ▶▶See p846.

**Primary adrenocortical insufficiency** (Addison's disease) is rare (~0.8/100,000), but can be fatal. Destruction of the adrenal cortex leads to glucocorticoid (cortisol) and mineralocorticoid (aldosterone) deficiency (see fig 1). Signs are capricious: it is 'the unforgiving master of non-specificity and disguise'.[51] You may diagnose a viral infection or anorexia nervosa in error (K⁺ is ↓ in the latter but ↑ in Addison's).

**Cause** 80% are due to autoimmunity in the UK. *Other causes:* TB (commonest cause worldwide), adrenal metastases (eg from lung, breast, renal cancer), lymphoma, opportunistic infections in HIV (eg CMV, *Mycobacterium avium*, p411); adrenal haemorrhage (▶▶Waterhouse-Friderichsen syndrome p728; antiphospholipid syndrome; SLE), congenital (late-onset congenital adrenal hyperplasia).

**Symptoms** Often diagnosed late: lean, tanned, tired, tearful ± weakness, anorexia, dizzy, faints, flu-like myalgias/arthralgias. *Mood:* depression, psychosis, low self-esteem.[12] *GI:* nausea/vomiting, abdominal pain, diarrhoea/constipation. *Think of Addison's in all with unexplained abdominal pain or vomiting.* Pigmented palmar creases & buccal mucosa (↑ACTH; cross-reacts with melanin receptors). Postural hypotension. Vitiligo. ▶▶Signs of critical deterioration (p846): Shock (↓BP, tachycardia), T°↑, coma.

**Tests** Na⁺↓ & K⁺↑ (due to ↓mineralocorticoid), glucose ↓ (due to ↓cortisol). Also: uraemia, Ca²⁺↑, eosinophilia, anaemia. Δ: *Short ACTH stimulation test (Synacthen® test):* Do plasma cortisol before and ½h after tetracosactide (Synacthen®) 250µg IM. Addison's is excluded if 30min cortisol >550nmol/L. Steroid drugs may interfere with assays: ask lab. NB: in pregnancy and contraceptive pill, cortisol levels may be reassuring but falsely↑, due to ↑cortisol-binding globulin. *Also* •*ACTH:* In Addison's, 9AM ACTH is ↑ (>300ng/L: inappropriately high). It is low in secondary causes •*21-Hydroxylase adrenal autoantibodies:* +ve in autoimmune disease in >80% •*Plasma renin & aldosterone:* To assess mineralocortocoid status. AXR/CXR: Any past TB, eg upper zone fibrosis or adrenal calcification? If no autoantibodies, consider further tests (eg adrenal CT) for TB, histoplasma, or metastatic disease.

**Treatment** Replace steroids: ~15-25mg *hydrocortisone* daily, in 2-3 doses, eg 10mg on waking, 5mg lunchtime. Avoid giving late (may cause insomnia). Mineralocorticoids to correct postural hypotension, Na⁺↓, K⁺↑: *fludrocortisone* PO from 50-200µg daily. Adjust both on clinical grounds. If there is a poor response, suspect an associated autoimmune disease[1] (check thyroid, do coeliac serology: p280).

*Steroid use:* Warn against abruptly stopping steroids. Emphasize that prescribing doctors/dentists/surgeons *must* know of steroid use: give *steroid card*, advise wearing a bracelet declaring steroid use. Add 5-10mg hydrocortisone to daily intake before strenuous activity/exercise. Double steroids in febrile illness, injury or stress. Give out syringes and in-date IM hydrocortisone, and show how to inject 100mg IM if vomiting prevents oral intake (seek medical help; admit for IV fluids if dehydrated).

**Follow-up** Yearly (BP, U&E); watch for autoimmune diseases (pernicious anaemia[et al]).[2]

**Prognosis (treated)** Adrenal crises and infections do cause excess deaths: mean age at death for men is ~65yrs (11yrs < estimated life expectancy; women ~3yrs).

**Secondary adrenal insufficiency** The commonest cause is iatrogenic, due to long-term steroid therapy leading to suppression of the pituitary-adrenal axis. This only becomes apparent on withdrawal of the steroids. Other causes are rare and include hypothalamic-pituitary disease leading to ↓ACTH production. Mineralocorticoid production remains intact, and there is no hyperpigmentation as ↓ACTH.

1 Adrenal destruction also causes depletion of adrenal androgens. These may have an effect on quality of life. However, studies on replacement of dehydroepiandrosterone (DHEA), a precursor of sex hormone synthesis, in adrenal failure have been inconclusive.
2 Autoimmune polyglandular syndromes types 1-4: 1 Monogenic syndrome (AIRE gene on chromosome 21); signs: candidiasis, hypoparathyroidism+Addison's. 2 (Schmidt syndrome) Adrenal insufficiency+ autoimmune thyroid disease ± DM ± pleuritis/pericarditis 3 Autoimmune thyroid disease + other autoimmune conditions but *not* Addison's. 4 Autoimmune combinations not included in 1-3 above.

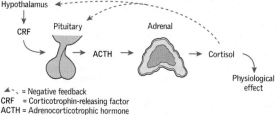

Fig 1. Pathways involved in adrenal function.

"Typical day—wakes up at 11.30, still feels tired, then will have some breakfast and usually fall asleep on the couch. The most energy req. activity in last 1 month is—cooking herself a pasta meal. Then, totally exhausted will sleep more in pm, then eat some dinner. Goes to bed at 11pm—latest. Not able to concentrate...Used to weigh 45kg. Now weighs 42kg."[52]

Placed on a page about Addison's disease, we might think there are sufficient clues to raise the suspicion of Addison's (even though her electrolytes were not particularly awry, and her pigmentation was barely perceptible). But change the context to our last busy clinic. We are a little distracted. The memory of Addison's is fading. Who among us will hear the alarm bell ring?

**Primary hyperaldosteronism** is excess production of aldosterone, independent of the renin-angiotensin system, causing ↑sodium and water retention, and ↓renin release. Consider if the following features: hypertension, hypokalaemia or alkalosis in someone not on diuretics. Sodium tends to be mildly raised or normal.

*Symptoms:* Often asymptomatic or signs of hypokalaemia (p688): weakness (even quadriparesis), cramps, paraesthesiae, polyuria, polydipsia. BP↑ but not always.

*Causes:* ~⅔ are due to a solitary aldosterone-producing adenoma[1] (*Conn's syndrome*). ~⅓ are due to bilateral adrenocortical hyperplasia. Rare causes: adrenal carcinoma or glucocorticoid-remediable aldosteronism (GRA). In GRA, the ACTH regulatory element of the 11β-hydroxylase gene fuses to the aldosterone synthase gene, increasing aldosterone production, and bringing it under the control of ACTH.

*Tests:* U&E, renin and aldosterone (see BOX, ideally not on diuretics, hypotensives, steroids, K+, or laxatives for 4wks). Do not rely on a low K+, as >20% are normokalaemic. For GRA (suspect if there is a family history of early hypertension), genetic testing is available.

*Treatment:* •*Conn's:* Laparoscopic adrenalectomy. Spironolactone (25-100mg/24h PO) for 4wks pre-op controls BP and K+. •*Hyperplasia:* Treated medically: spironolactone, amiloride, or eplerenone (a newer selective aldosterone receptor antagonist, which doesn't cause gynaecomastia).•*GRA:* dexamethasone 1mg/24h PO for 4wks, normalizes biochemistry but not always BP. If BP is still ↑, use spironolactone as an alternative.•*Adrenal carcinoma:* Surgery ± post-operative adrenolytic therapy with mitotane—prognosis is poor.

**Secondary hyperaldosteronism** Due to a high renin from ↓renal perfusion, eg in renal artery stenosis, accelerated hypertension, diuretics, CCF or hepatic failure.

**Bartter's syndrome** This is a major cause of congenital (autosomal recessive) salt wasting—via a sodium and chloride leak in the loop of Henle via a defective channel. Presents in childhood with failure to thrive, polyuria and polydipsia. BP is *normal*. Sodium loss leads to volume depletion, causing ↑renin and aldosterone production, leading to hypokalaemia and metabolic alkalosis, ↑urinary K+ and Cl-. *Treatment:* K+ replacement, NSAIDs (to inhibit prostaglandins), and ACE-i.

## Phaeochromocytoma

Rare catecholamine-producing tumours. They arise from sympathetic paraganglia cells (=phaeochrome bodies), which are collections of chromaffin cells. They are usually found within the adrenal medulla. Extra-adrenal tumours (paragangliomas) are rarer, and often found by the aortic bifurcation (the organs of Zuckerkandl). Phaeochromocytomas *roughly* follow the 10% rule: 10% are malignant, 10% are extra-adrenal, 10% are bilateral, and 10% are familial. They are a dangerous but treatable cause of hypertension (in <0.1%). *Associations:* ~90% are sporadic; 10% are part of hereditary cancer syndromes (p215), eg thyroid, MEN-2a and 2b, neurofibromatosis, von Hippel-Lindau syndrome (succinate dehydrogenase subunit mutations). *Classic triad:* Episodic headache, sweating, and tachycardia (±BP↑, ↓ or ↔, BOX).

**Tests** WCC↑ •Plasma + 3 × 24h urines for free metadrenaline and normetadrenaline (better than catecholamines and vanillylmandelic acid[53]) ± clonidine suppression test if borderline.•*Localization:* Abdominal CT/MRI, or meta-iodobenzylguanidine (MIBG= chromaffin-seeking isotope) scan (can find extra-adrenal tumours, p752).

**Treatment** *Surgery,* α-blockade pre-op: phenoxybenzamine (α-blocker) is used before β-blocker to avoid crisis from unopposed α-adrenergic stimulation, β-block too if heart disease or tachycardic. *Consult the anaesthetist. Post-op:* Do 24h urine metadrenalines 2wks post-op, monitor BP (risk of BP↓↓). ▶▶*Emergency R̥:* p847. If malignant, chemotherapy or therapeutic radiolabelled MIBG may be used. *Follow-up:* Lifelong: malignant recurrence may present late, genetic screening.

---

**1** Tumours from the zona glomerulosa, zona fasciculata, or zona reticularis associate with syndromes of ↑ mineralocorticoids, glucocorticoids, or androgens respectively, usually; remember 'GFR=miner GA'.

## Hypertension: a common context for hyperaldosteronism tests

Think of Conn's in these contexts: •Hypertension associated with hypokalaemia •Refractory hypertension, eg despite ≥3 antihypertensive drugs •Hypertension occurring before 40yrs of age (especially in women).

The approach to investigation remains controversial, but the simplest is to look for a suppressed renin and ↑ aldosterone (may be normal if there is severe hypokalaemia). CT or MRI of the adrenals is done to localize the cause. This should be done after hyperaldosteronism is proven, due to the high number of adrenal incidentalomas. If imaging shows a unilateral adenoma, **adrenal vein sampling** may be done (venous blood is sampled from both adrenals). If one side reveals increased aldosterone production compared with the other (>3-fold difference), an adenoma is likely, and surgical excision is indicated. If no nodules or bilateral nodules are seen think about adrenal hyperplasia or GRA.

►NB: renal artery stenosis is a more common cause of refractory ↑BP and ↓K⁺ (p308).

## Features of phaeochromocytoma (often episodic and often vague)

Try to diagnose before death: suspect if BP hard-to-control, accelerating or episodic.
• *Heart:* Pulse ↑; palpitations/VT; dyspnoea; faints; angina; MI/LVF; cardiomyopathy.[1]
• *CNS:* Headache; visual disorder; dizziness; tremor; numbness; fits; encephalopathy; Horner's syndrome (paraganglioma); subarachnoid/CNS haemorrhage.
• *Psychological:* Anxiety; panic; hyperactivity; confusion; episodic psychosis.
• *Gut:* D&V; abdominal pain over tumour site; mass; mesenteric vasoconstriction.
• *Others:* Sweats/flushes; heat intolerance; pallor; T°↑; backache; haemoptysis.

Symptoms may be precipitated by straining, exercise, stress, abdominal pressure, surgery, or by agents such as β-blockers, IV contrast agents, or the tricyclics. The site of the tumour may determine precipitants, eg if pelvic, precipitants include sexual intercourse, parturition, defecation, and micturition. Adrenergic crises may last minutes to days. Suddenly patients feel "as if about to die"—and then get better, or go on to develop a stroke or cardiogenic shock. On examination, there may be no signs, or hypertension ± signs of heart failure/cardiomyopathy (±paradoxical shock, similar to Takotsubo's [1]), episodic thyroid swelling, glycosuria during attacks, or terminal haematuria from a bladder phaeochromocytoma.

---

**1** *Takotsubo cardiomyopathy* (=stress- or catecholamine-induced cardiomyopathy/broken heart syndrome) may cause sudden chest pain mimicking MI, with ↑ST segments, and its signature apical ballooning on echo (also ↓ ejection fraction) occurring during catecholamine surges. It is a cause of MI in the presence of normal arteries. The stress may be medical (SAH, p482) or psychological.

Endocrinology

**Hirsutism** is common (10% of women) and usually benign. It implies hair growth in women, in the male pattern. Causes are familial, idiopathic or are due to ↑ androgen secretion by the *ovary* (eg polycystic ovarian syndrome, ovarian cancer, *OHCS* p281), the *adrenal gland* (eg late-onset congenital adrenal hyperplasia, *OHCS* p251, Cushing's syndrome, adrenal cancer), or *drugs* (eg steroids). *Polycystic ovarian syndrome (PCOS)* causes secondary oligo- or amenorrhoea, infertility, obesity, acne and hirsutism (*OHCS* p252). Ultrasound: bilateral polycystic ovaries. Blood tests: ↑testosterone (if ≥6nmol/L, look for an androgen-producing adrenal or ovarian tumour), ↓sex-hormone binding globulin, ↑LH:FSH ratio (not consistent), TSH, lipids. Metformin may restore cycles and fertility, and helps insulin resistance (consider OGTT, p198). Address any feelings of lack of conformity to society's perceived norms of feminine beauty. A multifaceted approach helps distress and improves sexual self-worth.

*Management:* What else is going on in her life that makes it worse *now*? Be supportive!
• Local measures: Shaving; laser photoepilation; wax; creams, eg **eflornithine**, or electrolysis (expensive/time-consuming, but effective); bleach (1:10 hydrogen peroxide).

• Oestrogens help, so consider the combined Pill (*OHCS* p302)—Yasmin® is one choice as its progestogen, **drospirenone**, is an antimineralocorticoid. If no real help after 6-8 months, try co-cyprindiol (its anti-androgen is **cyproterone acetate**; it's not licensed as a simple contraceptive. SE: depression).[54]

• **Metformin** and **spironolactone** are sometimes tried.[55] Healthy eating is important.
• **Clomifene** is used for infertility (a fertility expert should prescribe).

**Virilism** Onset of amenorrhoea, clitoromegaly, deep voice, temporal hair recession + hirsutism. Look for an androgen-secreting adrenal or ovarian tumour.

**Gynaecomastia** (ie abnormal amount of breast tissue in men; may occur in normal puberty). Oestrogen/androgen ratio↑ (*vs* galactorrhoea in which prolactin is↑). *Causes:* Hypogonadism (see BOX), liver cirrhosis (oestrogens↑), hyperthyroidism, tumours (oestrogen-producing, eg testicular, adrenal; HCG-producing, eg testicular, bronchial); drugs: oestrogens, spironolactone, digoxin, testosterone, marijuana; if stopping is impossible, consider testosterone if hypogonadism ± anti-oestrogen (tamoxifen).

**Erectile dysfunction** (ED=impotence) Erections result from nitric oxide (NO) induced cyclic guanosine monophosphate (cGMP) build-up. cGMP-dependent protein kinase activates large-conductance, Ca²⁺-activated K⁺ channels so hyperpolarizing and relaxing vascular and trabecular smooth muscle cells, allowing engorgement.

ED is common after 50yrs, and often multifactorial. A psychological facet is common (esp. if ED occurs only in some situations, if onset coincides with stress, and if early morning 'incidental' erections still occur: these also persist in early organic disease).
*Organic causes:* The big 3: smoking, alcohol and diabetes (∴ reduce NO +autonomic neuropathy). Also: *endocrine:* hypogonadism, hyperthyroidism, ↑prolactin; *neurological:* cord lesions, MS, autonomic neuropathy; *pelvic surgery*, eg bladder-neck, prostate; *radiotherapy; atheroma; renal* or *hepatic failure; prostatic hyperplasia; penile anomalies*, eg post-priapism, or Peyronie's (p722); *drugs:* digoxin, β-blockers, diuretics, antipsychotics, antidepressants, oestrogens, finasteride, narcotics.
*Workup:* After a full sexual and psychological history do: U&E, LFT, glucose, TFT, LH, FSH, lipids, testosterone, prolactin ± Doppler. Is penile arterial pressure enough for inflow? Is penile sensation OK (if not, ?CNS problem). Is the veno-occlusive mechanism OK?
*R:* •Treat causes •Counselling •Oral phosphodiesterase (PDE5) inhibitors ↑cGMP. Erection isn't automatic (depends on erotic stimuli). Sildenafil 25-100mg ½-1h pre-sex (food and alcohol upset absorption). *SE:* headache (16%), flushing (10%), dyspepsia (7%), stuffy nose (4%); transient blue-green tingeing of vision (inhibition of retinal PDE6).*CI:* See BOX. Tadalafil (long t½) 10-20mg ½-36h pre-sex. Don't use >once daily. SE: headache, dyspepsia, myalgia; ?no visual SEs. Vardenafil (5-20mg).•Vacuum aids (ideal for penile rehabilitation after radical prostatectomy; partners may receive unnatural sensations), intracavernosal injections, transurethral pellets, and prostheses (inflatable or malleable; partners may receive unnatural sensations).•Corpus cavernosum tissue engineering (eg on acellular collagen scaffolds) is in its infancy.

## Contraindications[ci]/cautions to Viagra® and other oral ED agents

- Concurrent use of nitrates[ci]
- BP↑↑ or systolic ≤90mmHg[ci] arrhythmia
- Degenerative retinal disorders,[ci] eg retinitis pigmentosa (for sildenafil)
- Unstable angina[ci] Stroke <6mths ago[ci]
- Myocardial infarction <90d ago[ci]
- Bleeding; peptic ulcer (sildenafil)
- Marked renal or hepatic impairment

**Other cautions** ▶Angina (especially if during intercourse).
- Peyronie's disease or cavernosal fibrosis.
- Risk of priapism (sickle-cell anaemia, myeloma, leukaemia).
- Concurrent complex antihypertensive regimens.
- Dyspnoea on minimal effort (sexual activity may be unsupportable).

Use in coronary artery disease has been a question, but is probably OK.[56]

*Interactions:* Nitrites[ci]; cytochrome p450 (CYP3A) inducers: macrolides, protease inhibitors, theophyllines, azole antifungals, rifampicin, phenytoin, carbamazepine, phenobarbital, grapefruit juice (↑bioavailability). Caution if α-blocker use; avoid vardenafil with type 1A (eg quinidine; procainamide) and type 3 anti-arrhythmics (sotalol; amiodarone)—as well as nitrates as above.

## Male hypogonadism

Hypogonadism is failure of testes to produce testosterone, sperm, or both. Features: small testes, ↓libido, erectile dysfunction, loss of pubic hair, ↓muscle bulk, ↑fat, gynaecomastia, osteoporosis, mood↓. If prepubertal: ↓virilization; incomplete puberty; eunuchoid body; reduced secondary sex characteristics. Causes include:

**Primary hypogonadism** is due to testicular failure, eg from •Local trauma, torsion, chemotherapy/irradiation •Post-orchitis, eg mumps, HIV, brucellosis, leprosy •Renal failure, liver cirrhosis or alcohol excess (toxic to Leydig cells) •Chromosomal abnormalities, eg Klinefelter's syndrome (47XXY)—delayed sexual development, small testes and gynaecomastia. Anorchia is rare.

**Secondary hypogonadism** ↓Gonadotropins (LH & FSH), eg from •Hypopituitarism •Prolactinoma •Kallman's syndrome—isolated gonadotropin releasing hormone deficiency, often with anosmia and colour blindness •Systemic illness (eg COPD; HIV; DM) •Laurence-Moon-Biedl and Prader-Willi syndromes (*OHCS* p648 & p652) •Age.

*R:* (p224) If total testosterone ≤8nmol/L, on 2 mornings (or <15 if LH↑ too) and muscle bulk↓, testosterone may help, eg 1% dermal gel (Testogel®). Heart,[57] bladder and sexual function may perk up in age-related hypogonadism. Beware medicalizing ageing! **CI:** Ca²⁺↑; nephrosis; polycythaemia; prostate, breast° or liver ca. Monitor PSA.

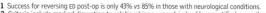

1 Success for reversing ED post-op is only 43% *vs* 85% in those with neurological conditions.
2 Criteria include marked disruption to relationships or mood, judged by a certified prescriber.

Hypopituitarism entails ↓secretion of anterior pituitary hormones (figs 1 & 2). They are affected in this order: growth hormone (GH), gonadotropins: follicle-stimulating hormone (FSH) and luteinizing hormone (LH), prolactin (PRL), thyroid-stimulating hormone (TSH), and adrenocorticotrophic hormone (ACTH). Panhypopituitarism is deficiency of all anterior hormones, usually caused by irradiation, surgery, or pituitary disease.

**Causes** are at 3 levels: 1 *Hypothalamus:* Kallman's syndrome (p223), tumour, inflammation, infection (meningitis, TB), ischaemia. 2 *Pituitary stalk:* Trauma, surgery, mass lesion (craniopharyngioma, p226), meningioma, carotid artery aneurysm. 3 *Pituitary:* Tumour, irradiation, inflammation, autoimmunity,[1] infiltration (haemochromatosis, amyloid, metastases), ischaemia (pituitary apoplexy, p226; DIC;[2] Sheehan's syndrome[3]).

**Features** are due to:

1 **Hormone lack:** •*GH lack:* Central obesity, atherosclerosis, dry wrinkly skin, strength↓, balance↓, wellbeing↓, exercise ability↓, cardiac output↓, osteoporosis, glucose↓. •*Gonadotropin (FSH; LH) lack:* ♀: Few, scant, or no menses (oligomenorrhoea or amenorrhoea), fertility↓, libido↓, osteoporosis, breast atrophy, dyspareunia. ♂: Erectile dysfunction, libido↓, muscle bulk↓, hypogonadism (↓hair, all over; small testes; ejaculate volume↓; spermatogenesis↓). •*Thyroid lack:* As for hypothyroidism (p212). •*Corticotropin lack:* As for adrenal insufficiency (p218). NB: no ↑skin pigmentation as ↓ACTH. •*Prolactin lack:* Rare: absent lactation.

2 **Causes:** eg pituitary tumour (p226), causing mass effect, or hormone secretion with ↓secretion of other hormones—eg prolactinoma, acromegaly, rarely Cushing's.

**Tests** (The triple stimulation test is now rarely done.)
• *Basal tests:* LH and FSH (↓ or ↔), testosterone or oestradiol (↓); TSH (↓ or ↔), T₄ (↓); prolactin (may be ↑, from loss of hypothalamic dopamine that normally inhibits its release), insulin-like growth factor-1 (IGF-1; ↓—used as a measure of GH axis, p230), cortisol (↓). Also do U&E (Na↓ from dilution), Hb↓ (normochromic, normocytic).
• *Dynamic tests:* 1 Short Synacthen® test: (p218) to assess the adrenal axis. 2 Insulin tolerance test (ITT): Done in specialist centres to assess the adrenal and GH axes. CI: epilepsy, heart disease, adrenal failure. Consult lab first. It involves IV insulin to induce hypoglycaemia, causing stress to ↑cortisol and GH secretion. It is done in the morning (water only taken from 22:00h the night before). Have 50% glucose and hydrocortisone to hand and IV access. Glucose must fall below 2.2mmol/L and the patient should become symptomatic when cortisol and GH are taken). Normal: GH >20mU/L, and peak cortisol >550nmol/L.
3 Arginine + growth hormone releasing hormone test.
4 Glucagon stimulation test is alternative when ITT is contraindicated.
• *Investigate cause:* MRI scan to look for a hypothalamic or pituitary lesion.

**Treatment** involves hormone replacement and treatment of underlying cause.
• *Hydrocortisone* for 2° adrenal failure (p218) ▶before other hormones are given.
• *Thyroxine* if hypothyroid (p212, but TSH is useless for monitoring).
• *Hypogonadism* (for symptoms and to prevent osteoporosis). ♂: Options include *testosterone enanthate* 250mg IM every 3 weeks, daily topical gels or buccal mucoadhesive tablets. Patches are also used.[4] ♀: (premenopausal) *Oestrogen:* Transdermal oestradiol patches, or contraceptive pill (exceeds replacement needs) ± *testosterone* or *dehydroepiandrosterone* (DHEA, in hypoandrogenic women; a small amount may improve wellbeing and sexual function, and help bone mineral density and lean body mass).
• *Gonadotropin* therapy is needed to induce fertility in both men and women.
• *Growth hormone* (BOX). Refer to an endocrinologist for insulin tolerance testing.

---

1 Autoimmune hypophysitis (=inflamed pituitary) mimics pituitary adenoma. It may be triggered by pregnancy or immunotherapy blocking CTLA-4. No pituitary auto-antigen is yet used diagnostically.
2 Snake bite is a common cause in India (eg when associated with acute renal failure).
3 Sheehan's syndrome is pituitary necrosis after postpartum haemorrhage.
4 Testogel® (50mg testosterone in 5g of gel) is applied in a thin film. 100mg/d may be needed (approach by 25mg increments). Use on clean, dry, healthy skin (shoulders, arms, abdomen), as soon as sachet is opened. Allow to dry for 5min. Wash hands after use, avoid shower/bath for at least 6h. Avoid skin contact with gel sites to prevent testosterone transfer to others (esp pregnant women and children).

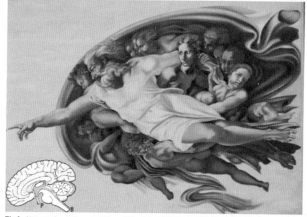

Fig 1. Neuroendocrinology: emotions ⇄ thoughts ⇄ actions. As Michelangelo foretold (in his *Creation of Adam*) 'all gods and demons that have ever existed are within us as possibilities, desires, and ways of escape'. Within the dark red vault of our skull we see human and god-like forms reaching out, as thoughts escape into actions—with legs extending into our brainstem (B) and a fist pushing from our hypothalamus into the pituitary stalk (P).⁵⁸ Frank Lynn Meshberger Above the pituitary we have thoughts, ideas, impulses, and neurotransmitters. Below we have hormones. Between is the realm of neuroendocrinology—the neurosecretory cells which turn emotions into the releasing factors for the pituitary hormones (fig 2).

Image courtesy of Gary Bevans.

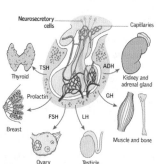

Fig 2. Neuroregulation and integration of endocrine axes makes us who we are—and who we are and what we do feeds back into our hormonal milieu. Multifactorial disruptions within the growth hormone (GH), luteinizing hormone (LH)-testosterone, adrenocorticotropin (ACTH)-cortisol and insulin axes play a major role in healthy maturation and ageing. But it is a truism to say that good health depends on the right balance and feedback loops. The myth of the pituitary as the 'conductor of the orchestra' is exploded by the placenta—that maverick organ with its heavy metal drowning out anything that the pituitary can do (p231).⁵⁹

## Using somatropin (GH) in those >25yrs old  (see nice.org.uk)

Somatotropin addresses problems of ↑fat mass, ↓bone mass, ↓lean body mass (muscle bulk), ↓exercise capacity and problems with heat intolerance. NB: increased abdominal fat results in reduced insulin sensitivity and dyslipidaemia.

Somatotropin uses DNA technology to mimic human GH. It can be used in known GH deficiency, eg peak GH response of <9mu/L (3ng/mL) during ITT—if there is impaired quality of life and treatment for other pituitary deficiencies is under way.

**Self-injection** 0.15-0.3mg/d (max 1mg/d); needs lessen with age. Dose titration (1ˢᵗ 3 months of therapy) is done by an endocrinologist. SE: oedema, carpal tunnel syndrome, myalgia, CCF, BP↑, ICP↑ (rare). IGF-1 levels rise with GH replacement. ↑IGF-1 is linked with ↑risk of neoplasia. CI: malignancy, pregnancy, renal transplant.

Somatotropin can be stopped after 9 months if quality of life scores do not improve by 7 points or more. *Using GH in children*: See OHCS p180.

*Endocrinology*

Pituitary tumours (almost always benign adenomas) account for 10% of intracranial tumours (see figs 1 & 2). They may be divided by size: a microadenoma is a tumour <1cm across, and a macroadenoma is >1cm. There are 3 histological types:

1 *Chromophobe*—70%. Many are non-secretory,[1] some cause hypopituitarism. Half produce prolactin (PRL); a few produce ACTH or GH. Local pressure effect in 30%.
2 *Acidophil*—15%. Secrete GH or PRL. Local pressure effect in 10%.
3 *Basophil*—15%. Secrete ACTH. Local pressure effect rare.

Symptoms are caused by pressure, hormones (eg galactorrhoea), or hypopituitarism (p224). FSH-secreting tumours can cause macro-orchidism in men, but are rare.

**Features of local pressure** Headache, visual field defects (bilateral temporal hemianopia, due to compression of the optic chiasm), palsy of cranial nerves III, IV, VI (pressure or invasion of the cavernous sinus; fig 3). Also, diabetes insipidus (DI) (p232; more likely from hypothalamic disease); disturbance of hypothalamic centres of T°, sleep, and appetite; erosion through floor of sella leading to CSF rhinorrhoea.

**Tests** MRI defines intra- and supra-sellar extension; accurate assessment of visual fields; screening tests: PRL, IGF-1 (p230), ACTH, cortisol, TFTs, LH/FSH, testosterone in ♂, short Synacthen® test. Glucose tolerance test if acromegaly suspected (p230). If Cushing's suspected, see p217. Water deprivation test if DI is suspected (p232).

**Treatment** Start hormone replacement as needed (p224). Ensure steroids are given before levothyroxine, as thyroxine may precipitate an adrenal crisis. For Cushing's disease see p217, prolactinoma p228, acromegaly p230.

• *Surgery (fig 4):* Most pituitary surgery is trans-sphenoidal, but if there is supra-sellar extension, a trans-frontal approach may be used. For prolactinoma, 1st-line treatment is medical with a dopamine agonist, p228. *Pre-op:* Ensure hydrocortisone 100mg IV/IM. Subsequent cortisol replacement and reassessment varies with local protocols: get advice. *Post-op:* Retest pituitary function (p224) to assess replacement needs. Repeating dynamic tests for adrenal function ≥6 weeks post-op.

• *Radiotherapy:* (eg stereotactic) Good for residual or recurrent adenomas (good rates of tumour control and normalization of excess hormone secretion).[60]

**Post-op** Recurrence may occur late after surgery, so life-long follow-up is required. Fertility should be discussed: this may be reduced post-op due to ↓ gonadotrophins.

**Pituitary apoplexy** Rapid pituitary enlargement from a bleed into a tumour may cause mass effects, cardiovascular collapse due to acute hypopituitarism, and death. Suspect if acute onset of headache, meningism, ↓GCS, ophthalmoplegia/visual field defect, especially if there is a known tumour (may present like subarachnoid haemorrhage). ℞: Urgent steroids (hydrocortisone 100mg IV) and meticulous fluid balance ± cabergoline (dopamine agonist, if prolactinoma) ± surgery; find the cause, eg a predisposition to thrombosis, from antiphospholipid syndrome.

**Craniopharyngioma** Not strictly a pituitary tumour: it originates from Rathke's pouch so is situated between the pituitary and 3rd ventricle floor. They are rare, but are the commonest childhood intracranial tumour. Over 50% present in childhood with growth failure; adults may present with amenorrhoea, ↓libido, hypothalamic symptoms (eg diabetes insipidus, hyperphagia, sleep disturbance) or tumour mass effect. *Tests:* CT/MRI (calcification in 50%, may also be seen on skull x-ray). *Treatment:* Surgery ± post-op radiation; test pituitary function post-op.

| **Classification by hormone secreted** (may be revealed by immunohistology) | | | |
|---|---|---|---|
| PRL only (→prolactinoma) | 35% | ACTH (→Cushing's disease) | 7% |
| GH only (→acromegaly) | 20% | LH/FSH/TSH | ≥1%[2,61] |
| PRL and GH | 7% | No obvious hormone | 30% |

1 If <1cm, usually 'incidentaloma'; most non-functioning macroadenomas are revealed by mass effect and/or hypopituitarism. Here, recurrence after surgery is common, so follow carefully with MRIs.

2 Sensitive methods of TSH measurement have improved recognition of TSH-secreting tumours. These are now more frequently found at microadenoma stage, medially located, and *without* associated hormone hypersecretion. In these tumours, somatostatin analogues (p230) are very helpful.

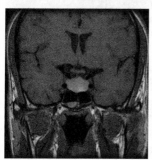

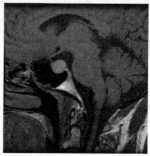

**Fig 1.** Sagittal T1 weighted MRI of the brain (no gadolinium contrast) showing a lesion in the pituitary fossa, most likely a haemorrhagic pituitary adenoma. Differential diagnosis includes a Rathke's cleft cyst.

**Fig 2.** Coronal T1 weighted MRI of the brain (no gadolinium contrast) showing a lesion in the pituitary fossa (see fig 1).

Figs 1 & 2 courtesy of Norwich Radiology Dept.

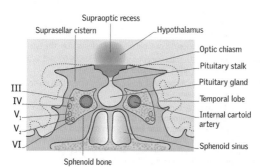

**Fig 3.** The pituitary gland's relationships to cranial nerves III, IV, V, and VI.

Reproduced from Turner & Wass, *Oxford Handbook of Endocrinology & Diabetes* (2009), with permission from Oxford University Press.

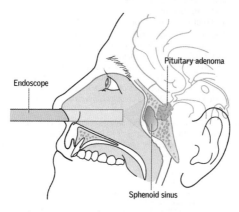

**Fig 4.** Endoscopic surgery is now possible for pituitary surgery.

Endocrinology

This is the commonest hormonal disturbance of the pituitary. It presents earlier in women (menstrual disturbance) but later in men (eg with erectile dysfunction and or mass effects). Prolactin stimulates lactation.[et al 12] Raised levels lead to hypogonadism, infertility and osteoporosis, by inhibiting secretion of gonadotropin releasing hormone (hence ↓LH/FSH and ↓testosterone or oestrogen).

**Causes of raised plasma prolactin** (PRL; >390mu/L) PRL is secreted from the anterior pituitary and release is inhibited by dopamine produced in the hypothalamus. Hyperprolactinaemia may result from 1 Excess production from the pituitary, eg prolactinoma. 2 Disinhibition, by compression of the pituitary stalk, reducing local dopamine levels or 3 Use of a dopamine antagonist. A PRL of 1000-5000mu/L may result from any, but >5000 is likely to be due to a prolactinoma, with macroadenomas (>10mm) having the highest levels, eg 10,000-100,000.

- *Physiological:* Pregnancy; breastfeeding; stress. (Acute rises occur post-orgasm.)[1]
- *Drugs (most common cause):* Metoclopramide; haloperidol; α-methyldopa; oestrogens; ecstasy/MDMA;[2] antipsychotics (a reason for 'non-compliance': sustained hyperprolactinaemia may cause ↓libido, anorgasmia, and erectile dysfunction).
- *Diseases: Prolactinoma:* micro- or macroadenoma; *Stalk damage:* pituitary adenomas, surgery, trauma; *Hypothalamic disease:* craniopharyngioma, other tumours; *Other:* hypothyroidism (due to ↑TRH), chronic renal failure (↓excretion).

**Symptoms** ♀: Amenorrhoea or oligomenorrhoea; infertility; galactorrhoea. Also: libido↓, weight↑, dry vagina. ♂: Erectile dysfunction, ↓facial hair, galactorrhoea. May present late with osteoporosis or local pressure effects from the tumour (p226).

**Tests** Basal PRL: non-stressful venepuncture between 09.00 and 16.00h. Do a pregnancy test, TFT, U&E. MRI pituitary if other causes are ruled out.

**Management** Refer to a specialist endocrinology clinic. Dopamine agonists (bromocriptine or cabergoline) are 1st-line.

*Microprolactinomas:* A tumour <10mm on MRI (~25% of us have asymptomatic microprolactinomas). **Bromocriptine**, a dopamine agonist, ↓PRL secretion, restores menstrual cycles and ↓tumour size. Dose is titrated up: 1.25mg PO; increase weekly by 1.25-2.5mg/d until ~2.5mg/12h. SE: nausea, depression, postural hypotension (minimize by giving at night). If pregnancy is planned♀, use barrier contraception until 2 periods have occurred. If subsequent pregnancy occurs, stop bromocriptine after the 1st missed period. An alternative dopamine agonist is **cabergoline**: more effective and fewer SE, but there are less data on safety in pregnancy. NB: ergot alkaloids (bromocriptine and cabergoline) can cause fibrosis (eg echocardiograms are needed). Trans-sphenoidal surgery may be considered if intolerant of dopamine agonists. It has a high success rate, but there are risks of permanent hormone deficiency and prolactinoma recurrence, and so it is usually reserved as a 2nd-line treatment.

*Macroprolactinomas:* A tumour >10mm diameter on MRI. As they are near the optic chiasm, there may be ↓acuity, diplopia, ophthalmoplegia, visual-field loss, and optic atrophy. Treat initially with a dopamine agonist (bromocriptine if fertility is the goal). Surgery is rarely needed , but consider if visual symptoms or pressure effects which fail to respond to medical treatment. Bromocriptine, and in some cases radiation therapy, may be required post-op as complete surgical resection is uncommon. If pregnant, monitor closely ideally in a combined endocrine/antenatal clinic as there is ↑risk of expansion.

**Follow-up** Monitor PRL. If headache or visual loss, check fields (? do MRI). Medication can be decreased after 2yrs, but recurrence of hyperprolactinaemia and expansion of the tumour may occur, and so these patients should be monitored carefully.

---

1 The prolactin increase (♂ and ♀) after coitus is ~400% greater than after masturbation; post-orgasmic prolactin is part of a feedback loop decreasing arousal by inhibiting central dopaminergic processes. The size of post-orgasmic prolactin increase is a neurohormonal index of sexual satisfaction.
2 MDMA also ↑oxytocin; prolactin + oxytocin are thought to mediate post-orgasmic wellbeing.

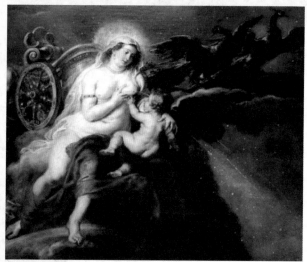

**Fig 1.** Galactorrhoea can be prolific enough to create medium-sized galaxies (bottom right). In the *Birth of the Milky Way* Hera is depicted by Rubens in her chariot, being drawn through the night sky by ominous black peacocks. Between journeys, she enjoyed discussing difficult endocrinological topics with her husband Zeus (who was also her brother), such as whether women or men find sexual intercourse more enjoyable. Hera inclined to the latter—and it is on this flimsy evidence, and her gorgeous galactorrhoea, that we diagnose her hyperprolactinaemia (which is known to decrease desire, lubrication, orgasm, and satisfaction). In the end, this issue was settled, in favour of Zeus's view, by Tiresias, who had unique insight into this intriguing question: every time this soothsayer saw two snakes entwined, (s)he changed sex, so coming to know a thing or two about gender and pleasure. This is a primordial example of an 'N of 1' trial, where the subject is his or her own control. Generalizability can be a problem with this methodology.

Image courtesy of the Prado Museum.[62]

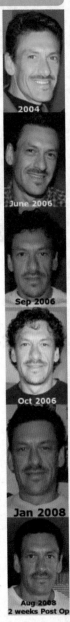

Endocrinology

This is due to ↑secretion of GH (growth hormone) from a pituitary tumour (99%) or hyperplasia, eg via ectopic GH-releasing hormone from a carcinoid tumour. ♀:♂≈1:1. Incidence:UK 3/million/yr. ~5% are associated with MEN-1 (p215). GH stimulates bone and soft tissue growth through ↑secretion of insulin-like growth factor-1 (IGF-1).

**Symptoms** Acroparaesthesia (*akron*=extremities); amenorrhoea; libido↓; headache; ↑sweating; snoring; arthralgia; backache; fig 1: "My rings don't fit, nor my old shoes, and now I've got a wonky bite (malocclusion) and curly hair. I put on lots of weight, all muscle and looked good for a while; now I look so haggard".

**Signs** (BOX) often predate diagnosis by >4yrs. If acromegaly occurs before bony epiphyses fuse (rare), gigantism occurs.

**Complications** (may present with CCF or ketoacidosis).
• Impaired glucose tolerance (~40%), DM (~15%).
• Vascular: BP↑, left ventricular hypertrophy (±dilatation/CCF), cardiomyopathy, arrhythmias. There is ↑risk of ischaemic heart disease and stroke (?due to ↑BP ± insulin resistance and GH-induced increase in fibrinogen and decrease in protein S).
• Neoplasia: colon cancer risk↑; colonoscopy may be needed.[63]

**Acromegaly in pregnancy** (Subfertility is common) Pregnancy may be normal; signs and chemistry may remit. Monitor glucose.

**Tests** ↑Glucose, ↑Ca²⁺ and ↑PO₄³⁻. *GH:* Don't rely on random GH as secretion is pulsatile and during peaks acromegalic and normal levels overlap. GH also ↑ in: stress, sleep, puberty, and pregnancy. Normally GH secretion is inhibited by high glucose, and GH hardly detectable. In acromegaly GH release fails to suppress.
• If basal serum GH is >0.4µg/L (1.2mIU/L) and/or if IGF-1↑ (p224), an oral glucose tolerance test (OGTT) is needed. [2000 Consensus statement] If the lowest GH value during OGTT is above 1µg/L (3mIU/L), acromegaly is confirmed. With general use of very sensitive assays, it has been said that this cut-off be decreased to 0.3µg/L (0.9mIU/L).[64] *Method:* Collect samples for GH glucose at: 0, 30, 60, 90, 120, 150min. Possible false +ves: puberty, pregnancy, hepatic and renal disease, anorexia nervosa, and DM.
• MRI scan of pituitary fossa. • Look for hypopituitarism (p224).
• Visual fields and acuity. • ECG, echo. Old photos if possible.

**Treatment** Aim to correct (or prevent) tumour compression by excising the lesion, and to reduce GH and IGF-I levels to at least a 'safe' GH level of <2µg/L (<6mIU/L). A 3-part strategy: 1 Transsphenoidal surgery is often 1ˢᵗ-line. 2 If surgery fails to correct GH/IGF-I hypersecretion, try somatostatin analogues (SSA) and/or radiotherapy, SSA being generally preferred. Example: **octreotide** (Sandostatin Lar®, given monthly IM), or **lanreotide** (Somatuline LA®). SE: pain at the injection site; gastrointestinal: abdominal cramps, flatulence, loose stools, ↑gallstones; impaired glucose tolerance. 3 The GH antagonist **pegvisomant** (recombinant GH analogue) is used if resistant or intolerant to SSA. It suppresses IGF-1 to normal in 90%, but GH levels may rise; rarely tumour size increases, so monitor closely. *Radiotherapy:* If unsuited to surgery or as adjuvant; may take years to work. *Follow-up:* Yearly GH, IGF-1↓OGTT; visual fields; vascular assessment. BMI; photos (fig 2,3).

**Prognosis** May return to normal (any excess mortality is mostly vascular). 16% get diabetes with SSAs vs ~13% after surgery.

2004

June 2006

Sep 2006

Oct 2006

Jan 2008

Aug 2008
2 weeks Post Op

Fig 1.  Acromegaly. Courtesy of Omar Rio.[65]

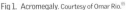

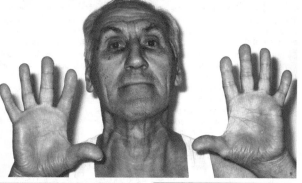

Endocrinology

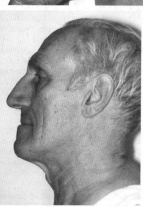

Figs 2 & 3. Coarsening of the face and ↑ growth of hands and mandible (prognathism).

### Signs of acromegaly

- ↑Growth of hands (fig 2; may be spade-like), jaw (fig 3) and feet (sole may encroach on the dorsum)
- Coarsening face; wide nose
- Big supraorbital ridges
- Macroglossia (big tongue)
- Widely spaced teeth
- Puffy lips, eyelids, and skin (oily and large-pored); also skin tags
- Scalp folds (*cutis verticis gyrata*; ∴ expanding but tethered skin)
- Skin darkening (fig 2)
- Acanthosis nigricans (fig 6, p565)
- Laryngeal dyspnoea (fixed cords)
- Obstructive sleep apnoea
- Goitre (↑ thyroid vascularity)
- Proximal weakness + arthropathy
- Carpal tunnel signs in 50%, p507
- Signs from any pituitary mass: hypopituitarism ± local mass effect (p226; vision↓; hemianopia); fits.

### ☼ Dysmorphia,[1] personal identity, and acromegaly

We might have devoted this box to a grotesque homunculus depicting the signs of acromegaly: all disconnected lips, hands, feet, brows, and noses. But our integrative ethics disallow this, and ask us instead to see if acromegaly can reveal something universal about our patients and ourselves. What is it like to feel in the grip of some 'alien puberty' or 'empty pregnancy'? These analogies are physiological as well as metaphorical.[2,3] The changes of acromegaly are not so insidious that the patient thinks all is fine: there is often partial knowledge and a few dark thoughts on looking into the mirror. Even when we lay our lives end-to-end for inspection (fig 1), changes are subtle. It can take the observations of others to force us to come face-to-face with the truth of our new unfolding self. In one patient the comment was "So are you pregnant again?" "Why do you ask?" "Because your nose is as big as it was when you were last pregnant". So here we have the well-known 'physiological acromegaly of pregnancy'[2] predating the pathological, as the carnival of personal identity moves from helter-skelter to roller-coaster.

1 Morpheus, the god of sleep, has the ability to take on any human form and to appear in dreams.
2 GH variants made by the placenta rise exponentially until 37wks' gestation; pituitary GH gradually drops to near-undetectable levels. 'Gestational acromegaly' probably develops to foster fetoplacental growth; its side-effects include facial oedema, carpal tunnel symptoms, and nose enlargement.
3 Puberty sees GH- and gonad-mediated rises in bone and muscle mass + other 'acromegalic' effects.

This is the passage of large volumes (>3L/day) of dilute urine due to impaired water resorption by the kidney, because of reduced ADH secretion from the posterior pituitary (cranial DI) or impaired response of the kidney to ADH (nephrogenic DI). See fig 1.

**Symptoms** Polyuria; polydipsia; dehydration; symptoms of hypernatraemia (p686). *Polydipsia can be uncontrollable and all-consuming*, with patients drinking anything and everything to hand: in such cases, if beer is on tap, disaster will ensue!

**Causes of cranial DI** •*Idiopathic* (≤50%) •*Congenital:* defects in ADH gene, DIDMOAD[1] •*Tumour* (may present with DI + hypopituitarism): craniopharyngioma, metastases, pituitary tumour •*Trauma:* temporary if distal to pituitary stalk as proximal nerve endings grow out to find capillaries in scar tissue and begin direct secretion again •Hypophysectomy •*Autoimmune* hypophysitis (p224) •*Infiltration:* histiocytosis, sarcoidosis •*Vascular:* haemorrhage[3] •*Infection:* meningoencephalitis.

**Causes of nephrogenic DI** •Inherited •*Metabolic:* low potassium, high calcium •*Drugs:* lithium, demeclocycline •Chronic renal disease •Post-obstructive uropathy.

**Tests** U&E, $Ca^{2+}$, glucose (exclude DM), serum and urine osmolalities. Serum osmolality estimate ≈ $2 \times (Na^+ + K^+)$ + urea + glucose (all in mmol/L). Normal plasma osmolality is 285-295mOsmol/kg, and urine can be concentrated to more than twice this concentration. Significant DI is excluded if urine to plasma (U:P) osmolality ratio is more than 2:1, provided plasma osmolality is no greater than 295mOsmol/kg. In DI, despite raised plasma osmolality, urine is dilute with a U:P ratio <2. In primary polydipsia there may be dilutional hyponatraemia—and as hyponatraemia may itself cause mania, be cautious of saying "It's water intoxication from psychogenic polydipsia".

**Diagnosis** The *water deprivation test* aims to test the ability of kidneys to concentrate urine for diagnosis of DI, and then to localize the cause. See BOX.

NB: it is often difficult to differentiate primary polydipsia from partial DI.

ΔΔ: DM; diuretics or lithium use; *primary polydipsia*—this causes symptoms of polydipsia and polyuria with dilute urine. Its cause is poorly understood;[4] it may be associated with schizophrenia or mania (±Li+ therapy), or, rarely, hypothalamic disease (neurosarcoid; tumour; encephalitis; brain injury; HIV encephalopathy). As part of this syndrome, the kidneys may lose their ability to fully concentrate urine, due to a wash-out of the normal concentrating gradient in the renal medulla.

**Treatment** *Cranial DI:* Find the cause—MRI (head); test anterior pituitary function (p224). Give desmopressin, a synthetic analogue of ADH (eg Desmomelt® tablets).

*Nephrogenic:* Treat the cause. If it persists, try bendroflumethiazide 5mg PO/24h. NSAIDs lower urine volume and plasma Na+ by inhibiting prostaglandin synthase: prostaglandins locally inhibit the action of ADH.

▶▶**Emergency management** • Do urgent plasma U&E, and serum and urine osmolalities. Monitor urine output carefully and check U&E twice a day initially.

• IVI to keep up with urine output. If severe hypernatraemia, do not lower Na+ rapidly as this may cause cerebral oedema and brain injury. If Na+ is ≥170, use 0.9% saline initially—this contains 150mmol/L of sodium. Aim to reduce Na+ at a rate of less than 12mmol/L per day. Use of 0.45% saline can be dangerous.

• Desmopressin 2μg IM (lasts 12-24h) may be used as a therapeutic trial.

---

1 DIDMOAD is a rare autosomal recessive disorder: Diabetes Insipidus, Diabetes Mellitus, Optic Atrophy and Deafness (also known as Wolfram's syndrome).
2 Suspect neurosarcoidosis if CSF protein↑ (seen in 34%), facial nerve palsy (25%), CSF pleocytosis (23%), diabetes insipidus (21%), hemiparesis (17%), psychosis (17%), papilloedema (15%), ataxia (13%), seizures (12%), optic atrophy (12%), hearing loss (12%), or nystagmus (9%).
3 Sheehan's syndrome is pituitary infarction from shock, eg postpartum haemorrhage. It is rare.
4 Most of us could drink 20L/d and not be hyponatraemic; some get hyponatraemic drinking 5L/d; they may have Psychosis, Intermittent hyponatraemia, and Polydipsia (PIP syndrome), ?from ↑intravascular volume leading to ↑atrial natriuretic peptide, p131, hence natriuresis and hyponatraemia.

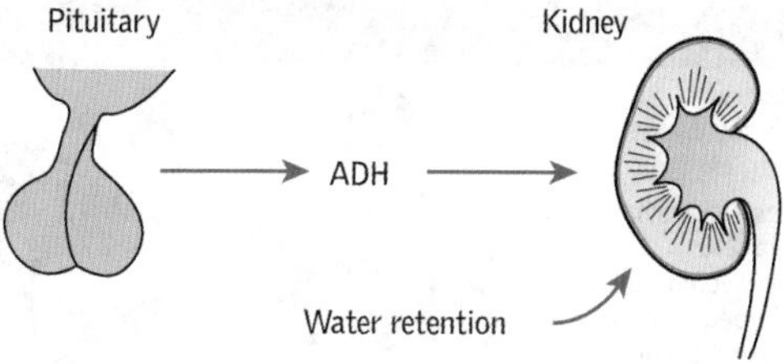

Fig 1. Pathway of renal regulation. ADH=antidiuretic hormone=ADV=antidiuretic vaso-pressin=arginine vasopressin=AVP. The essential role of ADH V2 and AQP2 (aquaporin 2) receptors in water homeostasis is clear now we know that mutations in their genes cause nephrogenic diabetes insipidus such that the kidney is unable to concentrate urine in response to ADH.

## The 8-hour water deprivation test

This test aims to determine whether the kidneys continue to produce dilute urine despite dehydration, and then to localize the cause. Do not do the test before establishing that urine volume is >3L/d (output less than this with normal plasma $Na^+$ and osmolality excludes significant disturbance of water balance).

• Stop test if *urine* osmolality >600mOsmol/kg in Stage 1 (DI is excluded).
• Free fluids until 07.30. Light breakfast at 06.30, no tea, no coffee, no smoking.

**Stage 1** Fluid deprivation (0–8h): for diagnosis of DI. Start at 08.00.

• Empty bladder, then no drinks and only dry food.
• Weigh hourly. If >3% weight lost during test, order urgent serum osmolality. If >300mOsmol/kg, proceed to Stage 2. If <300, continue test.
• Collect urine every 2h; measure its volume and osmolality.
• Venous sample for osmolality every 4h.
• Stop test after 8h (16.00) if urine osmolality >600mOsmol/kg (ie normal).

**Stage 2** Differentiate cranial from nephrogenic DI.

• Proceed if urine still dilute—ie urine osmolality <600mOsmol/kg.
• Give desmopressin 2µg IM. Water can be drunk now.
• Measure urine osmolality hourly for the next 4h.

### Interpreting the water deprivation test

| | |
|---|---|
| Normal | Urine osmolality >600mOsmol/kg in Stage 1 U:P ratio >2 (normal concentrating ability). |
| Primary polydipsia | Urine concentrates, but less than normal, eg >400–600mOsmol/kg. |
| Cranial DI | Urine osmolality increases to >600mOsmol/kg *after* desmopressin (if equivocal an extended water deprivation test may be tried (no drinking from 18:00 the night before)). |
| Nephrogenic DI | No increase in urine osmolality after desmopressin. |

## Contents

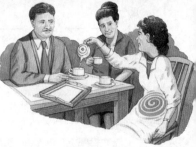

Fig 1. Families are rarely what they seem: Otto, Aurelia and Sylvia seem to be having a nice cuppa, but Warren (the son and brother) is absent, Otto's leg is missing, Aurilia is beside herself with anxiety, and neither is fully aware of the turmoil spiraling out of control in their unstable daughter, Sylvia. How the gut weaves in and out of our patients' stories is one of gastroenterology's perpetually fascinating and significant riddles. So whenever you are presented with an image in gastroenterology, ask what is missing, and try to work out the forces which are perpetuating or relieving symptoms (pathogenesis *versus* salutogenesis). This is all very helpful, but it can never be relied on to tame or predict what happens next. So what *did* happen next? See opposite to find out.

**Relevant pages in other chapters:** *Signs & symptoms:* Abdominal distension (p57); epigastric pain (p57); flatulence (p58); guarding (p62); heartburn (p244); hepatomegaly (p63); LIF & LUQ pain (p57); palmar erythema (p33); rebound tenderness (p62); regurgitation (p59); RIF & RUQ pain (p57); skin discolouration (p28); splenomegaly (p606); tenesmus (p59); vomiting (p56); waterbrash (p606); weight loss (p29).
*Surgical topics:* Contents to *Surgery* (p566). *Haematology:* Iron-deficiency (p320). *Infections:* Viral hepatitis (p406).
*Radiology:* The plain abdominal film (AXR) (p740); radiological GI procedures (p756).
*Emergencies:* Upper GI bleeding (p830); acute liver failure (p806).

*We thank Simon Campbell (Consultant Gastroenterologist, Manchester Royal Infirmary), who is our Specialist Reader for this chapter, and our Junior Readers, Rona Zhao and Sarah Cochrane, for their contribution.*

We learn about gastroenterological diseases as if they were separate entities, independent species collected by naturalists, each kept in its own dark matchbox—collectors' items collecting dust in a desiccated world on a library shelf. But this is not how illness works. Otto had diabetes, but refused to see a doctor until it was far advanced, and an amputation was needed. He needed looking after by his wife Aurelia. But she had her children Warren and Sylvia to look after too. And when Otto was no longer the bread-winner, she forced herself to work as a teacher, an accountant, and at any other job she could get. Otto's illness manifested in Aurelia's duodenum—as an ulcer. The gut often bears the brunt of other people's worries. Inside every piece of a gut is a lumen[1]—the world is in the gut, and the gut is in the world. But the light does not always shine. So when the lumen filled with Aurelia's blood, we can expect the illness to impact on the whole family. Her daughter knows where blood comes from ('straight from the heart ... pink fizz'). After Otto died, Sylvia needed long-term psychiatric care, and Aurelia moved to be near her daughter. The bleeding duodenal ulcer got worse when Sylvia needed electroconvulsive therapy. The therapy worked and now, briefly, Sylvia, before her own premature death, is able to look after Aurelia, as she prepares for a gastrectomy.

The story of each illness told separately misses something; but even taken in its social context, this story is missing something vital—the poetry, in most of our patients lived rather than written—tragic, comic, human, and usually obscure—but in the case of this family not so obscure. Welling up, as unstoppable as the bleeding from her mother's ulcer, came the poetry of Sylvia Plath.[2]

**1** *Lumen* is Latin for light (hence its medical meaning of a tubular cavity open to the world at both ends), as well as being the SI unit of light flux falling on an object—ie the power to transilluminate. All doctors have this power, whether by insightfully interpreting patients' lives and illnesses to them, or by acts of kindness—even something so simple as bringing a cup of tea.

**2** *...And here you come, with a cup of tea*
  *Wreathed in steam.*
  *The blood jet is poetry,*
  *There is no stopping it.*
  *You hand me two children, two roses.*   Sylvia Plath: *Kindness*: Collected Poems; 1981; Faber
  Source: katemoses.com/books/w_chronology.html

Gastroenterology

'*There's a lot of people in this world who spend so much time watching their health that they haven't the time to enjoy it*' Josh Billings (1818-85).

Recent UK government guidelines emphasize simply eating less (eg 2600 calories/d for men and 2080 for women) rather than specifying dietary content,[2] recognizing that there are no good or bad foods, and no universally good or bad diets. Don't consider diet independently of desired lifestyle; and don't assume we all want to be thin, healthy, and live forever. If we are walking to the South Pole, our bodies need as much energy-rich fat as possible. But if we are sedentary, the converse may *not* be true. After decades of research, we still don't know who should eat what, or when. Are 3 meals a day healthier than 1? Is fat harmful if weight is normal? Is a balanced diet (see BOX) best? Should we eat 3, 5, 7, or 9 fruits daily? (one recommendation for men, but some studies find no benefit beyond 3).[3] Are green vegetables (or yellow?) better than fruits? (maybe, for preventing diabetes).[4]

The traditional answer to these questions (the more fruit the better) may be wrong because of complex interactions between eating and health. All diets have unintended consequences: eg the 'good' antioxidant epicatechin (a flavonoid) in dark chocolate is annulled by taking milk at the same time.[5] Randomized trials show that low-carbohydrate Atkins-type diets (↑fat and ↑protein) improve lipid profiles and insulin resistance (possible SEs of renal problems and ↑Ca²⁺ excretion[6,7] may have been over-played,[8] but note that bowel flora is changed in a way that is ?carcinogenic).[9] To complicate matters, diet is also confounded by lifestyle—while some studies show vegetarians may be less likely to die from ischaemic heart disease,[10] is this effect because vegetarians in the UK are more likely to be non-smokers?[11] Do vitamin/antioxidant supplements help? β-carotene and vitamins A & E may increase mortality.[12,13]

**Current recommendations must take into account 3 facts:**
• Obesity costs health services as much as smoking—1 in 4 UK adults is obese.[14]
• Diabetes mellitus is burgeoning: in some places prevalence is >7% (p198).
• Past advice has not changed eating habits in large sections of the population.

**Advice is likely to focus on the following:**
*Body mass index (BMI; BOX 3):* aim for 20-25. Controlling quantity may be more important than quality. In hypertension, eating the 'right' things lowered BP by 0.6mmHg and controlling weight caused a 3.7mmHg reduction in 6 months.[15 RTC]
*Oily fish:* Rich in omega-3 fatty acid (eg mackerel, herring, pilchards, salmon—but benefits are not fully substantiated).[16] If tinned fish, avoid those in unspecified oils. Nuts are good too: walnuts lower cholesterol (polyunsaturates:saturates=7:1, ie very good). Soya protein lowers cholesterol, low-density lipoproteins, and triglycerides.
*Refined sugar:* (See BOX for its deleterious effects.) Use fruit to add sweetness. Have low-sugar drinks: a 330mL can of non-diet carbonated soft drink can have up to 10 teaspoons (40g) of refined sugar. Don't add sugar to drinks or cereals. (In a thin, active, elderly, normoglycaemic person, sugar may be no great evil.)
*Eat enough fruit and fibre:* See BOX 1 and *reduce salt intake.*
*Enjoy moderate alcohol use (adults <65yrs):* ♀: ≤14U/wk; ♂: ≤21U/wk (controversial)—taken regularly (no binges!). Alcohol inhibits platelet aggregation and is antioxidant (∴ cardioprotective). There is no evidence that spirit or beer drinkers should switch to wine. If LDL cholesterol is ≥5.25mmol/L, benefits are more likely.[17]

▶*Avoid this diet if:* •<5yrs old •Need for low residue (eg Crohn's, UC, p274) or special diet (coeliac disease, p280) •Weight loss is expected. *Emphasis may be different in:* Dyslipidaemia (p704); DM (p198); obesity; constipation (p248); liver failure (p258); chronic pancreatitis (p280); renal failure (less protein)(p296); BP↑.[18]

**Difficulties** It is an imposition to ask us to change our diet (children often refuse point-blank); a more subtle approach is to take a food we enjoy (crisps) and make it healthier (eg low-salt crisps made from jacket potatoes and fried in sunflower oil).

## Traditional low-fat nutritional advice: the balance of good health

A low-fat diet may not only be for the sake of good health, as it can also help control symptoms, eg from gallstones, and while it is unrealistic to expect all our patients' troubles to drift away as the weight comes off, we can offer the incentive of an improvement in both symptoms and health as encouragement.

**Starchy foods** Bread, rice, pasta, potatoes, etc. form the main starch energy source (wholemeal/unprocessed is recommended).

**Fibre** (Mainly non-starch polysaccharide, NSP) 14g/1000kcal is recommended for children and adults. Fibre is claimed to ↓risk of vascular disease, diabetes, breast cancer,[19] and obesity—as well as constipation and piles. Soluble fibre improves insulin sensitivity (non-diabetics and diabetics). If obese, fibre supplements may aid weight loss.[20] Prebiotic fibres might enhance immunity.[21] ↑Fluid intake with diets high in NSP, eg 8 cups (1-2½ pints) daily. Warn about bulky stools. Phytate in NSP can ↓$Ca^{2+}$ and iron absorption, so restrict main intake to 1 meal a day. Iron availability in bread depends on how it is leavened. Modern methods (eg the Chorleywood process, which depends on very fast agitation) decrease iron availability compared with leavening dough slowly.[22]

**Fruit and vegetables** eg >6 pieces of fruit (with skins)[23] or portions of pulses, beans, or lightly cooked greens per day (aims to ↓vascular and cancer deaths).[24]

**Meat and alternatives** Meat should be cooked without additional fat. Lower fat alternatives, such as white meat (poultry, without skin), white fish, and vegetable protein sources (eg pulses, soya) are encouraged.

**Dairy foods** Low-fat semi-skimmed milk/yoghurt; Edam or cottage cheese.

**Fat and sugary foods** Avoiding extra fat in cooking is advised ('grill, boil, steam, or bake, but don't fry'). Fatty spreads (eg butter) are kept to a minimum and snack foods (crisps, sweets, biscuits, and cake) are avoided.

## Losing weight—why and how?

**The risks of too much sugar** Excess sugar causes caries, diabetes, obesity—which itself contributes to osteoarthritis, cancer,[25] hypertension,[26] and increased oxidative stress—so raising cardiovascular mortality[27] and much more.

**Losing weight** Motivational therapy. Consider referral to a dietician—a needs-specific diet may be best. In conjunction with exercise and diet strategies, targeted weight-loss can also be achieved successfully with psychotherapy.[28]

**Drugs or surgery for obesity?** The most desirable treatment for obesity is still primary prevention, but pharmacotherapy does work.[29] *Orlistat* lowers fat absorption (hence SE of oily faecal incontinence)—see *OHCS* p530.[1] *Surgery:* See p628.

## Calculating body mass index

BMI=(weight in kg)/(height in m)$^2$

| BMI | State | Some implications within the categories |
|---|---|---|
| <18.5 | Underweight | <17.5 is one of the criteria for anorexia nervosa |
| 18.5-25 | On target | |
| 25-30 | Overweight | Weight loss should be considered |
| 30-40 | Obesity | >32 is unsuitable for day-case general surgery |
| >40 | Extreme/morbid obesity | >40 is an indication for bariatric surgery |

Caveats: BMI does not take into account the distribution of body fat, and is harder to interpret for children and adolescents. ►Waist circumference >94cm in men and >80cm in women reflects omental fat and correlates better with risk than does BMI. BMI is still a valid way of comparing nations: average BMI in the USA in 2005 was 28.7. In Japan, it was 22. A nation can be lean without being poor. If other nations adopted the lifestyle of the USA, this would be equivalent to adding a billion people to the planet in terms of sustainability.[30] For more details on ethnic variations, see p199.

1 Research continues into the hormones involved in obesity—eg the satiety-inducing **leptin** and the hunger-inducing **ghrelin**.

Gastroenterology

The diagnosis will often come out of your patient's mouth, so open it! So many GI investigations are indirect...now is your chance for direct observation.

**Leucoplakia** (fig 1) is an oral mucosal white patch that will not rub off and is not attributable to any other known disease. It is a premalignant lesion, with a transformation rate, which ranges from 0.6% to 18%.[32] Oral hairy leucoplakia is a shaggy white patch on the side of the tongue seen in HIV, caused by EBV. ▶When in doubt, refer all intra-oral white lesions (see BOX).

**Aphthous ulcers** (fig 2) 20% of us get these shallow, painful ulcers on the tongue or oral mucosa that heal without scarring. *Causes of severe ulcers:* Crohn's and coeliac disease; Behçet's (p708); trauma; erythema multiforme; lichen planus; pemphigus; pemphigoid; infections (herpes simplex, syphilis, Vincent's angina, p726). ℞: *Minor ulcers:* avoid oral trauma (eg hard toothbrushes or foods such as toast) and acidic foods or drinks. **Tetracycline** or antimicrobial mouthwashes (eg chlorhexidine). *Severe ulcers:* Possible therapies include systemic corticosteroids (eg oral **prednisolone** 30-60mg/d PO for a week) or thalidomide (absolutely contraindicated in pregnancy)[33] ▶Biopsy any ulcer not healing after 3 weeks to exclude malignancy; refer to an oral surgeon if uncertain.

**Candidiasis (thrush; fig 3)** causes white patches or erythema of the buccal mucosa. Patches may be hard to remove and bleed if scraped. *Risk factors:* Extremes of age; DM; antibiotics; immunosuppression (long-term corticosteroids, including inhalers; cytotoxics; malignancy; HIV). ℞: *Nystatin* suspension 100,000U (1mL swill and swallow/6h) or *amphotericin* lozenges. *Fluconazole* for oropharyngeal thrush.

**Cheilitis (angular stomatitis)** Fissuring of the mouth's corners is caused by denture problems, candidiasis, or deficiency of iron or riboflavin (vitamin $B_2$). (fig 2, p321)

**Gingivitis** Gum inflammation ± hypertrophy occurs with poor oral hygiene, drugs (phenytoin, ciclosporin, nifedipine), pregnancy, vitamin C deficiency (scurvy, p278), acute myeloid leukaemia (p350), or Vincent's angina (p726).

**Microstomia** (fig 4) The mouth is too small, eg from thickening and tightening of the perioral skin after burns or in epidermolysis bullosa (destructive skin and mucous membrane blisters ± ankyloglossia) or systemic sclerosis (p554).

**Oral pigmentation** Perioral brown spots characterize Peutz-Jeghers' (p722). Pigmentation anywhere in the mouth suggests Addison's disease (p218) or drugs (eg antimalarials). Consider malignant melanoma. *Telangiectasia:* Systemic sclerosis; Osler-Weber-Rendu syndrome (p722). *Fordyce glands* (creamy yellow spots at the border of the oral mucosa and the lip vermilion) are sebaceous cysts, common and benign. *Aspergillus niger* colonization may cause a black tongue.

**Teeth** (fig 5) A blue line at the gum-tooth margin suggests lead poisoning. Prenatal or childhood tetracycline exposure causes a yellow-brown discolouration.

**Tongue** This may be furred or dry (xerostomia) in dehydration, if on tricyclics,[etc1] after radiotherapy, in Crohn's disease, Sjögren's (p724) and Mikulicz's syndrome.[34] (p720)

*Glossitis* means a smooth, red, sore tongue, eg caused by iron, folate, or $B_{12}$ deficiency (fig 1, p329). If local loss of papillae leads to ulcer-like lesions that change in colour and size, use the term **geographic tongue** (harmless migratory glossitis).

*Macroglossia:* The tongue is too big. Causes: myxoedema; acromegaly; amyloid. (p364) A *ranula* is a bluish salivary retention cyst to one side of the frenulum, named after the bulging vocal pouch of frogs' throats (genus *Rana*).

*Tongue cancer* typically appears on tongue edge as a raised ulcer with firm edges and environs. Main risk factors: smoking and alcohol.[2] Examine under the tongue and ask patient to deviate his extended tongue sideways. Spread: anterior ⅓ of the tongue drains to the submental nodes; middle ⅓ to the submandibular nodes; posterior ⅓ to the deep cervical nodes (see BOX, p600). *Treatment:* Radiotherapy or surgery. 5yr survival (early disease): 80%. ▶When in doubt, refer tongue ulcers.

1 Drugs causing xerostomia: ACE-i, antidepressants; antihistamines; antipsychotics; antimuscarinics/anticholinergics; bromocriptine; diuretics; loperamide; nifedipine; opiates; prazosin; prochlorperazine. etc.
2 Betel nut (*Areca catechu*) chewing, common in South Asia, may be an independent risk factor.[8]

## White intra-oral lesions

- Idiopathic keratosis
- Leucoplakia
- Lichen planus
- Poor dental hygiene
- Candidiasis
- Squamous papilloma
- Carcinoma
- Hairy oral leucoplakia
- Lupus erythematosus
- Smoking
- Aphthous stomatitis
- Secondary syphilis

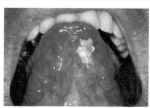

**Fig 1.** Leucoplakia on the underside of the tongue. It is important to refer leucoplakia because it is premalignant.

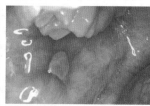

**Fig 2.** An aphthous ulcer inside the cheek. The name is tautological: *aphtha* in Greek means ulceration.

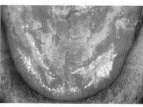

**Fig 3.** White fur on an erythematous tongue caused by oral candidiasis. Oropharyngeal candidiasis in an apparently fit patient may suggest underlying HIV infection.

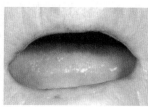

**Fig 4.** Microstomia (small, narrow mouth), eg from hardening of the skin in scleroderma which narrows the mouth. It is cosmetically and functionally disabling.[a]

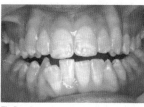

**Fig 5.** White bands on the teeth can be caused by excessive fluoride intake.

Gastroenterology

Dysphagia is difficulty in swallowing and always needs investigating urgently to exclude malignancy (unless of short duration, and associated with a sore throat).

**Causes** Oral, pharyngeal, or oesophageal? Mechanical or motility related? (See BOX.)

**5 key questions to ask**

1 Was there difficulty swallowing solids **and** liquids from the start? (See BOX.)
 **Yes:** motility disorder (esp if non-progressive, eg achalasia, CNS, or pharyngeal causes).
 **No:** Solids then liquids: suspect a stricture (benign or malignant).
2 Is it difficult to make the swallowing movement?
 **Yes:** Suspect bulbar palsy, especially if patient coughs on swallowing.
3 Is swallowing painful (odynophagia)?
 **Yes:** Suspect cancer, oesophageal ulcer (benign or malignant), *Candida* (eg immunocompromised or poor steroid inhaler technique) or spasm.
4 Is the dysphagia intermittent or is it constant and getting worse?
 **Intermittent:** Suspect oesophageal spasm.
 **Constant and worsening:** Suspect malignant stricture.
5 Does the neck bulge or gurgle on drinking?
 **Yes:** Suspect a pharyngeal pouch (see OHCS p573).

**Signs** Is the patient cachectic or anaemic? Examine the mouth; feel for supraclavicular nodes (left supraclavicular node = Virchow's node—suggests intra-abdominal malignancy); look for signs of systemic disease, eg systemic sclerosis (p554), CNS disease.

**Tests** FBC (anaemia). U&E (dehydration); CXR (mediastinal fluid level, no gastric bubble, aspiration). Upper GI endoscopy ± biopsy—in high dysphagia, precede by barium swallow (fig 1) for pharyngeal pouch (± ENT opinion). 2nd-line: video fluoroscopy to identify dysmotility, eg achalasia. Oesophageal manometry if barium swallow is normal.

**Specific conditions** *Oesophagitis* p244. *Diffuse oesophageal spasm* causes intermittent dysphagia ± chest pain. Barium swallow: abnormal contractions, eg corkscrew oesophagus.[1] *Achalasia:* The lower oesophageal sphincter fails to relax (due to degeneration of the myenteric plexus), causing dysphagia (for fluids and solids), regurgitation, substernal cramps, and ↓weight. CXR: fluid level in dilated oesophagus (eg above heart); barium swallow: dilated tapering oesophagus. Treatment: endoscopic balloon dilatation, or Heller's cardiomyotomy—then proton pump inhibitors (PPIs, p244). Botulinum toxin injection if a non-invasive procedure is needed (repeat every few months).[57] Calcium channel blockers and nitrates also relax the sphincter. Longstanding achalasia may cause oesophageal cancer. *Benign oesophageal stricture:* Caused by gastro-oesophageal reflux (GORD, p244), corrosives, surgery, or radiotherapy. Treatment: endoscopic balloon dilatation. *Oesophageal cancer:* (p620). Associations: ♂, GORD,[38] tobacco, alcohol, Barrett's oesophagus (p709), achalasia, tylosis (palmar hyperkeratosis), Paterson-Brown-Kelly (Plummer-Vinson) syndrome (post-cricoid dysphagia, upper oesophageal web + iron-deficiency). *CNS causes:* Ask for help from a speech rehab specialist.

## Nausea and vomiting Exclude pregnancy! (other causes: p56)

**Regurgitation or vomiting?** The former is effortless (unassociated with nausea).

**What's in your vomit?** "Coffee grounds" ≈ GI bleeding; recognizable food ≈ gastric stasis; feculent ≈ small bowel obstruction or bacterial overgrowth.

**Timing** Morning ≈ pregnancy or ICP↑; 1h post food ≈ gastric stasis/gastroparesis (DM); vomiting that relieves pain ≈ peptic ulcer; preceded by loud gurgling ≈ GI obstruction. Vomiting only when your mother-in-law visits suggests a different line of enquiry.

**Tests** *Bloods:* FBC, U&E, LFT, $Ca^{2+}$, glucose, amylase. *ABG:* A metabolic (hypochloraemic) alkalosis from loss of gastric contents (pH >7.45, ↑$HCO_3^-$) indicates severe vomiting. *Plain AXR* if suspected bowel obstruction (p742). *Upper GI endoscopy* (p256) if persistent vomiting. Consider head CT in case ICP↑. Identify and **treat** underlying causes if possible.

**Treatment** See TABLE. Be pre-emptive, eg pre-op for post-op symptoms. Try the oral route first. 30% need a 2nd-line anti-emetic, so be prepared to prescribe more than one, but avoid drugs in pregnancy and children. Give IV fluids with K+ replacement if severely dehydrated or nil-by-mouth, and monitor electrolytes and fluid balance.

1 Non-propulsive contractions manifest as tertiary contractions or 'corkscrew oesophagus' (fig 4, p757) and suggest a motility disorder and may lead to ↓acid clearance.[6] Symptoms and radiology may not match. *Nutcracker oesophagus* denotes distal peristaltic contractions >180mmHg. It may cause pain,[6] relieved by nitrates, sublingual **nifedipine**, or smooth muscle relaxants (sildenafil, p316).[t]

## Causes of dysphagia

| **Mechanical block** | **Motility disorders** |
|---|---|
| Malignant stricture (fig 1) | Achalasia (see opposite) |
|   Oesophageal cancer | Diffuse oesophageal spasm |
|   Gastric cancer | Systemic sclerosis (p554) |
|   Pharyngeal cancer | Neurological bulbar palsy (p511) |
| Benign strictures |   Pseudobulbar palsy (p511) |
|   Oesophageal web or ring (p240) |   Wilson's or Parkinson's disease |
|   Peptic stricture |   Syringobulbia (p520) |
| Extrinsic pressure |   Bulbar poliomyelitis (p432) |
|   Lung cancer |   Chagas' disease (p438) |
|   Mediastinal lymph nodes |   Myasthenia gravis (p516) |
|   Retrosternal goitre | |
|   Aortic aneurysm | **Others** |
|   Left atrial enlargement | Oesophagitis (p244; reflux or *Candida*/HSV) |
| Pharyngeal pouch | Globus (="I've got a lump in my throat": try to distinguish from true dysphagia) |

**Gastroenterology**

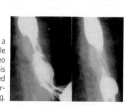

Fig 1. A malignant lower oesophageal stricture on a barium swallow. Its shouldered edges lead to an 'apple core' effect with an irregular mucosal pattern. On video fluoroscopy there would be no peristalsis visible in this segment. Benign strictures would have a more funnelled appearance with a normal mucosal pattern. Note the normal gastro-oesophageal junction. ©Dr Stephen Golding.

### The marshmallow test

To a thoughtful marshmallow eater the question "Is your dysphagia worse with solids or liquids?" is tricky, as marshmallows neatly span this great divide. Never mind: leave it all to the endoscopist to sort out? Not really: endoscopy is poor at assessing dynamic events such as swallowing. In anyone with complicated swallowing problems it is much better to coat a marshmallow with barium and follow its progress at fluoroscopy. Where are the hold-ups and how many swallows does it take before the oesophagogastric junction is successfully negotiated? [42]

### Remembering your anti-emetics

One way of recalling anti-emetics involves using (simplified) pharmacology.

| Receptor | Antagonist | Dose | Notes |
|---|---|---|---|
| H$_1$ | *Cyclizine* | 50mg/8h PO/IV/IM | GI causes |
| | *Cinnarizine* | 30mg/8h PO | Vestibular disorders |
| D$_2$ | *Metoclopramide* | 10mg/8h PO/IV/IM | GI causes; also prokinetic |
| | *Domperidone* | 60mg/12h PR<br>20mg/6h PO | Also prokinetic |
| | *Prochlorperazine* | 12.5mg IM;<br>5mg/8h PO | Vestibular/GI causes |
| | *Haloperidol* | 1.5mg/12h PO | Chemical causes, eg opioids |
| 5HT$_3$ | *Ondansetron* | 4mg/8h IV slowly | Doses can be much higher for, eg, emetogenic chemotherapy |
| Others | *Hyoscine hydro-bromide* | 200–600µg SC/IM | Antimuscarinic ∴ also anti-spasmodic and antisecretory (don't prescribe with a prokinetic) |
| | *Dexamethasone* | 6-10mg/d PO/SC | Unknown mode of action; an adjuvant |
| | *Midazolam* | 2-4mg/d SC (syringe driver) | Unknown action; anti-emetic effect outlasts sedative effect [43] |

►All antidopaminergics can cause dystonias and oculogyric crisis, especially in younger patients.

**War** The stomach is a battle ground between the forces of attack (acid, pepsin, *Helicobacter pylori*, bile salts) and defence (mucin secretion, cellular mucus, bicarbonate secretion, mucosal blood flow, cell turnover).[44] Gastric antisecretory agents, eg $H_2$ receptor antagonists (H2RAs), and proton pump inhibitors (PPIs) may only work if you have optimized cytoprotection (antacids and sucralfate work this way). Success may depend on you being not just a brilliant general, but also a tactician, politician, and diplomat. Plan your strategy carefully with the FLOWCHART (fig 1). As in any war, neglecting psychological factors can prove disastrous (see R: below). The aim is not outright victory but *maintaining the balance of power* so all may prosper.

**Symptoms** Epigastric pain often related to hunger, specific foods, or time of day ± bloating, fullness after meals, heartburn (retrosternal pain + reflux); tender epigastrium. **Alarm** symptoms: Anaemia (iron deficiency); loss of weight; anorexia; recent onset/progressive symptoms; melaena/haematemesis; swallowing difficulty.

**H. pylori**[1] (BOX 1). *If ≤55yrs old* test for *H. pylori*; treat if +ve. 'Test and treat,'[2] eg lansoprazole 30mg/24h PO for 4wks reduces symptoms and recurrence more than acid suppression alone. ▶*If ≥55* (and *new* dyspepsia not from NSAID use and persisting for >4-6wks) *or alarm symptoms*, refer for urgent endoscopy (p256).

**Duodenal ulcer** (DU, fig 1 p255) is 4-fold commoner than GU. *Major risk factors:* *H. pylori* (90%); drugs (NSAIDs; steroids; SSRI).[45] *Minor:* ↑Gastric acid secretion; ↑gastric emptying (↓duodenal pH); blood group O; smoking. The role of stress is debated.
*Symptoms:* Epigastric pain typically before meals or at night, relieved by eating or drinking milk. 50% are asymptomatic; others experience recurrent episodes.
*Signs:* Epigastric tenderness. *Diagnosis:* Upper GI endoscopy (stop PPI 2wks before). Test for *H. pylori*. Measure gastrin concentrations when off PPIs if Zollinger-Ellison syndrome (p730) is suspected. ΔΔ: Non-ulcer dyspepsia; duodenal Crohn's; TB; lymphoma; pancreatic cancer (p276). *Follow-up:* None; if good response to R (eg PPI).

**Gastric ulcers** (GU) occur mainly in the elderly, on the lesser curve. Ulcers elsewhere are more often malignant. *Risk factors:* *H. pylori* (~80%); smoking; NSAIDs; reflux of duodenal contents; delayed gastric emptying; stress, eg neurosurgery or burns (Cushing's or Curling's ulcers). *Symptoms:* Asymptomatic or epigastric pain (related to meals ± relieved by antacids) ± weight↓. *Tests:* Upper endoscopy to exclude malignancy (stop PPI >2wks before, see FLOWCHART); multiple biopsies from ulcer rim and base (histology, *H. pylori*) and brushings (cytology). Repeat endoscopy (eg if perforation or bleeding) to check healing (biopsy if suspicious of gastric ca).

**R:** *Lifestyle:* Purge stress[46] by creating opportunities for people to move from disease into health through dialogue and reflection on their lives—eg would he/she see benefit in ↓alcohol and tobacco use? Both will help. Avoid any aggravating foods.
*H. pylori eradication:* Triple therapy[3] is 80-85% effective at eradication.
*Drugs to reduce acid:* PPIs are effective, eg *lansoprazole* 30mg/24h PO for 4 (DU) or 8 (GU) wks. $H_2$ blockers have a place (*ranitidine* 300mg each night PO for 8wks).
*Drug-induced ulcers:* Stop drug if possible. PPIs may be best for treating and preventing GI ulcers and bleeding in patients on NSAID or antiplatelet drugs. Misoprostol is an alternative with different SE.[47] If symptoms persist, re-endoscope, recheck for *H. pylori*, and reconsider differential diagnoses (eg gallstones). *Surgery:* p626.

**Complications** Bleeding ▶▶(p252), perforation ▶▶(p608), malignancy, gastric outflow↓.

**Functional (non-ulcer) dyspepsia** Treatment is hard. *H. pylori* eradication, only after a +ve result) *may* help, but long-term effects of such a strategy are unknown. Some evidence favours PPIs and psychotherapy. PPI SE aren't negligible.[12] Antacids, antispasmodics, $H_2$ blockers, misoprostol, prokinetic agents, sucralfate, or tricyclics have less evidence.[48] Bismuth preparations are an interesting and ancient option (eg DeNol® 120mg/12h), having healing and anti-*Helicobacter* properties; it's available over-the-counter, avoiding medicalization. It turns stools black.

---

1 *H. pylori* is the commonest bacterial pathogen found worldwide (>50% of the world population over 40yrs has it).[45] It's a **class I carcinogen** causing gastritis (p253), duodenal/gastric ulcers & gastric cancer/ lymphoma (MALT, p356), also associated with coronary artery disease, B12 and iron deficiency.
2 PPI SE reflect lack of gastric acid: gastroenteritis; B12↓ (also osteoporosis, alopecia, photosensitivity; LFT↑).

## $^{13}$C breath test is the most accurate non-invasive *Helicobacter* test

| Invasive tests | CLO test | Sensitivity | 95% | Specificity | 95% |
|---|---|---|---|---|---|
| | Histology | | 95% | | 95% |
| | Culture | | 90% | | 100% |
| Non-invasive | $^{13}$C breath test | | 95% | | 95% |
| | Stool antigen | | 95% | | 94% |
| | Serology | | 92% | | 83% |

Every breath we exhale leaves our own unique breathprint on the world: nitrogen, oxygen, $CO_2$ vapour, and ~250 volatile substances that give useful information about our state of health to scientists and lovers—kisses are faster but less reliable than spectrometers, which can inform about GI diseases, asthma, organ rejection, and cancer.[10]

### Differential diagnosis of dyspepsia

- Non-ulcer dyspepsia
- Oesophagitis/GORD
- Duodenal/gastric ulcer
- Gastric malignancy
- Duodenitis
- Gastritis (p253)

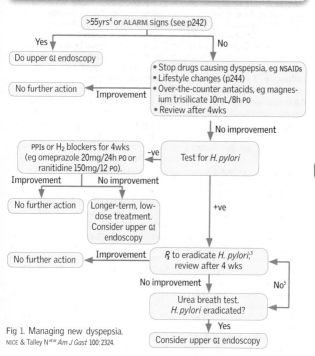

Fig 1. Managing new dyspepsia.
NICE & Talley N *et al* Am J Gast 100:2324.

Why not start everyone on a PPI straight away? Simple measures are safer (more and more PPI SE are reported). Also, PPIs and ranitidine cause false -ve breath tests and antigen tests: stop for >2wks before (>4wks for bismuth and antibiotics).[52] ► See NICE.

**3** *H. pylori* eradication (NICE/BNF): **either** PAC500 regimen (full dose PPI, amoxicillin 1g, clarithromycin 500mg) twice daily **or** PMC250 (full dose PPI, metronidazole 400mg, clarithromycin 250mg) twice daily for 7d. PPIs: omeprazole 20mg/12h; lansoprazole: 30mg/12h. **Resistant infections:** tripotassium dicitratobismuthate (De Noltab® 2 twice daily ½h before food[13]) + PPI + 2 antibiotics for 14d. Bismuth causes black stools: warn the patient! NB: you may need to continue the PPI if the ulcer is large or bleeds.[13]
**4** Some experts recommend endoscopy if >45yrs old.
**5** Don't treat +ve cases of *H. pylori* more than twice. If still +ve, do endoscopy.

Gastroenterology

GORD is common, and is said to exist when reflux of stomach contents (acid ± bile)[1] causes troublesome symptoms (≥2 heartburn episodes/wk) and/or complications.[34] If reflux is prolonged, it may cause oesophagitis (fig 1), benign oesophageal stricture, or Barrett's oesophagus (fig 2 and p709; it is pre-malignant). Causes: lower oesophageal sphincter hypotension, hiatus hernia (see below), loss of oesophageal peristaltic function, abdominal obesity, gastric acid hypersecretion, slow gastric emptying, overeating,[34] smoking, alcohol, pregnancy, surgery in achalasia, drugs (tricyclics, anticholinergics, nitrates), systemic sclerosis, *Helicobacter pylori*? ●※[2]

**Symptoms** *Oesophageal:* Heartburn (burning, retrosternal discomfort after meals, lying, stooping or straining, relieved by antacids); belching; acid brash (acid or bile regurgitation); waterbrash (↑↑salivation: "My mouth fills with saliva"); odynophagia (painful swallowing, eg from oesophagitis or ulceration). *Extra-oesophageal:* Nocturnal asthma, chronic cough, laryngitis (hoarseness, throat clearing), sinusitis.[55]

**Complications** Oesophagitis, ulcers, benign stricture, iron-deficiency. *Metaplasia →dysplasia→neoplasia:* GORD may induce Barrett's oesophagus (p709; distal oesophageal epithelium undergoes metaplasia from squamous to columnar—this intestinal metaplasia looks velvety, fig 2). 0.6-1.6%/yr of those with low-grade Barrett's progress to oesophageal cancer[56] (higher if 2 histologists concur: diagnosing low-grade dysplasia is tricky: the Prague criteria should be used).[57] Length of lesion matters less than histology. Overall risk of adenocarcinoma in GORD is <1 in 1000/yr. *Histology: Gastric metaplasia:* low risk of malignant change. *Intestinal metaplasia*—2-yrly surveillance. *Low-grade dysplasia*—90% get adenocarcinoma within 6yrs. *High-grade dysplasia:* 50% have adenocarcinoma already.

**ΔΔ** Oesophagitis from corrosives, NSAIDs, herpes, *Candida*; duodenal or gastric ulcers or cancers; non-ulcer dyspepsia; sphincter of Oddi malfunction; cardiac disease.

**Tests** Endoscopy if: symptoms for >4wks; persistent vomiting; GI bleeding/iron deficiency; palpable mass; age >55; dysphagia; symptoms despite treatment; relapsing symptoms; weight↓. Barium swallow may show hiatus hernia. 24h oesophageal pH monitoring ± manometry help diagnose GORD when endoscopy is normal.

**Treatment** ℞ *Encourage:* Raising the bed head ± weight loss; smoking cessation; small, regular meals. "Get to know your own disease, and learn tricks that work for you..."*Avoid:* Hot drinks, alcohol, citrus fruits, tomatoes,[58] onions, fizzy drinks, spicy foods, coffee, tea, chocolate, and eating <3h before bed. Avoid drugs affecting oesophageal motility (nitrates, anticholinergics, $Ca^{2+}$ channel blockers—relax the lower oesophageal sphincter) or that damage mucosa (NSAIDs, $K^+$ salts, bisphosphonates).

*Drugs:* Antacids, eg *magnesium trisilicate mixture* (10mL/8h), or alginates, eg *Gaviscon Advance®* (10-20mL/8h PO) relieve symptoms. For oesophagitis, try a PPI, eg *lansoprazole* 30mg/24h PO[59] PPIs are better than $H_2$ blockers. If unresponsive, try twice-daily PPI. Metoclopramide as mono- or adjunctive therapy is discouraged![60]

*Surgery* (eg laparoscopic) aims to ↑resting lower oesophageal sphincter pressure. Consider in severe GORD (confirm by pH-monitoring/manometry) if drugs are not working. Atypical symptoms (cough, laryngitis) are less likely to improve with surgery compared to patients with typical symptoms. Options are many, eg Nissen fundoplication, p626; HALO® or Stretta radiofrequency ablation of the gastro-oesophageal junction if high-grade dysplasia (and maybe low-grade too).[61]

**4 grades** *Los Angeles classification of GORD* Minor diffuse changes (erythema, oedema; friability) are not included, and the term **mucosal break** (a well-demarcated area of slough/erythema) is used to encompass the old terms erosion & ulceration:[62]

1 ≥1 mucosal break(s) <5mm long not extending beyond 2 mucosal fold tops.
2 Mucosal break >5mm long limited to the space between 2 mucosal fold tops.
3 Mucosal break continuous between the tops of 2 or more mucosal folds but which involves less than 75% of the oesophageal circumference.
4 Mucosal break involving ≥75% of the oesophageal circumference.

1 Bile reflux may be as important as acid; bile is alkaline; it may respond to sucralfate (2g/12h PO), domperidone or metoclopramide. Roux-en-Y diversion may be needed (p624).[63]
2 H. pylori eradication may not influence the course of GORD. ●※ but may help symptoms.[65]

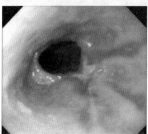

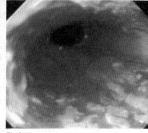

Fig 1. Upper GI endoscopy showing longitudinal mucosal breaks in severe oesophagitis.

Fig 2. Barrett's oesophagus.

Figs 1 & 2 ©Dr A Mee.

## Hiatus hernia

**Sliding hiatus hernia** (80%) is where the gastro-oesophageal junction slides up into the chest—see fig 3. Acid reflux often happens as the lower oesophageal sphincter becomes less competent in many cases.

**Rolling hiatus hernia** (20%) is where the gastro-oesophageal junction remains in the abdomen but a bulge of stomach herniates up into the chest alongside the oesophagus—see figs 3 and 4. As the gastro-oesophageal junction remains intact, gross acid reflux is uncommon.

*Clinical features* Common: 30% of patients >50yrs, especially obese women. 50% have symptomatic gastro-oesophageal reflux.

*Imaging* Barium swallow is the best diagnostic test; upper GI endoscopy visualizes the mucosa (?oesophagitis) but cannot reliably exclude a hiatus hernia.

*Treatment* Lose weight. Treat reflux symptoms. Surgery indications: intractable symptoms despite aggressive medical therapy, complications (see opposite). It is advised to repair rolling hiatus hernia prophylactically (even if asymptomatic) as it may strangulate, which needs prompt surgical repair (which has a high mortality and morbidity rate).

Sliding hernia — Diaphragm

Rolling hernia — Peritoneal sac

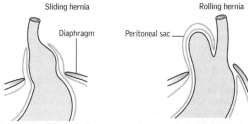

Fig 3. Hiatus hernia—sliding and rolling.

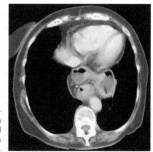

Fig 4. CT chest (IV contrast) showing the rolling components of a hiatus hernia anterior to the oesophagus. Between the oesophagus and the vertebral column on the left-hand side is the aorta. ©Dr S Golding.

Gastroenterology

Diarrhoea≈decreased stool consistency[66] from water, fat (steatorrhoea), or inflammatory discharge. Watery diarrhoea is osmotic, secretory (eg microscopic colitis),[1] or 'functional' (typically from irritable bowel syndrome). Laxative-induced diarrhoea is often osmotic. Steatorrhoea is characterized by ↑gas, offensive smell, and floating, hard-to-flush stools—giardiasis (p436) and coeliac disease (p280) are classic examples. Inflammatory diarrhoea (Crohn's, UC) has blood and pus in the stool. Invasive bacteria and parasites also produce inflammation.

**History** Work (is he a chef?—don't work until an infective cause is ruled out) *Acute or chronic?* If acute (<2wks) suspect gastroenteritis—any risk factors? HIV; achlorhydria, eg PA, p328, or on acid suppressants, eg PPI? Travel? Diet change? Contact with D&V? Any fever/pain? Chronic diarrhoea alternating with constipation suggests irritable bowel (p276). Weight↓, nocturnal diarrhoea and anaemia mandate close follow-up (UC/Crohn's[etc]?).

*Bloody diarrhoea: Campylobacter, Shigella/Salmonella* (p426), *E. coli*, amoebiasis (p436), UC, Crohn's, colorectal cancer (p618), colonic polyps, pseudomembranous colitis, ischaemic colitis (p622). Fresh PR bleeding: p631.

*Mucus* occurs in IBS(p276), colorectal cancer, and polyps. *Frank pus* suggests IBD, diverticulitis, or a fistula/abscess. White cells are microscopically *absent* in amoebiasis, cholera, *E. coli* and viruses.

*Explosive:* Eg cholera; giardia; yersinia (p422); rotavirus. *Large bowel:* (*Salmonella, Shigella, C. diff & entamoeba).* Watery stool ± blood/mucus; pelvic pain relieved by defecation; tenesmus; urgency. *Small bowel symptoms:* Periumbilical (or RIF) pain not relieved by defecation.

**Look for** Dehydration—dry mucous membranes, ↓skin turgor; capillary refill >2s; shock (►►think of cholera, p426). Any fever, weight↓, clubbing, anaemia, oral ulcers (p238), rashes or abdominal mass or scars? Any goitre/hyperthyroid signs? Do rectal exam for masses (eg rectal cancer) or impacted faeces (if you don't put your finger in, you'll put your foot in it by missing this diagnosis which responds to codeine!)

- **Blood** *FBC:* MCV↓/Fe deficiency, eg coeliac or colon ca; MCV↑ if alcohol abuse or B₁₂ absorption↓, eg in coeliac or Crohn's; eosinophilia if parasites. *ESR/CRP↑:* Infection, Crohn's/UC, cancer. *U&E:* K⁺↓≈severe D&V. *TSH↓:* Thyrotoxicosis. *Coeliac serology:* p280.
- **Stool** *MC&S:* Bacterial pathogens, ova cysts, parasites *C. diff* toxin (see BOX). *Faecal fat excretion* or ¹³C-hiolein (highly labelled triolein) breath test (nicer and reliable) if symptoms of chronic pancreatitis, malabsorption, or steatorrhoea.[67]
- **Rigid sigmoidoscopy** With biopsy of normal and abnormal looking mucosa: ~15% of patients with Crohn's disease have macroscopically normal mucosa.
- **Colonoscopy/barium enema** (malignancy? colitis?) ►Avoid in acute episode. If normal, consider small bowel radiology (eg Crohn's) ± ERCP (chronic pancreatitis).

**Management** Treat causes. Food handlers: no work until stool samples are -ve. If a hospital outbreak, wards may need closing. *Oral rehydration* is better than IV, but if impossible, give 0.9% saline + 20mmol K⁺/L IVI. ►If dehydrated and bloody diarrhoea for ≥2wks, IV fluids may well be needed. *Codeine phosphate* 30mg/8h PO or *loperamide* 2mg PO after each loose stool (max 16mg/day) ↓stool frequency (avoid in colitis; both may precipitate toxic megacolon).[68] Avoid antibiotics unless infective diarrhoea is causing systemic upset (fig 1) to avoid selecting resistant strains. *Antibiotic-associated diarrhoea[3]* may respond to probiotics (eg lactobacilli).

---

1 Think of this in any chronic diarrhoea; do biopsy (may be +ve on normal looking colonic mucosa—reported as 'lymphocytic' or 'collagenous' colitis). Prognosis: good. *Budesonide* is 1ˢᵗ-line, then 5-aminosalycics (p273), *bismuth* (eg Pepto-Bismol®), or *loperamide*.
2 Vasoactive intestinal polypeptide-secreting tumour; suspect if K⁺↓ and acidosis; Ca²⁺↑; Mg²⁺↓
3 Erythromycin is prokinetic, others cause overgrowth of bowel organisms, or alter bile acids.

**Common causes**
- Gastroenteritis
- Parasites/protozoa
- IBS (p276)
- Colorectal cancer
- Crohn's; UC; coeliac

**Less common causes**
- Microscopic colitis[1]
- Chronic pancreatitis
- Bile salt malabsorption
- Laxative abuse
- Lactose intolerance
- Ileal/gastric resection
- Overflow diarrhoea
- Diverticular disease
- Bacterial overgrowth
- *C. difficile* (BOX)

**Non-GI or rare causes**
- Thyrotoxicosis
- Autonomic neuropathy
- Addison's disease
- Ischaemic colitis
- Tropical sprue •Pellagra
- Gastrinoma •VIPoma[2]
- Carcinoid •Amyloid

**Drugs** (many, see BNF)
- Antibiotics[3] •PPI
- Propranolol •NSAIDs
- Cytotoxics •Digoxin
- Laxatives •Alcohol

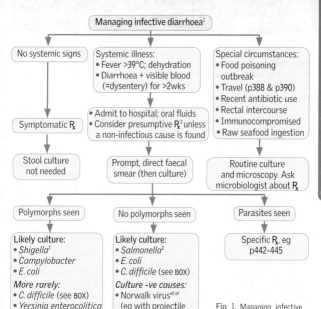

Fig 1. Managing infective diarrhoea.

---

### *Clostridium difficile*: the cause of pseudomembranous colitis

*C. difficile* is a Gram +ve 'superbug' whose spores are contagious (faecal-oral or from the environment, where spores can live for ages and are hard to eradicate).

*Signs:* T°↑; colic; mild diarrhoea—or serious bloody diarrhoea with systemic upset—CRP↑↑, WCC↑↑, albumin↓, and colitis (with yellow adherent plaques on inflamed non-ulcerated mucosa—the pseudomembrane) and multi-organ failure.

*Asymptomatic carriage:* 1-3% of all adults (∴ broad-spectrum/IV antibiotic use).

*Predictors of fulminant C. diff colitis:* >70yrs; past *C. diff* infection; use of antiperistaltic drugs; Girotra's triad: 1 Increasing abdominal pain/distention and diarrhoea 2 Leukocytosis >18,000 3 Haemodynamic instability.[69] *Deaths:* 6500/yr[uk].

*Toxins:* Tissue culture, ELISA, and PCR help defect *C. difficile* toxins (CDT). Some strains produce no toxin and are non-pathogenic; most produce toxins A and B. Some strains are hypervirulent, eg NAP1/027.

*R:* Stop the causative antibiotic (if possible). Treatment is not usually needed if asymptomatic (use of antibiotics for *C. difficile* is controversial). If symptomatic, give **metronidazole** ≤400mg/8h PO for ≤10d (**vancomycin** 125mg/6h PO is better in severe disease; if complications, up to 2g/day).[70]

▶Urgent colectomy may be needed if toxic megacolon, LDH↑, or if deteriorating.

*Recurrent disease:* Repeat metronidazole once only (overuse causes irreversible neuropathy). NB: probiotics may prevent recurrences (*Saccharomyces boulardii* 500mg/12h PO, unless immunosuppressed or CVP line *in situ*). Administration of stools (via NGT or colonoscope) from healthy subjects may have a role.[70]

*Preventing spread:* Meticulous cleaning, use of disposable gloves, not using rectal thermometers, hand-washing, and ward protocols (eg 'bare below elbows').

---

1 Be aware of your local pathogens, and be prepared to close wards and hospitals if contagion is afoot.
2 Prompt specific R: eg ciprofloxacin 500mg/12h PO for 6d may be needed before sensitivities are known. Metronidazole is also tried, as giardia is a common cause of watery diarrhoea (no leukocytes) in travellers.

Gastroenterology

Constipation reflects ↑transit time or pelvic dysfunction, eg a rectocele.[1] 30% of us feel we are constipated (only 15% meet the Rome criteria, BOX).[1] ♀:♂≈2:1. Doctors' chief concerns are to find pointers to major pathology, eg constipation + rectal bleeding≈cancer; constipation + distension + active bowel sounds≈stricture/GI obstruction; constipation + menorrhagia≈hypothyroidism,[etc].

**The patient** Ask about frequency, nature, and consistency of stools. Is there blood or mucus in/on the stools? Is there diarrhoea alternating with constipation (eg IBS, p276)? Has there been recent change in bowel habit? Any pain?[1] Ask about diet and drugs. ▶PR examination can be essential. Refer the patient if there are atypical features, eg weight↓, abdominal pain, and anaemia (signs of colorectal ca).

**Tests** (?None in young, mildly affected patients.) Indications for investigation: age >40yrs; change in bowel habit; associated symptoms (weight↓, PR mucus or blood, tenesmus). *Blood:* FBC, ESR, U&E, $Ca^{2+}$, TFT. *Sigmoidoscopy* and biopsy of abnormal mucosa. *Barium enema/colonoscopy* if suspected colorectal malignancy. Transit studies; anorectal physiology; biopsy for Hirschprung's[etc] are occasionally needed.

**Treatment** Often reassurance, drinking more, and diet/exercise advice (p237) is all that is needed. Treat causes (BOX). A high-fibre diet is often advised, but may cause bloating without helping constipation.[2] ▶Only use drugs if these measures fail, and try to use them for short periods only.[2] Often, a stimulant such as **senna** ± a bulking agent is more effective and cheaper than agents such as *lactulose*.[2] *Bulking agents* ↑faecal mass, so stimulating peristalsis. They must be taken with plenty of fluid and may take a few days to act. CI: difficulty in swallowing; GI obstruction; colonic atony; faecal impaction. *Bran* powder 3.5g 2-3 times/d with food (may hinder absorption of dietary trace elements if taken with every meal).[3] *Ispaghula husk*, eg 1 Fybogel® 3.5g sachet after a meal, mixed in water and swallowed promptly (or else it becomes an unpleasant sludge). *Methylcellulose*, eg Celevac® 3-6 500mg tablets/12h with ≥300mL water. *Sterculia*, eg Normacol® granules, 10mL sprinkled on food daily. *Stimulant laxatives* increase intestinal motility, so do not use in intestinal obstruction or acute colitis. Avoid prolonged use as it **may** cause colonic atony and hypokalaemia (but there are no good long-term data). Abdominal cramps are an important SE. Pure stimulant laxatives are *bisacodyl* tablets (5-10mg at night) or suppositories (10mg in the mornings) and *senna* (2-4 tablets at night). *Docusate sodium* and *danthron*[3] (=dantron) have stimulant and softening actions. *Glycerol* suppositories act as a rectal stimulant. *Sodium picosulfate* (5-10mg up to 12h beforehand) is useful for rapid bowel evacuation prior to procedures. *Stool softeners* are particularly useful when managing painful anal conditions, eg fissure. *Arachis oil* enemas lubricate and soften impacted faeces. *Liquid paraffin* should not be used for a prolonged period (SE: anal seepage, lipoid pneumonia, malabsorption of fat-soluble vitamins). *Osmotic laxatives* retain fluid in the bowel. *Lactulose*, a semisynthetic disaccharide, produces osmotic diarrhoea of low faecal pH that discourages growth of ammonia-producing organisms. *Macrogol* (eg Movicol®) is another example. It is useful in hepatic encephalopathy (initial dose: 30-50mL/12h). SE: bloating, so its role in treating constipation is limited. *Magnesium salts* (eg magnesium hydroxide; magnesium sulfate) are useful when rapid bowel evacuation is required. *Sodium salts* (eg Microlette® and Micralax® enemas) should be avoided as they may cause sodium and water retention. *Phosphate enemas* are useful for rapid bowel evacuation prior to procedures.

**If laxatives don't help** (eg after 6 months) A multidisciplinary approach with behaviour therapy, habit training ± sphincter biofeedback may help. $5HT_4$ agonists inducing peristalsis by systemic (not luminal) means include **prucalopride**.[4]

---

**1** *Rectocele:* front wall of the rectum bulges into the back wall of the vagina. **Levator ani syndrome:** chronic rectal pain without detectable organic cause, worse on walking and defecation. It may be reproduced by coccygeal traction (on PR) with a specific trigger point on the levator muscle.
**2** Risks of laxative abuse are overemphasized ('cathartic colon' is a questionable entity); stimulant laxatives may be used chronically on those who do not respond to bulk or osmotic laxatives alone.[5]
**3** Danthron causes colon & liver tumours in animals, so reserve use for the very elderly or terminally ill.

## 4 definitions of constipation

≤2 bowel actions/wk—or less often than the person's normal habit—or passed with difficulty, straining, or pain—or with a sense of incomplete evacuation.

## Making constipation glamorous

The best way to make something glamorous is to associate it with somewhere beautiful, immortal, and seductive, so now we have the famous Rome criteria—named after 'the eternal city'.

## The Rome criteria

Constipation: the presence of ≥2 symptoms during bowel movements (BMs):
• Straining for ≥25% of BMs
• Lumpy or hard stools in ≥25% of BMs
• Sensation of incomplete evacuations for ≥25% of BMs
• Sensation of anorectal obstruction or blockage for ≥25% of BMs
• Manual manoeuvres to facilitate at least 25% of BMs (eg digital evacuation, support of the pelvic floor)
• Fewer than 3 BMs per week

Chronicity entails constipation for the last 90 days, with onset ≥6 months ago.

## ✿ Rome feeds anal fixations[76]

▶Applying the Rome criteria teaches us to be obsessive about our bowels—a prime example of medicalizing our way into two diseases for the price of one—or, quite often, none, as it is possible to be healthy and pass stools only weekly.

As well as moving beyond the traditional oral, anal and phallic stages of development, we propose that doctors must also move beyond their stage of obsessive counting, before they can be of real service to their patients.[77]

## All roads lead away from Rome

Most people declaring themselves to be constipated do so in flagrant disregard of the Rome criteria,[78] perhaps on the grounds that you cannot tell someone they are not hungry just because they eat more than 2 meals a day.

Ironically, the highest prevalence of constipation is in nursing homes, the one place where Rome cannot penetrate may be as inmates may be too demented to report sensations of anal blockage.[79] This is an example of **vicarious constipation**, ie leading your life painfully slowly, through the bowels of another.

## Causes of constipation

### General
• Poor diet ± lack of exercise
• Poor fluid intake/dehydration
• Irritable bowel syndrome
• Old age
• Post-operative pain
• Hospital environment (↓privacy; having to use a bed pan)
• Distant, squalid, or fearsome toilets

### Anorectal disease (esp. if painful)
▶▶ Anal or colorectal cancer
• Fissures (p632), strictures, herpes
• Rectal prolapse
• Proctalgia fugax (p632)
• Mucosal ulceration/neoplasia
• Pelvic muscle dysfunction/levator ani syndrome[1]

### Intestinal obstruction
▶▶ Colorectal carcinoma (p618)
• Strictures (eg Crohn's disease)
• Pelvic mass (eg fetus, fibroids)
• Diverticulosis (rectal bleeding is a commoner presentation)
• Pseudo-obstruction (p613)

### Metabolic/endocrine
• Hypercalcaemia (p690)
• Hypothyroidism (rarely *presents* with constipation)
• Hypokalaemia (p688)
• Porphyria
• Lead poisoning

### Drugs (pre-empt by diet advice)
• Opiates (eg morphine, codeine)
• Anticholinergics (eg tricyclics)
• Iron
• Some antacids, eg with aluminium
• Diuretics, eg furosemide
• Calcium channel blockers

### Neuromuscular (slow transit from decreased propulsive activity)
• Spinal or pelvic nerve injury (eg trauma, surgery)
• Aganglionosis (Chagas' disease, Hirschsprung's disease)
• Systemic sclerosis
• Diabetic neuropathy

### Other causes
• Chronic laxative abuse (rare—diarrhoea is commoner)
• Idiopathic slow transit
• Idiopathic megarectum/colon
✿ Psychological, eg anorexia nervosa, depression, or abuse as a child.

NB: constipation is unlikely to be the sole symptom of serious disease, so be reassuring (if PR, ESR & TSH are ↔).

Jaundice (icterus) refers to yellowing of skin, sclerae, and mucosae from ↑plasma bilirubin (visible at ≥60µmol/L—not always easy to spot if mild, fig 1). Jaundice is classified by the site of the problem (pre-hepatic, hepatocellular, or cholestatic/obstructive) or by the type of circulating bilirubin (conjugated or unconjugated). Kernicterus=unbound bilirubin deposited in infant basal ganglia (→opisthotonus).

**Unconjugated hyperbilirubinaemia** As unconjugated bilirubin is water insoluble, it does not enter urine, resulting in unconjugated (acholuric) hyperbilirubinaemia.

*Overproduction:* Haemolysis (p332, eg malaria/DIC, etc); ineffective erythropoiesis.

*Impaired hepatic uptake:* Drugs (contrast agents, rifampicin), right heart failure.

*Impaired conjugation:* Eponymous syndromes: Gilbert's, p714; Crigler-Najjar, p710.

*Physiological neonatal jaundice* is caused by a combination of the above, OHCS p115.

**Conjugated hyperbilirubinaemia** *Hepatocellular dysfunction:* There is hepatocyte damage, usually with some cholestasis. *Causes: Viruses:* hepatitis (A, B, C[etc] p406); CMV (p404); EBV (p401); drugs (see TABLE); alcohol; cirrhosis (see BOX); liver metastases/abscess; haemochromatosis; autoimmune hepatitis (AIH); septicaemia; leptospirosis; syphilis; $\alpha_1$-antitrypsin deficiency (p264); Budd-Chiari (p710); Wilson's disease (p269); failure to excrete conjugated bilirubin (Dubin-Johnson & Rotor syndromes, p712-24); right heart failure; toxins, eg carbon tetrachloride; fungi (fig 3).

*Impaired hepatic excretion (cholestasis):* Primary biliary cirrhosis; primary sclerosing cholangitis; drugs (BOX); common bile duct gallstones; pancreatic cancer; compression of the bile duct, eg lymph nodes at the porta hepatis; cholangiocarcinoma; choledochal cyst; Caroli's disease;[1] biliary atresia; Mirrizi's syndrome (obstructive jaundice from common bile duct compression by a gallstone impacted in the cystic duct, often associated with cholangitis). As conjugated bilirubin is water soluble, it is excreted in urine, making it dark. Less conjugated bilirubin enters the gut and the faeces become pale. When severe, it can be associated with an intractable pruritus which is best treated by relief of the obstruction.

**The patient** *Ask* about blood transfusions, IV drug use, body piercing, tattoos, sexual activity, travel abroad, jaundiced contacts, family history, alcohol use, and all medications (eg old drug charts; GP records). *Examine* for signs of chronic liver disease (p260), hepatic encephalopathy (p259), lymphadenopathy, hepatomegaly, splenomegaly, ascites and a palpable gallbladder (if seen with painless jaundice the cause is not gallstones—Courvoisier's law').[2] Pale stools + dark urine ≈ cholestatic jaundice.

**Tests** See p260 for screening tests in suspected liver disease.[3] *Urine:* Bilirubin is absent in pre-hepatic causes (=acholuric jaundice); in obstructive jaundice, urobilinogen is absent. *Haematology:* FBC, clotting, film, reticulocyte count, Coombs' test and haptoglobins for haemolysis (p330), malaria parasites (eg if unconjugated bilirubin/fever); Paul Bunnell (EBV). *Chemistry:* U&E, LFT[2] (bilirubin—unconjugated & conjugated), ALT, AST, alk phos, γ-GT, total protein, albumin.[10] If AST >1000, it's probably viral hepatitis. Paracetamol levels. *Microbiology:* Blood and other cultures; leptospira & hepatitis A, B, C serology[etc]. *Ultrasound:* Are the bile ducts dilated >6mm (obstruction)? Are there gallstones, hepatic metastases or a pancreatic mass? ERCP (p756) if bile ducts are dilated and LFT not improving. MRCP (p756) or endoscopic ultrasound (EUS) if conventional ultrasound shows gallstones but no definite common bile duct stones. *Liver biopsy* (p256) if bile ducts are normal. Consider abdominal CT/MRI if abdominal malignancy is suspected.

**What to do?** ▸▸ *Treat the cause promptly.* A stone causing mild jaundice today may be causing fatal pancreatitis or ascending cholangitis tomorrow. If it's malaria, you may only have a few hours. If the liver is failing (ascites, encephalopathy[etc]; p258), get help from a hepatologist; do INR. In post-hepatic causes, is stenting needed?

---

1 Multiple segmental cystic or saccular dilatations of intrahepatic bile ducts with congenital hepatic fibrosis. It may present in 20yr-olds, with portal hypertension±recurrent cholangitis/cholelithiasis.
2 Pancreatic or gall bladder cancer is more likely, as stones would have fibrosed the GB (∴ unexpandable).
3 Albumin & INR are the best indicators of hepatic synthetic function. ↑Transaminases (ALT, AST) indicate hepatocyte damage. ↑Alk phos suggests obstructive jaundice, but also occurs in hepatocellular jaundice, malignant infiltration, pregnancy (placental isoenzyme), Paget's disease, and childhood (bone isoenzyme).

Fig 1. It's easy to miss mild jaundice, especially under fluorescent light, so take your patient to the window, and as you both gaze at the sky, use the opportunity to broaden the horizons of your enquiries ... where have you been ... where are you going ... who are you with ... what are you taking ...? ☜In the gaps, your patient may tell you the diagnosis—alcohol or drug abuse, sexual infections/hepatitis, or worries about the side-effects of their TB or HIV medication or a spreading cancer "from this lump here which I haven't told anyone about yet." Reproduced from *Clinical Skills, Second Edition*, by T.A. Roper, ©OUP.

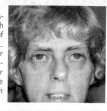

## The pathway of bilirubin metabolism

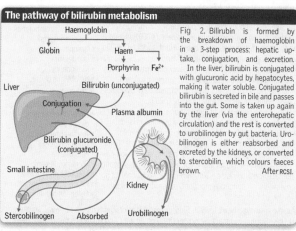

Fig 2. Bilirubin is formed by the breakdown of haemoglobin in a 3-step process: hepatic uptake, conjugation, and excretion.

In the liver, bilirubin is conjugated with glucuronic acid by hepatocytes, making it water soluble. Conjugated bilirubin is secreted in bile and passes into the gut. Some is taken up again by the liver (via the enterohepatic circulation) and the rest is converted to urobilinogen by gut bacteria. Urobilinogen is either reabsorbed and excreted by the kidneys, or converted to stercobilin, which colours faeces brown. After RCSI.

## Causes of jaundice in a previously stable patient with cirrhosis

• Sepsis (esp. UTI, pneumonia, or peritonitis)
• Malignancy: eg hepatocellular carcinoma
• Alcohol; drugs (BOX)
• GI bleeding

*Signs of decompensation:* Ascites; dilated abdominal veins; CNS signs; oedema.

## Examples of drug-induced jaundice  (Look for an eosinophilia ± WCC↑/DRESS)★

| Haemolysis | • Antimalarials (eg dapsone) | |
|---|---|---|
| Hepatitis | • Paracetamol overdose (p856) | • Sodium valproate |
| | • Isoniazid, rifampicin, pyrazinamide | • Halothane |
| | • Monoamine oxidase inhibitors | • Statins |
| Cholestasis | • Flucloxacillin (may be weeks after R) | • Sulfonylureas |
| | • Fusidic acid, co-amoxiclav, nitrofurantoin | • Prochlorperazine |
| | • Steroids (anabolic; the Pill) | • Chlorpromazine |

★DRESS = drug rash with eosinophilia & systemic symptoms (fever, dyspnoea etc)[81]

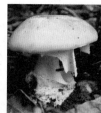

Fig 3. *Amanita phalloides* (Latin for 'phallic toadstool'; also known as the 'death cap') is a lethal cause of jaundice. It is the most toxic mushroom known. After ingestion (its benign appearance is confusing), amatoxins induce hepatic necrosis, eg with liver failure. Some have been treated successfully by transplantation.

©Ian Herriott. NB: don't use this image for identification!

Gastroenterology

**Haematemesis** is vomiting of blood. It may be bright red or look like coffee grounds. **Melaena** (Greek *melas* = black) means black motions, often like tar, and has a characteristic smell of altered blood. Both indicate upper GI bleeding.

Take a brief history and examine to assess severity. *Ask about* past GI bleeds; dyspepsia/known ulcers; known liver disease or oesophageal varices (p254); dysphagia; vomiting; weight loss. Check drugs (see MINIBOX) and alcohol use. Is there serious comorbidity (bad prognosis), eg cardiovascular disease, respiratory disease, hepatic or renal impairment, or malignancy? *Look for* signs of chronic liver disease (p260) and do a PR to check for melaena. Is the patient shocked? ►"Do you feel faint when you sit up?" Also:

| Common causes |
| --- |
| • Peptic ulcers |
| • Mallory-Weiss tear |
| • Oesophageal varices |
| • Gastritis/gastric erosions |
| • Drugs (NSAIDs, aspirin, steroids, thrombolytics, anticoagulants) |
| • Oesophagitis |
| • Duodenitis |
| • Malignancy |
| • No obvious cause |

| Rare causes |
| --- |
| • Bleeding disorders |
| • Portal hypertensive gastropathy |
| • Aorto-enteric fistula[2] |
| • Angiodysplasia |
| • Haemobilia |
| • Dieulafoy lesion[3] |
| • Meckel's diverticulum |
| • Peutz-Jeghers' syndrome |
| • Osler-Weber-Rendu synd. |

• Peripherally shut down/cool and clammy; capillary refilling (CR) time >2s—urine output <½ mL/kg/h.
• ↓GCS (tricky to assess in decompensated liver disease) or signs of encephalopathy (p259).
• Poor urine output, eg <25mL/h or <½mL/kg/h.
• Tachycardic (pulse >100bpm, and JVP not raised).
• Systolic BP <100mmHg; postural drop >20mmHg.
• Do the *Rockall score* (TABLE). Alternative: the *Glasgow Blatchford score (GBS)*—if GBS≈0, admission can be avoided—ie Hb ≥130g/L (or ≥120g/L if ♀); systolic BP ≥110mmHg; pulse <100/min; urea <6.5mmol/L; no melaena or syncope + no past/present liver disease or heart failure.

**Acute management** (p830). Skill in resuscitation determines survival, so get good at this! Summary: start by protecting the airway and giving high-flow $O_2$, then:
►► Insert 2 large-bore (14-16G) IV cannulae and take blood for FBC (an early Hb may be normal because haemodilution has not yet taken place), U&E (↑urea out of proportion to creatinine is indicative of a massive blood meal), LFT, clotting, and crossmatch 4-6 units (give 1 unit for each 10g/L that the Hb is less than 140g/L).
►► Give IV fluids (p831) to restore intravascular volume while waiting for blood to be crossmatched.[82] In a dire emergency—ie haemodynamically deteriorating despite fluid resuscitation measures—give group O Rh-ve blood.
►► Insert a urinary catheter and monitor hourly urine output.
►► Organize a CXR, ECG, and check ABG.
►► Consider a CVP line to monitor and guide fluid replacement.
►► Transfuse (with crossmatched blood if needed) until haemodynamically stable.
►► Correct clotting abnormalities (vitamin K (p258), FFP, platelets).
►► Monitor pulse, BP, and CVP (keep >5cmH2O) at least hourly until stable.
►► Omeprazole, eg 80mg as a bolus dose IV then continuous IVI at 8mg/h for 3d.[83, 84]
►► Arrange an urgent *endoscopy*, preferably at a dedicated endoscopy unit.[85, 86 1]
►► Inform surgeons of severe bleeds on admission—if endoscopic control fails, surgery may be needed—or emergency mesenteric angiography/embolization.

**Further management** ►Anatomy is important in assessing risk of rebleeding. Posterior DUs are highest risk as they are nearest to the gastroduodenal artery.
• Re-examine after 4h and ask about the need for FFP if >4 units transfused.
• Hourly pulse, BP, CVP, urine output (4hrly if haemodynamically stable may be OK).
• Transfuse to keep Hb >100g/L; always keep 2 units of blood in reserve.
• Check FBC, U&E, LFT, and clotting daily.
• Keep nil by mouth for 24h. Allow clear fluids after 24h and light diet after 48h, as long as there is no evidence of rebleeding (BOX and p254).

1 National Confidential Enquiry into Patient Outcome & Death (NCEPOD) says that in 7% endoscopy is too late.
2 A patient with an aortic graft repair and upper GI bleeding is considered to have an aorto-enteric fistula until proven otherwise: CT abdomen is usually required as well as endoscopy.
3 A Dieulafoy lesion is the rupture of an unusually big arteriole, eg in the fundus of the stomach.

## Gastritis

*Causes:* Alcohol, NSAIDs, *H. pylori*, reflux/hiatus hernia, atrophic gastritis, granulo-mas (Crohn's; sarcoidosis), CMV, Zollinger-Ellison & Ménétrier's disease (p730 & 720).
*Presentation:* Epigastric pain, vomiting; haematemesis. *Δ:* Endoscopy + biopsy.
*Prevention:* Give PPI gastroprotection with NSAIDs; this also prevents bleeding from acute stress ulcers/gastritis so often seen with ill patients (esp. burns) on ITU.
*Treatment:* Ranitidine or PPI; eradicate *H. pylori* as needed (p243). Triple thera-py now often fails: quadruple R with bismuth subcitrate may be needed. Trox-ipide 100mg/8h PO improves gastric mucus. Endoscopic cautery may be needed.

## Rockall risk-scoring for upper GI bleeds

| | 0 pts | 1 pt | 2 pts | 3 pts |
|---|---|---|---|---|
| **Pre-endoscopy** | | | | |
| Age[I] | <60yrs | 60–79yrs | ≥80yrs | |
| Shock: systolic BP & pulse rate[I] | BP >100mmHg Pulse <100/min | BP >100mmHg Pulse >100/min | BP <100mmHg | |
| Comorbidity[I] | Nil major | | Heart failure; ischae-mic heart disease | Renal failure Liver failure | Metast-ases |
| **Post-endoscopy** Diagnosis[F] | Mallory-Weiss tear; no lesion; no sign of recent bleeding | All other diagnoses | Upper GI malig-nancy | |
| Signs of recent haemorrhage on endoscopy[F] | None, or dark red spot | | Blood in upper GI tract; adherent clot; visible vessel | |

I These criteria make up the initial Rockall score.[87] F Added to the initial score, these criteria give the final Rockall score. Other scores have been compared prospectively—the Glasgow Blatchford score (GBS, see opposite), an age-extended GBS (EGBS), the Baylor bleeding score, and the Cedars-Sinai Medical Centre predictive index. The EGBS is the most promising but needs validating. No scoring system seems to accurately predict patients' 30-day mortality, or rebleeding.[88] See the non-parametric paradox p10, for one reason why. The table below is the most optimistic attempt to do so, but your patient may not behave as predicted.

## Prediction of rebleeding and mortality from the Rockall score[89]

Rockall scores help predict risk of rebleeding and mortality after upper GI ble-eding.[90] An initial score >6 is said to be an indication for surgery, but decisions relating to surgery are rarely taken on the basis of Rockall scores alone (p254).

| Score | Mortality with initial scoring | Mortality after endoscopy |
|---|---|---|
| 0 | 0.2% | 0% |
| 1 | 2.4% | 0% |
| 2 | 5.6% | 0.2% |
| 3 | 11.0% | 2.9% |
| 4 | 24.6% | 5.3% |
| 5 | 39.6% | 10.8% |
| 6 | 48.9% | 17.3% |
| 7 | 50.0% | 27.0% |
| 8+ | - | 41.1% |

## Management of peptic ulcer bleeds based on endoscopic findings

**High-risk**[91] *Active bleeding or non-bleeding visible vessel:* Admit patient to a monitored bed or ICU and perform endoscopic haemostasis (eg Endoclip).[92] Start PPI by IVI (opposite). H₂ blockers and somatostatin (octreotide) have no role. If haemodynamically stable start oral intake of clear liquids 6h after endoscopy. Change to oral PPI after 72h. Eradication therapy if *H. pylori* is present.

*Adherent clot:* Remove at endoscopy and ensure haemostasis; treat as above.

**Low-risk** *Flat, pigmented spot or clean base:* There is no need for endoscopic haemostasis. Consider early hospital discharge after endoscopy if the patient has an otherwise low clinical risk and safe home environment. Treat with a PPI (p242). Initiate oral intake with a regular diet 6h after endoscopy in stable pa-tients. Initiate treatment if positive for *H. pylori* (p243).

**Endoscopy** should be arranged after resuscitation, within 4h of a suspected variceal haemorrhage, or when bleeding is ongoing within 24h of admission (fig 1). It can: •Identify bleeding sites •Help estimate risk of rebleeding •Aid treatment—sclerotherapy, variceal banding (fig 2), or argon plasma coagulation (for superficial lesions).[93] *Endoscopic signs associated with risk of rebleeding:* Active arterial bleeding (80% risk); visible vessel (50% risk); adherent clot/black dots (30% risk).

**Rebleeding** 40% of rebleeders die of complications. Identify high-risk patients (TABLE, p253) and monitor closely for signs of rebleeding. IVI of *omeprazole* has a preventive role. Get help; inform a surgeon at once if: • Haematemesis with melaena •↑Pulse rate •↓CVP (assess via JVP or CVP line) •↓BP •↓Urine output.

**Indications for surgery** (p626) ▶Contact the surgical team at the onset.
• Severe bleeding or bleeding despite transfusing 6U if >60yrs (8U if <60yrs).
• Active or uncontrollable bleeding at endoscopy—or rebleeding.
• Initial Rockall score ≥3 or final Rockall score >6 (but see TABLE, p253).

**Oesophageal varices** *Pathogenesis:* Progressive liver fibrosis + regenerative nodules produce contractile elements in the liver's vascular beds→Portal hypertension→Splanchnic vasodilation→Increased cardiac output→Salt and water retention→Hyperdynamic circulation/increased portal flow→Formation of collaterals between the portal and systemic systems, eg in the lower oesophagus and gastric cardia→Gastro-oesophageal varices develop once portal pressure (measured by hepatic venous pressure gradient) is >10mmHg→If >12mmHg variceal bleeding may be brisk→Death (more likely if clotting problems and advanced cirrhosis).[94] 6-week mortality depends on severity of liver disease (~0% for Child A; ~30% for Child C).[94] Rebleeding is common and is worse with large varices. NB: varices may also be found in the stomach, around the umbilicus (*caput medusae* is rare), and in the rectum.

**Causes of portal hypertension** *Pre-hepatic:* Thrombosis (portal or splenic vein). *Intra-hepatic:* Cirrhosis (80% in UK); schistosomiasis (commonest worldwide); sarcoid; myeloproliferative diseases; congenital hepatic fibrosis. *Post-hepatic:* Budd-Chiari syndrome (p710); right heart failure; constrictive pericarditis; veno-occlusive disease. *Risk factors for variceal bleeds:* ↑Portal pressure, variceal size, endoscopic features of the variceal wall (eg haematocystic spots) and Child-Pugh score ≥8 (p261).[95]

**Suspect varices as a cause of GI bleeding** if there is alcohol abuse or cirrhosis. Look for signs of chronic liver disease, encephalopathy, splenomegaly, ascites, hyponatraemia, coagulopathy, and thrombocytopenia.

**Prophylaxis** *Primary:* ~30% of cirrhotics with varices bleed—reducible to 15% by: 1 Non-selective β-blockade (propranolol 40-80mg/12h PO) 2 Repeat endoscopic banding ligation. Which is better in cirrhosis? Studies give conflicting answers.[96, 97] Deaths related to bleeding are similar (~7%), but ligation is riskier. Endoscopic sclerotherapy is not used as complications (eg stricturing) may outweigh benefits.[98]

*Secondary:* After a 1st variceal bleed, 60% rebleed within 1yr. Options are 1 & 2 as above + transjugular intrahepatic porto-systemic shunt (TIPS)[1] for varices resistant to banding (surgical shunt if TIPS is impossible for technical reasons). Endoscopic banding may be better than sclerotherapy (↓bleeding rates; fewer complications).[99]

**Acute variceal bleeding** Get help at the bedside from your senior.
▶▶Resuscitate until haemodynamically stable (avoid saline). If very anaemic, transfuse to Hb of 80g/L. NB: over-resuscitating may augment bleeding.
▶▶Correct clotting abnormalities with *vitamin K* (p258), FFP and platelet transfusions. Studies on Factor VIIa failed to show benefit in terms of mortality.
▶▶Start IVI of *terlipressin*, eg 1-2mg/6h for ≤3d; relative risk of death ↓ by 34%.[100] Somatostatin analogues are alternatives (less used in the UK).[101, 102]
▶▶Endoscopic banding (fig 2) or sclerotherapy should be tried (banding may be impossible because of limited visualization).
▶▶If bleeding uncontrolled, a Minnesota tube or Sengstaken-Blakemore tube (see BOX) should be placed by someone with experience; get an anaesthetist's help.

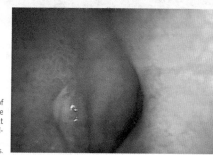

Fig 1. Endoscopy image of a duodenal ulcer (p235). See also 'Lumen', p235 for what can happen when such ulcers bleed.

©Dr Jon Simmons.

## Balloon tamponade with a Sengstaken-Blakemore tube

In life-threatening variceal bleeding, this can buy time for transfer to a specialist liver centre or for surgical decompression.[1] It uses balloons to compress gastro-oesophageal varices. Before insertion, inflate balloons with a measured volume (120-300mL) of air giving pressures of 60mmHg (check with sphygmomanometer).

- Deflate, and clamp exits; then pass the lubricated tube (try to avoid sedation) and inflate the gastric balloon with the predetermined volume of air. Cooling the tube beforehand probably doesn't make it any easier to pass.[103]
- ▶ Check position with a portable x-ray before inflating the oesophageal balloon.
- Check pressures (should be 20-30mmHg greater than on the trial run). This phase of the procedure is dangerous: do not over-inflate the balloon because of the risk of oesophageal necrosis or rupture.
- Tape to patient's forehead to ensure the gastric balloon impacts gently on the gastro-oesophageal junction.
- Place the oesophageal aspiration channel on continuous low suction and arrange for the gastric channel to drain freely.
- Leave *in situ* until bleeding stops. Remove after <24h.

Various other techniques of insertion may be used, and tubes vary in structure. ▶Do not try to pass one yourself if you have no or little experience: ask an expert; if unavailable, transfer urgently to a specialist liver centre.

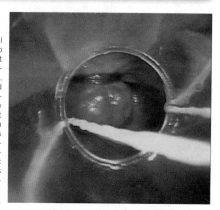

Fig 2. Endoscopic variceal banding involves sucking up a varix into the transparent banding chamber, then placing an elastic band around it. After a few days the banded varix starts to slough, leaving scar tissue in a shallow ulcer. Preventing recurrent variceal bleeds demands a combination of β-blockers and endoscopic band ligation. TIPS (transjugular intrahepatic porto-systemic shunts)[1] are for when this has not worked (or will probably not work, 'early TIPS').

©Dr Jon Simmons.

1 TIPS shunts blood away from the portal circulation through an artificial side-to-side porto-systemic anastomosis in the liver; also used in uncontrolled variceal haemorrhage. Patients with associated renal failure, decreased cardiac preload, and decreased cardiac performance benefit most from TIPS.[104]

Gastroenterology

►Consent is needed for all these procedures; see p570. SBE/IE prophylaxis isn't usually needed, but if neutropenic, immunocompromised, or partially draining possibly infected bile, antibiotics may be used (eg **ciprofloxacin** 750mg PO 1h pre-op).[105]

**Upper GI endoscopy** *Indications:* BOX 1. *Pre-procedure:* Stop PPIs, etc 2wks pre-op if possible (∴ pathology-masking). Nil by mouth for 4h before. Don't drive for 24h if sedation is used. *Procedure:* Sedation, eg *midazolam* 1-5mg slowly IV (to remain conscious; if deeper sedation is needed, *propofol* via an anaesthetist (narrow therapeutic range)); nasal prong O₂ (eg 2L/min; monitor respirations & ECG, not just oximetry). The pharynx is sprayed with local anaesthetic before the endoscope is passed. Continuous suction must be available to prevent aspiration. *Complications:* Sore throat; amnesia from sedation; perforation (<0.1%); cardiorespiratory arrest (<0.1%). Bleeding can be a big problem (eg with sphincterotomies); get help if on clopidogrel or warfarin (stop 5d pre-op, start LMWH, p344, 48h later; restart warfarin on day 5).

**Duodenal biopsy** is the gold standard for diagnosing coeliac disease (p280). It is also useful in investigating unusual causes of malabsorption, eg giardiasis, lymphoma, Whipple's disease, amyloid, or microscopic colitis (p246).

**Sigmoidoscopy** views the rectum + sigmoid colon to splenic flexion. Do rigid or flexible sigmoidoscopy before barium enema in suspected cancer. Flexible sigmoidoscopes gain the best access (→splenic flexure), but ~25% of cancers are still out of reach. It can be used therapeutically (±insertion of a flatus tube) for decompression of sigmoid volvulus (BOX, p613). *Preparation:* Give a *phosphate enema*. *Procedure:* Learn from an expert; do PR exam first. Do biopsies—macroscopic appearances may be normal, eg IBD, amyloidosis, microscopic colitis.

**Colonoscopy** *Indications:* TABLE 2. *Preparation:* Stop iron 1wk pre-op; low residue diet 1-2d pre-op. Clear fluids but no solid food after lunch on the day before. *Sodium picosulfate* (Picolax®) 1 sachet for morning & afternoon on the day before. *Procedure:* Do PR first. Sedation (see above) and analgesia are given before a flexible colonoscope is passed and guided around the colon. *Complications:* Abdominal discomfort; incomplete examination; haemorrhage after biopsy or polypectomy; perforation (0.1%). See figs 2-6. Post-op: no alcohol, and advise against operating machinery for 1 day.

**Video capsule endoscopy (VCE)** "The best way to evaluate obscure GI bleeding (p320) and to detect small bowel Crohn's".[106] Do small bowel imaging (eg contrast) or patency capsule test ahead of VCE if patient has abdominal pain or symptoms suggesting small bowel obstruction. It surpasses CT enterography in finding small flat bowel bleeding lesions, and can detect oesophageal problems despite rapid transit. See BSG guidelines.[107]

Fig 1. Capsule endoscopy.

*Pre-op:* Clear fluids only the evening before then nil by mouth as for colonoscopy. *Procedure:* A capsule (fig 1) transmits video via radio to pads on the skin. Movies are stored in a device worn on the belt. Normal activity can take place for the day. *Complications:* Capsule retention in 1% (endoscopic or surgical removal is needed); obstruction, incomplete exam (eg battery failure, slow transit, achalasia). *Problems:* No therapeutic options; poor localization of lesions; may miss cancers (still a problem with newer devices, eg PillCam COLON 2—sensitivity only 77%).[108, 109]

**Liver biopsy** Route: *percutaneous* if INR OK, or *transjugular* with fresh frozen plasma. *Indications:* LFT↑, chronic viral, alcoholic or autoimmune hepatitis; suspected cirrhosis or liver cancer; biopsy of hepatic lesions; PUO. *Pre-op:* Nil by mouth for 8h. Are INR <1.5 and platelets >100×10⁹/L? Give analgesia. *Procedure:* Sedation may be given. Do under US/CT guidance; the liver borders are percussed out and where there is dullness in the mid-axillary line in expiration, *lidocaine* 2% is infiltrated down to the liver capsule. Breathing is rehearsed and a needle biopsy is taken with the breath held in expiration. Afterwards lie on the right side for 2h, then in bed for 4h; do pulse and BP regularly. *Complications:* Local pain; pneumothorax; bleeding (<0.5%); death (<0.1%).

## Indications for upper GI endoscopy

| Diagnostic indications | Therapeutic indications |
|---|---|
| Haematemesis | Treatment of bleeding lesions |
| New dyspepsia (if ≥55yrs old, p242) | Variceal banding and sclerotherapy |
| Gastric biopsy (?cancer) | Stricture dilatation |
| Duodenal biopsy | Stent insertion, laser therapy |
| Persistent vomiting | Argon plasma coagulation for suspected vascular abnormality |
| Iron deficiency (cancer, hiatus hernia^etc) | |

## Indications for colonoscopy

| Diagnostic indications | Therapeutic indications Stents |
|---|---|
| Rectal bleeding—when settled, if acute | Haemostasis (eg by clipping vessel) |
| Iron-deficiency anaemia (bleeding cancer) | Bleeding angiodysplasia lesion (argon |
| Persistent diarrhoea | beamer photocoagulation—delivers |
| Biopsy of lesion seen on barium enema | energy via gas in an ionized plasma) |
| Assessment or suspicion of IBD | Volvulus untwisting (decompression) |
| Colon cancer surveillance | Pseudo-obstruction    Polypectomy |

*Sherlock Holmes:* A blood culture done for SBE grows *Strep bovis*...S.H. astounds Watson by inserting his colonoscope to apprehend a hidden but deadly cancer—the known but arcane portal of entry ('translocation') of this otherwise rare bug.

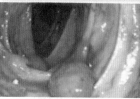

Fig 2. A big polyp seen on colonoscopy. An advantage of colonoscopy over barium enema is the ability to biopsy or intervene at the same time—in this case, polypectomy.

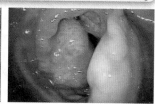

Fig 3. Colonoscopy image of an adenocarcinoma—p618. Compared with a colonic polyp (fig 2), the carcinoma is irregular in shape and colour, larger and more aggressive.

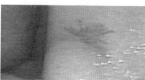

Fig 4. Angiodysplasia lesion seen at colonoscopy. Bleeding may be brisk. R: Endoscopic obliteration. See p630. It is associated with aortic stenosis (Heyde's syndrome).[110]

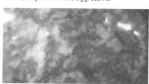

Fig 5. Colonic mucosa in active UC (p272); it is red, inflamed and friable (bleeds on touching). Signs of severity: mucopurulent exudate, mucosal ulceration ± spontaneous bleeding. If quiescent, there may only be a distorted or absent mucosal vascular pattern.

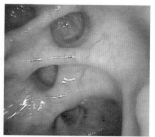

Fig 6. Colonoscopy image showing diverticulosis (p630). Navigating safely through the colon, avoiding the false lumina of the diverticula, can be a challenge. Don't go there if diverticula are inflamed (diverticulitis): perforation is a big risk. *Other CI to colonoscopy:* MI in last month; ischaemic colitis (*OHGH*, p165).

Figs 2 & 4 courtesy of Dr Anthony Mee.
Figs 3, 5 & 6 courtesy of Dr J Simmons.

More images: gastrosource.com/kisweb/atlas.htm

**Definitions** Liver failure may occur suddenly in the previously healthy liver = **acute hepatic failure**. More often it occurs as a result of decompensation of chronic liver disease = **acute-on-chronic hepatic failure**. **Fulminant hepatic failure** is a clinical syndrome resulting from massive necrosis of liver cells leading to severe impairment of liver function: **hyperacute** = encephalopathy (BOX 2) within 7d of onset of jaundice; **acute** = within 8-28d; **subacute** = within 5-26wks. There is decreasing risk of cerebral oedema as the onset of encephalopathy is increasingly delayed.

**Causes** *Infections:* Viral hepatitis (esp B, C, CMV), yellow fever, leptospirosis. *Drugs:* Paracetamol overdose, halothane, isoniazid. *Toxins:* Amanita phalloides mushroom (fig 3, p251), carbon tetrachloride. *Vascular:* Budd-Chiari synd. (p710), veno-occlusive disease. *Others:* Alcohol, primary biliary cirrhosis, haemochromatosis, autoimmune hepatitis, α₁-antitrypsin deficiency, Wilson's disease, fatty liver of pregnancy (*OHCS* p26), malignancy, HELLP syndrome (Haemolysis, Elevated Liver enzymes and Low Platelets; it is usually associated with pre-eclampsia) (*OHCS* p26).

**Signs** Jaundice, hepatic encephalopathy (see BOX 2), *fetor hepaticus* (smells like pear drops), asterixis/flap (p50), constructional apraxia (cannot copy a 5-pointed star?). Signs of chronic liver disease (p260) suggest acute-on-chronic hepatic failure.

**Tests** *Blood:* FBC (?infection,[1] ?GI bleed), U&E,[2] LFT, clotting (↑PT/INR), glucose, paracetamol level, hepatitis, CMV and EBV serology, ferritin, α₁-antitrypsin, caeruloplasmin, autoantibodies (p268). *Microbiology:* Blood culture; urine culture; ascitic tap for MC&S of ascites—neutrophils >250/mm³ indicates spontaneous bacterial peritonitis (p260). *Radiology:* CXR; abdominal ultrasound; Doppler flow studies of the portal vein (and hepatic vein in suspected Budd-Chiari syndrome, p710). *Neurophysiology:* EEG, evoked potentials (and neuroimaging) have a limited role.[111]

**Management** ▶▶Beware sepsis, hypoglycaemia, GI bleeds/varices & encephalopathy:
• Nurse with a 20° head-up tilt in ITU. Protect the airway with intubation and insert an NG tube to avoid aspiration and remove any blood from stomach.
• Insert urinary and central venous catheters to help assess fluid status.
• Monitor T°, respirations, pulse, BP, pupils, urine output hourly. Daily weights.
• Check FBC, U&E (BOX 2), LFT, and INR daily.
• 10% glucose IV, 1L/12h to avoid hypoglycaemia. Do blood glucose every 1-4h.
• Treat the cause, if known (eg GI bleeds, sepsis, paracetamol poisoning, p856). N-acetylcysteine probably does not help in non-paracetamol liver failure.[112]
• If malnourished, get dietary help: good nutrition can decrease mortality (eg carbohydrate-rich foods)[113] Give *thiamine* and *folate* supplements (p728).
• Treat seizures with *lorazepam* (p836).[114]
• Haemofiltration or haemodialysis, if renal failure develops (BOX 2).
• Try to avoid sedatives and other drugs with hepatic metabolism (BOX and *BNF*).
• Consider PPI as prophylaxis against stress ulceration, eg *omeprazole* 40mg/d IV/PO.
• Liaise early with nearest transplant centre regarding appropriateness—BOX 4.

**Treat complications** *Cerebral oedema:* On ITU: 20% *mannitol* IV; hyperventilate.

*Ascites:* Restrict fluid, low-salt diet, weigh daily, diuretics (p260).

*Bleeding: Vitamin K* 10mg/d IV for 3d, platelets, FFP + blood as needed ± endoscopy.

*Blind ℞ of infection: Ceftriaxone* 1-2g/24h IV, **not** gentamicin (↑risk of renal failure).

*↓Blood glucose:* If ≤2mmol/L or symptomatic, ℞ 50mL of 50% glucose IV; check often.

*Encephalopathy:* Avoid sedatives; 20° head-up tilt in ITU; *lactulose* 30-50mL/8h + regular enemas to ↓numbers of nitrogen-forming gut bacteria; aim for 2-4 soft stools/d.

**Worse prognosis if:** grade III-IV encephalopathy, age >40yrs, albumin <30g/L, ↑INR, drug-induced liver failure, late-onset hepatic failure worse than fulminant failure.

1 Neutrophilic leucocytosis need not mean a secondary infection: alcoholic hepatitis may be the cause.
2 Urea is synthesized in the liver, so is a poor test of renal function in liver failure; use creatinine instead.

## Prescribing in liver failure

Avoid drugs that constipate (opiates, diuretics—↑risk of encephalopathy), oral hypoglycaemics, and saline-containing IVIs. *Warfarin* effects are enhanced. *Hepatotoxic drugs include:* Paracetamol, methotrexate, isoniazid, azathioprine, phenothiazines, oestrogen, 6-mercaptopurine, salicylates, tetracycline, mitomycin.

## Hepatic encephalopathy: letting loose some false neurotransmitters

As the liver fails, nitrogenous waste (as ammonia) builds up in the circulation and passes to the brain, where astrocytes clear it (by processes involving the conversion of glutamate to glutamine). This excess glutamine causes an osmotic imbalance and a shift of fluid into these cells—hence cerebral oedema.[115] Grading:

I Altered mood/behaviour; sleep disturbance (eg reversed sleep pattern); dyspraxia ("Please copy this 5-pointed star"); poor arithmetic. No liver flap.

II Increasing drowsiness, confusion, slurred speech ± liver flap, inappropriate behaviour/personality change (ask the family—don't be too tactful).

III Incoherent; restless; liver flap; stupor, but not coma, which defines grade IV

▶What else could be clouding consciousness? Hypoglycaemia; sepsis; trauma; postictal.

## What is hepatorenal syndrome (HRS)?

Cirrhosis + ascites + renal failure ≈ HRS—*if other causes of renal impairment have been excluded*. Abnormal haemodynamics causes splanchnic and systemic vasodilatation, but renal *vasoconstriction*. Bacterial translocation, cytokines and mesenteric angiogenesis cause splanchnic vasodilatation, and altered renal autoregulation is involved in the renal vasoconstriction.

**Types of HRS:** *HRS I* is a rapidly progressive deterioration in circulatory and renal function (median survival <2wks), often triggered by other deteriorating pathologies. *Terlipressin* replenishes hypovolaemia. Haemodialysis may be needed.

*HRS 2* is a more steady deterioration (survival ~6 months). Transjugular intrahepatic portosystemic stent shunting is the best option for most (TIPS, p255).

**Other factors in cirrhosis** may contribute to poor renal function (p261).

**Transplants** Liver transplant may be required. After >8–12wks of pre-transplant dialysis, some may be considered for combined liver-kidney transplantation.[116, 117]

## King's College Hospital[UK] criteria for liver transplantation

| Paracetamol-induced liver failure | Non-paracetamol liver failure |
|---|---|
| • Arterial pH <7.3 24h after ingestion | • PT >100s |
| Or all of the following: | Or 3 out of 5 of the following: |
| • Prothrombin time (PT) >100s | 1 Drug-induced liver failure |
| • Creatinine >300μmol/L | 2 Age <10 or >40yrs old |
| • Grade III or IV encephalopathy | 3 >1wk from 1st jaundice to encephalopathy |
| | 4 PT >50s |
| | 5 Bilirubin ≥300μmol/L [118] |

Fulfilling these criteria predicts poor outcome in acute liver failure. Transplants are **cadaveric** (heart-beating or non-heart-beating)[1] or from **live donors** (right lobe)—**valid donor consent** is a problem. See p263 for indications in chronic disease. Refer earlier rather than later, eg when ascites is refractory or after a 1st episode of bacterial peritonitis. CI: active sepsis; ↓life-expectancy (≤2yrs[e]) from concurrent diseases; psychosocial factors precluding immunosuppression.

---

1 There is renewed interest in (and an increased number of) non-heart-beating cadaveric donors.[119]

**Gastroenterology**

Cirrhosis (Greek *kirrhos* = yellow) implies irreversible liver damage. Histologically, there is loss of normal hepatic architecture with bridging fibrosis and nodular regeneration.

**Causes** Most often chronic alcohol abuse, HBV, or HCV infection. Others: see BOX 1.

**Signs** May be none (just ↑LFT) or decompensated end-stage liver disease. *Chronic liver disease:* Leuconychia: white nails with lunulae undemarcated, from hypoalbuminaemia; Terry's nails—white proximally but distal ⅓ reddened by telangiectasias;[120] clubbing; palmar erythema; hyperdynamic circulation; Dupuytren's contracture; spider naevi (fig 1); xanthelasma; gynaecomastia; atrophic testes; loss of body hair; parotid enlargement; hepatomegaly, or small liver in late disease.

**Complications** *Hepatic failure:* Coagulopathy (↓factors II, VII, IX, & X causes ↑INR); encephalopathy—ie liver flap (asterixis) + confusion/coma; hypoalbuminaemia (oedema, leuconychia); sepsis (pneumonia; septicaemia); spontaneous bacterial peritonitis (SBP); hypoglycaemia. *Portal hypertension:* Ascites (fig 2); splenomegaly; portosystemic shunt including oesophageal varices (± life-threatening upper GI bleed) and *caput medusae* (enlarged superficial periumbilical veins). HCC: ↑risk.

**Tests** *Blood:* LFT: ↔ or ↑bilirubin, ↑AST, ↑ALT, ↑alk phos, ↑γGT. Later, with loss of synthetic function, look for ↓albumin ± ↑PT/INR. ↓WCC & ↓platelets indicate hypersplenism. *Find the cause:* Ferritin, iron/total iron-binding capacity (p262); hepatitis serology; immunoglobulins (p264); autoantibodies (ANA, AMA, SMA, p555); α-feto protein (p270); caeruloplasmin in patients <40yrs old (p269); α₁-antitrypsin (p264). *Liver ultrasound + duplex* may show a small liver or hepatomegaly, splenomegaly, focal liver lesion(s), hepatic vein thrombus, reversed flow in the portal vein, or ascites. *MRI:* Caudate lobe size↑, smaller islands of regenerating nodules, and the presence of the right posterior hepatic notch are more frequent in alcoholic cirrhosis than in virus-induced cirrhosis.[121] MRI scoring systems based on spleen volume, liver volume, and presence of ascites or varices/collaterals can quantify severity of cirrhosis in a way that correlates well with Child grades (see BOX 3).[122] *Ascitic tap* should be performed and fluid sent for urgent MC&S—neutrophils >250/mm³ indicates spontaneous bacterial peritonitis (see below for treatment). *Liver biopsy* (p256) confirms the clinical diagnosis.

**Management** *General:* Good nutrition is vital. Alcohol abstinence (p282). Avoid NSAIDs, sedatives, and opiates. *Colestyramine* helps pruritus (4g/12h PO, 1h after other drugs). Consider ultrasound ± α-fetoprotein every 3–6 months to screen for HCC, p270.[123] *Specific:* For hepatitis-induced cirrhosis see p406. High-dose *ursodeoxycholic acid* in PBC (p266) may normalize LFT, but may have no effect on disease progression.[124] *Penicillamine* for Wilson's disease (p269). *Ascites:* Bed rest, fluid restriction (<1.5L/d), low-salt diet (40–100mmol/d). Give *spironolactone* 100mg/24h PO; ↑dose every 48h, to 400mg/24h—it counters deranged renin-angiotensin-aldosterone (RAA) axis. Chart daily weight and aim for weight loss of ≤½kg/d. If response is poor, add *furosemide* ≤120mg/24h PO; do U&E (watch Na⁺) often. Therapeutic paracentesis with concomitant albumin infusion (6–8g/L fluid removed) may be tried. *Spontaneous bacterial peritonitis (SBP):* ►Must be considered in any patient with ascites who deteriorates suddenly (may be asymptomatic). Common organisms are *E. coli, Klebsiella,* and streps.[125] ℞: eg *cefotaxime* 2g/6h or *tazocin*® 4.5g/8h (see datasheet) for 5d or until sensitivities known (+ *metronidazole* 500mg/8h IV if recent instrumentation to ascites). Give prophylaxis for high-risk patients (↓albumin, ↑PT/INR, low ascitic albumin) or those who have had a previous episode: eg *norfloxacin* 400mg PO daily continued until death, transplant, or ascites resolves.[126] *Renal failure:* See BOX 4.

**Prognosis** Overall 5yr survival is ~50%. Poor prognostic indicators: encephalopathy; serum Na⁺ <110mmol/L; serum albumin <25g/L; ↑INR.

**Liver transplantation** is the only definitive treatment for cirrhosis (p263). This increases 5yr survival from ~20% in end-stage disease to ~70%.[127]

Fig 1. Spider naevi consist of a central arteriole, from which numerous vessels radiate (like the legs of a spider). These fill from the centre as opposed to telangiectasias that fill from the edge. They occur most commonly in skin drained by the superior vena cava. Up to 5 are said to be normal (they are common in young ♀). Causes include liver disease, contraceptive steroids, and pregnancy (ie changes in oestrogen metabolism).

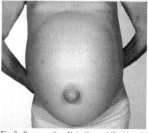

Fig 2. Gross ascites. Note the umbilical hernia (p615) and a mild degree of gynaecomastia. There are veins visible on the anterior abdominal wall, though they are not in the pattern of *caput medusae*.

## Causes of cirrhosis

(cryptogenic in up to 20%)

- Chronic alcohol abuse
- Chronic HBV or HCV infection[1]
- Genetic disorders: haemochromatosis (p262); α₁-antitrypsin deficiency (p264); Wilson's disease (p269)
- Hepatic vein events (Budd-Chiari, p710)
- Non-alcoholic steatohepatitis (NASH)
- Autoimmunity: primary biliary cirrhosis (p266); primary sclerosing cholangitis (p266); autoimmune hepatitis (p268)
- Drugs: eg amiodarone, methyldopa, methotrexate

## Is cirrhosis becoming decompensated? ►►Prepare to make an arrest...

Cirrhosis may lie in wait for years before committing one of its 3 great crimes against the person: jaundice, ascites, or encephalopathy. There are almost always accomplices who, if arrested *now*, may stop a killing from unfolding.[2] These usual suspects are: ►dehydration ►constipation ►covert alcohol use ►infection (eg spontaneous peritonitis, see above) ►opiate over-use—or ►an occult GI bleed. If all have alibis, think of portal vein thrombosis, and call in the Chief Inspector.

## Child-Pugh grading of cirrhosis and risk of variceal bleeding

Grade A = 5-6, grade B = 7-9, grade C >10. Risk of variceal bleeding is much higher if score is >8. The grading can also be used to predict mortality[2] and quantify need for liver transplantation (p263). NB: all such scoring systems come with the 'non-parametric health warning', see p10.

|  | 1 point | 2 points | 3 points |
|---|---|---|---|
| Bilirubin (µmol/L) | <34 | 34-51 | >51 |
| Albumin (g/L)[128] | >35 | 28-35 | <28 |
| Prothrombin time (seconds > normal) | 1-3 | 4-6 | >6 |
| Ascites | none | slight | moderate |
| Encephalopathy (p259) | none | 1-2 | 3-4 |

## Cirrhosis and deteriorating renal function

In cirrhosis, ↓hepatic clearance of immune complexes leads to their trapping in the kidney (∴ IgA nephropathy ± hepatic glomerulosclerosis). HCV can cause cryoglobulinaemia ± membranoproliferative glomerulonephritis; HBV may cause membranous nephropathy ± PAN. Membranoproliferative glomerulonephritis can occur in α₁-antitrypsin deficiency.[129] See p259 for hepatorenal syndrome.

1 Clues as to which patients with chronic HCV will get cirrhosis: platelet count ≤140 x 10⁹/L, globulin/albumin ratio ≥1, and AST/ALT ratio ≥1—100% +ve predictive value but lower sensitivity (~30%).[130]
2 If Child-Pugh grade C, then 1yr survival is 42% and 5yr survival is 21% (vs 84 and 44% for grade A).

This is an inherited disorder of iron metabolism in which ↑ intestinal iron absorption leads to iron deposition in joints, liver, heart, pancreas, pituitary, adrenals and skin. Middle-aged men are more frequently and severely affected than women, in whom the disease tends to present ~10yrs later (menstrual blood loss is protective).

**Genetics** HH is one of the commonest inherited conditions in those of Northern European (especially Celtic) ancestry (carrier rate of ~1 in 10 and a frequency of homozygosity of ~1 in 200–400). The gene responsible for most HH is called HFE, found on the short arm of chromosome 6. The 2 major mutations are termed C282Y and H63D. C282Y accounts for 60–90% of HH, and H63D accounts for 3–7%, with compound heterozygotes accounting for 1–4%. Penetrance is unknown but is <100%.[131]

**The patient** *Early on:* Nil—or tiredness; arthralgia (2nd+3rd MCP joints + knee pseudo-gout); erections↓. *Later:* Slate-grey skin pigmentation; signs of chronic liver disease (p260); hepatomegaly; cirrhosis; dilated cardiomyopathy; osteoporosis.[132] *Endocrinopathies:* DM ('bronze diabetes' from iron deposition in pancreas); hypogonadism (p224) from pituitary dysfunction↓ (*not* from testicular iron deposition, but may be via cirrhosis, esp. if drinks >60g/d of alcohol); hyporeninaemic hypoaldosteronism[133]

**Tests** *Blood:* ↑LFT, ↑serum ferritin (>1mg/L is very suggestive, but *any* inflammatory process can ↑ferritin); transferrin saturation >45%.[1] Glucose (?DM). HFE genotype.

*Images:* Chondrocalcinosis [et al] (fig 1). Liver MRI: Fe overload (sensitivity 84-91%).

*Liver biopsy:* Perl's stain quantifies iron loading[2] and assesses disease severity.

*ECG/ECHO* if cardiomyopathy suspected.

**Management** *Venesect* ~1 unit/1-3wks, until ferritin ≤50μg/L (may take 2yrs). Iron will continue to accumulate, so maintenance venesection is needed for life (1u every 2-3 months to maintain haematocrit <0.5, ferritin <100μg/L, and transferrin saturation <40%). Consider desferrioxamine (p336) if intolerant of this. *Monitor:* LFT and glucose/diabetes (p198). Hb[A1c] levels may be falsely low as venesection ↓the time available for Hb glycosylation.[134]

*Over-the-counter drugs:* Ensure vitamin preparations [etc] contain no iron.

*Diet:* A well-balanced low-iron diet may help. Tea, coffee or red wine with meals ↓iron absorption, but fruit/fruit juice (high in vit. c) and white wine ↑absorption.

*Screening:* Serum ferritin and genotype. ►Screen 1st-degree relatives by genetic testing even if they are asymptomatic and have normal LFT (in young people LFT may be normal).[135] Prevalence of iron overload in asymptomatic C282Y homozygotes is ≤0.5%. How many will go on to develop iron overload is unknown.

**Prognosis** Venesection returns life expectancy to normal if non-diabetic and non-cirrhotic (and liver histology *can* improve). Arthropathy may improve or worsen. Gonadal failure is irreversible. ►If cirrhosis, 22-30% get hepatocellular cancer, especially if: age >50yrs (risk ↑×13), HBsAg +ve (risk ↑×5), or alcohol abuse (risk ↑×2).[136, 137]

**Secondary haemochromatosis** may occur if many transfusions (~40L in total) have been given.[138] To reduce need for transfusions, find out if the haematological condition responds to erythropoietin or marrow transplantation before irreversible effects of iron overload become too great. See iron management in thalassaemia, p336.

---

**1** In heterozygotes, biochemical tests may be normal or show mild ↑ in transferrin saturation or ferritin.
**2** The HII aims to separate HH from other causes of hepatic siderosis (eg HBV; alcoholic cirrhosis). HII in μmol iron/gram liver/year = [iron concentration (μg iron per gram dry weight of liver)/55.846 (atomic weight of Fe)]/patient's age. HII >1.9 in a non-cirrhotic liver strongly suggests HH. ►*Caveats:* •~7% of those with HH have an HII <1.9. Using a threshold hepatic iron concentration of 71μmol/g as well as HII can detect most of these.[139] • Cirrhotic livers can rapidly accumulate iron in non-HH liver disease making HII >1.9. Some say that an HII cut-off of ~4.2 is best in diagnosing HH in cirrhotics.[140] • Iron is not uniformly distributed in the liver (sampling variation). • Correlation among HII, phenotypic HH, and genotypic HH is not 100%.

## A bit about iron metabolism

60% of body iron is in haemoglobin, and erythropoiesis requires ~5-30mg iron/day—provided by macrophages (recycling of haeme iron after phagocytosis of old RBCs). Intestinal iron absorption (1-2mg/day) compensates for daily iron losses.

Red meats, liver, seafoods, enriched breakfast cereals and pulses and some spices (eg paprika) are iron-rich. Most dietary iron is $Fe^{3+}$, which is reduced by low gastric pH and ascorbic acid (vitamin C) to better-absorbed $Fe^{2+}$. Absorption occurs mainly in the duodenum and jejunum, though very small amounts are absorbed in the stomach and ileum. Iron requirements are greater for women (menstrual loss), when growing, in pregnancy, and in chronic infection.

Hepcidin, a peptide synthesized in hepatocytes, secreted in plasma, is a negative regulator of gut iron absorption and haeme iron recycling by macrophages. Hepcidin synthesis is stimulated by iron and repressed by iron deficiency and by ↑ marrow erythropoiesis[141] (eg in anaemia, bleeding, haemolysis, dyserythopoiesis or erythropoietin injections). A defect in activation of hepcidin normally triggered by iron excess causes haemochromatosis whereas a defect in hepcidin repression is responsible for an iron refractory iron deficiency anaemia.

In HH the total body iron is up to 10-fold that of a normal person, with loading found particularly in the liver and pancreas (×100). Hepatic disease classically starts with fibrosis, progressing to cirrhosis as a late feature.

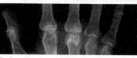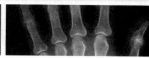

Fig 1. Haemochromatosis causes stressed joints to deteriorate faster than resting joints: the 2nd and 3rd MCP joints have osteophytes and narrowed joint spaces compared to the normal hand (right image) in this man who only used his dominant hand for his production line job.

From 'Haemochromatosis arthropathy & repetitive trauma', C Morgan, D Smith, 2012, with permission BMJ Publishing Group.

## Liver transplantation in chronic liver disease     (for acute, see p259)

The first liver transplantation was in Denver, USA, in 1963. Now 800-1000 are done each year in the UK and Ireland. The limiting step for the procedure is often the waiting-list for a donor organ (live or cadaveric—see p259). The indications for transplantation in chronic disease (see TABLE) are generally because of advanced cirrhosis (p260), the grading of which has been used as a selection criterion.[1]

**Indications**
- Advanced cirrhosis secondary to:
  - Alcoholic liver disease
  - Hepatitis (B & C—or autoimmune)
  - Primary biliary cirrhosis (p266)
  - Wilson's disease (p269)
  - $\alpha_1$-antitrypsin deficiency (p264)
  - Primary sclerosing cholangitis (p266)
- Hepatocellular cancer (1 nodule <5cm or 2-3 nodules <3cm)

**Contraindications**
- Extrahepatic malignancy
- Multiple tumours
- Severe cardiorespiratory disease
- Systemic sepsis
- HIV infection
- Non-compliance with drug therapy

The post-op period involves 12-24h on ITU, with enteral feeding starting as soon as possible and close monitoring of LFT. Immunosuppression examples: *ciclosporin* or *tacrolimus* + *azathioprine* or *mycophenolate mofetil* + *prednisolone*. Hyperacute rejection is a result of ABO incompatibility. Acute rejection (T-cell mediated, at 5-10d): the patient feels unwell with pyrexia and tender hepatomegaly—often managed by altering the immunosuppressives. Other complications: sepsis (esp. Gram -ve and CMV), hepatic artery thrombosis, chronic rejection (at 6-9 months), disease recurrence,[142] and, rarely, graft-versus-host disease.[143] Average patient survival at 1yr ~80% (5yr survival 60-90%; depends on the pre-op disease). Poor pre-transplant renal function may predict poor outcome.[144]

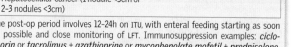

**1** The Model for End-stage Liver Disease (MELD) helps crack the conundrum of who should get a transplant.[145]

A1AT deficiency is an inherited conformational disease[1] that can be fatal. It commonly affects lung (emphysema) and liver (cirrhosis and hepatocellular cancer, HCC) and can present in homozygous or heterozygous forms. A1AT is a glycoprotein and one of a family of serine protease inhibitors made in the liver that control inflammatory cascades. Deficiency is called a serpinopathy. It makes up 90% of serum $\alpha_1$-globulin on electrophoresis (p701). A1AT deficiency is the chief genetic cause of liver disease in children. In adults, its lack is more likely to cause emphysema. Lung A1AT protects against tissue damage from neutrophil elastase—a process that is also induced by cigarette smoking (p176). *Associations:* HCC (p270), asthma, pancreatitis, gallstones, Wegener's▪ (p728). *Prevalence:* ~1:4000 (higher in Caucasians).

**Genetics** The gene for this autosomal recessive disorder is found on chromosome 14; carrier frequency of 1:10. Genetic variants are typed by electrophoretic mobility as **medium** (M), **slow** (S), or **very slow** (Z). S and Z types are due to single amino acid substitutions at positions 264 and 342, respectively. These result in ↓production of $\alpha_1$-antitrypsin (S=60%, Z=15%). The normal genotype is PiMM, the homozygote is PiZZ; heterozygotes are PiMZ and PiSZ (at low risk of developing liver disease).

**The patient** Symptomatic patients usually have the PiZZ genotype: dyspnoea from emphysema; cirrhosis; cholestatic jaundice. Cholestasis often remits in adolescence.

**Tests** Serum $\alpha_1$-antitrypsin ($\alpha_1$AT) levels↓, usually (eg <11µmol/L or <75% of lower limit of normal, which is ~0.9g/L; labs vary). Note the 'usually'. Because A1AT is part of the acute-phase response, inflammation may hide a low level. Unless you do genotyping, you will inevitably mis-label some cirrhosis as cryptogenic.[146] *Liver biopsy:* (p256) Periodic acid Schiff (PAS) +ve; diastase-resistant globules. *Phenotyping* by isoelectric focusing requires expertise to distinguish SZ and ZZ phenotypes. Phenotyping can miss null phenotypes. *Prenatal diagnosis* is possible by DNA analysis of chorionic villus samples obtained at 11-13wks' gestation. DNA tests are likely to find greater use in the future. Measuring lung density with CT may be better than lung function tests at predicting disease progression and mortality.[147]

**Management** ☼Do some joined-up thinking with GP, lung and liver specialists and geneticists (who else in the family needs testing?). Supportive R̊: for emphysema and liver disease may be sufficient for some. Quit smoking. Giving IV A1AT pooled from human plasma is expensive and useless according to some, but COPD exacerbations *may* be prevented (no good randomized trials).[148,149] *Liver transplantation* is needed in decompensated cirrhosis. *Inhaled A1AT* has been tried in lung disease.

**Prognosis** Some patients have life-threatening symptoms in childhood, whereas others remain asymptomatic and healthy into old age. Worse prognosis if male, a smoker, or obese.[150] Emphysema is the cause of death in most, liver disease in ~5%. In adults, cirrhosis ± HCC affect 25% of A1AT-deficient adults >50yrs.

---

### Some screening tests for chronic liver disease

- HBV and HCV serology (p406).
- Iron studies for haemochromatosis: ↑ferritin, ↑iron, ↓TIBC (p262).
- $\alpha_1$-antitrypsin deficiency (plasma for genetics): see above.
- Wilson's disease: ↓serum copper, ↓caeruloplasmin (p269).
- PBC: ↑AMA (p266).
- PSC: ANA, p-ANCA and IgM may be ↑; AMA -ve (p266).
- AIH (autoimmune hepatitis): ↑ANA + ↑ASMA; ↑IgG (p268).
- Immunoglobulins: IgA (↑ in alcoholic liver disease); IgG (↑ in AIH) and IgM (↑ in PBC).
- HCC: ↑ α-fetoprotein (p270).
- Conjugated and unconjugated bilirubin (for Gilbert's disease).

---

1 Serpinopathies entail inappropriate conformational change and self-association (polymerization) of a serpin molecule. Kinetic instability of serpin Z $\alpha_1$-antitrypsin promotes abnormal aggregation. How this causes injury is unclear, but in the lung it involves ↓antiprotease protection on airway epithelial surfaces.[151]

## Approaches to abnormal liver function tests (LFTs)

Abnormal LFT can be found in ~17% of the asymptomatic general population. Also, remember that a normal LFT does not exclude liver disease.

### Tests of hepatocellular injury or cholestasis

*Aminotransferases* (AST, ALT) are released in the bloodstream after hepatocellular injury. ALT is more specific for hepatocellular injury (but also expressed in kidney and muscle). AST is also expressed in the heart, skeletal muscle, and RBCs.[152]

*Alkaline phosphatase* may originate from liver, bone (so raised in growing children), placenta, kidney, intestine, and WCC.[152]

*Gamma-glutamyltransferase* (GGT; γGT) is present in liver, pancreas, renal tubules and intestine—but not bone, so it helps tell if a raised alk phos is from bone (GGT↔) or liver (GGT↑). NB: it is not specific to alcohol damage to the liver.

**Tests of hepatic function** Serum albumin, serum bilirubin, PT (INR).

**Hepatocellular predominant liver injury** AST & ALT↑. Evaluate promptly, eg history from family ("Could he be consuming ↑alcohol?"); ultrasound for fatty liver, metastases,[etc] viral serology (hepatitis A, B, C,[etc] and Monospot®, p401).

*Alcoholic liver disease:* AST/ALT ratio is typically 2:1 or more. When the history is not reliable, normal alk phos, GGT↑ and macrocytosis suggest this condition.[153]

*Acute viral hepatitis:* AST & ALT↑; bilirubin may be ↔. NB: AST may be ↑↑, p406 & p283.

*Chronic viral hepatitis:* AST & ALT↑; HBV & C are a leading cause worldwide.

*Autoimmune hepatitis (AIH)* occurs mainly in young and middle-aged females with concomitant autoimmune disorders (eg rheumatological or thyroiditis).[154]

*Fatty infiltration of the liver* (p269) is probably the chief cause of mildly raised LFTs in the general population. Risk factors for non-alcoholic fatty liver disease (steatohepatitis): obesity, DM, ↑lipids. It's a diagnosis of exclusion. One study found that in 83% of patients with elevated AST and ALT whose serum evaluation was otherwise negative, biopsy revealed steatosis of no prognostic significance. In 10% biopsy was normal—a reminder that mildly raised LFTs need not mean pathology.[155] Although US, CT, or MRI may help, biopsy is the gold standard.[156,157]

*Ischaemic hepatitis* can be seen in conditions when effective circulatory volume is low (eg MI, hypotension, haemorrhage). AST and ALT are ↑, as well as LDH.[158]

*Drug-induced hepatitis:* As no specific serology identifies most culprits, a good history is vital. Paracetamol overdose causes most acute liver failure in the UK.

**Cholestasis predominant liver injury** Alk phos and GGT↑; AST and ALT mildly↑.

**Management** For each specific diagnosis, manage accordingly. If asymptomatic and other tests are -ve, try lifestyle modification. R: Help reduce weight and alcohol use (p282 & OHCS p513); control DM & dyslipidaemia; stop hepatotoxic drugs.

**Follow-up** Repeat tests after a few months; if still ↑, do US (±abdominal CT). If diagnosis still unclear, get help: is biopsy needed?; consider α₁-antitrypsin levels, serum caeruloplasmin (Wilson's disease), coeliac serology, ANA and ASMA (AIH, p268).[155]

*Essence:* Interlobular bile ducts are damaged by chronic autoimmune granulomat-ous[1] inflammation causing cholestasis which may lead to fibrosis, cirrhosis, and por-tal hypertension. *Cause:* Unknown environmental triggers (?pollutants, xenobiotics, non-pathogenic bacteria) + genetic predisposition (eg IL12A locus) leading to loss of immune tolerance to self-mitochondrial proteins. *Antimitochondrial antibodies (AMA)* are the hallmark of PBC. *Prevalence:* ≤4/100,000. ♀:♂ ≈ 9:1. **Risk ↑ if:** +ve fam-ily history (seen in 1-6%); many UTIs; smoking; past pregnancy; other autoimmune diseases; ↑ use of nail polish/hair dye. *Typical age at presentation:* ~50yrs.

**The patient** Often asymptomatic and diagnosed after finding ↑alk phos on routine LFT. Lethargy, sleepiness, and pruritus may precede jaundice by years. *Signs:* Jaun-dice; skin pigmentation; xanthelasma (p704); xanthomata; hepatosplenomegaly. *Complications:* Those of cirrhosis (p260); osteoporosis is common. Malabsorption of fat-soluble vitamins (A, D, E, K) due to cholestasis and ↓ bilirubin in the gut lumen results in osteomalacia and coagulopathy; HCC (p270, so check AFP twice-yearly).

**Tests** *Blood:* ↑Alk phos, ↑γGT, and mildly ↑AST & ALT; late disease: ↑bilirubin, ↓albumin, ↑prothrombin time. 98% are AMA M2 subtype +ve, eg in a titre of 1:40 (see above). Other autoantibodies (p555) may occur in low titres (see BOX). Immunoglobulins are ↑ (esp. IgM). TSH & cholesterol ↑ or ↔. *Ultrasound:* Excludes extrahepatic cholestasis. *Biopsy:* Not usually needed (unless drug-induced cholestasis or hepatic sarcoidosis need excluding); look for granulomas around bile ducts ± cirrhosis. Liver granuloma *ΔΔ:* sarcoidosis, PBC, TB, parasites/schistosomiasis, brucellosis, & drug reactions.

**Treatment** *Symptomatic:* Pruritus: try *colestyramine* 4-8g/24h PO; *naltrexone* and *rifampicin* may also help. Diarrhoea: *codeine phosphate*, eg 30mg/8h PO. Osteo-porosis prevention: p696. *Specific: Fat-soluble vitamin prophylaxis:* vitamin A, D and K. Consider high-dose *ursodeoxycholic acid (UDCA)*. If baseline bilirubin >24μmol/L,[159] it may improve survival and delay transplantation.❧ SE: weight↑. Predictors of a good response to UDCA: alk phos normalizing or reducing to <40% of baseline; bilirubin falling to <17μmol/L.[159] *Monitoring:* Regular LFT; ultrasound; AFP. *Liver transplanta-tion* (p263) is for end-stage disease (eg bilirubin >100μmol/L) or intractable pruritus. Histological recurrence in the graft: ~17% after 5yrs; although graft failure can occur as a result of recurrence, it is rare and unpredictable.

**Prognosis** Once jaundice develops, survival is <2yrs without transplantation.[160]

## Primary sclerosing cholangitis (PSC)

PSC entails progressive cholestasis with bile duct inflammation and strictures (figs 1, 2).

**Symptoms/signs** Pruritus ± fatigue; if advanced: ascending cholangitis, cirrhosis and end-stage hepatic failure. *Associations:* • ♂sex • HLA-A1; B8; DR3 • AIH (BOX) (p268); >80% of Northern European patients also have inflammatory bowel disease (IBD), usually ul-cerative colitis (UC) of the whole colon. IBD often presents before PSC. Despite typically inactive colitis, risk of colorectal malignancy is paradoxically much increased.

**Cancers** Bile duct, gallbladder, liver and colon cancers are more common, so do yearly colonoscopy + ultrasound; consider cholecystectomy for gallbladder polyps.[2]

**Tests** ↑Alk phos, then ↑bilirubin; hypergammaglobulinaemia and/or ↑IgM; AMA -ve, but ANA, SMA, and ANCA may be +ve; see BOX and p555. ERCP (fig 1) distinguishes large duct from small duct disease. *Liver biopsy* shows a fibrous, obliterative cholangitis.

**Treatment** *Liver transplant* is the mainstay for end-stage disease; recurrence oc-curs in up to 30%; 5yr graft survival is >60%. Prognosis is worse for those with IBD, as 5-10% develop colorectal cancer post-transplant.[160] *Ursodeoxycholic acid* may protect against colon cancer and improve LFT (histological benefit is less clear). High doses, eg 25-30mg/kg/d, may be harmful. *Colestyramine* 4-8g/24h PO for pruritus (*naltrexone* and *rifampicin* may also help). Antibiotics for bacterial cholangitis.

---

**1** Other causes of liver granulomas: TB, sarcoid, infections with HIV (eg toxoplasmosis, CMV, mycobacteria), PAN, SLE, Wegener's❦, lymphoma, syphilis, isoniazid, quinidine, carbamazepine, allopurinol. Signs: PUO; LFT↑.
**2** Usually GB polyps are an incidental finding on ultrasound, and they can often be left if <1cm diameter, but in PSC they are much more likely to become malignant.[161]

### Testing for autoantibodies—overlapping, nested mine-fields

The conditions opposite and on the next page all include the measurement of autoantibodies—with their varying sensitivities and specificities—as part of an investigative work-up. Quite often such a work-up shows strange overlap conditions between apparently different diseases: strange until we realize that it is the concept of a uniquely demarcated disease which is odd. The body knows no diseases, only pain and death. It is our own minds which force the unnatural construct of a unitary disease on unsuspecting and innocent cells and bodies.

For example, autoimmune hepatitis (AIH) overlaps with inflammatory bowel disease and PSC.[162] Doing antimitochondrial, antinuclear, antismooth muscle, antiliver kidney microsomal type 1, antiliver cytosol type 1, perinuclear antineutrophil nuclear, and antisoluble liver antigen antibodies sometimes helps, and sometimes mystifies things further.[163] As ever, management should be individualized dependent on liver histology, serum immunoglobulin levels, autoantibodies, the degree of biochemical cholestasis, cholangiography, and the mood of the day.

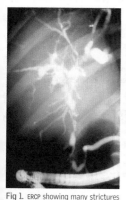

Fig 1. ERCP showing many strictures in the biliary tree with a characteristic 'beaded' appearance. MRCP (fig 2) is more cost effective.

© Dr Anthony Mee (fig 1) & ©Norwich Radiology Department (fig 2).

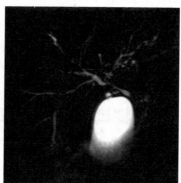

Fig 2. MRCP showing features of PSC. The intrahepatic ducts show multifocal strictures. (MRCP = magnetic resonance cholangiopancreatography). Strictures can be hard to differentiate from cholangiocarcinoma (coexistence of UC may promote this development). Stenting may be needed.

An inflammatory liver disease of unknown cause[1] characterized by suppressor T-cell defects with autoantibodies directed against hepatocyte surface antigens. Classification is by autoantibodies (see TABLE). AIH predominantly affects young or middle-aged women (bimodal, ie 10–30yrs—or >40yrs old). Up to 40% present with acute hepatitis and signs of autoimmune disease, eg fever, malaise, urticarial rash, polyarthritis, pleurisy, pulmonary infiltration, or glomerulonephritis. The remainder present with gradual jaundice or are asymptomatic and diagnosed incidentally with signs of chronic liver disease. Amenorrhoea is common and disease tends to attenuate during pregnancy. *Complications:* Those associated with cirrhosis (p260) and drug therapy.

**Tests** Serum bilirubin, AST, ALT and alk phos all usually ↑, hypergammaglobulinaemia (esp. IgG), +ve autoantibodies (see TABLE). Anaemia, WCC↓, and platelets↓ indicate hypersplenism. *Liver biopsy* (p256): mononuclear infiltrate of portal and periportal areas and piecemeal necrosis ± fibrosis; cirrhosis≈worse prognosis. MRCP (p756) helps exclude PSC if alk phos disproportionately ↑.

**Diagnosis** depends on excluding other diseases (no lab test is pathognomonic). Diagnostic criteria based on IgG levels, autoantibodies, and histology in the absence of viral disease are helpful.[164] Sometimes diagnosis is a challenge—there is overlap with other chronic liver disease: eg PBC (p266), PSC (p266) and chronic viral hepatitis[165]

### Classifying autoimmune hepatitis: types I-III

I  Seen in 80%. Typical patient: ♀<40yrs. Antismooth muscle antibodies (ASMA) +ve in 80%.[166] Antinuclear antibody (ANA) +ve in 10%. IgG↑ in 97%. Good response to immunosuppression in 80%. 25% have cirrhosis at presentation.

II  Commoner in Europe than USA. More often seen in children, and more commonly progresses to cirrhosis and less treatable. Antiliver/kidney microsomal type 1 (LKM1) antibodies +ve. ASMA and ANA -ve.

III  Like type I but ASMA and ANA -ve. Antibodies against soluble liver antigen (SLA) or liver-pancreas antigen.

**Management** *Immunosuppressant therapy: Prednisolone* 30mg/d PO for 1 month; ↓by 5mg a month to a maintenance dose of 5–10mg/d PO. Corticosteroids can sometimes be stopped after 2yrs but relapse occurs in 50–86%. *Azathioprine* (50–100mg/d PO) may be used as a steroid-sparing agent to maintain remission. Remission is achievable in 80% of patients within 3yrs. 10- and 20yr survival rates are >80%.[167] SE are a big problem (p370)—partly ameliorated by a switch to *budesonide*, eg in non-cirrhotic AIH.[168]

*Liver transplantation* (p263) is indicated for decompensated cirrhosis or if there is failure to respond to medical therapy, but recurrence may occur. It is effective (actuarial 10yr survival is 75%).

**Prognosis** appears not to matter whether symptomatic or asymptomatic at presentation (10yr survival ~80% for both). The presence of cirrhosis at presentation reduces 10yr survival from 94% to 62%. Overlap syndromes: AIH-PBC (primary biliary cirrhosis) overlap is worse than AIH-AIC (autoimmune cholangitis).

### Associations of autoimmune hepatitis

| | |
|---|---|
| •Pernicious anaemia | •Autoimmune haemolysis |
| •Ulcerative colitis | •Diabetes mellitus |
| •Glomerulonephritis | •PSC (p266) |
| •Autoimmune thyroiditis | •HLA A1, B8, and DR3 haplotype |

**1** Hepatotropic viruses (eg measles, herpes viruses) and some drugs appear to trigger AIH in genetically predisposed individuals exposed to a hepatotoxic *milieu intérieur*. Viral interferon can inactivate cytochrome P-450 enzymes (∴ ↓ metabolism of ex- or endogenous hepatotoxins). Putative examples of exogenous agents: monosodium glutamate (MSG; E621) and aspartame (E951), which, if regularly consumed in excess, may promote formation of salt bridges between amino acids. These compounds then act as autoantigens causing CD4 T-helper cell activation.[169-170]

# Non-alcoholic fatty liver disease (NAFLD) Prevalence: up to 30%

Fatty liver entails ↑fat in hepatocytes (steatosis) ± inflammation (steatohepatitis). The cause is often alcohol, but if a patient presents with LFT↑ (typically ALT↑) or a fatty liver on ultrasound, consider NAFLD if they drink <18u/wk (<9u in women). It may (rarely) progress to hepatic fibrosis ± hepatocellular cancer (all-cause mortality is hardly affected).[171] *Typical patient:* Middle-aged obese ♀. *Risk factors:* DM; dyslipidaemia; parenteral feeding; jejuno-ileal bypass; Wilson's disease; drugs (eg amiodarone, methotrexate, tetracycline). *Δ:* Biopsy may be needed. *Treatment:* Control risk factors. Bariatric surgery helps. No drug is of proven benefit. *Follow-up:* LFT; glucose.

# Wilson's disease/hepatolenticular degeneration

Wilson's disease is a rare (3/100,000) inherited disorder of biliary copper excretion with too much copper (Cu) in liver and CNS (basal ganglia, eg globus pallidus hypodensity ± putamen cavitation). It is treatable, so screen all youngsters with cirrhosis.

**Genetics** It is an autosomal recessive disorder of a gene on chromosome 13 that codes for a copper transporting ATPase, ATP7B. Many mutations are known (>200) with HIS1069GLU being the commonest in European populations.

**Physiology** Total body copper content is ~125mg. Intake≈3mg/day (absorbed in proximal small intestine). In the liver, copper is incorporated into caeruloplasmin. In Wilson's disease, intestinal copper absorption and transport into the liver are intact, while copper incorporation into caeruloplasmin in hepatocytes and its excretion into bile are impaired. Therefore, copper accumulates in liver, and later in other organs.

**Signs** Children present with *liver disease* (hepatitis, cirrhosis, fulminant liver failure); young adults often start with *CNS signs*: tremor; dysarthria; dysphagia; dyskinesias; dystonias; purposeless stereotyped movements (eg hand clapping); dementia; parkinsonism; micrographia; ataxia/clumsiness.
*Mood:* Depression/mania; labile emotions; libido↑↓; personality change. ►Ignoring these may cause years of needless misery. ☺Often the doctor who is good at combining the analytical and integrative aspects will be the first to make the diagnosis.
*Cognition:* Memory↓; quick to anger; slow to solve problems; IQ↓; delusions; mutism.
*Kayser-Fleischer (KF) rings:* Copper in iris (see 6 below); they are not invariable.
*Also:* Haemolysis; blue lunulae (nails); arthritis; hypermobile joints; grey skin.

**Tests** ►Equivocal copper studies need expert interpretation.
1 *Urine:* 24h copper excretion is *high*, eg >100μg/24h (normal <40μg).
2 *LFT↑:* Non-specific (but ALT >1500 is *not* part of the picture).
3 *Serum copper:* Typically <11μmol/L.
4 *Serum caeruloplasmin↓:* <200mg/L (<140mg/L is pathognomonic).
   • *Falsely low caeruloplasmin:* Protein-deficiency states (eg nephrotic syndrome, malabsorption); any chronic liver disease can cause ↓synthesis.
   • *Falsely high caeruloplasmin:* Caeruloplasmin is an 'acute phase reactant', so sometimes high in inflammation/infection and pregnancy.
5 *Molecular genetic testing* can confirm the diagnosis.
6 *Slit lamp exam:* KF rings: in iris/Descemet's membrane (fig 1 OHCS p448).
7 *Liver biopsy:* ↑Hepatic copper (Cu >250μg/g dry weight); hepatitis; cirrhosis.
8 *MRI:* Degeneration in basal ganglia, fronto-temporal, cerebellar and brainstem.[172]

**Management** *Diet:* Avoid eating foods with a high copper content (eg liver, chocolate, nuts, mushrooms, legumes, and shellfish). Copper content of atypical water sources (eg well water) should be analysed. *Drugs:* Lifelong *penicillamine* (500mg/6-8h PO for 1yr, maintenance 0.75-1g/d). SE: nausea, rash, WCC↓, Hb↓, platelets↓, haematuria, nephrosis, lupus. Monitor FBC and urinary Cu and protein excretion. Say "report sore throat, T°↑, or bruising at once" in case WCC/platelets↓↓. Stop if WCC <2.5×10⁹/L or platelets falling (or <120×10⁹/L). *Alternative: Trientine dihydrochloride* 600mg/6-12h PO (SE: rash; sideroblastic anaemia). *Liver transplantation* (p263) if severe liver disease. *Screen siblings* as asymptomatic homozygotes need treating.

*Prognosis:* Pre-cirrhotic liver disease is reversible; CNS damage is less so. There are no clear clinical prognostic indicators.[173] Fatal events: liver failure, bleeding, infection.

Gastroenterology

The commonest (90%) liver tumours are secondary (metastatic) tumours, eg from breast, bronchus, or the gastrointestinal tract (see TABLE 2). Primary hepatic tumours are much less common and may be benign or malignant (see TABLE 1).

**Symptoms** Fever, malaise, anorexia, weight↓, RUQ pain (∵ liver capsule stretch). Jaundice is late, except with cholangiocarcinoma. Benign tumours are often asymptomatic. Tumours may rupture causing intraperitoneal haemorrhage.

**Signs** Hepatomegaly (smooth, or hard and irregular, eg metastases, cirrhosis, HCC). Look for signs of chronic liver disease (p260) and evidence of decompensation (jaundice, ascites). Feel for an abdominal mass. Listen for a bruit over the liver (HCC).

**Tests** *Blood:* FBC, clotting, LFT, hepatitis serology, α-fetoprotein[1] (↑ in 50–80% of HCC, though it is an uncertain prognostic indicator[174] may be normal if tumour <3cm). *Imaging:* US or CT to identify lesions and guide biopsy. MRI is better at distinguishing benign from malignant lesions. Do ERCP (p756) and biopsy if cholangiocarcinoma is suspected. *Liver biopsy* (p256) may achieve a histological diagnosis; ►careful multidisciplinary discussion is required if potentially resectable, as seeding along the biopsy tract can occur. If the lesion could be a metastasis, find the primary, eg by CXR, mammography, endoscopy, colonoscopy, CT, MRI, or marrow biopsy.

**Liver metastases** signify advanced disease. Treatment and prognosis vary with the type and extent of primary tumour. Chemotherapy may be effective (eg lymphomas, germ cell tumours). Small, solitary metastases may be amenable to resection (eg colorectal cancer).[175] In most, treatment is palliative. *Prognosis:* Often <6 months.

**Hepatocellular carcinoma (HCC)** Primary hepatocyte neoplasia accounts for 90% of primary liver cancers; it is common in China & Africa (40% of cancers vs 2% in UK). *The patient:* Fatigue, appetite↓, RUQ pain, weight↓, jaundice, ascites, haemobilia.[1] ♂:♀≈3. *Causes:* HBV is the leading cause (esp. if >2.3×10⁴ virions/mL; this is quite a low level so most are at risk; p406). HCV;[2] AIH (p268); cirrhosis (alcohol, haemochromatosis, PBC); non-alcoholic fatty liver; aflatoxin; *Clonorchis sinensis*; anabolic steroids. *Δ:* 4-phase CT (delayed wash-out of contrast in a suspect mass); MRI; biopsy. *Treatment:* Resecting solitary tumours <3cm across ↑ 3yr survival to 59% from 13%; but ~50% have recurrence by 3yrs.[3] Liver transplant gives a 5yr survival rate of 70%.[4] Percutaneous ablation, tumour embolization (TACE[5]), and sorafenib are options.[176,177] *Prevention:* ►HBV vaccination (BOX) ►Don't reuse needles ►Screen blood ►↓Aflatoxin exposure (sun-dry maize).[178] *AFP and ultrasound (eg 6-monthly screen):* Consider if at ↑ risk: eg Africans; older Asians; cirrhosis from HBV; family history of HCC.[179,180]

**Cholangiocarcinoma** (biliary tree cancer); ~10% of liver primaries. *Causes:* Flukes (*Clonorchis*, p445); PSC (screening by CA19-9 may be helpful, p266); biliary cysts; Caroli's disease, p250; HBV; HCV; DM;[181] biliary-enteric drainage surgery;[182] N-nitroso toxins.[183] *The patient:* Fever, abdominal pain (±ascites), malaise, ↑bilirubin; ↑↑alk phos. *Pathology:* Usually slow-growing. Most are distal extrahepatic or perihilar. *Management:* 70% are unsuited to surgery. Of those that are, 76% recur. **Surgery:** eg major hepatectomy + extrahepatic bile duct excision + caudate lobe resection. 5yr survival is ~30%.[184] Post-op complications include liver failure, bile leak and GI bleeding.[185] **Stenting** of an obstructed extrahepatic biliary tree, percutaneously or via ERCP (p756), improves quality of life. **Liver transplant** is rarely indicated (as tumour is >3cm, and intrinsic liver disease and mets are often present). *Prognosis:* ~5 months.

**Benign tumours** *Haemangiomas* are the commonest benign liver tumours. They are often an incidental finding on ultrasound or CT and don't require treatment. Avoid biopsy!! *Adenomas* are common. Causes: Anabolic steroids, oral contraceptive pill; pregnancy. Only treat if symptomatic, or >5cm.

---

1 Haemobilia is late in HCC. Think of bleeding into the biliary tree whenever Quinke's triad obtains: RUQ pain, upper GI haemorrhage, and jaundice. It may be life-threatening.
2 5yr cumulative risk if cirrhosis is present is 30% in Japan and 17% in USA.
3 Operative mortality: 1.6%.[181] Recurrence is more likely if histology showed neoplastic emboli in small vessels. Get early warning of recurrence by arranging imaging, eg if AFP >5.45µg/L (esp. if trend is rising).[181] Fibrolamellar HCC, which occurs in children and young adults, has a better prognosis.
4 Milan criteria for liver transplantation in HCC: 1 nodule <5cm or 2-3 nodules <3cm.
5 TACE=transarterial chemoembolization, eg with drug-eluting beads; it causes fever and abdo pain in 50%.

## Primary liver tumours

| Malignant (Prognosis—regardless of type—is poor) | Benign |
|---|---|
| HCC | Cysts |
| Cholangiocarcinoma | Haemangioma[1]; common, ♀:♂≈5:1 |
| Angiosarcoma | Adenoma |
| Hepatoblastoma | Focal nodular hyperplasia |
| Fibrosarcoma & hepatic gastrointestinal stromal | Fibroma |
| tumour (GIST[2], formerly leiomyosarcoma) | Benign GIST (=leiomyoma) |

## Origins of secondary liver tumours

| Common in men | Common in women | Less common (either sex) |
|---|---|---|
| Stomach | Breast | Pancreas |
| Lung | Colon | Leukaemia |
| Colon | Stomach | Lymphoma |
| | Uterus | Carcinoid tumours |

## Using vaccines to prevent hepatitis B, hepatitis B-associated cirrhosis, chronic hepatitis, and hepatic neoplasia

Use hepatitis B vaccine 1mL into deltoid; repeat at 1 & 6 months (child: 0.5mL × 3 into the anterolateral thigh). *Indications:* Everyone (WHO advice, even in areas of 'low' endemicity).[118] This is expensive, but not as expensive as trying to rely on the ultimately unsuccessful strategy of vaccinating at-risk groups (health workers, IV drug users, sexual adventurers, sex workers, those on haemodialysis, and partners of known HBe antigen +ve carriers). The immunocompromised and others may need further doses. Serology helps time boosters and finds non-responders (correlates with older age, smoking, and ♂ sex). ►Know your own antibody level!

| Anti-HBS (IU/L) | Actions and comments (advice differs in some areas) |
|---|---|
| >1000 | Good level of immunity; retest in ~4yrs. |
| 100-1000 | Good level of immunity; if level approaches 100, retest in 1yr. |
| <100 | Inadequate; give booster and retest. |
| <10 | Non-responder; give another set of 3 vaccinations. Retest; if <10 get consent to check hepatitis B status: HBsAg +ve means chronic infection; anti-HB core +ve represents past infection and immunity. If a non-responder is deemed susceptible to HBV, and has recently come in contact with risky bodily fluids, offer 2 doses of anti-hep B immunoglobulin. |

NB: protection begins some weeks after dose 1, so it won't work if exposure is recent; here, specific antihepatitis B immunoglobulin is best if not already immunized. Twinrix® is an alternative that protects against hepatitis A *and* HBV.

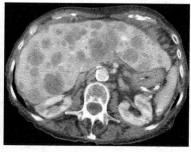

Fig 1. Axial CT of the liver after IV contrast showing many round lesions of varying size, highly suggestive of hepatic metastasis.
Courtesy of Norwich Radiology Dept.

1 Haemangiomas are hyperechoic on ultrasound; may be part of von Hippel-Lindau syndrome; may need surgery if diagnosis is uncertain (may be confused with HCC) or they are enlarging on 6-monthly US.
2 GISTs are mesenchymal tumours that are more likely to be found in the gut as a spherical mass arising from the muscularis propria, eg with GI bleeding. If unresectable, imatinib ↑2yr survival from 26% to 76%.

Gastroenterology

UC is a relapsing and remitting inflammatory disorder of the colonic mucosa. It may affect just the rectum (proctitis, as in ~50%) or extend to involve part of the colon (left-sided colitis, in ~30%) or the entire colon (pancolitis, in ~20%). It 'never' spreads proximal to the ileocaecal valve (except for backwash ileitis). *Cause:* Unknown;[1] there is some genetic susceptibility. *Pathology:* Hyperaemic/haemorrhagic granular colonic mucosa ± pseudopolyps formed by inflammation. Punctate ulcers may extend deep into the lamina propria—inflammation is normally not transmural. Mucosal disease differentiates it from Crohn's disease. *Histology:* See biopsy, below. *Prevalence:* 100–200/100,000. *Incidence:* 10–20/100,000/yr. ♀:♂ >1:1. Most present aged 15–30yrs. UC is 3-fold as common in non-smokers (the opposite is true for Crohn's disease)—symptoms may relapse on stopping smoking.

**Symptoms** Episodic or chronic diarrhoea (± blood & mucus); crampy abdominal discomfort; bowel frequency relates to severity (see TABLE); urgency/tenesmus≈rectal UC. Systemic symptoms in attacks: fever, malaise, anorexia, weight↓.

**Signs** May be none. In acute, severe UC there may be fever, tachycardia, and a tender, distended abdomen. *Extraintestinal signs:* Clubbing; aphthous oral ulcers; erythema nodosum (p275); pyoderma gangrenosum; conjunctivitis; episcleritis; iritis; large joint arthritis; sacroiliitis; ankylosing spondylitis; fatty liver; PSC (p266); cholangiocarcinoma; nutritional deficits; amyloidosis (p266).[189]

**Tests** *Blood:* FBC, ESR, CRP, U&E, LFT, blood culture.
*Stool MC&S/CDT* (p247) to exclude *Campylobacter, C. difficile, Salmonella, Shigella, E. coli,* amoebae.
*AXR:* No faecal shadows; mucosal thickening/islands (fig 2, p743); colonic dilatation (below). *Erect CXR:* Perforation. *Ba enema* (fig 1): Never do during severe attacks or for diagnosis.
*Colonoscopy* shows disease extent and allows biopsy (p256, fig 5)—look for inflammatory infiltrate; goblet cell depletion; glandular distortion; mucosal ulcers; crypt abscesses.

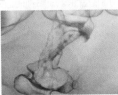

Fig 1. Ba enema: ulcers + loss of haustral pattern. ©OTM.

| Assessing severity in UC (Truelove & Witts criteria modified to include CRP)[190] | | | |
|---|---|---|---|
| Variable | Mild UC | Moderate UC | Severe UC |
| Motions/day | <4 | 4–6 | >6 |
| Rectal bleeding | Small | Moderate | Large |
| T°C at 6AM | Apyrexial | 37.1–37.8°C | >37.8°C |
| Resting pulse | <70 beats/min | 70–90 beats/min | >90 beats/min |
| Haemoglobin | >110g/L | 105–110g/L | <105g/L |
| ESR (do CRP too) | <30 (<16 might be better)[191] | | >30 (or CRP >45mg/L) |

**Complications** ►Perforation and bleeding are 2 serious dangers, also:
• Toxic dilatation of colon (mucosal islands, colonic diameter >6cm).
• Venous thrombosis: give prophylaxis to all inpatients (p344).[192] Colonic cancer: risk≈15% with pancolitis for 20yrs. Intra-epithelial neoplasms may occur in flat, normal-looking mucosa. To spot these, surveillance colonoscopy is done, eg 2–4yrs, with 4 random biopsies/10cm. Endomicroscopy (expensive!) may ↑ detection rates.[2]

**Inducing remission** *Mild UC:* • 5-ASA[3], eg sulfasalazine (SSZ) or mesalazine (=mesalamine) or olsalazine are the mainstay for remission-induction/maintenance. SSZ is cheapest and often as good (unless sulfa-allergic).[193] Once-a-day regimen: Mezavant XL®, 2 gastro-resistant 1.2g tabs once daily.[194]

• Steroids help remission induction, eg *prednisolone* ~20mg/d PO ± twice-daily steroid foams PR (eg *hydrocortisone* as Colifoam®), or *prednisolone* 20mg retention enemas (Predsol®).[4] If improving in 2wks, ↓steroids slowly. If not treat as moderate UC.

*Moderate UC:* If 4–6 motions/day, but otherwise well, try oral *prednisolone* 40mg/d for 1wk, then 30mg/d for 1wk, then 20mg for 4 more weeks + 5-ASA[3] (eg 4 Mezavent 1.2g tabs once daily) + twice-daily steroid enemas.[4] If improving, ↓steroids gradually. If no improvement after 2 weeks, treat as severe UC.

*Severe uc:* If unwell and ≥6 motions/d, admit for nil by mouth & IV hydration (eg 1L of 0.9% saline + 2L dextrose-saline/24h, + 20mmol K⁺/L for maintenance; less if elderly).

- *Hydrocortisone* 100mg/6h IV.
- Rectal steroids, eg *hydrocortisone* 100mg in 100mL 0.9% saline/12h PR.
- Monitor T°, pulse, and BP—and record stool frequency/character on a stool chart.
- Twice-daily exam: document distension, bowel sounds, and tenderness.
- Daily FBC, ESR, CRP, U&E ± AXR. Consider blood transfusion (eg if Hb <90–100g/L). NB: day 3 CRP >45 or bowels open >8×/day=85% chance of colectomy on this admission.
- Parenteral nutrition is only very rarely required (eg if severely malnourished).
- If improving in 5d, transfer to *prednisolone* PO (40mg/24h) with a 5-ASA (eg *sulfasalazine* 500mg/6h) to maintain remission.
- If on day 3 CRP >45 or >6 stools/d, ►►action is probably needed, eg colectomy or *rescue therapy* with *ciclosporin* or *infliximab*, which can avoid urgent colectomy in steroid-refractory patients (the need for elective colectomy in the long-term is not modified).[190][195]

**Topical therapies** Proctitis may respond to *suppositories* (*prednisolone* 5mg or *mesalazine*, eg Asacol® 250mg/8h or Pentasa® 1g at bedtime). Topical 5-ASAs work better than topical steroids.[196] Procto-sigmoiditis may respond to *foams* PR (20mg Predfoam®/12–24h or 5-ASA, eg Asacol® 1g/d); disposable applicators aid accurate delivery. Retention enemas may be needed in left-sided colitis.

**Surgery** This is needed at some stage in ~20%, eg *proctocolectomy + terminal ileostomy:* It may be possible to retain the ileocecal valve, and hence reduce liquid loss.[197] *Colectomy* with *ileo-anal pouch* later. *Surgical mortality:* 2–7%, higher if perforation. *Pouchitis* may improve with antibiotics (eg *metronidazole* + *ciprofloxacin* for 2wks) and immunosuppressants.[198]

| Indications: |
| --- |
| Perforation |
| Massive haemorrhage |
| Toxic dilatation |
| Failed medical therapy |

**It's time for immunomodulation if...** no remission comes with steroids, or if prolonged use is required. Agents: azathioprine, methotrexate, infliximab, adalimumab or calcineurin inhibitors (ciclosporin; tacrolimus).[199] Dose example: *Azathioprine* (2-2.5mg/kg/d PO after food).[200] Treat for several months, and monitor FBC every 4-6wks.

**Maintaining remission** All 5-ASAs ↓relapse rate from 80% to 20%—examples are *sulfasalazine, mesalazine,* and *olsalazine*.[4] Maintenance continues for life. *Sulfasalazine* (500mg/6h PO) is 1ˢᵗ-line.♦[*] SEs relate to sulfapyridine intolerance (headache, nausea, anorexia). Warn of SEs: T°↑, rash, haemolysis (►monitor FBC and U&E at start, then at 3 months, then annually), hepatitis, pancreatitis, paradoxical worsening of colitis, and reversible oligospermia.[201] Newer 5-ASAs (eg *mesalazine* 400-800mg/8h PO or *olsalazine* 500mg/12h PO) are as good at maintaining remission, have fewer SEs, but are more expensive. They are indicated in *sulfasalazine* intolerance and young men in whom fertility is a concern (less effect on sperm).[202]

---

### Diagnosing 'indeterminate colitis'

After full investigation, IBD may not obviously be Crohn's or UC. Indeterminate colitis more often resembles UC, and may be due to unrecognized variants of UC with transmural inflammation or skip lesions. Colectomy + pouch formation may be needed (see MINIBOX), though pouch failure rate is higher than in UC.[203]

---

1 Crohn's and UC *may* involve adhesin-expressing strains of *E. coli* capable of inducing interleukin-8 production and transepithelial migration of WBCs.[204]

2 Confocal laser endomicroscopy (CLE) makes real-time micron-scale live imaging and on-table decisions with less need for repeat procedures. With CLE we go beyond histology: we can watch capillary circulation, cellular death, and vascular and endothelial translocation. Proving that all this saving lives is hard.[205]

3 Sulfasalazine is a 5-aminosalicylic acid (5-ASA, the active ingredient) + sulfapyridine (carries 5-ASA to the colon, where it is cleaved off), mesalazine is 5-ASA and olsalazine is a dimer of 5-ASA that is also cleaved in the colon. Rare hypersensitivity reactions: worsening colitis, pancreatitis, pericarditis, nephritis.

4 *Budesonide* (Entocort®) enemas, 1 nocte, may have fewer SEs ∴ ↓suppression of plasma cortisol.[206]

Gastroenterology

A chronic inflammatory GI disease characterized by transmural granulomatous inflammation affecting any part of the gut from mouth to anus (esp terminal ileum (in ~70%) and proximal colon). Unlike UC, there is unaffected bowel between areas of active disease (skip lesions). *Cause:* Unknown.[1] Mutations of the NOD2/CARD15 gene ↑risk. *Prevalence:* 0.5–1/1000; less if Asian. ♀/♂ >1. *Incidence:* 5–10/100,000/yr. Presentation is mostly at ~20–40yrs. *Associations:* Altered cell-mediated immunity. Smoking ↑risk ×3–4; NSAIDs may exacerbate disease. *Classification:* Complex![2]

**Symptoms** Diarrhoea/urgency ("I get up at 4AM, go 5–6 times in the next 45mins..."), abdominal pain, weight loss/failure to thrive. Fever, malaise, anorexia. "I can be fine one minute, and deathly ill the next. The vomiting, the pain, the diarrhoea that smells so bad it could clear Grand Central Station in 0.5 seconds...I have even been attacked after I came out of the bathroom by 3 guys because I stunk up the place."

**Signs** Aphthous ulcerations; abdominal tenderness/mass; perianal abscess/fistulae/skin tags; anal strictures. *Beyond the gut:* (fig 1) clubbing, skin, joint & eye problems.

**Complications** Small bowel obstruction; toxic dilatation (colonic diameter >6cm, toxic dilatation is rarer than in UC); abscess formation (abdominal, pelvic, or ischiorectal); fistulae (present in ~10%), eg colovesical (bladder), colovaginal, perianal, enterocutaneous; perforation; rectal haemorrhage; colon cancer; fatty liver, PSC (p266); cholangiocarcinoma, renal stones, osteomalacia, malnutrition, amyloidosis.

**Tests** *Blood:* FBC, ESR, CRP, U&E, LFT, INR, ferritin, TIBC, B12, folate. *Stool* MC&S and CDT (p247) to exclude *C. difficile, Campylobacter, E. coli et al.* *Colonoscopy + rectal biopsy* even if mucosa looks normal (20% have microscopic granulomas). *Small bowel enema* detects ileal disease. *Capsule endoscopy* (p256, dummy patency capsule 1st that disintegrates if it gets stuck). *Barium enema* (rarely used): cobblestoning, 'rose thorn' ulcers ± colon strictures. *Colonoscopy* (fig 2) is preferred to barium enema to assess disease extent. *MRI* can assess pelvic disease and fistulae (as good as EUA). Small bowel MRI assesses disease activity and shows site of strictures.

Find out how your patient deals with what may be a brutal disease (no intimacy...no sex...no hope..."I live with this alone and will die alone"). With a collaborative approach, courage, attention to detail and a dose of humour, this can change. Help quit smoking. ▸*Optimize nutrition* (BOX). Assess severity: T°↑, pulse↑, ↑ESR, ↑WCC, ↑CRP + ↓albumin may merit admission (esp. if he looks ill). NB: the liver often switches to making CRP-type proteins rather than albumin. Specific options: aminosalicylates, steroids, immunosuppressants, TNF inhibitors, antibiotics, diet/supplements.

*Mild attacks:* (Symptomatic but systemically well). *Prednisolone* 30mg/d PO for 1wk, then 20mg/d for 4wks. See in clinic 3-weekly. If symptoms resolve, ↓prednisolone by 5mg every 2–4 weeks; stop steroids when parameters are normal (see also BOX).

*Severe:* Looks ill. Admit for IV steroids, nil by mouth, and IVI (eg 1L 0.9% saline + 2L dextrose-saline/24h, + 20mmol K⁺/L, less if elderly). *Hydrocortisone* 100mg/6h IV.
• Treat rectal disease: steroids, eg *hydrocortisone* 100mg in 100mL 0.9% saline/12h PR.
• *Metronidazole* 400mg/8h PO, or 500mg/8h IV, helps (esp. in perianal disease or superadded infection). SEs: alcohol intolerance; irreversible neuropathy.
• Monitor T°, pulse, BP, and record stool frequency/character on a stool chart.
• Physical examination daily. FBC, ESR, CRP, U&E, and plain AXR.
• Consider need for blood transfusion (if Hb <100g/L) and parenteral nutrition.
• If improving after 5d, transfer on to oral *prednisolone* (40mg/d). If not, *infliximab* and *adalimumab* have a role (esp. in fistulizing Crohn's). CI: CCF; infection. NICE 2010
• Consider abdominal sepsis complicating Crohn's disease especially if abdominal pain (ultrasound, CT & MRI are often required to assess this). Seek surgical advice.

*Perianal disease* occurs in about 50%. MRI and examination under anaesthetic (EUA) are an important part of assessment. Treatment includes oral antibiotics, immunosuppressant therapy ± *infliximab*, and local surgery ± seton insertion[207]

**1** Environmental agents are implicated. Genetics: colon involvement goes with ↑CARD15 gene expression in macrophages & intestinal epithelial cells.[208] Dysregulated immune responses might be primary or from infecting gut commensals, eg *Mycobacterium avium para*-TB;[208] *E. coli* adhesins, p273, may have a role.
**2** Vienna classification into 24 groups depending on age (> or <40yrs), site affected, and behaviour.

## Additional therapies in Crohn's disease (useful in ≤50% of patients)

**Azathioprine (AZA)** (2-2.5mg/kg/d PO) can be a used as a steroid-sparing agent, eg if steroid SEs, and if there are multiple/rapid relapses. It takes 6-10 weeks to work.[210] Steroids are so disappointing in the long term that *early combined immunosuppression* (azathioprine + infliximab ± steroids) is a tempting early option ('reversing the pyramid'). But evidence is scant; get expert advice.[211, 212]

**Sulfasalazine** Efficacy of 5-ASA in Crohn's is unproven but high-dose PENTASA post-op in patients with ileal resection may ↓recurrent disease.

**TNFα inhibitors** TNFα plays an important role in pathogenesis of Crohn's disease, therefore TNFα inhibitors, eg *infliximab* and *adalimumab*, can ↓disease activity. They counter neutrophil accumulation and granuloma formation, activate complement, and cause cytotoxicity to CD4+ T-cells, thus clearing cells driving the immune response. Response may be short-lived, but it may be repeated at 8wks. Trials have also shown it to be effective as maintenance therapy.[213] CI: Sepsis, ↑LFT >3-fold above top end of normal, concurrent *ciclosporin* or *tacrolimus*. SE: Rash. Avoid in people with known underlying malignancy.[214] TB may reactivate when on infliximab, so screen patients before starting the treatment (CXR, PPD). Cost per QALY: (see p10) £6700 (higher in fistulizing Crohn's).[215] According to SONIC trial, combined AZA and infliximab can ↑ efficacy of R at 12 months, but there are long-term safety issues (eg hepatosplenic T cell lymphomas).

**Methotrexate** A large randomized trial recommended 25mg IM weekly for remission induction, enabling complete withdrawal from steroids in patients with refractory Crohn's. NNT ≈ 5—see p669. There was no evidence for lower doses, and no substantial SE were found.[216] Methotrexate is contraindicated in pregnancy.

**Nutrition** Enteral is preferred (eg polymeric diet); consider TPN as a last resort. *Elemental diets* (E028®) contain amino acids and can give remission.[217, 218] **Low residue diets** help control Crohn's activity, but won't on their own give remission.

**Antibiotics** such as rifaximin EIR (extended intestinal release) 800mg/d PO gave a remission in one RCT.[219] **Probiotics** (eg lactobacilli): no randomized data.[220]

**IV immunoglobulin** Small series report rapid benefit (no randomized trials).[221]

**Surgery** 50-80% need ≥1 operation in their life. It never cures. In the severely affected, it can become a devastating cycle of deterioration. Indications: drug failure (most common); GI obstruction from stricture; perforation; fistulae; abscess. Surgical aims are: 1 to defunction (rest) distal disease, eg with a temporary ileostomy or 2 resection of the worst areas—but see short bowel syndrome, p582[222] Bypass and pouch surgery is **not** done in Crohn's (∴ ↑risk of recurrence).

**Poor prognosis if:** Age <30yrs (onset age is bimodal: peaks 20-30yrs and 60-70); steroids needed at 1st presentation; perianal disease; diffuse small bowel disease.

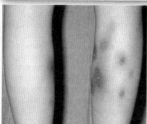

Fig 1. *Beyond the gut...* "I hate how this stupid illness is crippling me..." As well as erythema nodosum on the shins (above; also caused by sarcoid, drugs, streptococci and TB) Crohn's can associate with sero-ve arthritis of big joints, spondyloarthropathy, ankylosing spondylitis, sacroiliitis, pyoderma gangrenosum, conjunctivitis, episcleritis, and iritis.

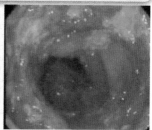

Fig 2. Deep fissured ulcers seen at coloscopy. The end result? "My family does not or will not even talk to me about the disease ... I don't know when urgency to race for the bathroom will happen so I don't go out and have been living a hermit life..." ©Dr A Mee.

IBS denotes a mixed group of abdominal symptoms for which no organic cause can be found. Most are probably due to disorders of intestinal motility or enhanced visceral perception (the 'brain-gut' axis: see BOX). Several diagnostic criteria exist that evaluate symptoms and their duration (eg Manning, Rome II/III),[223,224] but they are not always helpful in practice because of complex interactions between IBS and chronic pain syndromes (BOX).[225] *Prevalence:* 10–20%; age at onset: ≤40yrs; ♀:♂ ≥2:1.

**Diagnosis** Only diagnose IBS if abdominal pain (or discomfort) is either relieved by defecation *or* associated with altered stool form or bowel frequency (constipation and diarrhoea may alternate) *and* there are ≥2 of: urgency; incomplete evacuation; abdominal bloating/distension; mucous PR; worsening of symptoms after food. Other symptoms: nausea, bladder symptoms, backache. Symptoms are chronic (>6 months), and exacerbated by stress, menstruation, or gastroenteritis (post-infection IBS). *Signs:* Examination is often normal, but general abdominal tenderness is common. Insufflation of air during sigmoidoscopy (*not* usually needed) may reproduce the pain. *Think of other diagnoses if:* Age >40yrs (esp male); history <6 months; anorexia; weight↓; waking at night with pain/diarrhoea; mouth ulcers; abnormal CRP, ESR, Hb, coeliac serology. ▶Investigate PR bleeding urgently. **Management** See BOX.

## Carcinoma of the pancreas

*Epidemiology:* ≤2% of all malignancy; ~6500 deaths/yr (UK). UK incidence is rising. *Typical patient:* ♂ >60yrs old. *Risk factors:* Smoking, alcohol, carcinogens, DM, chronic pancreatitis, waist circumference↑ (ie adiposity);[226] and possibly a high fat and red or processed meat diet.[227] *Pathology:* Mostly ductal adenocarcinoma (metastasize early; present late). 60% arise in the pancreas head, 25% in the body, 15% tail. A few arise in the ampulla of Vater (ampullary tumour) or pancreatic islet cells (insulinoma, gastrinoma, glucagonomas, somatostatinomas (p215), VIPomas); both have a better prognosis. *Genetics:* ~95% have mutations in the KRAS2 gene.

**The patient** Tumours in the head of the pancreas present with **painless obstructive jaundice.** 75% of tumours in the body and tail present with epigastric pain (radiates to back and relieved by sitting forward). Either may cause anorexia, weight loss, diabetes or acute pancreatitis. *Rarer features:* Thrombophlebitis migrans (eg an arm vein becomes swollen and red, then a leg vein); Ca²⁺↑; marantic endocarditis; portal hypertension (splenic vein thrombosis); nephrosis (renal vein metastases). *Signs:* Jaundice + palpable gallbladder (Courvoisier's 'law', p250); epigastric mass; hepatomegaly; splenomegaly; lymphadenopathy; ascites.

**Tests** *Blood:* Cholestatic jaundice. CA 19-9↑ (p534) is non-specific, but helps assess prognosis. *Imaging:* US or CT can show a pancreatic mass ± dilated biliary tree ± hepatic metastases. They can guide biopsy and help staging prior to surgery/stent insertion. Compared to MRI and CT, EUS (endoscopic sonography) is most accurate for diagnosis and staging.[228] ERCP (p756) shows biliary tree anatomy and may localize the site of obstruction. ℞: Most ductal cancers present with metastatic disease; <20% are suitable for radical surgery. Don't automatically exclude if hepatic or mesenteric arteries are invaded; they can be reconstructed.[229] *Surgery:* Consider pancreatoduodenectomy (Whipple's, p279), eg if fit and with no metastases. Post-op morbidity is high (mortality <5%); non-curative resection confers no survival benefit. *Laparoscopic excision:* Tail lesions are easiest. *Post-op chemotherapy* delays disease progression. *Palliation of jaundice:* Endoscopic or percutaneous stent insertion may help jaundice and anorexia. Rarely, palliative bypass surgery is done for duodenal obstruction or unsuccessful ERCP. *Pain:* Disabling pain may need big doses of opiates (p576), or radiotherapy. Coeliac plexus infiltration with alcohol may be done at the time of surgery, or percutaneously. Referral to a palliative care team is essential.

**Prognosis** Often dismal (but keep up-to-date as chemotherapy is improving). Mean survival <6 months. 5yr survival: 3%ᵁᴷ. Overall 5yr survival after Whipple's procedure (p279) 5–14%. Prognosis is better if: tumour <3cm; no nodes involved; -ve resection margins at surgery; ampullary or islet cell tumours.[225]

## ☼Managing IBS

Make a *positive* diagnosis (OPPOSITE) but also try to exclude other diagnoses, so:
• If the history is classic, FBC, ESR, CRP, LFT & coeliac serology (p280) are sufficient.
• If ≥50yrs or any marker or organic disease (T▸t, blood PR, weight↓): colonoscopy.
• Have a low threshold for referring if family history of ovarian or bowel cancer.
• Excluding ovarian cancer may need serum CA-125 (OHCS p281; if >35 do US scan).
• If diarrhoea is prominent do: LFT; stool culture; B12/folate; anti-endomysial anti-bodies (coeliac, p280); TSH; consider referral ± barium follow-through (if symptoms suggest small bowel disease) ± rectal biopsy.

Further investigation should be guided by symptoms and include:
• Upper GI endoscopy (dyspepsia, reflux) or small bowel radiology (Crohn's).
• Duodenal biopsy (coeliac disease), eg if anti-endomysial antibodies +ve.
• Giardia tests, p436 (it often triggers IBS; antiparasitic R may not help)[230]
• ERCP (p756, eg chronic pancreatitis) or MRCP (p756) if active pancreatitis.
• Transit studies and anorectal physiological studies—rarely used.

**Refer if: 1** Diagnosis unsure **2** If changing symptoms in 'known IBS' **3** *To surgeon* if rectal mucosal prolapse **4** *To dietician* if food intolerance[1] **5** *To psycho- or hypno-therapist* if stress or depression (seen in ≥50%) or refractory symptoms (here, NICE favours cognitive therapy, OHCS p372) **6** *To gynaecologist* if cyclical pain, dyspareunia, dysmenorrhoea; CA-125↑; endometriosis (OHCS p288) often mimics IBS **7** *To dermatologist* if co-existing atopy (IBS is 3-fold more common in atopy)[231] **8** *To yourself* (wearing a different hat) or *pain clinic* if *chronic pain overlap syndromes* (fibromyalgia + chronic fatigue + chronic pelvic pain) or detrusor problems.

**R ⸪** Treatment is rarely 50% successful, so aim to make symptoms less intrusive by forging a *therapeutic alliance*. *Explanation* and *reassurance* are vital as is *interdisciplinary teamwork* (interdisciplinary implies a harmonized approach, not just multidisciplinary with each specialist ploughing his own furrow).[232] Ensure a healthy diet; fibre, lactose, fructose, wheat, starch, caffeine, sorbitol, alcohol and fizzy drinks may worsen symptoms. Probiotics and water-soluble fibre may be OK. Many IBS patients report food intolerance[2], but few clinicians consider food hypersensitivity to be a cause of IBS. No tests can identify food intolerance reliably.[NICE 2012] Dietary elimination and food challenge data are contradictory. Further R depends on which symptoms predominate:

• *Constipation:* The standard healthy diet (p236) may be problematic: ↑fibre intake can worsen flatulence/bloating; avoid insoluble fibre, such as bran (oats are better). *Bisacodyl* and *sodium picosulfate*[233] can help constipation. *Ispaghula* has non-fermentable water-soluble fibre—better than *lactulose* which ferments (↑gas production is hard to distinguish from bloating).[234]
• *Diarrhoea:* Avoid sorbitol sweeteners; try a bulking agent ± *loperamide* 2mg after each loose stool; max 16mg/d (NNT=5). SE: colic, bloating, ileus.
• *Colic/bloating:* Oral antispasmodics: *mebeverine* 135mg/8h (over the counter); *alverine citrate* 60-120mg/8h;[235] *dicycloverine* 10-20mg/8h.[236] Adding *simeticone* (=dimeticone; it's in Imodium Plus®) improves spasm.[237] Once-daily *Bacillus coagulans* GBI-30, *B. infantis* 35624, *E. coli* DSM17252 and *L. acidophilus.*[238, 239]
• *Psychological symptoms/visceral hypersensitivity:* Emphasize the positive! In 50% symptoms go or improve after 1yr; <5% worsen. Consider cognitive behaviour therapy (OHCS p372), hypnosis,[1] and tricyclics, eg *amitriptyline* 10-50mg at night (SE: dry mouth); explain that it's for chronic pain (± depression).[240, 241] NNT=6. Explain that all forms of abuse (sexual, physical, verbal) perpetuate IBS.

**The future** Interest is being expressed in modulating the brain-gut axis by 5-HT3 antagonists (eg alosetron; 2012 data show it can ↑ quality of life and ↓ restriction of daily activities in women with severe diarrhoea-predominant IBS, but it has a chequered regulatory history owing to SE, eg ischaemic colitis).[242]

---

**1** Food intolerance: dietary fibre and lactose (milk and dairy foods). Wheat resistant starch, caffeine, fructose, sorbitol, alcohol and fizzy drinks.
**2** 12wks of hypnosis helps abnormal sensory perception:[243] ▸Do not think of hypnosis as dubious; it is a neat way to influence the brain-gut axis, reducing doctor dependency and stopping patients from being patients (passive recipients of suffering). Benefits may last ≥5yrs.[244, 245]

▶Always consider that more than one nutritional disorder is likely to be present.

**Scurvy** is due to lack of vitamin C.[1] Is the patient poor, pregnant, or on an odd diet? *Signs:* 1 Listlessness, anorexia, cachexia (p29). 2 Gingivitis, loose teeth, and foul-breath (halitosis). 3 Bleeding from gums, nose, hair follicles, or into joints, bladder, gut. 4 Muscle pain/weakness. 5 Oedema.[246,247] *Diagnosis:* No test is completely satisfactory. WBC ascorbic acid↓. *R:* Dietary education; *ascorbic acid* ≥250mg/24h PO.

**Beriberi** There is heart failure with general oedema (wet beriberi) or neuropathy (dry beriberi) due to lack of vitamin $B_1$ (thiamine). For treatment and diagnostic tests, see Wernicke's encephalopathy (p728).

**Pellagra** = lack of nicotinic acid. Classical triad: diarrhoea, dementia, dermatitis (Casal's necklace) ± neuropathy, depression, insomnia, tremor, rigidity, ataxia, fits. It may occur in carcinoid syndrome and anti-TB drugs (isoniazid). It is endemic in China and Africa. *R:* Education, electrolyte replacement, *nicotinamide* 100mg/4h PO.[248] See BOX.

**Xerophthalmia** This vitamin A deficiency syndrome is a big cause of blindness in the Tropics. Conjunctivae become dry and develop oval/triangular spots (Bitôt's spots). Corneas become cloudy and soft. Give *vitamin A* (OHCS p450). ▶Get special help if pregnant: vitamin A embryopathy must be avoided. Re-educate and monitor diet.

## Carcinoid tumours

This is a specialized area! A diverse group of tumours of enterochromaffin cell (neural crest) origin, by definition capable of producing 5HT. Common sites: appendix (45%), ileum (30%) or rectum (20%).[2] They also occur elsewhere in the GI tract, ovary, testis, and bronchi. 80% of tumours >2cm across will metastasize (ie consider all as malignant). *Symptoms & signs:* Initially few. GI tumours can cause appendicitis, intussusception, or obstruction. Hepatic metastases may cause RUQ pain. Tumours may secrete bradykinin, tachykinin, substance P, VIP, gastrin, insulin, glucagon, ACTH (∴ Cushing's syndrome), parathyroid, and thyroid hormones. 10% are part of MEN-1 syndrome (p215); 10% occur with other neuroendocrine tumours.[249]

**Carcinoid syndrome** occurs in ~5% and implies hepatic involvement.

*Symptoms and signs:* Bronchoconstriction; paroxysmal flushing especially in upper body (± migrating weals); diarrhoea; CCF (tricuspid incompetence and pulmonary stenosis from 5HT-induced fibrosis). *CNS effects:* Many, eg enhanced ability to learn new stimulus–response associations.[250] ▶*Carcinoid crisis:* See BOX.

**Δ** 24h urine 5-hydroxyindoleacetic acid↑ (5HIAA, a 5HT metabolite; levels change with drugs and diet, eg bananas, avocado, walnuts, pineapple, coffee, chocolate: discuss with lab). CXR + chest/pelvis MRI/CT help locate primary tumours. Plasma chromogranin A (reflects tumour mass); [111]Indium octreotide scintigraphy (octreoscan);[251] and positron emission tomography (p753) also have a role. Echocardiography and BNP (p131) can be used to investigate carcinoid heart disease.[252] **ΔΔ:** GIST.[3]

*R: Carcinoid syndrome:* Octreotide (somatostatin analogue) blocks release of tumour mediators and counters peripheral effects. Alternative: *lanreotide*. Effects lessen over time. Other options: *loperamide* or *cyproheptadine* for diarrhoea;[253] *interferon-α* as add-in therapy◆[?] with *octreotide*.[254] *Tumour therapy:* Resection is the only cure for carcinoid tumours (fig 1), so it is vital to find the primary site (see above). At surgery, tumours are an intense yellow. Procedures depend on site, eg rectal carcinoid tumours <1cm can be resected endoscopically.[255] Debulking (eg enucleating), embolization, or radiofrequency ablation of hepatic metastases can ↓symptoms. Give *octreotide* cover to avoid precipitating a massive carcinoid crisis.

**Median survival** 5-8yrs (~3yrs if metastases are present, but may be up to 20yrs; so beware of giving up too easily, even in metastatic disease)[249]

---

1 That oranges and lemons prevent 'the scurvy' was noted by the naval surgeon James Lind in 1753.[216]
2 Some are never clinically detected: 1 in 300 autopsies have a small bowel carcinoid tumour.
3 Gastrointestinal stromal tumours (GISTs) are mesenchymal tumours arising from interstitial Cajal cells of the wall of the gut. They may co-exist with carcinoid tumours.[257]

## ▶▶Carcinoid crisis

When a tumour outgrows its blood supply or is handled too much during surgery, mediators flood out. There is life-threatening vasodilatation, hypotension, tachycardia, bronchoconstriction and hyperglycaemia. It is treated with high-dose *octreotide*, supportive measures and careful management of fluid balance (ie a central line is needed—see p789 for insertion technique).

## ⋮ Food mountains, the pellagra paradox, and the sorrow that weeping cannot symbolize[1]

'The sweet smell is a great sorrow on the land. Men who can graft the trees and make the seed fertile and big can find no way to let the hungry people eat their produce ... The works of the roots of the vines, of the trees, must be destroyed to keep up the price ...

There is a crime here that goes beyond denunciation. There is a sorrow here that weeping cannot symbolize. There is a failure here that topples all our success. The fertile earth, the straight tree rows, the sturdy trunks, and the ripe fruit. And children dying of pellagra must die because a profit cannot be taken from an orange. And coroners must fill in the certificates—died of malnutrition—because the food must rot, must be forced to rot.

The people come with nets to fish for potatoes in the river, and the guards hold them back; they come in rattling cars to get the dumped oranges, but the kerosene is sprayed. And they stand still and watch the potatoes float by, listen to the screaming pigs being killed in a ditch and covered with quicklime, watch the mountains of oranges slop down to a putrefying ooze; and in the eyes of the people there is a failure; and in the eyes of the hungry there is a growing wrath. In the souls of the people the grapes of wrath are filling and growing heavy, growing heavy for the vintage.'

How do John Steinbeck's grapes grow in our 21st-century soil? Too well; a double harvest, it turns out, as not only is much of the world starving, amid plenty (for those who can pay) but also there is a new 'sorrow in our land that weeping cannot symbolize': pathological 'voluntary' self-starvation, again amid plenty, in pursuit of the body-beautiful according to images laid down by media gods. If gastroenterologists had one wish it might not be the ending of all their diseases, but that humankind stand in a right relationship with Steinbeck's fertile earth, his straight trees, his sturdy trunks, and his ripe fruit.

## Whipple's procedure

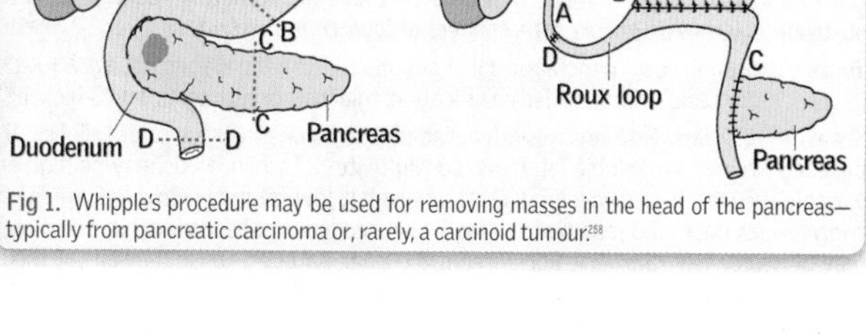

(a) Areas of reflection of different parts     (b) Post-operation

**Fig 1.** Whipple's procedure may be used for removing masses in the head of the pancreas—typically from pancreatic carcinoma or, rarely, a carcinoid tumour.[58]

---

1 J Steinbeck *The Grapes of Wrath*, chapter 25.

**Symptoms** Diarrhoea; ↓weight; lethargy; steatorrhoea (stool fat↑; hard to flush away) bloating.

**Deficiency signs** Anaemia (↓Fe, B₁₂, folate); bleeding disorders (↓vit κ); oedema (↓protein); metabolic bone disease (↓vit D); neurological features, eg neuropathy.

**Tests** FBC (↓ or ↑MCV); ↓Ca²⁺; ↓Fe; ↓B₁₂ + folate; ↑INR; lipid profile; coeliac tests (below). *Stool:* Sudan stain for fat globules; stool microscopy (infestation); α₁AT (p264), elastase. *Ba follow-through:* Diverticula; Crohn's; radiation enteritis. *Breath hydrogen analysis:* for bacterial overgrowth.¹ Take samples of end-expired air; give glucose; take more samples at ½h intervals; ↑exhaled hydrogen = overgrowth. *Endoscopy + small bowel biopsy, ERCP:* (p756) biliary obstruction; chronic pancreatitis. **Causes** See BOX.

*Tropical malabsorption* (*Giardia, Cryptosporidium, Isospora belli, Cyclospora cayetanensis*, microsporidia.) *Tropical sprue:* Villous atrophy + malabsorption occurring in the Far and Middle East and Caribbean—the cause is unknown. *Tetracycline* 250mg/6h PO + *folic acid* 15mg/d PO + optimum nutrition may help.²⁵⁹

## Coeliac disease

▶Suspect this in all those with diarrhoea + weight loss or anaemia (esp. if iron or B₁₂ ↓). It is a T-cell-mediated autoimmune disease of the small bowel in which prolamin (alcohol-soluble proteins in wheat, barley, rye ± oats) intolerance causes villous atrophy and malabsorption (including of bile acids).²,³ *Associations:* HLA DQ2 in 95%; the rest are DQ8; autoimmune disease; dermatitis herpetiformis. *Prevalence:* 1 in 300-1500 (commoner if Irish). *Typical age:* Any (peaks in infancy and 50-60yrs). ♀:♂ >1:1. There is a 10% prevalence in 1ˢᵗ-degree relatives and a 30% relative risk for siblings.

**Presentation** Stinking stools/steatorrhoea; diarrhoea; abdominal pain; bloating; nausea + vomiting; aphthous ulcers; angular stomatitis (p321, fig 2); weight↓; fatigue; weakness; osteomalacia; failure to thrive (children). ⅓ are asymptomatic.

**Diagnosis** Hb↓; RCDW↑ (p319); B₁₂↓, ferritin↓. Antibodies: α-gliadin, transglutaminase and anti-endomysial—an IgA antibody, 95% specific unless patient is IgA-deficient. Duodenal biopsy done at endoscopy (p256—as good as jejunal biopsy if ≥4 taken): subtotal villous atrophy, ↑intra-epithelial WBCs + crypt hyperplasia, **reversing** on gluten-free diet (along with ↓symptoms & antibodies). ▶Exclude coeliac in all labelled as IBS (p276).

**Treatment** Lifelong gluten-free diet (ie no prolamins)—patients become experts. Rice, maize, soya, potatoes, oats (≤50g/d),²⁶⁰ and sugar are OK. Gluten-free biscuits, flour, bread, and pasta are prescribable. Verify diet by endomysial antibody tests.

**Complications** Anaemia; 2° lactose-intolerance⁴; GI T-cell lymphoma (rare; suspect if refractory symptoms or ↓weight); ↑risk of malignancy (gastric, oesophageal, bladder, breast, brain); myopathies; neuropathies; hyposplenism; osteoporosis.

## Chronic pancreatitis

Epigastric pain 'bores' through to back, eg relieved by sitting forward or hot water bottles on epigastrium/back (look for *erythema ab igne*'s mottled dusky greyness); bloating; steatorrhoea; ↓weight; brittle diabetes. Symptoms relapse and worsen.

**Causes:** Alcohol; rarely: familial; cystic fibrosis; haemochromatosis; pancreatic duct obstruction (stones/tumour); ↑PTH; congenital (*pancreas divisum*).

**Tests** *Ultrasound ± CT* (pancreatic calcifications confirm the diagnosis), *MRCP + ERCP* (risks acute attack); *AXR:* speckled calcification; ↑glucose; breath tests, eg ¹³C-hiolien.²⁶¹

**Treatment** *Drugs:* Give analgesia (coeliac-plexus block may give brief relief);²⁶² lipase, eg Creon®; fat-soluble vitamins (eg Multivite®). Insulin needs may be high or variable (beware hypoglycaemia). *Diet:* No alcohol; low fat may help. Medium-chain triglycerides (MCT oil®) may be tried (no lipase needed for absorption, but diarrhoea may be worsened). *Surgery:* For unremitting pain; narcotic abuse (beware of this); weight↓: eg pancreatectomy or pancreaticojejunostomy (a duct drainage procedure).

**Complications** Pseudocyst; diabetes; biliary obstruction; local arterial aneurysm; splenic vein thrombosis; gastric varices; pancreatic carcinoma.

## Causes of gastrointestinal malabsorption

**Common in the UK** Coeliac disease; chronic pancreatitis; Crohn's disease.

**Rarer**

- ↓*Bile:* Primary biliary cirrhosis; ileal resection; biliary obstruction; colestyramine.
- *Pancreatic insufficiency:* Pancreatic cancer; cystic fibrosis.
- *Small bowel mucosa:* Whipple's disease (p730); radiation enteritis; tropical sprue; small bowel resection; brush border enzyme deficiencies (eg lactase insufficiency); drugs (metformin, neomycin, alcohol); amyloid (p364).
- *Bacterial overgrowth* (esp. in elderly); in jejunal diverticula; post-op blind loops. DM & PPI use are also risk factors. Try *metronidazole* 400mg/8h PO or *oxytetracycline* 250mg/6h. Don't confuse with afferent loop syndrome (p624).
- *Infection:* Giardiasis; diphyllobothriasis (B₁₂ malabsorption); strongyloidiasis.
- *Intestinal hurry:* Post-gastrectomy dumping; post-vagotomy; gastrojejunostomy.

## Deficiency syndromes and the sites of nutrient absorption

| Vitamin/nutrient | Site of absorption | Deficiency syndrome |
|---|---|---|
| A$^F$ | Small intestine | Xerophthalmia (p278) |
| B₁ (thiamine) | Small intestine | Beriberi (p278); Wernicke's encephalopathy (p728) |
| B₂ (riboflavin) | Proximal small intestine | Angular stomatis; cheilitis (p238) |
| B₆ (pyridoxine) | Small intestine | Polyneuropathy |
| B₁₂ | Terminal ileum | Macrocytic anaemia (p326); neuropathy; glossitis |
| C | Proximal ileum | Scurvy (p278) |
| D$^F$ | Jejunum as free vitamin | Rickets (p698); osteomalacia (p698) |
| E$^F$ | Small intestine | Haemolysis; neurological deficit |
| K$^F$ | Small intestine | Bleeding disorders (p338) |
| Folic acid | Jejunum | Macrocytic anaemia (p326) |
| Nicotinamide | Jejunum | Pellagra (p278) |
| **Mineral** | | |
| Calcium | Duodenum + jejunum | p690 |
| Copper | Stomach + jejunum | Menkes' kinky hair syndrome |
| Fluoride | Stomach | Dental caries |
| Iodide | Small intestine | Goitre; cretinism |
| Iron | Duodenum + jejunum | Microcytic anaemia (p320) |
| Magnesium | Small intestine | p693 |
| Phosphate | Small intestine | Osteoporosis; anorexia; weakness |
| Selenium | Small intestine | Cardiomyopathy (p693) |
| Zinc | Jejunum | Acrodermatitis enteropathica; poor wound healing (p693) |

$^F$ = fat-soluble vitamin, thus deficiency is likely if there is fat malabsorption.

1 Bacterial overgrowth proximal to the colon causes diarrhoea, abdominal pain, vitamin malabsorption and possibly malnutrition. Causes: old age, chronic pancreatitis; HIV; bacteria not killed by gastric acid (PPI; achlorhydria); fistulae; post-gastrectomy/Roux-en-Y; jejunal diverticula; amyloidosis; autonomic neuropathy. Diagnosis: breath test or culture of duodenal aspirate (>10⁵ colonies/mL). OHGH p226.

2 Bile acid malabsorption: too much bile getting to the colon causes watery diarrhoea. There is also bloating±gallstone formation. Causes: coeliac or Crohn's, post-cholecystectomy syndrome, or radiation enteritis. Δ: SeHCAT test (selenium homocholic acid taurine): OHGH p232. Ŗ: ↑Fluid intake (to ↓risk of forming oxalate stone); bile acid sequestrants (colestyramine; colestipol; colesevelam); vitamins A, D, E and K.²⁸⁴

3 Infectious causes have been implicated: eg *Candida albicans* could be one trigger. HWP1 has amino acid sequences identical to coeliac disease-related α-gliadin T-cell epitopes.²⁸⁵

4 Lactose intolerance (lactase↓ on brush border, OHGH p384) causes bloating, colic, wind and diarrhoea after milk products. Investigate with the lactose hydrogen breath test. Lactase can be replaced, if a lactose-free diet does not agree. Probiotics may have a role.²⁶³

An alcoholic is one whose repeated drinking leads to harm in work or social life. Intake ranges from binging to heavy daily use, and is usually tied in with other life or health issues. Other addictions may also be involved. Lifetime prevalence: ~10%♂ (♀≈4%). ▶Denial is a leading feature, so be sure to question relatives. Benefits of low dose alcohol (eg <20u/wk in men, <15u/wk in women, see p236) are unproven.

**CAGE questions** Ever felt you ought to cut down on your drinking? Have people annoyed you by criticizing your drinking? Ever felt bad or guilty about your drinking, eg if it led to you neglecting your responsibilities or to social or psychological harm? Ever had an eye-opener to steady nerves in the morning? Drinking to relieve withdrawal symptoms is a very telling sign. CAGE (yes to ≥2) helps detect dependency (sensitivity 43-94%; specificity 70-97%)[266] but accuracy does change according to background population. There are other screening methods: eg TWEAK (BOX 1); AUDIT[267]

**Organs affected** ▶Don't forget the risk of trauma while intoxicated.[268]
*The liver:* Normal in 50%; ɣGT↑ or ↑↑[1]—but may be ↑↑ in *any* type of liver inflammation, eg fatty liver, AIH (p268), HBV. *Fatty liver:* Acute/reversible, but may progress to cirrhosis if drinking continues (also seen in obesity, DM, and with amiodarone). *Alcoholic hepatitis:* BOX 2 & 3. 80% progress to cirrhosis (hepatic failure in 10%). *Cirrhosis* (p260): 5yr survival is 48% if drinking continues (if not, 77%). Biopsy: Mallory bodies ± neutrophil infiltrate (can be indistinguishable from NASH, p261).

*CNS:* Self neglect; ↓memory/cognition: high-potency vitamins IM may reverse it (p728; don't delay!); cortical atrophy; retrobulbar neuropathy; fits; falls; wide-based gait neuropathy; confabulation/Korsakoff's (p718) ± Wernicke's encephalopathy (p728).

*Gut:* Obesity; D&V; gastric erosions; peptic ulcers; varices (p254); pancreatitis (acute or chronic); cancer (many types); oesophageal rupture (∵ vomiting against a closed glottis; suspect if shock and surgical emphysema in the neck: Boerhaave's syndrome).

*Blood:* MCV↑; anaemia from: marrow depression, GI bleeding, alcoholism-associated folate deficiency, haemolysis; sideroblastic anaemia. See p320.

*Heart:* Arrhythmias; BP↑; cardiomyopathy; sudden death in binge drinkers.

**Withdrawal** starts 10-72h after last drink. *Signs:* Pulse↑; BP↓; tremor; confusion; fits; hallucinations (*delirium tremens*)—may be visual or tactile, eg animals crawling all over skin. Consider it in any new (≤3d) ward patient with acute confusion.

**Alcohol contraindications** Driving; hepatitis; cirrhosis; peptic ulcer; drugs (eg antihistamines, metronidazole); carcinoid; pregnancy (eg fetal alcohol syndrome—IQ↓, short palpebral fissure, absent philtrum, and small eyes).

**Management** *Alcohol withdrawal:* Admit; do BP + TPR/4h. Beware BP↓. For the 1st 3d give generous *chlordiazepoxide*, eg 10-50mg/6h PO, weaning over 7-10d (TABLE 2); alternative: *diazepam*. Vitamins may be needed (p728). *Prevention:* (OHCS p513): Alcohol-free beers; price may help promote low-risk drinking (see below). NB: there are no absolutes: risk is a continuum. *1u≈9g ethanol≈1 spirits measure≈1 glass of wine≈½pint of beer. Treating established alcoholics* may be rewarding, particularly if they really want to change. If so, group therapy or self-help (eg Alcoholics Anonymous) may be useful—especially if self-initiated and determined. Encourage the will to change. ✨Suggest: **1** Graceful ways of declining a drink, eg "I'm seeing what it's like to go without for a bit". **2** Not buying him- or herself a drink when it is his/her turn. **3** "Don't lift your glass to your lips until after the slowest drinker in your group takes a drink." **4** "Sip, don't gulp." Give follow-up and encouragement.

**Relapse** 50% will relapse soon after starting treatment. *Acamprosate* (p455)[269] may help intense anxiety, insomnia, and craving. CI: pregnancy, severe liver failure, creatinine >120μmol/L. SE: D&V, libido ↑ or ↓; dose example: 666mg/8h PO if >60kg and <65yrs old.[270] It should be started as soon as acute withdrawal is complete and continued for ~1yr. *Disulfiram* can be used to treat chronic alcohol dependence. It causes acetaldehyde build-up (like metronidazole) with extremely unpleasant effects to *any* alcohol ingestion—eg flushing, throbbing headache, palpitations. Care must be taken to avoid alcohol (eg toiletries, food, medicines) since severe reactions can occur. ▶Confer with experts if drugs are to be used.

## TWEAK screening questions[271]

| | |
|---|---|
| • Have you an increased tolerance of alcohol? | 2 points |
| • Do you worry about your drinking? | 2 points |
| • Have you ever had alcohol as an eye-opener in the morning? | 1 point |
| • Do you ever get amnesia after drinking alcohol? | 1 point |
| • Have you ever felt the need to c(k)ut down on your drinking? | 1 point |

A score of ≥2 suggests an alcohol problem. It may be more sensitive than the CAGE questionnaire in some populations (eg pregnant women).[272]

## Patterns of lab tests in alcoholic and other liver disease

| | AST | ALT | AST : ALT | MCV |
|---|---|---|---|---|
| Alcoholic liver disease | ↑↑ | ↑ | >2 | ↑↑ |
| Hepatitis C (HCV) | ↑ or ↔ | ↑↑ | <1* | ↔ |
| Non-alcoholic fatty liver disease | ↑ | ↑↑ | <1 | ↑ or ↔ |

*Ratio may reverse if cirrhosis develops. Reference intervals: p742. How to remember AST:ALT ratios...alcohol is the prime cause of any liver disease, but if ALT↑ more than anything else, you've got to think of ALTernative diagnoses.

## Managing alcoholic hepatitis [273, 274]

**The patient** Malaise; TPR↑; anorexia; D&V; tender hepatomegaly ± jaundice; bleeding; ascites. *Blood:* WCC↑; platelets↓ (toxic effect or ∴ hypersplenism); INR↑; AST↑; MCV↑; urea↑. ►Jaundice, encephalopathy or coagulopathy ≈ *severe* hepatitis.
- Most need hospitalizing; urinary catheter and CVP monitoring may be needed.
- Screen for infections ± ascitic fluid tap and treat for SBP (p260).
- Stop alcohol consumption: for withdrawal symptoms, if *chlordiazepoxide* by the oral route (see below) is impossible, try *lorazepam* IM.
- Vitamins: vit K: 10mg/d IV for 3d. Thiamine 100mg/d PO (high-dose B vitamins can also be given IV as *Pabrinex*®—1 pair of ampoules in 50mL 0.9% saline IVI over ½h; see Datasheet—have resuscitation equipment to hand).
- Optimize nutrition (35–40kcal/kg/d non-protein energy). Use ideal body weight for calculations, eg if malnourished.
- Don't use low-protein diets even if severe encephalopathy is present. Give >1.2g/kg/d of protein; this prevents encephalopathy, sepsis, and some deaths.
- Daily weight; LFT; U&E; INR. If creatinine↑, get help with this—HRS (p259). Na↓ is common, but water restriction may make matters worse.
- Prednisolone 40mg/d for 5d tapered over 3wks if Maddrey score >31 and encephalopathy.●☞ ►CI: sepsis; variceal bleeding. Maddrey Discriminant Factor (DF) = (4.6 × patient's prothrombin time in sec – control time) + bilirubin (µmol/L). This score roughly reflects mortality (the MELD score is an alternative). NB: prednisolone plus N-acetylcysteine may increase 1-month survival, but 6-month survival is not improved.[275]

*Prognosis:* Mild episodes hardly affect mortality; if severe, mortality ≈ 50% at 30d. 1yr after admission for alcoholic hepatitis, 40% are dead...a sobering thought.

## An example of a chlordiazepoxide-reducing regimen

| Day | AM | noon | PM | at night | total/d |
|---|---|---|---|---|---|
| 1 | 20mg | 20mg | 20mg | 20mg | 80mg |
| 2 | 20mg | 15mg | 15mg | 20mg | 70mg |
| 3 | 15mg | 15mg | 15mg | 15mg | 60mg |
| 4 | 15mg | 10mg | 10mg | 15mg | 50mg |
| 5 | 10mg | 10mg | 10mg | 10mg | 40mg |
| 6 | 10mg | 5mg | 5mg | 10mg | 30mg |
| 7 | 5mg | 5mg | 5mg | 5mg | 20mg |
| 8 | 5mg | – | – | 5mg | 10mg |
| 9 (final day) | – | – | – | 5mg | 5mg |

►*Caveats:* higher doses for 1st few days for severe withdrawal; there may still be mild withdrawal symptoms at day 3. Have a 5mg dose written for PRN use.

---

**1** Gamma GT is ↑ in 52% of alcoholics; it is also ↑ in 50% of those with non-alcoholic fatty livers. Its best use is not in diagnosing alcoholism but in seeing if a raised alk phos is likely to be from liver, not bone.[276]

**Contents**

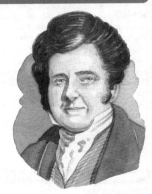

Fig 1. Richard Bright (1789-1858). Richard Bright began his career as a philosophy and economics student in Edinburgh, but quickly switched to medicine. He finished his training in London where he began research into kidney diseases. He is known as the father of modern nephrology, describing 'Bright's disease' or the combination of protein in the urine, hypertension and oedema, and deducing from autopsy studies that this was due to kidney disease. He inspired future generations to find treatments beyond that of blood letting to reduce blood pressure.

*Relevant pages in other chapters: Symptoms and signs:* Frequency (p64); loin pain (p57); oedema (p29); oliguria (p65); polyuria (p65).

*Surgery:* Renal stones (p640); renal & urological ca (p646); urinary retention (p644); incontinence (p650).

*Clinical chemistry:* Kidney function (p682); ►Creatinine clearance and eGFR (p683); Urate and the kidney (p694).

*Emergencies:* Management of acute kidney injury (p848).

*Also:* Vasculitis (p558); polyarteritis nodosa (p558); genitourinary TB (p289); immunosuppressives (p370); biochemistry of renal function (p682); electrolyte physiology (p688); Na⁺ (p686); K⁺ (p688); calcium (p690); urate and the kidney (p694); osteomalacia (p698); urinary tract imaging (p758); catheters (p776).

*In OHCS:* Gynaecological urology (*OHCS* p306); bacteriuria and pyelonephritis in pregnancy (*OHCS* p28); obstetric causes of acute tubular necrosis (*OHCS* p28); chronic kidney disease in pregnancy (*OHCS* p28); UTI in children (*OHCS* p174); urethral valves (*OHCS* p132); horseshoe kidney (*OHCS* p132); ectopic kidney (*OHCS* p132); hypospadias (*OHCS* p132); Wilms' nephroblastoma (*OHCS* p133); kidney disease in children (*OHCS* p176); nephritis and nephrosis in children (*OHCS* p178); Potter's syndrome (*OHCS* p132).

*We thank our Specialist Readers Dr Andrew Fry and Dr Andrew Mooney, and our Junior Reader Tom Georgiou, for their contribution to this chapter.*

**R**enal disease presents with rather few clinical syndromes—listed from 1 to 7 below. One underlying pathology may have a variety of clinical presentations, and vice versa, but patients will generally present with:

1 *Renal pain and dysuria:* Renal pain is usually a dull ache, constant and in the loin. It may be due to renal obstruction (look for swelling ± tenderness), pyelonephritis, acute nephritic syndrome, polycystic kidneys, or renal infarction. **Renal (ureteric) colic** is severe waxing and waning loin pain radiating to the groin or thigh, eg with fever and vomiting. It is caused by a renal stone, clot, or a sloughed papilla. **Urinary frequency** with dysuria (pain on voiding) suggests a UTI.

2 *Oliguria and polyuria:* Oliguria is a urine output of <0.5mL/kg/h. *Pathological* causes: Pre-renal, ie ↓perfusion; intrinsic renal, ie renal parenchymal disease; post-renal, ie obstruction. Polyuria is the voiding of abnormally high volumes of urine, usually from high fluid intake—or diabetes mellitus, diabetes insipidus (p232), hypercalcaemia, renal medullary disorders (urine concentrating ability is impaired).

3 *Acute kidney injury (AKI)* (previously termed acute renal failure or ARF). Indicates significant decline in renal function occurring over hours or days. AKI usually occurs secondary to a circulatory dysfunction (hypotension, hypovolaemia, sepsis) or urinary obstruction. Primary renal disease is a less common cause.

4 *Proteinuria and nephrotic syndrome:* Normal protein excretion is <150mg/d, as the glomerular basement membrane prevents passage of high-molecular-weight proteins (eg albumin) into urine. Nephrotic syndrome = proteinuria >3g/d, hypoalbuminaemia, oedema. Nephrotic range proteinuria (>3g/d) is almost always a sign of glomerular disease. Urine dipstick is unreliable for quantifying protein excretion; use spot protein:creatinine ratio or albumin:creatinine ratio on an early morning MSU.

5 *Haematuria:* Blood in the urine may arise from anywhere in the renal tract. Take haematuria seriously, as it may be the only sign of GU malignancy (esp if >40yrs old and a smoker). However, in the majority of cases it has a benign cause (eg infection, renal stones). The question of who to refer haematuria patients to (urologist or nephrologist) is answered on p286.

6 *Chronic kidney disease (CKD)* is defined as irreversible, substantial, and longstanding loss of renal function. It is classified according to glomerular filtration rate (GFR): see p683. There is often a poor correlation between symptoms and severity of renal disease. Progression may be so insidious that patients attribute symptoms to age or a minor illnesses. **Referral to renal services is based on local guidelines, but as a general rule refer if CKD stage 3 or more (p300),[1] ie GFR <60mL/min,** *if other features are present:*
 • GFR is falling progressively
 • Non-visible (microscopic) haematuria
 • Urine protein:creatinine ratio (PCR)↑,p286
 • Unexplained anaemia, hyperkalaemia, or calcium or phosphate imbalance
 • Suspected systemic illness (eg SLE)
 • BP uncontrolled despite taking 3 drugs.
 Refer *urgently* if GFR 15–29 (same-day if <15) even if *no* other features present.

7 *Silence:* Serious renal failure may cause **no symptoms at all.** This is why we check U&Es before surgery and other major interventions. The silence of renal disease creeps up on us (doctors and patients). Do not dismiss odd chronic symptoms such as fatigue or 'not being quite with it' without considering checking renal function. *Microalbuminuria* is a silent harbinger of serious renal and cardiovascular risk. It is described on p314. In one study, 30% of those with type 2 diabetes mellitus died within ~5 years of developing microalbuminuria. This is partly preventable by use of ACE-i.

Perform dipstick urinalysis whenever you suspect renal disease. This is a crude way of checking whether the urine contains anything that it shouldn't, eg protein, blood, glucose. Abnormalities can reflect renal tract or systemic disease and usually require further investigation. Proteinuria particularly requires formal quantification.

**Proteinuria** Consensus is now to avoid 24h collections (costly, inaccurate) and use albumin:creatinine ratio (ACR) or protein:creatinine ratio (PCR) on a random urine sample, ideally an early morning sample as this avoids orthostatic proteinuria. ACR is preferred to PCR, especially in diabetics.[2]

| Conversion factors | | |
|---|---|---|
| ACR mg/mmol | PCR mg/mmol | Protein excretion g/24h |
| 30 | 50 | 0.5 |
| 70 | 100 | 1 |

Normal ACR is <2.5 (men) or <3.5 (women). Transient rises to ~5 can occur with fever or exercise. Causes of raised ACR/PCR: glomerular or tubular disease (eg nephrotic syndrome, p302), DM, amyloidosis, ↑BP, interstitial nephritis, heavy metals, multiple myeloma (though dipsticks do not detect light chains), pregnancy, CCF. *Microalbuminuria:* Ultra-sensitive dipsticks are now available to measure microalbuminuria (albumin excretion 30–300mg/24h). Causes: DM, ↑BP, minimal change GN.

**Haematuria** Blood in the urine may arise from anywhere in the renal tract. It is classified as visible (VH—previously known as macroscopic, frank) or non-visible (NVH—found on dipstick or microscopy). Non-visible is subdivided into symptomatic (sNVH—with LUTS: dysuria, hesitancy, urgency, p644) and asymptomatic (aNVH). Dipstick of fresh urine is more sensitive than MSU, which has a high false -ve rate, therefore no need to confirm every positive dip with microscopy.[3] However, MC&S of urine is useful for further analysis of cause. Patients with one episode of VH, one of sNVH or persistent aNVH require further assessment.

- Exclude transient causes: (UTI, vigorous exercise, menstruation).
- Check creatinine/eGFR, proteinuria (spot ACR or PCR) and BP.
- Painless VH usually means bladder cancer (p648); refer urgently.
- In aNVH or if systemic symptoms, consider FBC, ESR, CRP, blood film, clotting (NB do not simply attribute haematuria to anticoagulants/antiplatelet agents).[3]
- Urine MC&S to look for infection, malignant/inflammatory cells, casts, crystals.
- USS and rapid referral to nephrology if rapid decline in GFR or haematuria with proteinuria, casts or dysmorphic cells. Red cell casts ≈ glomerular bleeding.

| Who to refer and to whom? | | |
|---|---|---|
| | Urology | Nephrology |
| VH | All patients, any age | <40yrs, cola-coloured urine, recent infection, eg URTI |
| sNVH | All patients, any age | |
| aNVH | Persistent, >40yrs | <40yrs with BP >140/90, eGFR <60mL/min, ACR >30 or PCR >50 |

All others should be monitored in primary care with annual review of urine dip, BP, eGFR and proteinuria (ACR/PCR); refer if above features appear. *Causes: Renal:* neoplasia, glomerulonephritis (often IgA nephropathy, p300), tubulointerstitial nephritis, polycystic kidney disease, papillary necrosis, infection (pyelonephritis), trauma. *Extrarenal:* Calculi, infection, neoplasia, trauma (eg from catheter). Some drugs can cause haematuria: eg, captopril, cephalosporins, ciprofloxacin, furosemide, NSAIDs. Ask about risk factors for renal tract cancer (smoking, chronic analgesic use, toxin exposure). *Imaging:* AXR is no longer used for primary assessment of stones; CTKUB is first choice investigation (see p758). NB Not all women with recurrent UTI + haematuria need cystoscopy, but have a good reason not to (Reynard's rule).[4]

**Others** *Glucose* DM, pregnancy, sepsis, renal tubular damage. *Ketones:* Starvation, ketoacidosis. *Leucocytes:* UTI, vaginal discharge. *Nitrites:* UTI, high-protein meal. *Bilirubin:* Obstructive jaundice. *Urobilinogen:* Pre-hepatic jaundice. *Specific gravity:* Normal range (NR): 1.000–1.030. *pH:* NR: 4.5–8 (acid–base balance: p684).

Figs on p287 reproduced from Davison *et al*, *Oxford Textbook of Clinical Nephrology*, OUP

## Urinalysis

**Using dipsticks** Store dipsticks in a closed container in a cool, dry place, not refrigerated. If improperly stored, or past expiry date, do not use. Dip the dipstick briefly in urine, run edge of strip along container and hold strip horizontally. **Read at the specified time**—check instructions. For haematuria, etc. see p286.

**Urine specific gravity** (SG) is not a good measure of osmolality. Causes of low SG (<1.003): diabetes insipidus, renal impairment. Causes of high SG (>1.025): diabetes mellitus, adrenal insufficiency, liver disease, heart failure, acute water loss.

### Sources of error in interpreting dipstick results

*Bilirubin:* False +ve: phenothiazines. False –ve: urine not fresh, rifampicin.

*Urobilinogen:* False –ve: urine not fresh. Normally present in urine due to metabolism of bilirubin in the gut by bacteria and subsequent absorption. Excess may give a false +ve test for prophobilinogen.

*Ketones:* L-dopa affects colour (false +ve). 3-Hydroxybutyrate gives a false –ve.

*Blood: False +ve dipstick haematuria:* haemoglobinuria, dehydration, myoglobinuria (eg in rhabdomyolysis), porphyria, phenindione, phenolphthalein, or contamination with menstrual blood.
*False –ve:* low urinary pH, air-exposed dipsticks.

*Urine glucose:* Depends on the test strips used, some can give false +ve but can give false +ve to peroxide, chlorine; and false –ve with ascorbic acid, salicylate, L-dopa.

*Protein: False +ve:* urine pH>7.5; concentrated urine; frank haematuria; presence of penicillin, sulfonamides, pus, semen or vaginal secretions.
*False –ve:* dilute urine; non-albumin urinary proteins.

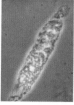
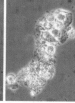
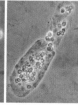
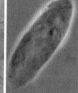

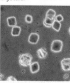
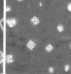
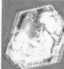
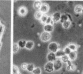

Fig 1 granular cast; Fig 2 (below) uric acid crystals.
Fig 3 white cell cast; Fig 4 (below) calcium oxalate crystals.
Fig 5 red cell cast; Fig 6 (below) cystine crystal.
Fig 7 hyaline cast; Fig 8 (below) white cells.

## Urine microscopy

Usually done by local laboratory. Put a drop of fresh, unspun urine on the slide, cover with a coverslip and examine under low and high power, looking for red and white cells, bacteria, casts and crystals. Some example images are shown above. When interpreting laboratory results remember:
• >10/mm³ white cells in an unspun specimen is abnormal, often from UTI, see p288.
• >2/mm³ red cells is abnormal, see haematuria.
• Casts are cylindrical bodies formed in the lumen of distal tubules, and can be waxy, granular, hyaline or cellular. Some types can indicate specific diseases.
• Crystals are common in old or cold urine and may not signify pathology. They are important in stone formers.

Renal medicine

**Definitions** *Bacteriuria:* Bacteria in the urine; may be asymptomatic or sympto-matic. *UTI:* The presence of a pure growth of >10⁵ organisms per mL of fresh MSU. *Lower UTI:* urethra (urethritis), bladder (cystitis), prostate (prostatitis). *Upper UTI:* renal pelvis (pyelonephritis). Up to a third of women with symptoms have negative MSU (= abacterial cystitis or the urethral syndrome).

**Classification** UTIs may be **uncomplicated** (normal renal tract + function) or **com-plicated** (abnormal renal/GU tract, voiding difficulty/obstruction, ↓renal function, im-paired host defences, virulent organism, eg *Staph. aureus*). For urethritis, see p418.

**Risk factors** ♀, sexual intercourse, exposure to spermicide in ♀ (by diaphragm or condoms), pregnancy, menopause; ↓*host defence* (immunosuppression, DM); *urinary tract:* obstruction (p642), stones, catheter, malformation. NB: in pregnancy, UTI is common and often asymptomatic, until serious pyelonephritis or premature delivery (± fetal death) supervenes, so do routine dipstick in pregnancy. Urine in catheterized bladders is almost always infected—CSUs and R̥ are pointless unless the patient is ill.

**Organisms** *E. coli* is the main organism (75-95% in the community but >41% in hospital). Occasionally other enterobacteriaceae such as *Proteus mirabilis* and *Klebsiella pneumonia,* and other bacteria such as *Staphylococcus saprophyticus.*

**Symptoms**
• *Acute pyelonephritis:* High fever, rigors, vomiting, loin pain and tenderness, oligu-ria (if acute kidney injury).
• *Cystitis:* Frequency, dysuria, urgency, haematuria, suprapubic pain.
• *Prostatitis:* Flu-like symptoms, low backache, few urinary symptoms, swollen or tender prostate on PR. Treatment: see p647.

**Signs** Fever, abdominal or loin tenderness, foul-smelling urine. Occasionally distend-ed bladder, enlarged prostate. NB: see *Vaginal discharge,* p418.

**Tests** If symptoms are present, dipstick the urine; treat empirically if nitrites or leu-cocytes are +ve while awaiting sensitivities on an MSU. If dipstick is -ve but patient symptomatic, send an MSU for lab MC&S to confirm this. Send a lab MSU anyway if male, a child (*OHCS* p174; do ultrasound), pregnant, immunosuppressed or ill. A pure growth of >10⁵ organisms/mL is diagnostic. If <10⁵ organisms/mL and pyuria (eg >20 WBCs/mm³), this may still be significant; treat if symptomatic. Cultured organisms are tested for sensitivity to a range of antibiotics; check local sensitivity patterns (p378).

*Causes of sterile pyuria:* ►TB
• Treated UTI <2 weeks prior
• Inadequately treated UTI
• Appendicitis
• Calculi; prostatitis
• Bladder tumour
• UTI with fastidious culture requirement
• Papillary necrosis (eg DM or analgesic excess)
• Tubulointerstitial nephritis
• Polycystic kidney
• Chemical cystitis (eg cyclophosphamide)

*Blood tests:* FBC, U&E, CRP, and blood cultures if systemically unwell ('urosepsis'). Consider fasting glucose and PSA (wait 6 months, as UTI causes false +ves).

*Imaging:* Consider USS and referral to urology for assessment (CTKUB, cystoscopy, urodynamics) for UTI in children; men; if failure to respond to treatment; recurrent UTI (>2/year); pyelonephritis; unusual organism; persistent haematuria.

**Prevention of UTI** Drink more water. Antibiotic prophylaxis, continuously or post-coital, ↓UTI rates in females with many UTIs. Self-treatment with a single antibiotic dose as symptoms start is an option. Drinking 200-750mL of cranberry or lingo berry juice a day, or taking cranberry concentrate tablets, ↓risk of symptomatic recurrent infection in women by 10-20%[5] (may inhibit adherence of bacteria to bladder uroepi-thelial cells; avoid if taking warfarin). There is no evidence that post-coital voiding, or pre-voiding, or advice on wiping patterns in females is of benefit.[6]

## Features of genitourinary tuberculosis

None is specific, so have a high index of suspicion in sterile pyuria and those with risk factors (esp. if HIV+ve), look for a high ESR/CRP, ask about past lung TB (but often there is no history). In one study of 100 males with GU TB 67% of symptoms appeared acutely.[7]

- Dysuria (eg in 50% of those with prostate TB)
- Flank pain (59%; a cold abscess in the flank is a rare presentation)
- Perineal pain (40%)
- Mycobacteriuria 38% (early-morning sample)
- Scrotal fistula 12%
- Leucocytes in urine 85% , eg 'sterile pyuria'; (78% in prostatic secretions)
- Haematuria in 53%

## What is the predictive value of urinary symptoms and dipstick for diagnosing UTI?

This is a controversial area, with a meta-analysis of 70 studies concluding that in the general population, a combination of negative nitrite and leucocyte tests on dipstick was sufficient to rule out UTI.[8]

A dipstick positive for either leucocytes or nitrites has a sensitivity of 75% and specificity of 82% in predicting urinary tract infection.[9] However, a strong specific history (eg dysuria, frequency) has a 90% positive predictive value and warrants treatment even if dipstick is negative. Symptoms should respond in a few hours of starting therapy,[10] so if ongoing despite adequate course of treatment consider: resistant or unusual organism, causes of sterile pyuria (p288), STI.

## Managing UTI[11]

▶Drink plenty of fluids; urinate often (don't 'hold on').

**Management of bacterial UTI in adult non-pregnant women**
- Consider empirical treatment for presumed *E. coli* in otherwise healthy women who present with lower UTI: local sensitivities vary but consider trimethoprim 200mg/12h PO or nitrofurantoin, eg 50mg/6h PO for 3-6d (if normal renal function), amoxicillin 500mg/8h PO. Alternative: cefalexin 1g/12h (if eGFR >40). 2nd line: co-amoxiclav PO (7d course). The latter 2 may cause problems with *C. difficile*. If there is no response, do a urine culture.
- In case of vaginal itch or discharge consider vaginal examination and swabs for other diagnoses, eg thrush, chlamydia, other STIs.
- In non-pregnant women with upper UTI, take a urine culture and treat with, eg co-amoxiclav 1.2g/8h IV, then oral when afebrile, complete 7d course. Avoid nitrofurantoin as it does not achieve effective concentrations in urine. Resistance to trimethoprim is common. Non-pregnant women with asymptomatic bacteriuria do not need antibiotics so screening is not recommended.

**Managing bacterial UTI in pregnant women** Get expert help. Any bacteriuria (symptomatic or asymptomatic) should be treated with an antibiotic. Dipstick and urine culture should be repeated at each antenatal visit.

**Managing bacterial UTI in adult men**
- Take UTI in men seriously as it often results from an anatomical or functional anomaly. Therefore, all men with symptoms of upper UTI, recurrent UTI or who fail to respond to antibiotic therapy should be referred to a urologist. Also consider prostatitis, epididymitis and chlamydial infection.
- Bacterial UTI in men may need a 2wk course of a quinolone, such as levofloxacin (if no response, think of prostatitis and treat for 4wks).
- Antibiotic therapy of asymptomatic bacteriuria in elderly men (>65yrs old) is not recommended, as it does not reduce morbidity or mortality while it increases the risk of adverse events such as rashes or GI problems.

Renal medicine

### Definition

The term acute renal failure (ARF) has now been changed to acute kidney injury (AKI). This allows us to consider AKI as a spectrum of damage from a mild deterioration in function to severe injury requiring renal replacement therapy (RRT), as even small rises in creatinine increase the risk of mortality.[12] It is defined as a rapid reduction in kidney function over hours to days, as measured by serum urea and creatinine, and leading to a failure to maintain fluid, electrolyte and acid–base homeostasis.[13] AKI is common, occurring in up to 18% of hospital patients, and is an independent risk factor for mortality. The Kidney Diseases: Improving Global Outcomes (KDIGO) guidelines[14] suggest the following criteria for diagnosing AKI:

- Rise in creatinine >26μmol/L in 48hrs
- Rise in creatinine >1.5 × baseline (best figure in last 3/12)
- Urine output <0.5mL/kg/h for >6 consecutive hours.

Recently several staging systems for AKI have been brought in to try to standardize care. All use serum creatinine and urine output to categorize patients. Although creatinine is not the best biomarker for monitoring AKI, no other potential biomarker has yet proven better for predicting outcome. Having incorporated several staging systems, the UK Renal Association recommends using KDIGO staging of AKI:

| KDIGO staging system for AKI | | |
|---|---|---|
| | **Serum creatinine (sCr) criteria** | **Urine output criteria** |
| 1 | Increase >26μmol/L in 48h OR increase > 1.5 × baseline | <0.5mL/kg/h for >6 consecutive hours |
| 2 | Increase 2-2.9 × baseline | <0.5mL/kg/h for >12h |
| 3 | Increase >3 × baseline OR >354 μmol/L OR commenced on RRT irrespective of stage | <0.3mL/kg/h for >24h or anuria for 12h |

It is important to consider the risk of AKI in all patients being admitted to hospital. A 2009 NCEPOD report: *Adding Insult to Injury*[15] identified many deficiencies in care of patients with AKI, including poor recognition and management. Given the high incidence and increased mortality, all hospital admissions should be assessed for the risk of developing AKI. Risk factors are shown below:

| Risk factors for developing AKI | |
|---|---|
| • Age >75 | • Diabetes |
| • Chronic kidney disease | • Drugs (esp newly started) |
| • Cardiac failure | • Sepsis |
| • Peripheral vascular disease | • Poor fluid intake/increased losses |
| • Chronic liver disease | • History of urinary symptoms |

**Causes:** Commonest are ischaemia, sepsis and nephrotoxins, although prostatic disease causes up to 25% in some studies and has the best prognosis.[16]

1 *Pre-renal* (40-70%) due to renal hypoperfusion, eg hypotension (any cause, including hypovolaemia, sepsis), renal artery stenosis ± ACE-i.

2 *Intrinsic renal* (10-50%) may require a renal biopsy for diagnosis:
   - Tubular—acute tubular necrosis (ATN) is the commonest renal cause of AKI, often a result of pre-renal damage or nephrotoxins such as drugs (eg aminoglycosides), radiological contrast (see p293), and myoglobinuria in rhabdomyolysis. Also crystal damage (eg ethylene glycol poisoning, uric acid), myeloma, ↑$Ca^{2+}$.
   - Glomerular—autoimmune such as SLE, HSP, drugs, infections, primary glomerulonephritides are important not to miss (see p300)
   - Interstitial—drugs, infiltration with, eg lymphoma, infection, tumour lysis syndrome following chemotherapy
   - Vascular—vasculitis, malignant ↑BP, thrombus or cholesterol emboli from angiography, HUS/TTP (p308), large vessel occlusion, eg dissection or thrombus

3 *Post-renal* (10-25%) caused by urinary tract obstruction:
   - Luminal—stones, clots, sloughed papillae
   - Mural—malignancy (eg ureteric, bladder, prostate), BPH, strictures
   - Extrinsic compression—malignancy (esp pelvic), retroperitoneal fibrosis.

## Assessment of the patient with AKI

**Assessment** ▶ Make sure you know about the renal effects of all drugs taken.

▶▶ All assessment should include basic ABCDE approach, and as part of C:
- Assess volume status—check BP, JVP, skin turgor, capillary refill (<2s), urine output (catheterize).
- Check an urgent K⁺ on a venous blood specimen and an ECG to check for life-threatening hyperkalaemia (see p293).

*History:* check for risk factors (see BOX), comorbidities, ask about previous renal disease, recent fluid intake and losses, new drugs including chemotherapy, systemic features such as rash, joint pain, fevers. Other systems—productive cough, haemoptysis, GU or GI symptoms, etc.

*Examination:* Full systemic examination. Specific features to look for include a palpable bladder, palpable kidneys (polycystic disease), abdominal/pelvic masses, renal bruits (signs of renovascular disease), rashes.

*Bedside tests:* Always, always dip the urine. See p236. Dipstick can suggest infection (leucocytes + nitrites), glomerular disease (blood + protein). Microscopy for casts, crystals and cells. Culture for infection. Consider Bence Jones protein.

*Blood tests:* U&E, FBC, LFT, clotting, CK, ESR, CRP. Consider ABG for acid base assessment. Culture blood if signs of infection. Consider blood film and renal immunology if systemic cause suspected: immunoglobulins and paraprotein electrophoresis, complement (C3/C4), autoantibodies (ANCA, ANA, anti-GBM, esp if haemoptysis, see p300, p555) and ASOT.

*Imaging:* A renal USS can help to distinguish obstruction and hydronephrosis, and look for abnormalities such as cysts, small kidneys, masses, as well as assess corticomedullary differentiation (reduced in chronic kidney disease). Complete anuria is unusual in AKI and if present suggests an obstructive cause. In elderly men this should be considered prostatic and can often be relieved by catheterization. If catheterization does not resolve anuria and you suspect obstruction above the prostate, get an urgent USS to check for hydronephrosis and consider an urgent CTKUB (does not require contrast), which can show obstructing masses or calculi. Consider CXR if signs of fluid overload.

### Is the injury acute or the damage chronic?
Suspect chronic if small kidneys (<9cm) on USS, anaemia, low Ca²⁺, high PO₄³⁻, but the only definite sign of chronic disease is previous blood results showing high creatinine/low GFR.

### When to refer to a nephrologist (and what they would like to know):
- Firstly assess the patient, correct pre- and post-renal factors, and treat urgent problems such as hyperkalaemia and pulmonary oedema.
- *Always refer*: Hyperkalaemia in an oligoanuric patient, hyperkalaemia or fluid overload unresponsive to medical ℞, urea >40mmol/L ± signs of uraemia such as pericarditis, patients with suspected glomerulonephritis (blood and protein on urinalysis) or systemic disease. *Consider referral*: No obvious reversible cause, creatinine >300 or rising >50µmol/L per day.
- *What they want to know*: The history and timecourse, U&E results—esp K⁺, urine dipstick, drugs, fluid balance and current volume status (see p681).

### Indications for dialysis (RRT p298) (discuss with a nephrologist EARLY)
▶▶ Refractory pulmonary oedema
▶▶ Persistent hyperkalaemia (K⁺ >7mmol/L)
▶▶ Severe metabolic acidosis (pH<7.2 or base excess <10)
▶▶ Uraemic complications such as encephalopathy or
▶▶ Uraemic pericarditis (pericardial rub)
▶▶ Drug overdose—BLAST: Barbituates, Lithium, Alcohol (and ethylene glycol), Salicylates, Theophyline, see p766.

### General measures

- *Assess volume status:* look for ↓urine volume, non-visible JVP, poor tissue turgor, ↓BP, ↑pulse. Signs of fluid overload: ↑BP, ↑JVP, lung crepitations, peripheral oedema, gallop rhythm on cardiac auscultation.
- *Aim for euvolaemia:*[17] if difficult balance with risk of fluid overload, consider titrating input hourly, by matching previous hours output + 25mL/h for insensible losses. This is not usually practical outside of an HDU setting as it requires intensive nursing input. If euvolaemic review balance daily, over 24-hour period aim to match input to loss (urine, vomit, diarrhoea, drains) + 500mL for insensible loss (more if T°↑). ►Avoid K⁺-containing fluids unless hypokalaemic.
- *Stop nephrotoxic drugs:* (See 'sick day rules' BOX) eg NSAIDs, ACE inhibitor, gentamicin, amphotericin. Stop metformin if creatinine is >150mmol/L, see p200. Check and adjust doses of renally excreted drugs (ask your pharmacist for the *Renal Drug Handbook*, a weighty but valuable tome!).
- *Monitoring:* Consider transfer to intensive care or high-dependency unit (ICU/HDU).
  - Check pulse, BP, JVP, and urine output hourly (insert a urinary catheter). Consider inserting a CVP line if on HDU/ICU.
  - Daily U&Es.
  - Daily fluid balance chart and daily weight.
- *Nutrition* is vital in the critically unwell patient: aim for normal calorie intake (more if catabolism ↑↑, eg burns, sepsis) and protein ∼0.5g/kg/d. If oral intake is poor, consider nasogastric nutrition early (parenteral if NGT impossible, p588).

### Treat underlying cause

- *Pre-renal:* Correct volume depletion with appropriate fluids, treat sepsis with antibiotics, consider referral to ICU for inotropic support if signs of shock (see p804).
- *Post-renal:* Catheterize and consider CT of renal tract (CTKUB) and urology referral if obstruction likely cause. If signs of obstruction and hydronephrosis on CT/USS then discuss with urology regarding cystoscopy and retrograde stents or nephrostomy insertion; this buys time to allow treatment of cause of obstruction, eg stone, mass.
- *Intrinsic renal:* ►Refer early to nephrology if concern over tubulointerstitial or glomerular pathology, any signs of systemic disease, multi-organ involvement (eg pulmonary-renal, hepatorenal syndromes) or indications for dialysis (see p291).

### Manage complications

- Hyperkalaemia (see BOX p293).
- Pulmonary oedema (see BOX p293).
- Uraemia—may require dialysis if severe or complications, eg encephalopathy, pericarditis, contact renal team. Otherwise symptomatic management.
- Acidaemia—may require dialysis, consider sodium bicarbonate orally or IV if in HDU/ICU setting, discuss with nephrology before initiating.

### Renal replacement therapy

Options in AKI include haemodialysis and haemofiltration, both require large-bore venous access (eg internal jugular line). Haemodialysis is usually done intermittently and allows good clearance of solutes in short periods but requires the patient to be haemodynamically stable. If patients are stable enough for ward-based care this is usually the modality of choice. Patients on the ICU are often filtered, as the fluid shifts are much less significant and therefore BP is less likely to drop. However, filtration is much slower at clearing solutes, and is usually performed continuously while the patient is in established renal failure (p298).

### Prognosis

Prognosis depends on early recognition and intervention,[18] as the more prolonged the insult, the less likely full recovery of function. Mortality can be as high as 80% depending on the cause: burns (80%); trauma/surgery (60%); medical illness (30%); obstetric/poisoning (10%).

## Hyperkalaemia (also p848)

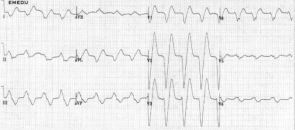

Fig 1. ECG showing severe hyperkalaemia; note broadening of QRS complexes.

**ECG changes** (in order): Tall 'tented' T waves; small or absent P wave; increased PR interval; widened QRS complex; 'sine wave' pattern; asystole.
Immediate treatment:

▶▶ 10mL of 10% calcium gluconate IV via a big vein over 2min, repeated as necessary until ECG improves. This is cardioprotective but does not affect K⁺ level.

▶▶ Intravenous insulin + glucose: see p849. Insulin stimulates intracellular uptake of K⁺, lowering serum K⁺ by 1–2mmol/L over ~60min.

▶▶ Salbutamol nebulizers work in the same way as insulin/glucose but high doses are required (10–20mg) and tachycardia can limit use.

▶▶ If venous bicarbonate low (ie patient is acidotic) giving IV sodium bicarbonate (eg 50mL of 8.4% NaHCO₃ as an infusion or bolus into a big vein) can help to drive K⁺ into cells, though the effect is unpredictable.

All of these measures are **temporary** and only **buy time** to definitively lower K⁺, via either renal clearance (eg relieving obstruction with catheter or correcting pre-renal failure with fluids) or haemodialysis/filtration if the patient is oligoanuric.

## Pulmonary oedema

(also p812)

• Sit up and give high-flow O₂ •Venous vasodilator, eg diamorphine 2.5mg IV (+antiemetic, eg cyclizine 50mg IV). •Furosemide 80–250mg IV either as IVI over 1h or boluses titrated to response (larger doses are needed in renal failure). •If no response, urgent haemodialysis or haemofiltration is needed. •Consider continuous positive airway pressure ventilation (CPAP). •IV nitrates also have a role (p813).

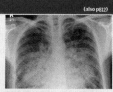

Fig 2. Severe pulmonary oedema.

## Prevention of AKI—'Sick-day rules'

It is far easier and better for the patient to try to prevent AKI than manage it once established. Up to 30% of cases are preventable. If a patient is admitted acutely unwell, do a risk assessment for AKI, and if they are high risk consider:
**Reviewing drugs**: Continuing usual medications can be catastrophic if a patient is high risk—diarrhoea and vomiting, third space losses, eg pancreatitis, poor intake, sepsis or other cause of hypotension (ie most surgical patients in the immediate post-op period for any significant surgery!). *Withhold/avoid:* Diuretics, ACE inhibitors, antihypertensives if BP low (NB do not stop β-blockers acutely, consider ↓dose), metformin if creatinine rising (risk of lactic acidosis), NSAIDs, nephrotoxic antibiotics (eg gentamicin, nitrofurantoin). *Use with caution:* Opiates can accumulate in renal failure, start with lower dose and build up to patient's pain threshold, keep naloxone handy. **Contrast:** Acutely unwell patients often have multiple contrast CT scans and procedures. This is an important cause of AKI, see p307 & 762. Ensure patient is well hydrated, eg 1L 0.9% saline over 12 hours pre and post procedure.

**Definition** Impaired renal function for >3 months based on abnormal structure or function, or GFR <60mL/min/1.73m² for >3 months with or without evidence of kidney damage. Classification: 5 stages (BOX). Symptoms usually only occur once stage 4 is reached (GFR <30). End-stage renal failure (ESRF) is defined as GFR <15 mL/min/1.73m² or need for renal replacement therapy (RRT—dialysis or transplant).[19]

**Causes**

1 *Diabetes*: 20% UK, 43% USA. Type II >> type I
2 *Glomerulonephritis:* commonly IgA nephropathy, also rarer disorders, eg mesangiocapillary GN, systemic disorders, eg SLE, vasculitis
3 *Unknown:* up to 20% in the UK have no obvious cause of CKD, many of these present late with small, shrunken kidneys where a biopsy would be uninformative
4 Hypertension or renovascular disease
5 Pyelonephritis and reflux nephropathy

Rarer causes include obstructive uropathy, which commonly causes AKI but is often reversible, chronic interstitial nephritis (eg myeloma, amyloid), and following previous AKI. Adult polycystic kidney disease (APKD) is the commonest inherited cause of CKD, rare inherited disorders include Alport's syndrome and Fabry's disease (p712).

**Screening** Intervening early in CKD can reduce the progression to ESRF and so screening is recommended for at-risk patients with:
• Diabetes mellitus
• Hypertension
• Cardiovascular disease (IHD, peripheral vascular disease, cerebrovascular disease)
• Structural renal disease, known stones or BPH
• Recurrent UTIs or those with childhood history of vesicoureteric reflux
• Multisystem disorders which could involve the kidney, eg SLE
• Family history of ESRF or known hereditary disease, eg APKD
• Opportunistic detection of haematuria or proteinuria

Some guidelines also suggest routine screening in those >60yrs, although this is debatable, as many elderly people fall into CKD stage 3 but have little or no progression over many years. Is there a benefit to labelling them with a disease?

**History** When assessing a patient with known/suspected CKD, try to identify:
• *Possible cause*: ask about previous UTIs, LUTS (lower urinary tract symptoms, p644), PMH of ↑BP, DM, IHD, systemic disorder, renal colic. Check drug history and family history (draw tree if positive). Systems review: always be on the lookout for more than is immediately obvious, possible rare causes, symptoms suggestive of systemic disorder or malignancy.
• *Current state*: uraemic symptoms such as anorexia, vomiting, restless legs, fatigue, weakness, pruritus, bone pain. In women ask about amenorrhoea, in men impotence. Symptoms become more common with progression through CKD stages 4 and 5 but if slow onset many patients remain asymptomatic. Check for oliguria, dyspnoea, ankle swelling.

**Examination** See p295 for examining patients with known CKD. In first presentation look for pallor, uraemic tinge to the skin (yellowish), purpura, excoriations, ↑BP, cardiomegaly, signs of fluid overload and possible cause, eg ballotable polycystic kidneys. If untreated patients can present in extremis with severe uraemia and hyperkalaemia causing arrhythmias, encephalopathy, seizures or coma.

**Tests** *Blood:* Hb (normochromic, normocytic anaemia), ESR, U&E, glucose (DM), ↓Ca²⁺, ↑PO₄³⁻, ↑ alk phos (renal osteodystrophy).↑PTH if CKD stage 3 or more (p214).
*Urine:* Dipstick, MC&S, albumin: creatinine ratio or protein:creatinine ratio (p286).
*Imaging:* USS to check size, anatomy and corticomedullary differentiation. In CKD kidneys are usually small (<9cm) but can be enlarged in infiltrative disorders (amyloid, myeloma), APKD and DM. If asymmetrical consider MAG3 renogram to look at contribution of each kidney to overall function.
*Histology:* Consider renal biopsy if rapidly progressive disease or unclear cause and normal sized kidneys.

### Examining the patient with known CKD/ESRF

You are looking for:
1 Cause of ESRF/CKD, eg polycystic kidneys, signs of IHD, DM
2 Current mode of renal replacement therapy (RRT) and any complications, eg transplant + skin malignancy from immunosuppression
3 Previous types of RRT and any complications, eg arteriovenous fistula + parathyroidectomy scar

*Periphery:* Hypertension, arteriovenous fistula (thrill, bruit, has it been recently needled?), signs of previous transplant—bruising from steroids, skin malignancy from immunosuppression.

*Face:* Pallor of anaemia, yellow tinge of uraemia, gum hypertrophy from ciclosporin, cushingoid appearance from steroids.

*Neck:* Current or previous tunnelled line insertion (if removed, look for a small scar over internal jugular, and a larger scar in 'breast pocket' area from the exit site), scar from parathyroidectomy.

*Abdomen:* PD catheter or sign of previous catheter (small midline scar just below umbilicus and small round scar to side of midline from exit site), signs of previous transplant (hockey-stick scar, palpable mass), ballotable polycystic kidneys ± liver.

*Elsewhere:* Signs of diabetic neuropathy, retinopathy, cardiovascular or peripheral vascular disease.

### Classifying renal impairment in chronic kidney disease (CKD)²ₙₒₑ

This is based on presence of kidney damage and GFR, irrespective of diagnosis.

| Stage | GFR (mL/min) | Notes |
|---|---|---|
| 1 | >90 | Normal or ↑GFR with other evidence of renal damage* |
| 2 | 60-89 | Slight ↓GFR with other evidence of renal damage* |
| 3 A | 45-59 | Moderate ↓GFR with or without evidence of other renal |
| 3 B | 30-44 | damage* |
| 4 | 15-29 | Severe ↓GFR with or without evidence of renal damage* |
| 5 | <15 | Established renal failure |

*Proteinuria, haematuria, or evidence of abnormal anatomy or systemic disease. One reason to classify renal impairment is to motivate secondary prevention, eg to 'mandate' ACE-i or ARB if BP >140/85 especially if proteinuria is present or stage ≥3.

*Problems using MDRD formula to grade renal disease by eGFR (see p683):*

▶Remember that the eGFR is only a screening test and, especially in mild renal impairment, may underestimate renal function.

### Monitoring renal function

Some patients with CKD lose renal function at a constant rate, so one can plot the reciprocal creatinine as a straight line, parallel to the fall in GFR. However, there is much individual variation in progression, so any plot is of limited use.[20] Rapid decline in renal function greater than expected may be due to: infection, dehydration, uncontrolled ↑BP, metabolic disturbance (eg $Ca^{2+}$↑), obstruction, nephrotoxins (eg drugs). Intervention at this point may delay ESRF. Registry data show that the mean estimated GFR at which dialysis is commenced is ~8mL/min.

*Why does falling GFR matter?* 1 Good renal function is essential for an optimum *milieu intérieur.* 2 A falling GFR is an *independent* risk factor for cardiovascular disease; ▶*this is the chief cause of death from renal failure.*

Estimating GFR is difficult and notoriously inaccurate. If in doubt, calculate using 24 hour creatinine clearance or radioisotope clearance. See p683 for details.

Mild-moderate CKD is usually managed in general practice or by other physicians caring for the patient (eg diabetologists). Refer early to a nephrologist if the patient meets any of the following criteria:

- Stage 4 and 5 CKD
- Moderate proteinuria (ACR >70mg/mmol, see p286) unless due to DM and already appropriately treated
- Proteinuria with haematuria
- Rapidly falling eGFR (>5mL/min/1.73m² in 1yr, or >10mL/min/1.73m² within 5yrs)
- ↑BP poorly controlled despite ≥4 antihypertensive drugs at therapeutic doses
- Known or suspected rare or genetic causes of CKD
- Suspected renal artery stenosis

Management of patients can be split into four main approaches:

**1 Investigation**
- *Identifying and treating reversible causes*: relieve obstruction, stop nephrotoxic drugs, deal with high Ca²⁺ and cardiovascular risk (stop smoking, achieve a healthy weight), tight glucose control in DM.

**2 Limiting progression/complications**
- *BP:* Even a small BP drop may save significant renal function.[21] Target BP is <130/80 (<125/75 if diabetic or ACR >70).[22] Choice of drug as per local guidance; in diabetic kidney disease, even with normal BP, treat with an ACE-i or ARB.[23]
- *Renal bone disease* (risk of osteodystrophy or adynamic bone disease): Check PTH and treat if raised.[24] PO₄³⁻ rises in CKD, which ↑PTH further, and also precipitates in the kidney and vasculature. Restrict diet, give binders (eg Calcichew®) to ↓ gut absorption. Vit D analogues (eg alfacalcidol) and Ca²⁺ supplements ↓bone disease and hyperparathyroidism (2° and 3°, p214).[1]
- *Cardiovascular modification:* In CKD stages 1 and 2, risk from cardiovascular death is higher than the risk of reaching ESRF. Give statins (p704) to CKD patients with raised lipids as per guidelines for any patient. Give aspirin also (CKD is not a contraindication to the use of low-dose aspirin, but beware of risk of bleeding).
- *Diet:* Multidisciplinary team care is essential and all patients should be reviewed by a dietician for advice on a healthy, moderate protein diet, K⁺ restriction if hyperkalaemic, and avoidance of high phosphate foods (eg milk, cheese, eggs).

**3 Symptom control**
- *Anaemia:* Check haematinics and replace iron/B₁₂/folate if necessary. If still anaemic consider recombinant human erythropoietin. There are many formulations, all of which should increase Hb in an iron, B₁₂ and folate replete patient. If Hb falls despite this, and no infection, haemolysis, or blood loss, etc. suspect red cell aplasia (anti-epo antibodies). Stop at once and get help from haematology. Keep Hb 100–120g/L; above this risks IV access thrombosis, ↑BP, MI).[25]
- *Acidosis:* Consider sodium bicarbonate supplements for patients with low serum bicarbonate; this not only improves symptoms but may slow progression of CKD.[26] Caution in patients with hypertension, as sodium load can ↑BP.
- *Oedema:* High doses of loop diuretics may be needed (eg furosemide 250mg–2g/24h ± metolazone 5–10mg/24h PO each morning), and restriction to fluid and sodium intake.
- *Restless legs/cramps:* Check ferritin (low levels worsen symptoms), clonazepam (0.5–2mg daily) or gabapentin (p508) may help. Quinine sulfate (300mg nocte) can help with cramps.

**4 Preparation for renal replacement therapy (RRT)**
- See p298.

---

**1** Alfacalcidol and calcitriol (=1,25-dihydroxycholecalciferol) help by ↓parathyroid hormone, but greatly ↑ intestinal Ca²⁺ and PO₄³⁻ absorption and bone mineral mobilization, leading to PO₄³⁻↑ and Ca²⁺↑ (risks vascular calcification). New vit D analogues (eg paricalcitol weekly IV[27]) retain suppressive action on PTH and gland growth, but have less effect on Ca²⁺ and PO₄³⁻ absorption, and help cardiovascular status.[28]

## Renal biopsy

Most acute kidney injury is due to pre-renal causes or acute tubular necrosis, and recovery of renal function typically occurs over the course of a few weeks. Renal biopsy should be performed only if knowing histology will influence management. Once chronic kidney disease is established, the kidneys are small, there is a higher risk of bleeding from biopsy, and the results are usually unhelpful. Biopsies should only be carried out by physicians trained in the procedure, but the following information can be helpful if you are managing the pre- or post-biopsy patient.

*Indications for renal biopsy:* Unexplained acute kidney injury or chronic kidney disease, acute nephritic syndromes, unexplained proteinuria and haematuria, systemic diseases associated with kidney dysfunction, suspected transplant rejection (p299) or to guide treatment.[29]

*Pre-procedure:* Check FBC, clotting, group and save. The physician performing the procedure should obtain written informed consent. Ultrasound to delineate anatomy. Stop anticoagulants (aspirin 1 week, warfarin 2-3 days, low molecular weight heparin 24 hours).

*Contraindications:* • Abnormal clotting • Hypertension >160/>90mmHg • Single kidney (except for renal transplants) • Chronic kidney disease with small kidneys (<9cm) • Uncooperative patient • Horseshoe kidney • Renal neoplasms.

*Post-procedure:* Bed rest for a minimum of 6h. Monitor pulse, BP, symptoms, and urine colour. Bleeding is the main complication; most occurs within 8h, although it may be delayed by up to 72h. Macroscopic haematuria occurs in ~10%, although blood transfusion is only needed in ~1-2%. Aspirin or warfarin can be restarted the next day if procedure uncomplicated.

## Prescribing in renal failure

Relate dose modification to GFR, and the extent to which a drug is renally excreted. This is significant for aminoglycosides (gentamicin, p767), cephalosporins, and a few other antibiotics (p378-381), heparin, lithium, opiates, and digoxin.

▶Never prescribe in renal failure before checking how its administration should be altered. Loading doses (eg digoxin) should not be changed. If the patient is on dialysis (peritoneal or haemodialysis), dose modification depends on how well it is eliminated by dialysis.

The best text to consult is the *Renal Drug Handbook*, an invaluable text detailing dose modification for almost any drug you could want to use. Most pharmacies and all hospitals should have a copy so speak to your pharmacist.

Mean GFR at start of dialysis is usually about 8-10mL/min. Preparation is vital, and an MDT approach with psychological, nursing, dietetic and medical input can help patients make difficult decisions. The 'best' form of renal replacement therapy (RRT) is transplantation, but it involves major surgery and is not always successful. Dialysis, whether it be haemo- or peritoneal, can maintain stability but has many complications. For some patients no form of RRT is acceptable. *Conservative management*, particularly in the very elderly or those with significant comorbidities, is not an unreasonable option, and allows the focus of care to be on symptom control and delaying progression of disease. If a patient chooses active RRT then there are two main options aside from transplantation:

**Haemodialysis (HD)** Blood is passed over a semi-permeable membrane against dialysis fluid flowing in the opposite direction, thus blood is always meeting a less-concentrated solution and diffusion of small solutes occurs down the concentration gradient. Larger solutes do not clear as effectively.[30] Ultrafiltration creates a negative transmembrane pressure and is used to clear excess fluid.

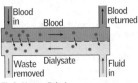

Fig 1. Haemodialysis.

*Problems:* Disequilibrium syndrome, hypotension, time consuming, access problems (arteriovenous fistula: thrombosis, stenosis, steal syndrome; tunnelled venous access line: infection, blockage, recirculation of blood).

**Haemofiltration** Water is cleared across the dialysis membrane using positive pressure to drag small and larger size solutes into the waste by convection. The ultrafiltrate is replaced with an appropriate volume of fluid either before (pre-dilution) or after (post-dilution) the membrane, with less haemodynamic instability than haemodialysis.

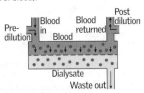

Fig 2. Haemofiltration.

**Peritoneal dialysis (PD)** Uses the peritoneum as a semi-permeable membrane. A Tenckhoff catheter is inserted into the peritoneal cavity and fluid infused, allowing solutes to diffuse slowly across. Ultrafiltration can be achieved by adding osmotic agents such as glucose to the fluid. It is simple to perform, can be carried out continuously and at home, and so allows the patient more freedom. There are multiple regimens that can be tailored to the patient's needs.

*Problems:* PD peritonitis, exit site infection, loss of membrane function over time (which can lead to technical failure and need to switch to alternative form of RRT).

**Complications of RRT** Annual mortality is ~20%, mostly due to *cardiovascular disease:* MI and CVA are much commoner in dialysis patients, thought due to a combination of hypertension and calcium/phosphate dysregulation. *Protein-calorie malnutrition* is common in HD and is associated with ↑morbidity and mortality. *Renal bone disease:* high bone turnover, renal osteodystrophy and osteitis fibrosa (due to ↑PTH). *Infection:* Uraemia causes granulocyte dysfunction. Sepsis-related mortality is 100- to 300-fold greater in dialysis patients than general population. *Amyloid* accumulates in long-term dialysis patients and may cause carpal tunnel syndrome, arthralgia, and fractures. *Malignancy* is commoner in dialysis patients; this may be related to the cause of ESRF, eg urothelial tumours in analgesic nephropathy.

**Stopping dialysis** Dialysis exerts a big toll on quality of life, and it may all become too much, eg if very old[31] or there is comorbidity (eg psychiatric or mobility issues). 8-20% of deaths in dialysis patients are due to its withdrawal.[32] ►Good palliative care allows a good death and mitigates discomfort caused by uraemia. Good communication in the renal team, clear protocols and living wills help the big ethical dilemma.[33]

## Renal transplantation

This is the treatment of choice for end-stage renal failure (ESRF). However, a transplant involves major surgery, long-term immunosuppression and a number of potential complications, and patients must be physically and psychologically suitable for a transplant. Anaesthetic assessment is key, with cardiac testing and investigation of other systems as appropriate, eg lung function testing.

**Absolute contraindications** Active infection, cancer (if >5yrs ago and considered cured, may be considered for transplant), severe comorbidity.

**Types of graft** *DCD:* Donor after cardiac death, patients who do not meet criteria for brainstem death, retrieval of organs only begins when cardiac output has ceased. High risk of delayed graft function due to long warm ischaemic time. *DBD:* Donor after brainstem death, patients who meet criteria for brainstem death and therefore remain on cardiorespiratory support for retrieval. Much reduced risk of delayed graft function. *LD:* Living donor grafts give much better outcomes, with planned surgery and minimal ischaemic time. Can be related (parent, sibling) or unrelated (spouse, friend). All live donor transplants must be assessed by an Independent Assessor from the Human Tissue Authority before permission can be given to the surgical centre to go ahead with transplantation. For all donors this involves a psychological assessment ensuring they understand the risks of transplantation.

### Immunosuppression

*Induction:* Conventional induction is with anti-IL-2R monoclonal antibody basiliximab; however, many centres are now using alemtuzumab (Campath®), which provides broad immunosuppression and allows a steroid-free maintenance regimen. This is particularly useful in patients with diabetes, but trials are ongoing.

*Maintenance:* Most patients are maintained on triple therapy of a calcineurin inhibitor (CNI, tacrolimus or ciclosporin), an antimetabolite (azathioprine or mycophenolate) and prednisolone.

### Complications

*Surgical:* Bleed, thrombosis, infection, urinary leaks, lymphocele, hernia.

*Delayed graft function:* Affects up to 40% of grafts, far more common in DCD. Usually ATN in graft due to ischaemia-reperfusion injury.

*Rejection:* Can be acute or chronic. Acute is divided into humoral (antibody mediated) or cellular (far commoner); usual treatment for either is high dose IV methylprednisolone and an intensification of immunosuppression. Antibody-mediated rejection often requires plasma exchange in addition to clear donor-specific antibodies. Chronic allograft nephropathy is the new terminology for chronic rejection. It is thought to be a combination of chronic, low-grade antibody response plus vascular changes and the effects of CNIs. It generally does not respond to treatment but sometimes progression can be slowed by switching CNI to sirolimus.

*Drug toxicity:* Neurological (tremor, confusion with CNIs), new onset diabetes after transplant (NODAT), gum hypertrophy and hirsutism (ciclosporin), agranulocytosis and hepatitis (antimetabolites).

*Infection:* Increased risk of all infections, but opportunists and viral infections particularly due to poor T cell response. HSV, *Candida*, *Pneumocystis jirovecii*, CMV.

*Malignancy:* 5-fold increased risk of cancer with immunosuppression, particularly skin and viral associated. Women should have regular cervical smears, EBV-associated post-transplant lymphoproliferative disorder is particularly problematic.

*Cardiovascular disease:* Probably due to drug effects, the leading cause of death in transplant patients. ↑BP in >50% of transplants, probably due in part to donor vascular disease in the graft, plus immunosuppressants.

**Prognosis** Current figures show 1-year graft survival ranges from 91% (DCD) to 96% (LD), and patient survival from 96% (DCD) to 99% (LD). 10-year graft survival is 60% from DCD, up to 80% from a living donor. Figures are improving year on year.[34]

Renal medicine

The glomerulonephritides are a common cause of ESRF in adults. Many people find the glomerulonephritides complex, confusing and the list of diseases difficult to remember. However, with renal disease, remember the names for the glomerulonephritides are often descriptive, relating to the histology or cause. It is simpler to think in terms of the presentation, and then your list of possible causes reduces to a more manageable one. Glomerulonephritis simply means inflammation of the glomeruli and nephrons; when you remember this you can appreciate what the consequences of this inflammation are:

• Damage to the glomerulus restricts blood flow, leading to compensatory ↑BP
• Damage to the filtration mechanism allows protein and blood to enter the urine
• Loss of the usual filtration capacity leads to acute kidney injury

Depending on the degree of inflammation and damage, and what it is caused by, patients therefore present with a spectrum of disease:

1 Blood pressure: normal to malignant hypertension
2 Urine dipstick: *proteinuria* mild→nephrotic; *haematuria* mild→macroscopic
3 Renal function: normal to severe impairment

**Presentation:** Many patients present with specific syndromes:

| Syndrome | BP | Urine | GFR |
|---|---|---|---|
| Nephrotic (p302) | Normal-mild ↑ | Proteinuria >3.5g/day | Normal-mild ↓ |
| Nephritic | Moderate-severe ↑ | Haematuria (mild-macro) | Moderate-severe ↓ |

**Causes:** generally considered primary (no underlying drive to disease) or secondary (to infection, autoimmunity or malignancy) and tend to present with similar syndromes.

| Syndrome | Common primary causes | Common secondary causes |
|---|---|---|
| Nephrotic | Membranous<br>Minimal change<br>FSGS (p303)<br>Mesangiocapillary GN | Diabetes<br>SLE (class V nephritis)<br>Amyloid<br>Hepatitis B/C |
| Nephritic | IgA nephropathy<br>Mesangiocapillary GN | Post streptococcal<br>Vasculitis<br>SLE (other classes of nephritis)<br>Anti-GBM disease (Figs 1 & 2)<br>Cryoglobulinaemia |

**Tests:** looking for degree of damage and potential cause. *Blood:* FBC, U&E, LFT, ESR, CRP; immunoglobulins, electrophoresis, complement (C3, C4); autoantibodies (p555): ANA, ANCA, anti-dsDNA, anti-GBM; blood culture, ASOT, HBsAg, anti-HCV (p406). *Urine:* RBC casts, MC&S, Bence Jones protein, ACR (see p286). *Imaging:* CXR, renal ultrasound.

*Renal biopsy* (p297) will give the most information and is where many of the complex names arise. Generally it is reported as follows: what is affected (mesangial cells, capillaries, basement membrane, endothelium), how much of the kidney is involved (focal vs diffuse), how much of the glomerulus is involved (segemental vs global), and what is seen on immunofluorescence (deposition of Igs, complement, immune complexes or pauci immune) and electron microscopy.

**General management** ► Early referral to a nephrologist. Keep BP <130/80, or <125/75 if proteinuria >1g/d. Include an ACE-i or ARB as these have proven benefits in reducing proteinuria and preserving renal function; however, there is no additional benefit from dual therapy. [35]

## Specific types of glomerulonephritis

**IgA nephropathy:** Commonest GN in the developed world. Most present with macro- or microscopic haematuria; occasionally nephritic syndrome. *Typical patient:* Young man with episodic macroscopic haematuria, recovery is often rapid between attacks. There is ↑IgA, possibly due to infection, which forms immune complexes and deposits in mesangial cells. *Renal biopsy:* Mesangial proliferation, immunofluorescence (IF) shows deposits of IgA and C3. *R:* BP control with ACE-i. With nephritic presentation immunosuppression may slow decline of renal function. *Prognosis:* Worse if ↑BP, male, proteinuria or renal failure at presentation. 20% of adults develop ESRF over ~20yrs.

**Henoch-Schönlein purpura (HSP)** is a systemic variant of IgA nephropathy, causing a small vessel vasculitis. *Features:* Purpuric rash on extensor surfaces (typically on the legs), flitting polyarthritis, abdominal pain (GI bleeding) and nephritis. *Diagnosis:* Usually clinical. Confirmed with positive IF for IgA and C3 in skin or renal biopsy (identical to IgA nephropathy). *Treatment:* Same as IgA nephropathy. *Prognosis:* 15% nephritic patients → ESRF; if both nephritic and nephrotic syndrome, 50% →ESRF.

**Systemic lupus erythematous (SLE):** ~⅓ of patients with SLE will have evidence of renal disease with vascular, glomerular, and tubulointerstitial damage. Split into class I-IV (increasing severity) and class V (membranous). Requires early treatment.

**Anti-glomerular basement membrane (GBM) disease** (figs 1 and 2): Also known as Goodpasture's disease, caused by auto-antibodies to type IV collagen, an essential component of the GBM. Type IV collagen is also found in the lung and pulmonary haemorrhage can occur, especially in smokers. Present with haematuria/nephritic syndrome, AKI may occur within days of onset of symptoms. If R (plasma exchange, steroids ± cytotoxics) is started early, full recovery is possible and relapses are rare. Renal prognosis is poor if dialysis-dependent at presentation.

**Post-streptococcal GN** (a diffuse proliferative GN) occurs 1-12 weeks after a sore throat or skin infection. A streptococcal antigen is deposited on the glomerulus, causing a host reaction and immune complex formation. *Presentation:* Usually nephritic syndrome. *Renal biopsy:* Not usually done unless atypical presentation. Inflammatory reaction affecting mesangial and endothelial cells, IF: IgG and C3 deposits. *Serology:* ↑ASOT, ↓C3. *Treatment:* Supportive; >95% recover renal function.

**Rapidly progressive GN (RPGN):** The most aggressive GN, with potential to cause ESRF over days. There are different causes; all have the biopsy finding of crescents affecting most glomeruli. RPGN is classified pathologically into 3 categories:[36]
- Immune complex disease (~45% of cases): eg post-infectious, SLE, IgA/HSP
- Pauci-immune disease (~50% of cases, 80-90% ANCA +ve): granulomatosis with polyangiitis (GPA, previously known as Wegener's*—c-ANCA +ve, p728), microscopic polyangiitis (MPA—P-ANCA +ve), Churg-Strauss syndrome, p710.
- Anti-GBM disease (~3%): Goodpasture's disease p714.

*Clinically:* AKI ± systemic features (eg fever, myalgia, weight loss, haemoptysis). Pulmonary haemorrhage is the commonest cause of death in ANCA +ve patients. *Treatment:* Aggressive immunosuppression with high-dose IV steroids and cyclophosphamide ± plasma exchange. *Prognosis:* 5-year survival 80%.

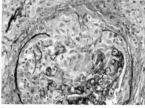

Fig 1. Crescentic GN: a proliferation of epithelial cells and macrophages with rupture of Bowman's capsule, in this patient caused by anti-GBM (Goodpasture's) disease (p714).

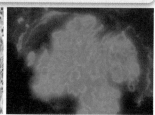

Fig 2. Immunofluorescence for IgG, showing linear staining characteristic of anti-GBM disease.

Figs 1 & 2 courtesy of Dr I. Roberts.

Renal medicine

▶If there is oedema, dipstick MSU for protein to avoid missing renal disease.

**Definition** The nephrotic syndrome is a triad of:
• Proteinuria >3.5g/24h (ACR >250mg/mmol)
• Hypoalbuminaemia (<25g/L, usually much lower)
• Oedema

Severe hyperlipidaemia (total cholesterol >10mmol/L) is often present.[37]

**Causes** Nephrotic syndrome is not a diagnosis, therefore the underlying cause should always be sought. It can be due to primary renal disease or secondary to a number of systemic disorders.
• *Primary causes:* Minimal change disease, membranous nephropathy, focal segmental glomerulosclerosis (FSGS), mesangiocapillary GN (MCGN).
• *Secondary causes:* Hepatitis B/C (usually membranous, hep C can cause MCGN), SLE (class V lupus nephritis causes a membranous pattern), diabetic nephropathy, amyloidosis, paraneoplastic (usually membranous pattern) or drug related (again usually membranous—NSAIDs, penicillamine, anti-TNF, gold).

**Pathophysiology** Injury to the podocyte appears to be the main cause of proteinuria, podocytes wrap around the glomerular capillaries and maintain the filtration barrier, preventing large molecular weight proteins from entering the urine. Effacement of the foot processes or loss of podocytes can cause heavy protein loss.

**Assessment** Patients present with pitting oedema, which can be severe and rapid onset, occurring in dependent areas and areas of low tissue resistance, eg periorbitally. *History:* Ask about acute or chronic infections, drugs, allergies, systemic symptoms suggestive of autoimmunity or malignancy. *Signs:* Urine dip shows ++++ protein, albumin is low, BP is usually normal or mildly increased, renal function is usually normal or mildly impaired. *Differential diagnosis:* CCF (↑JVP, pulmonary oedema, mild proteinuria) or liver disease (↓albumin).

▶Refer to a nephrologist for further assessment and renal biopsy.
• In children minimal change GN is the commonest cause of nephrotic syndrome and a trial of steroids causes resolution in 90%. Biopsy is avoided in children unless no response to steroids or if clinical features suggest another cause, eg age <1yr, family history, extrarenal disease (eg arthritis, rash, anaemia), renal failure, haematuria.
• All adults should undergo a biopsy as well as full assessment (see under tests for GN, p300). Renal biopsy is more difficult in patients with nephrotic syndrome because of gross oedema and a hypercoagulable state.

**Complications**
• *Susceptibility to infection* (eg cellulitis, *Streptococcus* infections and spontaneous bacterial peritonitis) happens in up to 20% of adult patients because of ↓serum IgG, ↓complement activity, and ↓T cell function (due in part to loss of immunoglobulin in urine and also to immunosuppressive treatments).
• *Thromboembolism:* (Up to 40%): eg DVT/PE, renal vein thrombosis. This hypercoagulable state is partly due to ↑clotting factors and platelet abnormalities.
• *Hyperlipidaemia:* ↑Cholesterol and triglycerides, thought to be due to hepatic lipoprotein synthesis in response to low oncotic pressure.

**Treatment**
1 *Reduce oedema:* Loop diuretics, eg furosemide are used, often high doses are needed. Gut oedema may prevent oral absorption so IV route is useful. Check daily weight (aim for 0.5-1kg loss/day) and daily U&Es. Fluid restrict to 1L/day and salt restrict while giving diuretics.
2 *Reduce proteinuria:* ACE-i or ARB should be started in all patients.
3 *Reduce risk of complications:* Anticoagulate if nephrotic range proteinuria, start a statin to reduce cholesterol (although often resolves spontaneously when cause treated), treat infections promptly and vaccinate (pneumovax II®, p160; flu).
4 *Treat underlying cause:* Find and treat underlying infections, malignancy or systemic disease. Stop causative drugs. Some primary causes do respond to specific therapies.

**Minimal change** Commonest cause of nephrotic syndrome in children (76%, and 20% of nephrotic adults). In adults it can be idiopathic or in association with drugs (NSAIDs) or paraneoplastic (usually Hodgkin's lymphoma). *Biopsy:* Normal under light microscopy (hence the name). Electron microscopy shows effacement of the podocyte foot processes. ℞: 90% of children and 70% of adults undergo remission with steroids, but the majority relapse. Spontaneous remission can occur, and suggests the benefit of steroids is to hold disease until the poorly understood underlying process abates.[38] Frequently relapsing or steroid-dependent disease is treated with cyclophosphamide or ciclosporin/tacrolimus. *Prognosis*: ~1% → ESRF.

**Membranous nephropathy** Accounts for 20-30% of nephrotic syndrome in adults; 2-5% in children. Mostly idiopathic, but can be associated with malignancy, hepatitis B, drugs (gold, penicillamine, NSAIDs) and autoimmunity (thyroid, SLE). *Biopsy:* Diffusely thickened GBM with IgG and C3 subepithelial deposits on immunofluorescence (IF). *Treatment:* Secondary involves treating the underlying cause, proteinuria often remits with, eg control of hepatitis B viraemia. In idiopathic membranous, treatment involves general measures such as ACE/ARB and diuretics. Spontaneous complete remission occurs in up to 30% and partial remission in 24-40% by 5 years. However, with the discovery that antibodies directed against the phospholipase A2 receptor are found in up to 80% of patients with idiopathic membranous nephropathy, interest is growing in immunosuppressive therapy. Trials are ongoing into the use of the modified Ponticelli regimen (alternating IV steroids with chlorambucil/cyclophosphamide), historically results have been variable. In patients who are anti-PLA2 antibody positive, rituximab, an anti-CD20 monoclonal antibody, is also being trialled.

**Mesangiocapillary GN** Previously divided into type I, II and III, now a more aetiology-based approach divides into **immune complex** (IC) mediated and **complement** mediated. *IC mediated* is driven by circulating immune complexes, which deposit in the kidney and activate complement via the classical pathway. An underlying cause can be found in most cases, eg hepatitis C, SLE and monoclonal gammopathies. *Complement mediated* is less common and involves persistent activation of the alternative complement pathway, eg C3 nephritic factor. Patients can have extra-renal manifestations, eg Drusen in the retina. *Biopsy:* mesangial and endocapillary proliferation, a thickened capillary basement membrane, double contouring (tramline) of the capillary walls. IF can show Ig staining, complement staining or light chains depending on cause. Electron microscopy shows electron dense deposits. *Treatment:* underlying cause as priority, ACE/ARB for all. Immunosuppression if rapid progression of disease with steroids ± cyclophosphamide if rapid deterioration in renal function. Given the role of complement, it is possible that new complement-targeted therapies such as eculizumab may be trialled. *Prognosis:* poor where no underlying cause can be found. In patients who reach ESRF (usually idiopathic disease) it can recur in transplants and lead to graft loss.

**Focal segmental glomerulosclerosis (FSGS)** may be primary (idiopathic) or secondary (vesicoureteric reflux, IgA nephropathy, Alport's syndrome (*OHCS* p638), vasculitis (p558), sickle-cell disease, heroin use). HIV is associated with the collapsing subtype (poor prognosis). *Presentation:* Usually nephrotic syndrome or proteinuria. ~50% have impaired renal function. *Biopsy:* Some glomeruli have scarring of certain segments (ie focal sclerosis). IF: IgM and C3 deposits in affected areas. ℞: Responds to corticosteroids in ~30%. Cyclophosphamide or ciclosporin are considered if steroid-resistant. *Prognosis:* Untreated most progress to ESRF. Spontaenous remission probably <10%. Longer courses of treatment lead to response in up to 70%; however, those presenting with abnormal renal function have much poorer prognosis, 30-50% → ESRF. It recurs in approx. 20% of transplanted kidneys, and may respond to plasma exchange.

Renal medicine

### Loop diuretics, eg furosemide, bumetanide

*Mechanism:* Block the $Na^+/K^+/2Cl^-$ co-transporter in the thick ascending limb of the Loop of Henle, hence increase the solute load of the filtrate and reduce water resorption. *Effects:* Significant loss of water and $Na^+Cl^-$. $Ca^{2+}$, $K^+$ and $H^+$ excretion is also increased. *Clinical use:* They are readily absorbed from the GI tract, and given orally they act within 1 hour. IV the peak effect is seen within 30 minutes so they are useful in treating acute pulmonary oedema. Widely used in peripheral oedema (heart failure, ascites). They can also be used to treat severe hypercalcaemia. *Side effects:* Hypokalaemic metabolic alkalosis (because of $K^+$ and $H^+$ excretion), hypovolaemia, ototoxicity, allergic reactions.

### Thiazide diuretics, eg bendroflumethiazide, indapamide, metolazone

*Mechanism:* They inhibit the $Na^+Cl^-$ transporter in the distal convoluted tubule. They also decrease $Na^+Cl^-$ resorption and hence increase water loss. *Effects:* Moderate $Na^+$ and $Cl^-$ excretion. They result in low urine $Ca^{2+}$ by increasing urinary $Ca^{2+}$ resorption (the opposite effect of loop diuretics). They can cause profound hypokalaemia due to excessive $K^+$ loss. Excretion of uric acid is reduced, and $Mg^{2+}$ is increased. *Use:* Their action begins within 1-2 hours after ingestion, and lasts for 12-24 hours. Useful in ↑BP, long-term treatment of oedema (eg heart failure). They can reduce renal stone formation in patients with idiopathic hypercalciuria by decreasing urine calcium concentrations. *Side effects:* Hypokalaemia, hyponatraemia, hypomagnesaemia, metabolic alkalosis, hyperglycaemia, increased serum lipid and uric acid levels (thiazide diuretics are contraindicated in gout).

### Potassium-sparing diuretics

*Mechanism:* Spironolactone and eplerenone are aldosterone antagonists and hence inhibit the sodium-retaining action of aldosterone. Amiloride and triamterene block sodium channels in collecting tubules. Both types decrease $K^+$ excretion. *Effects:* They increase $Na^+$ excretion and decrease $K^+$ and $H^+$ excretion, there is a mild associated diuresis. The onset of action of spironolactone is very slow, and takes several days to have its full effect. Amiloride has a much faster onset and a duration of action of only 12-16 hours. *Use:* Usually used to control the $K^+$ wasting caused by loop diuretics or thiazides and are given as combination therapy. Spironolactone and eplerenone have significant benefits in hyperaldosteronism (↑serum aldosterone. Primary = Conn's, rare. Secondary occurs in cirrhosis and heart failure). *Side effects:* Hyperkalaemia is common, metabolic acidosis can occur. Anti-androgenic effects (eg gynaecomastia) are seen with spironolactone, as is GI upset.

### Osmotic diuretics

Mannitol is a solute that is freely filtered at the glomerulus but poorly reabsorbed from the tubule, so it remains in the lumen and holds water by osmotic effect. The reduction in water reabsorption occurs in the proximal tubule and loop of Henle and also slightly increases $Na^+$ loss. *Effects:* Mannitol can reduce brain volume and intracranial pressure by osmotically extracting water from the tissue into the blood. *Use:* Haemolysis, rhabdomyolysis, reducing intra-ocular and intra-cranial pressures. *Side-effects:* ↑$Na^+$, headache, nausea, vomiting. In patients who are unable to form urine the transient expansion of the extracellular fluid when water is extracted from intra-cellular fluid can cause pulmonary oedema.

### Carbonic anhydrase inhibitors

such as acetazolamide act on the proximal tubule to increase excretion of bicarbonate and consequently sodium, potassium and water. This causes alkalinization of the urine and hence a mild metabolic acidosis. They are not used as diuretics but are still available for use in *glaucoma* to reduce the formation of aqueous humour. It is also used by climbers (as Diamox®) to increase respiration (the body's attempt is to clear the acidosis) and hence improve acclimatization to altitude and reduce the risk of acute mountain sickness (with its rare but deadly complications of high-altitude pulmonary and cerebral oedema).

---

1 Principal source: *Pharmacology*. Authors: HP Rang, MM Dale, JM Ritter, PK Moore. Fifth Edition. 2003 Churchill Livingstone.

2 $Na^+$ = sodium, $Cl^-$ = chloride, $K^+$ = potassium, $Ca^{2+}$ = calcium, $Mg^{2+}$ = magnesium, $H^+$ = hydrogen ion.

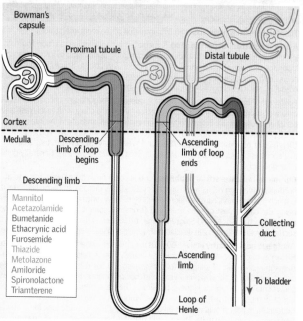

**Fig 1.** The nephron and sites of action of diuretics.

**Proximal convoluted tubule** This segment reabsorbs amino acids, glucose, and numerous cations. It is also responsible for 60–70% of the total reabsorption of Na⁺. Bicarbonate is reabsorbed by means of the enzyme carbonic anhydrase; this process can be inhibited by carbonic anhydrase inhibitors (eg acetazolamide). Some drugs that are used in treating gout affect uric acid transport in this segment.

**Thick ascending limb of the loop of Henle** Na⁺/K⁺/2Cl⁻ co-transporter (which is the target of loop diuretics) acts in this segment. It is also a major site of calcium and Mg reabsorption. 20–30% of the filtered sodium is reabsorbed in this segment.

**Distal convoluted tubule** 5–8% of sodium reabsorption occurs in this segment. Calcium is also reabsorbed in this segment under the control of PTH.

**Cortical collecting tubule** In this segment Na⁺ is reabsorbed accompanied by an equivalent excretion of K⁺ or H⁺ ions into urine. Therefore this segment is the main site of urine acidification and K⁺ excretion. This is also the site of action of the potassium-sparing diuretics.

**Tubulointerstitial nephritis (TIN)** Inflammation of the renal interstitium.

**Acute interstitial nephritis (AIN)** is mediated by an immune reaction to drugs, infections or autoimmune disorders. *Drugs:* NSAIDs, antibiotics; diuretics; also allopurinol, omeprazole, phenytoin, among others. *Infections*: Staphs, Streps, *Brucella*, *Leptospira*, several viruses. *Immune disorders*, eg SLE, sarcoid—or *no obvious cause*. ►Take a full drug history including over-the-counter and herbal preparations.

*Features:* Usually mild renal impairment; raised ↑BP/oliguria are uncommon (indicate worse prognosis). Drug reactions: often 'allergic' picture with fever, rash and peripheral eosinophilia. Biopsy shows inflammatory cell infiltrate in the interstitium. *R:* stop/treat causative agent. If renal function does not improve within a week then trial of prednisolone 1mg/kg/24h for 4 weeks may improve prognosis but the evidence base is poor and trials have had mixed results. *Prognosis:* Generally good if caught early.

**Chronic tubulointerstitial nephritis (CIN)** is common in disorders leading to abnormal anatomy, eg reflux nephropathy, cystic kidney disease. In normal kidneys it is much less common, causing about 3% ESRF in the UK, with analgesic nephropathy being the commonest cause. Drugs and toxins are common causes, autoimmune diseases such as SLE, RA and Sjögren's rarer; often seen in haematological disorders such as myeloma, light chain disease and sickle cell disease, so investigate for these.

**Analgesic nephropathy** in the 1950s-70s was the commonest cause of AKI and CKD. History is of chronic, heavy analgesic use, usually NSAIDs, commoner in women. Patients may complain of loin pain (papillary necrosis) but it is often silent until late CKD. Urinalysis can show sterile pyuria and mild proteinuria but may be normal. USS shows small and irregular kidneys. IVU shows the classic 'cup and spill' appearance but CT without contrast is more sensitive.[39] Biopsy shows CIN. *R:* Stop/treat cause. Sudden flank pain should prompt an ultrasound or CT urogram to look for obstruction from a sloughed papilla. There is an ↑ risk of atherosclerosis in these patients.

**Aristolochic acid** is a nephrotoxin found in plants endemic to areas along the River Danube (*Balkan herb nephropathy*) and some Chinese medicine (*Chinese herb nephropathy*). It can cause CIN in genetically susceptible individuals. *Clinical features:* There is a long duration between exposure and disease presentation. Patients are usually normotensive, ↑BP only develops with ESRF.[40] There is an ↑ risk of urothelial tumours, reported in up to 40%.[41]

**Urate nephropathy** *Acute crystal nephropathy:* AKI due to uric acid precipitation within the tubules. It is most often due to tumour lysis syndrome, seen in haematological malignancies after chemotherapy, which leads to overproduction of uric acid.[42] The renal parenchyma appears bright on USS. Plasma urate is often markedly raised with urinary birefringent crystals on microscopy. *R:* p346: keep well hydrated, allopurinol pre-chemo, urinary alkalinization with sodium bicarbonate (↑solubility of uric acid). *Chronic urate nephropathy:* Much reduced incidence with improved diet and earlier treatment of gout with allopurinol. Hyperuricaemic nephropathy is associated with several familial disorders including familial juvenile gout and xanthinuria.

**Hypercalcaemia** can cause AKI whatever the cause (myeloma, sarcoid, malignancy, nephrocalcinosis, etc). Reduce the calcium acutely with rehydration and IV bisphosphonates (see p691) but ultimately treat the underlying cause.

**Radiation nephritis** is renal impairment following radiotherapy and occurs acutely (<1 year) or can have a chronic onset (years later). *Signs:* ↑BP, proteinuria, progression to ESRF. Biopsy shows interstitial fibrosis. *R:* Strict BP control, nil specific. *Prevention:* During radiotherapy, ensure adequate shielding (or exclusion) of renal areas.

Many agents may be toxic to the kidneys and cause acute kidney injury (AKI), usually by direct acute tubular necrosis, or by causing interstitial nephritis. Examples are shown (not an exhaustive list and idiosyncratic reactions are possible).

- Analgesics (NSAIDs)
- Antimicrobials: gentamicin, sulfonamides, penicillins, rifampicin, amphotericin, aciclovir
- Anticonvulsants: lamotrigine, valproate, phenytoin
- Other drugs: omeprazole, furosemide, thiazides, ACE-i and ARBs, cimetidine, lithium, iron, calcineurin inhibitors, cisplatin
- Anaesthetic agents: methoxyflurane, enflurane
- Radiocontrast material
- Crystals: urate
- Toxins: aristolochia, cadmium, lead, arsenic, ethylene glycol
- Haemoglobin in haemolysis, myoglobin in rhabdomyolysis
- Proteins: Igs in myeloma, light chain disease
- Bacteria: streptococci, legionella, brucella, mycoplasma, chlamydia, TB, salmonella, campylobacter
- Viruses: EBV, CMV, HIV, polyoma virus, adenovirus, measles
- Other: leptospirosis, syphilis, toxoplasma, leishmania

**Aminoglycosides** (gentamicin, amikacin, streptomycin) are well-recognized nephrotoxins. Typically give mild non-oliguric AKI, 1–2wks into therapy. Risk is ↑by old age, renal hypoperfusion, pre-existing CKD, high dosage/prolonged treatment, and co-administration of other nephrotoxins. Recovery may be delayed or incomplete. Single bolus doses of aminoglycosides can be as effective as multiple doses in treating infection and less nephrotoxic. ►Check levels p766!

**Radiocontrast nephropathy** is a very common cause of iatrogenic AKI with IV contrast radiological studies. Risk factors are diabetes mellitus, high doses of contrast medium, hypovolaemia, other nephrotoxic agents, and previous CKD. *Prevention is key*: stop nephrotoxic agents peri-procedure, and pre-hydrate with IV 0.9% sodium chloride in patients with risk factors. ►Follow local protocols and inform radiology, who may use less nephrotoxic medium. See p763.

**Rhabdomyolysis** results from skeletal muscle breakdown, with release of its contents into the circulation, including myoglobin, $K^+$, $PO_4^{3-}$, urate and creatine kinase (CK). Complications include ↑$K^+$ and AKI: myoglobin is filtered by the glomeruli and precipitates, obstructing renal tubules. *Causes:* Many, including post-ischaemia; eg embolism, clamp on artery during surgery, trauma: prolonged immobilization (eg after falling), burns, crush injury, excessive exercise, uncontrolled seizures; drugs and toxins: statins, alcohol, ecstasy, heroin, snake bite, carbon monoxide, neuroleptic malignant syndrome (p855); infections: Coxsackie, EBV, influenza; metabolic: $K^+$↓, $PO_4^{3-}$↓, myositis, malignant hyperpyrexia (p574); inherited muscle disorders: McArdle's disease (p718), Duchenne's muscular dystrophy (p514). *Clinical features:* Often of the cause, with muscle pain, swelling, tenderness, and red-brown urine. *Tests:* Plasma CK >1000iU/L (often >10,000iU/L). MI must be excluded as a cause (troponin negative). Visible myoglobinuria (tea- or cola-coloured urine) occurs when urinary myoglobin exceeds 250µg/mL (normal <5ng/mL)[G] Urine is +ve for blood on dipstick but *without* RBC on microscopy. *Others:* $K^+$↑, $PO_4^{3-}$↑↑, $Ca^{2+}$↓ (enters muscle), urate↑. AKI occurs 12–24 hours later, and DIC is associated (p346). Compartment syndrome can result from muscle injury. *Treatment:* Urgent treatment for hyperkalaemia (p849). IV fluid rehydration is a priority to prevent AKI: maintain urine output at 300mL/h until myoglobinuria has ceased; initially up to 1.5L fluid/h may be needed. If oliguric, CVP monitoring is useful to prevent fluid overload. IV sodium bicarbonate is used to alkalinize urine to pH >6.5, to stabilize a less toxic form of myoglobin. Dialysis may be needed. Ideally manage patient in HDU/ICU setting to allow early detection of deterioration and regular bloods and monitoring. Prognosis is good if treated early.

Hypertension often causes renal problems (eg CKD, p296, and sometimes AKI eg in malignant hypertension or pre-eclampsia[1]) and most renal diseases can cause hypertension (esp. diabetic nephropathy, glomerulonephritis, chronic interstitial nephritis, polycystic kidneys and renovascular disease).

**Renovascular disease** (Fig 1) Defined as stenosis of the renal artery or one of its branches. *Causes:* Atherosclerosis (in 80%: >50yrs, arteriopaths: often co-existent IHD, stroke or peripheral vascular disease), fibromuscular dysplasia (10%, younger ♀). Rarer: Takayasu's arteritis, antiphospholipid syndrome, post-renal transplant, thromboembolism, external compression. *Signs:* ↑BP resistant to treatment; worsening renal function after ACE-i/ARB in bilateral renal artery stenosis; 'flash' pulmonary oedema (sudden onset, without LV impairment on cardiac echo). Abdominal ± carotid or femoral bruits, and weak leg pulses may be found. *Tests:* USS: renal size asymmetry (affected side is smaller), disturbance in renal blood flow on Doppler US. CT/MR angiography are more sensitive. Renal angiography is 'gold standard', but do after CT/MR as it is invasive (p759). *R:* Comprehensive antihypertensive regimens (p134), transluminal angioplasty ± stent placement or revascularization surgery. Best medical management is probably superior to revascularization in atherosclerotic disease, see the ASTRAL trial.[44]

**Haemolytic uraemic syndrome (HUS)** HUS is characterized by *microangiopathic haemolytic anaemia* (MAHA): intravascular haemolysis + red cell fragmentation. Endothelial damage triggers thrombosis, platelet consumption and fibrin strand deposition, mainly in renal microvasculature. The strands cause mechanical destruction of passing RBCs. Thrombocytopenia and AKI result. *Causes:* 90% are from *E. coli* strain O157 ('O' denotes the somatic antigen, as opposed to H, the flagellar antigen). This produces a verotoxin that attacks endothelial cells. This typically affects young children in outbreaks (more common than sporadically) after eating undercooked contaminated meat. *Signs:* Abdominal pain, bloody diarrhoea, and AKI. *Tests:* Haematuria/proteinuria. Blood film: fragmented RBC (schistocytes, p330); ↓platelets, ↓Hb. Clotting tests are normal. *R:* Seek expert advice. Dialysis for AKI may be needed. Plasma exchange is used in severe persistent disease. *Prognosis:* Worse in non-*E. coli* cases. Mortality 3–5%, good prognosis if caught early.

**Thrombotic thrombocytopenic purpura (TTP fig 2)** There is an overlap between TTP and HUS, and many physicians consider them a spectrum of disease. All patients have MAHA (severe, often with jaundice) and low platelets. Other features can include AKI, fluctuating CNS signs (eg seizures, hemiparesis, ↓consciousness, ↓vision) and fever. The classic description included the full 'pentad' of features, but with the advent of plasma exchange this is rarely seen. Mortality is higher than childhood HUS and can be >90% if untreated, though reduced to ~20% with plasma exchange. *Pathophysiology:* There is a genetic or acquired deficiency of a protease (ADAMTS13) that normally cleaves multimers of von Willebrand factor (vWF). Large vWF multimers form, causing platelet aggregation and fibrin deposition in small vessels, leading to microthrombi. *Causes:* Idiopathic (40%), autoimmunity (eg SLE), cancer, pregnancy, drug associated (eg quinine), bloody diarrhoea prodrome (as childhood HUS), haematopoietic stem cell transplant. ▶*It is a haematological emergency: get expert help.* *Tests:* As HUS. *R:* Urgent plasma exchange may be life-saving. Steroids are the mainstay for non-responders, although new therapies such as eculizumab (monoclonal antibody targeting terminal complement pathway C5) have shown promising results in case reports,[45] though seem to be more effective in children than adults.[46] Trials are ongoing. Because thrombotic thrombocytopenic purpura is uncommon, a high index of suspicion is required for rapid diagnosis and prompt initiation of plasma-exchange treatment. ▶The unexplained occurrence of thrombocytopaenia and anaemia should prompt immediate consideration of the diagnosis and evaluation of a peripheral blood smear for evidence of microangiopathic haemolytic anaemia.

---

1 Pre-eclampsia is an example. In later pregnancy, this causes hypertension, oedema and proteinuria which may lead to AKI and stroke; see OHCS p48 and remember that finding out if your patient is pregnant is vital!

## Diabetes mellitus and the kidney

Diabetes is best viewed as a vascular disease with the kidney as one of its chief targets for end-organ damage. The single most important intervention in the long-term care of DM is the control of BP, to protect the heart, the brain, and the kidney. Renal damage may be preventable with good BP and glycaemic control.

In *type 1 DM* nephropathy is rare in the first 5yrs, after 10yrs annual incidence rises to a peak at 15yrs, then falls again. Those who have not developed nephropathy at 35yrs are unlikely to do so. In *type 2 DM* around 10% have nephropathy at diagnosis and up to half will go on to develop it over the next 20yrs. 20% of people with type 2 DM will develop ESRF.

►Everyone with DM should be screened annually for microalbuminuria.

*Microalbuminuria* (30–300mg albumin/24h) gives early warning of impending renal problems and is also a strong independent risk factor for cardiovascular disease. Standard dipsticks do not detect this, so use specialized dipsticks or estimate using an albumin : creatinine ratio of >2.5 in men or >3.5 in women.

Those who are positive should be started on an ACE-i (p109) or angiotensin-2 receptor blockers (ARB), *irrespective* of blood pressure as these reduce intra-glomerular pressure and hence proteinuria. *SE:* U&E↑ (monitor K⁺ and creatinine periodically; stop if there is a rise in creatinine of >20%), cough (with ACE-i). Usually, ACE-i are first-line and ARBs for ACE-i-intolerant individuals. There is currently insufficient evidence that ACE-i and ARB are of additive benefit.[47] In one study, the combination of telmisartan and ramipril was associated with more adverse events without an increase in benefit.[48] ►Example of target BP in DM *if no proteinuria:* 130/80; *if microalbuminuria/proteinuria* is present, aim 125/75mmHg.

Is microalbuminuria reversible? If caught early and managed vigorously:
• Tight glycaemic control
• Tight BP control with ACE/ARB
• Manage CV risk: stop smoking, reduce cholesterol, consider aspirin

See p314 for more detail on diabetes and the kidney.

## Cholesterol emboli

Cholesterol emboli may be released from atheromatous plaques (often aorta) which lodge in the distal microcirculation (eg renal vessels, peripheral circulation, gut) to cause ischaemia. An inflammatory response leads to fever, myalgia and ↑eosinophils. *Risks:* Atheroma, ↑cholesterol, aortic aneurysm, thrombolysis, arterial catheterization, eg during interventional radiological procedures. *Signs:* Fever, uncontrolled ↑BP, livedo reticularis (p559), oliguria, AKI, gangrene, GI bleeds. *R:* Haemodynamic monitoring, nutritional and metabolic support, dialysis when indicated. Statins are also tried (p704); avoid anticoagulants and instrumentation. *Prognosis:* Often progressive and fatal; some regain renal function after dialysis.

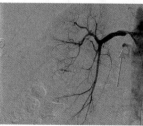

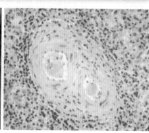

Fig 1. Renal angiogram showing renal artery stenosis.

Courtesy of Dr Edmund Godfrey.

Fig 2. Thrombi in small arterioles due to fibrin and platelet deposition, characteristic of TTP.

Courtesy of Prof Christine Lawrence.

Renal medicine

**Renal tubular acidosis (RTA)** is a metabolic acidosis due to impaired acid secretion by the kidney. There is a hyperchloraemic metabolic acidosis with normal anion gap (p684). There are 4 types, type 3 RTA is a rare combination of types 1 and 2.

**Type 1 (distal) RTA** is due to an inability to excrete $H^+$ and generate acidic urine in the distal tubule, even in states of metabolic acidosis. *Causes:* Inherited disorders, acquired include SLE, Sjögren's and drug related (amphotericin). *Features:* Include rickets (+ growth failure) or osteomalacia, due to buffering of $H^+$ with calcium in bone. Nephrocalcinosis with renal calculi, leading to recurrent UTIs, is due to a combination of hypercalciuria, ↓urinary citrate (reabsorbed as a buffer for $H^+$) and alkaline urine: all favour calcium phosphate stone formation. *Tests:* Urine pH >5.5 despite metabolic acidosis. *Treatment:* Oral sodium bicarbonate or citrate. Complications are mostly from renal calculi—ESRF may result from nephrocalcinosis.

**Type 2 (proximal) RTA** is due to a 'bicarbonate leak': a defect in $HCO_3^-$ reabsorption in the proximal tubule resulting in excess $HCO_3^-$ in the urine (pH <5.5) leading to a metabolic acidosis. Type 2 RTA is often associated with a more generalized tubular defect (Fanconi syndrome, below), and is rarer than type 1. Hypokalaemia is common, due to the osmotic diuretic effect of ↓$HCO_3^-$ reabsorption, causing ↑flow rate to distal tubule ∴ ↑$K^+$ excretion. *Diagnosis:* IV sodium bicarbonate load: there is a high fractional excretion of $HCO_3^-$ (>15%). *Treatment:* High doses of bicarbonate (>10mmol/kg/day) are required.

**Type 4 (hyperkalaemic) RTA** is due to 'hyporeninaemic hypoaldosteronism'. Hypoaldosteronism causes hyperkalaemia and acidosis (↓$K^+$ and $H^+$ excretion). *Causes:* Addison's, diabetic nephropathy, interstitial nephritis (SLE, chronic obstruction), drugs ($K^+$-sparing diuretics, β-blockers, NSAIDs, ciclosporin). *Treatment:* Remove any cause. Fludrocortisone 0.1mg, furosemide or Calcium Resonium® are used to control $K^+$.

**Fanconi syndrome** = proximal tubular dysfunction leading to loss of amino acids, glucose, $PO_4^{3-}$ and $HCO_3^-$ in urine. This causes dehydration, metabolic acidosis, osteomalacia/rickets and electrolyte abnormalities. *Causes:* Congenital—idiopathic, cysteinosis, Wilson's disease (p269), tyrosinaemia, Lowe syndrome. Acquired—heavy metal poisoning (lead, mercury, cadmium, platinum, uranium), drugs (gentamicin, cisplatin, ifosfamide), light chains (myeloma, amyloid), Sjögren's. *Treatment:* Remove any cause and replace losses. $K^+$, sodium bicarbonate, $PO_4^{3-}$ and vitamin D supplements are used.

**Cystinosis** (fig 1) There is accumulation of cystine in lysosomes due to an autosomal recessive defect. Cystine deposits cause Fanconi syndrome, visual impairment, myopathy, hypothyroidism and progression to ESRF <10yrs. *Treatment:* As Fanconi syndrome. Oral cysteamine ↓intralysosomal cystine and delays ESRF, but is poorly tolerated. Renal cystinosis does not recur after transplant; extra-renal disease progresses.

**Hereditary hypokalaemic tubulopathies**

- *Bartter syndrome:* p220; Low $K^+$, metabolic alkalosis, hypercalciuria. Inherited mutation in the co-transporter targeted by LOOP diuretics, so a similar pattern of metabolic abnormalities. Usually present in infancy. Replace $K^+$ and consider indomethacin, a prostaglandin synthesis inhibitor, which can resolve abnormalities.
- *Gitelman syndrome:* Low $K^+$, metabolic alkalosis, hypocalciuria and low $Mg^{2+}$. Inherited mutation in the co-transporter targeted by THIAZIDE diuretics, so a similar pattern of metabolic abnormalities. Usually present later than Bartter's with muscle cramps, weakness and low BP. Replace $Mg^{2+}$, may also require $K^+$ supplementation.

Check 24h urine for $Na^+$, $K^+$, $Ca^{2+}$, urea, creatinine ± protein excretion. Take blood simultaneously for creatinine to calculate creatinine clearance (p683; eGFR may mislead). Patients should be managed at a specialist centre.[49]

## Causes of renal tubular acidosis

**Type 1 (distal)**
- Idiopathic (usually inherited, AD or AR forms)
- Genetic associations (eg Marfan's, Ehlers-Danlos syndrome)
- Autoimmune disease commonest cause in adults (eg SLE, Sjögren's)
- Nephrocalcinosis (eg hypercalcaemia, medullary sponge kidney)
- Tubulointerstitial disease (eg chronic pyelonephritis, chronic interstitial nephritis, obstructive uropathy, renal transplant rejection)
- Drugs (eg lithium, amphotericin)

**Type 2 (proximal)**
- Idiopathic
- Fanconi syndrome
- Tubulointerstitial disease (eg myeloma, interstitial nephritis)
- Drugs (eg lead or other heavy metals, acetazolamide, out-of-date tetracycline)

*Renal medicine*

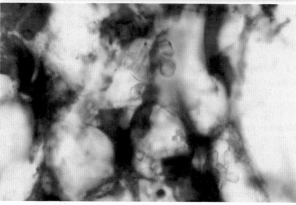

**Fig 1.** Cystine crystals in the bone marrow, found in cystinosis. Crystals accumulate in most tissues, especially the kidneys.

Courtesy of Professor Christine Lawrence.

### Autosomal dominant polycystic kidney disease (APKD)

*Prevalence:* 1:1000. 85% of patients have mutations in PKD1 (chromosome 16) and reach ESRF by 50s. Remainder have mutation in PKD2 (chromosome 4) and have a slower course, reaching ESRF by 70s. Can be clinically silent for many years so family screening is important. *Signs:* Renal enlargement with cysts, abdominal pain ± haematuria (haemorrhage into a cyst), cyst infection, renal calculi, BP↑, progressive renal failure. *Extrarenal:* liver cysts, intra-cranial aneurysm→SAH (subarachnoid haemorrhage, see p482), mitral valve prolapse, ovarian cysts and diverticular disease. *R̩:* Monitor U&E. ↑BP should be treated aggressively, with target levels of <130/80mmHg[50] (ACE-i are best choices). Treat infections, dialysis or transplantation for ESRF, genetic counselling. Pain may be helped by laparoscopic cyst removal or nephrectomy. ↑Water intake, ↓Na⁺ intake, and avoiding caffeine may also help.[51] *Screening for PKD:* Genetic testing for PKD1 is difficult as the gene is large and there are hundreds of described mutations. USS screening offers good sensitivity and specificity depending on age. Age 18-39yrs >3 unilateral or bilateral cysts, 40-59yrs >2 cysts in each kidney, >60yrs >4 cysts in each kidney have good sensitivity and specificity and a positive predictive value close to 100%.[52] Genetic screening for some PKD2 mutations is available in specialist centres. *Screening for SAH* with magnetic resonance angiography may be done in 1ˢᵗ-degree relatives of those with SAH + ADPKD. Some screen with no family history, especially for certain occupations (eg pilots).

### Autosomal recessive polycystic kidney disease (See fig 1 and OHCS p132).

Prevalence 1:40,000, chromosome 6. *Signs:* Variable, many present in infancy with multiple renal cysts and congenital hepatic fibrosis. There is currently no specific therapy. Genetic counselling of family members is important.

### Medullary cystic disease

Inherited disorder with tubular loss and medullary cyst formation. The juvenile (autosomal recessive) form accounts for 10-20% of ESRF in children. The adult form (autosomal dominant) is rare. *Signs:* Shrunken kidneys, cysts restricted to the renal medulla, salt wasting, polyuria, polydipsia, enuresis (↓urine concentrating ability), failure to thrive, renal impairment → ESRF.[53] *Extrarenal:* retinal degeneration, retinitis pigmentosa, skeletal changes, cerebellar ataxia, liver fibrosis.

### Renal phakomatoses

(neuroectodermal syndromes). *Tuberous sclerosis:* OHCS p638. A complex autosomal dominant disorder with hamartoma formation in skin, brain, eye, kidney, and heart caused by genes on chromosomes 9 (TSC1) & 16 (TSC2). *Signs are variable:* •Skin: adenoma sebaceum, angiofibromas (see images in OHCS p639), 'ash leaf' hypomelanic macules, shagreen patches (sacral plaques of shark-like skin), periungual fibroma •IQ↓ •Epilepsy. *Von Hippel-Lindau syndrome* (p726) is the chief cause of inherited renal cancers. *Cause:* Germline mutations of the VHL tumoursuppressor gene (also inactivated in most sporadic renal cell cancers).[54]

### Alport syndrome

OHCS p638. *Prevalence:* 1:5000. ~85% of cases are X-linked, due to mutations in the COL4A5 gene, which encodes the $\alpha_5$ chain of type IV collagen.[55] *Signs:* Haematuria, proteinuria and progressive renal insufficiency. Patients often exhibit systemic manifestations, eg sensorineural deafness and ocular defects (eg lenticonus: bulging of lens capsule seen on slit-lamp examination).[56] *Pathology:* Thickened GBM with 'splitting'. Type IV collagen is the antigen in anti-GBM disease (Goodpasture's disease), hence there is a risk of anti-GBM glomerulonephritis post-renal transplant. *R̩:* None specific, as for CKD.

### Fabry's disease See p712.

### Hyperoxaluria

can be primary (inherited enzyme defect) or secondary: increased intake (rhubarb, spinach, tea), increased intestinal resorption due to ileal disease or short bowel syndrome. *Presents* with oxalate renal stones and nephrocalcinosis. *Treatment:* ↑fluid intake, reduce oxalate in diet, calcium supplements. Liver transplant is curative in primary hyperoxaluria and can be combined with renal transplant.

### Cystinuria

not to be confused with cystinosis. Manifests with cysteine renal stones. *Treatment:* ↑Fluid intake, urine alkalinization with potassium citrate.

## Genetics: triumphs and disasters

As soon as genetics solves one problem, others appear. You might think that the application of science to medicine is an undisputed boon. Petty has provided a compelling counter-example.[57] A man with adult polycystic kidney disease due to a known PKD1 mutation is in end-stage renal failure. A transplant from a matched, living, related, unaffected donor is highly desired. There are problems in his family, but he persuades his adult children to have genetic testing to see if there are eligible donors. Each is apparently happy to donate a kidney to his/her father.

A can of worms is opened when one son realizes that he is the only child who can offer a good match—and that his brother is carrying the same mutation as his estranged father (there is a 50:50 chance of passing on the PKD gene). The eligible son would rather save his kidney to help his brother than his father. Old animosities resurface, and the family is in turmoil. How will you feel if the father dies of a complication of dialysis, and both his sons feel guilty forever? We should not be too surprised at all this: often in medicine bad comes out of our good intentions. How can we make good come out of bad? By remembering this example, and not doing tests lightly, and by making genetic counselling as professional as possible, so complications can be foreseen and disasters pre-empted. Furthermore, do not have unreasonable expectations about what genetic counselling can do. The number of diseases being found to have a significant genetic component is increasing faster than geneticists can formulate rational guidelines for screening.[58]

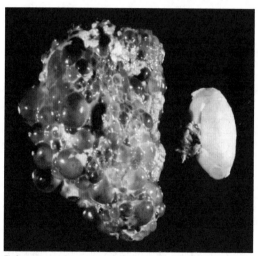

**Fig 1.** A polycystic kidney (left) compared with a normal sized kidney (right). The progressive increase in size often leads to abdominal discomfort, and there may be haemorrhage into a cyst causing haematuria, or infection.

Courtesy of the PKD Foundation.

**Amyloidosis** (p364) can cause proteinuria, nephrotic syndrome or progressive renal failure. *Diagnosis:* US: large kidneys; biopsy: see p364. *Treatment:* p364.

**Diabetes** This is one of the commonest causes of ESRF in the UK, accounting for ~18%. There are a number of mechanisms contributing to progression of diabetic ne-phropathy, one of the microvascular complications of diabetes. Early on, glomerular and tubular hypertrophy occur, increasing GFR transiently, but ongoing damage from advanced glycosylation end-products (AGE—caused by non-enzymatic glycosylation of proteins from chronic hyperglycaemia) triggers more destructive disease. These AGE trigger an inflammatory response leading to deposition of type IV collagen and mesangial expansion, eventually leading to arterial hyalinization, thickening of the mesangium and glomerular basement membrane and nodular glomerulosclerosis (Kimmelstiel-Wilson lesions). Progression generally occurs in four stages:

1 *GFR elevated:* early in disease renal blood flow increases, increasing the GFR and leading to microalbuminuria. As sugars are controlled, this falls back to normal.

2 *Glomerular hyperfiltration:* in the next 5-10yrs mesangial expansion gradually occurs and hyperfiltration at the glomerulus is seen without microalbuminuria.

3 *Microalbuminuria:* as soon as this is detected it indicates progression of dis-ease, GFR may be raised or normal. This lasts another 5-10yrs.

4 *Nephropathy:* GFR begins to decline and proteinuria increases.

Patients with type 2 DM may present at the later stages having had undetected hyperglycaemia for many years before diagnosis. See p309 for treatment.

**Infection** Associated nephropathies are common causes of renal disease. *Glom-erulonephritis* occurs with many bacterial, viral and parasitic infections, including post-streptococcal, hepatitis B or C, HIV, SBE/IE, shunt nephritis, visceral abscess, syphilis, malaria, schistosomiasis and filiariasis. *Vasculitis* (p558) may occur with hepatitis B or C, post-streptococcal or staphylococcal septicaemia. *Interstitial ne-phritis:* Seen with bacterial pyelonephritis, viral (CMV, HIV, hepatitis B, hantavirus), fungal and parasitic (leishmaniasis, toxoplasmosis) infections.

**Malignancy** *Direct effects:* Renal infiltration (leukaemia, lymphoma), obstruction (pelvic tumours), metastases. *Indirect:* Hypercalcaemia, nephrotic syndrome, acute renal failure, amyloidosis, glomerulonephritis. *Treatment associated:* Nephrotoxic drugs, tumour lysis syndrome, radiation nephritis.

**Myeloma** (p362) is characterized by excess production of monoclonal antibody ± light chains, which are excreted and detected in ⅔ of cases as Bence Jones proteinu-ria. Myeloma kidney is due to blockage of tubules by casts, consisting of light chains. The light chains have a direct toxic effect on tubular cells, causing acute tubular necrosis. *Features:* AKI, CKD, amyloidosis (may cause proteinuria and nephrotic syn-drome), hypercalcaemic nephropathy. *Treatment:* Ensure fluid intake of 3L/day to prevent further impairment. Dialysis may be required in AKI. It might be possible to remove light chains by plasma exchange using special filters.

**Rheumatological diseases** *Rheumatoid arthritis (RA)* NSAIDs may cause inter-stitial nephritis. Penicillamine and gold can cause membranous nephropathy. AA amyloidosis (p364) occurs in ~15% of RA (often asymptomatic). *SLE* involves the glom-erulus in 40-60% of adults, causing acute or chronic disease. Proteinuria and ↑BP are common. Histological patterns range from minimal change to crescentic GN. Con-sider a renal biopsy if blood/protein on urine dipstick or deteriorating renal function. ℞: ACE-i if proteinuria. Corticosteroids and immunosuppressants (cyclophosphamide or mycophenolate) are used if biopsy shows aggressive glomerulonephritis (p556). *Systemic sclerosis* (p554) may affect the kidney, especially in diffuse disease. 'Renal crisis' presents with AKI + accelerated hypertension. ℞: ACE-i if ↑BP or in renal crisis. Di-alysis or transplant may be required. ANCA associated vasculitis (AAV) often involves the kidney and can cause ESRF; see p558.

**Hyperparathyroidism** Clinical features are from hypercalcaemia: p306.

**Sarcoidosis** may involve the kidney, often by abnormal calcium metabolism (p186). Interstitial nephritis and rarely glomerulonephritis are also associated.

Mostly we commute to work each day driven by motives we would rather not look at too deeply. But one renal physician used a red canoe to commute each day from his houseboat to the hospital. He could have been a very rich man but instead Belding Scribner gave his invention away, and continued his modest existence. He invented the Scribner shunt—a U of teflon connecting an artery to a vein, so allowing haemodialysis to be something that could be repeated as often as needed. Before Scribner, glass tubes had to be painfully inserted into blood vessels, which would be damaged by the procedure so that haemodialysis could only be done for a few cycles. Clyde Shields was his first patient with end-stage renal failure to receive the shunt—on 9 March 1960—and said that his first treatment 'took so much of the waste I'd stored up out of me that it was just like turning on the light from darkness'.[59] Scribner took something that was 100% fatal and overnight turned it into a condition with a 90% survival. In so doing he laid the foundations for a branch of bioethics because not everyone could have the treatment immediately. This is the branch of ethics that is to do with who gets what—ie distributive justice. In Scribner's day, this was decided by the famous 'Life and Death Committee' which had the unenviable job of choosing who would survive by placing people in order of precedence.

Scribner has said that his inventions sprang from his empathy for patients, including himself. 'I was a sickly child' he said, and at various times he needed a heart-lung machine, a new hip, and donated corneas. He was the sort of man whose patients would inspire him to worry away at their problems during the day—and then to awake at night with a brilliant solution.

On 19 June 2003, his canoe was found afloat but empty—and like those ancient Indian burial canoes found at Wiskam which have been polished to an unimaginable lustre by the action of the shifting sands around the Island of the Dead, so we polish and cherish the image of this man who gave everything away to help others.

## Contents

Fig 1. Here we see Los, the first haematologist, working naked, alone, and at night, hammering a red cell into shape, in his Laboratory of the Imagination. ☼"For every space larger than a red globule of Man's blood is visionary, and is created by the Hammer of Los: and every Space smaller than a Globule of Man's blood opens into Eternity."[1] When we ourselves are working alone and at night, hammering away at some difficult problem, we all need a Haematologist to show us how to move effortlessly from the macro to the micro, and from reductionist to integrative world views.

Image from the *Song of Los*, William Blake.

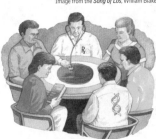

Fig 2. The new methodology: teamwork in action, as haematologist, geneticist, and lab staff deal with a troublesome spherocyte. ×3000

**Topics elsewhere:** Haemolytic uraemic syndrome (p308); normal values (p769).

**Read this!** D Nathan *Genes, Blood, and Courage*. <sup>Harvard University Press</sup> Dayem Saif, a 6-year-old with a stature of a 2-year-old, has an Hb of 1.5g/L—as low as his chance of survival with thalassaemia. This story about lab medicine and its stormy application at the bedside is *so* worth reading when feeling hemmed in by difficult patients, for it shows that there are no difficult patients, only difficult times. The book portrays the vital nature of the doctor-patient relationship, and warns us against labelling people—unless the label is a poem: Dayem Saif is Arabic for *Immortal Sword*.

*We thank our Specialist Reader Dr Drew Provan, and our Junior Reader Sarah Hickin, for their contribution to this chapter.*

## On the taking of blood and of holidays

This is not one of those pages about how you should be kind to the patient, explain in full what you are about to do, talk him or her through venepuncture, label the bottles carefully, and make a plan for communicating the results. Be all this as it may, there is something else that needs communicating about the *act* of taking blood. It is partly to do with the fact that as blood is life, and, because, as Ruskin taught us, 'there is no wealth but life', we are led to the conclusion that what is special about taking blood is that for once *we* are being given something valuable by the patient. What is this wealth? The answer is *time*. For while the blood is flowing into our tube we cannot be disturbed. We are excused from answering our bleeps, and from making polite conversation (a few grunts in reply to patients' enquires about the colour of their blood is quite sufficient)—and we can indulge in that almost unimaginable luxury, at least as far as life on the wards is concerned, of *reflecting on our own thoughts*. Accepting this sacred time as a sort of hypnotic holiday is excellent. For however many nights we have been awoken, and through however many wards we have traipsed to this bedside, this little holiday will be worth an hour's sleep—if our mind is furnished and ready to empty itself of all objectivity.

The best and most watched-for sight during venepuncture is when a chance characteristic of flow sets the jet of blood streaming into our tube into countless bouncing globules. Before coalescing again, these globules jostle together like the overcrowded chain of events that led us to this bedside. During this time, allow your own thoughts to coalesce into a more peaceful order if you can, and let William Blake help you banish objectivity, for he knew some truths about haematology unknown to strictly rational practitioners of this art:

> The Microscope knows not of this nor the Telescope: they alter
> The ratio of the Spectator's Organs but leave Objects untouch'd
> For every space larger than a red globule of Man's blood
> Is visionary, and is created by the Hammer of Los:[1]
> And every Space smaller than a Globule of Man's blood opens
> Into Eternity of which this vegetable Earth is but a shadow.
> The red Globule is the unwearied Sun by Los created
> To measure Time and Space to mortal Men ...

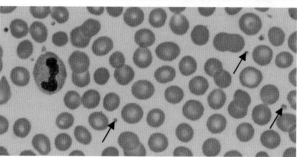

**Fig 3.** A blood film, with a neutrophil, normal red cells, and platelets (arrows).
©Prof. K Lewandowski & Dr H Jastrow.

**1** Los, the *globe of fire*, is a symbol used by Blake to encompass the exultant energy of creation, the poetic imagination, and the burning brightness where all his noble images were pounded out of eternity and compounded into the most compressed verse and art we have (*see* P Ackroyd 1996 *Blake*, Minerva). These lines are from his poem *Milton*, section 29, lines 17-24, page 516 in OUP's *Blake: Complete Writings*, edited (1925-1969) by Geoffrey Keynes, the surgeon, who, incidentally, led the way to lumpectomy for breast cancer, in preference to the much-hated radical mastectomy.

Anaemia is defined as a low haemoglobin (Hb) concentration, and may be due either to a low red cell mass or increased plasma volume (eg in pregnancy). A low Hb (at sea level) is <135g/L for men and <115g/L for women. Anaemia may be due to reduced production or increased loss of RBCs and has many causes. These will often be distinguishable by history, examination, and inspection of the blood film.

**Symptoms** Due to the underlying cause or to the anaemia itself: fatigue, dyspnoea, faintness, palpitations, headache, tinnitus, anorexia—and angina if there is pre-existing coronary artery disease.

**Signs** May be absent even in severe anaemia. There may be pallor (eg conjunctivae, although this is not a reliable sign; see fig 1). In severe anaemia (Hb <80g/L), there may be signs of a hyperdynamic circulation, eg tachycardia, flow murmurs (ejection-systolic loudest over apex), and cardiac enlargement; or retinal haemorrhages (rarely). Later, heart failure may occur: here, rapid blood transfusion may be fatal.

**Types of anaemia** The first step in diagnosis is to look at the mean cell volume (MCV, *normal* MCV is 76–96 femtolitres, $10^{15}$ fL = 1L).

*Low MCV—microcytic anaemia* (correlates with mean cell Hb ≤27 picograms).
1 Iron-deficiency anaemia (IDA, most common cause): p320.
2 Thalassaemia (suspect if the MCV is 'too low' for the Hb level and the red cell count is ↑). Definitive diagnosis needs DNA analysis, although finding a normal $Hb_{A2}$ with normal ferritin in a very microcytic picture is suggestive of possible alpha thalassaemia trait. See p336.
3 Sideroblastic anaemia (very rare): p320.

**NB:** the last two are conditions where there is an accumulation of iron, and so tests will show serum iron↑, ferritin↑, and a low total iron-binding capacity (TIBC).

*Normal MCV (normocytic anaemia)*

| | |
|---|---|
| 1 Acute blood loss | 5 Hypothyroidism (or ↑MCV) |
| 2 Anaemia of chronic disease (or ↓MCV) | 6 Haemolysis (or ↑MCV) |
| 3 Bone marrow failure | 7 Pregnancy |
| 4 Renal failure | |

If wcc↓ or platelet↓, suspect marrow failure: see p358.

*High MCV (macrocytic anaemia)*

| | |
|---|---|
| 1 $B_{12}$ or folate deficiency | 5 Myelodysplastic syndromes |
| 2 Alcohol excess—or liver disease | 6 Marrow infiltration |
| 3 Reticulocytosis (p322, eg with haemolysis) | 7 Hypothyroidism |
| 4 Cytotoxics, eg hydroxycarbamide | 8 Antifolate drugs (eg phenytoin) |

*Haemolytic anaemias* do not fit into the above classification as the anaemia may be normocytic or, if there are many young (hence larger) RBCs and reticulocytes, macrocytic (p330). Suspect if there is a reticulocytosis (>2% of RBCs; or reticulocyte count >100×10⁹/L), mild macrocytosis, haptoglobin↓, bilirubin↑ and urobilinogen↑. Often mild jaundice (but no bilirubin in urine as haemolysis causes pre-hepatic jaundice).

**Does he need a blood transfusion?** Usually No!—unless there is severe acute anaemia (one review suggests that transfusion is not essential for *most* patients unless Hb <70g/L). If there is an acute cause (eg haemorrhage with active peptic ulcer), transfusion up to 80g/L is sometimes needed. Chronic anaemia is better tolerated, and it is important to ascertain the cause, eg in iron-deficiency anaemia, iron supplements will raise the haemoglobin in a safer and less costly way.

In severe anaemia with heart failure, transfusion is vital to restore Hb to a safe level, eg 60–80g/L, but must be done with great care. Give packed cells *slowly* with 10–40mg furosemide IV/PO with alternate units (dose depends on previous exposure to diuretics; do not mix with blood). Check for rising JVP and basal crackles. If CCF gets worse, stop and treat. If immediate transfusion is essential, a 2-3 unit exchange transfusion can be tried, removing blood at the same rate as it is transfused (get help).

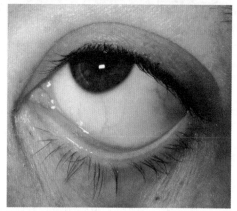

Fig 1. 'Conjunctival pallor', *the* classic sign of anaemia, is a confusing term as the conjunctiva is translucent, transmitting the colour of structures under it. The 'pallor' refers to the vasculature on the inner surface of the lid which is lacking Hb.

It is this colour  but it should be:

## Red cell distribution width (RCDW or RDW)

If all the red cells in a sample are about the same size, the graph of their volumes is narrow, as occurs in health. But in mixed anaemias the graph is broad, and an abnormal RCDW may be the first hint of such an anaemia. In coeliac disease, for example, poor absorption of iron (MCV↓) *and* folate (MCV↑) may occur, with microcytes and macrocytes circulating simultaneously, so the RCDW is raised. Anisocytosis (p322) is the visual analogue of this. RCDW = the standard deviation of MCV divided by the mean MCV, multiplied by 100. Reference interval: 11.5-14.6%. If the MCV is high and the RCDW is *normal*, the cause is likely to be alcohol, liver disease or a marrow problem (chemotherapy or aplastic anaemia).

This is common (seen in up to 14% of menstruating women).

*Causes:* •Blood loss, eg menorrhagia or GI bleeding[1] (upper p252; lower p631).
• Poor diet may cause IDA in babies or children (but rarely in adults), those on special diets, or wherever there is poverty.
• Malabsorption (eg coeliac disease) is a cause of refractory IDA.
• In the Tropics, hookworm (GI blood loss) is the most common cause.

*Signs:* Chronic IDA (signs now rare): koilonychia (fig 1 and p32), atrophic glossitis, angular cheilosis (fig 2), and, rarely, post-cricoid webs (Plummer-Vinson syndrome).

*Tests:* Microcytic, hypochromic anaemia with anisocytosis and poikilocytosis (figs 3 & 4). ↓MCV, ↓MCH and ↓MCHC. Confirmed by ferritin↓ (also serum iron↓ with ↑total iron-binding capacity—TIBC, but these are less reliable). ↑Red cell protoporphyrin. NB: ferritin is an acute phase protein and ↑ with inflammation, eg infection, malignancy. Serum transferrin receptors are also ↑ in IDA but are less affected by inflammation. If MCV↓, and good history of menorrhagia, oral iron may be started without further tests. Otherwise investigate for GI blood loss: gastroscopy, sigmoidoscopy, barium enema or colonoscopy, stool microscopy for ova if hookworm, etc. is a possibility. Faecal occult blood is not recommended as sensitivity is poor.
► *Iron deficiency with no obvious source of bleeding mandates careful GI workup.*[1]

*Treatment:* Treat the cause. Oral iron, eg ferrous sulfate 200mg/8h PO. SE: nausea, abdominal discomfort, diarrhoea or constipation, black stools. Hb should rise by 10g/L/week, with a modest reticulocytosis (ie young RBC, p322). Continue until Hb is normal and for at least 3 months, to replenish stores. Intravenous iron is almost never needed, but may be indicated if the oral route is impossible or ineffective, eg functional iron deficiency in chronic renal failure, where there is inadequate mobilization of iron stores in response to the acute demands of erythropoietin therapy.

The usual reason that IDA fails to respond to iron replacement is that the patient has rejected the pills. Negotiate on concordance issues (p3). Is the reason for the problem GI disturbance? Altering the dose of elemental iron with a different preparation may help. There may be continued blood loss, malabsorption, anaemia of chronic disease; or there is misdiagnosis, eg when thalassaemia is to blame.

## The anaemia of chronic disease (secondary anaemia)

It is the commonest anaemia in hospital patients (the 2^nd commonest anaemia, after IDA, worldwide).[3] *3 problems* (in which the polypeptide, hepcidin, plays a key role): 1 Poor use of iron in erythropoiesis 2 Cytokine-induced shortening of RBC survival 3 ↓Production of and response to erythropoietin.

*Causes:* Many, eg chronic infection, vasculitis, rheumatoid, malignancy, renal failure.
*Tests:* Mild normocytic anaemia (eg Hb >80g/L), ferritin normal or ↑. Do blood film, B_{12}, folate, TSH and tests for haemolysis (p330) as anaemia is often multifactorial.[4]
*Treatment:* Treating the underlying disease more vigorously may help (eg in 60% of patients with RA). Erythropoietin (p296) is effective in raising the haemoglobin level (SE: flu-like symptoms, hypertension, mild rise in the platelet count and thromboembolism). It is also effective in raising Hb and improving quality of life in those with malignant disease.[5] Iron given parenterally can safely overcome the functional iron deficiency. Inhibitors of hepcidin and inflammatory modulators show promise.[6]

## Sideroblastic anaemia

Microcytic anaemia does not equal iron deficiency! 20% of older people with an MCV <75fL are not iron deficient. ►*Think of sideroblastic anaemia whenever a microcytic anaemia is not responding to iron.*[7] Do a ferritin; look at a film (hypochromia) and a marrow (figs 5 & 6) to look for disease defining sideroblasts. ℞: Remove the cause. Pyridoxine may help ± repeated transfusion for severe anaemia.

---

1 In one study, 11% presenting to their GP with IDA had GI carcinoma.[2] Consider both upper and lower GI investigation as in another study, 29% (n=89) had abnormalities on both.[3]

## Interpreting plasma iron studies

|  | Iron | TIBC | Ferritin |
|---|---|---|---|
| Iron deficiency | ↓ | ↑ | ↓ |
| Anaemia of chronic disease | ↓ | ↓ | ↑ |
| Chronic haemolysis | ↑ | ↓ | ↑ |
| Haemochromatosis | ↑ | ↓ (or ↔) | ↑ |
| Pregnancy | ↑ | ↑ | ↔ |
| Sideroblastic anaemia | ↑ | ↔ | ↑ |

TIBC: total iron binding capacity.

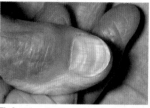

**Fig 1.** Koilonychia. Spoon-shaped nails, found in iron-deficiency anaemia.

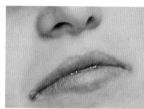

**Fig 2.** Angular cheilosis, ulceration at the side of the mouth, in iron deficiency. Also a feature of vitamin $B_{12}$ and $B_2$ (riboflavin) deficiency, and glucagonoma (p215). Courtesy of Dr Joseph Thompson: AskAnOrthodontist.com.

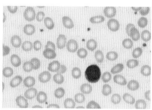

**Fig 3.** Microcytic hypochromic cells in iron-deficiency anaemia.

Courtesy of Prof. Krzysztof Lewandowski.

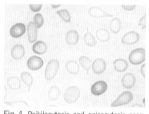

**Fig 4.** Poikilocytosis and anisocytosis seen, eg, in iron-deficiency anaemia.

Courtesy of Prof. Christine Lawrence (figs 4 & 5).

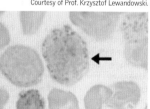

**Fig 5.** Ring sideroblasts in the marrow, with a perinuclear ring of iron granules, found in sideroblastic anaemia. It is characterized by ineffective erythropoiesis, leading to ↑iron absorption, iron loading in marrow ± haemosiderosis (endocrine, liver and heart damage due to iron deposition). It may be congenital (rare, x-linked) or acquired, eg idiopathic as one of the myelodysplastic/myeloproliferative diseases, but it can follow chemotherapy, anti-TB drugs, irradiation, alcohol or lead excess.

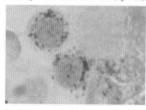

**Fig 6.** Two ringed sideroblasts showing how the distribution of what we take to be perinuclear mitochondrial ferritin can vary.[10] The problem in congenital sideroblastic anaemia is disordered mitochondrial haem synthesis, >15% marrow ring sideroblasts and <5% blasts is required for a diagnosis of refractory anaemia with ring sideroblasts/sideroblastic anaemia.[11]

Courtesy of Prof. Tangün and Dr Köroğlu.

▶Many haematological (and other) diagnoses are made by careful examination of the peripheral blood film. It is also necessary for interpretation of the FBC indices.

*Anisocytosis* is variation in RBC size, eg megaloblastic anaemia, thalassaemia, IDA.

*Acanthocytes:* (fig 1) Spicules on RBCs (∵ unstable RBC membrane lipid structure); causes: splenectomy; alcoholic liver disease; abetalipoproteinaemia; spherocytosis.

*Basophilic RBC stippling:* (fig 2) Denatured RNA found in RBCs, indicating accelerated erythropoiesis or defective Hb synthesis. Seen in lead poisoning, megaloblastic anaemia, myelodysplasia, liver disease, haemoglobinopathy, eg thalassaemia.

*Blasts:* Nucleated precursor cells. They are not normally in peripheral blood, but are seen in myelofibrosis, leukaemia and malignant infiltration by carcinoma.

*Burr cells (echinocytes):* RBC projections (less marked than in acanthocytes); fig 3.

*Cabot rings:* Seen in: pernicious anaemia; lead poisoning; bad infections (fig 9).[12]

*Dimorphic picture:* Two populations of red cells. Seen after treatment of Fe, B12, or folate deficiency, in mixed deficiency (↓Fe with ↓B12 or folate), post-transfusion, or with primary sideroblastic anaemia, where a clone of abnormal erythroblasts produce abnormal red cells, alongside normal red cell production.

*Howell-Jolly bodies:* DNA nuclear remnants in RBCs, which are normally removed by the spleen (fig 8). Seen post-splenectomy and in hyposplenism (eg sickle-cell disease, coeliac disease, congenital, UC/Crohn's, myeloproliferative disease, amyloid). Also in dyserythopoietic states: myelodysplasia, megaloblastic anaemia.

*Hypochromia:* (p320). Less dense staining of RBCs due to ↓Hb synthesis, seen in IDA, thalassaemia, and sideroblastic anaemia (iron stores unusable, p320).

*Left shift:* Immature neutrophils are sent out of the marrow, eg in infection, p325.

*Leukoerythroblastic film:* Immature cells (myelocytes, promyelocytes, metamyelocytes, normoblasts) ± tear-drop RBCs from marrow infiltration/infection (malignancy; TB; brucella; visceral leishmaniasis;[13] parvovirus B19)—or in UC[14] or haemolysis.

*Leukaemoid reaction:* A marked leucocytosis (WCC >50×10⁹/L). Seen in severe illness, eg with infection or burns, and also in leukaemia.

*Pappenheimer bodies:* (fig 5) Granules of siderocytes containing iron. Seen in lead poisoning, carcinomatosis, and post-splenectomy.

*Poikilocytosis* is variation in RBC shape, eg in IDA, myelofibrosis, thalassaemia.

*Polychromasia:* RBCs of different ages stain unevenly (young are bluer). This is a response to bleeding, haematinic replacement (ferrous sulfate, B12, folate), haemolysis, or marrow infiltration. Reticulocyte count is raised.

*Reticulocytes:* (normal range: 0.8–2%; or <85×10⁹/L) (fig 6). Young, larger RBCs (contain RNA) signifying active erythropoiesis. Increased in haemolysis, haemorrhage, and if B12, iron or folate is given to marrow that lack these.

*Right shift:* Hypermature white cells: hypersegmented polymorphs (>5 lobes to nucleus) seen in megaloblastic anaemia, uraemia, and liver disease. See p326, fig 1.

*Rouleaux formation:* (fig 7) Red cells stack on each other (it causes a raised ESR; p366). Seen with chronic inflammation,[16] paraproteinaemia and myeloma.

*Spherocytes:* Spherical cells found in hereditary spherocytosis and autoimmune haemolytic anaemia. See p332.

*Schistocytes:* Fragmented RBCs sliced by fibrin bands, in intravascular haemolysis (p332, fig 4). Look for microangiopathic anaemia, eg DIC (p346), haemolytic uraemic syndrome, thrombotic thrombocytopenic purpura (TTP; p308), or pre-eclampsia.

*Target cells:* (also known as Mexican hat cells, fig 8 and fig 3, p337) These are RBCs with central staining, a ring of pallor, and an outer rim of staining seen in liver disease, hyposplenism, thalassaemia—and, in small numbers, in IDA.

*Tear-drop RBCs:* Seen in extramedullary haemopoiesis; see leukoerythroblastic film.

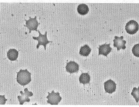

Fig 1. Acanthocytosis.

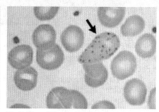

Fig 2. Basophilic stippling.

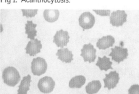

Fig 3. Burr cells: the cause may be renal or liver failure, or an EDTA storage artefact.

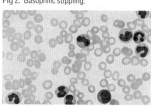

Fig 4. Left shift: presence of immature neutrophils in the blood. See p322.

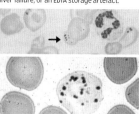

Fig 5. Pappenheimer bodies.

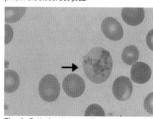

Fig 6. Reticulocytes. RNA in RBCs; supravital staining (azure B; cresyl blue) is needed.

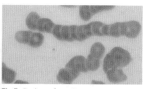

Fig 7. Rouleaux formation.

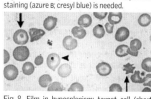

Fig 8. Film in hyposplenism: target cell (short arrow), acanthocyte (long arrow) and a Howell-Jolly body (arrow head).

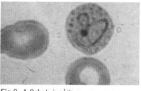

Fig 9. A Cabot ring.[1][15]

Figs 1, 6 & 7 ©Dr N Medeiros; figs 2 & 8 ©Prof. Barbara Bain & Massachusetts Medical Society; figs 3 & 5 (top) ©Prof. Christine Lawrence; fig 4 ©Prof. Krzysztof Lewandowski; figs 5 (bottom) & 9 ©Crookston Collection.

**1** Cabot 'figure-of-eight' rings may be microtubules from mitotic spindles. It is easy to confuse them with malaria parasites, p385 (especially if stippling gives a 'chromatin dot' artefact, as here).
Richard Clarke Cabot (1868–1939) liked diagnostic challenges: it was he who founded the dastardly hard but beautifully presented weekly clinicopathological exercises of the Massachusetts General Hospital which have made the *New England Journal of Medicine* so famous among discerning clinical detectives.
You may forget all about his rings—but not his aphorisms—for example: ►*"Before you tell the truth to the patient, be sure you know the truth, and that the patient wants to hear it."*[15]

Haematology

**Neutrophils** (figs 1 & 6) $2-7.5 \times 10^9$/L (40–75% of white blood cells: but absolute values are more meaningful than percentages).

*Increased in* (ie *neutrophilia*):
• Bacterial infections.
• Inflammation, eg myocardial infarction, polyarteritis nodosa.
• Myeloproliferative disorders.
• Drugs (steroids).
• Disseminated malignancy.
• Stress, eg trauma, surgery, burns, haemorrhage, seizure.

*Decreased in* (ie *neutropenia*—see p346)
• Viral infections.
• Drugs, eg post chemotherapy, cytotoxic agents, carbimazole, sulfonamides.
• Severe sepsis.
• Neutrophil antibodies (SLE, haemolytic anaemia)—↑ destruction.
• Hypersplenism (p367), eg Felty's syndrome (p712).
• Bone marrow failure—↓ production (p358).

**Lymphocytes** (fig 2) $1.5-4.5 \times 10^9$/L (20–45%).

*Increased in* (ie *lymphocytosis*):
• Acute viral infections.
• Chronic infections, eg TB, *Brucella*, hepatitis, syphilis.
• Leukaemias and lymphomas, especially chronic lymphocytic leukaemia.

Large numbers of abnormal ('atypical') lymphocytes are characteristically seen with EBV infection: these are T cells reacting against EBV-infected B cells. They have a large amount of clearish cytoplasm with a blue rim that flows around neighbouring RBCs. See fig 1, p401. Other causes of 'atypical' lymphocytes: see p401.

*Decreased in* (ie *lymphopenia*):
• Steroid therapy; SLE; uraemia; Legionnaire's disease; HIV infection; marrow infiltration; post chemotherapy or radiotherapy.

T-lymphocyte subset reference values: CD4 count: 537-1571/mm³ (low in HIV infection). CD8 count: 235-753/mm³; CD4/CD8 ratio: 1.2-3.8.

**Eosinophils** (fig 3) $0.04-0.4 \times 10^9$/L (1–6%).[17]

*Increased in* (ie *eosinophilia*):
• Drug reactions, eg with erythema multiforme, p564.
• Allergies: asthma, atopy.
• Parasitic infections (especially invasive helminths).
• Skin disease: especially pemphigus, eczema, psoriasis, dermatitis herpetiformis.

Also seen in malignant disease (including lymphomas and eosinophilic leukaemia), PAN, adrenal insufficiency,[18] irradiation, Löffler's syndrome (p718), and during the convalescent phase of any infection.

*The hypereosinophilic syndrome (HES)* is a severe disease of unknown cause, in which an ↑ eosinophil count (>$1.5 \times 10^9$/L for >6 weeks) leads to end-organ damage (endomyocardial fibrosis/restrictive cardiomyopathy, skin lesions, thromboembolic disease, lung disease, neuropathy, and hepatosplenomegaly). $R$: Oral steroids ± mepolizumab (an anti-interleukin-5 monoclonal antibody). If FIP1L1-PDFRA genotype, diagnose myeloproliferative HES/eosinophilic leukaemia (imatinib is 1st choice).[19]

**Monocytes** (fig 4) $0.2-0.8 \times 10^9$/L (2–10%). *Increased in* (ie *monocytosis*): Post chemo- or radiotherapy, chronic infections (eg malaria, TB, brucellosis, protozoa), malignant disease (including M4 and M5 acute myeloid leukaemia (p350), and Hodgkin's disease), myelodysplasia.

**Basophils** (fig 5) $0-0.1 \times 10^9$/L (0–1%). *Increased in* (ie *basophilia*): myeloproliferative disease, viral infections, IgE-mediated hypersensitivity reactions (eg urticaria, hypothyroidism), and inflammatory disorders (eg UC, rheumatoid arthritis).

Haematology

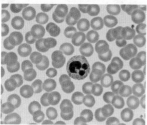

Fig 1. Neutrophil. These ingest and kill bacteria, fungi and damaged cells.

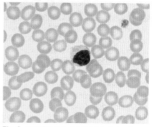

Fig 2. Lymphocyte: divided into T & B types, which have important roles in cell-mediated immunity & antibody production.

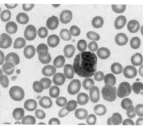

Fig 3. Eosinophil: these mediate allergic reactions and defend against parasites.

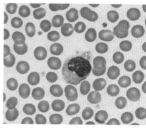

Fig 4. Monocyte: precursors of tissue macrophages.

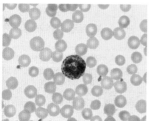

Fig 5. Basophil. The cytoplasm is filled with dark staining granules, containing histamine, myeloperoxidase and other enzymes. On binding IgE, histamine is released from the basophil.

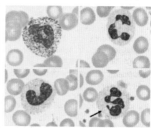

Fig 6. Variations on a neutrophil theme. Top left: 'toxic granulation': ie a neutrophil with coarse, deeply-staining granules (compare with the neutrophil to its right). This is a response to pregnancy or infection. Other neutrophil responses to infection include:
- Left shift: immature neutrophils are released with few lobes to their nuclei. A 'band form' has no lobes and may be shaped like a horseshoe (bottom left).
- Vacuoles in the cytoplasm (the most specific sign of bacterial infection).
- Döhle bodies: inconspicuous grey-blue areas of cytoplasm (residual ribosomes).

Up to 17% of neutrophils from females show a drumstick-shaped Barr body (arrow). It is the inactivated X chromosome.

Figs 1-5 courtesy of Prof. Krzysztof Lewandowski; Fig 6 courtesy of Prof. Tangün and Dr Köroğlu.

Macrocytosis (MCV >96fL) is common, often due to alcohol excess without any accompanying anaemia. Although only ~5% are due to $B_{12}$ deficiency, pernicious anaemia is the most common cause of a macrocytic anaemia in Western countries. $B_{12}$ and folate deficiency are megaloblastic anaemias. A megaloblast is a cell in which nuclear maturation is delayed compared with the cytoplasm. This occurs with $B_{12}$ and folate deficiency, as they are both required for DNA synthesis.

**Causes of macrocytosis**
• *Megaloblastic:* (fig 1) $B_{12}$ deficiency, folate deficiency, cytotoxic drugs.
• *Non-megaloblastic:* Alcohol, reticulocytosis (eg in haemolysis), liver disease, hypothyroidism, pregnancy.
• *Other haematological disease:* Myelodysplasia (fig 2), myeloma, myeloproliferative disorders, aplastic anaemia.

**Tests:** $B_{12}$ and folate deficiency result in similar blood film and bone marrow biopsy appearances.
*Blood film:* Hypersegmented polymorphs (fig 1) in $B_{12}$ and folate deficiency (target cells if liver disease; see fig 8, p323 and fig 3, p337).
*Other tests:* LFT (include γGT), TFT, serum $B_{12}$ and serum folate (or red cell folate—a more reliable indicator of folate status, as serum folate only reflects *recent* intake).
*Bone marrow biopsy* is indicated if the cause is not revealed by the above tests. It is likely to show one of the following 4 states:
  1 Megaloblastic.
  2 Normoblastic marrow (eg in liver disease, hypothyroidism).
  3 Abnormal erythropoiesis (eg sideroblastic anaemia, p320, leukaemia, aplasia).
  4 Increased erythropoiesis (eg haemolysis).

**Folate** is found in green vegetables, nuts, yeast and liver; it is synthesized by gut bacteria. Body stores can last for 4 months. Maternal folate deficiency causes fetal neural tube defects. It is absorbed by duodenum/proximal jejunum. *Causes of deficiency:*
• Poor diet, eg poverty, alcoholics, elderly.
• Increased demand, eg pregnancy or ↑cell turnover (seen in haemolysis, malignancy, inflammatory disease and renal dialysis).
• Malabsorption, eg coeliac disease, tropical sprue.
• Drugs, alcohol, anti-epileptics (phenytoin, valproate), methotrexate, trimethoprim.

*Treatment:* Assess for an underlying cause, eg poor diet, malabsorption. Treat with folic acid 5mg/day PO for 4 months, ►never without $B_{12}$ unless the patient is known to have a normal $B_{12}$ level, as in low $B_{12}$ states it may precipitate, or worsen, subacute combined degeneration of the cord (p328). In pregnancy prophylactic doses of folate (400µg/day) are given from conception until at least 12wks; this helps prevent spina bifida, as well as anaemia. NB: if ill (eg CCF) with megaloblastic anaemia, it may be necessary to treat before serum $B_{12}$ and folate results are known. Do tests then treat with large doses of hydroxocobalamin, eg 1mg/48h IM—see *BNF*, with folic acid 5mg/24h PO. Blood transfusions are very rarely needed, but see p318.

**Folate and ischaemic heart disease** Previous observational studies have indicated that higher homocysteine concentrations are associated with a greater risk of coronary heart disease. It has been suggested that folic acid supplementation may have a role in prevention of cardiac disease by lowering homocysteine levels. However, trials are disappointing (further studies awaited).[20] One meta-analysis also showed no causal relationship between high homocysteine concentrations and coronary heart disease risk in Western populations.[21]

**Folate and cognition** If borderline folate deficiency (as shown by ↑homocysteine), 800µg folic acid/d for 3yrs has been found to benefit cognition.[22] The FACIT trial 2007

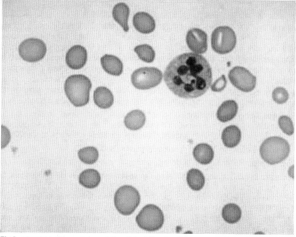

**Fig 1.** Megaloblastic anaemia: peripheral blood film showing many macrocytes and one hyper-segmented neutrophil (normally there should be ≤5 segments).

Courtesy of Professor Barbara Bain © 2005 Massachusetts Medical Society.

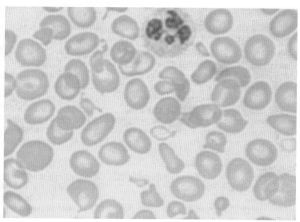

**Fig 2.** Oval macrocytes seen here in myelodysplastic syndromes. Note aniso- and poikilocytosis with small fragmented cells (schistocytes). NB: B12 and folate deficiencies also cause oval macro-cytes, but macrocytes caused by alcohol and liver disease are usually round.

Courtesy of Prof. Tangün and Dr Köroğlu.

Vitamin B12 is found in meat, fish, and dairy products, but not in plants. Body stores are sufficient for 4yrs. It is protein-bound and released during digestion. B12 then binds to intrinsic factor in the stomach, and this complex is absorbed in the terminal ileum. In B12 deficiency, synthesis of thymidine, and hence DNA, is impaired, so RBC production is slow. *Causes of deficiency:* •Dietary (eg vegans) •Malabsorption: *stomach* (lack of intrinsic factor): pernicious anaemia, post gastrectomy; *terminal ileum:* ileal resection, Crohn's disease, bacterial overgrowth, tropical sprue, tapeworms (*diphyllobothrium*) •Congenital metabolic errors.

**Features** *General:* Symptoms of anaemia (p318), 'lemon tinge' to skin due to combination of pallor (anaemia) and mild jaundice (due to haemolysis), glossitis (beefy-red sore tongue; fig 1), angular cheilosis (also known as stomatitis, p320).

*Neuropsychiatric:* Irritability, depression, psychosis, dementia.

*Neurological:* Paraesthesiae, peripheral neuropathy. Also:

*Subacute combined degeneration of the spinal cord:* Onset is insidious (*subacute*) with peripheral neuropathy due to ↓B12. There is a *combination* of symmetrical posterior (dorsal) column loss, causing sensory and LMN signs, and symmetrical corticospinal tract loss, causing motor and UMN signs (p450). Joint-position and vibration sense are often affected first leading to ataxia, followed by stiffness and weakness if untreated. The classical triad is: •Extensor plantars (UMN) •Absent knee jerks (LMN) •Absent ankle jerks (LMN). It may present with falls at night-time, due to a combination of ataxia and reduced vision, which is also seen with ↓B12. Pain and temperature sensation may remain intact even in severe cases, as the spinothalamic tracts are preserved. ▸Neurological signs of B12 deficiency can occur without anaemia.

**Pernicious anaemia** (PA) This is caused by an autoimmune atrophic gastritis, leading to achlorhydria and lack of gastric intrinsic factor secretion.

**Incidence** 1:1000; ♀:♂≈1.6:1; usually >40yrs; higher incidence if blood group A.

**Associations** Other autoimmune diseases (p555): thyroid disease (~25%), vitiligo, Addison's disease, hypoparathyroidism. Carcinoma of stomach is ~3-fold more common in pernicious anaemia, so have a low threshold for upper GI endoscopy.

**Tests** •Hb↓ (30–110g/L) •MCV↑ •WCC and platelets ↓ if severe •Serum B12↓[1] •Reticulocytes ↓ or normal as production impaired •Hypersegmented polymorphs (p326) •Megaloblasts in the marrow •Specific tests for PA: 1 Parietal cell antibodies: found in 90% with PA, but also in 3–10% without. 2 Intrinsic factor (IF) antibodies: specific for pernicious anaemia, but lower sensitivity. These target B12 binding sites (in 50%) or bind binding sites (in 35%).

**Treatment** Treat the cause if possible. If a low B12 is due to malabsorption, injections are required. Replenish stores with hydroxocobalamin (B12) 1mg IM alternate days, eg for 2wks (or, if CNS signs, until improvement stops). Maintenance: 1mg IM every 3 months for life (child's dose: as for adult). If the cause is dietary, then oral B12 can be given after the initial acute course (see BOX). Initial improvement is heralded by a transient marked reticulocytosis and hence ↑MCV, after 4-5 days.

**Practical hints** •Beware of diagnosing PA in those under 40yrs old: look for GI malabsorption (small bowel biopsy, p280).

• Watch for hypokalaemia as treatment becomes established.

• Transfusion is best avoided, but PA with high output CCF may require exchange transfusion (p318), after doing tests for FBC, folate, B12, and marrow sampling.

• As haemopoiesis accelerates on treatment, additional iron may be needed.

• Hb rises ~10g/L per week; WCC and platelet count should normalize in 1wk.

**Prognosis** Supplementation usually improves peripheral neuropathy within the first 3-6 months, but has little effect on cord signs. Patients do best if treated as soon as possible after the onset of symptoms: don't delay!

1 Plasma B12 levels are normal in many patients with subclinical B12 deficiency. See BOX.

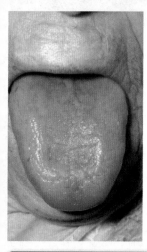

Fig 1. B12 deficiency glossitis; other causes: iron (or Zn) deficiency, pellagra, contact dermatitis/ specific food intolerances, Crohn's disease, drugs (minocycline, clarithromycin, some ACE-i). Glossitis may be the presenting feature of coeliac disease or alcoholism. Tongue TB: ulcers, fissure tuberculoma, or diffuse glossitis[23]

## When a low B12 is not due to pernicious anaemia

B12 deficiency is common, eg up to 15% of older people. If untreated, it can lead to megaloblastic anaemia and irreversible CNS complications. In the UK, the usual regimen is regular (eg 3-monthly) IM hydroxocobalamin (1mg). Elsewhere, *high-dose oral B12 regimen* (cyanocobalamin 1mg/day) is standard, less costly, and obviates the need for repeat visits to nurses. This use is not yet licensed in the UK[24] Passive absorption of B12 occurs throughout the gut—but only 1-2% of an oral dose is absorbed this (non-terminal ileum) way. The dietary reference range is ~2μg/d.

That a low B12 is not due to PA can usually be determined by serology testing for parietal cell and intrinsic factor antibodies (but -ve in 50% of those with PA), and plasma response to oral B12, and IM B12 if no response to oral doses. The oral dose may be given as cyanocobalamin 50-150μg/daily, between meals (in the NHS, mark the prescription 'SLS', p223, to justify/communicate this special indication). This *low-dose regimen* is often sufficient for B12 deficiency of dietary origin[25] NB: foods of non-animal origin contain no B12 unless fortified or contain bacteria. This information is important for vegans and their breastfed offspring.

*Non-dietary, non-autoimmune causes of a low B12:* Crohn's and coeliac disease; after gastric surgery; acid-suppressors (eg ranitidine); metformin; pancreatic insufficiency; false-low reading (seen in ≥20% so do 2 readings in isolated low B12). NB: normal serum B12 is documented in overt deficiency, which is confusing. Measuring holotranscobalamin and homocysteine or methylmalonic acid (↑ if B12 low) may be better, but have their own problems, and are non-standard tests.

NB: Schilling tests are not done as the radioisotope they use is not available.

Haemolysis is the premature breakdown of RBCs, before their normal lifespan of ~120d. It occurs in the circulation (*intravascular*) or in the reticuloendothelial system, ie macrophages of liver, spleen and bone marrow (*extravascular*). In sickle-cell anaemia, lifespan may be as short as 5d. Haemolysis may be asymptomatic, but if the bone marrow does not compensate sufficiently, a haemolytic anaemia results.

An approach is first to confirm haemolysis and then find the cause—try to answer these 4 questions:

**1** *Is there increased red cell breakdown?*
- ↑Anaemia with normal or ↑MCV.
- ↑Bilirubin: unconjugated, from haem breakdown (pre-hepatic jaundice).
- ↑Urinary urobilinogen (no urinary conjugated bilirubin).
- ↑Serum lactic dehydrogenase (LDH), as it is released from red cells.

**2** *Is there increased red cell production?*
- ↑Reticulocytes, causing ↑MCV (reticulocytes are large immature RBCs) and polychromasia.

**3** *Is the haemolysis mainly extra- or intravascular?*
Extravascular haemolysis may lead to splenic hypertrophy and splenomegaly. Features of intravascular haemolysis are:
- ↑Free plasma haemoglobin: released from RBCs.
- Methaemalbuminaemia: some free Hb is broken down in the circulation to produce haem and globin; haem combines with albumin to make methaemalbumin.
- ↓Plasma haptoglobin: mops up free plasma Hb, then removed by the liver.
- Haemoglobinuria: causes red-brown urine, in absence of red blood cells.
- Haemosiderinuria: occurs when haptoglobin-binding capacity is exceeded, causing free Hb to be filtered by the renal glomeruli, absorption of free Hb via the renal tubules and storage in the tubular cells as haemosiderin. This is detected in the urine in sloughed tubular cells by Prussian blue staining ~1 week after onset (implying a chronic intravascular haemolysis)

**4** *Why is there haemolysis?* Causes are on p332.

**History** Family history, race, jaundice, dark urine, drugs, previous anaemia, travel.

**Examination** Jaundice, hepatosplenomegaly, gallstones (pigmented, due to ↑bilirubin from haemolysis), leg ulcers (due to poor blood flow).

**Tests** FBC, reticulocytes, bilirubin, LDH, haptoglobin, urinary urobilinogen. Thick and thin films for malaria screen if history of travel. The blood film may show polychromasia and macrocytosis due to reticulocytes, or point to the diagnosis:
- Hypochromic microcytic anaemia (thalassaemia).
- Sickle cells (sickle-cell anaemia).
- Schistocytes (fig 4, p333; microangiopathic haemolytic anaemia).
- Abnormal cells in haematological malignancy.
- Spherocytes (hereditary spherocytosis or autoimmune haemolytic anaemia).
- Elliptocytes (fig 7, p333; hereditary elliptocytosis).
- Heinz bodies, 'bite' cells,[2] (glucose-6-phosphate dehydrogenase deficiency).

**Further tests**
- Direct antiglobulin (Coombs) *test* (DAT, fig 1) identifies red cells coated with antibody or complement. A +ve result indicates an immune cause of the haemolysis.
- RBC lifespan may be determined by *chromium labelling* and the major site of RBC breakdown may also be identified. This test is rarely done now.

The cause may now be obvious, but further tests may be needed. Membrane abnormalities are identified on the film and can be confirmed by *osmotic fragility* testing. *Hb electrophoresis* will detect haemoglobinopathies. *Enzyme assays* are reserved for situations when other causes have been excluded.

---

**1** See Provan D, *Oxford Handbook of Clinical and Laboratory Investigation*, 3e, OUP.
**2** On passing through the spleen, Heinz bodies may be removed, leaving an RBC with 'a bite taken out of it'. See p333 fig 2.

## Direct Coombs test / Direct antiglobulin test

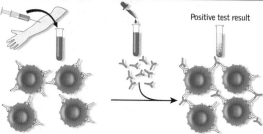

Blood sample from a patient with immune mediated haemolytic anaemia: antibodies are shown attached to antigens on the RBC surface.

The patient's washed RBCs are incubated with antihuman antibodies (Coombs reagent).

Positive test result

RBCs agglutinate: antihuman antibodies form links between RBCs by binding to the human antibodies on the RBCs.

## Indirect Coombs test / Indirect antiglobulin test

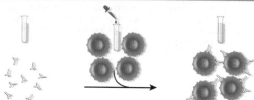

Recipient's serum is obtained, containing antibodies (Ig's).

Donor's blood sample is added to the tube with serum.

Recipient's Ig's that target the donor's red blood cells form antibody-antigen complexes.

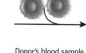

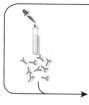

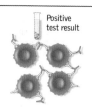

Positive test result

Anti-human Ig's (Coombs antibodies) are added to the solution.

Agglutination of red blood cells occurs, because human Ig's are attached to red blood cells.

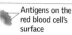

|  | Antigens on the red blood cell's surface |
| --- | --- |
| Y | Human anti-RBC antibody |
| Y | Antihuman antibody (Coombs reagent) |

**Fig 1.** The *direct* Coombs test detects antibodies on RBCs. The *indirect* Coombs test is used in pre-natal testing and before blood transfusion. It detects antibodies against RBCs that are free in serum: serum is incubated with RBCs of known antigenicity. If agglutination occurs, the indirect Coombs test is positive.

With kind permission of Aria Rad.

Haematology

**Acquired**—these are divided into immune and non-immune causes.

1 *Immune-mediated and direct antiglobulin test +ve* (Coombs test, p331):

- *Drug-induced* Causing formation of RBC autoantibodies from binding to RBC membranes (eg penicillin) or production of immune complexes (eg quinine).

- *Autoimmune haemolytic anaemia (AIHA;* fig 1): Mediated by autoantibodies causing mainly extravascular haemolysis and spherocytosis. Classify according to optimal binding temperature to RBCs: *Warm AIHA:* IgG-mediated, bind at body T° 37°C. ℞: Steroids/immunosuppressants (± splenectomy). *Cold AIHA:* IgM-mediated, bind at ↓T° (<4°C), activating cell-surface complement. Causes a chronic anaemia made worse by cold, often with Raynaud's or acrocyanosis. ℞: Keep warm. Chlorambucil may help. *Causes:* Most are idiopathic; 2° causes of warm AIHA include lymphoproliferative disease (CLL, lymphoma), drugs, autoimmune disease, eg SLE. Cold AIHA may follow infection (mycoplasma; EBV).

- *Paroxysmal cold haemoglobinuria* is seen with viruses/syphilis. It is caused by Donath-Landsteiner antibodies sticking to RBCs in the cold, causing self-limiting complement-mediated haemolysis on rewarming. *Isoimmune:* Acute transfusion reaction (p359); haemolytic disease of newborn.[26]

2 *Direct antiglobulin/Coombs –ve AIHA:* (2% of all AIHA) Autoimmune hepatitis; hepatitis B & C; post flu and other vaccinations; drugs (piperacillin, rituximab).[27]

3 *Microangiopathic haemolytic anaemia (MAHA):* A mechanical disruption of RBCs in circulation, causing intravascular haemolysis and schistocytes (figs 4 & 5). *Causes* include haemolytic-uraemic syndrome (HUS), TTP (p308), DIC, pre-eclampsia, eclampsia. Treat the underlying disease; transfusion or plasma exchange may be needed.

4 *Infection:* Malaria (p394): RBC lysis and 'blackwater fever' (haemoglobinuria).

5 *Paroxysmal nocturnal haemoglobinuria (Marchiafava-Micheli disease)* is a rare acquired stem cell disorder, with haemolysis (esp. at night→haemoglobinuria, fig 1, p719), marrow failure + thrombophilia. Visceral thrombosis (hepatic, mesenteric, renal and CNS veins) and pulmonary emboli predict poor outcome.[28] Δ: Urinary haemosiderin +ve. RBCs are sensitive to complement-mediated lysis due to abnormal surface glucosylphosphatidylinositol shown by cellular immuno-phenotyping. Ham's test +ve (*in vitro* acid-induced lysis, rarely done). ℞: Anticoagulation. Eculizumab has a role, so stem cell transplantation is less needed.

**Hereditary** Is there a defect in RBC enzymes, red cell membrane, or Hb?

1 *Enzyme defects:*

- *Glucose-6-phosphate dehydrogenase (G6PD) deficiency* ^X-linked is the chief RBC enzyme defect, affecting 100 million (mainly males) in the Mediterranean, Africa (G6PD-A), Middle/Far East (G6PD Canton is the main variant in China).[29] Most are asymptomatic, but may get oxidative crises due to ↓glutathione production, precipitated by drugs (eg primaquine, sulfonamides, aspirin), exposure to *Vicia fava* (broad beans/favism), or illness. In attacks, there is rapid anaemia and jaundice. *Film:* bite- and blister-cells (figs 2 & 3). Δ: Enzyme assay (>8wks after crisis as young RBCs may have enough enzyme so results may seem normal). ℞: Avoid precipitants (eg, henna, fig 8); transfuse if severe.

- *Pyruvate kinase deficiency* ^Autosomal recessive ↓ATP production causes ↓RBC survival. Homozygotes have neonatal jaundice; later, haemolysis with splenomegaly ± jaundice. Δ: Enzyme assay. ℞: Often not needed; splenectomy may help.

2 *Membrane defects:* All are Coombs –ve; all need folate; splenectomy helps some.

- *Hereditary spherocytosis* ^Autosomal dominant Prevalence: 1:3000. Less deformable spherical RBCs, so trapped in spleen→extravascular haemolysis. *Signs:* Splenomegaly, jaundice. Δ: Mild if Hb >110g/L & reticulocytes <6%; film: fig 6. ↑Bilirubin (→gallstones).

- *Hereditary elliptocytosis* ^Autosomal dominant Film: fig 7. Mostly asymptomatic (somewhat protects from malaria). 10% display a more severe phenotype (± death *in utero*).

- *Hereditary ovalocytosis and stomatocytosis* are rarer. Refer to a haematologist.

3 *Haemoglobinopathy:* • Sickle-cell disease (p334). • Thalassaemia (p336).

**Factors exacerbating haemolysis** Infection leads to ↑haemolysis. The anaemia may be exacerbated by parvoviruses (*OHCS* p142), producing a cessation of marrow erythropoiesis, ie aplastic anaemia, with no reticulocyte formation (p358).

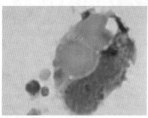

Fig 1. Autoimmune haemolytic anaemia: antibody-coated red cells undergoing phagocytosis by monocytes.

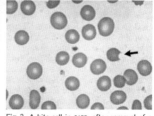

Fig 2. A bite-cell in G6PD, after removal of a Heinz body by the spleen; these are formed from denatured Hb during oxidative crises.

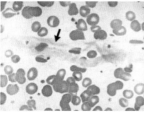

Fig 3. Blister-cells (arrows) in G6PD, following removal of Heinz bodies. Also contracted red cells (arrowheads).

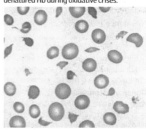

Fig 4. Microangiopathic anaemia, eg from DIC: numerous cell fragments (schistocytes) are present.

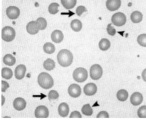

Fig 5. Fibrin strands, deposited in HUS and TTP (p308), slicing up RBCs (microangiopathy). Mechanical heart valves also slice up RBCs.

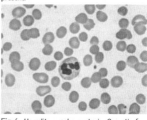

Fig 6. Hereditary spherocytosis. Osmotic fragility tests: RBCs show ↑fragility in hypotonic solutions.

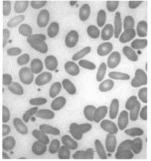

Fig 7. Hereditary elliptocytosis.

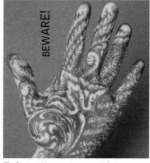

Fig 8. Avoid henna use in G6PD deficiency!

Fig 1 © Prof C Lawrence; figs 2-7 © Prof B Bain ©Massachusetts Medical Society.
Fig 8 © Catherine Cartwright-Jones (artist) and Roy Jones (photographer).

Haematology

Sickle-cell anaemia is an autosomal recessive disorder causing production of abnormal β globin chains. An amino acid substitution in the gene coding for the β chain (Glu → Val at position 6) results in the production of HbS rather than HbA. HbA₂ and HbF are still produced. It is common in people of African origin. The homozygote (SS) has sickle-cell *anaemia* (HbSS), and heterozygotes (HbAS) have sickle-cell *trait*, which causes no disability (and protects from *falciparum* malaria) except in hypoxia, eg in unpressurized aircraft or anaesthesia, when vaso-occlusive events may occur, so all those of African descent need a sickle-cell test pre-op. Symptomatic sickling also occurs in heterozygotes with genes coding other Hb variants (eg HbC leading to HbSC, or β-thalassaemia trait leading to HbS/βthal).

**Pathogenesis** HbS polymerizes when deoxygenated, causing RBCs to deform, producing sickle cells, which are fragile and haemolyse, and also block small vessels.

**Prevalence** 1:700 people of African heritage.

**Tests** Haemolysis is variable. Hb ≈ 60–90g/L, ↑reticulocytes 10–20%, ↑bilirubin. *Film:* sickle cells and target cells (fig 1). *Sickle solubility test:* +ve, but does not distinguish between HbSS and HbAS. *Hb electrophoresis:* Confirms the diagnosis and distinguishes SS, AS states, and other Hb variants. ►Aim for diagnosis *at birth* (cord blood) to aid prompt pneumococcal prophylaxis (vaccine, p160 ± penicillin V).

**Signs/symptoms** Chronic haemolysis is usually well tolerated (except in crises; BOX). *Vaso-occlusive 'painful' crisis:* Common, due to microvascular occlusion. Often affects the marrow, causing severe pain, triggered by cold, dehydration, infection or hypoxia. Hands and feet are affected if <3yrs old leading to *dactylitis*. Occlusion may cause *mesenteric ischaemia*, mimicking an acute abdomen. CNS infarction occurs in ∼10% of children, leading to *stroke*, *seizures* or *cognitive defects*. Transcranial Doppler ultrasonography indicates risk of impending stroke, and blood transfusions can prevent this by reducing HbS[30] Also *avascular necrosis* (eg of femoral head), *leg ulcers* (fig 2) and low-flow *priapism* (also seen in CML, may respond to hydration, α-agonists, eg phenylephrine, or aspiration of blood + irrigation with saline; if for >12h prompt cavernosus-spongiosum shunting can prevent later impotence).[31]
*Aplastic crisis:* This is due to parvovirus B19, with sudden reduction in marrow production, especially RBCs. Usually self-limiting <2wks; transfusion may be needed.
*Sequestration crisis:* Mainly affects children as the spleen has not yet undergone atrophy. There is pooling of blood in the spleen + liver, with organomegaly, severe anaemia and shock. Urgent transfusion is needed.

**Complications** •Splenic infarction occurs before 2yrs old, due to microvascular occlusion, leading to ↑susceptibility to infection (40% of childhood sickle deaths are caused this way); zinc supplements may help[32,33] •Poor growth •Chronic renal failure •Gallstones •Retinal disease •Iron overload (BOX 2) or blood-borne infection after repeated transfusion[34] •Lung damage: hypoxia→fibrosis→pulmonary hypertension, partly prevented by incentive spirometry: 10 maximal inspirations/2h[35]

**Management of chronic disease** ►Get help from a haematologist.
• Hydroxycarbamide if frequent crises. Dose example: 20mg/kg/d if eGFR >60mL/min.[1]
• Splenic infarction leads to hyposplenism. Prophylaxis, in terms of antibiotics and immunization, should be given (p367).
• Febrile children risk septicaemia: repeated admission may be avoided by outpatient ceftriaxone (eg 2 doses, 50mg/kg IV on day 0 and 1). Admission may still be needed, eg if Hb <50g/L, WCC <5 or >30 × 10⁹/L, T° >40°C, severe pain, dehydration, lung infiltration. Seek expert advice.
• Bone marrow transplant can be curative but remains controversial.

**Prevention** Genetic counselling; prenatal tests (OHCS p152-3). Parental education can help prevent 90% of deaths from sequestration crises.[36]

---

**1** Long-term hydroxycarbamide causes ↑production of fetal haemoglobin (HbF), ↓Hb polymerization, hence fewer painful crises, chest symptoms, admissions, blood transfusions + ↓mortality by 40%.[37,38] This may result from fewer episodes of marrow ischaemia and embolization. Nitric oxide is raised.

## Managing sickle-cell crises[39]

▶ Seek expert help early.

- Give *prompt*, generous analgesia, eg IV opiates (see p576).
- Crossmatch blood. FBC, reticulocytes, blood cultures, MSU ± CXR if T°↑ or chest signs.
- Rehydrate with IVI and keep warm. Give $O_2$ by mask if $P_aO_2$↓ or $O_2$ sats <95%.
- 'Blind' antibiotics (eg cephalosporin, p382) if T° >38°, unwell, or chest signs.
- Measure PCV, reticulocytes, liver, and spleen size twice daily.
- Give blood transfusion if Hb or reticulocytes fall sharply. Match blood for the blood group antigens Rh(C, D, E) and Kell, to prevent alloantibody formation. This helps oxygenation, and is as good as exchange transfusion (reserved for those who are rapidly worsening: it is a process where blood is removed and donor blood is given in stages),[40] Indications: severe chest crisis, suspected CNS event or multiorgan failure—when the proportion of HbS should be reduced to <30%.

*The acute chest syndrome:* Entails pulmonary infiltrates involving complete lung segments, causing pain, fever, tachypnoea, wheeze, and cough. It is serious. Incidence: ~0.1 episodes/patient/yr. 13% in the landmark Vichinsky study needed ventilation, 11% had CNS symptoms, and 9% of those over 20 years old died. Prodromal painful crisis occur ~2.5 days before any abnormalities on CXR in 50% of patients. The chief causes of the infiltrates are fat embolism from bone marrow or infection with *Chlamydia*, *Mycoplasma*, or viruses.[41] ℞: $O_2$, analgesia, blind antibiotics (cephalosporin + macrolide) until culture results known. Bronchodilators (eg salbutamol, p175) have proved to be effective in those with wheezing or obstructive pulmonary function at presentation. Blood transfusion (exchange if severe). *Take to ITU if $P_aO_2$ cannot be kept above 9.2kPa (70mmHg) when breathing air.*

*Patient-controlled analgesia* (example with paediatric doses) First try warmth, hydration, and oral analgesia: ibuprofen 5mg/kg/6h (codeine 1mg/kg/4-8h PO up to 3mg/kg/d may also be tried, but is less effective). If this fails, see on the ward and offer prompt morphine by IVI—eg 0.1mg/kg. Start with morphine 1mg/kg in 50mL 5% glucose, and try a rate of 1mL/h, allowing the patient to deliver extra boluses of 1mL when needed. Do respiration and sedation score every ¼h + $O_2$ sats if chest/abdominal pain.[42] Liaise with the local pain service.

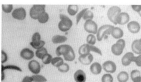 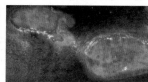

**Fig 1.** Sickle-cell film: there are sickle cells, target cells, and a nucleated red cell.

**Fig 2.** Leg ulcers in sickle-cell disease.

Figs 1 & 2 ©Prof. C Lawrence.

### ☺A 7-year-old tells us what it's like to have sickle-cell disease

"I have been hospitalized over 50 times for complications from this disease. To keep it controlled I started having monthly transfusions. After repeated transfusions my body began to get too much iron so I had to start getting infusions. I was taking the medication desferal[1] which my mummy had to insert a needle in my belly hooked up to a pump which I had to carry on my back in my neat Spiderman backpack. I was hooked up to the machine for 10 hours a day 5 days a week but it was okay I still got to play!!! I suffered from pain crisis which makes my legs and back hurt like someone is hitting me with a hammer.

You may notice that I may move slow or look tired when it is time for my blood transfusion. That is because the transfusions are like a heartbeat for my body, without it I can't survive. When I'm in pain the only thing that helps is morphine... I tell my mummy when she's crying I WILL BE OK!!"

1 This was necessary until a once-daily oral iron chelator came along: deferasirox (Exjade®).

The thalassaemias are genetic diseases of unbalanced Hb synthesis, with under-production (or no production) of one globin chain (see BOX). Unmatched globins precipitate, damaging RBC membranes, causing their haemolysis while still in the marrow. They are common in areas from the Mediterranean to the Far East.

**The β thalassaemias** are usually caused by point mutations in β-globin genes on chromosome 11, leading to ↓β chain production (β⁺) or its absence (β⁰). Various combinations of mutations are possible (eg β⁰/β⁰, β⁺/β⁺, or β⁺/β⁰).

**Tests** FBC, MCV, film, iron, HbA₂, HbF, Hb electrophoresis. MRI can monitor myocardial siderosis from iron overload.[43]

*β thalassaemia minor or trait (eg β/β⁺; heterozygous state):* This is a carrier state, and is usually asymptomatic. Mild, well-tolerated anaemia (Hb >90g/L) which may worsen in pregnancy. MCV <75fL, HbA₂ >3.5%, slight ↑HbF. Often confused with iron-deficiency anaemia.

*β thalassaemia intermedia* describes an intermediate state with moderate anaemia but not requiring transfusions. There may be splenomegaly. There are a variety of causes including mild homozygous β thalassaemia mutations, eg β⁺/β⁺, or co-inheritance of β thalassaemia trait with another haemoglobinopathy, eg HbC thalassaemia (1 parent has the HbC trait, and the other has β⁺). Sickle-cell β⁺ thalassaemia produces a picture similar to sickle-cell anaemia.

*β thalassaemia major (Cooley's anaemia)* denotes abnormalities in both β-globin genes, and presents in the 1ˢᵗ year, with severe anaemia and failure to thrive. Extramedullary haemopoiesis (RBCs made outside the marrow) occurs in response to anaemia, causing characteristic head shape, eg skull bossing (figs 1 & 2) and hepatosplenomegaly (also due to haemolysis). There is osteopenia (may respond to zoledronic acid).[44] Skull x-ray shows a 'hair on end' sign due to ↑marrow activity. Life-long blood transfusions are needed, with resulting iron overload/deposition seen after ~10yrs as endocrine failure (pituitary, thyroid, pancreas→diabetes mellitus), liver disease, and cardiac toxicity. The film shows very hypochromic, microcytic cells + target cells + nucleated RBCs. HbF↑↑, HbA₂ variable, HbA absent.

**Treatment** ▶Promote fitness; healthy diet. Folate (±carnitine) supplements help.[45]
• Regular (~2–4 weekly) life-long transfusions to keep Hb >90g/L, to suppress the ineffective extramedullary haematopoiesis and to allow normal growth.
• Iron-chelators to prevent iron overload. Oral deferiprone + desferrioxamine sc twice weekly.[46] SE: pain, deafness, cataracts, retinal damage, ↑risk of *Yersinia*. Alternative: deferasirox (p334). NB: iron overload is a big problem causing hypothyroidism, hypocalcaemia,[47] hypogonadism (men may get help from testosterone gel).[48]
• Large doses of ascorbic acid also increase urinary excretion of iron.
• Splenectomy if hypersplenism persists with increasing transfusion requirements (p367)—this is best avoided until >5yrs old due to risk of infections.
• Hormonal replacement or treatment for endocrine complications, eg diabetes mellitus, hypothyroidism. Growth hormone treatment has had variable success.[49]
• A histocompatible marrow transplant can offer the chance of a cure.[50]

**Prevention** Approaches include genetic counselling or antenatal diagnosis using fetal blood or DNA, then 'therapeutic' abortion.

**The α thalassaemias** (fig 3) There are two separate α-globin genes on each chromosome 16 ∴ there are four genes (termed αα/αα). The α thalassaemias are mainly caused by gene deletions. If all 4 α genes are deleted (--/--), death is *in utero* (*Bart's hydrops*). Here, HbBarts (γ₄) is present, which is physiologically useless. HbH disease occurs if 3 genes are deleted (--/-α); there may be moderate anaemia and features of haemolysis: hepatosplenomegaly, leg ulcers and jaundice. In the blood film, there is formation of β₄ tetramers (=HbH) due to excess β chains, Hb-Barts, HbA and HbA₂. If 2 genes are deleted (--/αα or -α/-α), there is an asymptomatic carrier state, with ↓MCV. With one gene deleted, the clinical state is normal.

## Structure of haemoglobin

The three main types of Hb in adult blood are:

| Type | Peptide chains | % in adult blood | % in fetal blood |
|------|----------------|------------------|------------------|
| HbA | $\alpha_2\,\beta_2$ | 97 | 10-50 |
| HbA$_2$ | $\alpha_2\,\delta_2$ | 2.5 | Trace |
| HbF | $\alpha_2\,\gamma_2$ | 0.5 | 50-90 |

Adult haemoglobin (HbA) is a tetramer of 2 α- and 2 β-globin chains each containing a haem group. In the first year of life, adult haemoglobin replaces fetal haemoglobin (HbF).

It might be thought that because the molecular details of the thalassaemias are so well worked out they represent a perfect example of the reductionist principle at work: find out *exactly* what is happening *within* molecules, and you will be able to explain all the manifestations of a disease. But this is not so. We have to recognize that two people with the identical mutation at their β loci may have quite different diseases. Co-inheritance of other genes and conditions (eg α thalassaemia) is part of the explanation, as is the efficiency of production of fetal haemoglobin. The reasons lie beyond simple co-segregation of genes promoting the formation of fetal Hb. The rate of proteolysis of excess α-globin chains may also be important—as may mechanisms that have little to do with genetic or molecular events. So the lesson the thalassaemias teach is more subtle than the reductionist one: it is that if you want to understand the *whole* picture, you must look at every level: genetic, molecular, physiological, social, and cultural. Each level influences the other, without necessarily determining them.

*Haematology*

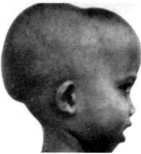

Fig 1. β thalassaemia major: bossing due to extramedullary haematopoiesis.

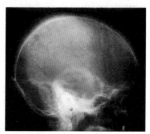

Fig 2. β thalassaemia major: skull x-ray.
©Dr E van der Enden (fig 1)
©Crookston collection (fig 2).

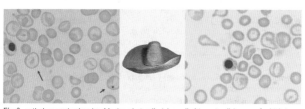

Fig 3. α thalassaemia showing Mexican hat cells (also called target cells)—one of which is arrowed on the left panel. Note also the tear-drop cell on the right panel, and the 2 normoblasts (nucleated red cells, one on each panel). The shorter *arrow* on the left panel points to a Howell-Jolly body. Note that the cells which are not Mexican hats are rather small (microcytic). There is also poikilocytosis (*poikilos* is Greek for varied—so this simply means that the vessels holding the haemoglobin are of varied shape).

Courtesy of Prof. Tangün and Dr Köroğlu.

After injury, 3 processes halt bleeding: vasoconstriction, gap-plugging by platelets, and the coagulation cascade (fig 1). Disorders of haemostasis fall into these 3 groups. The pattern of bleeding is important—vascular and platelet disorders lead to prolonged bleeding from cuts, bleeding into the skin (eg easy bruising and purpura), and bleeding from mucous membranes (eg epistaxis, bleeding from gums, menorrhagia). Coagulation disorders cause delayed bleeding into joints and muscle.

1 **Vascular defects** *Congenital:* Osler-Weber-Rendu syndrome (p722), connective tissue disease (eg Ehlers-Danlos syndrome, OHCS p642, pseudoxanthoma elasticum). *Acquired:* Senile purpura, infection (eg meningococcal, measles, dengue fever), steroids, scurvy (perifollicular haemorrhages), Henoch-Schönlein purpura (p716), painful bruising syndrome—women who develop tingling under the skin followed by bruising over limbs/trunk, resolving without treatment.

2 **Platelet disorders** *Decreased marrow production:* Aplastic anaemia (p358), megaloblastic anaemia, marrow infiltration (eg leukaemia, myeloma), marrow suppression (cytotoxic drugs, radiotherapy). *Excess destruction: Immune:* Immune thrombocytopenic purpura (ITP, below), other autoimmune causes, eg SLE, CLL, drugs, eg heparin, viruses; *Non-immune:* DIC (p346), thrombotic thrombocytopenic purpura (TTP) or HUS (p308), sequestration (in hypersplenism). **ITP** is caused by antiplatelet autoantibodies. It is acute (usually in children, 2wks after infection with sudden self-limiting purpura: OHCS p197) or chronic (seen mainly in women). Chronic ITP runs a fluctuating course of bleeding, purpura (esp. dependent pressure areas), epistaxis and menorrhagia. There is no splenomegaly. *Tests in ITP:* ↑megakaryocytes in marrow, antiplatelet autoantibodies often present. ℞: None if mild. If symptomatic or platelets <20 × 10⁹/L, prednisolone 1mg/kg/d, and reduce after remission; aim to keep platelets >30 × 10⁹/L—takes a few days to work. If relapse, splenectomy cures ≤80%. If this fails: immunosuppression, eg azathioprine or cyclophosphamide. Platelet transfusions are not used (except during splenectomy or life-threatening haemorrhage) as these are quickly destroyed by the autoantibodies. IV immunoglobulin may temporarily raise the platelet count, eg for surgery, pregnancy. Eltrombopag is a new oral thrombopoietin-receptor agonist that stimulates thrombopoiesis. *Poorly functioning platelets:* Seen in myeloproliferative disease, NSAIDs, and urea↑.

3 **Coagulation disorders** *Congenital:* Haemophilia, von Willebrand's disease (p726). *Acquired:* Anticoagulants, liver disease, DIC (p346), vitamin K deficiency.

**Haemophilia A** Factor VIII deficiency; inherited in an X-linked recessive pattern in 1:10,000 male births—usually due to a 'flip tip' inversion in the factor VIII gene in the X chromosome. There is a high rate of new mutations (30% have no family history). *Presentation* depends on severity and is often early in life or after surgery/trauma—with bleeds into joints leading to crippling arthropathy, and into muscles causing haematomas (↑ pressure can lead to nerve palsies and compartment syndrome). *Diagnose* by ↑APTT and ↓factor VIII assay. *Management:* Seek expert advice. Avoid NSAIDs and IM injections (fig 2). *Minor bleeding:* pressure and elevation of the part. Desmopressin (0.3µg/kg/12h IVI over 20min) raises factor VIII levels, and may be sufficient. *Major bleeds* (eg haemarthrosis): ↑factor VIII levels to 50% of normal. *Life-threatening bleeds* (eg obstructing airway) need levels of 100%, eg with recombinant factor VIII. *Genetic counselling:* OHCS p154.

**Haemophilia B (Christmas disease)** Factor IX deficiency (inherited, X-linked recessive); behaves clinically like haemophilia A.

**Acquired haemophilia** is a bleeding diathesis causing big mucosal bleeds in males and females caused by suddenly appearing autoantibodies that interfere with factor VIII.[51] *Tests:* APPT↑; VIII autoantibody↑; factor VIII activity <50%. ℞: Steroids.

**Liver disease** produces a complicated bleeding disorder with ↓synthesis of clotting factors, ↓absorption of vitamin K, and abnormalities of platelet function.

**Malabsorption** leads to less uptake of vitamin K (needed for synthesis of factors II, VII, IX, and X). Treatment is IV vitamin K (10mg) or FFP for acute haemorrhage.

Haematology

Extrinsic System        Intrinsic System

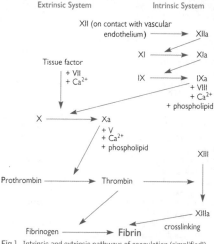

XII (on contact with vascular
endothelium) ⟶ XIIa

XI ⟶ XIa

Tissue factor
+ VII
+ Ca²⁺

IX ⟶ IXa
+ VIII
+ Ca²⁺
+ phospholipid

X ⟶ Xa
+ V
+ Ca²⁺
+ phospholipid

XIII

Prothrombin ⟶ Thrombin ⟶

XIIIa

Fibrinogen ⟶ Fibrin    crosslinking

Fig 1. Intrinsic and extrinsic pathways of coagulation (simplified!)

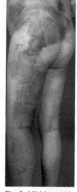

Fig 2. Mild haemoph-
ilia after an IM injection.
►Give vaccines etc SC!
©Crookston collection 53

## Fibrinolysis

**The fibrinolytic system** causes fibrin dissolution and acts via the generation of plasmin. The process starts with the release of tissue plasminogen activator (t-PA) from endothelial cells, a process stimulated by fibrin formation. t-PA converts inactive plasminogen to plasmin which can then cleave fibrin, as well as several other factors. t-PA and plasminogen both bind fibrin thus localizing fibrinolysis to the area of the clot.

### Mechanism of fibrinolytic agents

Alteplase (=rt-PA=Actilyse®; from recombinant DNA) is a fibrinolytic enzyme imitating t-PA, as above. Plasma $t\frac{1}{2} \approx 5$min.

Streptokinase is a streptococcal exotoxin and forms a complex in plasma with plasminogen to form an activator complex, which forms plasmin from unbound plasminogen. Initially there is rapid plasmin formation which can cause uncontrolled fibrinolysis. Plasminogen is rapidly consumed in the complex and then plasmin is only produced as more plasminogen is synthesized. The activator complex binds to fibrin, so producing some localization of fibrinolysis.

There are 3 sets of questions to be answered:

**1 Is there an emergency?**—needing immediate resuscitation or senior help?
- Is the patient about to exsanguinate (dizzy on sitting up, shock, coma, p800)?
- Is there hypovolaemia (postural hypotension, oliguria)?
- Is there CNS bleeding (meningism, CNS, and retinal signs)?
- Is there an underlying condition which escalates this apparently minor bleeding into an evolving catastrophe? For example:
  - Bleeding in pregnancy or the puerperium
  - GI bleeding in a jaundiced man (ie coagulation factors already depleted)
  - Bleeding in someone who is already anaemic (esp if other comorbidities).

**2 Why is the patient bleeding?** Is bleeding normal, given the circumstances (eg surgery, trauma, parturition), or does the patient have a bleeding disorder (BOX 1)?
- Is there a secondary cause, eg drugs (warfarin), alcohol, liver disease, sepsis?
- Is there unexplained bleeding, bruising, or purpura?
- Past or family history of excess bleeding, eg during trauma, dentistry, surgery?
- Is the pattern of bleeding indicative of vascular, platelet, or coagulation problems (p338)? Are venepuncture or old cannula sites bleeding (DIC, p346)? Look for associated conditions (eg with DIC).
- Is a clotting screen abnormal? Check FBC, platelets, PT, APTT and thrombin time. Consider D-dimers, bleeding time, and a factor VIII assay.

**3 In cases of bleeding disorders, what is the mechanism?** To help find the answer do FBC, film, and coagulation tests (citrate tube; false results if under-filled):
- *Prothrombin time (PT):* Thromboplastin is added to test the *extrinsic system.* PT is expressed as a ratio compared to control [International Normalized Ratio (INR), normal range = 0.9-1.2]. It tests for abnormalities in factors I, II, V, VII, X. Prolonged by: warfarin, vitamin K deficiency, liver disease, DIC.
- *Activated partial thromboplastin time (APTT):* Kaolin is added to test the intrinsic system. Tests for abnormalities in factor I, II, V, VIII, IX, X, XI, XII. Normal range 35-45s. Prolonged by: heparin treatment, haemophilia, DIC, liver disease.
- *Thrombin time:* Thrombin is added to plasma to convert fibrinogen to fibrin. Normal range: 10-15s. Prolonged by: heparin treatment, DIC, dysfibrinogenaemia.
- *D-dimers* are a fibrin degradation product, released from cross-linked fibrin during fibrinolysis (p339). This occurs during DIC, or in the presence of venous thromboembolism—deep vein thrombosis (DVT) or pulmonary embolism (PE). D-dimers may also be raised in inflammation, eg with infection or malignancy.
- *Bleeding time* tests haemostasis. It is done by making two small incisions into the skin of the forearm. Normal time to haemostasis: ≤10min.[51] NB: this is rarely done, as it is operator dependent; consider the PFA-100 instead (BOX 2).

**Interpretation**
- *Platelets:* If low, do FBC, film, clotting.
- *PT:* If long, look for liver disease or anticoagulant use.
- *APTT:* If long, consider liver disease, haemophilia (VIII or IX deficiency), or heparin.
- *Bleeding time:* Raised in von Willebrand's disease (p726), platelet disorders, and if on low- but not full-dose aspirin.[52]
- If both PT and APTT are very raised, with low platelets, and ↑D-dimers, consider DIC.

**Management** depends on the degree of bleeding. If shocked, resuscitate (p804). If bleeding continues in the presence of a clotting disorder or a massive transfusion, discuss the need for FFP and platelets with a haematologist. In ITP (p338), steroids ± IV immunoglobulin may be used. Especially in pregnancy (OHCS p88), consult an expert. Is there overdose with anticoagulants (p854)? In haemophiliac bleeds, *consult early* for coagulation factor replacement. *Never* give IM injections. Pre-op considerations: see BOX 3.

| Disorder | INR | APTT | Thrombin time | Platelet count | Bleeding time | Notes |
|---|---|---|---|---|---|---|
| Heparin | ↑ | ↑↑ | ↑↑ | ↔ | ↔ | |
| DIC | ↑↑ | ↑↑ | ↑↑ | ↓ | ↑ | ↑D-d, p346 |
| Liver disease | ↑ | ↑ | ↔/↑ | ↔/↓ | ↔/↑ | AST↑ |
| Platelet defect | ↔ | ↔ | ↔ | ↔ | ↑(↑) | |
| Vit κ deficiency | ↑↑ | ↑ | ↔ | ↔ | ↔ | |
| Haemophilia | ↔ | ↑↑ | ↔ | ↔ | ↔ | see p338 |
| von Willebrand's | ↔ | ↑↑ | ↔ | ↔ | ↑(↑) | see p726 |
| Special tests may be available (factor assays: ►consult a haematologist). | | | | | | |

## PFA-100: an alternative to the bleeding test

The PFA-100® (Platelet Function Analyzer-100) mimics the clotting process. To do the test, a tube of fresh blood is drawn and a portion put into a test cartridge. A vacuum draws blood through a thin glass tube coated with collagen and with either adrenaline or ADP, which activates the platelets in the moving sample and promotes platelet aggregation. The time it takes for a clot to form inside the glass tube and prevent further flow is measured as a closure time (CT). An initial screen is done with collagen/adrenaline. If the CT is normal, it is unlikely that a platelet dysfunction exists. The collagen/ADP test can confirm an abnormal collagen/adrenaline test. If both are abnormal, it is likely that there is platelet dysfunction and further testing for inherited or acquired bleeding disorders is indicated. If the collagen/ADP test is normal, then the abnormal collagen/adrenaline test may be due to aspirin ingestion.[53]

## Is this pre-op patient at risk of excessive bleeding?

Take a bleeding history! The more structured this is the better.[54] If excessive, prolonged, or unexplained bleeding in the past, or if on agents known to affect haemostasis, or if the liver is suspect, or there is a condition such as lupus, or if bleeding might be disastrous, further tests may be indicated after discussion with a haematologist: INR, FBC, film, aPPT, PFA-100 (see above) and von Willebrand factor (vWF: Ag). In one pre-op study the bleeding history was +ve in 11%, and tests showed impaired haemostasis in 40% of these. ~98% of these are detectable by PFA-100.[55]

*Haematology* (side margin)

▶Blood should only be given if strictly necessary *and there is no alternative*. Outcomes are often *worse* after a transfusion.

• Know and use local procedures to ensure that the right blood gets to the right patient at the right time.

• Take blood for crossmatching from only one patient at a time. Label immediately. This minimizes risk of wrong labelling of samples.[1]

• When giving blood, monitor TPR and BP every ½h.

• Do not use giving sets which have contained dextrose or Gelofusine®.

**Group-and-save (G&S) requests** Know your local guidelines for elective surgery. Having crossmatched blood to hand may not be needed if a blood sample is already in the lab, with group determined, without any atypical antibodies (ie G&S).

**Products** *Whole blood:* (rarely used) Indications: exchange transfusion; grave exsanguination—use crossmatched blood if possible, but if not, use 'universal donor' group O Rh-ve blood, changing to crossmatched blood as soon as possible. ▶Blood even <2d old has no effective platelets. *Red cells:* (packed to make haematocrit ~70%) Use to correct anaemia or blood loss. 1u ↑Hb by 10-15g/L. In anaemia, transfuse until Hb ~80g/L. *Platelets:* (p358) Not usually needed if not bleeding or count is >20 × $10^9$/L. 1u should ↑platelet count by >20 × $10^9$/L. Failure to do so suggests refractoriness—discuss with haematologist. If surgery is planned, get advice if <100 × $10^9$/L. *Fresh frozen plasma (FFP):* Use to correct clotting defects: eg DIC (p346); warfarin overdosage where **vitamin K** would be too slow; liver disease; thrombotic thrombocytopenic purpura (p308). It is expensive and carries all the risks of blood transfusion. Do not use as a simple volume expander. *Human albumin solution* is produced as 4.5% or 20% protein solution and is for use as protein replacement. 20% albumin can be used temporarily in the hypoproteinaemic patient (eg liver disease; nephrosis) who is fluid overloaded, without giving an excessive salt load. Also used as replacement in abdominal paracentesis (p779). *Others* Cryoprecipitate (a source of fibrinogen); coagulation concentrates (self-injected in haemophilia); immunoglobulin (*anti-D, OHCS* p9).

**Complications of transfusion**[5][6] ▶Management of acute reactions: see BOX 1.

• *Early (within 24h):* Acute haemolytic reactions (eg ABO or Rh incompatibility); anaphylaxis; bacterial contamination; febrile reactions (eg from HLA antibodies); allergic reactions (itch, urticaria, mild fever); fluid overload; transfusion-related acute lung injury (TRALI, ie ARDS due to antileucocyte antibodies in donor plasma).

• *Delayed (after 24h):* Infections (eg viruses: hepatitis B/C, HIV; bacteria; protozoa; prions); iron overload (treatment, p336); graft-versus-host disease; post-transfusion purpura—potentially lethal fall in platelet count 5-7d post-transfusion requiring specialist treatment with IV immunoglobulin and platelet transfusions.

**Massive blood transfusion** This is defined as replacement of an individual's entire blood volume (>10u) within 24h. Complications: platelets↓; $Ca^{2+}$↓; clotting factors↓; K⁺↑; hypothermia.

**Transfusing patients with heart failure** If Hb ≤50g/L with heart failure, transfusion with packed red cells is vital to restore Hb to a safe level, eg 60-80g/L, but must be done with great care. Give each unit over 4h with *furosemide* (eg 40mg slow IV/PO; don't mix with blood) with alternate units. Check for ↑JVP and basal lung crackles; consider CVP line. If CCF gets worse, and immediate transfusion is vital, try a 2-3u exchange transfusion, removing blood at same rate as transfused.

*Autologous transfusion* There is a role for patients having their own blood stored pre-op for later use. *Erythropoietin (EPO,* p296) can increase the yield of autologous blood in normal people. Intraoperative cell salvage with retransfusion is also being used more often—especially in cardiac, vascular and emergency surgery.[5][7] Cost-analysis shows that it may be worthwhile on an economic basis alone.[58]

---

**1** Other methods to avoid mishaps: electronic bar code readers; bedside ABO agglutination test on a card✍ (used in France; where this is linked with other methods, 99.65% reliability is achieved).[19]

## Transfusion reactions

All UK blood products are now leucocyte-depleted (white cells <5×10⁶/L) so as to reduce the incidence of complications such as alloimmunization to HLA class I antigens and febrile transfusion reactions. Does giving paracetamol and anti-histamines before the transfusion prevent even more serious reactions? Probably not (although some mild fevers may be prevented).[60]

| | |
|---|---|
| *Acute haemolytic reaction*<br>(eg ABO incompatibility) Agitation, T°↑ (rapid onset), ↓BP, flushing, abdominal/chest pain, oozing venepuncture sites, DIC. | STOP transfusion. Check identity and name on unit; tell haematologist; send unit + FBC, U&E, clotting, cultures, & urine (haemoglobinuria) to lab. Keep IV line open with 0.9% saline. Treat DIC (p346). |
| *Anaphylaxis*<br>Bronchospasm, cyanosis, ↓BP, soft tissue swelling. | STOP the transfusion. Maintain airway and give oxygen. Contact anaesthetist. ▶▶See p806. |
| *Bacterial contamination*<br>T°↑ (rapid onset), ↓BP, and rigors. | STOP the transfusion. Check identity against name on unit; tell haematologist and send unit + FBC, U&E, clotting, cultures & urine to lab. Start broad-spectrum antibiotics. |
| *TRALI* (See p342) Dyspnoea, cough; CXR 'white out' | STOP the transfusion. Give 100% O₂. ▶▶Treat as ARDS, p178. Donor should be removed from donor panel. |
| *Non-haemolytic febrile transfusion reaction*<br>Shivering and fever usually ½–1h after starting transfusion. | SLOW or STOP the transfusion. Give an antipyretic, eg *paracetamol* 1g. Monitor closely. If recurrent, use WBC filter. |
| *Allergic reactions*<br>Urticaria and itch. | SLOW or STOP the transfusion; *chlorphenamine* 10mg slow IV/IM. Monitor closely. |
| *Fluid overload*<br>Dyspnoea, hypoxia, tachycardia, ↑JVP and basal crepitations. | SLOW or STOP the transfusion. Give oxygen and a diuretic, eg *furosemide* 40mg IV initially. Consider CVP line. |

## Blood transfusion and Jehovah's Witnesses

These patients are likely to refuse even vital transfusions on religious grounds.[1] These views must be respected, but complex issues arise if the patient is a child, or (perhaps) an adult who lives a sheltered life, who may not be able to give or with-hold consent in an informed way—see p554. When in doubt, apply to the Court. Judges tend to take a narrow view on this, acting as if any immediate benefit to life must trump putative benefits in any life hereafter.[2] How can refusal be informed, it might be argued, if only the physical (and not the metaphysical) consequences of transfusion can be foreseen?

Even if metaphysical considerations are put to one side, it is a question whether giving a transfusion against consent could amount to a degrading act or torture, against which the European Convention on Human Rights gives absolute, inalien-able protection. ▶Some patients may not want to forsake their principles but would not mind too much being told what to do, thereby not being the means of their child's destruction, while being true to their beliefs. It is possible to hold two incompatible beliefs at the same time.[1]

---

**1** Accepting transfusion implies **self-expulsion** from the church, but it is no longer a '**disfellowshipping event**' with active expulsion.[61,62] This tenet is based on (among others) the biblical verse "*no soul of you shall eat blood*" (Leviticus 17:12).
**2** V Wason 1998 Court Order (High Court Family Division) Re L (A Minor), June 1-10.

**Haematology**

### Main indications

- *Therapeutic:* Venous thromboembolic disease: DVT and PE.
- *Prophylactic:* Prevention of DVT/PE in high-risk patients (p369), eg post-op.
  Prevention of stroke, eg in chronic AF or prosthetic heart valve.

**Heparin** *1 Low molecular weight heparin (LMWH)* Given sc. Molecular weight ~5000 Daltons (Da), eg dalteparin, enoxaparin, tinzaparin. Inactivates factor Xa (but not thrombin). T½ is 2- to 4-fold longer than standard heparin, and response is more predictable, and so only needs to be given once or twice daily, and no laboratory monitoring is usually required. It has replaced unfractionated heparin (UFH) as the preferred option in the prevention and treatment of venous thromboembolism and in acute coronary syndrome. See *BNF* for doses. It accumulates in renal failure: lower doses are used for prophylaxis, or UFH for therapeutic doses.

*2 Unfractionated heparin (UFH)* IV or SC. ~13,000 Daltons. A glycosaminoglycan, which binds antithrombin (an endogenous inhibitor of coagulation), increasing its ability to inhibit thrombin, factor Xa, and IXa. Rapid onset and has a short T½. Monitor and adjust dose with APTT (p340) BOX 3 and below.

*SE for both:* ↑Bleeding (eg at operative site, gastrointestinal, intracranial), heparin-induced thrombocytopenia (HIT), osteoporosis with long-term use. HIT and osteoporosis are less common with LMWH than UFH. Beware hyperkalaemia.

*CI:* Bleeding disorders, platelets <60×10⁹/L, previous HIT, peptic ulcer, cerebral haemorrhage, severe hypertension, neurosurgery.

**Warfarin** is used orally once daily as long-term anticoagulation. The therapeutic range is narrow, varying with the condition being treated (BOX 1 & BOX 2)—and is measured as a ratio compared with the standard INR. Warfarin inhibits the reductase enzyme responsible for regenerating the active form of vitamin K, producing a state analogous to vit K deficiency. *CI:* Peptic ulcer, bleeding disorders, severe hypertension, pregnancy (teratogenic, see *OHCS* p640). Use with caution in the elderly and those with past GI bleeds. In the UK, warfarin tablets are 0.5mg (white), 1mg (brown), 3mg (blue), or 5mg (pink). ▶Interactions: p768.

**Others** Fondaparinux is a pentasaccharide Xa inhibitor and may be used in place of LMWH for prophylaxis in certain situations. Factor Xa inhibitors (rivaroxaban and apixaban) and direct thrombin inhibitors (dabigatran, p125) are new oral anticoagulants that do not need monitoring—but they have not yet displaced warfarin.[13]

**Beginning therapeutic anticoagulation** (follow local guidelines, and see BNF). For treatment of venous thromboembolism, LMWH or UFH are used initially, and warfarin is given in combination usually from day 1. Heparin should be continued until INR has reached target therapeutic range (see BOX) *and* until day 5, as warfarin has an initial prothrombotic effect.
- *LMWH* Dose according to weight (see *BNF*).

*UFH IV infusion:* Give heparin 5000iu IV bolus over 30min (10,000iu in severe PE).
- Prepare syringe pump: with 0.9% saline.
- Infuse heparin at a rate of 18 units/kg/h. Check APTT at 6h, aim for APTT ratio 1.5-2.5 (see BOX). Measure APTT daily or 10h after dose change.

*Warfarin* is given daily; start with 10mg stat at 18.00. Do INR 16h later.
- If INR <1.8 (as is likely) the 2ⁿᵈ dose of warfarin is 5 or 10mg at 18.00 (24h after first dose). Give the lower dose if >60yrs, liver disease, or cardiac failure. But if INR >1.8 (warfarin sensitivity; rare) give just 0.5mg.
- Do INR daily for 5d and adjust dose (see BOX 2—use 5mg, not 10mg dose 3 if over 60, or liver disease, or cardiac failure).
- Stop heparin after 5d and when INR >2 for 2d. Tell lab when stopped.
- Measure INR on alternate days until stable, then weekly or less often.

**Antidotes** If UFH overdose: stop infusion. If there is bleeding, protamine sulfate counteracts UFH: discuss with a haematologist. Warfarin: see BOX 2.

## Warfarin guidelines and target levels for INR[1]

- Pulmonary embolism and DVT. Aim for INR of 2-3; 3.5 if recurrent.
- Atrial fibrillation[2]: for stroke prevention (p124). Target INR 2-3. An alternative is aspirin (but less effective), if the risk of bleeding with warfarin is high (eg falls with risk of intracranial bleed, or difficulty with monitoring). Target INR 2-3.
- Prosthetic metallic heart valves: for stroke prevention. Target INR 3-4.

### Duration of anticoagulation in DVT/PE

- If the cause will go away (eg post-op immobility):
  - At least 6 weeks for below knee DVT.
  - At least 3 months for above knee DVT or PE.
- At least 6 months if no cause found.
- Indefinitely for identified, enduring causes, eg thrombophilia (p368).

## Warfarin dosage and what to do when the INR is much too high

Below is a rough guide to warfarin dosing for target INR of 2-3; see text opposite.

| INR | <2 | 2 | 2.5 | 2.9 | 3.3 | 3.6 | 4.1 |
|---|---|---|---|---|---|---|---|
| 3rd dose | 10mg | 5mg | 4mg | 3mg | 2mg | 0.5mg | 0mg |
| Maintenance | ≥6mg | 5.5mg | 4.5mg | 4mg | 3.5mg | 3mg | * |

*Miss a dose; give 1-2mg the next day; if INR >4.5, miss 2 doses.

*When the INR is much too high:*                                  (see also *BNF*)

| INR 4.5-6 | Reduce warfarin dose or omit. Restart when INR <5. |
|---|---|
| 6-8 | Stop warfarin. Restart when INR <5. |
| >8, no or minor bleed, or epistaxis | If no bleeding: stop warfarin. 0.5-2.5mg vitamin K (oral) if risk factors for bleeding. Check INR daily. |
| Any major bleed (including intracranial haemorrhage) | Stop warfarin. Give prothrombin complex concentrate 50units/kg; discuss with haematologist. If unavailable, give FFP (15mL/kg≈1L for a 70kg man). Also give 5-10mg vitamin K IV slowly. |

Vitamin K may take some hours to work and can cause prolonged resistance when restarting warfarin, so avoid if possible when long-term anticoagulation is needed. Prothrombin complex concentrate contains a concentrate of factor IX, and provides a more complete and rapid reversal of warfarin than FFP.

## IV heparin dosing

| APTT ratio | >5 | 4-5 | 3-4 | 2.5-3 | 1.5-2.5 | 1.2-1.4 | <1.2 |
|---|---|---|---|---|---|---|---|
| Change rate (iu/h) by | -500* | -300 | -100 | -50 | 0 | +200 | +400 |

*Stop for 1 hour then recheck APTT. Reduce dose by 500iu/h and restart if <5.

1 Brit. Committee for Standards in Haematology. Guidelines on Oral Anticoagulation (Warfarin): 3e 2005.
2 For QALY-based decision analysis on who needs warfarin in AF, see R Thomson *Lancet* 355 956.

Leukaemia divides into 4 main types depending on the cell line involved:

| | Lymphoid | Myeloid |
|---|---|---|
| Acute | Acute lymphoblastic leukaemia (ALL) | Acute myeloid leukaemia (AML) |
| Chronic | Chronic lymphocytic leukaemia (CLL) | Chronic myeloid leukaemia (CML) |

These patients (esp. AML) fall ill suddenly and deteriorate fast, eg with: ▶▶Infection ▶▶Bleeding (R: platelets ± FFP) and ▶▶Hypervisosity (p366). Take nonspecific confusion/drowsiness or just "I feel a bit ill today" *seriously* (may be dead tomorrow): do blood cultures, glucose U&E, LFT, $Ca^{2+}$ and clotting. Consider CNS bleeding—CT/MRI if in doubt. With any new patient, find out the agreed aim of treatment: cure; prolonging disease-free survival; or palliation with minimal toxicity? Direct your efforts accordingly; get help if lack of clarity here.

**Neutropenic regimen** (for when neutrophil count ≤0.5 × 10⁹/L). ▶Close liaison with a microbiologist and haematologist is vital. Abide by infection control procedures! Use a *risk-assessment tool* (eg MASCC, see BOX).[64]
• Full barrier nursing if possible. Hand-washing is vital. Use a side room.
• Avoid IM injections (danger of an infected haematoma).
• Look for infection (mouth, axilla, perineum, IVI site). Take swabs.
• Check: FBC, platelets, INR, U&E, LFT, LDH, CRP. Take cultures (blood × 3—peripherally ± Hickman line; urine; sputum, stool if diarrhoea). CXR if clinically indicated.
• Wash perineum after defecation. Swab moist skin with chlorhexidine. Avoid unnecessary rectal examinations. Oral hygiene (eg hydrogen peroxide mouth washes/2h) and *Candida* prophylaxis are important (p238).
• TPR (vital signs) 4-hrly. High-calorie diet; avoid foods with high risk of microbial contamination. Vases containing cut flowers pose a *Pseudomonas* risk.

**Use of antibiotics in neutropenia** ▶Treat any known infection promptly.
• If t° >38°C or t° >37.5°C on 2 occasions, >1h apart, or the patient is toxic, assume septicaemia and start blind combination therapy—eg piperacillin-tazobactam—p378(+ vancomycin, p381, if Gram +ve organisms suspected or isolated, eg Hickman line sepsis). Check local preferences. Continue until afebrile for 72h or 5d course, and until neutrophils >0.5×10⁹/L. If fever persists despite antibiotics, think of CMV, fungi (eg *Candida; Aspergillus*, p440) and central line infection.
• Consider treatment for *Pneumocystis* (p411, eg co-trimoxazole, ie trimethoprim 20mg/kg + sulfamethoxazole 100mg/kg/day PO/IV in 2 daily doses). Remember TB.

**Other dangers** •*Tumour lysis syndrome:* Caused by a massive destruction of cells leading to K⁺↑, urate↑ and renal injury. *Risk↑* if: LDH↑, creatinine↑, urate↑, WCC >25×10⁹/L.[65] *Prevention:* high fluid intake + allopurinol pre-cytotoxics. For those at high risk of cell lysis, recombinant uricase (rasburicase) may be given. Seek advice.
• *Hypervisosity:* (p366). If WCC >100×10⁹/L WBC thrombi may form in brain, lung, and heart (leukostasis). Avoid transfusing before lowering WCC, eg with hydroxycarbamide or leukopheresis, as viscosity rises (risk of leukostasis↑).
• *DIC:* Widespread activation of coagulation, from release of procoagulants into the circulation with consumption of clotting factors and platelets, with ↑risk of bleeding. Fibrin strands fill small vessels, haemolysing passing RBCs, and fibrinolysis is also activated. *Causes:* Malignancy, sepsis, trauma, obstetric events: OHCS p88. *Signs:* (fig 1) Bruising, bleeding anywhere (eg venepuncture sites), renal failure. *Tests:* Platelets↓; PTT↑; APTT↑; fibrinogen↓ (correlates with severity); fibrin degradation products (D-dimers) ↑↑. Film: broken RBCs (schistocytes). R: Treat the cause. Replace platelets if <50×10⁹/L, cryoprecipitate to replace fibrinogen, FFP to replace coagulation factors. Heparin is controversial. Activated protein C reduces mortality in DIC with severe sepsis or multi-organ failure.[66] The use of all-transretinoic acid (ATRA) has significantly reduced the risk of DIC in acute promyelocytic leukaemia (the commonest leukaemia associated with DIC).
• *Preventing sepsis:* Fluoroquinolone (eg ciprofloxacin) before neutropenia gets serious; granulocyte colony stimulators¹ are of limited use (NICE says often not cost effective).[67] Herpes, pneumocystis and CMV (valganciclovir) prophylaxis have a role.[68]

---

1 Neutrophil production: genetically engineered recombinant human granulocyte-colony stimulating factor (G-CSF)—glycosylated lenograstim and non-glycosylated filgrastim. Follow guidelines/expert advice.

If the total score is ≥21, risk of septic complications is low (home-care is ?ok):

- Solid tumour or lymphoma with no previous fungal infection   4
- Outpatient status at onset of fever (not needing admission)   3
- Age <60yrs   2
- Burden of illness:   Mild (or no) symptoms   5
                    Moderate symptoms   3
                    Severe symptoms   0
- No hypotension (systolic BP >90mmHg)   5
- No COPD   4
- No dehydration   3

Although recommended by NICE, scores can never be validated for 2 reasons:

**1** You can never be *sure* a vital variable has not been left out of the score (why is CRP ignored, when its failure to fall after starting antibiotics is known to predict treatment failure?).[69]

**2** There are many ways to reach a score of 10 (say), some with severe symptoms, some with none, for example—they won't all have the same prognosis (the non-parametric paradox, p10, ie the score produces only numerals, not true numbers, and these numerals cannot be added, multiplied, divided, or even ranked).

Haematology

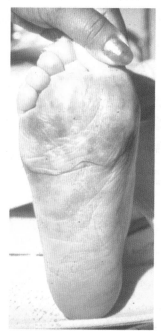

**Fig 1.** The appearance of disseminated intra-vascular coagulation (DIC) on the sole.
Courtesy of the Crookston collection.

This is a malignancy of lymphoid cells, affecting B or T lymphocyte cell lines, arresting maturation and promoting uncontrolled proliferation of immature blast cells, with marrow failure and tissue infiltration. It is thought to develop from a combination of genetic susceptibility (eg with translocations, and gains and losses of whole chromosomes[1]) + an environmental trigger. Ionizing radiation, eg x-rays, during pregnancy, and Down's syndrome are important associations.[70] It is the commonest cancer of childhood, and is rare in adults. CNS involvement is common.

**Classification** is based on 3 systems:

1 *Morphological* The FAB system (French, American, British) divides ALL into 3 types (L1, L2, L3) by microscopic appearance. Provides limited information (figs 1-4).
2 *Immunological* Surface markers are used to classify ALL into:
   • Precursor B-cell ALL • T-cell ALL • B-cell ALL.
3 *Cytogenetic* Chromosomal analysis. Abnormalities are detected in up to 85%, which are often translocations. Useful for predicting prognosis, eg poor with Philadelphia (Ph) chromosome (below), and for detecting disease recurrence.

**Signs and symptoms** (fig 5) are due to:
• Marrow failure: Anaemia ($\downarrow$Hb), infection ($\downarrow$WCC), and bleeding ($\downarrow$platelets).
• Infiltration: Hepato- and splenomegaly, lymphadenopathy—superficial or mediastinal, orchidomegaly, CNS involvement—eg cranial nerve palsies, meningism.

*Common infections:* Especially chest, mouth, perianal and skin. Bacterial septicaemia, zoster, CMV, measles, candidiasis, *Pneumocystis* pneumonia (p410).

**Tests** • Characteristic blast cells on blood film and bone marrow. WCC usually high.
• CXR and CT scan to look for mediastinal and abdominal lymphadenopathy.
• Lumbar puncture should be performed to look for CNS involvement.

**Treatment** ☺ Educate and motivate: without this, many may shy away from the responsibilities of self-care, to their detriment.[71] Interactive video games help.[72]
• *Support:* Blood/platelet transfusion, IV fluids, allopurinol (prevents tumour lysis syndrome). Insert a subcutaneous port system/Hickman line for IV access.[73]
• *Infections:* These are dangerous, due to neutropenia caused by the disease and treatment. Immediate IV antibiotics for infection. Start the neutropenic regimen (p346): prophylactic antivirals, antifungals and antibiotics, eg co-trimoxazole to prevent *Pneumocystis* pneumonia (p346), but beware: can worsen neutropenia.
• *Chemotherapy:* Patients are entered into national trials. A typical programme is:
   *Remission induction:* eg vincristine, prednisolone, L-asparaginase + daunorubicin.
   *Consolidation:* High-medium-dose therapy in 'blocks' over several weeks.
   *CNS prophylaxis:* Intrathecal (or high-dose IV) methotrexate ± CNS irradiation.
   *Maintenance:* Prolonged chemotherapy, eg mercaptopurine (daily), methotrexate (weekly), and vincristine + prednisolone (monthly) for 2yrs. Relapse is common in blood, CNS, or testis (examine these sites at follow-up). More details: OHCS p194.
• *Matched related allogeneic marrow transplantations* once in 1st remission is the best option in standard-risk younger adults (?too many SE if older).[74, 75]

*Haematological remission* means no evidence of leukaemia in the blood, a normal or recovering blood count, and <5% blasts in a normal regenerating marrow.

**Prognosis** Cure rates for children are 70-90%; for adults only 40% (higher when imatinib/rituximab, p353, are used). Poor prognosis if: adult, male, Philadelphia chromosome (p352): BCR-ABL gene fusion due to translocation of chromosomes 9 and 22, presentation with CNS signs, Hb$\downarrow$[76] or WCC >100×10$^9$/L or B-cell ALL. PCR is used to detect minimal residual disease, undetectable by standard means. Prognosis is poor if seen in high amounts at presentation or during remission. Prognosis in relapsed Ph-negative ALL is poor (improvable by marrow transplant).[77]

**Personalized treatment** ▶*One size does not fit all!*[78] Aim to tailor therapy to the exact gene defect, and according to individual metabolism. Monoclonal antibodies, gene-targeted retinoids, cytokines, vaccines, and T-cell infusions are relevant here.[79] Biomarkers, eg thiopurine methyltransferase, can predict toxicity from thiopurines.

---

1 Eg t(12;21) ETV6-RUNX1, t(1;19) TCF3-PBX1, t(9;22) BCR-ABL1—and rearrangement of MLL.

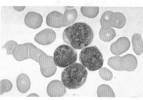

**Fig 1.** Blood film in ALL, L1 subtype. Small blasts with scanty cytoplasm.

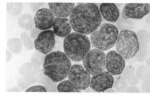

**Fig 2.** Bone marrow in ALL, L1 subtype.

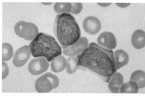

**Fig 3.** Blood film in ALL, L2 subtype. Larger blast cells with greater morphological variation and more abundant cytoplasm.

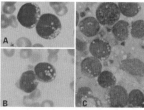

**Fig 4.** ALL L3. Blasts with vacuolated basophilic cytoplasm. A and B: blood films. C: lymph node.

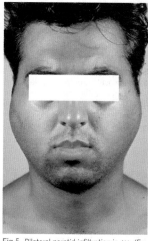

**Fig 5.** Bilateral parotid infiltration in ALL. (Enlarged salivary glands are also seen in mumps, HIV, bulimia, myxoedema, etc., p596.)

Figs 1, 2, 3, and 5 courtesy of Prof. Christine Lawrence; fig 4 courtesy of Prof. Tangün & Dr Köroğlu.

This neoplastic proliferation of blast cells is derived from marrow myeloid elements. It progresses rapidly (death in ~2 months if untreated; ~20% 3yr survival after R̲).

**Incidence** The commonest acute leukaemia of adults (1/10,000/yr; increases with age). AML can be a long-term complication of chemotherapy, eg for lymphoma. Also associated with myelodysplastic states (BOX), radiation, and syndromes, eg Down's.

**Morphological classification** There is much heterogeneity.[1] Now based on WHO histological classification, which is complex and requires specialist interpretation. It recognizes the important prognostic information from cytogenetics and molecular genetics.[1] 5 types:

1 AML with recurrent genetic abnormalities.
2 AML multilineage dysplasia (eg 2° to pre-existing myelodysplastic syndrome).
3 AML, therapy related.
4 AML, other.
5 Acute leukaemias of ambiguous lineage (both myeloid and lymphoid phenotype).

**Symptoms** •*Marrow failure:* Symptoms of anaemia, infection or bleeding. DIC occurs in acute promyelocytic leukaemia, a subtype of AML, where there is release of thromboplastin. Use of all-transretinoic acid with chemotherapy ↓risk of DIC (p346). •*Infiltration:* Hepatomegaly and splenomegaly, gum hypertrophy (fig 3), skin involvement. CNS involvement at presentation is rare in AML.

**Diagnosis** WCC is often ↑, but can be normal or even low. Blast cells may be few in the peripheral blood, so diagnosis depends on bone marrow biopsy. Differentiation from ALL may be by microscopy (figs 1, 2, 4; Auer rods are diagnostic of AML), but is now based on immunophenotyping and molecular methods. Cytogenetic analysis (eg type of mutation) affects treatment recommendations, and guides prognosis.[1]

**Complications** •Infection is the major problem, related to both the disease and during treatment. Be alert to septicaemia (p346). Infections may be bacterial, fungal or viral, and prophylaxis is given for each during therapy. *Pitfalls:* AML itself causes fever, common organisms present oddly, few antibodies are made, rare organisms—particularly fungi (esp. *Candida* or *Aspergillus*). •Chemotherapy causes ↑plasma urate levels (from tumour lysis)—so give allopurinol with chemotherapy, and keep well hydrated with IV fluids. •Leukostasis (p346) may occur if WCC ↑↑.

**Treatment** •*Supportive care* As for ALL. Walking exercises can relieve fatigue.[80]

•*Chemotherapy* is very intensive, resulting in long periods of marrow suppression with neutropenia + platelets↓. The main drugs used include *daunorubicin* and *cytarabine*, with ~5 cycles given in 1-week blocks to get a remission (RAS mutations occur in ~20% of patients with AML and enhance sensitivity to cytarabine).[81]

•*Bone marrow transplant (BMT)* Pluripotent haematopoietic stem cells are collected from the marrow. *Allogeneic* transplants from HLA-matched siblings or matched unrelated donors (held on international databases) are indicated during 1st remission in disease with poor prognosis. The idea is to destroy leukaemic cells and the immune system by cyclophosphamide + total body irradiation, and then repopulate the marrow by transplantation from a matched donor infused IV. BMT allows the most intensive chemotherapy regimens because marrow suppression is not an issue. Ciclosporin ± methotrexate are used to reduce the effect of the new marrow attacking the patient's body (graft vs host disease).

*Complications:* Graft vs host disease (may help explain the curative effect of BMT); opportunistic infections; relapse of leukaemia; infertility.

*Prognosis:* Lower relapse rates ~60% long-term survivors, but significant mortality of ~10%. Autologous BMT where stem cells are taken from the patient themselves, is used in intermediate prognosis disease, although some studies suggest better survival rates with intensive chemotherapy regimens.

*Autologous mobilized peripheral blood stem cell transplantation* may offer faster haemopoietic recovery and less morbidity.[82]

•Supportive care, or lower-dose chemotherapy for disease control, may be more appropriate in elderly patients, where intensive therapies have poorer outcomes.

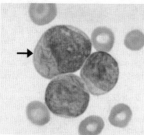

Fig 1. Auer rods (crystals of coalesced granules) found in AML myeloblast cells.

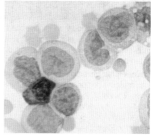

Fig 2. AML with monoblasts and myeloblasts on the peripheral blood film.

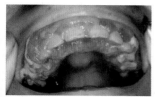

Fig 3. Gum hypertrophy in AML.

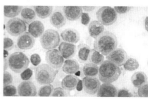

Fig 4. Marrow in AML: multiple monoblasts.

Images on this page are courtesy of Professor Christine Lawrence.

## Myelodysplastic syndromes (MDS, myelodysplasia)

These are a heterogeneous group of disorders that manifest as marrow failure with risk of life-threatening infection and bleeding. Most are primary disorders, but they may also develop secondary to chemotherapy or radiotherapy. 30% transform to acute leukaemia. *Tests:* Pancytopenia (p358), with ↓reticulocyte count. Marrow cellularity is usually increased due to ineffective haematopoiesis. Ring sideroblasts may also be seen in the marrow (fig 5, p321). There are different subtypes, grouped according to WHO classification.

*Treatment:*
• Multiple transfusions of red cells or platelets as needed.
• Erythropoietin ± human granulocyte colony stimulating factor (G-CSF) may lower transfusion requirement.
• Immunosuppressives are also used, eg ciclosporin or antithymocyte globulins.
• Curative allogeneic stem cell transplantation is one option—often inappropriate owing to age-related comorbidities—most are >70yrs old.
• Thalidomide analogues such as lenalidomide have a role, eg in low-risk MDS with 5q deletions. Hypomethylating agents (eg azacytidine and decitabine) have a role in symptomatic MDS (these target epigenetic changes in MDS).

*Prognosis:* Median survival: from 6 months to 6 years according to disease type.

1 4 types of heterogeneity: morphology, immunophenotype, cytogenetics, and molecular abnormality. Genome-wide technologies enable an ever more detailed molecular analysis of AML and this feeds into risk stratification of AML. Epigenetic and other profiling reveals more and more biomarkers, eg mutations in the genes encoding DNA (cytosine-5)-methyltransferase 3α (DNMT3A).[1]

CML is characterized by an uncontrolled clonal proliferation of myeloid cells (fig 1). It accounts for 15% of leukaemias. It is a myeloproliferative disorder (p360) having features in common with these diseases, eg splenomegaly. It occurs most often between 40–60yrs, with a slight male predominance, and is rare in childhood.

**Philadelphia chromosome** (Ph) Present in >80% of those with CML. It is a hybrid chromosome comprising reciprocal translocation between the long arm of chromosome 9 and the long arm of chromosome 22—t(9;22)—forming a fusion gene BCR/ABL on chromosome 22, which has tyrosine kinase activity. Those without Ph have a worse prognosis. Some patients have a masked translocation—cytogenetics do not show the Ph, but the rearrangement is detectable by molecular techniques.

**Symptoms** Mostly chronic and insidious: weight↓, tiredness, fever, sweats. There may be features of gout (due to purine breakdown), bleeding (platelet dysfunction), and abdominal discomfort (splenic enlargement). ~30% are detected by chance.

**Signs** Splenomegaly (>75%)—often massive. Hepatomegaly, anaemia, bruising (fig 2).

**Tests** WBC↑↑ (often >100×10$^9$/L) with whole spectrum of myeloid cells, ie ↑neutrophils, myelocytes, basophils, eosinophils. Hb↓ or normal, platelets variable. Urate↑, B$_{12}$↑. Neutrophil alk phos score↓ (seldom performed now). Bone marrow is hypercellular. Ph found on cytogenetic analysis of blood or bone marrow.

**Natural history** Variable, median survival 5–6yrs. There are 3 phases: *chronic*, lasting months or years of few, if any, symptoms → *accelerated phase*, with increasing symptoms, spleen size, and difficulty in controlling counts → *blast transformation*, with features of acute leukaemia ± death. **Treatment** See BOX.

## Chronic lymphocytic leukaemia (CLL)

Accumulation of mature B cells that have escaped programmed cell death and undergone cell-cycle arrest in the G0/G1 phase is the hallmark of CLL. It is the commonest leukaemia (>25%; incidence: ~4/100,000/yr). ♂:♀≈2:1. Mutations, trisomies and deletions (eg del17p13) influence risk; pneumonia may be a triggering event.[84]

| Rai stage: | 0 | Lymphocytosis alone | Median survival >13yrs |
|---|---|---|---|
| | I | Lymphocytosis + lymphadenopathy | 8yrs |
| | II | Lymphocytosis + spleno- or hepatomegaly | 5yrs |
| | III | Lymphocytosis + anaemia (Hb <110g/L) | 2yrs |
| | IV | Lymphocytosis + platelets <100 × 10$^9$/L | 1yr |

**Symptoms** Often none, presenting as a surprise finding on a routine FBC (eg done pre-op). May be anaemic or infection-prone. If severe: weight↓, sweats, anorexia.

**Signs** Enlarged, rubbery, non-tender nodes (fig 3). Splenomegaly, hepatomegaly.

**Tests** ↑Lymphocytes—may be marked (fig 4). Later: autoimmune haemolysis (p332), marrow infiltration: ↓Hb, ↓neutrophils, ↓platelets.

**Complications** 1 Autoimmune haemolysis. 2 ↑Infection due to hypogammaglobulinaemia (=↓↓IgG), bacterial, viral especially herpes zoster. 3 Marrow failure.

**Natural history** Some remain in *status quo* for years, or even regress. Usually nodes slowly enlarge (± lymphatic obstruction). Death is often due to infection (commonly pneumococcus, haemophilus, meningococcus, *Candida* or aspergillosis), or transformation to aggressive lymphoma (Richter's syndrome).

**Treatment** Consider drugs if: •Symptomatic •Immunoglobulin genes (IgVH) are unmutated •17p deletions (consider intensive ℞). *Fludarabine + cyclophosphamide + rituximab* if 1$^{st}$ line[85] (there is synergism).[86] *Bendamustine, alemtuzumab,* and *ofatumumab* may have a role (the latter is "not cost effective").[87,88]-NICE *Steroids* help autoimmune haemolysis. *Radiotherapy* helps treat lymphadenopathy and splenomegaly. *Supportive care:* Transfusions, IV human immunoglobulin if recurrent infection. *Relapsed disease:* One option is rituximab + dexamethasone (R-DEX). R-DEX can also be used to debulk before a *stem-cell transplant.*[89]

**Prognosis** ⅓ never progress, ⅓ progress slowly, and ⅓ progress actively. CD23 and β2 microglobulin correlate with bulk of disease and rates of progression.

## 35

## Treating CML

CML is the first example of a cancer where knowledge of the genotype has led to a rationally designed drug—*imatinib* (Glivec®), a specific BCR-ABL tyrosine kinase inhibitor, which has transformed therapy over the last 10yrs.[90]

More potent 2nd-generation BCR-ABL inhibitors: *dasatinib, nilotinib, bosutinib* and *ponatinib*. Dasatinib and nilotinib allow more patients to achieve deeper, more rapid responses associated with improved outcomes[91] (NICE says that dasatinib is often not cost-effective).[92] Imatinib SE: usually mild: nausea, cramps, oedema, rash, headache, arthralgia. May cause myelosuppression. Dasatinib has been used in imatinib-resistant blast crises. *Hydroxycarbamide* is also used.

Those with lymphoblastic transformation may benefit from treatment as for ALL. Treatment of myeloblastic transformation with chemotherapy rarely achieves lasting remission, and allogeneic transplantation offers the best hope.

*Stem cell transplantation* Allogeneic transplantation from an HLA-matched sibling or unrelated donor offers the only cure, but carries significant morbidity and mortality. Guidelines suggest that this approach should be used 1st line only in young patients where mortality rates are lower. Other patients should be offered imatinib. Patients are then reviewed annually to decide whether to continue imatinib, or to offer combination therapy or stem cell transplantation.

The role of autologous transplantation, if any, in CML remains to be defined.

Haematology

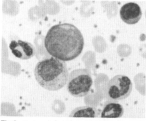

Fig 1. CML: numerous granulocytic cells at different stages of differentiation.

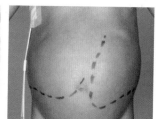

Fig 2. Hepatosplenomegaly in CML.

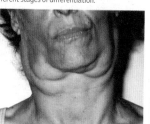

Fig 3. Bilateral cervical lymphadenopathy in CLL.

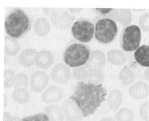

Fig 4. CLL: many lymphocytes and a 'smear' cell: a fragile cell damaged in preparation.

Figs 2 and 4 courtesy of Professor Christine Lawrence.

Haematology

Lymphomas are disorders caused by malignant proliferations of lymphocytes. These accumulate in the lymph nodes causing lymphadenopathy, but may also be found in peripheral blood or infiltrate organs. Lymphomas are histologically divided into Hodgkin's and non-Hodgkin's types. In Hodgkin's lymphoma, characteristic cells with mirror-image nuclei are found, called Reed-Sternberg cells (figs 1, 2, 3).

**Incidence** 2 peaks of incidence: young adults[1] and elderly. ♂:♀ ≈ 2:1. Risk↑ if: an affected sibling; EBV (p401); SLE; post-transplantation;[93] westernization;[93] obese.[94]

**Symptoms** Often presents with enlarged, painless, non-tender, 'rubbery' superficial lymph nodes, typically cervical (60–70%), also axillary or inguinal nodes (fig 4). Node size may increase and decrease spontaneously, and nodes can become matted. 25% have constitutional upset, eg fever, weight loss, night sweats, pruritus, and lethargy. There may be alcohol-induced lymph node pain. Mediastinal lymph node involvement can cause features due to mass effect, eg bronchial or SVC obstruction (p526), or direct extension, eg causing pleural effusions. *Pel-Ebstein fever* implies a cyclical fever with long periods (15–28 days) of normal or low temperature: it is, at best, rare.[2]

**Signs** Lymph node enlargement. Also, cachexia, anaemia, spleno- or hepatomegaly.

**Tests** *Tissue diagnosis:* Lymph node excision biopsy if possible. Image-guided needle biopsy, laparotomy or mediastinoscopy may be needed to obtain a sample. *Bloods* FBC, film, ESR, LFT, LDH, urate, $Ca^{2+}$. ↑ESR or ↓Hb indicate a worse prognosis. LDH is raised as it is released during cell turnover. PET (p753) also has an uncertain role.[95]

**Staging** (Ann Arbor system) Influences treatment and prognosis. Done by CXR, CT/PET of thorax, abdo, pelvis ± marrow biopsy if B symptoms, or stage III–IV disease.

　I　Confined to single lymph node region.
　II　Involvement of two or more nodal areas on the same side of the diaphragm.
　III　Involvement of nodes on both sides of the diaphragm.
　IV　Spread beyond the lymph nodes, eg liver or bone marrow.

Each stage is either 'A'—no systemic symptoms other than pruritus; or 'B'—presence of B symptoms: weight loss >10% in last 6 months, unexplained fever >38°C, or night sweats (needing change of clothes). 'B' indicates worse disease. Localized extra-nodal extension does not advance the stage, but is indicated by subscripted 'E', eg I-AE.

**Chemoradiotherapy** Radiotherapy[2] ± short courses of chemotherapy for stages I-A and II-A (eg with ≤3 areas involved). Longer courses of chemotherapy for II-A with >3 areas involved through to IV-B. 'ABVD': Adriamycin, Bleomycin, Vinblastine, Dacarbazine (+ radiotherapy in younger patients) cures ~80% of patients.[96] More intensive regimens are used if poor prognosis or advanced disease.[3] In relapsed disease, high-dose chemotherapy with peripheral stem-cell transplants may be used, involving autologous (or occasionally allogeneic) transplantation of peripheral blood progenitor cells to restore marrow function after therapy.[97]

*Complications of treatment:* See p528-9: Radiotherapy may ↑ risk of second malignancies—solid tumours (especially lung and breast, also melanoma, sarcoma, stomach and thyroid cancers), ischaemic heart disease, hypothyroidism and lung fibrosis due to the radiation field. Chemotherapy SE include myelosuppression, nausea, alopecia, infection. AML (p350), non-Hodgkin's lymphoma and infertility may be due to both chemo- and radiotherapy—see p531.

**5-year survival** Depends on stage and grade: >95% in I-A lymphocyte-predominant disease; <40% with IV-B lymphocyte-depleted.

**Emergency presentations** Infection; SVC obstruction—JVP↑, sensation of fullness in the head, dyspnoea, blackouts, facial oedema (seek expert help; see p526).

---

1 HL is the leading cause of malignancy if aged 15-24yrs (+ gonadal germ-cell tumours♂ and melanoma).[18]
2 Pel-Ebstein fever is dismissed by Richard Asher (*Talking Sense*) as existing only thanks to its exotic name (the 1885 patients of Dr P Pel had no histology, and fevers in Hodgkin's are *usually* non-specific). Another unfair reason for consigning it to myth is that the paper proving its relation to cyclical changes in node size doesn't come up in literature searches as Wilhelm *Ebstein* was spelled *Epstein* throughout.[8]
3 Eg BEACOPP (bleomycin/etoposide/doxorubicin/cyclophosphamide/vincristine/procarbazine/prednisone). In IIB, III, or IV, BEACOPP gives better initial control, but 7yr event free survival is similar: 78% *vs* 71%.[100] *Radiotherapy* can be guided by PET: extended field is no better (and has more SE) than involved field.[101]

| Classification (in order of incidence) | Prognosis |
|---|---|
| *Classical Hodgkin's lymphoma* | |
| Nodular sclerosing | Good |
| Mixed cellularity* | Good |
| Lymphocyte rich | Good |
| Lymphocyte depleted* | Poor |

NB: nodular lymphocyte predominant Hodgkin's is recognized as a separate entity, behaving as an indolent B-cell lymphoma.
*Higher incidence and worse prognosis if HIV +ve.

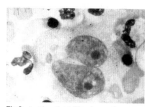

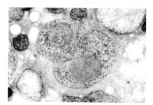

Fig 1. A Reed-Sternberg cell with 2 nuclei, characteristic of Hodgkin's lymphoma.
Courtesy of Professor Christine Lawrence.

Fig 2. Another Reed-Sternberg cell.
Courtesy of the Crookston collection.

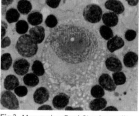

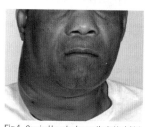

Fig 3. Mononuclear Reed-Sternberg cell in a lymph node.

Fig 4. Cervical lymphadenopathy in Hodgkin's disease.
©Prof. Tangün and Dr Köroğlu

Haematology

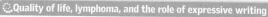

## Quality of life, lymphoma, and the role of expressive writing

Being treated for Hodgkin's disease is arduous. Our job is often to give encouragement—the more this is personalized for our individual patient the better.

One method is to encourage our patients to write about their experiences. In one study this gave clear-cut benefits in lymphoma patients. Participants report positive responses to writing, and post-writing half said that writing changed their thoughts about their illness in a positive way (this increased on subsequent follow-up). Textual analysis identifies themes related to experiences of positive change, transformation, and self-affirmation through reflection.[102,103] These techniques are akin to those used in post-traumatic stress—and remind us that some of our treatments are as destabilizing to our patients as any shipwreck, rape, or earthquake. See http://mylymphomastory.com for how to avoid self-pity despite the odds. "I can whine, I can complain, I can moan, and b*tch, about all of the above, but I won't.... The true feat isn't escaping death, rather, learning how to live."

Sometimes narrating lymphoma experiences reveals bitterness, loss of control, and a feeling that life has been rendered void.[104] Here our role is to receive these negatives and to try to keep the channels of communication open, as dialogue is the only validated means of filling these voids. The need to enhance support networks and bolster social ties may trump all our pharmacological imperatives.[105]

Haematology

This includes all lymphomas without Reed-Sternberg cells (p354)—a diverse group. Most are derived from B-cell lines; diffuse large B-cell lymphoma (DLBCL) is commonest.[106] Not all centre on nodes (extranodal tissues generating lymphoma include mucosa-associated lymphoid tissue, eg gastric MALT, below). Incidence has doubled since 1970 (to 1:10,000). *Causes:* Immunodeficiency—drugs; HIV (usually high-grade lymphoma from EBV transformed cells, p401); HTLV-1, p376; *H.pylori*; toxins; congenital.

**The patient** • Nodal disease (75% at presentation): superficial lymphadenopathy.
• Extranodal disease (25%)—*Skin:* T-cell lymphomas: Sézary syndrome (p598 & fig 1).
*Oropharynx:* Waldeyer's ring lymphoma causes sore throat/obstructed breathing.
*Gut:* 1 *Gastric MALT* is caused by *H.pylori*, and may regress with its eradication (p401). Symptoms: like gastric Ca, with systemic features (fever, sweats). MALT usually involves the antrum, is multifocal, and metastasizes late.
2 *Non-MALT gastric lymphomas* (60%) are usually diffuse large-cell B lymphomas—high-grade and not responding well to *H.pylori* eradication.
3 *Small-bowel lymphomas* are IPSID (immunoproliferative small intestine disease), MALT or enteropathy/coeliac-associated intra-epithelial T-cell lymphoma—presents with diarrhoea, vomiting, abdominal pain, and weight↓. Poor prognosis.
*Other possible sites:* Bone, CNS, and lung.
• Systemic symptoms—fever, night sweats, weight loss (less common than in Hodgkin's lymphoma) and indicates disseminated disease).
• Pancytopenia from marrow involvement—anaemia, infection, bleeding (↓platelets).

**Tests** *Blood:* FBC, U&E, LFT. ↑LDH≈worse prognosis, reflecting ↑cell turnover. *Marrow and node biopsy* for classification (a complex, changing quagmire, based on the WHO system of high- or low-grade). *Staging* Ann Arbor system (p354)—CT/MRI of chest, abdomen, pelvis. Send *cytology* of any effusion; LP for CSF cytology if CNS signs.

**Diagnosis/management** is multidisciplinary, synthesizing details from clinical evaluation, histology, immunology, molecular genetics, and imaging. *Generally:*
• Low-grade lymphomas are indolent, often incurable and widely disseminated. Include: follicular lymphoma, marginal zone lymphoma/MALT, lymphocytic lymphoma (closely related to CLL and treated similarly), lymphoplasmacytoid lymphoma (produces IgM = Waldenström's macroglobulinaemia, p364). *See* fig 2.
• High-grade lymphomas are more aggressive, *but often curable.* There is often rapidly enlarging lymphadenopathy with systemic symptoms. Include: Burkitt's lymphoma (childhood disease with characteristic jaw lymphadenopathy; figs 3 & 4), lymphoblastic lymphomas (like ALL), diffuse large B-cell lymphoma.

**Treatment** Depends on disease subtype. *Low grade:* If symptomless, none may be needed. Radiotherapy may be curative in localized disease. *Chlorambucil* is used in diffuse disease. Remission may be maintained by using α-*interferon* or *rituximab* (see below). *Bendamustine* is effective both with rituximab and as a monotherapy in rituximab-refractory patients.[107] *High grade:* (eg large B-cell lymphoma, DLBCL), 'R-CHOP' regimen: *Rituximab Cyclophosphamide, Hydroxy-daunorubicin, vincristine (Oncovin®)* and *Prednisolone.* Granulocyte colony-stimulating factors (G-CSFs) help neutropenia—eg filgrastim or lenograstim (at low doses it may be cost-effective).[108]

**Survival** Histology is important. Prognosis is worse if at presentation: • Age >60yrs • Systemic symptoms • Bulky disease (abdominal mass >10cm) • ↑LDH • Disseminated disease. Typical 5-yr survival for treated patients: ~30% for high-grade and >50% for low-grade lymphomas, but the picture is very variable.

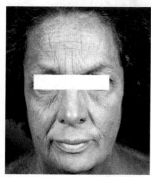

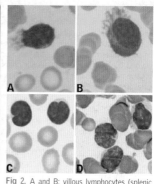

**Fig 1.** Cutaneous τ-cell lymphoma, which has caused severe erythroderma (Sézary syndrome) in a Caucasian woman.

Courtesy of Prof. Christine Lawrence.

**Fig 2.** A and B: villous lymphocytes (splenic marginal zone lymphoma). C: 'buttock cells' with cleaved nuclei (follicular lymphoma). D: Sézary cells with convoluted nuclei.

Courtesy of Prof. Tangün & Dr Köroğlu.

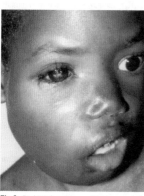

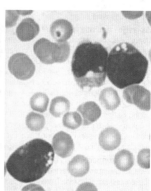

**Fig 3.** Burkitt's lymphoma, with characteristic jaw lymphadenopathy.

Courtesy of Dr Tom D Thacher.

**Fig 4.** Burkitt's lymphoma, with 3 basophilic vacuolated lymphoma cells.

Courtesy of Prof. Barbara Bain
©2005 Massachusetts Medical Society.

### The role of rituximab in untreated follicular lymphoma

Rituximab kills CD20+ve cells by antibody-directed cytotoxicity ± apoptosis induction. It also sensitizes cells to CHOP. It is cost-effective when used with:
- Cyclophosphamide, vincristine and prednisolone (CVP)
- Cyclophosphamide, doxorubicin, vincristine and prednisolone (CHOP)
- Cyclophosphamide, doxorubicin, etoposide, prednisolone & interferon-α (CHVPi)
- Mitoxantrone, chlorambucil and prednisolone (MCP)
- Chlorambucil.                                    NICE (2012 for STAGES III & IV)

It also has a role in maintaining remission, and in relapsed disease.

The marrow is responsible for haemopoiesis. In adults, this normally takes place in the central skeleton (vertebrae, sternum, ribs, skull) and proximal long bones. In some anaemias (eg thalassaemia), increased demand induces haematopoiesis beyond the marrow (extramedullary haematopoiesis), in liver and spleen, causing organomegaly. All blood cells arise from an early pluripotent stem cell, which divides in an asymmetrical way to produce another stem cell and a progenitor cell committed to a specific cell line. Committed progenitors further differentiate into myeloid or lymphocyte lineages, before their release into the blood as mature cells.

**Pancytopenia** is reduction in all the major cell lines: red cells, white cells and platelets. Causes are due to: 1 ↓*marrow production:* Aplastic anaemia, infiltration (eg acute leukaemia, myelodysplasia, myeloma, lymphoma, solid tumours, TB), megaloblastic anaemia, paroxysmal nocturnal haemoglobinuria (p332), myelofibrosis (p360), SLE. 2 ↑*peripheral destruction:* Hypersplenism.

**Agranulocytosis** implies that granulocytes (WBCs with neutrophil, basophil or eosinophil granules, fig 1) have stopped being made. Neutropenia (wcc ≤0.5×10⁹/L) may declare itself early as a sore throat (eg 2wks after starting the drug)[109] before some fatal infection: this is why we warn patients starting drugs causing agranulocytosis[1] "Report *any* fever". (Do FBC! Look at the result!! Stop the drug!!!) Granulocyte colony stimulating factor (G-CSF) + barrier nursing + neutropenia regimens (p346) may work.[110]

**Aplastic anaemia** is a rare stem cell disorder leading to pancytopenia and hypoplastic marrow (the marrow stops making cells). Presents with features of anaemia (↓Hb), infection (↓wcc) or bleeding (↓platelets). *Incidence:* ~5 cases per million/year. *Causes:* Most cases are autoimmune, triggered by drugs (viruses, eg parvovirus, hepatitis) or irradiation. May also be inherited, eg Fanconi anaemia (p712). *Tests:* Marrow examination is needed for the diagnosis. *Treatment:* Support the blood count (below). Asymptomatic patients don't need much except for supportive treatment (neutropenic regimen, p346). The treatment of choice in young patients who are severely affected is an allogeneic marrow transplantation from an HLA-matched sibling, which can be curative. Otherwise, immunosuppression with ciclosporin and antithymocyte globulin may be effective, although it is not curative in most. There is no clear role for G-CSF (p356).[111]

**Marrow support** Red cells survive for ~120d, platelets for ~8d, and neutrophils for 1-2d, so early problems are mainly from neutropenia and thrombocytopenia.

1 *Red cell transfusion:* Transfusing 1U should raise Hb by ~10-15g/L (p342). Transfusion may drop the platelet count (you may need to give platelets before or after).

2 *Platelets:* Traumatic bleeds, purpura and easy bruising occur if platelets <50×10⁹/L. Spontaneous bleeding may occur if platelets <20×10⁹/L, with intracranial haemorrhage rarely. Platelets are stored at room temperature (22°C; not in the fridge). In marrow transplant or if severely immunosuppressed, platelets may need irradiation before use to prevent transfusion-associated graft-versus-host disease (GVHD). Platelets must be ABO compatible. They are not used in ITP (p338). Indications: •Platelets <10×10⁹/L •Haemorrhage (eg DIC, p346) •Before invasive procedures (eg biopsy, lumbar puncture) to increase count to >50×10⁹/L. 4U of platelets should raise the count to >40×10⁹/L in adults; check dose needed with lab.

3 *Neutrophils:* Use a 'neutropenic regimen' if the count is 0.5×10⁹/L. See p346.

**Bone marrow biopsy** gives diagnostic information where there are abnormalities in the peripheral blood; it is also an important staging test in the lymphoproliferative disorders. Ideally take an aspirate *and* trephine usually from the posterior iliac crest (aspirates can be taken from the anterior iliac crest or sternum). The aspirate provides a film which is examined by microscope. The trephine is a core of bone which allows assessment of bone marrow cellularity, architecture and the presence of infiltrative disease (eg neoplasia). Coagulation disorders may need to be corrected pre-biopsy. Apply pressure afterwards (lie on that side for 1-2h if platelets are low).

---

1 Carbimazole, procainamide, sulfonamides, gold, clozapine, dapsone (antibody damage to stem cells).

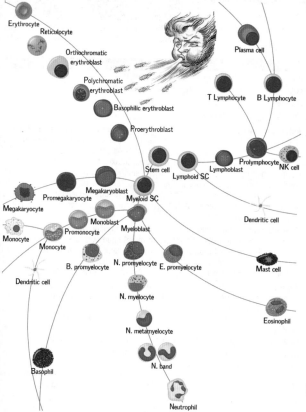

Erythrocyte

Reticulocyte

Orthochromatic erythroblast

Polychromatic erythroblast

Basophilic erythroblast

Proerythroblast

Plasma cell

T Lymphocyte   B Lymphocyte

Stem cell

Lymphoblast

Lymphoid SC

Prolymphocyte   NK cell

Megakaryoblast

Promegakaryocyte   Myeloid SC

Megakaryocyte

Monoblast

Promonocyte   Myeloblast

Dendritic cell

Monocyte

Monocyte

B. promyelocyte   N. promyelocyte   E. promyelocyte

Mast cell

Dendritic cell

N. myelocyte

Eosinophil

N. metamyelocyte

Basophil

N. band

Neutrophil

Fig 1. *Haemopoiesis and Sod's Law*. When we contemplate a diagram like this (of seemingly galactic complexity) we, being doctors, think "What can go wrong?" With a sinking feeling we realize that every arc is an opportunity for multiple disasters. Perhaps, using the Hammer of Los (p316) and our own ingenuity we might occasionally complete these pathways without Sod intervening (Sod's law states that if something can go wrong, it will—here Sod's tubercular breath is seen blowing the red cell line off course—TB is a famous cause of leukoerythroblastic anaemia). When we realize that *every day* each of us makes 175 billion red cells, 70 billion granulocytes, and 175 billion platelets[112] we sense that Sod is smiling to himself with especial relish. *Anything* can go wrong. *Everything* can go wrong. This latter we call *aplastic anaemia*. *Agranulocytosis* is when the Southerly arcs go wrong; thrombocytopenia when the West-pointing arcs go wrong. To the East we have the *lymphocytes* and their B- and T-cell complexities. *Anaemia* lies in the North of this diagram. And as for bleeding—how could our predecessors bear to waste a single drop of this stuff on purpose? Our minds are reeling at 175 billion red cells per day—but this is just when the system is idling. When we bleed, throughput can rise by an order of magnitude—if Sod is turning a blind eye are there are sufficient haematinics (eg iron, B₁₂ and folate) to allow maximum haemopoiesis?

Figure ©Aria Rad.

These are caused by proliferation of a clone of haematopoietic myeloid stem cells in the marrow. While the cells proliferate, they also retain the ability to differentiate into RBCs, WBCs or platelets.

| Classification is by the cell type which is proliferating | | |
|---|---|---|
| RBC | → | Polycythaemia rubra vera (PRV) |
| WBC | → | Chronic myeloid leukaemia (CML, p352) |
| Platelets | → | Essential thrombocythaemia |
| Fibroblasts | → | Myelofibrosis |

**Polycythaemia** may be relative (↓plasma volume, normal RBC mass) or absolute (↑RBC mass). *Relative polycythaemia* may be acute and due to dehydration (eg alcohol or diuretics). A more chronic form exists which is associated with obesity, hypertension, and a high alcohol and tobacco intake. *Absolute polycythaemia* is distinguished by red cell mass estimation using radioactive chromium ($^{51}Cr$) labelled RBCs. Causes are primary (*polycythaemia rubra vera*) or secondary due to hypoxia (eg high altitudes, chronic lung disease, cyanotic congenital heart disease, heavy smoking) or inappropriately ↑erythropoietin secretion (eg in renal carcinoma, hepatocellular carcinoma).

**Polycythaemia rubra vera** This is a malignant proliferation of a clone derived from one pluripotent marrow stem cell. A mutation in JAK2 (JAK2 V617F) is present in >90%. The erythroid progenitor offspring are unusual in not needing erythropoietin to avoid apoptosis (p511). There is excess proliferation of RBCs, WBCs, and platelets, leading to hyperviscosity and thrombosis. Commoner if >60yrs old.

*Signs* May be asymptomatic and detected on FBC, or present with vague signs due to hyperviscosity (p366): headaches, dizziness, tinnitus, visual disturbance. Itch after a hot bath, and erythromelalgia, a burning sensation in fingers and toes, are characteristic. Examination may show facial plethora and splenomegaly (in 60%). Gout may occur due to ↑urate from RBC turnover. Features of arterial (cardiac, cerebral, peripheral) or venous (DVT, cerebral, hepatic) thrombosis may be present.

*Investigations:* • FBC: ↑RCC, ↑Hb, ↑HCT, ↑PCV, often also ↑WBC and ↑platelets • B₁₂↑ • Marrow shows hypercellularity with erythroid hyperplasia • Neutrophil alkaline phosphatase (NAP) score is ↑ (↓ in CML) • ↓serum erythropoietin • Raised red cell mass on $^{51}Cr$ studies and splenomegaly, in the setting of a normal $P_aO_2$, is diagnostic.

*Treatment:* Aim to keep HCT <0.45 to ↓risk of thrombosis. In younger patients at low risk, this is done by venesection. If higher risk (age >60yrs, previous thrombosis), **hydroxycarbamide** (=hydroxyurea) is used. α-interferon is preferred in women of childbearing age. Low-dose aspirin 75mg daily PO is also given.◆

*Prognosis:* Variable, many remain well for years. Thrombosis and haemorrhage (due to defective platelets) are the main complications. Transition to myelofibrosis occurs in ~30% or acute leukaemia in ~5%. Monitor FBC every 3 months.

**Essential thrombocythaemia** A clonal proliferation of megakaryocytes leads to persistently ↑platelets, often >1000 × 10⁹/L, with abnormal function, causing bleeding or arterial and venous thrombosis, and microvascular occlusion—headache, atypical chest pain, light-headedness, erythromelalgia (fig 1). Exclude other causes of thrombocytosis (see BOX). *Treatment:* Low-dose aspirin 75mg daily.◆ Hydroxycarbamide is given to ↓platelets if >60yrs old or if previous thrombosis.

**Myelofibrosis** There is hyperplasia of megakaryocytes which produce platelet-derived growth factor, leading to intense marrow fibrosis and myeloid metaplasia (haemopoiesis in the spleen and liver)→massive hepatosplenomegaly. *Presentation:* Hypermetabolic symptoms: night sweats, fever, weight loss; abdominal discomfort due to splenomegaly; or bone marrow failure (↓Hb, infections, bleeding). *Film:* Leukoerythroblastic cells (nucleated red cells, p322); characteristic teardrop RBCs (see fig 2). Hb↓. Bone marrow trephine for diagnosis (fig 3). *Treatment:* Marrow support (see p358). Allogeneic stem cell transplant may be curative in young people but carries a high risk of mortality. *Prognosis:* Median survival 4-5 years.

## Causes of thrombocytosis

↑Platelets >450 × 10⁹/L may be a reactive phenomenon, seen with many conditions including:
- Bleeding
- Infection
- Chronic inflammation, eg collagen disorders
- Malignancy
- Trauma
- Post-surgery
- Iron deficiency

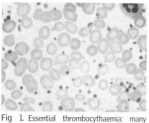

Fig 1. Essential thrombocythaemia: many platelets seen.

© Prof. Christine Lawrence.

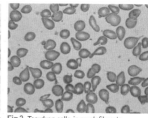

Fig 2. Teardrop cells, in myelofibrosis.

© Dr Nivaldo Medeiros.

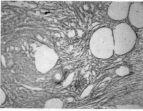

Fig 3. Marrow trephine in myelofibrosis: the streaming effect is caused by intense fibrosis. **Other causes of marrow fibrosis:** any myeloproliferative disorder, lymphoma, secondary carcinoma, TB, leukaemia, and irradiation.

© Professor Christine Lawrence.

Haematology

PCDs are due to an abnormal proliferation of a single clone of plasma or lympho-plasmacytic cells leading to secretion of immunoglobulin (Ig) or an Ig fragment, causing the dysfunction of many organs (esp kidney).[1] The Ig is seen as a mono-clonal band, or paraprotein, on serum or urine electrophoresis (see below).

**Classification** is based on immunoglobulin (Ig) product—IgG in ~⅔; IgA in ~⅓; A very few are IgM or IgD. Other Ig levels are low ('immunoparesis', causing ↑susceptibility to infection). In ~⅔, urine contains Bence Jones proteins, which are free Ig light chains of kappa (κ) or lambda (λ) type, filtered by the kidney.

**Incidence** 5/100,000. Peak age: 70yrs. ♂:♀≈1. Afro-Caribbeans:Caucasians≈2:1.

**Symptoms** ►Do serum protein electrophoresis & ESR on all over 50 with back pain.
• *Osteolytic bone lesions* causing backache, pathological fractures (eg long bones or ribs) and vertebral collapse. *Hypercalcaemia* may be symptomatic (p690). Lesions are due to ↑osteoclast activation, from signalling by myeloma cells.
• *Anaemia, neutropenia, or thrombocytopenia* may result from marrow infiltration by plasma cells, leading to symptoms of anaemia, infection and bleeding.
• *Recurrent bacterial infections* due to immunoparesis, and also because of neu-tropenia due to the disease and from chemotherapy.
• *Renal impairment* due to light chain deposition (p314 & p364) seen in up to 20% at diagnosis—mainly caused by precipitation of light chains with the Tamm-Hors-fall protein in the distal loop of Henle.[113] Also, monoclonal immunoglobulins induce changes in glomeruli. A rare type of damage is deposits of light chains in the form of AL-amyloid and subsequent nephrosis[114] (and other systemic problems, p364).

**Tests** FBC—normocytic normochromic anaemia, film—rouleaux formation (p322), persistently ↑ESR or PV (p366), ↑urea and creatinine, ↑Ca²⁺ (in ~40%), alk phos usu-ally ↔ unless healing fracture. Marrow[et al]—figs 1-4. *Screening test:* Serum and urine electrophoresis. β₂-microglobulin (as a prognostic test). *Imaging:* x-rays: lytic 'punched-out' lesions, eg pepper-pot skull, vertebral collapse, fractures or osteoporo-sis. CT or MRI may be useful to detect lesions not seen on XR. *Diagnostic criteria:* BOX.

**Treatment**[115] *Supportive:* • Bone pain should be treated with analgesia (avoid NSAIDs due to risk of renal impairment). Give all patients a *bisphosphonate* (clod-ronate, zolendronate or pamidronate), as they reduce fracture rates and bone pain. Local radiotherapy can help rapidly in focal disease. Orthopaedic procedures (vertebroplasty or kyphoplasty) may be helpful in vertebral collapse. • Anaemia should be corrected with *transfusion*, and *erythropoietin* may be used. • Renal failure: rehydrate, and ensure adequate fluid intake of 3L/day to prevent further renal impairment by light chains. Dialysis may be needed in acute renal failure • Infections: Treat rapidly with broad-spectrum antibiotics until culture results are known. Regular IV *immunoglobulin infusions* may be needed if recurrent.

*Chemotherapy:* If unsuitable for intensive R₂, *melphalan + prednisolone* is used. This can control disease for ~1yr, reducing paraprotein levels and bone lesions. Adding *bortezomib* increases the time to relapse.[116] In due course, disease may become uncon-trollable and resist treatment. Adding *thalidomide* (a teratogenic immunomodulator) improves event-free survival, eg in the elderly.[117] SE: birth defects; drowsiness; neuropa-thy; neutropenia; sepsis; orthostatic hypotension; thromboembolism (aspirin, or full anticoagulation is probably wise if risk ↑, eg hyperviscosity, or other comorbidities).[118] In fitter people, a more vigorous approach is used (high-dose therapy and stem-cell rescue, HDT) the VAD type regimen: *Vincristine, Adriamycin* and *Dexamethasone*. Autologous stem cell transplant may then be done, which improves survival but is not curative. Allogeneic transplantation can be curative in younger patients, but carries ↑risk of mortality (~30%). Thalidomide or bortezomib may be tried in relapsed disease. NB: *lenalidomide* is similar to thalidomide and, being a bit more potent, may have a role,[119] as may *bendamustine* (it drives cell death by promoting mitotic catastrophe in melphalan-resistant myeloma cells).[120]

**Prognosis** Worse if: >2 osteolytic lesions, β₂-microglobulin >5.5mg/L, Hb <11g/L; albumin <30g/L.[121] Cause of death: infection; renal failure (transplants have a role).[122]

---

1 Toxic and inflammatory effects of monoclonal free light chains (FLCs) affect kidney proximal tubule cells; intratubular casts also form via interaction with Tamm-Horsfall proteins.

## 36

## Myeloma diagnosis

Have a high index of suspicion, ▸eg in bone pain or back pain which is not improving, do an ESR and film and electrophoresis. Diagnostic criteria:

1 Monoclonal protein band in serum or urine electrophoresis
2 Plasma cells ↑ on marrow biopsy
3 Evidence of end-organ damage from myeloma:
   • Hypercalcaemia
   • Renal insufficiency
   • Anaemia
4 Bone lesions: a skeletal survey after diagnosis detects bone disease: x-rays of chest; all of spine; skull; pelvis ± Tc-99m MIBI and PET (p754)

## Causes of bone pain/tenderness

• Trauma/fracture (steroids ↑risk)
• Myeloma and other primary malignancy, eg plasmacytoma or sarcoma
• Secondaries (breast, lung, prostate[etc.])
• Osteonecrosis, eg from microemboli[1]
• Osteomyelitis/periostitis (eg syphilis)
• Hydatid cyst (bone is a rare site)
• Osteosclerosis, eg from hepatitis C
• Paget's disease of bone
• Sickle cell anaemia
• Renal osteodystrophy
• CREST syndrome/Sjögren's syndrome
• Hyperparathyroidism.

*Tests:* PSA, ESR, Ca$^{2+}$, LFT, electrophoresis.
*Treatment:* Treat the cause; bisphosphonates & NSAIDs may control symptoms.

**Haematology** (side margin)

## Complications of myeloma

• *Hypercalcaemia* (p690). This occurs with active disease, eg at presentation or relapse. Rehydrate vigorously with IV saline 0.9% 4-6L/d (careful fluid balance). IV bisphosphonates, eg zolendronate or pamidronate, are useful for treating hypercalcaemia acutely.
• *Spinal cord compression* (p470). Occurs in 5% of those with myeloma. Urgent MRI if suspected. Treatment is with dexamethasone 8-16mg/24h PO and local radiotherapy.
• *Hyperviscosity* (p366) causes reduced cognition, disturbed vision, and bleeding. It is treated with plasmapheresis to remove light chains.
• *Acute renal injury* is treated with rehydration. Urgent dialysis may be needed.

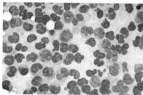

Fig 1. Myeloma bone marrow: many plasma cells with abnormal forms.

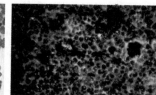

Fig 2. Marrow section in myeloma, stained with IgG kappa monoclonal antibody.

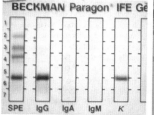

Fig 3. An IgG kappa paraprotein monoclonal band (immunofixation electrophoresis; a control sample has run on the left).

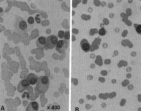

Fig 4. Plasma cells in myeloma. A: marrow smear; B: peripheral smear. Note rouleaux formation of red cells (p322 & p362).

1 Avascular necrosis from sickle-cell anaemia, sepsis, antiphospholipid syndrome, fat emboli.
Figs 1-3 courtesy of Prof. Christine Lawrence; fig 4 courtesy of Prof. Tangün and Dr Köroğlu.

Paraproteinaemia denotes presence in the circulation of immunoglobulins produced by a single clone of plasma cells. The paraprotein is recognized as a monoclonal band (M band) on serum electrophoresis.[1] There are 6 major categories:

1 *Multiple myeloma:* See p362.

2 *Waldenström's macroglobulinaemia:* This is a lymphoplasmacytoid lymphoma producing a monoclonal IgM paraprotein. Hyperviscosity is common (p366), with CNS and ocular symptoms. Lymphadenopathy and splenomegaly are also seen. ↑ESR, with IgM paraprotein on serum electrophoresis. ℞: None if asymptomatic. Chlorambucil, fludarabine or combination chemotherapy may be used. Plasmapheresis[1] for hyperviscosity (p366).

3 *Primary amyloidosis:* See below.

4 *Monoclonal gammopathy of uncertain significance* (MGUS) is common (3% >70yrs). There is a paraprotein in the serum but no myeloma, 1° amyloid, macroglobulinaemia or lymphoma, with no bone lesions, no Bence Jones protein and a low concentration of paraprotein, with <10% plasma cells in the marrow. Some develop myeloma or lymphoma. Refer to a haematologist (?for marrow biopsy).[123]

5 *Paraproteinaemia in lymphoma or leukaemia:* Eg seen in 5% of CLL.

6 *Heavy chain disease:* This is where neoplastic cells produce free Ig heavy chains. α chain disease is the most important, causing malabsorption from infiltration of small bowel wall. It may progress to lymphoma.

## Amyloidosis[11]

*Amyloid...the amorphous fibrillar protein*

This is a group of disorders characterized by extracellular deposits of a protein in abnormal fibrillar form, resistant to degradation. The following are the systemic forms of amyloidosis. Amyloid deposition is also a feature of Alzheimer's disease, type 2 diabetes mellitus and haemodialysis-related amyloidosis.

*AL amyloid (primary amyloidosis)* Proliferation of plasma cell clone→amyloidogenic monoclonal immunoglobulins→Fibrillar light chain protein deposition→Organ failure →Death. Associations: myeloma (15%); Waldenström's, lymphoma. Organs involved:
• Kidneys: glomerular lesions—proteinuria and nephrotic syndrome
• Heart: restrictive cardiomyopathy (looks 'sparkling' on echo), arrhythmias, angina
• Nerves: peripheral and autonomic neuropathy; carpal tunnel syndrome
• Gut: macroglossia (big tongue), malabsorption/weight↓, perforation, haemorrhage, obstruction, and hepatomegaly
• Vascular: purpura, especially periorbital—a characteristic feature (fig 1).

℞: Optimize nutrition; oral melphalan + prednisolone extends median survival from 13 months following diagnosis to 17 months.[124] High-dose IV melphalan with autologous peripheral blood stem cell transplantation may be better.

*AA amyloid (secondary amyloidosis)* Here amyloid is derived from serum amyloid A, an acute phase protein, reflecting chronic inflammation in rheumatoid arthritis, UC/Crohn's, familial Mediterranean fever, and chronic infections—TB, bronchiectasis, osteomyelitis. It affects kidneys, liver, and spleen (fig 2), and may present with proteinuria, nephrotic syndrome or hepatosplenomegaly. Macroglossia is not seen; cardiac involvement is rare.[2] ℞: manage the underlying condition optimally.

*Familial amyloidosis* (autosomal dominant, eg from mutations in transthyretin, a transport protein produced by the liver). Usually causes a sensory or autonomic neuropathy ± renal or cardiac involvement. Liver transplant can cure.

**Diagnosis** is made with biopsy of affected tissue, and positive Congo Red staining with red-green birefringence under polarized light microscopy. The rectum or subcutaneous fat are relatively non-invasive sites for biopsy and are +ve in 80%.

**Prognosis** Median survival is 1-2 years. Patients with myeloma and amyloidosis have a shorter survival than those with myeloma alone.

---

1 Electro*phoresis* and plasma*pheresis* look as though they should share endings, but they do not: Greek *phoros* = *bearing* (*esis* = *process*), but *aphairesis* is Greek for *removal.*
2 Murmurs; low voltage ECG, ventricular hypertrophy, diastolic dysfunction.[125]

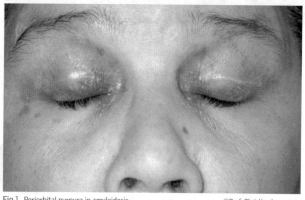

Fig 1. Periorbital purpura in amyloidosis.

©Prof. Christine Lawrence.

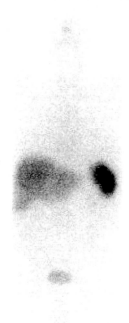

Fig 2. Areas of amyloid deposition in liver and spleen in amyloidosis (isotope scan). ©OTM/OUP.

Haematology

In many labs, this has replaced the ESR, as it is less affected by anaemia and results can be produced in 15min. The PV is affected by the concentration of large plasma proteins and is raised in the same conditions as the ESR. Both PV and ESR are raised in chronic inflammation and are less affected by acute changes <24h in duration. The CRP is more sensitive in acute change (see p701).

## Hyperviscosity syndrome

Blood is made to move! Our beautiful images seem to deny this, as if haematology were just a branch of histology. So what are the intrinsic disorders of flow? If blood viscosity rises there may be a few telltale signs before the quick becomes dead, eg lethargy; confusion; cognition↓; CNS disturbance; chest pain; abdominal pain; faints; visual disturbance (eg vision↓, amaurosis fugax, retinopathy—eg engorged retinal veins, haemorrhages, exudates; and a blurred disc as seen in fig 1a). The visual symptoms ('slow-flow retinopathy') are like 'looking through a watery car windscreen'

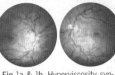

Fig 1a & 1b. Hyperviscosity syndrome.

(fig 1b). Other causes of slow-flow retinopathy: carotid disease and Takayasu's disease (p726). Also hyperviscosity may cause spontaneous GI or GU bleeding.

*Causes of high blood viscosity:* Very high red cell count (haematocrit >50, eg polycythaemia rubra vera), white cell count (>100×10⁹/L, eg leukaemia), or plasma components—usually immunoglobulins, in myeloma or Waldenström's macroglobulinaemia (p364, as IgM is larger and so ↑ viscosity more than the same amount of IgG). Drugs: oral contraceptives, diuretics, IV Ig, erythropoietin, chemotherapy, radio-contrast media.

*Treatment:* Urgent treatment is needed which depends on the cause. Venesection is done in polycythaemia. Leukopheresis in leukaemias to remove white cells. Plasmapheresis in myeloma and Waldenström's: blood is withdrawn via a plasma exchange machine, the supernatant plasma from this is discarded, and the RBCs returned to the patient after being resuspended in a suitable medium.

## Erythrocyte sedimentation rate (ESR) Normal range: ≤20mm/h.

The ESR is a sensitive but non-specific indicator of the presence of disease. It measures how far RBCs fall through a column of anticoagulated blood in 1h. It is really a length (eg 35mm in the 1st hour)—not a rate[126] If certain proteins cover red cells, these cause RBCs to stick to each other in columns so they fall faster (the same phenomenon as rouleaux on the blood film, p322). The main causes of a raised ESR are any inflammation, eg infection, rheumatoid arthritis, malignancy, myocardial infarction; or anaemia or a macrocytosis.

In those with a slightly raised ESR, the best plan is probably to wait a month and repeat it. There is a group of patients whose vague symptoms would have prompted nothing more than reassurance—were it not for a markedly raised ESR (>100mm/h)—and in whom there are no pointers to specific disease. The same advice does not hold true for these, where there is a 90% predictive value for disease. In practice, most have signs pointing to the cause. In one survey, serious underlying disease later found included myeloma, giant cell arteritis, abdominal aneurysm, metastatic prostatic carcinoma, leukaemia, and lymphoma. Therefore, it would be wise (after history and examination) to consider these tests: FBC, plasma electrophoresis, U&E, PSA, chest and abdominal imaging, ± biopsy of bone marrow or temporal artery.

ESR also rises with age. A simple, reliable way[127] to allow for this is to calculate the upper limit of normal, using the Westergren method, to be (for men) age in years ÷ 2. For women, the formula is (years + 10) ÷ 2. This is only a rough guide as some workers find no difference between men and women between the ages of 70 and 90yrs old[128] NB: some conditions *lower* the ESR, eg polycythaemia (due to ↑red cell concentration), microcytosis, and sickle-cell anaemia. Even a slightly raised ESR in these patients should prompt one to ask: "*What else is the matter?*"

## The spleen and splenectomy

The spleen was a mysterious organ for many years; we now know that it plays a vital immunological role by acting as a reservoir for lymphocytes, and in dealing with bacteraemias. Splenomegaly is a commonish problem and its causes are divided into *massive* (into the RIF) and *moderate*.

**Causes of massive splenomegaly** CML, myelofibrosis, malaria (hyperreactive malarial splenomegaly), leishmaniasis, 'tropical splenomegaly' (idiopathic—Africa, south-east Asia), and Gaucher's syndrome.

**Moderate splenomegaly:** See p606. •Infection (eg EBV, endocarditis, TB, malaria, leishmaniasis, schistosomiasis) •Portal hypertension (liver cirrhosis) •Haematological (haemolytic anaemia, leukaemia especially CML, lymphoma) •Connective tissue disease (RA, SLE) •Others: sarcoidosis, primary antibody deficiency (OHCS p198), idiopathic.

Splenomegaly can be uncomfortable and may lead to *hypersplenism*: pancytopenia as cells become trapped in the spleen's reticuloendothelial system, with symptoms of anaemia, infection, or bleeding. Splenectomy may be required if severe.

When faced with a mass in the left upper quadrant, it is vital to recognize the spleen: •Dull to percussion •It enlarges towards the RIF •It moves down on inspiration •You may feel a medial notch •'You can't get above it' (ie the top margin disappears under the ribs). The last three features differentiate the spleen from an enlarged left kidney. Abdominal USS or CT are used to image the spleen. When hunting the cause for enlargement look for lymphadenopathy and liver disease, eg: FBC, ESR, LFT ± liver, marrow, or lymph node biopsy.

**Splenectomy** Main indications: splenic trauma, hypersplenism, autoimmune haemolysis: in ITP (p338) or warm autoimmune haemolytic anaemia (p332), congenital haemolytic anaemias. Splenectomy was historically performed for staging in Hodgkin's disease, but CT and MRI have replaced this role. Mobilize early post-splenectomy as transient ↑platelets predisposes to thrombi. A characteristic blood film is seen following splenectomy, with Howell-Jolly bodies, Pappenheimer bodies and target cells (see p322).

▶*The main problem post-splenectomy is lifelong increased risk from infection.* The spleen contains macrophages which filter and phagocytose bacteria. Post-splenectomy infection is caused most commonly by encapsulated organisms: *Streptococcus pneumoniae*, *Haemophilus influenzae*, and *Neisseria meningitidis*. Reduce this risk by giving:[128]

1 Immunizations:
   • Pneumococcal vaccine (p160), at least 2 weeks pre-op to ensure good response, or as soon as possible after emergency splenectomy, eg after trauma. Re-immunize every 5–10yrs. Avoid in pregnancy.
   • *Haemophilus influenzae* type b vaccine (Hib, see p391).
   • Meningococcal C vaccine.
   • Annual influenza vaccine (p402).
2 Life-long prophylactic oral antibiotics (phenoxymethylpenicillin). Erythromycin if penicillin allergic.
3 Patient-held cards alerting health professionals to the infection risk.
4 Pendants or bracelets to alert medical staff.
5 Advice to seek medical attention if any signs of infection.
6 Urgent hospital admission if infection develops, for treatment with broad-spectrum antibiotics.
7 If travelling abroad, warn of risk of severe malaria and advise meticulous prophylaxis, with nets, repellent, and medication.

The above advice also applies to hyposplenic patients, eg in sickle-cell anaemia or coeliac disease.

Haematology

Thrombophilia is an inherited or acquired coagulopathy predisposing to thrombosis, usually venous: DVT or PE (venous thromboembolism: VTE). Special precautions are needed in *surgery*, *pregnancy*, and *enforced rest*. Risk is also increased by obesity, immobility, trauma (accidents or surgery), and malignancy. NB: thrombocytosis and polycythaemia may also cause thrombosis (p360). See BOX. Note only ~50% of patients with thrombosis and a +ve family history have an identifiable thrombophilia on routine tests: others may have abnormalities that are as yet unidentified.

**Inherited** • *Activated protein c (APC) resistance/factor V Leiden:* Chief cause of inherited thrombophilia. Present in ~5% of the population, although most will not develop thrombosis. Usually associated with a single point mutation in factor V (Factor V Leiden), so that this clotting factor is not broken down by APC. Risk of DVT or PE is raised 5-fold if heterozygous for the mutation (50-fold if homozygous). Thrombotic risk is increased in pregnancy and those on oestrogens (*OHCS* p33, p257 & p303).

• *Prothrombin gene mutation:* Causes high prothrombin levels and ↑thrombosis due to down-regulation of fibrinolysis, by thrombin-activated fibrinolysis inhibitor.

• *Protein c & s deficiency:* These vitamin κ-dependent factors act together to cleave and so neutralize factors V & VIII. Heterozygotes deficient for either protein risk thrombosis. Skin necrosis also occurs (esp. if on warfarin). Homozygous deficiency for either protein causes neonatal purpura fulminans—fatal, if untreated.

• *Antithrombin deficiency:* Antithrombin is a co-factor of heparin, and inhibits thrombin. Less common, affects 1:500. Heterozygotes' thrombotic risk is greater than protein c or s deficiency by ~4-fold. Homozygosity is incompatible with life.

**Acquired** Causes: 3rd generation progesterones[1] in contraceptive Pills (see TABLE for risk of thrombosis) and the antiphospholipid syndrome (APL: p556) when serum antiphospholipid antibodies are found (lupus anticoagulant ± anticardiolipin antibody), predisposing to venous *and* arterial thrombosis, thrombocytopenia, and recurrent fetal loss in pregnancy. In most it is a primary disease, but it is also seen in SLE.

| Risk of thrombosis associated with the Pill | |
|---|---|
| Not on Pill | 5:100,000 |
| 2nd gen. Pill[1] | 15:100,000 |
| 3rd gen. Pill[1] | 25:100,000 |
| Pregnancy | 60:100,000 |

**What tests?** Ask the lab. Do FBC, film, clotting (PT, thrombin time, APTT, fibrinogen) ± APC resistance test, lupus anticoagulant and anticardiolipin antibodies, and assays for antithrombin and proteins c & s deficiency (± DNA analysis by PCR for the Factor V Leiden mutation if APC resistance test is +ve, and for prothrombin gene mutation).

**When?** Ideally while well, not pregnant, and not anticoagulated for 1 month.

**Who?** Typically, do tests (eg antiphospholipid antibodies) in those who have had unprovoked DVT or PE if unsure as to whether to stop anticoagulation. See MINIBOX.

**Who not?** Already on lifelong anticoagulation (eg after PE). 1st-degree relatives of people with a history of DVT/PE or thrombophilia except in special circumstances.[129]

**What's the benefit of testing?** Often none! And cost/QALY is often ≥£20,000. So be sparing in requesting these tests, which can cause significant worry to patients.[130]

**Treatment** Treat acute thrombosis as standard—heparin, then warfarin to target INR of 2–3 (p345). If recurrence occurs with no other risk factors, lifelong warfarin should be considered. Recurrence whilst on warfarin should be treated by increasing target INR to 3–4. In antithrombin deficiency, high doses of heparin may be needed so liaise with a haematologist. In protein c or s deficiency, monitor treatment closely as skin necrosis may occur with warfarin.

**Prevention** Lifelong anticoagulation is not needed if asymptomatic, but advise of ↑ risk of VTE with the Pill or HRT, and counsel as regards to the best form of contraception. Warn about other risk factors for VTE. Prophylaxis may be needed in pregnancy, eg in antiphospholipid syndrome. Get expert help: aspirin and, sometimes, prophylactic heparin are used (*OHCS* p33), as warfarin is teratogenic. Prophylactic SC heparin may also be indicated in high-risk situations, eg pre-surgery.

**1** Desogestrel is an example. Risk of thrombosis is ~doubled with Pills containing this, *vs* levonorgestrel. Part of this effect is due to ↓ free protein S found with desogestrel (24 *vs* 33u/dL).[131,132]

Haematology

## Other risk factors for thrombosis

| Arterial | Venous |
|---|---|
| • Smoking | • Surgery |
| • Hypertension | • Trauma |
| • Hyperlipidaemia | • Immobility |
| • Diabetes mellitus | • Pregnancy, oral contraceptive pill, HRT |
| | • Age |
| | • Obesity |
| | • Varicose veins |
| | • Other conditions: heart failure, malignancy, inflammatory bowel disease, nephrotic syndrome, paroxysmal nocturnal haemoglobinuria (p332). |

For thrombophilia in pregnancy, see *OHCS* p33; for anticoagulant use in pregnancy and thromboprophylaxis, see *OHCS* p16.

### Consider special tests if:
• Arterial thrombosis or MI at <50yrs old (eg for APL)
• Venous thrombosis at <40yrs with no risk factors
• Familial VTE or with oral contraceptives/pregnancy
• Unexplained recurrent VTE
• Unusual site, eg mesenteric or portal vein thrombosis
• Recurrent fetal loss (≥3)
• Neonatal thrombosis

Haematology

As well as being used in leukaemias and cancers, these are used in organ and marrow transplants, rheumatoid arthritis, psoriasis, chronic hepatitis, asthma, SLE, vasculitis (eg Wegener's•, giant cell arteritis, polymyalgia, PAN), inflammatory bowel and other diseases (so this page could figure in almost any chapter).

**Prednisolone** Steroids can be life-saving, but bear in mind:
• Certain conditions may be made worse by steroids, eg TB, hypertension, chicken-pox, osteoporosis, diabetes: here careful monitoring is needed.
• Growth retardation may occur in young patients, and the elderly frequently get more side-effects from treatment.
• Interactions: [Prednisolone]↓ by anti-epileptics (below) and rifampicin.
• Avoid pregnancy (may cause fetal growth retardation). If breastfeeding and prednisolone >40mg/day, see BNF.

Minimize side-effects by using the lowest dose possible for the shortest period of time. Give doses in the morning, and alternate days if possible, to minimize adrenal suppression. Before starting long-term treatment (>3 weeks, or repeated courses) observe these guidelines:
• Explain about not stopping steroids suddenly. Collapse may result, as endogenous production takes time to restart. ►►See p846.
• Inform about the need to consult a doctor if unwell, and increase the dose of steroid at times of illness/stress (eg flu or pre-op).
• Encourage to carry a steroid card saying dose taken, and the reason.
• You *must* warn patients about the listed side-effects if they are receiving long-term treatment (over 6 weeks' worth): see BOX.
• Avoid over-the-counter drugs, eg NSAIDs: aspirin and ibuprofen (↑risk of DU).
• Prevent osteoporosis if long-term use (p696): exercise, bisphosphonates, calcium and vitamin D supplements, smoking cessation advice.

Do not stop long-term steroids abruptly as adrenal insufficiency may occur. Once a daily dose of 7.5mg/day of prednisolone is reached, withdrawal should be gradual. Patients on short-term treatment (<3 weeks) can be stopped immediately, unless they have had repeated courses of steroids, a history of adrenal suppression, greater than 40mg daily, or doses at night, where withdrawal should be gradual.

**Azathioprine** SE: p549. *Interactions:* mercaptopurine and azathioprine (which is metabolized to mercaptopurine) are metabolized by xanthine oxidase (XO). So azathioprine toxicity results if XO inhibitors are co-administered (eg allopurinol).

**Ciclosporin** This is a calcineurin inhibitor, as is tacrolimus which works in a similar way. It has an important role in reducing rejection in organ and marrow transplant. The main SE is dose-related nephrotoxicity. Do blood levels.
• Other SE: gum hyperplasia, tremor, BP↑ (stop if ↑↑), oedema, paraesthesiae, confusion, seizures, hepatotoxicity, lymphoma, skin cancer—avoid sunbathing.
• Monitor U&E and creatinine every 2 weeks for the first 3 months, then monthly if dose >2.5mg/kg/d (every 2 months if less than this). ►Reduce the dose if creatinine rises by >30% on 2 measurements *even if the creatinine is still in normal range*. Stop if the abnormality persists. Also monitor LFT.
• Interactions are legion: [ciclosporin]↑ by: ketoconazole, diltiazem, verapamil, the Pill, erythromycin, grapefruit juice. [ciclosporin]↓ by: barbiturates, carbamazepine, phenytoin, rifampicin. Avoid concurrent nephrotoxics: eg gentamicin. Concurrent NSAIDs augment hepatotoxicity—monitor LFT.

**Methotrexate** An antimetabolite. Inhibits dihydrofolate reductase, which is involved in the synthesis of purines and pyrimidines. See p549.

**Cyclophosphamide** An alkylating agent. SE: marrow suppression (monitor FBC), nausea, infertility, teratogenic, haemorrhagic cystitis due to an irritative urinary metabolite. There is a slight ↑risk of later developing bladder cancer or leukaemia.

## Side-effects of steroid use

| System: | Adverse reactions: |
|---|---|
| Gastrointestinal | Pancreatitis |
| | Candidiasis |
| | Oesophageal ulceration |
| | Peptic ulceration |
| Musculoskeletal | Myopathy |
| | Osteoporosis |
| | Fractures |
| | Growth suppression |
| Endocrine | Adrenal suppression |
| | Cushing's syndrome |
| CNS | Aggravated epilepsy |
| | Depression; psychosis |
| Eye | Cataracts; glaucoma |
| | Papilloedema |
| Immune | Increased susceptibility to and severity of infections, eg chickenpox |

Steroids can also cause fever and ↑wcc↑; steroids only rarely cause leucopenia.

Explain side-effects in terms that patients understand: document this and your plans to prevent osteoporosis if steroid use is going to be long term. Because the risks are mostly long term, you can use your judgement about when to explain about each side-effect. Because steroids can be life-saving, explaining everything all at once in a graphic way may result in your patient being very well informed, but dead.

## Contents

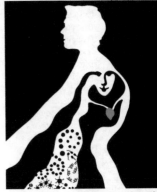

Fig 1. Infections seduce us into 3 beautiful but dangerous beliefs—that we can say that the cause of any communicable disease:

1 Is often simple and unitary, suggesting that simple 'magic bullet' treatments will work.
2 Determines the features of the disease more than host factors or social *milieu*.
3 Can be killed, leading to diseases being conquered by applying ever more reductionist science (microscopes, PCR,etc).

As we shall see, the 3 great infections diseases (TB, malaria, and HIV) test these ideas to destruction and show their enduring nature by requiring 3 older principles: ☙co-evolution, ☙co-operation, and ☙compromise.

An example: prospective studies show that after infective diarrhoea, some people recover fast while others get irritable bowel symptoms for years—predicated by their mental state at the time of infection. Don't blame the pathogen; don't blame the patient: don't blame anyone. Instead look for networks of interrelating causes interacting with random events.

The image is of the poet Rupert Brooke (1887-1915), before he died of the mosquito bite described in BOX 1: a random event witnessed by the hidden heart and face concealed in the image—his 'pulse in the eternal mind', seen here bidding us to act *now*, to right the wrongs for which infectious diseases are so infamous.

**Topics elsewhere** *Infections causing cancer* (H×9)—*viruses:* HPV→ca cervix + head & neck ca (OHCS p570); HHV-4/EBV→nasopharyngeal ca + lymphoma (p356); HHV-8→Kaposi sarcoma (p716); HTLV-1→leukaemia; HBV & HCV→HCC (p270)—*helminths,* eg *Schistosoma haematobium*→bladder cancer (p646)—bacteria *Helicobacter*→stomach ca (p620).¹
*See also:* Surgical prophylaxis (p572); SBE/IE (p144); pneumonia (p160-6); lung abscess (p164); lung fungi (p168); UTI (p288); encephalitis (p834); ▶▶meningitis (p832).

*We thank Dr Chris Conlon, our Specialist Reader, and Sinead Taylor, our Junior Reader.*

## ☼Death by septicaemia: two incompatible views

1 "Everything is for the best in the best of all possible worlds". *Candide. Voltaire*
   This is guaranteed (according to belief) either, in a graceful way, by God's good-ness (and his always beneficent if mysterious ways) or by the messy ways of natural selection (the weak are rooted out so that the strong may flourish).

2 "Preventable death is a tragic waste for which nothing can compensate and from which we can look for no crumb of comfort." As Henry James said on learning of the death by septicaemia of Rupert Brooke (fig 1) "I have no philoso-phy, nor piety, no art of reflection, no theory of compensation to meet things so hideous, so cruel, and so mad, they are just unspeakably horrible and irreme-diable to me and I stare at them with angry and almost blighted eyes". *Henry James*

We cite the infectious anger of this old Master to motivate us to do whatever it takes to stop these lives slipping through our fingers.[1] And as we look out at our burning world through his pupils we see how his *"almost"* blighted eyes reveal a tantalizing hint of resilience—on which we found this chapter.

### Getting the balance right in infectious diseases (ID)

It is not possible for any ID chapter to be constructed so that it has the right bal-ance throughout the world. Many of our readers come from communities where tetanus and malaria are daily problems—whereas, in UK consulting rooms, chest, GU, and ENT infections are likely to dominate.

In parts of Africa, ~70% of hospitalized patients are HIV+ve,[2] and most cannot even begin to mount an immune response to approach the classic descriptions be-loved of standard textbooks (eg there is meningitis without meningism; pneumonia without fever[etc]), and here medicine is, it seems, no more than the pathology of im-munosuppression. In Western hospital specialist ID practice, the chief problems are:
- Respiratory tract infections (p160–p168, and *Emergencies*, p826)
- Hospital-acquired infections, eg p392, p162, p420 (MRSA), p247 (C. difficile)
- Immunocompromise, eg HIV (p408–p415) and febrile neutropenia (p346)
- Infections associated with general surgery (p572 & p578)
- Infections in intensive care unit patients (examples on p382 & p441)
- Osteomyelitis (OHCS p696) and prosthetic joint infections (OHCS p707)
- Illness in a returning traveller (p388).

All these would be trumped by pandemic flu, if highly pathogenic (p402). But in all areas and at all times, the pitfalls are the same: not taking time to find out about your patient—where he has been, what his hobbies are (and his work), and with whom he or she has had contact. Always have a high index of suspi-cion for TB, and always remember that ID rarities are often very treatable.

Know your local emerging diseases (p387) and your local multiresistant organ-isms; remember that it is possible to have more than one infection. ▶*Two heads are better than one: so when in doubt, get help.* The best help is often from good microbiology and imaging departments. In many places these are impossible luxu-ries: a chest x-ray can cost more than the entire yearly health budget allocated to each patient.[3] If this is your predicament, try not to give up: bring your microscope to the bedside (p383) and campaign for better times.

### Notifiable diseases[UK] Inform the Public Health Consultant

| | | |
|---|---|---|
| Anthrax | Malaria | Rubella |
| Cholera | Measles | Scarlet fever |
| Diphtheria | Meningococcal sepsis | Tetanus |
| Dysentery (amoebiasis, typhoid/paratyphoid) | Mumps Ophthalmia neonatorum | Tuberculosis Typhus |
| Encephalitis | Plague | Viral haemorrhagic fevers, |
| Food poisoning | Poliomyelitis | eg yellow fever; lassa fever |
| Leprosy; Leptospirosis | Rabies; Relapsing fever | Whooping cough/pertussis |

(UK Health Protection Agency www.hpa.org.uk. 020 7759 2700; webteam@hpa.org.uk)

---

1 If you feel small and insignificant in the face of this challenge, remember that the mosquito that killed Rupert Brooke on his way to Gallipoli in 1915 was smaller still. See also: www.survivingsepsis.org.

Infectious diseases

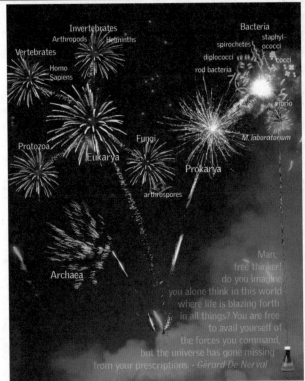

Fig 1. What is life? A thing of dynamism, fragility, beauty, danger, and evanescence, gushing forth from a single source, to be sure. But here the certainties end: what does it take to be alive? Are viruses and prions alive?[1 4-6] How many branches are there on our tree?[2 7-9] The harder we look, the more complexities we find. With the recent creation of synthetic bacteria (*Mycoplasma laboratorium*, seen here on the right issuing from its own domain) even the surety of a single common ancestor disappears into smoke.

Because micro-organisms get us up at night and kill our friends (p373) we think of them as bad. This is a big mistake. Kill off micro-organisms and the whole show fizzles out. Micro-organisms gave us the DNA and organelles needed for reading and digesting this page. Even killing a single pathogen might be a mistake: Sod's Law (see p359) will probably ensure that something worse will come to inhabit the vacated ecospace. So the whole affair is like one of our dear, complex geriatric patients: prod one part of her system and events ripple out in an unending stream of unintended consequences, played out under the stars (above), which themselves are evolving, and which donate and receive our primordial elements (p732).

Photo © David Meads.

**1** If a thing is organic and converts nutrients into progeny it is alive. If not, it is either non-living, dead, dying, or male. The average mind is surprised to learn that long before birth, baby girls have their full complement of eggs for the next generation; but for biologists this fact just illustrates Aristotle's dictum that the defining essence of life is that it has a plan for its own survival and continuity.
**2** Kingdoms are *not* the top categories. Think of 3 grand domains: **Archaea, Bacteria** (Eubacteria), and **Eukarya.** Archaea are like bacteria, having no cell nucleus or organelles, but as they have an independent evolutionary history they form a domain of their own. Eukarya have chromosomes and organelles and give rise to plants, animals, and fungi. Single-celled eukaryotes (protists) loom large in this chapter: plasmodia (malaria), trypanosoma (sleeping sickness), amoebae and giardia (p436).

### Examples of pathogens from various types of bacteria

This table is not exhaustive; it is simply a guide for the forthcoming pages.

**Gram-positive cocci**
Staphylococci (including MRSA, p420):
 coagulase +ve, eg *Staph. aureus*
 coagulase -ve, eg *Staph. epidermidis*
Streptococci (see fig 2 and p420):
 β-haemolytic streptococci, eg *Strep.
 pyogenes* Lancefield group A
 α-haemolytic streptococci
  *Strep. mitior, Strep mutans*
  *Strep. pneumoniae* (pneumococcus)
  *Strep. sanguis*
 Enterococci (non-haemolytic):
  *E. faecalis* (not a typical strep)
 Anaerobic streptococci
**Gram-positive bacilli (rods)**
Aerobes
 *Bacillus anthracis* (anthrax: p420)
 *Corynebacterium diphtheriae* (p421)
 *Listeria monocytogenes* (p421)
 *Nocardia* species
Anaerobes:
 Clostridium
  *C. botulinum* (botulism: p421)
  *C. perfringens* (gas gangrene: p421)
  *C. tetani* (tetanus: p424)
  *C. difficile* (diarrhoea, p247)
Actinomyces: *Actinomyces
 israelii* (p421), *A. naeslundii*,
 *A. odontolyticus, A. viscosus*
**Intracellular bacteria:** (o=obligate)
Chlamydia ° (p416, p162, OHCS p286)
 *C. trachomatis:* Tropical eye disease
  trachoma (OHCS p450)=serovars A-C
  GU/cervicitis (p417)=serovars B-K[10]
  lymphogranuloma ven. (p416)= L1-3[11]
 *Chlamydophila psittaci* (p162)
 *Chlamydophila pneumoniae* (p162)
*Coxiella burnetii* ° (p434)
*Bartonella* ° and *Ehrlichia* ° (p434)
*Rickettsia* ° (typhus, p435)
*Legionella pneumophila* (p162)

**Gram-negative cocci**
Neisseria: *Neisseria meningitidis* (meningitis, septicaemia)
 *N. gonorrhoea* (gonorrhoea, p418)
Moraxella: *Moraxella
 catarrhalis* (pneumonia, p423)
**Gram-negative bacilli (rods)**
*Escherichia coli*
*Shigella* species (p426)
*Salmonella* species (p426)
*Citrobacter freundii; C. koseri*
*Klebsiella pneumoniae; K. oxytoca*
*Enterobacter aerogenes; E. cloacae*
*Serratia marascens; Proteus mirabilis*
*Morganella morganii*
Providencia species; *Yersinia (Y. pestis,
 Y. enterocolitica, Y. paratuberculosis)*
*Pseudomonas aeruginosa* (p422)
*Haemophilus influenzae* (p422)
*Brucella* species (p423)
*Bordetella pertussis* (p422)
*Pasteurella multocida* (p447)
*Vibrio cholerae* (p426)
*Campylobacter jejuni* (p390)
Enterobacteriaceae (p390 & p422)
**Anaerobes:**
*Bacteroides* (wound infections, p572)
*Fusobacterium*
*Helicobacter pylori* (p242)
**Mycobacteria:** *M. tuberculosis* (TB, p398)
*M. bovis & M. leprae* (leprosy, p428)
Atypical mycobacteria: Suspect if imm-
 uncompromised
*M. avium intracellulare* (p411)
*M. scrofulaceum*    *M. kansasii*
*M. malmoense*      *M. marinum*
*M. xenopi*        *M. gordonae*
*M. smegmatis, M. phlei, M. flavescens*
**Spirochetes** (p430): *Borrelia burgdorferi* (Lyme dis., p430); *Bor. recurrentis*
*Treponema* (syphilis; yaws; pinta)
*Leptospira* (Weil's dis.; canicola fever)

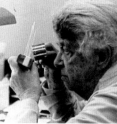

**Fig 2** Streptococci are grouped by haemolytic pattern (α, β, or non-haemolytic) or by Lancefield antigen (A-G), or by species. Rebecca Lancefield (1895-1981) is shown here with her hand lens, typing streps with a variety of M protein-specific[1] antibodies mixed with a streptococcal extract by detecting the precipitin in a pipette. Her lab became known as the Scotland Yard of Streptococcal Mysteries after she found that the most grievous crimes of the streptococcus almost always involve M as a secret accomplice. Although she arrested M on many occasions, M outlived her, and still stalks our wards and clinics.[12]
©Dr V Fischetti, Rockefeller University, NY.

**1** M proteins prevent neutrophils from engulfing streps unless a neutralizing antibody is present; hence repeated strep infections are common—immunity to one strep doesn't help with other types, eg streps with M 1, 3, 4, 5, 12, 14, 18, 19 & 24 cause throat infection—M 2, 49, 57, 59, 60 & 61 cause impetigo.[13]

Infectious diseases

## DNA viruses A) *Double-stranded DNA*

| | |
|---|---|
| **Papovavirus** | Papilloma virus: human warts |
| | JC virus: progressive multifocal leucoencephalopathy, PML |
| **Adenovirus** | >30 serotypes; 10% of viral respiratory disease |
| | 7% of viral meningitis |
| **Human herpes viruses (HHV)** | Alphaherpesvirusᵅ (eg neurotropic), betaᵝ (eg epithelio-tropic) and gammaherpesvirusᵞ (lymphotropic): |

* Herpes simplex virus (HSV) 1 & 2 (HHV-1 & HHV-2, p400)
* Herpes (varicella) zoster virusᵅ (HHV-3, p400)
* Cytomegalovirusᵝ—CMV, also called HHV-5, (p404)
* Herpes virus 6ᵝ & 7ᵝ (HHV-6 & 7): roseola infantum (mild, *OHCS* p143); also post-transplant, like CMV
* Epstein-Barr virus (EBV) (HHV-4, p401)ᵞ
* Infectious mononucleosis (glandular fever)
* Burkitt's lymphoma; nasopharyngeal carcinoma

HHV-8: Kaposi's sarcoma (p716)

Fig 1. Oral herpes (HSV1 or 2).

| | |
|---|---|
| **Pox viruses** | (1) Variola: smallpox (eradicated in 1979; some stocks left) |
| | (2) Vaccinia, cowpox |
| | (3) Orf, cutaneous pustules, caught from sheep |
| | (4) Molluscum contagiosum, pearly umbilicated papules, typically seen in children or with HIV |
| **Hepatitis B virus** | See p406 |

### B) *Single-stranded DNA*

| | |
|---|---|
| **Erythrovirus (=parvovirus)** | Erythema infectiosum (fifth disease, *OHCS* p142) 'slapped cheek' appearance ± aplastic crises |

## RNA viruses A) *Double-stranded RNA*

| | |
|---|---|
| **Reovirus** | Eg rotavirus (p390), infantile gastroenteritis |

### B) *Positive single-stranded RNA*

| | | |
|---|---|---|
| **Picornavirus** | 1 | Rhinovirus, common cold (>90 serotypes) |
| | 2 | Enteroviruses (eg echoviruses) are a leading cause of meningo-encephalitis/acute flaccid paralysis[14] |
| | i | Coxsackie A (meningitis, gastroenteritis); Coxsackie B (pericarditis, Bornholm disease) |
| | ii | Hepatitis A virus; iii Echovirus (30% of viral meningitis) |
| | iv | Enterovirus EV71 (hand, foot and mouth disease, *OHCS* p143) |
| | v | Poliovirus, p432 |
| **Coronavirus** | | Eg Urbani SARS-associated coronavirus (Dr Urbani described it and died in an outbreak in Vietnam in 2003); ▶p163. |
| **Togavirus** | | 1 Rubella 2 Alphavirus 3 Flavivirus (yellow fever, dengue, hepatitis C) |

### C) *Negative single-stranded RNA*

| | |
|---|---|
| **Orthomyxovirus** | Influenza A, B, C (p402) |
| **Paramyxovirus** | Parainfluenza, mumps, measles, respiratory syncytial virus |
| **Arenavirus** | Lassa fever (p388 & p432), some viral haemorrhagic fevers, lymphocytic-choriomeningitis virus (LCM) |
| **Rhabdovirus** | Rabies (p432) |
| **Bunyavirus** | Some viral haemorrhagic fevers |

### D) *Retroviruses* (RNA viruses using reverse transcriptase to make DNA)

**Human immunodeficiency virus**—HIV-1, HIV-2. Types A & B predominate in UK (p408)
**Human T-lymphotropic virus** HTLV-1-4; zoonotic transmission of simian T-lymphotropic viruses (STLVs) from other primates to humans.[15] *HTLV-I* is mostly asymptomatic, but 1-5% develop ATLL (adult T-cell leukaemia/lymphoma). Endemic clusters: southern Japan, Gabon, French Guyana and Colombia.[16] *HTLV-2* may be passed on by transfusions, injecting drug users, or sexually. Also seen in Amerindians and Pygmies. It may cause tropical spastic paraparesis (p520). *HTLV-3 & 4:* Prevalent in primate hunters in Cameroon.

Most travel-related illness is not from infections, but due to accidents, violence, MI, etc. Most infections are due to ignorance or indiscretions. ▶*Advice to travellers is more important than vaccination:* eg simple hygiene, malaria prophylaxis, and protective measures (eg safer sex). *Malaria* is a big killer; see p396 for prevention. *Rabies:* vaccinate before travelling if post-exposure vaccination is unlikely to be available (or their activities mean risk is ↑—or if they will be in a rabies area for >1month); seek immediate attention if bitten (wash the wound well); see p432. For *cholera* and *traveller's diarrhoea,* see p426 & p390.[17]

## Vaccines for travellers[18]

| Routine vaccination | Selective use for travellers | Mandatory vaccination |
|---|---|---|
| Diphtheria, tetanus, pertussis | Meningococcal disease | Yellow fever (in some countries) |
| Hepatitis B[1] | Hepatitis A | Meningococcal disease & polio[4] |
| Haem. influenzae B | Cholera | |
| BCG,[2] HPV (for girls) | Japanese encephalitis[3] | |
| Influenza | Rabies | |
| MMR | Tick-borne encephalitis | |
| Pneumococcal disease | Typhoid fever | |
| Poliomyelitis | Yellow fever[3] | |
| Rotavirus (for babies) | | |
| Varicella | | |

1 Routine for certain age groups or risk factors, selective for general travellers.
2 No longer routine in most industrialized countries.
3 These vaccines are included in some routine immunization programmes.
4 Required by Saudi Arabia for pilgrims; updates—see www.who.int/wer.

If only one attendance is possible, all is not lost (make up *en route*): malaria *prophylaxis/advice:* p396. Suggested vaccines: *Africa:* Meningitis, typhoid, diphtheria, tetanus, polio, hepatitis A ± yellow fever. *Asia:* Typhoid, diphtheria, tetanus, polio, hepatitis A. Consider rabies and Japanese encephalitis. *Meningitis and Hajj pilgrimage to Saudi Arabia:* All >2yrs old must be vaccinated against meningococcal meningitis with quadrivalent vaccine (serogroups A, C, Y & W135); must be <3yrs ago but not within the last 10 days. If 3 months–2yrs of age, give 2 doses of the A vaccine separated by 3 months.
*S. America:* Typhoid, diphtheria, tetanus, hepatitis A±yellow fever±rabies.
*Travel if immunocompromised:* Avoid live vaccines. Hepatitis B vaccine: p271.

**Preventing traveller's diarrhoea** *Water:* If in doubt, boil all water. Chlorination is OK, but doesn't kill amoebic cysts (get tablets from pharmacies). Filter water before purifying. Distinguish between simple gravity filters and water purifiers (which also attempt to sterilize chemically). Choose a unit that is verified by bodies such as the London School of Hygiene and Tropical Medicine (eg the MASTA[19] *Travel Well Personal Water Purifier*). Make sure that all containers are disinfected. Try to avoid surface water and intermittent tap supplies. In Africa assume that all unbottled water is unsafe. With bottled water, ensure the rim is clean & dry. Avoid ice. Other water-borne diseases include schistosomiasis (p445).

*Food:* Avoid salads and peel your own fruit. If you cannot wash your hands, discard the part of the food that you are holding (with bananas, careful unzipping obviates this precaution).[17] Hot, well-cooked food is best (>70°C for 2min is no guarantee; many pathogens survive boiling for 5min, but few last 15min).[20]

*Chemoprophylaxis:* Prophylactic antibiotics are not needed in healthy people, but those, eg with Crohn's/UC or immunosuppression should get prophylactic antibiotics. Bismuth salicylate can (to some extent) prevent traveller's diarrhoea. Ciprofloxacin 500mg/12h PO for 72h[21] + loperamide can give ~90% protection.

Infectious diseases

**Notes**
S=usually sensitive
2=S, but may be 2nd choice
?=may be resistant (esp. if hospital-acquired)
R=resistance likely
0=not appropriate

Sources: Medline and GAT (Sanford)

| | Amoxicillin/ ampicillin | Cefepime[12] | Cefotaxime[13] | Ciprofloxacin | Co-amoxiclav | Colistin[24] | Erythromycin[25] | Flucloxacillin | Gentamicin | Imipenem/ meropenem | Metronidazole | Penicillin | Tetracyclines | Ticarcillin/piperacillin/ azlocillin | Trimethoprim | Vancomycin/ teicoplanin |
|---|---|---|---|---|---|---|---|---|---|---|---|---|---|---|---|---|
| *Staph aureus* (MRSA, see p420) | R | S | S | ? | S | 0 | ? | S | S | 2 | R | R | ? | R if MRSA | ? | S |
| *Strep pneumoniae* | ? | S | S | ? | ? | 0 | ? | ? | R | 2 | R | ? | ? | 0 | ? | S |
| *Strep pyogenes* | ? | S | S | ? | ? | 0 | ? | S | R | 2 | R | ? | ? | 0 | ? | S |
| *Enterococcus faecalis* | ? | S | R | R | S | 0 | R | R | S | 2 | R | R | R | 2 | ? | S |
| *N. gonorrhoea* (p418) | ? | ? | ? | R[17] | ? | 0 | R[17] | 0 | 0 | 2 | R | ? | 2 | 0 | R | 0 |
| *N. meningitidis* | ? | S | S | ? | ? | 0 | 0 | 0 | 0 | 2 | R | ? | 0 | 0 | R | R |
| *H. influenza* | ? | S | S | S | ? | 0 | R | 0 | 2 | R | S | ? | S | 0 | S | R |
| *E. coli*[23] (UTI, nitrofurantoin p381) | R | S | ? | ? | ? | 0 | R | R | S | 2 | R | R | 2 | 2R | ? | ? |
| *E. coli* ESBL[29] extended spectrum beta lactamase | R | ? | R | R | R | R | 2 | R | R | ?S | R | R | R | R | R | R |
| *Klebsiella* ESBL | R | ? | S | ? | R | 2 | R | R | S | 2 | R | R | ? | 2R | ? | ? |
| *Proteus mirabilis* | R | S | S | S | S | 0 | R | R | S | 2 | R | R | R | 2R | R | ? |
| *Serratia* species[28] | R | ? | S | S | R | 0 | R | R | S | 2 | R | R | R | R | ? | ? |
| *Pseudomonas aeruginosa*[30] | R | S | R | ? | R | 2 | R | R | ? | 2 | R | R | R | R | ? | R |
| *Acinetobacter baumannii*[30] | R | R | R | R | R | 2 | R | R | R[31] | p423 | R | R | R | R | R | R |
| *Bacteroides fragilis* | R | R | R | R | R | 0 | ? | R | R | 2 | S | R | R | R | R | R |
| *Clostridium difficile* | 0 | 0 | 0 | 0 | 0 | 0 | 0 | 0 | 0 | 0 | S | 0 | 0 | 0 | 0 | S |

| **Penicillin-based antibiotics** | *Usual adult dose:* | *In renal failure:* |
|---|---|---|
| **Amoxicillin** Uses as for ampicillin but better absorbed PO. For IV therapy, use ampicillin. | 250–500mg/8h PO 1g/8h in recurrent or severe pneumonia | ↓Dose if cc <10 (cc=creatinine clearance, mL/min) |
| **Ampicillin** Broader spectrum than penicillin; more active against Gram −ve rods, but β-lactamase sensitive. Amoxicillin is better absorbed PO. | 500mg/4–6h IM/IV Listeria: 2g/4h IVI for 10d | ↓If cc <10, give doses every 12–24h |
| **Benzylpenicillin = penicillin G** Most streps, meningococcus, gonococcus, syphilis, gas gangrene, anthrax, actinomycosis, and many anaerobes. | 300–600mg/6h IV, 2.4g/4h in meningitis. If dose >1.2g, inject at rate <300mg/min | Anaphylaxis risk <1:100,000; huge doses cause Na+±± fits in renal failure |
| **Co-amoxiclav** = amoxicillin 250 or 500mg + clavulanic acid 125mg confers β-lactamase resistance so broader spectrum, but LFT may rise. | 1 tab/8h PO IV form: p382. NB: May contribute to *C. diff* infections♦※ | If eGFR 10–30, give 1 tab/12h; if eGFR <10, 1 tab (250+125)/24h |
| **Flucloxacillin** For Gram +ve β-lactamase producers (staphylococci). | 250–500mg/6h PO ½h before food. 0.5–2g/6h IV | Dose unaltered if eGFR >10 |
| **Phenoxymethylpenicillin(=pen. V)** Like pen. G but poorly absorbed; use as prophylaxis or to complete IV course. | 250–500mg/6h PO; take ½h before food | In severe renal failure, give doses every 12h |
| **Piperacillin** Very broad spectrum, including anaerobes, *Pseudomonas*, staphs (not MRSA or coagulase −ve). Reserve only for those with severe infection. May be used with aminoglycosides (but not in the same IVI). | Tazocin®= tazobactam 500mg + piperacillin 4g: dose: 4.5g/8h IV over 3–5min | Max dose of Tazocin® if eGFR <20: 4.5g/12h |
| **Procaine penicillin (= procaine benzylpenicillin)** Depot injection; good for syphilis; only available on a named patient basis in the UK. | Syphilis: p431 | Dose unaltered in renal failure. Resistance in GC is a problem, p418[37] |
| **Ticarcillin** Very broad spectrum, eg *Pseudomonas*, *Proteus*. Use with an aminoglycoside; more active than azlocillin or piperacillin. | Timentin®=3g ticarcillin +200mg clavulanic acid. Dose: 3.2g/8h IVI (/4h in severe infections) | If eGFR 30–60 1g/8h. If eGFR 10–30 0.8g/12h |

**Spectrum** Many cephalosporins are active against staphs (including β-lactamase producers), streps (except group D, *Enterococcus faecalis and faecium*), pneumococci, *E. coli*, some *Proteus*, *Klebsiella*, *Haemophilus*, *Salmonella*, and *Shigella*. 2nd-generation drugs (cefuroxime, cefamandole) are active against some *Neisseria* and *Haemophilus*. 3rd-generation drugs (cefotaxime, ceftazidime, ceftriaxone) have better activity against Gram -ve organisms. Ceftazidime has less Gram +ve activity (esp. against *Staph aureus*) and is used in *Pseudomonas* infections.

**Uses** Oral cephalosporins (cefaclor, cefalexin, cefuroxime axetil) have a role in UTI, pneumonia, and otitis media, but are not 1st-line (unless penicillin-allergic; but 10% will also be cephalosporin allergic). Their major use is parenteral, eg in surgical prophylaxis or post-op infection. 3rd-generation drugs (eg ceftriaxone) may be used in septicaemia. **SE:** Hypersensitivity; warfarin potentiation.

| Antibiotic | Adult dose | Notes   For body surface area calculation, see *BNF* |
|---|---|---|
| Cefaclor | 250mg (max 1g)/8h PO | No dose change in RF |
| Cefalexin | 500mg/8h PO | Max 3g/d if eGFR 40-50 (1.5g/d if eGFR 10-40; 750mg/d if eGFR <10) |
| | Max: 1.5g/6h PO | |
| Cefepime[4th] | 1-2g/12h IVI | Good activity against *Pseudomonas*, enterobacter, other resistant Gram -ve organisms and *S. aureus*. If CC 10-50: 1-2g/12h; if CC ≤10: 1g/24h |
| Cefpirome[4th] | 1-2g/12h IV over 5min | Broad spectrum, used in polymicrobial infection; pyelonephritis; pneumonia. Not for MRSA (p420) or bacteroides. Good against enterobacter.[32] In renal failure, get help, eg load with 1-2g, then if CC 20-50: 500mg-1g/12h; if CC 5-20: 500mg-1g/24h |
| Cefixime | Syrup: ½-1yr: 3.75mL (75mg)/d | Syrup = 100mg/5mL. Active against streps, coliforms, *Haemophilus*, *Proteus* and anaerobes. Staphylococci, *E. faecalis*, and *Pseudomonas* are resistant. Lower dose if eGFR <20. |
| | 1-4yrs: 5mL/d | |
| | 5-10yrs: 10mL/d | |
| | Adults: 200mg/12-24h | |
| Cefotaxime[3rd] | 1-2g/6-12h IVI/IM; max 3g/6h (gonorrhoea: 500mg stat) | Broad spectrum for serious infections only (pneumonia, meningitis). Unreliable activity against *Pseudomonas*. If eGFR <5 give 1g stat, then halve dose. |
| Cefradine | 250-500mg/6h PO or 500mg-1g/12h PO | Less active than cefuroxime. Halve normal dose if eGFR 5-20. |
| Ceftazidime[3rd] | UTI: 500mg-1g/12h IM/IV | Broad spectrum, incl. most *Pseudomonas* but less effective against Gram +ves; for serious infections only; may help in blind R̠ of neutropenic sepsis[33] (cefepime is better).[34] Reduce dose if eGFR <50. |
| | Other: 1-2g/8h | |
| | Max: 3g/12h if elderly | |
| | Route: IV/IM (avoid IM if dose >1g) | |
| Ceftriaxone[3rd] | 1-4g daily IM/IV over 3min; give ≤1g at each IM site. Use IVI, not IV, if dose >1g | Many Gram +ve and -ve infections. Used in meningitis (p382), pre-colonic surgery, and gonorrhoea. No activity against *Listeria*, enterococci, and *Pseudomonas*. If eGFR <10 ↓ dose, eg limit dose to 2g/d and check levels |
| Cefuroxime | 250-500mg/12h PO | Broad spectrum and good Gram -ve activity. Used in: surgical prophylaxis; cholecystitis;[35] post-op infections; severe pneumonia. Give 750mg per 12h if eGFR 10-20. |
| | 750mg-1.5g/8h IV/IM | |
| | Max IV: 1.5g/6h | |

*Abbreviations:* RF = renal failure; CC = creatinine clearance; CCM = CC/1.73m² body area; 4th= 4th-generation cephalosporin; not all are available in the UK; 3rd= 3rd-generation. Source: GAT and *BNF* 2013. eGFR = estimated GFR mL/min/1.73m².

Infectious diseases

Infectious diseases

| Antibiotic (and uses) | Adult dose examples | Notes cc=creatinine clearance, mL/min |
|---|---|---|
| **Amikacin** See gentamicin. Use ideal weight, p446. | 7.5mg/kg/12h IV; (~50% 12-18h if cc 10-50). | Resistance growing, but less common than for gentamicin |
| **Azithromycin** See clarithromycin, may be good against *N. gonorrhoeae*.[37] | 500mg/24h PO for 3d. | SE: see erythromycin. Caution if eGFR <10. |
| **Chloramphenicol** Rarely used 1st-line. May be used in typhoid fever & *Haemophilus* infection. Also in blind R̃ of meningitis if patient allergic to both penicillins and cephalosporins. Avoid in lactation and late pregnancy. | 12.5mg/kg/6h PO or IV; 25mg/kg/6h may be used in septicaemia or meningitis | SE (rare): marrow aplasia (check FBC often), neuritis, GI upset. Avoid long or repeated courses and in liver impairment or if cc <10mL/ min. *Interactions*: warfarin, rifampicin, phenytoin, sulfonylureas, phenobarbital. |
| **Ciprofloxacin** Used in adult cystic fibrosis, typhoid, *Salmonella, Campylobacter*, prostatitis, and serious or resistant infections. Avoid overuse. | 250-750mg/12h PO 200-400mg/12h IVI over ≥½h (over 1h, if 400mg used). | Good oral antipseudomonal agent. β-lactamase-resistant. If eGFR <30 ↑ dose interval to /24h. SE: D&V; rash; tendon rupture (esp. if >60yrs or on steroids); potentiates theophylline. |
| **Clarithromycin** A macrolide, like erythromycin, used for: *S. aureus*, streptococci, *Mycoplasma, H. pylori, Chlamydia*, MAI (p411). | 250-500mg/12h PO for 7-14d. *H. pylori*: 500mg/ 12h PO for 1wk as triple therapy (p243). MAI may need 12wks (p411). | Halve dose if eGFR <30. *Interactions*: statins, ergot, warfarin, carbamazepine, theophyllines, zidovudine; never use with pimozide. |
| **Clindamycin** Active against Gram +ve cocci including penicillin resistant staph, and anaerobes. | 150-300mg/6h PO; max 450mg/6h PO. 0.2-0.9g/ 8h IV or IM (by IVI only, if >600mg used) | Stop if diarrhoea occurs (pseudomembranous colitis, p247). Used in staph. bone/ joint infection. |
| **Co-trimoxazole** Sulfamethoxazole 400mg + trimethoprim 80mg. 1st choice in *Pneumocystis jiroveci* (p410), toxoplasmosis and nocardia. NB: can act against *S. aureus*. | 960mg-1.44g/12h PO/ IVI; see *Pneumocystis* (p410). | SE (mostly ∵ sulfonamide, elderly at ↑risk): jaundice; Stevens-Johnson, fig 1 p725; marrow depression; folate↓. If eGFR 15-30, halve dose. CI: G6PD deficiency. |
| **Daptomycin** Used only in Gram +ve infections, eg staph septicaemia, right-sided endocarditis, but not pneumonia as it binds surfactant. | 6mg/kg IVI over 30min once daily (every 48h if eGFR ≤30). | A new lipopeptide antibiotic occurring in soil saprotrophails. SE: BP↓, SVT, CCF, myalgia, CK↑ (in up to 10%), LFT↑, INR↑, platelets↓↑, hyperglycaemia. |
| **Doxycycline** Used in travellers' diarrhoea, *Chlamydia*, leptospirosis, syphilis, and brucellosis. | 200mg PO on 1st day then 100mg/24h; max 200mg/d in severe infections. | As for tetracycline, but may be used in renal failure. |
| **Ertapenem** Broad-spectrum carbapenem antibiotic used in bad aerobic Gram-ve infections (not *Pseudomonas*) and some staphs (not MRSA). | 1g IVI over 30min daily, or 1g diluted with 3.2mL of 1% lidocaine IM. | SE: few; as with many antibiotics, *Clostridium difficile* colitis is reported. Max 500mg/d if eGFR <30. |
| **Erythromycin** Macrolide, used in penicillin allergy. Used 1st line in atypical pneumonia, p162. | 250-500mg/6h PO (≤4g/d in *Legionella*). 6.25-12.5mg/kg/6h IVI (adult and child). | SE: D&V; phlebitis in IV use. *Interactions*: statins, warfarin, theophylline, ergotamine, carbamazepine. |
| **Fusidic acid/sodium fusidate** Anti-staph agent (incl. some MRSA, p420); used in osteomyelitis. | 500mg/8h PO. | Combine with another antistaphylococcal drug. SE: GI upset, reversible changes in LFTs. |

| Antibiotic (and uses): | Adult dose examples | Notes (eg use in renal failure) |
|---|---|---|
| **Gentamicin** Spectrum is wide but poor against streps & anaerobes, so use with a penicillin ± metronidazole. Synergy with ampicillin against enterococci. For serious Gram –ve infections. | ▶p766. *Once-daily IV dose* over 15min: 5mg/kg$^{LBW}$ (7mg if very ill). Plasma levels *not* needed if only one stat dose used, eg in UTI. Use LBW, lean body weight, p446. | **Avoid:** prolonged use, concurrent furosemide, use in pregnancy/myasthenia gravis. ▶Do U&E often. SE: oto- and nephrotoxicity. |
| **Imipenem** (+cilastatin) Very broad spectrum: Gram +ve and –ve organisms, anaerobes and aerobes. β-lactam stable. | 250–500mg/6h IVI. High doses risk seizures. | Pregnancy/lactation: avoid. SE: fits; D&V; myoclonus, eosinophilia, WCC↓, Coombs' +ve; LFT abnormal. See package insert, eg if <70kg. If eGFR <70, reduce dose; see datasheet. |
| **Linezolid** An oxazolidinone antibiotic used against MRSA, VISA, and VRE. | 600mg/12h PO/IVI over 1h if eGFR >30 SE: D&V, gastritis, T°↑, tinnitus, neuropathy, WCC↓. | May cause pancytopenia if ≥2wks' use; monitor FBC and visual acuity. CI: BP↑↑, phaeochromocytoma, carcinoid, thyrotoxicosis |
| **Meropenem** See imipenem. | ½–1g/8h IVI, max 2g/8h (1g/12h if eGFR 26–50). | Causes fewer seizures than imipenem. |
| **Metronidazole** 1$^{st}$ choice *vs* anaerobes, *Gardnerella*, *Entamoeba histolytica*, and *Giardia lamblia*; use PO in *C. difficile*. | 400mg/8h PO. PR dose: 1g/8h for 3d then 1g/12h. IVI dose: 500mg/8h for ≤10d. Pregnancy/breast-feeding: avoid high doses. | Disulfiram reaction with alcohol; interacts with warfarin, phenytoin, cimetidine; care if LFT↑. SE: irreversible neuropathy (prolonged dosing). |
| **Minocycline** Spectrum is wider than tetracycline's. | 100mg/12h PO. Monitor LFT. | As tetracycline, but more SE (hepatitis, pneumonitis). |
| **Nitrofurantoin** UTI. | 50mg/6h PO with food. | Good *vs E.coli*. CI: eGFR <60. |
| **Oxytetracycline** | 250–500mg/6h PO. | See tetracycline. |
| **Rifampicin**$^{UK}$ = **rifampin**$^{US}$ Mycobacteria, prophylaxis in meningitis contacts. | Dose example: 600mg/d PO before breakfast. See TB, p398. | Caution in liver disease. Interferes with contraceptive Pill. See p398. |
| **Teicoplanin** See vancomycin, but not given PO. | IV/IM: 400mg/12h for 3 doses, then 400mg/24h. | If eGFR 40–60, use normal dose but every 48h from day 4. |
| **Tetracycline** Used in chronic bronchitis; 1$^{st}$ line in *Chlamydia*, Lyme disease, mycoplasma, brucellosis, rickettsia. | 250–500mg/6h PO 1h before food. 500–1000mg/24h IVI (not if liver disease). IV preparation not available in UK. | Avoid if <12yrs old, in pregnancy, and if CC ≤50. Absorption ↓by iron, milk, and antacids. SE: photosensitivity, D&V. |
| **Tobramycin** As gentamicin; better against *Pseudomonas*. | 1mg/kg/8h IVI or slow IV/IM. Dose↓ in renal failure. | Monitor levels (peak <10mg/L; trough <2mg/L); reduce dose if CC ≤50. |
| **Trimethoprim** Used in UTI, COPD. Dose in prophylaxis: 100mg/24h PO. | 200mg/12h PO (100mg/12h PO if eGFR <15; if eGFR 15–30, halve dose from day 3). | SE: depressed marrow, D&V. CC 10–50: ½ dose after day 3. CC 10–15, ½ dose. |
| **Vancomycin** PO: *C. difficile* if severe infection (p247) or metronidazole is contraindicated; IV: MRSA or other Gram +ve organisms (not *Erysipelothrix* species). | 125mg/6h PO; 1g/12h IVI over 100min; do peak level 2h post-IVI, eg after dose 3; aim for <30mg/L and ≤10mg/L pre-dose 4. | In renal failure, get help; nomograms are available. SE: renal and ototoxicity. Do not overuse (↑risk of multiple resistance). |

*Abbreviations:* MRSA, p420; VISA: vancomycin-intermediate resistance *S. aureus*; VRE: vancomycin-resistant enterococci.

Infectious diseases

*History:* A good history may reveal the source of infection: ask about respiratory, GI and GU symptoms; any travel or possible immunocompromise? *Signs* (variable!) T°↑ (or ↓); pulse↑; respiratory rate↑; BP↓ (eg ≤90/70mmHg); look for localizing signs.

*Tests:* If time allows and not too ill, culture all possible sources before treating (blood, sputum, urine, faeces, skin/wound swabs, CSF, aspirates). Do FBC, ESR, CRP, U&E, LFT, clotting, serology, malaria film, acute phase serum. Save serum for virology (compare with convalescent sample in ~2wks), CXR, ABG if indicated. MSU/dipstick.

*Prognosis:* Poor if very old or young, BP↓, WCC↓, $P_aO_2$↓, DIC, hypothermia.

*Treatment:* ►►Get help (eg if you cannot get an IV access; antibiotics *must* be up and running within 1h of telltale signs of serious sepsis). Follow local guidelines. Suspect MRSA, so have a low threshold for using vancomycin (also useful if penicillin allergic). Change antibiotic in the light of sensitivities. Give drugs IV (over ≥5min) if severely ill (eg for ~2 days, then change to PO if possible). If in doubt, ask an infection specialist.

**Common fatal errors** Nurses not reporting worsening vital signs; doctor not reacting, or wasting time trying in vain for IV access (p775); pharmacy slow to supply antibiotics; unsuitable antibiotic used; not acting on results of lab data.

| Infection | Treatment examples (be aware of local guidelines) |
|---|---|
| **Septicaemia (bloodstream infection)** | |
| From urinary tract sepsis | Co-amoxiclav 1.2g/8h (=amoxicillin 1g+clavulanic acid 200mg) IV over 3min + gentamicin IV 5mg/kg *once daily* is typical max dose; p767 |
| From intra-abdominal sepsis | Ceftazidime 2g/8h IM/IV + metronidazole 500mg/8h IVI |
| ►►From *Meningococcus* sepsis | Cefotaxime 2g/6h (p833) or ceftriaxone 2g/12h IV over 30min |
| From skin or bone source | Flucloxacillin 1g/6h IV |
| Unknown cause | Co-amoxiclav 1.2g/8h IV+gentamicin 5-7mg/kg once daily, p767 + metronidazole 500mg/8h IVI |
| ►►With neutropenia (consider the MASCC score, p347) | Tazocin® =piperacillin 4g with tazobactam 500mg 4.5g/8h IV over ~4min + gentamicin (as above). |
| **Pneumonia** | |
| Mild community-acquired | Amoxicillin 500mg/8h PO |
| Possible atypical pneumonia | Add erythromycin 500mg/6h PO |
| Severe community-acquired | Co-amoxiclav as above + erythromycin 12.5mg/kg/6h IV; see legionellosis, p162 |
| Hospital-acquired | Ceftazidine (above) or Tazocin® 4.5g/8h IV |
| **Meningitis (p832)** | |
| *Meningococcus* *Pneumococcus* *Haemophilus* | ►►Ceftriaxone 2g/12h IV over 3min or cefotaxime, p833 (or benzylpenicillin 1.2g IV stat if outside hospital) |
| *Listeria* | Add ampicillin 2g/4h IVI and gentamicin, p381 |
| If HSV encephalitis possible | Add aciclovir 10mg/kg/8h IVI (if eGFR >50) |
| **Endocarditis (p145)** | |
| **Osteomyelitis/septic arthritis** | Flucloxacillin 1g/6h IV slowly |
| UTI (simple) | Trimethoprim 200mg/12h PO |
| **Cellulitis** | Flucloxacillin (p378) |
| **Wound infection** | Await swab result; if ill, flucloxacillin 1g/6h slow IV |

### Using a side-room laboratory (near-patient testing)

The main advantage of doing your own lab work is that it enables you to have intelligent chats with lab staff, and to encourage their diligence (lab staff make errors out of boredom; amateurs make errors out of ignorance). The great thing is to understand the sources of error—and allow for them at the bedside.[17] Be aware of health and safety issues. Where available, good dipstick or test-kit technology can be used, eg Optimal® for malaria diagnosis.

**Urine** Get used to microscoping your own urines. Labs are often too busy to do this well, and sometimes careful microscopy pays great dividends. See p290. Dipstick analysis is OK but misses casts, etc (p286) and cannot distinguish streps from rods. If dipstick +ve for leucocytes, nitrites, blood, or protein, send for culture and testing for antibiotic sensitivities. If +ve for glucose, suspect diabetes (do fasting plasma glucose). If heavily +ve for protein, do 24h protein collection.

**Blood** Use precautions: all specimens could be HBV, HCV, or HIV +ve. To make a *thick blood film* (malaria diagnosis), use fresh whole blood: a small blob should be spread out untidily to cover ~1cm², thinly enough for watch hands to be seen through. The untidiness helps the microscopist, giving areas of varying thickness, some of which will be ideal for what is often a tricky task. Label and allow to dry. To make a *thin blood film*, put 1 small drop of blood near one end of the slide. Take another slide, place its end in the drop of blood, angled at 45°. Push the slide away from you to spread the blood into a thin film (practice makes perfect!). Allow the film to dry, fix in methanol for 5s, then stain as follows.

*Leishman's stain:* Cover with 10 drops. After 30s add 20 drops of water. Leave for 15min. Pick up the slide with forceps (to avoid purple fingers) and rinse in fast-flowing tap water—for 1s only. Allow to dry. Examine under oil immersion. Note red cell morphology. Do a differential white count. Polymorphs have lobed nuclei. Lymphocytes are small (just larger than red cells) and round, having little cytoplasm. Monocytes are larger than lymphocytes, but similar, with kidney-shaped nuclei. Eosinophils are like polymorphs, but have prominent pink-red cytoplasmic granules. Basophils are rare, and have blue granules—images: p325. Learn to use a white cell counting chamber—don't expect to rival lab accuracy.

*Field's stain* is easy to use and gives good quick results for malaria, trypanosomes & filaria. Dip the slide in solution A for 5s then solution B for 3s. Dip in tap water for 5s after each staining. Stand to dry. Examine thick film for >5min before saying "no malaria". **NB:** ward *serology tests*, eg *Para*Sight F® are available for *P. falciparum*, but cannot replace microscopy as they are not 100% sensitive[38] and parasites are not quantified (needed to plan treatment). New, cheap, pocket microscopes such as the Newton (NM1) have a role here, as does PCR[39,40]

**Pus (Gram stain)** Make a smear; fix by gentle heat. Flood slide with cresyl violet for 30s. Wash in running water. Flood with Lugol's iodine for 30s. Wash with running water. Decolourize with acetone for 1-3s until no blue colour runs out. Counterstain for 30s with neutral red or safranin. Wash and dry. Gram +ve organisms appear blue-black; Gram -ve ones look red, but are easier to miss.

**Near-patient chemistry** In one sense this is less taxing than the above tests—the skill lies in the people who made the reagents easy to use. A problem is quality control and the black box effect: when we put a strip into a machine, eg to measure cardiac enzymes, we cannot see the workings of the black box: it just gives a deceptively accurate-looking figure. Frequent calibration of equipment is only a partial answer to this. It is only after you have spent a long time trying to get good results from near-patient analysers, comparing paired samples with the lab, that one appreciates the reproducibility and reliability of the formal lab. ►Speed of reporting is useless if you cannot trust the results.

Infectious diseases

▶Always consider this when there are evasive answers or unexplained findings, especially in younger patients. Ask direct questions: "Do you use any drugs?"; "Have you ever injected drugs? "; "Does your partner use any drugs? "; "Do you share needles? "; "Have you ever had an HIV test?"; "How do you finance your drugs?" List drugs used, and prescribed drugs, with names of prescriber.

*Behavioural clues:*
• Temporary resident seen by GP: "Just passing through your area".
• Demands analgesia/anti-emetics. Knows pharmacopoeia well: "I just need some pethidine for my renal colic/sickle-cell crisis".
• Erratic behaviour on the ward; unexplained absences; mood swings.
• Unrousable in the mornings; agitation from day 2.
• Heavy smoking; strange smoke smells (cannabis, cocaine, heroin).

*Physical clues:*
• Acetone or glue smell on breath (solvent abuse).
• Small pupils (opiates), reversed by naloxone.
• Needle tracks on arms, groin, legs, between toes; IV access hard.
• Abscesses and lymphadenopathy in nodes draining injection sites.
• Signs of drug-associated illnesses (endocarditis, p144; AIDS, p410; viral hepatitis).

| Common and possible presentations in drug abusers | |
|---|---|
| Unconscious | p800<br>Benzodiazepines—if in ITU consider flumazenil 0.2mg IV over 15s then 0.1mg/min as needed, to 1mg (2mg if on ITU). |
| Psychosis or agitation | Ecstasy (p855), LSD, amphetamine, anabolic steroids, benzodiazepines. Haloperidol may help (p11). |
| Asthma or dyspnoea | Is there opiate-induced pulmonary oedema?<br>NB: asthma may follow the smoking of heroin. |
| Lung abscess | Right-sided endocarditis (Staph) until proved otherwise. |
| PUO | Is it endocarditis, eg with no cardinal signs (p144)? |
| Fever/PUO/shivering/headache | Do blood cultures; start, eg gentamicin (p381 & p766). |
| Hyperpyrexia | See phenothiazine poisoning, p855. |
| Abscesses | If over injection site, then often of mixed organisms.<br>Eg on injecting suspended tablets into groin. |
| DVT | Any compression damage (compartment syndrome)? Do CK. |
| Pneumonia | Pneumococcus, haemophilus, TB, pneumocystis (p410). |
| Tachyarrhythmia | (If young); cocaine, amphetamines, endocarditis. |
| Jaundice | Hepatitis A, B, or C; anabolic steroids (cholestasis). |
| 'Glandular fever' | May be presentation of HIV seroconversion illness. |
| Osteomyelitis | Including spinal. Staph. aureus/Gram -ve organisms. |
| Constipation | If severe, opiate abuse may be the cause. |
| Blindness | Consider fungal ophthalmitis ± endocarditis. |
| Runny nose | Opiate withdrawal (+ colic/diarrhoea, yawns, lacrimation, dilated pupils, insomnia, piloerection, myalgia, mood↓; can occur in neonates if mother is an opiate abuser); cocaine use. |
| Neuropathies | (and any odd CNS signs) Consider solvent abuse. |
| Infarctions | (eg of spinal cord, brain, heart) Suspect cocaine use. |

| **IV drug abuse and infectious disease** | |
|---|---|
| **Vocabulary** The 1st step in helping a recreational drug user is to communicate.... | |
| Amphetamines | May be called speed; whiz; Billy; pink champagne |
| Amyl nitrate | Goldrush; poppers; snappers |
| Barbiturates | Barbs; idiot pills |
| Synthetic cannabis-like drugs | Annihilator |
| Cocaine | Coke; Charlie; uncle; the white; the nice; snow; crack |
| Dihydrocodeine | DFs |
| Drug-induced sleep | Gauching; nodding; going on the nod |
| Drug intoxication | Stoned; off it; bladdered; ripped; wiped out; off my box |
| Heroin | Smack; the nasty; gear; brown; skag; hit; Harry; junk |
| Ecstasy (MDMA) | E; X; echo; disco biscuit; love drug; XTC; snow[41] |
| Heroin with ecstasy | Party pack (2-for-1 deal when pusher's business is low) |
| Filter | Bud/cigarette tip, for drawing drugs through before use |
| GBL (γ-butyrolactone) | Nail varnish remover (deadly if used with alcohol) |
| Injecting | Mainlining; hitting/jacking up; cranking; having a dig |
| (subcutaneous/IM/failed) | (skin popping/muscle popping/failed) |
| (subclavian) | (pocket shot). NB: febrile reaction is a 'bad hit'[41] |
| Ketamine | Special K (Home Office class C drug, like cannabis); a 'K hole' is a dissociative state (hole in consciousness, p489)—may be a ketamine prelude to 'ego death' |
| LSD | Acid; trips; cardboard; tabs; microdots (2mm tabs) |
| Marijuana | Weed; pot; draw; ganja; grass; resin; Mary; hash; skunk |
| Methadone | Mud; juice (implies liquid methadone) |
| Methylenedioxyamphetamine | MDA; snowball (like MDMA but more psychedelic)[42] |
| Needles | Spikes; nails (tools=syringes) |
| Obtaining drugs | Score (selling drugs=deal) |
| PCP | Angel dust; KJ; ozone; missile |
| Prostitution | Working the block; on the game; flogging one's golly |
| Prostitute's client | Mush; punter |
| Shooting gallery | Hygienic supervised surroundings for injecting |
| Shoplifting | Grafting |
| Smoking heroin | Chasing the dragon (bonging=smoking cocaine) |
| Syringes | Works; tools (barrel of a syringe=gun) |
| Temazepam | Temazies |
| Tourniquet | Key |
| Wanted by police | 'On me toes'; keeping head down |
| White heroin | China white |
| Withdrawing from opiates | Turkeying; clucking |
| Zopiclone | Zim-zims |

**Helping IV drug users (IDUs) on the ward** ►Fully assess any severe cutaneous infection (± imaging of deeper structures). Anthrax and other serious infections (eg IE/SBE) present this way in IDUs. Take blood cultures; vancomycin + ciprofloxacin + clindamycin may be needed.[43]

- Drug users everywhere face stigma, mistreatment, alienation from medical services (that's you?)● and violation of their human rights. It's so easy to think... IV drug abusers? It's their fault...I'm busy...they are beneath my consideration.
- A non-judgemental approach will help cooperation and may avoid self-discharge.
- Establish firm rules of acceptable ward behaviour. NSAIDs help with pain relief.
- In general, don't prescribe benzodiazepines. Methadone may be needed if opiate addicts develop bad withdrawal signs or symptoms in hospital. Get help.
- Encourage safe-sex; support schemes giving new needles to drug users (recently outlawed in the USA for some reason, where many share needles).
- Encourage regular HIV tests (9% are HIV +ve;[USA] most have no regular serology).[44]
- Don't just think "HIV": ~10 million IV drug abusers are thought to be hepatitis C +ve (ie 80%); 6 million are hep B core antigen +ve;[45] 3 million are HIV +ve.[46]
- Commercial sex workers need STD screen, speculum exam (OHCS p242) + cervical cytology/HPV screen as carcinoma in situ is common (OHCS p273). Screen for syphilis (p431), HIV (p408) and hepatitis B (vaccination, p271). Use gloves. Liaise with GP.

Infectious diseases

Contrary to Gustave Flaubert, most fevers are not caused by plums, melons, April sunshine, etc,[47] but by our immune responses to self-limiting viral infections resulting in production of interferons and cytokines. PUO in adults is defined as a temperature >38.3°C for >3wks with no obvious source despite appropriate investigations (eg after 3 days in the hospital or after 3 outpatient visits).[48] Signs of bacteraemia include confusion, renal failure, neutrophilia, ↓plasma albumin,[49] and ↑CRP (p701).

**Causes**[49] Infection (23%); connective tissue diseases (22%); tumours (20%); drug fever (3%); miscellaneous (14%). PUOs resist diagnosis in 25% of patients.

- *Infections* Abscesses (lung, liver, subphrenic, perinephric, pelvic); empyema; bacteria (*Salmonella, Brucella, Borrelia, Leptospira*, p430); rheumatic fever; SBE/IE (may be culture -ve, eg Q fever); TB (CXR may be normal, so culture sputum and urine); other granulomas (actinomycosis, toxoplasmosis); *parasites* (eg amoebic liver abscess, malaria, schistosomiasis, trypanosomiasis); fungi; typhus.[50] Asking "Where have you been" is vital: find an expert on that area, or else you will miss diagnoses you may have never heard of, eg melioidosis (*Burkholderia*, p447, the chief cause of fatal bacteraemic pneumonia in parts of SE Asia).
- *Neoplasms* Especially *lymphomas* (any pattern: Pel-Ebstein fever, p354, is rare). Occasionally *solid tumours* (GI; renal cell). Patients may be unaware of fever.
- *Connective tissue disease* Rheumatoid arthritis, polymyalgia rheumatica, Still's disease, giant cell arteritis, SLE, PAN, Kawasaki disease.
- *Others* Drugs (T°↑ may occur months after starting but remits within days of stopping; eosinophilia is a clue); pulmonary embolism; stroke; Crohn's; ulcerative colitis; sarcoid; amyloid; familial Mediterranean fever—recurrent polyserositis (peritonitis, pleurisy) + fevers, abdominal pain, and arthritis; treat with colchicine; cause: gene defect, eg at 16p13;[51] hyper IgD syndrome (periodic prolonged fevers, large joint arthritis, lymphadenopathy, abdominal pain, skin rash, and ↑IgD (>100u/mL)).[52]

**Examples of intermittent fevers** Always think of malaria; septicaemia (eg from diverticular disease); UTI; pelvic inflammatory disease; IE/SBE; TB; filarial fever—and rarities, eg: amyloid; *Brucella*; occult thromboembolism;[53] Castleman's disease.[54]
- *Daily spikes:* Abscess; TB;[55] schistosomiasis. *Twice-daily spikes:* Leishmaniasis.[56]
- *Saddleback fever* (eg fever for 7d, then normal for 3d): Colorado tick fever; *Borrelia; Leptospira;* dengue; Legionnaire's disease;[57] *Ehrlichia*[58](p434).
- *Longer periodicity:* Pel-Ebstein (eg from lymphoma, p354).
- *Remitting* (diurnal variation, not dipping to normal): Amoebiasis; malaria; *Salmonella;* Kawasaki disease; CMV; TB.[59]

**History** Work; hobbies; sexual activities; eating raw animals; drug abuse; immunosuppression; distant travel (▶p388); animal/people contacts; bites; cuts; surgery; rashes; diarrhoea; drugs (eg non-prescription); immunization; sweats; weight↓; lumps; and itching.

**Examine** Teeth; rectum; vagina; skin lesions; nodes; liver; spleen (p606); nails; heart; joints; temporal arteries; retina (Roth spots, fig 1—caused by microinfarcts, eg from SBE/IE, hypertension, HIV, connective tissue disease, anaemia, Behçet's, viraemia, hypercoagulability).

**Symptom patterns** Dialogue with experts ± decision support to diagnose fever with any other symptom.

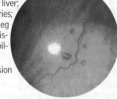

Fig 1. Roth spots.
©J Trobe.

Many diseases preoccupying infectious disease specialists are new or newly re-emerging: food-borne *E. coli*, waterborne *Cryptosporidium*, airborne Legionnaire's disease, blood-borne hepatitis c, and HIV have come to the fore in the last 30yrs. Why have these years been so tumultuous in the ID world? Greed and exploitation? Examples: 1 Each year we consume 4 centuries-worth of animal and plant life,[60] so promoting ecological instability. 2 Economic drive builds dams (↑breeding grounds for vectors by orders of magnitude) and forces land development, putting people closer to vectors, eg ticks, mosquitoes, and rodents. Intensive farming makes it easier for infectious agents to jump the species barrier—eg hantavirus (from rodents),[1] haemorrhagic fever viruses, arboviruses, Nipah and Hendra viruses, avian influenza, monkeypox virus, SARS (p163), and CJD, p710). Consider also these 10 interacting causes:[61]

1 Famine and war (± threats of bioterrorism, eg with anthrax and smallpox). Sound vector-control practices are impossible if wars are being fought.
2 Unprecedented movements of peoples, their animals and their parasites, mixing genes, cultures, customs, and behaviour, eg eating raw molluscs and crabs facilitates toxoplasma, trematode, cestode, and nematode zoonoses.
3 Microbial adaptation and change making antibiotics less successful.
4 Human susceptibility to infection (increased immunocompromise).
5 Climate change leading to shifting ecosystems and, in some places, economic disaster (p372) worsened if local populations have no immunity.
6 Warmer parts of Europe (eg Italy) are now seeing tropical diseases such as Chikungunya fever (a mosquito-borne disease commoner in Africa and Asia that can cause arthritis for weeks, but is usually self-limiting).[62]
7 Human demographics (economic development and land use)—and an increasing world population (rising at ~86 million per year).
8 Tourism and commerce. West Nile virus, for example, reached New York from its ancestral home in the Middle East on a bird carried by a ship or plane.[63] With SARS, the specific tourists, businessmen, and doctors who took the virus from Hong Kong to Hanoi, Singapore, and Toronto have been identified.[64]
9 Technology and industry—easy to blame, but also part of the solution. Food security for millions living on <$1/day depends on increasing rice yields through high-tech genetic manipulation to produce insect- and saline-resistant rice. Good crops from disease-free plants mean disease-free people.
10 Breakdown of public health measures with poverty and social inequality.

**Can we win against infectious diseases?** No! All we can do is live with them. To help us do this in ways that are not too destructive, we need robust public health surveillance institutions, sound vector-control policies, political will, quarantine laws, and, above all, openness and cooperation. SARS and its spread emphasize this in a graphic way: as the Chinese and other less-than-open societies have found out, when it comes to reporting infectious diseases, lying means dying.[2] Winning or losing is the wrong image: infectious diseases have made us who we are. The ability of genomes to produce and emit DNA/RNA sequences allows *horizontal* transmission of genes, and is one of the main motors of evolution.[65]

1 Hantaviruses cause hantavirus pulmonary syndrome (HPS) in the Americas and haemorrhagic fever with renal syndrome (HFRS) in Asia and Europe. In Scandinavia/North Europe, a milder form of HFRS occurs (nephropathica epidemica). HPS presents with acute respiratory failure (dyspnoea), renal failure, thrombocytopenia, and reactive lymphocytosis. Diagnosis: serology; PCR. Treatment: ensure fluid homeostasis. Extracorporeal membrane oxygenation in decompensated patients.[66]
2 This led to the sacking of health ministers and more transparent reporting methods. Problems remain—eg the slow reporting in 2008 of enterovirus EV71 outbreaks—an important cause of paralysis,[67] meningitis, brainstem encephalitis, and neurogenic pulmonary oedema/cardiogenic shock,[68] as well as self-limiting hand, foot & mouth disease (T°↑, mouth ulcers + palm and sole vesicles).

Infectious diseases

**Emergency help**[UK] Liverpool 0151 708 9393, London 020 7388 9600, Birmingham 0121 766 6611, Oxford 01865 225430, HPA 020 7759 2700. Travel details (where; prophylaxis; immunization; disease exposure) are **vital**, even if you cannot interpret yourself, so seek expert opinion *early*. ✆Have a good gossip with your patient to get to the truth while he is still conscious (vital clues, p446). Know your locally re-emerging diseases! Examples: TB, Lyme disease, leptospirosis, malaria, typhus, cholera, salmonella, hepatitis A, shigella, mumps, measles, brucellosis.[69] NB: a visit to the tropics doesn't preclude mundane fevers, eg flu. *Examine all over:* any bites/eschar, p435? Do serology, thick film and blood culture. **In every ill traveller, consider:**

1 ▸▸*Malaria* (p394-6): Fever, rigors, headaches, dizziness, flu symptoms, faints, diarrhoea, thrombocytopenia. *Complications:* anaemia, renal failure, pulmonary oedema, cerebral oedema. *Diagnosis:* serial thick and thin blood films.
2 *Typhoid* (p426): Presents with fever, relative bradycardia, abdominal pains, dry cough, constipation, lymphadenopathy, headache, splenomegaly ± rose spots (rare). *Complication:* GI perforation. *Diagnosis:* blood or marrow culture.
3 *Dengue fever (DF)* (p433): Presents with fever, headache, myalgia, rash (flushing or petechial), thrombocytopenia, and leucopenia. *Diagnosis:* serology.
4 *Amoebic liver abscess* (p436): T°↑, jaundice, RUQ pain. Do ultrasound.
5 *Also:* Travellers' diarrhoea ('turista'), taeniasis, cysticercosis and trichinosis (p442).

**Jaundice** Think of viral hepatitis, cholangitis, liver abscess, leptospirosis, typhoid, malaria, dengue fever, yellow fever, haemoglobinopathies.

**Gross splenomegaly** Malaria causing HMS,[1] visceral leishmaniasis (kala-azar).

**Diarrhoea & vomiting** (p390 & p246) *E. coli* (Travellers' diarrhoea) is commonest. Consider *Salmonella, Shigella, Campylobacter, Giardia lamblia, Vibrio cholerae*, etc. (p390). See p246 for general management. If diarrhoea is prolonged, consider protozoal infection of small bowel or tropical sprue (p280). In HIV: cryptosporidia, microsporidia, and *Isospora belli* (need special stains).

**Hepatosplenomegaly** p606 malaria; *Brucella*; typhoid; typhus (fig 1); leishmaniasis.

**Respiratory symptoms** Common respiratory pathogens (p162), typhoid, *Legionella*, TB, Q fever, histoplasmosis, Löffler's (p718), HIV ± pneumocystosis. Do CXR & $P_aO_2$.

**Arthritis** Gonococcus; septicaemia; viruses (Ross river, Chikungunya).[70]

**Erythema nodosum** (p564) Causes: streps, TB, leprosy, fungi, Crohn's disease, ulcerative colitis, sarcoidosis, pregnancy, drugs (sulfonamides, contraceptive steroids).

**Anaemia** Hookworm, malaria, kala-azar, haemolysis, malabsorption.

**Bleeding** (melaena, nose bleeds, haematuria, DIC/ARDS) Viral haemorrhagic fevers.

**Skin signs** • Purpura or any rash: meningococcaemia • Typhus ('eschar' =scab; fig 1) • Orf (pustules) • Leprosy (p428, anaesthetic, hypopigmented areas) • Tropical ulcers • Leishmaniasis (ulcers/nodules) • Onchocerciasis (itchy nodules) • Myiasis (nodules=larvae of insects) • Transitory migratory swellings: gnathostomiasis • Calabar swellings (loa loa, p443) • Scabies (itchy allergic rash + burrows, p416 & OHCS p608).

**Acute abdomen** Perforating typhoid ulcer, toxic megacolon in amoebic or bacillary dysentery, sickle-cell crisis, ruptured spleen.

**Rarities to consider** ▸ Ask about local emergency isolation policy & contact tracing.
*Rabies & yellow fever:* (p432); other CNS viral infections, eg encephalitis (p400; p834).
*Lassa fever:* (Nigeria, Sierra Leone, Liberia). *Signs:* Fever; exudative sore throat; face oedema; collapse. Δ: PCR/EM; serology. ℞: Isolate & refer. See VHF guidelines.[71]
*Marburg & Ebola virus:* (Sudan, Zaire, Kenya). Transmission: close contact/fluids; (maybe via air too).[72] *Signs:* T°↑, myalgia, D&V, pleuritic pain, hepatitis, shock, bleeding from any orifice/gums. A maculopapular rash appears on day 5-7 and desquamates in <5d.[73] Δ: PCR or electron microscopy; serology. ℞: Isolate and refer.[74]
*Other viruses causing haemorrhage:* Dengue, Crimea-Congo fever (CCHF, p446), haemorrhagic fever with renal syndrome, yellow fever. ▸ See p432.

1 HMS (hyper-reactive malarial splenomegaly/tropical splenomegaly syndrome) is a chronic condition *usually* only seen in endemic areas (IgM↑↑); acute malaria causes lesser splenomegaly.

## Some typical incubation times[75]

For fever with diarrhoea: p390

Incubation times are not set in stone: expect variability.

| <14 days | 14 days to 6wks | >6wks |
|---|---|---|
| **Undifferentiated fever** | | |
| Malaria | Malaria | Malaria |
| Typhoid | Typhoid | Hepatitis B or E |
| Leptospirosis | Leptospirosis | Kala-azar |
| Dengue fever | Hepatitis A or E | Lymphatic filariasis |
| Rickettsiae | Acute schistosomiasis | Schistosomiasis |
| Acute HIV infection | Acute HIV infection | Amoebic liver abscess |
| **Fever with CNS signs** | | |
| Malaria | | |
| Viral and bacterial meningitis and encephalitis | East African trypanosomiasis | Rabies |
| East African trypanosomiasis | Rabies | |
| Poliomyelitis | | |
| **Fever with chest signs** | | |
| Influenza | Tuberculosis | Tuberculosis |
| Legionellosis | Q fever | |
| Q fever | | |
| Acute histoplasmosis | | |
| SARS | | |

### Hitch-hiking to a Fools' Paradise

We think we are absolved of thinking of tropical diseases when the answer to "Where have you been?" is "Bournemouth" and in our blinkered way we carry on in our Fools' Paradise until disaster bites. It's not just a question of forgotten holidays or amnesic stopovers. Maybe our patient is an airport baggage-handler and has been bitten by a hitch-hiking mosquito: who knows? We never will if we don't ask. Even if there has been no travel to the tropics *global warming is ensuring that the tropics are travelling to us*. To the first writers of medical books, Paradise was just beyond the Far East, and the world was a disc surround by oceans of blue water. The world moves on, tarnished, tawdry, and trashed, and Paradise appears to be evolving with ever more serpents in the garden beguiling us with ambiguous answers to the great question: "Where have you been?"

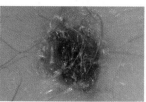

Fig 1. Dr Watson was treating this dentist's presumed septicaemia until Holmes went over his hindquarters with a lens, revealing this lesion. "I see you have been hunting bushbuck in the Eastern Cape again, Mr S—. This eschar is the tell-tale *tache noire* of typhus." Prompt **doxycycline** averted disaster. Elementary? We are all uneasy amalgams of dullness and brilliancy, jackal and hind, haunted and hunted, as well as hunting.

©M Seare.

Infectious diseases

Ingesting certain bacteria, viruses, and toxins is a common cause of D&V (p56 & p246). Contaminated food and water are common sources, but often no specific cause is found. Ask about details of food and water taken, cooking method, time until onset of symptoms, and whether fellow-diners were affected. Ask about swimming, canoeing, etc. NB: food poisoning is a notifiable disease (p373) in the UK.

| Organism/source | Incubation | Clinical features | Notes/sources of infection |
|---|---|---|---|
| Staph. aureus | 1–6h | D&V, P, hypotension | Meat |
| Bacillus cereus | 1–5h | D&V | Rice |
| Red beans | 1–3h | D&V | |
| Heavy metals, eg zinc | 5min–2h | V, P (?work exposure) | (Delayed fever ± flu-like features) |
| Scrombotoxin | 10–60min | D, flushing, sweating | Fish (NB may report hot mouth) |
| Mushrooms | 15min–24h | D&V, P, fits, coma (LFT↑↑) | Image: p251 (hepatic & renal failure) |
| Salmonella | 12–48h | D&V, P, fever, septicaemia | Meat, eggs, poultry |
| C. perfringens | 8–24h | D, P afebrile | Meat |
| C. botulinum | 12–36h | V, paralysis | Processed food |
| C. difficile | 1–7d | Bloody D, P, gut perforation; toxic megacolon; hospital-acquired (1000 deaths/yrUK) | Antibiotic-associated; getting more virulent (eg strain BI/NAP1 with 20-fold ↑ in toxin A and B production)[?] |
| Vibrio cholerae | 2h–5d | See p426 | Water* |
| Vib. parahaemolyticus | 12–24h | Profuse D; P, V | Seafood |
| Campylobacter | 2–5d | Bloody D, P, T°↑, peritonism | Milk, poultry, water* |
| Listeria | | Meningoencephalitis; "I've got flu"; miscarriages | Cheese, pâtés |
| E. coli type O157 | 12–72h | Cholera/typhoid-like;* | Haemolytic-uraemic sy., p308 |
| Y. enterocolitica | 24–36h | D, P, fever | Milk* |
| Cryptosporidium (fig1) | 4–12d | D in HIV | Cow→water→man |
| Giardia lamblia | 1–4wks | p436 (D, malabsorption) | *Nappies, cats,[?] dogs, crows[?] |
| Entamoeba histolytica | 1–4wks | See p436 | * |
| Noroviruses, eg Norwalk SRVS (small round structured virus) | 12–48h[?] mean≈34h | Fever, P, D & projectile V;[?] 'winter vomiting illness'. Δ: no leucocytes in faeces; PCR | *Fecal-oral (vomit is infectious); very contagious, and common. Infectious for ≤48h after symptoms resolve[?] |
| Rotavirus | 1–7d | D&V, fever, malaise | *(Vaccine available for infants aged from 6 weeks, 2 doses) |
| Shigella | 2–3d | Bloody D, P, fever | Any food |

V = vomiting; D = diarrhoea; P = abdominal pain. *May be food- or water-borne.

**Tests** *Stool microscopy/culture* if from abroad, an institution, or in day care, or an outbreak is suspected. In these circumstances culture of the food source may help.

**Prevention** Hygiene; if abroad, avoid unboiled/unbottled water, ice cubes, salads, and peel own fruit. Eat only freshly prepared hot food (or *thoroughly* rewarmed, p377).[20] Household water treatment and safe storage technologies can ↑ water quality and ↓ rates of diarrhoea, eg chlorine or solar disinfection, and ceramic or biosand filtration.[1 82]

**Management** Usually symptomatic. Maintain *oral fluid* intake (±oral rehydration sachets). For severe symptoms (but not in dysentery), give *anti-emetics*, eg *prochlorperazine* 12.5mg/6h IM + *antidiarrhoeals* (*codeine phosphate* 30mg PO/IM or *loperamide* 4mg stat, then 2mg after each loose stool). *Antibiotics are only indicated if systemically unwell, immunosuppressed or elderly*; resistance is common. *Cholera*: *tetracycline* reduces transmission.

*Salmonella*: *ciprofloxacin* 500mg/12h PO, 200–400mg/12h IVI over 60min (remember that antibiotic therapy in salmonella enteritis may ↑ number of chronic carriers). *Shigella and Campylobacter*: *ciprofloxacin* as above.

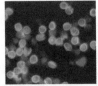

Fig 1. *Cryptosporidium* (immunofluorescence). It is a tiny protozoan (5µm) but a big cause of diarrhoea, esp in children in the 3rd world. It is life threatening if HIV+ve; self-limiting if CD4 ≥100; if <100, 14L of diarrhoea can be lost/d (bad news). It's a UK crime to sell water if >1 oocysts/10L. Spread: unboiled water; cattle. If found in stool, quantify excretion. If R needed, ask a microbiologist (R often fails); optimizing anti-HIV R may be the best approach.[83] Consider: nitazoxanide 0.5g/12h PO for 3d (if >12yrs).

©S Upton; Kansas Univ.

1 The top few cm of sand traps most organisms, which develop into a highly active food chain (the *biological layer*, which must remain partially wet). Further filtration occurs in the lower layers of sand.

*Active immunization* stimulates the immune system (humoral+cellular immunity). *Passive immunization* uses pre-formed antibody (nonspecific or antigen-specific). ▶Strengthening routine immunization is a global priority for us all. Most incompletely vaccinated children live in India (32%), Nigeria (14%), and Indonesia (7%).[2012 data]

| Age | Immunization (L=live vaccine) | (DoH[UK] 2012) |
|---|---|---|
| 2 months | **Pediacel®**, ie 5-in-1 diphtheria + tetanus + acellular pertussis + inactivated polio + haemophilus B (HiB); if prem, still give at 2 months; can give if ≤10 yrs if missed vacs; + **Prevenar 13®** (13-valent pneumococcal) | |
| 3 months | **Pediacel®** + **NeisVac-C®** or **Meningitec®** (Meningitis C vaccine) | |
| 4 months | **Pediacel®** + **Prevenar 13®** (pneumococcal) + **NeisVac-C** or **Meningitec®** | |
| 12 mths | **Menitorix®** (*H. influenzae* with meningitis C) | |
| 13 mths | **MMRvaxPro®**[L] or **Priorix®**[L] (measles, mumps and rubella) + **Prevenar 13®** | |
| 3¼-5yrs | **Repevax®** or **Infanrix-IPV®** (diphtheria, tetanus, pertussis and polio) + **Priorix®**[L] or **MMRvaxPro®**[L] | |
| 12-13yrs | **Gardasil®** 3 doses if ♀ separated by 1 then 6 mths (HPV/cervical ca, *OHCS* p272) | |
| 13-18⁺yrs | **Revaxis®** (low-dose diphtheria, tetanus, inactivated polio; can also be used for primary vaccination if >10yrs) | |
| Pregnant | Pertussis, 1 dose of **Repevax®** in 3rd trimester & influenza vaccine if indicated | |
| Any age | **BCG**[L] (not for everyone, since 2004 in UK) If ↑risk of TB, eg for all in high-risk areas (eg London), or in groups at ↑risk, eg TB contact, or (grand) parents or from high-prevalence country, ie >40/100,000/yr—or a visitor to such a country for >1 month. May start at 3d old. **Hepatitis B:** p271; universal (WHO advice) or if at ↑risk. MMRvaxPro® may be given at any age if the above is missed. One-off *pneumococcal vaccine* 23-valent Pneumovax II®±repeat if at ↑risk after >5yrs (eg splenectomy).[84] (**Prevenar 13®**×2, as above, if <2yrs old.) Yearly *flu vaccine* if caring for at-risk person or if chronic heart, chest, liver, or renal disease; DM; immunosuppression (eg HIV +ve, cirrhosis, on chemotherapy, or spleen function↓, eg ∴ coeliac or sickle-cell disease). **Revaxis®** booster. | |

▶*An acute febrile illness is a contraindication to any vaccine*. Give live vaccines either together or separated by ≥3wks. Caution with live vaccines in patients who are immune-deficient (transplants, cancer chemotherapy, steroids, HIV infection)—seek expert advice. ▶*Contraindications to vaccines:* see *OHCS* p151.

▶**Bacille Calmette-Guérin (BCG)** Live attenuated anti-TB vaccine (works in ≤80% for ~10yrs). Make a 7mm blanched weal between the top and middle ⅓ of arm (deltoid's insertion) or, for cosmesis, the upper, outer thigh. Expect to feel marked resistance as the injection goes in. If, while injecting, propagation of the weal stops, you are going too deep: re-insert the needle. A swelling appears after 2-6wks, developing into a papule or small ulcer. Avoid air-occluding dressings. SE: pain, local abscess, regional lymphadenitis (the most common SE. The risk is ↑ in infants aged <30d, so give a reduced dose of vaccine.) CI: immunosuppression, pregnancy, pyrexia, or eczema at vaccination site.[85] **T-spot-TB®/Mantoux test** (p398) Offer to those at risk of TB (see BCG, above). It is now not routinely needed for those <6yrs being referred for BCG on the above criteria. **Travel** p377. Get expert advice![1]

▶*Advice to travellers is more important than vaccination:* eg simple hygiene, malaria prophylaxis, and protective measures (mosquito nets, safe sex advice, etc).

**Immunization in special situations** If *splenectomized/hyposplenic (eg sickle cell):* meningitis vaccine; pneumococcal; HiB (above); annual flu vaccine. *Chronic lung, heart, liver or kidney disease, diabetes:* pneumococcal; annual flu vaccine.

**Further details** Rotavirus vaccination for all infants (UK DoH 2013). Hepatitis B (p271); flu (p403); pneumococcal (p160); meningococcal (ACWY Vax® = group A, C, W135 & Y®), for short-term use, eg travel abroad. NB: the common group B meningococcal (MenB) strains are not covered by current vaccines; reverse vaccinology (eg Bexsero®) is changing this.[2]

1 *Schools of tropical medicine:* London: 020 7636 8636; Liverpool: 0151 708 9393.
2 Depends on identifying genes coding for surface-exposed proteins, which are able to induce bactericidal antibodies against a broad range of B strains. Vaccine combining these proteins is being developed.

Infectious diseases

Nosocomial means hospital-acquired. Fever is common in hospitalized patients of all ages. Nosocomial fever usually results from exposure to pyrogens in the hospital environment or from a medical intervention. Nosocomial fever occurs in 2-30% of inpatients: most are bacterial infections.

**Definition** Two of the many commonly used definitions are as follows:
1 Oral temperature of ≥38.1°C developing ≥24h after admission and is recorded on ≥2 consecutive occasions in patients with no history of fever in the preceding week.
2 Oral temperature >38.0°C that occurs at least 48h after admission and is recorded on at least two occasions during any 48-hour period.

**Risk factors** Alcoholism, cerebrovascular disease, CCF, 'Do-not-resuscitate' status, faecal incontinence, foot ulcers, indwelling bladder catheter, indwelling IV catheter, malignancy, number of procedures before febrile illness, pressure ulcers.

**Causes** can be grouped into five clinical entities:
1 *Infections* (the most common cause): UTI, pneumonia (eg post-op), bacteraemia, skin and soft tissue infections, CNS infection, catheter-related, GI infection, peritonitis, sinusitis, upper respiratory or other self-limiting viral infection, diverticulitis, cholangitis, vascular infections, device-related colitis, tuberculosis.
2 *Inflammation:* Aspiration, ARDS, arthritis, autoimmune conditions, adrenal insufficiency, connective-tissue disorder, drug-induced fever, acalculous cholecystitis, phlebitis, procedure-related pancreatitis, haematoma, thrombosis, sickle-cell crisis, GI bleeding, graft-versus-host disease, IV contrast reaction.
3 *Ischaemia:* Stroke, MI, pulmonary embolism, bowel ischaemia.
4 *Malignancy:* Leukaemia, lymphoma, non-haematological cancer.
5 *Drug-induced fever* is another important cause.

**Approach** Nosocomial UTI is the most common cause in those on general medicine wards, whereas nosocomial pneumonia is the most common cause of nosocomial fever in ITU patients. The cause of nosocomial fever is often not apparent, especially when symptoms or obvious physical findings suggestive of a specific illness are absent. In such cases, follow these steps:
1 Get a detailed history and do a careful physical examination covering all systems including the skin. Elucidate the surgical history and procedures performed during hospitalization. Study the patient's medication list carefully (is it a drug fever?).
2 Initial lab and imaging studies should be non-invasive, inexpensive, and based on the findings of patient's history and physical examination: FBC, LFT, ESR, urinalysis, basic cultures (eg MSU, blood, swabs of suspect areas), CXR, ESR.
3 If the initial evaluation does not reveal the cause of nosocomial fever, more expensive and invasive studies may be needed. These studies should be based on clinical suspicion and the results of the initial studies. They include: US, CT scan, MRI, nuclear medicine scanning, and serology. These modalities, including directed biopsies where indicated, reduce the need for more invasive procedures. The use of radionuclide scanning, such as technetium $^{99m}$Tc, gallium-67, or indium-labelled leukocytes, is warranted for obscure inflammatory or neoplastic conditions that are not diagnosed by conventional imaging studies.

**Prevention** Nosocomial infections result in a 4-fold ↑ in mortality, highlighting the importance of preventive measures—see BOX.

▶Each country has its own risk profile, so get to know, and follow, local guidelines.

*Hand decontamination:* There must be written policies and procedures for hand washing. Jewellery must be removed before washing.

*Personal hygiene:* Nails must be clean and kept short. False nails should not be worn. Hair must be worn short or pinned up. Beard and moustaches must be kept trimmed short and clean. Wash hands before and after each patient contact. Alcohol-based hand gels are helpful (but do not kill *C. difficile* spores).

*Working clothes:* In the UK there is a bare-below-the-elbows policy—and no white coats owing to the theoretical risk of cross-infection for cuffs and wristwatches. In areas such as burn units or ITU (and on many ordinary UK wards), uniform trousers and a short-sleeved gown are required for men and women. In other units, women may wear a short-sleeved dress.

*Shoes:* In aseptic units and in theatre, wear dedicated easy-to-clean shoes.

*Caps:* In aseptic units, theatre, or performing selected invasive procedures, staff must wear caps or hoods which completely cover the hair.

*Masks:* Cotton wool or gauze masks don't catch microorganisms. Paper masks with synthetic material for filtration are better. Wear these masks in theatre, to care for immunocompromised patients or to puncture body cavities in order to protect the patient. In other situations, staff must wear masks to protect themselves (eg when caring for patients with airborne infections, or when performing bronchoscopy, etc). Patients with infections that may be transmitted by air must use surgical masks when outside their isolation room.

*Gloves:* Wear sterile gloves for surgery, care for immunocompromised patients, and invasive procedures entering body cavities. Non-sterile gloves should be worn for all patient contacts where hands are likely to be contaminated, or for any mucous membrane contact. Staff should wear non-sterile gloves to protect themselves while caring for patients with communicable disease transmitted by contact, or performing bronchoscopy, etc. Hands must be washed when gloves are removed or changed. Don't reuse disposable gloves!

*Safe injection practices:* •No unnecessary injections •Sterile disposable equipment •Prevent contamination of medications •Safe sharps disposal practices.

**Preventing transmission from the environment** Adequate methods for cleaning, disinfecting and sterilizing must be in place. Written policies/procedures must be developed for each facility, and updated regularly.

*Cleaning hospitals:* Routine cleaning is necessary to ensure that the hospital is visibly clean and free from dust and soiling. 90% of microorganisms are present within 'visible dirt', and the purpose of routine cleaning is to eliminate this dirt. Neither soap nor detergents have antimicrobial activity, and the cleaning process depends essentially on mechanical action. There are 4 hospital zones:

**Zone A:** no patient contact, eg administration, library—normal domestic cleaning.

**Zone B:** care of patients who are not infected, and not highly susceptible—clean by procedures that don't raise dust. Dry sweeping or vacuum cleaners are not recommended. Using detergent solution improves the quality of cleaning. Disinfect areas visibly contaminated by blood or body fluids prior to cleaning.

**Zone C:** infected patients (isolation wards)—clean with a detergent/disinfectant solution, with separate cleaning equipment for each room.

**Zone D:** highly susceptible patients (protective isolation) or protected areas, eg operating suites, delivery rooms, ITU, A&E and haemodialysis units—clean using a detergent/disinfectant solution and separate cleaning equipment.

All horizontal surfaces in zones B, C & D and in all toilets must be cleaned ≥daily.

**Microbial monitoring** aims to quantify cleaning rigour and to find organisms before they kill,[91] using swabs, sponges, contact plates, dip slides + enrichment broths and selective media (+PCR for quicker recognition of impending problems).

Clean→inspect→monitor→record→reclean (*all* areas, even hard to find ductwork).

▶Someone dies of malaria every few seconds; most are African children, but the old adage that older people in endemic areas have immunity and rarely get serious malaria is untrue: deaths are under-reported (~1.2 million/yr—a number that has been falling since 2004, owing to the Gates foundation [et al]). [82] Check for malaria in any sick patient from an endemic area (>3 billion are at risk). *Species:*[92] *P. vivax:* incubation 10–17d, '*benign tertian malaria*', fever spikes every 48h. *P. ovale:* similar to *P. vivax*, except untreated infection lasts less long. Both may produce true relapses by new invasion of the blood from latent hypnozoites in the liver, up to a few years after complete clearance of parasites from the blood[93] *P. malariae:* incubation 18–40d, recurs 72-hourly ('quartan'[1,4,7...]); may 'lie low' in the blood to recrudesce after 1–52yrs. It is rarely fatal but may cause glomerulonephritis. *P. falciparum:* incubation 7–10 days, symptoms recur 36–48hrly; fulminating disease. *P. knowlesi* is a rare emergent species (common in monkeys).[94] See also figs 2–6.

**Biology** Spread: fig 2 Plasmodium protozoa injected by ♀ *Anopheles* mosquitoes multiply in RBCs causing haemolysis, RBC sequestration and cytokine release. *Fever paroxysms* reflect synchronous release of flocks merozoites from mature schizonts (fig 2). 3 phases: 1 Shivering (≤1h): "I feel so cold." 2 Hot stage (2–6h): T≈41°C, flushed, dry skin; nausea/vomiting; headache. 3 Sweats (~3h) as T° falls.[95] *Protective factors:* G6PD lack; sickle-cell trait; melanesian ovalocytosis; some HLA B53 alleles enable T cells to kill parasite-infected hepatocytes in non-Europeans.

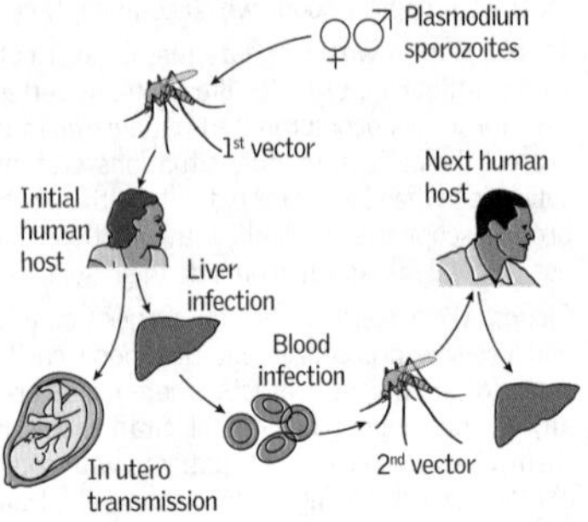

Fig 1. Malaria lifecycle.

(Labels: Plasmodium sporozoites; 1st vector; Initial human host; Liver infection; Blood infection; In utero transmission; Next human host; 2nd vector)

**Falciparum malaria** Mortality: eg 20%; higher if <3yrs old or pregnant.[1] 90% present within 1 month of the mosquito event, with prodromal headache, malaise, myalgia ± anorexia before the 1st fever paroxysm (±faints). There may be no pattern to fever spikes (esp . initially); *don't rely on periodicity to rule out any type of malaria!*

*Signs:* Anaemia, jaundice, and hepatosplenomegaly. No rash or lymphadenopathy.

*Complications: Anaemia* is common, eg from haemolysis of parasitized RBCs (often serious in children). *Thrombocytopenia.*

*5 grim signs:* 1↓Consciousness/coma (*cerebral malaria* ▶▶p397) 2Convulsions 3Coexisting chronic illness 4Acidosis (eg esp bad if HCO3⁻ <15mmol/L) 5Renal failure (eg from acute tubular necrosis). Multivariate analysis shows that other factors[2] are harder to relate to ↓survival in younger patients in an *independent* way.[96]

*Pregnancy:* ▶▶OHCS p27. Use chemoprophylaxis when pregnant in endemic areas.

**Diagnosis** Serial thin & thick blood films (needs much skill, don't always believe -ve reports, or reports based on thin film examination alone); if *P. falciparum,* you must know the level of parasitaemia. Rapid stick tests are available if microscopy cannot be performed or previously treated seriously ill patient: see p383 for ParaSight F®. Serology is not useful. Other tests: FBC (anaemia, thrombocytopenia), clotting (DIC, p346), glucose (hypoglycaemia), ABG/lactate (lactic acidosis), U&E (renal failure), urinalysis (haemoglobinuria, proteinuria, casts), blood culture to rule out septicaemia.

1 To prevent malaria deaths in pregnancy, intermittent preventive treatment is often used, but the standard 2-dose sulfadoxine-pyrimethamine regimen is often insufficient owing to resistance.[97]

2 •Extensor posture •Plantars ↑↑ •Dysconjugate gaze •Teeth-grinding (bruxism) •Hypoglycaemia (25% of children, 8% of adults; (it's also an SE of quinine) •Haemoglobinuria, ie '*blackwater fever*' •DIC •Plasma or CSF lactate >5mmol/L •Pulmonary oedema (ARDS, p178) •*Shock* may mean *algid malaria* from supervening bacterial sepsis, dehydration, or spleen rupture •Hyperparasitaemia (>5% of RBCs parasitized); if ≥20% or >10⁴/µL) of parasites are mature trophozoites or schizonts, prognosis is poor, even if few parasites seen (reflects critical mass of sequestered RBCs [98]); ditto if malaria pigment in >5% of neutrophils or Hb <50g/L. [99]

## Preventing malaria deaths (eradication or containment?)

Eradication attempts without good primary care (and a good vaccine) are likely to be counter-productive. 'Containment' public health measures entail political will + money for indoor antimosquito spraying, insecticide treated bednets, good antenatal/paediatric care, and reliable distribution of malaria drugs (no wars, no corruption). The US has led here (>$1bn over 5yrs) and will[100]

Bill & Melinda Gates Foundation; PMI: US President's malaria initiative

(a)  (b)  (c)  (d)

(e)  (f)  (g)  (h)

(i)  (j)  (k)  (l)

(m)  (n)  (o)  (p)

Fig 2. *P. ovale*. Plasmodia live in red cells: what a fantastic niche!—full of food and protected from prowling immunocytes. **a** is void—an unclaimed bag of food; **b-i** show trophozoites; **g**'s RBC is fimbriated and oval, giving the species its name; **k-n** are schizonts containing segmenting merozoites; **o** and **p** are ♀ and ♂ gametocytes. Having this marvellous knack of sexual reproduction (in the mosquito's gut) ensures the almost infinite variety of plasmodia, and their co-evolution with man.[101] With this in mind, it is interesting to note that the development of haemoglobin AS, CC, and AC genotypes and homozygous and heterozygous α-thalassaemia give significant protection only from *severe* malaria.[102]

After the Nicholson paintings in Oatney's *Primate Malarias*.

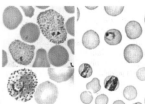

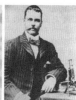

**Fig 3.** *P. vivax* ring forms partly hidden by Schuffner's dots.  **Fig 4.** *P. malariae* ring and band forms from 2 specimens.  **Fig 5.** *P. falciparum* sausage-like gametocytes in RBC ghosts.  **Fig 6.** Ronald Ross who first described the malaria lifecycle.

Fig 3 was stained and examined in the field (p383) by JML; figs 4–6©S Upton, Kansas Univ.

Infectious diseases

**Treatment** ▶If the patient has taken prophylaxis, don't use the same drug for treatment. If species unknown or mixed infection, treat as *P. falciparum*. Nearly all *P. falciparum* is resistant to chloroquine and in many areas also to Fansidar® (*pyrimethamine* + *sulfadoxine*). If in doubt, consider as resistant. *Chloroquine*[103] is 1st choice for benign malarias in most parts of the world, but chloroquine-resistant *P. vivax* occurs in Papua New Guinea, Indonesia, parts of Brazil, Colombia and Guyana.[104] Never rely on chloroquine if used alone as prophylaxis. See HPA (www.hpa.ork.uk).

*Treating uncomplicated P. ovale, P. vivax, & P. malariae:* Chloroquine base:[1] 10mg/kg (max 620mg), then 5mg/kg (max 310mg) at 6h, 24h and 48h. In resistant cases, try Malarone®, quinine, or Riamet®. Primaquine dose in *P. vivax*: 500µg/kg (max. 30mg) daily for 14d; *P. ovale*: 250µg/kg (max. 15mg) daily for 14d—given after chloroquine to treat liver stage and prevent relapse. Screen for G6PD deficiency first. CI: pregnancy. *P. malariae* does not need primaquine.

*Treating uncomplicated Falciparum malaria* (or if species is uncertain): As multidrug resistance to chloroquine, amodiaquine,[etc] is common, combination therapy, preferably containing artemisinin derivatives, is recommended by WHO.[105] •Artemether-lumefantrine (Riamet®2)—if >35kg: 4 tabs stat, then 4 tablets at 8, 24, 36, 48 and 60h.[106] •Artesunate-amodiaquine (Coarsucam®); if a fixed combination pill is available (AS 100mg + AQ 270mg), the dose is 2 pills/d for 3d. If aged 7-13yrs, it is 1 pill/d for 3d.[106] •Dihydroartemisinin-naphthoquine[107] •Dihydroartemisinin-piperaquine.[108] •Atovaquone-proguanil (Malarone®; 4 'standard' tablets once daily for 3 days) may also work. These are better than quinine regimens (eg 600mg quinine salt/8h PO for 7d, + doxycycline 100mg/24h or clindamycin 450mg/8h for 7d).[109] Artemisinins are OK in children and pregnancy (from 13 weeks; use quinine + clindamycin in 1st trimester).[110] The oral route is OK if able to swallow and no severe signs.

*Treating severe*[3] *Falciparum malaria:* IV R̴ is needed. Take to ITU. ▶▶See BOX.

*Other treatments:* Tepid sponging + paracetamol if necessary for fever. Transfuse if severe anaemia. Consider exchange transfusion if patient severely ill. Treat 'algid' malaria as malaria + bacterial shock (p778). Monitor TPR, BP, urine output, and blood glucose frequently. Daily parasite count, platelets, U&E, LFT.

**Prophylaxis for travellers** ▶*Prophylaxis does not give full protection.* Risks vary; get local advice. Avoid mosquitos: wear long-sleeves between dusk and dawn, use repellents (diethyltoluamide/DEET), long-lasting insecticidal bed-nets (US$5; last ~5yrs).

Except for Malarone® & mefloquine (below), take drugs from 1wk before travel (to reveal any SE) and continue for 4wks after return. None is required if just visiting cities of East Asia. There is no good protection for parts of SE Asia.[111]

*If little/no chloroquine resistance:* Proguanil 200mg/24h + chloroquine base 300mg/wk.

*If chloroquine-resistant P. falciparum:* Mefloquine 250mg/wk (18d before to 4wks after trip) or doxycycline 100mg/d (1d before to 4wks after) or atovaquone250mg + proguanil100mg (Malarone®) 1 tab/d (1d before travel to 7d after).[112] If poor medical care and not pregnant, carry standby treatment (eg Riamet®, Malarone®).

**Antimalarial SE** *Chloroquine:* headache, psychosis, retinopathy (in chronic use). *Fansidar®:* Stevens-Johnson syndrome, erythema multiforme, LFT↑, blood dyscrasias. *Primaquine:* Epigastric pain, haemolysis if G6PD-deficient, methaemoglobinaemia. *Malarone®:* Abdominal pain, nausea, headache, dizziness.

*Mefloquine:* Nausea, dizziness, dysphoria, insomnia, neuropsychiatric signs, long t½. Avoid mefloquine if: •Low risk of chloroquine-resistant malaria •Past or family history of epilepsy, psychosis •Need for delicate work (pilots[etc]) •Risk of pregnancy within 3 months of last dose. *Interactions:* Quinidine, halofantrine.

---

**1** 155mg chloroquine base ≈ 250mg chloroquine phosphate (PO).
**2** Dispersable formulation example for children with uncomplicated malaria: Coartem® (20mg artemether+120mg lumefantrine): 1 tab per dose if 5-14kg; 3 tabs/dose if 25-34kg; repeat if vomits within 1h.
**3** Prostration, consciousness↓, fits, respiratory distress, unable to drink, uncontrolled vomiting, macroscopic haemoglobinuria, jaundice, systolic BP ≤70mmHg, bleeding/DIC, inability to sit or stand.

## Severe *P. falciparum* malaria

Falciparum malaria is one of the great killers (mortality is ~100% in untreated severe malaria, 15–20% with treatment), so get expert help in anyone who could have travelled abroad particularly in the last few months, who is feverish with ↓consciousness. But fever is not *always* a feature of malaria, and signs may be unusual if prophylaxis has been given, and is partly effective. The central event in severe falciparum malaria is sequestration of parasitized erythrocytes in the microvasculature of vital organs. Death rate: ~1 million deaths/yr, worldwide.[113]

**Key questions** What is the parasite count, the plasma bicarbonate and the creatinine? Are there complications: shock (algid malaria), metabolic acidosis, hypoglycaemia, renal failure, or acute respiratory distress syndrome (ARDS, p178)?

**R:** (on ITU) *Always* take advice. The main goal is to prevent death. Check FBC, daily parasite count, platelets, U&E, LFT, plasma glucose. Degree of acidosis is an important determinant of outcome. Assess fluid balance meticulously. ▶▶*Start antimalarials in full dose as soon as possible*. Meta-analyses unequivocally favour parenteral artesunate over quinine for the treatment of severe malaria in adults and children and in different regions[114] of the world—so, give **artesunate** (if *immediately* available[1]) or **quinine** (dihydrochloride) 20mg salt/kg IVI (max 1.4g) over 4h, then after 8h give 10mg/kg (max 700mg) over 4h every 8h[2] Give IV until the patient can swallow; complete the course orally (see 'c' below). Monitor for hypoglycaemia. Alternative: **artemether** (3.2mg/kg followed by 1.6mg/kg daily); in the UK, artemether is not always available: get local advice. Don't wait for an ideal drug if a good alternative is to hand: delay is fatal.[115]

If swallowing OK and no complications (shock, ARDS, renal failure) give either:
a) **Artemether-lumefantrine** Riamet®, see p396.
b) **Malarone®** (atovaquone + proguanil; 4 tabs once daily for 3d with food).
c) **Quinine** (600mg salt/8h PO for 7d), with either **doxycycline** 200mg daily or **clindamycin** 450mg/8h for 7d PO.

### ITU monitoring in cerebral malaria

▶▶Fluid requirements vary widely; careful fluid management is critical. Haemofilter early if renal failure. Ventilate early if pulmonary oedema.

▶▶Consider exchange transfusion in very seriously ill patients if feasible.

▶▶Monitor blood lactate (or bicarbonate) and glucose: quinine may cause hypoglycaemia. Do LFT + clotting studies; crossmatch blood if haematocrit <20%.

▶▶Repeated U&E (and arterial blood gases if ARDS).

▶▶Arrange repeated skilled microscopy to monitor parasite counts.[116]

Expect at least a 75% decrease in the parasite count by 48h of treatment.

### Pitfalls

• Failure to take a full travel history (+stop-overs) and failure to check if the patient has already received treatment (can make the blood smear 'negative').
• Thinking that malaria in returning travellers is too rare (1000–2000/yr UK) or too exotic for today's work-a-day ward round or clinic, where "it's probably just flu".
• Delay in treatment while seeking lab confirmation.
• Failure to examine enough blood films before excluding the diagnosis.
• Belief that preventive drugs will work, when the parasite is often one step ahead.
• Not asking local experts about emerging patterns of drug resistance.
• Ignoring the possibility of counterfeit drugs (38% in one study from SE Asia).[117]
• No IV artesunate/quinine available *immediately*. (Quinidine is an alternative.[2])
• Not observing falciparum patients closely for the first few days.
• Forgetting that malaria is a big cause of coma, jaundice, anaemia & renal failure.

---

1 Artesunate dose 2.4mg/kg as a bolus at 0, 12 & 24h, then daily. It is not universally available.[118 RTC]
2 Do not give **quinine** loading doses if already definitely had quinine, quinidine or mefloquine in last 24h. Warn about tinnitus. If IV quinine is not available, **quinidine gluconate** is an alternative, eg a loading dose of 10mg/kg over 1–4h, then 0.02mg/kg/min IV by pump for 72h or until can swallow. ECG monitoring is essential when quinidine is given (not needed for quinine). Stop or ↓infusion if BP↓ or QTc prolonged by >25% (p90).

Infectious diseases

TB kills 2 million people/yr; it is the cause of death of most people with HIV. TB is one reason why the poor stay poor—and then die. If HIV+ve, risk↑ if: CD4↓; ESR↑; many co-infections; poor nutrition; high viraemia.[119] **UK incidence** ~8200/yr; 350 deaths/yr.

**Diagnosis** *Latent TB:* Do a Mantoux test. If +ve (or non-reliable) consider interferon-gamma testing (eg *Quantiferon TB Gold*® or *T-spot-TB*®, see below).

*Active TB:* If CXR suggests TB, take sputum samples (≥3, with one early morning sample, before starting treatment if possible) and send for MC&S for AFB (acid-fast bacilli resist acid on Ziehl-Neelsen (ZN) staining). If spontaneously produced sputum cannot be obtained, bronchoscopy and lavage may be needed.

*Active non-respiratory TB:* Try hard to get samples: sputum, pleura & pleural fluid, urine, pus, ascites, peritoneum, bone marrow or CSF. Send surgical samples for culture. Microbiologist should routinely do TB culture on these, even if it is not requested. All patients with non-respiratory TB should have a CXR to find coexisting respiratory TB. Incubate cultures for up to 12wks on Lowenstein-Jensen medium.

*PCR:* Allows rapid identification of rifampicin (and likely multidrug) resistance.

*Histology:* The hallmark is the presence of caseating granulomata.

*CXR signs:* Consolidation, cavitation, fibrosis, and calcification.

*Immunological evidence of TB* may be helpful: *Tuberculin skin test:* TB antigen is injected intradermally and the cell-mediated response at 48-72h is recorded. A +ve test indicates immunity. It may also indicate previous exposure or BCG. A strong +ve test probably means active TB. *False-ve tests* occur in immunosuppression (miliary TB, sarcoid, AIDS, lymphoma). *Quantiferon TB Gold*® and *T-spot-TB*® tests measure the delayed hypersensitivity reaction developed after contact with *M. tuberculosis*; they use specific, complex *M. tuberculosis* antigens and are better than older Mantoux tests, which rely on reactions to serial dilutions of TB antigen.[120]

**Treating pulmonary TB** (BOXES) ► If histology & clinical picture are consistent with TB, start R̟ without waiting for culture results, and continue even if these are -ve. Contact tracing and public health notification are essential.[121]

*Before R̟:* Stress importance of compliance/concordance (helps the patient & prevents resistance). Test colour vision (Ishihara chart) and acuity before and during treatment as ethambutol may cause (reversible) ocular toxicity. Check FBC, U&E, LFT. If pre-R̟ creatinine clearance=10-50mL/min: Rifampicin: ↓dose by 50%. Ethambutol: monitor U&E; avoid if possible. No dose change for ethionamide or isoniazid.

*Initial phase:* 8wks on 4 drugs (depending on susceptibilities): daily adult doses if >50kg: rifampicin 600mg; isoniazid 300mg; pyrazinamide 2g; ethambutol 15mg/kg.
► Patients often forget pills, so consider *Directly Observed Therapy* (DOT) as follows:
  1 *Rifampicin* 600-900mg (child 15mg/kg) PO 3 times/wk.
  2 *Isoniazid* 15mg/kg PO 3 times/wk, max 900mg + *pyridoxine* 10mg/24h (esp. if diabetic, chronic renal failure, HIV +ve or alcoholic) to prevent neuropathy.
  3 *Pyrazinamide* 2.5g PO (2g if <50kg) 3 times/wk (child 50mg/kg; max 2g).
  4 *Ethambutol* 30mg/kg PO 3 times a week for 8wks, or *streptomycin* (see BNF).

*Continuation phase* (16wks on 2 drugs) rifampicin and isoniazid at same doses. Rifinah 300® = rifampicin 300mg + isoniazid 150mg; get advice about resistance. Continue rifampicin. Consider steroids if meningeal or pericardial TB.

**Main side-effects** ► Seek help in renal or hepatic failure, or pregnancy.
Rifampicin: LFT↑ (small AST rise is OK, stop if bilirubin↑), platelets↓, orange discolouration of urine, tears and contact lens, inactivation of the Pill, flu symptoms.
Isoniazid: LFT↑, WCC↓, stop if neuropathy and give *pyridoxine* (50mg/8h PO).
Ethambutol: Optic neuritis (colour vision is the first to deteriorate).
Pyrazinamide: Hepatitis, arthralgia (CI: acute gout; porphyria).

**WHO's/G8 'stop TB' plan** Sputum smear microscopy*et al* for all as needed; directly observed therapy (DOT) in front of a health worker for 6 months.[122]

**Problems to overcome** ☺Stigma around TB ("It's dirty & means I may have HIV") ☺Lack of confidentiality[123] ☺No good primary care/active case detection ☺Poverty.

## Chemoprophylaxis for asymptomatic tuberculous infection

Immigrant or contact screening may identify asymptomatic TB; here, chemoprophylaxis may prevent disease progression. Prophylaxis entails one or two anti-TB drugs for shorter periods than for symptomatic disease (eg rifampicin and isoniazid for 3 months, or isoniazid alone for 6 months). Suitable patients for chemoprophylaxis include adults with documented recent tuberculin conversion, and some young immigrants (16-34yrs) who are T-spot-TB/Mantoux +ve, without prior BCG vaccination.[124] ►Seek expert advice, and see NICE guidance.[125] ►Start standard anti-TB *R* once any clinical or CXR evidence of active TB found.

## Some clinical features of TB
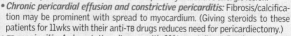
» Ask about recent contact with TB

- *Pulmonary TB:* This may be silent or present with cough, sputum, malaise, weight loss, night sweats, pleurisy, haemoptysis (may be massive), pleural effusion, or superimposed pulmonary infection. Investigation and treatment: see p398. An aspergilloma/mycetoma (p168) may form in the cavities.

- *Miliary TB:* Occurs following haematogenous dissemination. Signs may be non-specific or overwhelming. CXR: fig 1. Look for retinal TB too. Biopsy of lung, liver, lymph nodes, or marrow may yield AFB or granulomata.

- *Genitourinary TB:* May cause dysuria, frequency, loin/back pain, haematuria, sterile pyuria (p288; do 3 EMUs±renal US). Renal TB may spread to bladder, seminal vesicles, epididymis, or Fallopian tubes. Endometrial TB: OHCS p274.

- *Bone TB:* (OHCS p696) Look for vertebral collapse and Pott's vertebra, p722.

- *Skin TB (lupus vulgaris):* Look for jelly-like nodules, eg on face or neck.

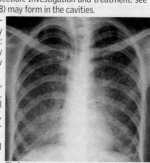
Fig 1. Miliary TB (nodular opacities).
©Dr Vijay Sadasivam, Radiologist, SKS Hosp, Salem, Tamil Nadu, India.

- *Peritoneal TB:* Abdominal pain; GI upset. Look for AFB in ascites (send large volume to lab); laparotomy may be needed.

- *Acute TB pericarditis:* Think of this as a primary exudative allergic lesion.

- *Chronic pericardial effusion and constrictive pericarditis:* Fibrosis/calcification may be prominent with spread to myocardium. (Giving steroids to these patients for 11wks with their anti-TB drugs reduces need for pericardiectomy.)

- *TB meningitis:* A devastating disease with 30% mortality.[126] *Prodrome:* Fever, headache, vomiting, abdominal pain, drowsiness, meningism, and delirium often worsening over 1-3wks (rarely many months) ± seizures (may be the only or 1ˢᵗ sign).[127] CNS signs: Tremor, papilloedema; cranial nerve palsies. *Diagnosis:* LP (p782—the 1ˢᵗ few LPs may be normal); TB PCR; look for immunosuppression (HIV) and TB elsewhere (CXR, etc). MRI + enhancement.[127] CT (obstructive hydrocephalus; basal enhancement; CNS tuberculomas).[128] ►►*Treat on suspicion:*[129] Isoniazid + rifampicin for 12 months, with pyrazinamide and streptomycin during the 1ˢᵗ 2 months is often used (OTM). *Ethambutol* or *ethionamide* are alternatives to streptomycin. Add *pyridoxine* 10-20mg/24h PO to regimens using isoniazid to prevent neuropathies.[130] In adults, daily single doses of 300mg of isoniazid, 600mg of rifampicin, and 2g of pyrazinamide are adequate. Higher doses aren't needed and are hepatotoxic. Always check sensitivities of the organism, and discuss the chances of multidrug-resistant TB with a microbiologist. TBM with resistance to isoniazid and rifampicin is likely to be fatal.[131] There is a role for dexamethasone (eg for 1ˢᵗ month),[132] but tuberculomas may start to appear surgically.[133, 134] Mannitol for ICP↑ (p841).[135] *Complications:* Hydrocephalus (may need surgery).[136] Cognition ↓.

## Why is the diagnosis of tuberculous so often missed?

Patients and doctors ignore cough, weight loss and haemoptysis,etc and are ignorant of risk factors: immersion in poverty, alcohol, tobacco, contact with TB, immunosuppression (eg HIV; DM; malignancy; extremes of age), and renal disease.[137] *Suspect TB continually*; take a good history, and don't expect CXRs to be typical!

Infectious diseases

**Herpes simplex virus (HSV)** Manifestations of primary infection:

1 *Genital herpes* can be a chronic, life-long infection. Majority of cases (esp. recurrent) are caused by HSV-2 (HSV-1 is taking over).[138] *Signs:* Flu-like prodrome, then grouped vesicles/papules develop around genitals, anus, or throat. These burst, forming shallow ulcers (heal in ~3wks). Also: urethral discharge ± dysuria (esp if ♀); urinary retention. *OHCS* p268. *Tests:* PCR. ℞: Give analgesia. *Aciclovir* 400mg/8h PO, *famciclovir* 250mg/8h PO (500mg/12h for 10d if immunocompromised[138]), or *valaciclovir* 500mg/12h for 5d (for longer if healing is incomplete). If frequent (≥6/yr) or severe recurrences, continuous *aciclovir* 400mg/12h PO, *famciclovir* 250mg/12h PO or *valaciclovir* 500mg/24h.[138] *Prevention:* Condoms, even for oral sex.

2 *Gingivostomatitis:* Ulcers filled with yellow slough appear in the mouth.

3 *Herpetic whitlow:* Abrasions allow virus to enter the finger, causing a vesicle.

4 *Herpes gladiatorum:* Vesicles wherever HSV is ground into the skin by force.

5 *Eczema herpeticum:* HSV infection of eczematous skin; usually children.

6 *Herpes simplex meningitis:* This is uncommon and usually self-limiting (typically HSV-2 in women during a primary attack).

7 *Systemic infection* may be mild but life-threatening if immunocompromised. Signs: fever, sore throat, lymphadenopathy, pneumonitis, and hepatitis.

8 *Herpes simplex encephalitis:* Spreads from cranial nerve ganglia, to frontal and temporal lobes. ►*Suspect if:* fever, fits, headaches, odd behaviour, dysphasia, hemiparesis, or coma or brainstem encephalitis, meningitis, or myelitis. Δ: Urgent PCR on CSF (it remains +ve ~5d after initiating ℞). CT/MRI or EEG: non-specific temporal lobe changes; brain biopsy is needed[140] if MRI cannot distinguish from glioma. Seek expert help: careful fluid balance to minimize cerebral oedema, p840; ►►*prompt* aciclovir, eg 10mg/kg/8h IV for ≥10d, saves lives (p834). Mortality: 19%.

9 *HSV keratitis:* Corneal dendritic ulcers. *Avoid steroids.* See *OHCS* p416.

*Tests:* Rising antibody titres in 1° infection; culture; PCR for fast diagnosis.

*Recurrent HSV:* Dormant HSV in ganglion cells may be reactivated by illness, immunosuppression, menstruation, or sunlight. Cold sores (perioral vesicles) are one manifestation. Aciclovir cream may be disappointing.

**Varicella zoster** Varicella (chickenpox; fig 1) is a contagious febrile illness with crops of blisters at various stages, eg on the back. Complications, eg purpura fulminans/DIC (get help; ►►may need heparin[141]), pneumonitis, and ataxia, are commoner in pregnancy and adults than in children.[142] Incubation: 11-21d. Infectivity: 4d before the rash until all lesions are scabbed (~1 week). *OHCS* p144. After infection, virus is dormant in dorsal root ganglia. Reactivation causes **shingles** (affects 20% at some time; eg if old or immunosuppressed). Pain in dermatomal distribution (p458, fig 1) precedes malaise and fever by some days. *Shingles* ℞: Treat

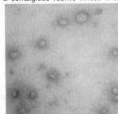
**Fig 1.** Chickenpox. ©Dr C Leung.

acute zoster, eg with *aciclovir* 800mg 5 times/d PO for 7d if eGFR >25; if immunocompromised: 10mg/kg/8h slowly IVI for 10d; alternative: *famciclovir*, or valaciclovir (1g/8h PO for 7d; it is aciclovir's prodrug—a 2012 meta-analysis says that post-herpetic neuralgia is less).[143] If conjunctiva affected, use 3% aciclovir ointment 5×/day. Beware iritis; test acuity often; say to report *any* visual loss at once. SE of aciclovir: GFR↓ (do U&E & LFT), vomiting, encephalopathy, urticaria. *Post-herpetic neuralgia (PHN)* in affected dermatomes can last years; it is hard to treat and can be intolerable.[1] Try amitriptyline (start with 10mg at night), topical lidocaine patches, or gabapentin (p508) ± carbamazepine, phenytoin, or topical capsaicin as a counter-irritant. Last resort: ganglion ablation. Refer to a pain clinic. ►In those ≥60yrs HZ vaccine prevents PHN in >60%.[1] Those 50-59yrs benefit too. CI: immunosuppression.

1 "Endless torture...10-fold worse than childbirth...hell on earth...all I can do is pray for death." So...vaccinate!

Epstein-Barr virus (EBV) infects 90% of people at some point during their lives.[144] Spread: saliva or droplet (presumed). Incubation 4–5wks. ☞ In early childhood it causes few symptoms, but adolescents/young adults may develop infectious mononucleosis. EBV also is associated with several cancers (stomach; nasal/ENT; lymphoma). EBV is a DNA herpesvirus with a predelection for B-lymphocytes, and causes proliferation of T cells ('atypical' mononuclear cells) which are cytotoxic to EBV-infected cells. The latter are 'immortalized' by EBV infection and can, very rarely, proliferate in a way indistinguishable from immunoblastic lymphoma in immunodeficient individuals (whose suppressor T cells fail to check multiplication of these B cells).

**The patient** Sore throat, T°↑, anorexia, malaise, lymphadenopathy (esp. posterior triangle of neck), palatal petechiae, splenomegaly, fatigue/↓mood (risk is ~5-6 times that of other common upper respiratory tract infections,[145] depending in part on features present at onset, eg less fit premorbidly, no delay in Monospot® becoming +ve, and need for bed rest).[146] Fatigue is also part of 'severe chronic active EBV infection', rare, eg with anaemia, platelets↓ & hepatosplenomegaly.[147] *Severe complications:* Meningoencephalitis, cerebellitis, Guillain-Barré, myeloradiculitis, cranial nerve lesions (eg VII, bilateral in 40%[148]), fulminant hepatitis, respiratory distress syndrome, severe thrombocytopenia/aplastic anaemia, acute renal failure, myocarditis.

**Blood film** Lymphocytosis and atypical lymphocytes (large, irregular nuclei, fig 1). These may occur in: viral infections (CMV, HIV, parvovirus, dengue); toxoplasmosis; typhus; leukaemia; lymphoma; drugs; lead poisoning.

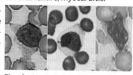

**Heterophil antibody test** (Monospot®, Paul-Bunnell) 90% show heterophil antibodies by 3wks, disappearing after ~3 months (≤1yr).[149] They agglutinate sheep RBC but are absorbed

Fig 1. Atypical lymphocytes flowing round RBCs; abundant cytoplasm (dark at contact points). ©JML & A Schneider.

(and thus agglutination is prevented) by ox RBC, but not guinea-pig kidney cells. This pattern distinguishes them from other heterophil antibodies. They don't react with EBV or its antigens. *False +ve Monospot® tests:* Hepatitis, rubella, parvovirus, lymphoma, leukaemia, malaria, ca of pancreas, and SLE.[150] If serology is difficult, try PCR.[151]

*Other false trails:* Older patients may have little pharyngitis or adenopathy, but more prolonged fever and LFT↑, often with no telltale lymphocytosis or atypical lymphocytes.[152] So, if Monospot -ve, they may be subjected to dangerous over-investigation unless you request EBV-specific IgM—implies current infection (IgG reflects past infection). PCR may reveal ↑↑serum EBV DNA levels and warn of fulminant infection.[153]

ΔΔ: Streptococci (colonization seen in 30% of EBV, so throat swabs often mislead), CMV (if pregnant do CMV serology, p404, as CMV in pregnancy has important implication), viral hepatitis, HIV seroconversion, toxoplasmosis, leukaemia, diphtheria.

**℞:** None usually needed. Patients may expect chronic fatigue when they hear the diagnosis; don't go along with this! ☺Be optimistic (avoid *vigorous* sport; spleen rupture is reported). Avoiding alcohol 'to protect the liver' is controversial. Steroids[154] ± aciclovir[155] (p400) are sometimes used for the severest signs, listed above.[156]

*Never give ampicillin or amoxicillin for sore throats as they often cause a severe rash in those with acute EBV infection (this does not indicate a life-long allergy).*

**EBV oncogenicity** Lymphoma[157] (eg post-transplant),[158] nasopharyngeal cancer (esp. in Asia), leiomyosarcoma[159] and oral hairy leucoplakia (p238; aciclovir-responsive). A vaccine to prevent EBV cancers is being developed.[160]

**Other EBV-associated diseases** Crescentic glomerulonephritis;[161] haemophagocytic syndrome (EBV over-activates T cells & macrophages, with over-production of cytokines, eg causing fatal coagulopathy[162]±central pontine myelinolysis).[163] The EBV Gianotti-Crosti rash (self-limiting papular acrodermatitis of childhood) consists of pale or red monomorphous 1-10mm papules and plaques placed symmetrically over extensor surfaces of limbs, buttocks, and face (also caused by streps, hep B, HIV, echo, Coxsackie, and respiratory syncytial viruses). forlag.fadl.dk/sample/derma/images/447.htm

Infectious diseases

This is the most important viral respiratory infection owing to its ubiquity, unpredictability, and complications (esp. if elderly). In a pandemic (see BOX) millions may die (1918 pandemic) or it may be global but milder (eg 1957). *Spread:* Droplets (to stop this, masks for medics must be well-fitted). *Incubation:* 1-4d. *Infectivity:* 1d before to 7d after symptoms start. *Immunity* is only to a strain that has already attacked you. *Symptoms:* T°↑, headache, malaise/mood↓, myalgia, prostration, nausea, vomiting, conjunctivitis/eye pain (± photophobia). *Δ:* Serology (paired sera; takes >2wks). *Culture* (1wk, from nasopharyngeal swabs). *PCR:* (eg 36h; sensitivity 94%; specificity ~100%).[163] *Complications:* Bronchitis (20%),[164] pneumonia (esp. staph), sinusitis, otitis media, encephalitis, pericarditis, Reye's syndrome (coma, LFT↑↓).

**Treatment** ▶Follow national guidelines. Bed rest ± paracetamol; if severe pneumonia, take to ITU to prevent shock/hypoxia (cover *strep pneumoniae* and resistant staphs, eg **co-amoxiclav & clarithromycin** or **doxycycline**).[165] Oseltamivir is a neuraminidase inhibitor used in influenza A & B, eg if >1yr old presenting with recent (<48h) symptoms typical of flu, when flu is circulating in the community. Dose (>13yrs old and eGFR >30): 75mg/12h PO for 5d. If 1-12yrs old, adjust dose according to body weight.[166] SE: D&V, dyspepsia, headache, insomnia, dizziness, conjunctivitis, epistaxis, rash; rarely hepatitis, Stevens-Johnson, p724 ± ?flawed reports of hallucinations in children.[167] Zanamivir is an inhaled neuraminidase inhibitor active against influenza A & B. It prevents viral release from infected cells and infection of adjacent cells. It is used to ↓symptoms in those >5yrs old with typical flu symptoms starting <48h ago (36h if a child)—when flu is circulating in the community.[166] Dose: 2 blisters (2×5mg)/12h for 5d (before any other inhalers). NB: inhalation is not an ideal route, eg if elderly. SE: bronchospasm; oropharyngeal oedema.[168] *Ensure the patient knows how to use the Diskhaler.* Note: drugs do not influence the course of flu by very much.

**Prevention** •*Hygiene:* see BOX. •Use whole *trivalent vaccine* (from inactivated virus), reserving split vaccine (fragmented virus) for those <13yrs old. It is made from current serotypes and takes <2wks to work. Use if risk↑: DM; COPD; asthma (not mild); heart, renal or liver failure; immunosuppression (eg splenectomy; steroid use); haemoglobinopathy; medical staff,☺ carers; ≥65yrs (esp. in institutions). Vaccinating all at risk poses logistic challenges in ageing populations. Dose: 0.5mL SC (once). In children repeat at 6wks (½ dose if <3yrs; *routine* vaccination of children might save 100 deaths/yr). SE: Pain/swelling; T°↑, headache. Guillain-Barré and pericarditis are rare. Efficacy is 'modest' (relative risk of pneumonia falls from 1 to 0.88 after vaccination in the elderly; all-cause mortality is slightly reduced).[169] •*Oseltamivir:* Prophylactic indications: formal notice that A or B is circulating *and* >1yr old *and* <48h since exposure *and* in at-risk group. It's not needed if vaccinated >2wks ago with well-matched vaccine *unless* living in rest- or nursing-home, etc when it can be used *whatever* vaccination status. Dose: 75mg/d (if 24-40kg, 60mg/d; 16-23kg, 45mg/d) all for ≥10d. Resistance is common in some A/H1N1, B and A/H5N1.

## The common cold (coryza)

Rhinoviruses are the main culprits (>80 strains), and cause a self-limiting nasal discharge (becoming mucopurulent over a few days). *Incubation:* 1-4d. *Complications:* (6% in children) Otitis media, pneumonia, febrile convulsions. R☺: Avoid medications! Encourage a "leave it to your own brilliant body" approach rather than getting into tangles with drugs or herbal extracts (*Echinacea*, OHCS p161), as any ↓in symptoms is almost negligible.[170] Zinc gluconate yields conflicting results in trials.[171,172] If nasal obstruction in infants hampers feeding, try 0.9% saline nose drops.

What to do if an ITU nurse or doctor declines vaccination for religious reasons, or to promote autonomy? The risk is fatal transmission to a vulnerable patient.[173] Force is unjustified, and exclusion from ITU may be impractical in under-staffed units. As ever, dialogue is the only way forward..

## The ART of making and delaying new pandemics

When an animal source of virus couples with human virus (reassortment[1]) to form a novel hybrid with efficient replication and person-to-person transmission, a pandemic is born. Millions of deaths only occur if no previous immunological exposure *and* the new strain is highly pathogenic. What can we do? Early clusters may be containable, but once transmission is established, quarantine is probably futile and the pandemic will become global! But strategic planning can help:

- Simulated exercises before the event to enhance preparedness.
- Stockpile vaccine (if it can be made in time), antivirals, and vital supplies. Masks (must be well-fitting) are recommended by WHO when health workers are within 1 metre of a probable case, eg on entering a room with such people.
- Seamless international cooperation with WHO and bodies like the European Centre for Disease Prevention, eg to cancel mass events and give information.
- Buy time in spreading epidemics by moving hosts (eg free range hens) indoors.
- Quarantine restrictions around clusters of animal infections, eg a 3km zone where entry and exit are banned, with movements restricted in a further 10km monitoring zone where checking of residents, and their hosts destroyed.[174]
- Social distancing: less travel; no mass events (discos, theatre, cinema, schools).[175]
- Self-isolation at 1st sign of illness. Personal hygiene: wash hands, don't sneeze into your hand (your elbow may be better); carry, use & bin tissues; use only once.

### Prevention, containment, health systems response, and communications

This 4-part response to highly pathogenic flu pandemics depends on how far we have progressed down the pandemic path. Preceding a pandemic there is an *interpandemic period—phase 1*: no new subtypes. *Phase 2*: new circulating animal virus arrives; and then a *pandemic alert period*. *Phase 3*: 'human infections with a new subtype, [with] rare instances of spread to a close contact'. *Phase 4*: 'small clusters of highly localized spread' (virus isn't well adapted to us). In *phase 5* there are large clusters of human-to-human spread. A *pandemic* is declared when efficient human transmission is happening in ≥3 WHO regions.

### How does pandemic influenza differ from seasonal influenza?

- Those with no immunity (eg the young) are at risk and prone to complications.
- Death rates are higher, depending on: 1 Numbers getting infected 2 Virulence factors (fig 1) 3 Host vulnerability 4 Preventive and treatment measures.
- Transmission is more efficient, occurring not only in autumn and winter.
- 2-3 waves of infection may occur; later waves may be more severe. Increased death rates are observed even in milder pandemics, over the next 3 winters.

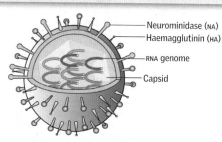

**Fig 1.** Influenza A. Orthomyxoviridae (RNA) have 2 genera: influenza A & B viruses—and influenza C, distinguished by antigenic differences between their nucleoproteins (NP) and matrix (M) proteins. Influenza B and C are almost exclusive to man. Influenza A infects birds and mammals; they are subtyped by surface glycoproteins (haemagglutinin, HA) and neuraminidase (NA). 15 HAs (H1 to 15) and 9 NAs (N1 to 9) are known. Pathogenicity is partly determined by HA glycosylation patterns and amino acids at HA cleavage sites.

**1** In genetic reassortment, 2 viral sources shuffle genetic material in someone with a dual infection. Also, simple stepwise single mutations can accumulate to produce new strains. Reassortment is a key factor in the long-term evolution of influenza A virus, including the periodic emergence of epidemic viruses.[176, 177]

Infectious diseases

The protozoan *Toxoplasma gondii* infects via the gut (poorly cooked meat; soil-contaminated vegetables), lung, or broken skin. Lifecycle: fig 1. In humans, the oocysts release trophozoites, which migrate widely (esp. to eye, brain, and muscle). Toxoplasmosis occurs worldwide. Infection is lifelong. HIV may reactivate it.

**The patient** ►*In any undiagnosed lymphadenopathy or any granulomatous uveitis or retinitis, think of toxoplasmosis, esp. if immunosuppressed (HIV, pregnancy).* Most infections are asymptomatic: in the UK >50% are infected by 70yrs. Symptomatic acquired toxoplasmosis resembles infectious mononucleosis, and is usually self-limiting. Eye infection, usually congenital, presents with posterior uveitis, eg in the 2nd decade of life, and may cause cataract. In the immunocompromised (eg AIDS), myocarditis, encephalitis, focal CNS signs, stroke or seizures can occur.

**Tests** Acute infection is confirmed by a 4-fold rise in antibody titre over 4wks or specific IgM (unreliable if HIV +ve). Reactivation of latent toxoplasmosis in HIV presents problems (you may need to look for toxoplasma antigen and IgG).[178] PCR may be rewarding.[179] Parasite isolation is difficult; lymph node or CNS biopsy may be diagnostic. CT: characteristic multiple ring-shaped contrast-enhancing CNS lesions.

**Treatment** Often not needed (get help).[180] If the eye is involved, or if immunocompromised, *pyrimethamine + sulfadiazine.* ►If pregnant, get help. Sampling of fetal cord blood at ~21wks for IgM indicates severe infection. For HIV, see p410.

**Prevention** Cook food to >63°C/145°F. Does this mean no rare meat? Perhaps only if you are immunocompromised; abandoning rare meat might not have much impact as vegetable sources still abound, and peeling and washing *everything* is impractical. Freezing meat may ↓infectivity. Wash hands after contact with soil.
*Advice in pregnancy/immunosuppression:* Don't change cat litter. Don't handle stray cats (esp. kittens).[181] Antenatal screening may be worthwhile in areas of high prevalence (eg in Riyadh 38% of antenatal samples are +ve for anti-T gondii IgG antibodies, indicating past exposure but not current risk).[182]

**Congenital toxoplasmosis** (OHCS p34) Abortion, seizures, choroidoretinitis (fig 2), hydrocephalus, microcephaly, cerebral calcification. Worse prognosis if early infection.

## Cytomegalovirus (CMV)

CMV (fig 2) is acquired by direct contact (doctors are at ↑risk),[183] blood transfusion, or organ transplantation. After acute infection, CMV becomes latent but the infection may reactivate at times of stress or immunocompromise. If immunocompetent, primary infection is usually asymptomatic, but an illness indistinguishable from glandular fever or acute hepatitis may occur. In transplant recipients or post marrow transplantation: fever > pneumonitis > colitis > hepatitis > retinitis (figs 3-5). In AIDS: retinitis > colitis > CNS disease ('>' means 'is commoner than').

**Diagnosis** of acute CMV infection is hard; virus growth is slow and there may be prolonged CMV excretion from past infection. Serology helps; specific IgM indicates acute infection (unreliable if HIV +ve). CMV PCR (including quantitative tests) of blood, CSF and bronchoalveolar lavage is available.

**Treat** only if serious infection (eg immunocompromised), with *ganciclovir* 5mg/kg/12h IV over 1h via central line, or oral *valganciclovir, foscarnet, cidofovir*. Immunization is being explored. CMV in HIV, see p410.

**Post-transplant prevention**[180] Weekly PCR for 14wks to detect CMV antigenaemia/viraemia; if +ve, get help; *ganciclovir* starting dose example: 5mg/kg/12h IV if eGFR OK). Use CMV-ve, irradiated blood if transfusing transplant, HIV, or leukaemia patients. Alternative strategy: pre-emptive anti-CMV Rx (can lead to improved graft survival).[184]

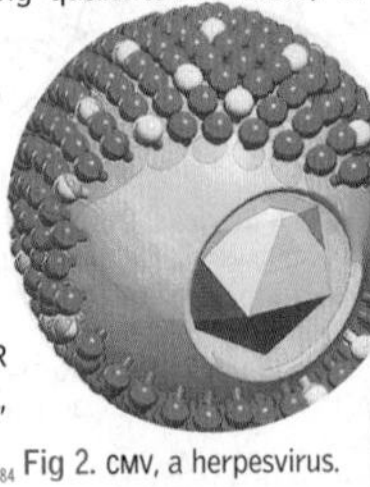

Fig 2. CMV, a herpesvirus.

**Congenital CMV** (OHCS p34) Jaundice, hepatosplenomegaly, and purpura. Chronic defects: IQ↓, cerebral palsy, epilepsy, deafness, and eye problems. There is no treatment.

### *Toxoplasma gondii:* a subtle parasite

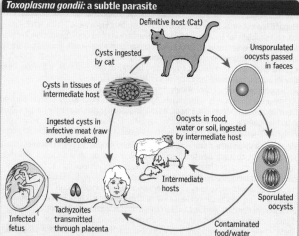

Fig 1. Oocysts in cat faeces can stay in the soil for months, where animals such as rats eat them. They get infected, and, under the direction of *Toxoplasma* in the amygdala, these rats lose their innate fear of cats, and so tend to get eaten. So parasites ensure their success by facilitating their jump from the intermediate to the definitive host. How does the parasite overwhelm the innate fear of cats? By causing a type of sexual attraction to the normally aversive cat odour (through limbic activity).

Data from Fernando Monroy; www2.nau.edu/~fpm/research/res.html

*Immunocompromised humans with toxoplasmosis may show these signs:*
• Confusion, seizures, and signs of brainstem or spinal cord injury.
• Meningoencephalitis + localizing signs (fever + headache → drowsiness → coma → death, eg over days or weeks). CSF: mild lymphocytic pleocytosis and protein↑. Abnormal MRI, eg multifocal myelin loss; microglial nodules; ring-enhancing lesions often at the grey-white junction with subcortical white matter perifocal oedema. Within large diffuse lesions look for discrete small haemorrhagic lesions. Contrast medium may reveal fine-beaded parallel lines or small discrete nodules traversing the white matter suggesting perivenous spread.[186]
• *Pseudotumour cerebri* syndrome (p502): transient intracranial hypertension.
• ICP↑/space-occupying mass mimicking a tumour or a brain abscess.
• Multiple mass lesions that can be the cause of hemisensory abnormalities, hemiparesis, cranial nerve palsy, aphasia, and tremors.
• Acute psychosis (rare; there may be no other signs of immunodeficiency).[187]
• In some areas, eg India, toxoplasmosis is *the* major HIV-associated CNS infection.[188]

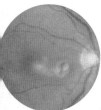

Fig 3. Retinal toxoplasmosis.

Fig 2 © K Radsak; 3-5 ©Prof Trobe.

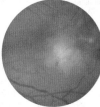

Fig 4. Ill-defined yellow infiltrates. ΔΔ: toxoplasmosis; herpes simplex/zoster; syphilis; sarcoidosis; leukaemia.

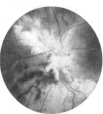

Fig 5. In HIV this 'mozzarella pizza' fundus means CMV retinitis. If CD4↓↓, re-examine in 2 days; ► is it progressing?

Infectious diseases

**Hepatitis A** RNA virus. *Spread:* Faecal–oral or shellfish. Endemic in Africa and S America, so a problem for travellers. Most infections are in childhood. *Incubation:* 2–6wks. *Symptoms:* Fever, malaise, anorexia, nausea, arthralgia—then: jaundice (rare in children) hepatosplenomegaly, and adenopathy. *Tests:* AST and ALT rise 22–40d after exposure (ALT may be >1000u/L), returning to normal over 5–20wks. IgM rises from day 25 and means recent infection. IgG is detectable for life.

*R̟:* Supportive. Avoid alcohol. Rarely, interferon-α for fulminant hepatitis.

*Active immunization* is with Havrix Monodose®, an inactivated protein derived from HAV. Dose: if >16yrs old, 1 IM dose (1mL to deltoid) gives immunity for 1yr (20yrs if further booster is given at 6 months). Use Havrix Monodose Junior® if 1–15yrs old. *Prognosis:* Usually self-limiting. Fulminant hepatitis is rare. Chronicity doesn't occur.

**Hepatitis B virus** (HBV, a DNA virus.) *Spread:* Blood products, IV drug abusers (IVDU), sexual, direct contact. *Deaths:* 1 million/yr. *Risk groups:* IV drug users and their sexual partners/carers; health workers; haemophiliacs; job exposure to blood (morticians/embalmers); haemodialysis (and chronic renal failure); the sexually promiscuous; foster carers; close family members of a carrier or case; staff or residents of institutions/prisons; babies of HBsAg +ve mothers; adopted child from endemic area. *Endemic in:* Far East, Africa, Mediterranean *et al*. *Incubation:* 1–6 months. *Signs:* Resemble hepatitis A but arthralgia and urticaria are commoner. *Tests:* HBsAg (surface antigen) is present 1–6 months after exposure. HBeAg (e antigen) is present for 1½–3 months after acute illness and implies high infectivity. HBsAg persisting for >6 months defines carrier status and occurs in 5–10% of infections; biopsy may be indicated unless ALT↔ and HBV DNA <2000iu/mL. Antibodies to HBcAg (anti-HBc) imply past infection; antibodies to HBsAg (anti-HBs) alone imply vaccination. HBV PCR allows monitoring of response to therapy. See fig1. *Vaccination:* p271. Passive immunization (specific anti-HBV immunoglobulin) may be given to non-immune contacts after high-risk exposure.

*R̟:* Avoid alcohol. Immunize sexual contacts. Refer all with chronic liver inflammation (eg ALT ≥30iu/L)⬥ for antivirals, eg pegylated (PEG) interferon alfa-2a, lamivudine, entecavir[189] adefovir. The aim is to clear HBsAg and ▶prevent cirrhosis and HCC (risk is ↑↑ if HBsAg and HBeAg +ve).[190] *Other complications:* fulminant hepatic failure, cholangiocarcinoma, cryoglobulinaemia.

**Hepatitis C virus (HCV)** RNA flavivirus. *Spread:* Blood: transfusion (thousands of UK cases; compensation is available), IV drug abuse, sexual, acupuncture. UK prevalence: >200,000.⬥[191] Early infection is often mild/asymptomatic. ~85% develop silent chronic infection; ~25% get cirrhosis in 20yrs—of these, ≤4% get hepatocellular cancer (HCC)/yr. ▶HCV is the chief reason for liver transplant in the West. *Risk factors for progression:* Male, older, higher viral load, use of alcohol, HIV, HBV. *Tests:* LFT (AST:ALT <1:1 until cirrhosis develops, p260), anti-HCV antibodies confirms exposure; HCV-PCR confirms on-going infection/chronicity; liver biopsy if HCV-PCR +ve to assess liver damage and need for treatment. Do HCV genotype (BOX 1).

*R̟:* BOX 2; quit alcohol. *Complications:* Glomerulonephritis; cryoglobulinaemia; thyroiditis; autoimmune hepatitis; PAN; polymyositis; porphyria cutanea tarda.

**Hepatitis D virus (HDV)** Incomplete RNA virus (needs HBV for its assembly). HBV vaccination prevents HDV infection. 5% of HBV carriers have HDV co-infection. It may cause acute liver failure/cirrhosis. *Tests:* Anti-HDV antibody (only ask for it if HBsAg +ve). *R̟:* As interferon-α has limited success, liver transplantation may be needed.

**Hepatitis E virus (HEV)** RNA virus. Similar to HAV; common in Indochina (commoner in older men and also commoner than hepatitis A in UK); mortality is high in pregnancy. It is associated with pigs. Epidemics occur (eg Africa). Vaccine is available in China (not Europe). Δ: Serology. *R̟:* Nil specific.

**Hepatitis G & GB** Parenterally transmitted. No good evidence they damage the liver.

**Other causes of hepatitis** Alcohol; drugs; toxins; EBV/CMV; leptospirosis; malaria; Q fever; syphilis; yellow fever; autoimmune hepatitis, p268; Wilson's (p269).

## Serological markers of HBV infection

| | Incubation | Acute | Carrier | Recovery | Vaccinated |
|---|---|---|---|---|---|
| LFT | | ↑↑↑ | ↑ | Normal | Normal |
| HBsAg | + | + | + | | |
| HBeAg | + | + | +/− | | |
| Anti-HBs | | | | + | + |
| Anti-HBe | | +/− | | | |
| Anti-HBc IgM | | + | +/− | | |
| Anti-HBc IgG | + | + | + | + | |

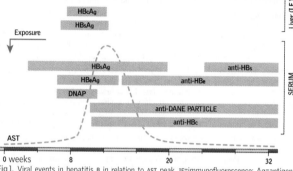

Fig 1. Viral events in hepatitis B in relation to AST. IF=immunofluorescence; Ag=antigen; HBs=hep.B surface; HBc=hep. B core; HBe=hep. B e antigen; DNAP=DNA polymerase.

## Protease inhibitors, ribavirin and PEGinterferon-α in HCV

The non-structural 3 serine protease inhibitors boceprevir and telaprevir are the first in a new class of directly acting antivirals against genotype 1 hepatitis C (HCV). When combined with pegylated interferon and ribavirin, these drugs greatly improve sustained virological response rates in treatment-naïve patients and those who have had past treatment failure on simpler treatment. Boceprevir binds to HCV non-structural 3 (NS3) active site; telaprevir binds NS3.4A. Treatment duration: 24-48wks (in specialist centres). Response rate: 40-70%. SE:[1] Efficacy is less if: •HCV genotype 4, 5, or 6 is involved •↑Viral load •Older patients •↑Delay before Rx starts •Black patients (vs Caucasians) •Men •HIV+ve.
NB: PEGylated interferon has an inert tail retarding its elimination (hence it is given SC once weekly). CI: •Interferon allergy •Autoimmune hepatitis •Severe liver dysfunction/decompensated cirrhosis •Age <3yrs •Severe or unstable heart disease in past 6 months •Past severe psychiatric conditions (esp. depression) •Pregnancy/lactation •Haemoglobinopathies (a contraindication to ribavirin).

*HIV and hepatitis C:* HCV prevalence is ~7% for sexually transmitted HIV and >90% for IV transmission. Untreated HIV may accelerate progress of HCV-induced liver fibrosis. Given the safety and efficacy of therapy, and the bad effects of chronic hepatitis C, consider all HIV/HCV co-infected patients for therapy.[192] *Re-infection* after clearance of virus (undetectable HCV RNA)—ie newly detectable HCV RNA accompanied by a switch in HCV genotype or clade—is quite common in HIV+ve men who have sex with men (eg 15 per 100 person-years), so re-test often.[193]

1 Severe drug reactions/rashes with eosinophilia and systemic symptoms. Anaemia may need erythropoietin alpha and decreased ribavirin doses (esp if cirrhosis). Transfusion is sometimes required.

*Infectious diseases*

HIV1, a retrovirus (p376), is responsible for most HIV infections. HIV2 causes a similar illness (?longer latent period). Over 30 million people are HIV +ve (2.5 million/yr; 2 million deaths/yr; most are in Africa (Africa has 25% of the world's disease burden, 3% of total health workforce, and 1% of wealth)).[94] In many areas, incidence is falling as using antivirals ↓infectivity by 96%.[195] There is increasing HIV transmission in eastern Europe & Middle East, where homosexuality is less accepted and driven underground. *UK prevalence:* ~100,000.[196] *UK incidence:* 6280/yr (in 2011); ♂:♀≈3:1[197]—heterosexual:gay or bisexual=42% *vs* 44%;[198] IV drug abusers: 2%; mother-baby: 3% (~600,000 child deaths/yr globally). Oral sex: 3-7%.[199,200]

**Immunology** HIV binds, via its gp120 envelope glycoprotein, to CD4 receptors on helper T lymphocytes, monocytes, macrophages, and neural cells. CD4 +ve cells migrate to the lymphoid tissue where the virus replicates, producing billions of new virions. These are released, and in turn infect new CD4 +ve cells. As infection progresses depletion or impaired function of CD4 +ve cells ↓immune function.

**Virology** RNA retrovirus; HIV1 has 9 subtypes or 'clades'. After cell entry, viral reverse *transcriptase* enzyme makes a DNA copy of the RNA genome. The viral *integrase* enzyme then integrates this into host DNA. The core viral proteins are initially synthesized as big polypeptides that are cleaved by viral *protease* enzymes into the enzymes and building blocks of the virus. The completed virions are then released by budding. The number of circulating viruses (viral load) predicts progression to AIDS.

**Stages** *Seroconversion (primary infection)* may be accompanied by a transient illness 2-6wks after exposure: fever, malaise, myalgia, pharyngitis, maculopapular rash or meningoencephalitis (rare). A period of *asymptomatic infection* follows but 30% have *persistent generalized lymphadenopathy (PGL)*, defined as nodes >1cm diameter at ≥2 extra-inguinal sites, persisting for 3 months or longer. Later, constitutional symptoms develop: T°↑, night sweats, diarrhoea, weight↓, ± minor opportunistic infections, eg oral candida, oral hairy leucoplakia, herpes zoster, recurrent herpes simplex, seborrhoeic dermatitis, tinea. This collection of symptoms and signs is referred to as the *AIDS-related complex (ARC)* and is regarded as a prodrome to AIDS. *AIDS:* HIV + an indicator disease (p410). CD4 usually ≤200 × 10⁶/L.

*Time-scales:* HIV→AIDS≈8yrs; ARC→AIDS≈2yrs; AIDS→death≈2yrs (without HARRT).[201]

*Which signs correlate best with HIV progression?* Chronic fever (odds ratio 5.6 *vs* those in whom HIV is not progressing); PGL (4.7); cough for >1 month (3.5); chronic diarrhoea (3.3); oral thrush (3.2); weight↓ by 10% in <1 month (2.9); TB (2.8); zoster (2.5).

**Diagnosis** Serum (or salivary) HIV-Ab by ELISA, eg confirmed by Western blot. In recent infection, HIV-Ab might be -ve (window period ~1-3wks after exposure); here, checking HIV RNA (PCR) or core p24 antigen in plasma, or repeating ELISA at 6wks and 3 months confirms diagnosis. 4th-generation kits can test for HIV-Ab and p24-Ag. Rapid test kits give results in 30min; but +ve results must be confirmed by ELISA. OraQuick ADVANCE® uses oral fluid, and may be bought over the counter, eg in UK/USA—sensitivity of 97.4%; specificity of 99.9% (untrained vs trained testers).[202] HIV subtypes A and B predominate in the UK; D is commoner in Africa; hybrid/recombinant types have a worse prognosis as they bind to immune cells more readily.

**Prevention** Blood screening; disposable equipment; antenatal antiretrovirals if HIV+ve±Caesarean birth ± bottle-feeding (may ↑mortality if hygiene poor); PEP (p412).

▶*A stop-HIV sexual manifesto:* ☺Good HIV information (TV, wind-up radios, eg in Africa; HIV issues in soap operas are influential).[203] ☺Accessible HIV tests with opt-out not opt-in when done in clinics[204] (expensive counselling just if +ve). ☺Good sexual negotiation skills. ☺Condoms for *all* sexual contact, or abstinence●❋ (very unreliable![205]—also "I'd rather be dead than abstain"[206]). ☺Reframing of our bodies as a route to intimacy rather than as instruments of gratification always entailing penetration. ☺Fewer sexual partners. NB: 3 *simultaneous* partners is *much* riskier than 6 serial partners. ☺↓Alcohol use (to avoid risky behaviour).

Good trials find that circumcision prevents ~65% of HIV (and herpes[207]) over 1½yrs.[208] It is not a reliable preventive: circumcised men must not behave as if they are safe.

## HIV, TB, poverty and multi- or extensively drug-resistant TB (MDR-TB; XDR-TB)

If your patient is HIV+ve and has cough, fever, night sweats, or weight loss, he has TB till proven otherwise (sensitivity: ~90%).[209] TB is a common, serious complication of HIV. ~40% of those with AIDS in the developing world have TB. Morbidity from HIV-TB leads to vicious spirals of decline: loss in productivity →failing economies→unbalanced health budgets→incomplete courses of TB drugs →selection of drug-resistant organisms→more TB deaths→ruin.[210]

New cases of MDR-TB: ~500,000/yr; mortality >20%.[211] *Other HIV-TB interactions:*

- Mantoux tests may be negative and the presentation of TB may be atypical.
- ↑Reactivation of latent TB (LTB).[1] Previous BCG vaccination does not prevent this.[212]
- Smears may be -ve or scanty[2] for TB; culture is vital to determine drug sensitivity.
- Normal or atypical CXR, eg lobar or bibasal pneumonia, hilar lymphadenopathy.
- Extrapulmonary and disseminated disease is much more common.
- TB treatment in poor countries entails a 4-drug initial phase (2 months of rifampicin, isoniazid, pyrazinamide & ethambutol) and a 2-drug continuation phase (4 months of rifampicin & isoniazid, or 6 months of isoniazid & ethambutol). HIV is known to increases case fatality and rates of recurrent TB after this regimen.[213]
- There is ↑toxicity (D&V, hepatitis, rash neuropathy) from combining anti-TB and anti-HIV drugs (eg stavudine, lamivudine & nevirapine as twice-daily generic tablet, often used in resource-poor/WHO HAART, p414). NB: it may be best to delay HAART until 1-2 months after TB ℞ is started (unless CD4 <100×10⁶/L).[213]
- As HAART reconstitutes CD4 counts, paradoxical worsening of TB symptoms may occur (the 'immune reconstitution inflammatory response', IRIS).[214]
- HIV may or may not necessitate prophylaxis with isoniazid (may prevent TB deaths in children),[215,216] but either way, regular clinical monitoring is vital.

►Directly observed treatment strategy (DOTS) prevents MDR-TB and XDR-TB.[217] In areas where resistance is common, DOTS-plus (use of 2nd-line drugs) may be a solution.[218]

►Respiratory isolation is vital if TB patients are near HIV +ve people. Nosocomial (hospital-acquired) and MDR-TB are major problems worldwide, affecting HIV +ve and HIV -ve people. Mortality is ~80% in patient-to-patient spread. Test TB cultures against 1st- and 2nd-line agents; 5+ drugs may be needed in MDR-TB:[219]

| First-line anti-TB agents: | | Second- or third-line agents:[220] | |
|---|---|---|---|
| Isoniazid | Streptomycin | Ofloxacin | Para-amino salicylic acid (PAS) |
| Rifampicin | Amikacin | Moxifloxacin | Clarithromycin |
| Pyrazinamide | Kanamycin | Cycloserine | Azithromycin |
| Ethambutol | Capreomycin | Ethionamide | Linezolid; meropenem; clavulanate |

**Reducing MDR-TB: chief goals** Early identification; full treatment; isolation.[221] So...

1 Early isolation of suspected TB. A suspicious CXR or past MDR-TB is enough.
2 Directly observe and confirm that patients take all drugs as prescribed.
3 Staff to use effective masks (also patients on leaving isolation rooms).
4 ZN staining available 24/7; do sputum induction/expectoration in isolation rooms.
5 Ensure that doors to isolation rooms have automatic closing devices.
6 Providing negative air pressure in isolation rooms.
7 Only stop isolation after ≥3 sputum samples are AFB -ve on culture for MDR-TB.
8 Frequent tuberculin skin surveillance tests for workers and contacts.

**Extensively drug-resistant tuberculosis (XDR-TB)** This most worrying strain (there may be no treatment options) is occurring in at least 45 countries. Most are in former Soviet Union and Africa.[211] It is associated with cumulative duration of past treatment with 2nd-line TB drugs.[222] Compulsory confinement is suggested[223,224] (not by proponents of Hippocratic medicine "I will put my patient's interests 1st!").

1 LTB implies no X-ray or clinical sign of active TB. 30% of the world's population has LTB.[225] Targeted testing and treatment of LTB in high-risk groups (eg born in endemic area or immunosuppressed) is advised in well-off countries. New tests for LTBI (QuantiFERON-TB; T-SPOT.TB) are better than tuberculin skin tests (too many false +ves and false -ves if immunosuppressed; a reaction >15mm is significant even if no risk factors).[226] ℞: 9 months of daily isoniazid in rich low-prevalence countries.[227]

2 Digestion/liquefaction + centrifugation/gravity sedimentation increases sensitivity by 13-33%.[228]

Infectious diseases

Most complications are either psychological or the result of suppression of T-cell-mediated immunity. ►Test all with newly diagnosed HIV for toxoplasma, CMV, hepatitis B/C, and syphilis—eg serology; tuberculin test.

For TB see p409; HHV-8/**Kaposi's sarcoma**[1] see p716; for **Leishmaniasis** see p439.

**Pulmonary** The lung is the most vulnerable organ; in developed countries bacterial pneumonia (esp. pneumococcal)[229] is commonest; elsewhere it is TB (p398 & p409) and *Pneumocystis jiroveci* pneumonia (PCP, fig 1)—the chief life-threatening fungal opportunistic infection (others: aspergillus, cryptococcus, histoplasma). Suspect it in anyone with cough/breathlessness or pneumothorax. CXR may be normal; CT: diffuse ground-glass opacity, consolidation, nodules, cysts.[230] Δ: Sputum (eg induced or via bronchoscopy and bronchoalveolar lavage.[231] R: high-dose co-trimoxazole (see BOX); special monitoring must be available; precede each dose by prednisolone 50mg (reduce after 5d, and tail off). *Primary prophylaxis:* If CD4 <200×10⁶/L: *co-trimoxazole* 480mg/24h PO or 960mg 3×/wk. Prophylaxis is essential after 1ˢᵗ attack until CD4 >200×10⁶/L.[232] Other pathogens: *M. avium intracellulare* (MAI); CMV. Also: HHV-8 (Kaposi's sarcoma, lymphoma)[1] and *lymphoid interstitial pneumonitis*.

**Gut** Oral pain may be caused by *candidiasis*, HSV or aphthous ulcers, or tumours. *Oral candida* R: *Nystatin* suspension 100,000U (1mL swill and swallow/6h). *Oesophageal* involvement causes dysphagia ± retrosternal discomfort—R: fluconazole, ketoconazole, or itraconazole PO for 1–2wks. Relapse is common. HSV and CMV also cause oesophageal ulcers (similar to *Candida*). *Anorexia/weight loss* is common, also LFT↑ and *hepatomegaly* from viral hepatitis, sclerosing cholangitis, drugs or MAI. *MAI* causes fever, night sweats, malaise, anorexia, weight↓, abdominal pain, diarrhoea, hepatomegaly, and anaemia. Δ: Blood cultures, biopsies (lymph node, liver, colon, bone marrow). R: *ethambutol + clarithromycin + rifabutin* (BOX). *Chronic diarrhoea* may be caused by bacteria (*Salmonella, Shigella, Campylobacter*, atypical mycobacteria, *C.difficile*), protozoa (*Cryptosporidium* p390, *Microsporidium, Isospora belli*, cyclospora), or viruses (CMV, adenovirus). *Perianal disease* may be from recurrent HSV ulceration, perianal warts, squamous cell cancer (rare). Kaposi's sarcoma (p716) and lymphomas can also affect the gut.

**Eye** CMV retinitis (acuity↓ ± blindness) may affect 45% of those with AIDS. Fundoscopy: characteristic 'mozzarella pizza' signs, fig 5 p405. *Treatment:* see BOX. Ganciclovir-containing intra-ocular implants, where available, can improve quality of life.[233] (NB: risk of post-op retinal detachment, one implant does not prevent disease in the other eye.) The need for maintenance therapy may be reviewed if CD4 ≥100×10⁶/L—eg after immune restoration by HAART (p414), if retinitis is inactive.[234]

**CNS** *Acute HIV* is associated with transient meningoencephalitis, myelopathy, and neuropathy. *Chronic HIV-associated neurocognitive disorder* (HAND)[143] comprises dementia and various encephalopathies (PML, p376). *Toxoplasma gondii* (p404) is the main CNS pathogen in AIDS, presenting with focal signs. CT/MRI shows ring-shaped contrast enhancing lesions. Treat with *pyrimethamine* (+*folinic acid*) + *sulfadiazine* or *clindamycin* for 6 months. Lifelong secondary prophylaxis is needed. Pneumocystis prophylaxis also protects against toxoplasmosis.[235] *Cryptococcus neoformans* (fig 2; and p440) causes a chronic meningitis, eg with no neck stiffness. R: See BOX. *Tumours* affecting the CNS include primary cerebral lymphoma, B-cell lymphoma. CSF JC virus PCR is useful in distinguishing PML from lymphoma.

**Psychological complications** HIV is *the* paradigm of a *biopsychosocial illness.* HIV is 100% preventable, yet very prevalent. Asking *why* tells us more about ourselves than about HIV.[236] Shame, sexual imperatives, pride and prejudice[237] keep HIV underground and multiplying. Imagine you are pregnant and HIV+ve, eg as a result of rape, and you will appreciate some of the psychological problems (p414). Being HIV+ve is associated with dissociation during sex ("I had no connection to what was going on...numb...unfeeling...I would try to say something but couldn't").[237] Appreciating some of these psychological complexities helps us realize why simplistic messages about safe sex so often fail. ☼*Farrant's injunction to HIV doctors: Extension of life without efforts to address patients' quality of life is not ethical.*[138]

| Infection | Treatment/side-effects/prophylaxis |
|---|---|
| *Tuberculosis* | The commonest and most lethal opportunistic infection: ℞: (p409). If no active infection, prophylaxis may be needed if significant exposure, or tuberculin skin test >5mm induration (*isoniazid* 300mg/day + *pyridoxine* 10–20mg/day PO; get expert local help, eg on how long to continue prophylaxis).[239] |
| *Pneumocystis jiroveci* <br>  <br> Fig 1. *P. jiroveci* (fluorescent stain × 1000). <br> © Subhash K Mohan. | *Co-trimoxazole* (=trimethoprim 1 part + 5 parts sulfamethoxazole) 120mg/kg/d IVI in 2-4 divided doses for 14–21d (SE: nausea, vomiting, fever, rash, myelosuppression) *or* *pentamidine isetionate* 4mg/kg/d by slow IVI for 14–21d (SE: BP↓, hyper- or hypoglycaemia, renal failure, LFT↑, myelosuppression, arrhythmias). *Prednisolone* 50mg/d PO (reducing dose) if severe hypoxia. Stop after 21d. 2ⁿᵈ-line agents: *Primaquine + clindamycin, pentamidine isetionate, atovaquone.* Secondary prophylaxis, eg *co-trimoxazole* 480mg/24h PO; same dose as 1° prophylaxis, essential after 1ˢᵗ attack. |
| *Candidiasis* <br> (See figs on p441) | *Local ℞: Nystatin* suspension 100,000u swill & swallow/6h. *Systemic ℞, if mucosal: Fluconazole* 50-100mg/d PO for 7-30d; *if invasive:* 400mg/d (continue according to response; SE: nausea, LFT↑, platelets↓) or *itraconazole* (SE: CCF, nausea, LFT↑). *Amphotericin B* (p169) is for severe systemic infection. Relapse is common. |
| *Toxoplasmosis* <br> (fig 3, p405) | *Indications for ℞:* Typical CNS features + lab data (CD4 <200 cells/µL, +ve toxoplasma IgG and ring-enhancing lesions on CT/MRI). *Acute phase: pyrimethamine* 200mg PO once, then 75mg/d + *sulfadiazine* 1.5g/6h PO + *leucovorin* (folinic acid) 5-20mg 3 times a week, continued for 1 week after stopping pyrimethamine (stop the latter 1 week after 'cure'). |
| *Cryptococcal meningitis* <br>  <br> Fig 2. *Cryptococcus.* <br> ©Dr M McGinnis. | Δ: India ink stain (fig 2); CSF culture; cryptococcal antigen in blood and CSF. NB: the capsule is an essential virulence factor for this yeast. *Amphotericin B* IV (p169) + *5-flucytosine.*[240] 20% mortality. Normalizing ICP (repeat LPs ± shunts) may help. Give secondary prophylaxis (fluconazole) until CD4 >150×10⁶/L and cryptococcal antigen −ve.[241] Mortality: 41%.[242] |
| *CMV retinitis* <br> (fig 4, p405) | Induction: *ganciclovir* eye implant. *Valganciclovir* 900mg /12h PO for 3wks, then 900mg/24h PO or *cidofovir*: start with 5mg/kg IV once weekly for 2wks (with probenecid and IV fluids), then reduce to alternate weekly doses. |
| *MAI Mycobacterium avium intracellulare* (=MAC, M. avium complex, p410). | *Clarithromycin* 500mg/12h + *ethambutol* 15mg/kg/d + *rifabutin* 300mg/d, all PO. Prophylaxis if CDC <50/mm³: *azithromycin* 1.2g/wk PO. |
| *Mycobacterium xenopi* | Best ℞ unknown; clarithromycin-rifampicin-ethambutol, with moxifloxacin as an alternative may be tried.[243] |
| *M. kansasii* | Isoniazid + rifampicin + ethambutol. |
| *Strep. pneumoniae* | Prophylaxis: 23-valent pneumococcal vaccine, p160.[239] |

**1** Human herpes virus 8 (HHV-8) is an oncogenic gamma-herpes virus (p376) described in 1994 in Kaposi's sarcoma (KS) lesions. HHV-8 is involved in multicentric Castleman's disease (MCD) and primary effusion lymphoma (PEL), both rare B-cell lymphomas. HHV-8-related tumours chiefly affect the immunocompromised. HAART ↓incidence of KS but not MCD or PEL. HHV-8-related diseases often affect the lung. MCD presents with fever and lymphadenopathy associated with interstitial lung disease without opportunistic infection. Urgent help may be needed. PEL signs: T°↑, lymphocytic-exudative pleural effusion (no pleural mass on CT). Therapy is complex (get help with special antiretroviral and chemotherapy regimens).[244]

Infectious diseases

▶Get comfortable talking about sex and sexuality, and requesting HIV tests. It's vital that you do—literally. If you find this difficult, get help (OHCS p328). Keep practising! NB: asking "Are you gay?" is not very helpful. If speaking to a man, ask about sex with other men, as many don't identify themselves as gay (esp. in repressive countries). Globally, men who have sex with men are 19-fold more likely to get HIV than others.[245]

Preventing HIV depends on us all promoting *lifelong* safer sex, condoms, fewer partners—and regular testing (esp. where rates of HIV are ↑). Videos + interactive discussions can double condom use; *100% condom programmes* also help.

☙Warn everyone about dangers of sexual tourism/promiscuity. Teach skills in sexual negotiation. Explain how alcohol can undermine safe sex messages.
☙Promote human rights so groups driving spread of HIV aren't driven underground.
☙Introduce drug users to needle exchange schemes ("Don't share needles").
☙Promote the work of STI clinics. Good control of other STIs ↓HIV incidence by 40%.
☙Encourage HIV testing, eg in pregnancy (±Caesarean sections if +ve, OHCS p23).[1]
☙Diagnose HIV *early*: have a high index of suspicion in all with TB, pneumonia, diarrhoea, meningitis, weight↓, lymphoma, severe fungal infections, or candida.[246]

**Pre- & post-exposure prophylaxis (PReP/PEP)** Follow guidelines and know drug locations. Seroconversion post-needle-stick: ~0.4% (HIV); 30% for hep B if HBeAg +ve.
• Wash well. If needle-stick, encourage bleeding; do not suck or immerse in bleach.
• Note name, address, and clinical details of donor.
• Report incident to occupational health and fill in an accident form.
• Store blood from both parties (HIV, HBV & HCV tests).
• Immunize (active and passive) against hepatitis B at once, if needed (p271).
• Counsel and test recipient at 3 and 6 months.
• Weigh risks by questioning donor; if HIV+ve, what is the CD4 and viral load count?
• Before prophylaxis, do a pregnancy test. Was the inoculum big? Was injury deep?

Start PEP in case of a significant exposure to blood or other high-risk fluid from an HIV+ve source, or any source at ↑risk of HIV infection. PEP is not indicated after low risk exposures (eg urine, vomit, saliva, faeces, unless they are visibly bloodstained). Start PEP as soon as possible (certainly within 48-72h), and continue for ≥28d. PEP is not needed if exposure >72h ago. Do *follow-up testing* at 12 and 24wks post- (or 24wks after cessation of PEP) and continue for at >12wks after the HIV exposure event (or for at least 12wks from when PEP was stopped). *Starter regimen:* One *Truvada®* tab (245mg *tenofovir* and 200mg *emtricitabine*) once a day plus two Kaletra® film-coated tabs (200mg *lopinavir* and 50mg *ritonavir*) twice a day. *Truvada®* + *Kaletra®* is the preferred regimen, but *Combivir®* + *Kaletra®* may be considered as an option if there are difficulties sourcing starter packs containing *Truvada®*.[247]

**Acute seroconversion** Early identification matters! Signs are like infectious mononucleosis (eg lymphadenopathy, myalgia, rash, headache; rarely meningitis); do tests if there are unusual signs, eg oral candidiasis, recurrent shingles, leucopenia, or CNS signs (antibody tests may be -ve but viral p24 antigen and HIV RNA levels are ↑ in early infection). As ever, the first best 'test' is to take a thorough history. If you do identify acute seroconversion illness, get expert help—and advise unambiguously on preventing transmission. It is not known if early therapy is worthwhile.[248]

**Other direct effects of HIV** Osteoporosis; dementia (the brain is a sanctuary for HIV—and HAART may not prevent dementia from developing):[249]

**When seeing HIV+ve people, ask...** •Have you been to an STD clinic? (STDs promote spread of HIV) •Using condoms? •Sharing needles? •Have you told your partner(s)? •What is your CD4 cell count/HIV-1 RNA level? Viral load helps plan start of antiretrovirals; CD4 <200, <100, and <50/mm³ prompt prophylaxis for *pneumocystis, toxoplasma*, and MAC (p410), respectively •What's your CMV & toxoplasma titre? (counsel to avoid infection, eg no undercooked meat; avoid cats,$^{etc}$) •Recent CXR? (eg TB; pneumocystosis) •Last cervical smear? (risk of neoplasia↑)[239] •Are you sad or depressed? ☙Are you taking time to nurture and teach family & friends? ▶Quality of life & drug efficacy relate to self-efficacy, social support and finding holistic benefits in disease.[250]

### HIV tests and counselling

Pre-test counselling doesn't need to be exhaustive. Testing is routine/'opt-out'[251] in antenatal and STI clinics, new patient medicals, etc. CDC recommends routine screening in healthcare settings for all aged 13-64yrs. If in doubt, get help from STI clinic.
- Determine level of risk (eg unprotected sex; sex overseas; male-male sex; rape).
- Discuss test benefits: partner protection; ↓vertical transmission; getting ℞.
- What are the difficulties? Will you tell family and friends? Explain possible effects on: job, mortgage, insurance (we have no obligation to disclose HIV status).
- Do post-test counselling (eg to re-emphasize ways to ↓risk exposure).

*Rapid point-of-care HIV tests* have big benefits, eg on labour ward. 2 rapid tests done in parallel ↑accuracy (blood is more sensitive than saliva: 98% *vs* 99.7%).[252]

*Home-use HIV tests* are starting to be used by sex partners to inform sexual decisions. Absence of counselling is a problem (or failure to use the post-test counselling phone number if one is provided),[253] as is delayed entry into HIV care. Research must be done to determine the best context for their use.[254]

*Counselling throughout life/safe sex:* Issues arise if sexual partners are HIV-discordant. If the woman is HIV-ve, the HIV+ve man is required to use condoms. If pregnancy is wanted, sperm washing to remove HIV can be successful.[255] n=635

Legal help may be needed on housing, next-of-kin, employment, and guardianship of children, and making a will. Making advance directives needs special skill. Domiciliary genitourinary teams, GP, and hospices all have a role.

### Aims of HAART (highly active antiretroviral therapy)

- HAART aims to suppress plasma HIV RNA concentrations below the limit of detection and restore immune function. This is not a cure as latent replication-competent provirus exists in resting CD4+ T lymphocytes and persistent (but cryptic) viral replication remains intact.[256] Lifelong suppression of plasma HIV RNA is problematic—hence the need for strategies to *eradicate* HIV.
- In theory, these effects can be helped by any therapy that blocks histone deacetylase 1 (HDAC1 mediates virion production). This is the rationale behind studies of HDAC1 blockers such as valproic acid—which has been shown to ↓frequency of resting cell infection (mean reduction 75%).[257]

 HAART must be part of a holistic, integrated, individualized care plan, proceeding with managing comorbidities, eg malnutrition, malaria, etc.[258]

### Monitoring HIV infection[259]

**Routine tests**
- CD4 T cell count (every 3-6 months). CD4 counts are expensive. A reasonable alternative is the TLC—the total lymphocyte count: a TLC of 1400/μL ≈ a CD4 count of 200/μL as far as risk of mortality from HIV goes.[260]
- HIV RNA (every 3-6 months).
- Serum U&E, HCO₃, Cl, creatinine, bilirubin (total + direct)/LFT (every 6-12 months).
- FBC differential (every 3-6 months).
- Fasting lipid profile and glucose (annually).

**Other tests** Pregnancy test; drug resistance testing.

### Indications for initiating antiretroviral therapy[259]

- History of an AIDS-defining illness or with a CD4 count ≤350 cells/μL.[261]
- Antiretroviral therapy should also be initiated in the following groups of patients regardless of CD4 count: pregnant women; patients with HIV-associated nephropathy; and patients co-infected with HBV when treatment is indicated for hepatitis B.
- Antiretroviral therapy may be considered in some patients with CD4 counts >350 cells/mm³ (high viral load, or when CD4 count is falling rapidly).

**1** Without interventions, rate of vertical transmission is 15-20%; prolonged breastfeeding doubles this, falling to <2% with antiretroviral prophylaxis, elective Caesars and bottle feeding.

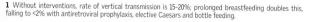

Infectious diseases

*Seek expert help early.* Ask if a once-daily regimen (below) is possible. Nonspecialists need to be aware of 4 things: **1** Drug interactions are important, so don't co-prescribe without computerized decision support (or prolonged reading of drug data). **2** Any new sign in your patient may be a side-effect or an effect of HIV itself. **3** Know baseline viral load, eg >100,000 *vs* 50 copies/mL now. Is the CD4 count rising? **4** Monitor: BP; U&E, glucose/lipids. HAART may cause renal failure±insulin resistance.

### Nucleoside reverse transcriptase inhibitors (NRTI)

*Zidovudine (AZT)* was the 1st anti-HIV drug. Dose: 250–300mg/12h PO or 1mg/kg/4h IV. SE: anaemia, WCC↓, GI disturbance, fever, rash, myalgia. Stop if ↑LFT, hepatomegaly, lactic acidosis. CI: anaemia, neutropenia, breastfeeding.

*Didanosine (DDI; Videx EC®)* 250mg/24h PO if eGFR >80 and wt <60kg; 400mg/24h if ≥60kg. SE: pancreatitis, neuropathy, urate↑, GI disturbance, retinal and optic nerve changes, liver failure. Stop if significant rise in LFT or amylase. CI: breastfeeding.

*Lamivudine (3TC)*[262] is well-tolerated. Dose: 150mg/12h PO, take without food. SE: see zidovudine, but less common. Stop if: ↑LFT; big liver; lactic acidosis; pancreatitis.

*Emtricitabine (FTC)* It is like lamivudine but is also active against hepatitis B[283]

*Stavudine (D4T)* 40mg/12h PO if ≥60kg; 30mg/12h if <60kg; stop if neuropathy or LFT↑.

*Tenofovir* 245mg/24h PO. SE: see lamivudine.

*Abacavir* 600mg/24h PO. SE: hepatitis, lactic acidosis, hypersensitivity syndrome (3–5%)—rash, fever, vomiting; may be fatal if rechalled.

### Protease inhibitors (PI) slow cell-to-cell spread, and lengthen the time to the first clinical event. PIs are often given with low-dose ritonavir (100mg/12h PO), which appears to enhance drug levels. All PIs are metabolized by the cytochrome p450 enzyme system so increase the concentrations of certain drugs by competitive inhibition of their metabolism[264] PIs can cause dyslipidaemia, hyperglycaemia/insulin resistance.

*Lopinavir/ritonavir (Kaletra®)* 400mg (+100mg ritonavir)/12h PO. SE: see saquinavir.

*Saquinavir* 1g/12h PO within 2h of a meal. SE: oral ulcers, paraesthesiae, myalgia, headache, dizziness, pruritus, rash, pancreatitis.

*Fosamprenavir; tipranavir; darunavir; atazanavir; indinavir.*

### Non-nucleoside reverse transcriptase inhibitors (NNRTI) These also may interact with drugs metabolized by the cytochrome p450 enzyme system[265]

*Nevirapine* 200mg/24h for 2wks, then 200mg/12h PO. Resistance emerges readily. SE: Stevens-Johnson syndrome, toxic epidermal necrolysis, hepatitis.

*Efavirenz* Dose: 600mg/24h PO. SE: rash, insomnia, dizziness. Avoid in pregnancy.

*Rilpivirine* A new NNRTI. Resistance may develop (+cross resistance to other NNRTI).

### Integrase strand transfer inhibitors (InSTIs) *Raltegravir; elvitegravir; dolutegravir*[266] May be combined with tenofovir lamivudine.[267] SE: GI upset; insomnia.

### CCR5 antagonists (CC-chemokine receptor 5) *Maraviroc* 300mg/12h PO.

### Once-a-day tablets On an empty stomach at night; those with InSTI may be best, eg
- **Kivexa®/Epzicom®** = abacavir + lamivudine;[268] may be given with dolutegravir. Others include:
- **Atripla®**=tenofovir, emtricitabine + efavirenz (causes psychiatric symptoms in 4%).
- **Stribild®**=elvitegravir + cobicistat + tenofovir + emtricitabine.
- **Eviplera®**=tenofovir, emtricitabine + rilpivirine. *Availability depends on location.*

 It's not all about drugs! There is no point in what we do if negatives outweigh positives, eg endless rounds of appointments; low/suicidal mood; poor body image; low self-esteem; guilt; discrimination; stigma; safe-sex conundrums; intercurrent infections; financial/insurance headaches; family conflict with soon-to-be-orphaned children. ►*Enable patients to become people in charge of their own destiny.* Treat low mood holistically. Make symptoms less intrusive. Randomized trials show that even one session of art therapy can achieve these ends.[269] Phone-delivered support[270] and conflict resolution workers *can* help. HIV+ve people can be involved in caring for other HIV people to mutual advantage.[271] This may help bridge cultural phenomena known to inhibit access to HIV services, eg machismo and marianism in Latino and other cultures.[271] (*Marianism* is excessive humility and willingness of women to sacrifice themselves, and to be submissive to their sexually wayward husbands; *machismo* is its hypermale homophobic counter-stereotype.)

## Golden rules in HAART (highly active antiretroviral therapy)

- Start HAART early, ideally before CD4 count <200 x 10⁶/L.
- Negotiate strict adherence; try to use once-daily regimens where available (eg Atripla® Stribild®). Harmonize pills with the patient's expectations and lifestyle.
- Is the patient suitable to include in an ongoing research trial?
- Aim for no more than twice-daily dosing, if possible.
- Use ≥3 drugs (minimizes replication and cross-resistance). No dual therapies.
- Monitor plasma viral load & CD4 count; *what seems like elimination of HIV often turns into reactivation when treatment stops.* Aim for undetectable viral loads 4 months after starting HAART. Suspect poor adherence if viral load rebounds.
- If viral loads remains high despite good adherence, if there is a consistent fall in CD4 count, or if new symptoms occur, change to a new combination of anti-HIV drugs and request resistance tests, eg genotyping for HIV reverse transcriptase/protease mutations (if available).
- Stay informed about new drugs, and emerging classes of drugs.

## Examples and problems with HAART regimens

- Typical regimen for HIV-1: efavirenz 600mg/24h PO with 2 NRTIs (eg lamivudine 300mg/24h PO + tenofovir disoproxil fumarate 245mg/24h PO). Monitor U&E, eg tenofovir 245mg/2d if eGFR 30-50; 245mg/3-4d if eGFR 10-30.
- To avoid NRTI SE (eg lipoatrophy) non-NRTI regimens may be tried, eg efavirenz + lopinavir + ritonavir.[272,273]
- Comorbidities: no ddI if pancreatitis. If polyneuropathy, avoid using d-drugs (ddI, ddC/dideoxycitidine, d4T). Type 2 DM may need insulin with PIs.
- Common initial regimens consist of two nucleoside analogues, combined with either a protease inhibitor, an NNRTI or a third nucleoside analogue.[274]
- In older patients (50-60yrs) getting a good immune response (IR=CD4↑ by >100/μL) is ∼30% less likely vs those <25yrs starting HAART; survival is also lower.[275]
- Managing highly antiviral-experienced patients is complicated by drug resistance (BOX 3), SEs, drug interactions and quality-of-life issues. So potent regimens need expert input to maximize activity against resistant virus.[276]
- Attempts to extend HAART are experimental, and non-standard (megaHAART, eg tenofovir + emtricitabine + efavirenz + raltegravir + maraviroc).[277]

## Drug-resistance and virologic failure

(HIV RNA >1000 copies/mL)

This is an increasing problem, partly related to complex interactions between the patient's genotype and problems with not taking HAART as prescribed.

In some studies, resistance to one or more HIV drug was >80%.[277] 24 important mutations have been detected in the protease coding region and 14 in the reverse transcriptase (RT) coding region.

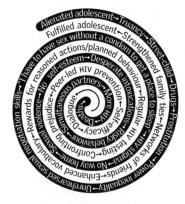

*Infectious diseases*

The UK top 10 STIs: genital warts, chlamydia, genital herpes, gonorrhoea, HIV, hepatitis B & C, pubic lice, syphilis, trichomonas. ▶Refer early to genitourinary medicine (GUM) clinic for microbiology tests, contact tracing and notification. Some clinics offer walk-in services and on-call services. Avoid antibiotics until seen in GUM clinic.

**UK incidence** is rising alarmingly, by >10%/yr, as safer sex practices are being ignored. Prevalence of chlamydia is ~11%$^{UK}$ (>104,000 new cases of genital *Chlamydia*); 22,320 cases of gonorrhoea, and >2250 cases of syphilis.[278] In the USA in 2010, there were 45,834 new cases of syphilis (vs 48,298 for HIV and 309,341 for gonorrhea).[279]

**History** Ask about timing of last intercourse; contraceptive method; sexual contacts; duration of relationship; sexual practices/orientations; past STI; menstrual and medical history; antimicrobial therapy. Are sexual negotiation skills up to scratch?

**Examination** Detailed examination of genitalia including inguinal nodes and pubic hair. Scrotum, subpreputial space, and male urethra. PR examination and proctoscopy (if indicated); PV and speculum examination.

**Signs** Vaginal/urethral discharge (p418), genital lesions: herpes (p400); syphilis (p431); *Chlamydia* (BOX); genital warts (OHCS p599); salpingitis (OHCS p286); lice (OHCS p608).

**Tests** Refer to GUM clinic. Urine: dipstick and MSU/MC&S. Ulcers: swabs for HSV culture (viral transport medium) and dark ground microscopy for syphilis (*T. pallidum*). Urethral smear for Gram stain/culture for *N. gonorrhoeae* (send quickly to lab in Stuart's medium); urethral swab for *Chlamydia* (free tests also available from UK chemists, see BOX). High vaginal or swab in Stuart's medium for microscopy/culture (*Candida, Gardnerella vaginalis*, anaerobes, *Trichomonas vaginalis*); special endocervical swab for *Chlamydia trachomatis*. *Chlamydia* (an obligate intracellular bacteria) is the trickiest STD to diagnose as it is asymptomatic, difficult to culture, and serology may be unhelpful as it cross-reacts with *C. pneumoniae*. Urine ligase chain reaction and PCR are quite good screening tests, with sensitivity >90%. Other tests: include *Chlamydia* antigen and nucleic acid probe assays.[280] *Blood tests:* Syphilis, hepatitis, and HIV serology after counselling.

**Follow-up** At 1wk and 3 months, with repeat smears, cultures, and syphilis serology.

**Scabies** (*Sarcoptes scabei*, an arachnid) Spread is common in families. *The patient:* Papular rash (on abdomen or medial thigh; itchy at night) + burrows (in digital web spaces and flexor wrist skin). *Incubation:* ~6wks (during which time sensitization to the mite's faeces and/or saliva occurs). Penile lesions produce red nodules. *Δ:* Tease a mite out of its burrow with a needle for microscopy (dropping oil and scraping with a scalpel may provide faeces or eggs). *R:* ▶Bedding, clothing, etc. of the patient and close contacts should be decontaminated (eg washing in hot water and drying in a hot dryer). Give written advice (OHCS p608). Apply 5% *permethrin* over whole body including scalp, face (avoid eyes), neck and ears (BNF). Do not forget the soles. Wash off after 8–12h; repeat after 7d; use 5% cream on hands if washed before the 8h elapses.[271]

Fig 1. *Sarcoptes scabei.*
©Prof S. Upton; Kansas Univ.

**Lymphogranuloma** *Signs:* Inguinal lymphadenopathy + ulceration. *Causes:* Lymphogranuloma venereum (*Chlamydia trachomatis*; serovar L2 causes proctitis too, eg in HIV +ve European men);[281] chancroid (*Haemophilus ducreyi*),[1] or granuloma inguinale (*Klebsiella* (*Calymmatobacterium*) *granulomatis*, ie donovanosis). The latter causes extensive, painless, fleshy red genital ulcers and pseudobuboes (inguinal nodes abscess), with possible elephantiasis ± malignant change. *Δ:* 'Closed safety-pin' inclusion bodies in cytoplasm of histiocytes. *R:* *Doxycycline* 100mg/12h PO until all lesions epithelialized—or *azithromycin*, *erythromycin*, or *tetracycline*.

---

1 In the Tropics, chancroid is a common cause of sexually acquired genital ulcers, typically with a granular, yellow base and ragged edges (± inguinal buboes, which may need draining via a wide-bore needle); the cause is *Haemophilus ducreyi*. WHO recommends erythromycin 500mg/6h PO for 7d, ceftriaxone 250mg IM (1 dose), or azithromycin 1g PO (1 dose). Chancroid facilitates spread of HIV.

## Chlamydia screening to prevent pelvic inflammatory disease

Genital *Chlamydia trachomatis* is the commonest STI in the UK (≥100,000 diagnoses in GUM clinics/yr). Highest rates are in those <24yrs old—implying long-term morbidity—salpingitis, infertility, and ectopic pregnancy in 2-4%.[282] Shame, embarrassment about discussing STIs with partners, lack of appointments, and having to be sensible are the main obstacles. ☻Dialogue is key; you can help by talking frankly with your patients about sex: see *OHCS* p328 for honing this skill. As part of implementing the UK National Chlamydia Screening Programme, UK high street pharmacies and GP surgeries offer free yearly chlamydia tests (self-administered) to those aged 16-24yrs (and if +ve, to their partners, of *any* age). Uptake of this service is patchy and it may be hard to sustain. Colleges, prisons, and armed forces are also targeted.[283] NB: only 0.5% of young adults respond to mass media campaigns inviting them in for screening.

Free home-based urine test kits may be distributed to garages, hairdressers, and supermarkets with results texted to mobile phones—removing the need to provide embarrassing samples at the doctor's surgery.

Walk-in STI clinics and late-opening GP clinics allow *prompt* treatment.

NICE advocates yearly opportunistic screening of young adults (eg with nucleic acid amplification tests on urine) *wherever* they present to primary care, irrespective of presenting symptoms.[284] This might halve the incidence of pelvic inflammatory disease. Issues about efficient contact tracing are unresolved. NB: there is no good evidence to support using screening to halt transmission, or to reduce rates of orchitis,♂ ectopic pregnancy or infertility.

First-void (early morning) urine may be the single best diagnostic specimen (for *C. trachomatis* and *M. genitalium*—another common STI) for detection by PCR. An additional endocervical specimen may also be needed.[285]

For genital chlamydial infection give azithromycin 1g PO as a single dose.

## ☻A holistic approach to sexual health

A simple reading of this chapter supports the fallacy that the pathogen is everything—that we are simply the unvarying terrain on which they wreak their havoc.

Claude Bernard was one of the first to point out that the terrain is more important than the pathogen—get the terrain right, and the pathogen loses its grip. Louis Pasteur embodied the pathogen theory of disease; nevertheless, his deathbed words were: "Bernard is right; the pathogen is nothing; the terrain is everything." Bernard had drunk a glassful of cholera to prove his point (no one quite knows how he survived but French physiologists are a tough lot).

So when we look at sexual infections we must look at the terrain *and* the pathogen—and ask questions such as how does this couple stay healthy (the science of 'salutogenesis'[286]) whereas another couple or triad keeps getting ill? Take thrush for example: always a commensal, but in some patients also a big problem. For the terrain to be optimum, nutrition and the immune system must be optimum too. If the subject has HIV, candida may become invasive—not because it changes but because the terrain changes—in this case probably HIV-related downregulation of anti-β-1,2-oligomannosidic epitopes (an epitope is a surface portion of an antigen capable of eliciting an immune response and of combining with the antibody produced to counter that response).[287]

Understand terrain (above) in its widest sense: it has local, individual, and social axes. Each of these merit interventions in our efforts to reduce sexual infections. Also note that one pathogen often alters the terrain for another—for example one sexual infection makes further infections more likely as inflamed surfaces offer juicy portals of entry. ☻So our job in infectious diseases is to get the terrain right. *If we simply focus on killing pathogens we will always fail.*

Infectious diseases

Infectious diseases

Non-offensive vaginal discharge may be physiological. Most that smell or itch are due to infection. Foul discharge may be due to a foreign body (eg forgotten tampons, or beads in children). ▶Discharges rarely resemble their classical descriptions. ▶Untreated GU inflammation ↑viral shedding of HIV-1 in semen 3-fold.

**Thrush** *(Candida albicans)* Thrush is the commonest cause of discharge and is classically described as white curds. The vulva and vagina may be red, fissured, and sore. The partner may be asymptomatic. *Risk factors:* Pregnancy, immunodeficiencies, diabetes, the Pill, antibiotics. *Δ:* Microscopy: strings of mycelium or oval spores. Culture on Sabouraud's medium. *R:* A single imidazole vaginal pessary, eg **clotrimazole** 500mg + cream for the vulva (and partners) is convenient. Alternative: 1 dose of **fluconazole** 150mg PO. Reassure that thrush is not necessarily sexually transmitted. Recurrent thrush: see *OHCS* p284.

*Trichomonas vaginalis* (TV) causes vaginitis + thin, bubbly, fishy smelling discharge. It is sexually transmitted. Exclude gonorrhoea (may coexist). The motile flagellate may be seen on wet film microscopy, or cultured (fig 1). *R:* **Metronidazole** 400mg/12h PO for 5 days or 2g PO stat. Treat the partner. If pregnant, use the 5-day regimen.

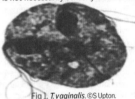

Fig 1. *T. vaginalis.* ©S Upton.

**Bacterial vaginosis** causes a fishy smelling discharge. The vagina is not inflamed. Itch is rare. Vaginal pH: >5.5, hence alteration of bacterial flora ± overgrowth of, eg *Gardnerella vaginalis, Mycoplasma hominis*, peptostreptococci, *Mobiluncus* and anaerobes, eg *Bacteroides* species with too few lactobacilli. There is ↑risk of pre-term labour ± amniotic infection. *Δ:* Stippled vaginal epithelial 'clue cells' on wet microscopy. Culture. *R:* **Metronidazole** 400mg/12h PO for 5d (probiotic *Lactobacillus* GR-1 and RC-14 for 28d ↑ cure rates),[288] or **clindamycin** cream.

**Gonorrhoea** *(Neisseria gonorrhoea)* (fig 2; GC) can infect any columnar epithelium (urethra, cervix, rectum, pharynx, conjunctiva). ♂: Urethral pus ± dysuria; tenesmus; proctitis ± discharge PR, eg if gay. ♀: Often asymptomatic (as is pharyngeal GC), or vaginal discharge, dysuria, proctitis. *Local complications:* Prostatitis, cystitis, salpingitis, Bartholinitis. *Systemic:* Septicaemia (petechiae + hand or foot pustules; arthritis; Reiter's• syndrome; SBE/ IE). *Obstetric:* Ophthalmia neonatorum^ND (*OHCS* p36). *Long-term:* Urethral stricture, fertility↓. *R:* Encourage safe sex; trace contacts (get help from GUM clinic); pro-

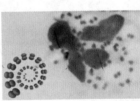

Fig 2. Pairs of gonococci in a neutrophil; their long axes lie parallel, as with lovers, and testicles (inset), reminding us that infertility from epididymo-orchitis is a leading complication. The time it takes to descend the spiral, from the sublime to the excruciating, is 2-10 days.
Spiral by Luke Famery.

mote sexual negotiation skills; purge abusive relationships. *Uncomplicated infection of cervix, urethra & rectum:* **Ceftriaxone** 500mg IM stat (or **cefixime** 400mg PO stat) + *R* for chlamydia (**azithromycin** 1g PO stat or **doxycycline** 100mg/12h PO for 7d).

**Non-gonococcal urethritis** (NGU) is commoner than GC. Discharge is thinner and signs less acute. Women (typically asymptomatic) may have cervicitis, urethritis, or salpingitis (pain, fever, infertility). Rectum and pharynx are not infected. *Organisms:* *C. trachomatis* (▶special swabs are needed, *OHCS* p286); *Ureaplasma urealyticum; Mycoplasma genitalium; Trichomonas vaginalis; Gardnerella*; Gram -ve and anaerobic bacteria; *Candida. Complications:* Similar to local complications of GC. *Chlamydia* may cause Reiter's syndrome and neonatal conjunctivitis. *R:* **Azithromycin** 1g PO stat, or **doxycycline** 100mg/12h PO for 7d. *Also:* **Erythromycin** 500mg/6h PO for 14d, or **ofloxacin** 400mg/24h for 7d. Trace contacts. Avoid intercourse during treatment and alcohol for 4wks.[289]

**Non-infective urethritis** Traumatic; chemicals; cancer; foreign body.

Emergence of antibiotic resistance is the third-most important obstacle in the perpetual and perpetually unwinnable war against infectious diseases. Other obstacles are poverty, ignorance, and corruption—and over-using antibiotics. Guidelines, which exist on local, regional, and national levels, help optimize therapy, but must be continually updated in the vain task of trying to keep up with pathogens. To monitor resistance patterns, infective isolates from different

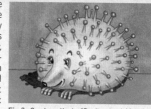

Fig 3. Say to patients: "Don't get prickly when your doctor denies you antibiotics for flu."

UK regions are tested against a variety of antibiotics to determine antibiotic sensitivities, as measured by the minimal inhibitory concentration (MIC) of drug required to prevent organism growth in culture. A rising MIC indicates drug resistance, and may prompt revision of the guidelines, but be sceptical of even the most up-to-date ones when events at the bedside so dictate.

One example is the emergence of ciprofloxacin resistance in *Neisseria gonor-rhoea*.[27] Resistance is now the rule rather than the exception. Historical data: in 2000, 2% of isolates were resistant; 3% in 2002; and 43% in 2006. 2012 data show that some strains are now resistant to penicillins, ceftriaxone, cefixime, cefotaxime, ciprofloxacin and tetracycline.[290] Another example: in 2004 only 4% of *E. coli* causing septicaemia were resistent to ciprofloxacin—now it is 21%.

National guidelines aim for chosen drugs to eliminate gonococcal infection in >95% of patients. Ciprofloxacin, previously 1st-line, now has to be replaced by cephalosporins (eg cefixime) in new guidelines.[291] Avoiding use of broad-spectrum antibiotics (eg cephalosporins, co-amoxiclav) may help reduce overall antibiotic resistance, but ill patients often need such drugs: a big dilemma.

**"A post-antibiotic era means an end to modern medicine as we know it..."**
So says WHO (2012),[292] commenting gloomily on emerging untreatable infections. When we hear these sorts of comments we should listen to Claude Bernard: if you cannot change the organism, change the terrain in which the organism appears to be flourishing.  This is an opportunity for combining reductionist (eg vaccination) and non-reductionist/integrative medicine, for example paying attention to populations, diet, hygiene and the role of the mind in preventing and managing infection. People get better from septicaemia without antibiotics thanks to a strong immune system. Psychoneuroimmunology is starting to understand how. We are not suggesting treating infections without antibiotics, we are simply saying that if no antibiotic works, that is not the end of the road.[293] Bedside medicine can rediscover its old roots, more or less successfully.

**Possible ways to try to stop or slow antibiotic resistance**[290]
- Discourage over-the-counter antibiotic availability.
- Don't use antibiotics for well patients with probable viral infections.
- Educate patients not to get prickly (fig 3) when their GP does not prescribe (this is the basis of a current amusing public health drive, linked to an annual European antibiotic awareness day (Nov 18th)).
- Whenever antibiotics are used, explain that the full course should be taken: "Don't keep a few in reserve to save for our next illness..."
- Tailor the antibiotic to the likely bacterium (p378).

Infectious diseases

**Staphylococci** When pathogenic, these are usually *Staph. aureus*. Often they infect skin, lids, or wounds. Severe *Staph. aureus* infections: pneumonia, osteomyelitis; septic arthritis; endocarditis; septicaemia. Production of β-lactamase which destroys many antibiotics (p378-70) is the main problem. *Staph. aureus* toxins cause food poisoning (p390) and toxic shock syndrome: shock, confusion, fever, a rash, diarrhoea, myalgia, CPK↑, platelets↓ (associated with the use of tampons). Deep *Staph.* infections need ≥4wks of *flucloxacillin* 500mg/6h IV. *Coagulase -ve staphs (CoNS): Staph. epidermidis (albus)* is usually only pathogenic if immunocompromised, or associated with foreign material (pacemakers, IV lines, or joint prosthesis). Removing the foreign material may well be needed.

*Methicillin-resistant Staph. aureus (MRSA)* is typically a hospital-acquired infection, causing pneumonia, septicaemia, wound infections, and death (risk ↑5-fold).[294] It accounts for ~6% of total hospital-acquired infection. There are ≥17 sub-types. NB: glycopeptide-resistant enterococci and *C. difficile* are bigger problems (p247). In the UK it is mandatory to record all infections. UK prevalence has fallen by 30% (to 1.7/100,000) since 2010 despite ward overcrowding and reluctance to close affected wards, perhaps due to better barrier-nursing facilities and improved hygiene (eg washing hands between patients). Carriage rates (nasal): 1-10%. Risk factors: HIV; dialysis; on ITU. MRSA is community-acquired in up to 40%. Whole genome sequencing helps track outbreaks, enabling prompt control. R: Discuss with a microbiologist. *Vancomycin* or *teicoplanin* are used, but strains with reduced sensitivity (vancomycin-intermediate *Staph. aureus* (VISA)—↓sensitivity to *both* drugs) have emerged. Here, consider *linezolid* (may be used 1st-line too),[295] or *daptomycin*. Prevention (p391):
• Isolate recently admitted patients with suspected MRSA. Group MRSA cases on one ward (impractical if hospital has to run at 100% capacity).
• Wash your hands and your stethoscope! (also TV remote controls, etc).
• Ask about the need for eradication (with *mupirocin*).
• Be meticulous in looking after intravascular catheters.
• Surveillance swabs of patients and staff in outbreak ± whole genome sequencing.
• Use gowns/gloves when dealing with infected or colonized patients. Masks may be needed during contact with MRSA pneumonia.

**Streptococci** Group A streps (eg *Strep. pyogenes*) are common pathogens, causing wound and skin infections (impetigo, erysipelas, *OHCS* p598), tonsillitis, scarlet fever[ND], necrotizing fasciitis (p662), toxic shock, or septicaemia. Late complications: rheumatic fever; glomerulonephritis. *Strep. pneumoniae* (pneumococcus, Gram +ve diplococcus) causes pneumonia, otitis media, meningitis and septicaemia. Resistance to penicillin is a problem. *Strep. sanguis, Strep. mutans,* and *Strep. mitior* ('viridans' group), *Strep. bovis* and *Enterococcus faecalis* all cause endocarditis. *Enterococcus faecalis* also causes UTI, wound infections, and septicaemia. *Strep. mutans* is a very common cause of dental caries. *Strep. milleri* forms abscesses, eg in CNS, lungs, and liver. Most streps are sensitive to penicillins, but *Enterococcus faecalis* and *Enterococcus faecium* may present some difficulties. They usually respond to a combination of *ampicillin* and an aminoglycoside, eg *gentamicin* (p381 & p767).

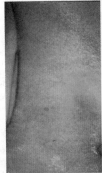
Fig 1. Ascending lymphangitis from strep-infected (diabetic) ankle ulcer. ©Prof A Huntley.

Vancomycin-resistant enterococci (VRE) have been reported. Some strains of VRE are sensitive to *teicoplanin* or *linezolid* (p381).

**Anthrax**[ND] *(Bacillus anthracis)* Occurs, eg in Africa, Asia, China, Eastern Europe, and Haiti. Spread is by handling infected carcasses or via contaminated cattle-feed; well-cooked meat poses no risk. *4 types: 1* Cutaneous *2* GI (eg GI bleeding) *3* Inhalational (dyspnoea) *4* 'Injectional' (eg from contaminated heroin).[296] Terrorists have used long-lasting anthrax spores as a biological weapon.[297] *Signs:* Common cutaneous form: local black skin pustule (→oedema (may be striking)→fever→regional lymphadenopathy→septicaemia (± hepatosplenomegaly/meningoencephalitis) in 20% (often fatal). *Tests:* CXR (wide mediastinum). Lab: large Gram +ve rod. PCR. ℞: (for inhalational anthrax) *Ciprofloxacin* 400 mg/12h IVI or *doxycycline* 100mg/12h PO/IV + *clindamycin* 1.2g/12h IVI; continue one or other for 60d depending on sensitivities. Get help. Post-exposure prophylaxis uses *doxycycline* or any *quinolone* (eg *ciprofloxacin, levofloxacin*) for 60d. *Prevention:* Immunize animals and humans at risk; enforce sound food-handling and carcass hygiene.[298]

**Diphtheria**[ND] is caused by *Corynebacterium diphtheriae* toxin. *Signs:* Tonsillitis ± a pseudomembrane over the fauces ± lymphadenopathy ('bull neck'). ENT details and antitoxin: OHCS p158. ℞: *Erythromycin* 12mg/kg/6h IVI. *Prevention:* p391. Give non-immune contacts *erythromycin* 500mg/6h PO for >7d; get lab help.

**Listeriosis** is caused by *Listeria monocytogenes*, a Gram +ve bacillus with an odd ability to multiply at low temperatures. Sources of infection include pâtés, raw vegetables/prepared salads (eg diced celery),[299] unpasteurized milk/soft cheeses (brie, camembert, blue vein types). It may cause non-specific flu-like illness, rash, or PUO, pneumonia, meningoencephalitis/ataxia, eg if immunocompromised or pregnant (where it may cause miscarriage or stillbirth), or neonatal[300] Δ: Culture blood, placenta, amniotic fluid, CSF + any expelled products of conception. ►*Take blood cultures in any pregnant patient with unexplained fever for ≥48h.* Serology, vaginal, and rectal swabs don't help (it may be a commensal here).℞: *Ampicillin* IV (*erythromycin* if allergic) + *gentamicin*; p378 & p381 for doses. *Prevention in pregnancy:* •Avoid soft cheeses, pâtés, and under-cooked meat. •Observe 'use by' dates and standing times if using microwaves. •Ensure reheated food is piping hot; throw away any left-overs.

**Clostridia** Tetanus p424. *C. perfringens* causes wound infections and gas gangrene ± shock or renal failure after surgery/trauma (p391) or more rarely infections (eg septicaemia with intravascular haemolysis or gas-forming liver abscess)[301] if immunosuppressed (malignancy, DM). ℞: Debridement is vital; *benzylpenicillin* 1.2-2.4g/4h IV + *clindamycin* 900mg/8h IVI, antitoxin and hyperbaric O₂ may also be used. Amputation may be necessary. Clostridia food poisoning (p390). *C. difficile:* Diarrhoea (pseudomembranous colitis following antibiotic therapy, p247).

*C. botulinum* spores are ubiquitous; germination/toxin production occurs in anaerobic, low-salt, low-sugar, low-acid, warm conditions. Transporting food, eg unrefrigerated sausages (*botulus* is Latin for sausage) may cause outbreaks in unconnected areas.[302] *C. botulinum* toxin blocks release of acetylcholine causing flaccid paralysis. It cannot spread from one person to another. 2 adult forms: food-borne and wound botulism. ►*Risk is high in IV drug abusers* if heroin is contaminated with *C. botulinum*. *Signs:* Afebrile, flaccid paralysis ('descending') dysarthria, dysphagia, diplopia, ptosis, then difficulty in holding the head up, then dropping things, then respiratory failure—and *no* sensory signs—9h-9 days[302,303] after ingestion.[304] Autonomic signs: dry mouth, fixed or dilated pupils. *Tests:* Find toxin in blood samples or, in wound botulism, identify *C. botulinum* in wound specimens by prompt referral to a reference lab. Samples include: serum, wound pus, swabs in anaerobic transport media.[305] ℞: Get help (on ITU). *Botulinum antitoxin* works if given early. Also give to those who have ingested toxin but are as yet asymptomatic. *C. botulinum* is sensitive to *benzylpenicillin* and *metronidazole*. In the UK, antitoxin is sourced via CDSC (020 7210 300)[306]

*Nocardia* species cause subcutaneous infection (eg Madura foot) in warm climes, and, if immunocompromised, abscesses (lung, liver, cerebral). Microscopy: branching chains of cocci. ℞: *Trimethoprim* 5mg/kg/8h IVI + *sulfamethoxazole* 25mg/kg/8h IVI for 3wks (do serum levels) then reduce + cefriaxone 1g/12h IV.

**Actinomycosis** is caused by *Actinomyces israelii*. Usually causes subcutaneous infections, forming sinuses with pus which contain sulfur granules—eg on the jaw (or IUCDs, OHCS p298). It may cause abdominal masses (may mimic appendix mass). ℞: *Ampicillin* 12.5mg/kg/6h for 30d then penicillin V for 100d. Liaise with surgeons.

*Infectious diseases*

**Enterobacteria** Some are normal gut commensals, others environmental organisms. They are a big cause of UTI and intra-abdominal sepsis (eg post-op and in the acute abdomen), and a common cause of septicaemia. Unusually, they may cause pneumonia (especially *Klebsiella*), meningitis, or endocarditis. They may be sensitive to **ampicillin** and **trimethoprim** but resistance is growing. Resistance of *K. pneumoniae* to **amikacin** is seen in 50% (in some places), **ceftazidime** (90%) and **tobramycin** (90%)[31] so **imipenem** may be needed. *Salmonella* & *Shigella* are discussed on p426.

***Pseudomonas aeruginosa*** is a serious pathogen (esp. nosocomial or if immunocompromised, and in cystic fibrosis). It causes pneumonia, septicaemia (risk ↑ if: immunosuppressed, recent antibiotic use, central venous or urinary catheter[307]), UTI, wound infection, osteomyelitis, and cutaneous infections. The main problem is its increasing antibiotic resistance. ℞: **Piperacillin** (p378) or **mezlocillin** + an aminoglycoside (p766). Ciprofloxacin, ceftazidime, and imipenem (p380) are also useful.

**Acinetobacter infections** (eg *A. baumannii*) This Gram –ve coccobacillus causes pneumonia ± septicaemia. Risk↑ if debilitated/hospitalized. Risk↑ if vascular catheter *in situ*, ventilator use/tracheostomy, enteral feeding, or recent use of 3ʳᵈ-generation cefalosporins or carbapenem. We carry it on our hands, and it inhabits ventilators. ITU outbreaks occur in summer. ℞: **Imipenem** ± aminoglycosides. Multidrug-resistance may require use of nephrotoxic **polymyxins** or **tigecycline**. *Infection control:* Clean the source; sterilize the reservoir, characterize transmission—and interrupt.[308]

***Yersinia pestis*** causes plague[ND], a disease of small animals and their fleas (fig 1) that can also infect us by flea bite, direct contact, or droplet. *Incubation:* 1-7d.

*Signs:* Flu-like symptoms, sudden fever, chills, head and body-aches, weakness, and nausea/vomiting. 3 types:

1 *Bubonic plague* is the most common form. *Yersinia pestis* enters the skin from the site of the bite and travels via lymphatics to the nearest node. Swollen nodes ('buboes') are very painful and can suppurate.

Fig 1. Rat flea: *Xenopsylla cheopis.* ©S Upton, Kansas Univ.

2 *Septicaemic plague* is a late complication.

3 *Pneumonic plague* is the worst kind and can be transmitted via droplets without involving fleas or animals. Untreated, it has a high mortality rate.

Δ: Phage typing of bacterial culture, or 4-fold ↑ in antibodies to F antigen.

℞: Isolate suspects; *streptomycin* up to 15mg/kg/12h IM for 10d. If in 1ˢᵗ ⅓ of pregnancy, **amoxicillin** 500mg/8h PO; if later, **co-trimoxazole** 480mg/12h PO. Children: co-trimoxazole.[209] Staying at home, quarantine (inspect daily for 1wk), insect sprays to legs/bedding, and avoiding dead animals helps stop spread.

*Vaccination* doesn't offer instant protection, so is not recommended for immediate protection in outbreaks. It is reserved for high-risk groups (eg lab personnel).[310]

***Yersinia enterocolitica*** In Scandinavia this typically causes a reactive, asymmetrical polyarthritis of weight-bearing joints; in America, it causes enteritis. It also causes uveitis, appendicitis, mesenteric lymphadenitis, myositis, glomerulonephritis, thyroiditis, colonic dilatation, ileitis/perforation, and septicaemia. Δ: Agglutination titres >1:160 mean recent infection. ℞: **Ciprofloxacin** 500mg/12h PO for 3-5d.

**Whooping cough[ND]** (*Bordetella pertussis*) After 1wk of catarrh, fever & cough, characteristic paroxysms of coughing & inspiratory whoops occur (esp. in children). Most recover well, but it may last months ("my 100-day cough"). Some (esp. babies <2 months old, hence too young to vaccinate) develop pneumonia ± subsequent bronchiectasis, fits & brain damage. Lymphocytosis is a telling sign in older patients. Pertussis is under-diagnosed: ▸have a high index of suspicion, and access to *pernasal swabs* (eg blue-topped; contact lab)—insert into the nostril and guide gently *horizontally* to the back of the nose. If obstruction is felt, reinsert via the other nostril. When resistance to the posterior pharyngeum is felt, withdraw and place in its transport medium. It can be stored (for <24h) at 4-8°C before transport.

℞: **Clarithromycin** dose (for 7d): adult=500mg/12h; neonate/child <8kg=7.5mg/kg/12h; 8-11kg=62.5mg/12h; 12-19kg=125mg/12h; 20-29kg=187.5mg/12h; 30-40kg=250mg/12h all PO. If pregnant: **erythromycin 500mg/6h.** *If macrolides not tolerated:* cotrimoxazole (p380; not if pregnant or neonatal). Exclude from school [etc] until treated for 5d. *Chemoprophylaxis* (same doses as R̊ above; HPA advice) if: baby <1yr and not fully vaccinated; those likely to transmit to such babies, eg mothers or >32wks pregnant, nursery workers; health workers (unless vaccinated in the last 5yrs); household contacts. Complete vaccination courses in these groups as needed. Pertussis vaccine (p391) is indicated at any time in pregnancy, eg with a 2nd dose after 28wks.[311]

NB: *immunization* (p391) hasn't controlled pertussis well: incidence in adults doubled recently over a 5yr period.[312] Immunity wanes 5yrs after dose 5, hence a growing case for vaccinating adults as above, esp. pregnant women, who then pass antibodies directly via the placenta to those who most need it, ie neonates.[313]

***Moraxella catarrhalis*** (Gram -ve diplococcus) is a cause of pneumonia, exacerbations of COPD, otitis media, sinusitis, and septicaemia. R̊: Clarithromycin 500mg/12h PO.

**Brucellosis** This zoonosis (p446) from contact with animals, their droplet exhalations or other products, eg unpasteurized goat (or human) milk. It is common in the Middle/Far East and Bosnia, eg in vets or farmers. *Cause:* B. melitensis (worst sort); B. abortus; B. suis/canis. *Symptoms* may be indolent and last years: eg PUO, sweats, malaise, anorexia, weight↓, hepatosplenomegaly, rash, D&V, myalgia, backache, arthritis, spondylodiscitis (fig 2),[314] sacroiliitis, bursitis, orchitis, TIA,[315] cranial palsies (II, VI, VII), urinary retention, depression, hallucinations.[316]

*Complications:* Osteomyelitis, SBE/IE (culture -ve; a big cause of brucella deaths),[317] abscesses (liver, spleen, lung, breast· psoas), meningoencephalitis, myelitis, aortitis.

Δ: Pancytopenia; blood culture (≥6wks; rapid culture systems exist, contact lab); serology: if titres equivocal (≥1:40 in non-endemic zones) do ELISA ± immunoradiometric assay. R̊: ~6wks ☙ *doxycycline* 100mg/12h PO + *rifamp-icin* + *gentamicin* (for 7d).[318] Oral pills might engender more relapses, a *big* problem, but not, ironically, if IM leads to ↑defaulting: either way, the best doctors negotiate ~100% concordance. *Surgery:* For abscesses or SBE/IE.

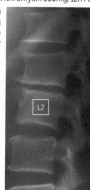

Fig 2. Loss of joint space between L1 & L2 + destruction of L2's anterior body.
©M Reeder; F McGuinness.

***Haemophilus influenzae*** typically affects unvaccinated children usually <4yrs old. It causes otitis media, acute epiglottitis, pneumonia, osteomyelitis, and septicaemia. In adults it may cause exacerbations of chronic bronchitis. R̊: Unreliably sensitive to ampicillin; cefotaxime is more reliable. Capsulated types tend to be much more pathogenic than non-capsulated types. ►Immunization: p391.

**Tularaemia** (*Francisella tularensis* Gram -ve bacillus; acquired by handling infected animal carcasses). It causes rash, fever, malaise, tonsillitis, headache, hepatospleno-megaly, and lymphadenopathy ± papules at sites of inoculation (eg fingers). *Complications:* Meningitis, osteomyelitis, SBE/IE, pericarditis, septicaemia. Δ: Contact local microbiologist for advice. Only use labs with safety cabinets for dangerous pathogens. Swabs and aspirates must be transported in approved containers. R̊: Gentamicin or tobramycin. Oral tetracycline may be good for chemoprophylaxis. *Prevention:* Find the animal vector; reduce human contact with it as far as possible. Vaccination may be possible for high-risk groups.

**Cat-scratch disease** Cause: Bartonella henselae (small, curved, Gram -ve rod or Afepilis felis—suggested by: 1 Recent cat scratch 2 Regional adenopathy (-ve tests for other causes, p29) 3 +ve cat scratch skin test antigen response 4 Microabscesses in nodes. If HIV+ve, skin lesions are like Kaposi's sarcoma. R̊: (Often not needed or unresponsive) Azithromycin,[319] or ciprofloxacin, rifampicin and co-trimoxazole.

See also *Spirochetes* p430; *Neisseria* p375; *Legionella* p162.

Infectious diseases

**Essence** Tetanospasmin, *Clostridium tetani's* exotoxin, causes muscle spasms and rigidity, cardinal features of tetanus (='to stretch').

**Incidence** ~50 people/yr in the UK. Mortality: 40% (80% in neonates).

**Pathogenesis** Spores of *C. tetani* live in faeces, soil, dust, and on instruments. A tiny breach in skin or mucosa, eg cuts, burns, ear piercing, banding of piles, may admit the spores. Diabetics are at risk. Spores then germinate and make the exotoxin. This travels up peripheral nerves and interferes with inhibitory synapses.

**The patient** *20% have no evidence of recent wounds.*[320] Signs appear from 1d to several months from the (often forgotten) injury. There is a prodrome of fever, malaise, and headache before classical features develop: *trismus* (=lockjaw; Greek *trismos* = grinding, hence difficulty in opening the mouth); *risus sardonicus* (a grin-like posture of hypertonic facial muscles); *opisthotonus* (fig 1); *spasms* (which at first may be induced by movement, injections, noise, etc, but later are spontaneous; they may cause dysphagia and respiratory arrest); autonomic dysfunction (arrhythmias ± wide fluctuations in BP).

**Differential diagnosis** is dental abscess (both cause trismus), rabies, phenothiazine toxicity, and strychnine poisoning. Phenothiazine toxicity usually only affects facial and tongue muscles (see p855).

**Poorer prognosis** Incubation <1wk;[320] trismus leads to spasms in <48h; neonates; elderly; post-infective; postpartum (a big cause of maternal mortality worldwide).

**Treatment** ►►Get help on ITU. ABC (may need tracheostomy and ventilation). Debride all wounds. Monitor ECG + BP + SpO₂ (keep >92%, eg with O₂ mask + reservoir); careful fluid balance.
- Human tetanus immunoglobulin (HTIG) 150 units/kg IM at multiple sites to neutralize toxin.
- Aim to keep the patient asleep but rousable to obey simple requests. **Diazepam** 5-20mg/8h PO (mild disease; much higher doses may be needed, eg 480mg/d)[328] or, to control spasms, 0.05-0.2mg/kg/h IVI (≤140mg/d) or phenobarbital 1.0mg/kg/h IM or IV + chlorpromazine 0.5mg/kg/6h IM (IV bolus is dangerous) starting 3h after the phenobarbital. If this fails to control the spasms, paralyse and ventilate (get anaesthetist's help). Dose example: pancuronium 2-4mg IV, then 1-2mg/h by IVI if needed; get expert help on ITU.[322]
- Metronidazole, eg 500mg/6h PO for 7d (?better than benzylpenicillin 1.2g/4h IV).

**Prevention** See BOX. Active immunization with tetanus toxoid is part of the 3-stage vaccine during the 1st year of life (eg Pediacel®, p391). Boosters are given on starting school and in early adulthood. Once 5 injections have been given, re-vaccinate only at the time of significant injury, and consider a final one-off booster at ~65yrs.[323] *Neonatal and maternal tetanus* are caused by unhygienic methods of delivery, abortion, or umbilical-cord care (eg on day 6-8 of life). 34 countries have not achieved WHO's global elimination target (eg with education and 2 doses of tetanus toxoid antenatally).[324] Mortality is high (eg 50% of infants).

*Primary immunization of adults:* 0.5mL tetanus toxoid IM repeated twice at monthly intervals. In the UK, the formulation is Revaxis®, p391.

*Secondary prevention:* See BOX.

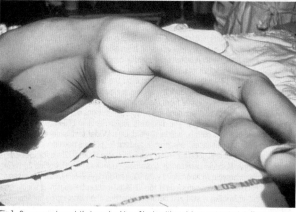

Fig 1. Spasm causing opisthotonus (arching of body with neck hyperextension). Differential diagnosis: tetanus, rabies, cerebral malaria, neurosyphilis, acute cerebral injury, catatonia.
© Courtesy of Centres for Disease Control and Prevention.

### Tetanus prophylaxis in wound management[325]

#### Clean, minor wounds
*Uncertain history of previous vaccination or fewer than 3 doses:* Give vaccine.
*3 or more previous doses:* No need to vaccinate unless vaccination status is incomplete or unknown.

**All other wounds** (wounds contaminated with dirt, faeces, soil, and saliva, puncture wounds, avulsions, and wounds caused by missiles, crushing, burns, and frostbite).

*Uncertain history of previous vaccination or fewer than 3 doses:* Give vaccine and tetanus immunoglobulin (TIG). The recommended dose of TIG for recent (<24h) wounds of average severity is 250 units IM (500 units if wound >24h old, and in burns or heavy contamination). When both tetanus vaccine and TIG are administered, use separate syringes and separate injection sites.

*Give tetanus vaccine* (p391) if born before 1961 or vaccination status is unknown, or immunosuppressed, or a past course was incomplete.

▶Hygiene education and wound debridement are of vital importance.

Infectious diseases

**Typhoid and paratyphoid** are caused by *Salmonella typhi* and *S. paratyphi* (types A, B, and C), respectively. (Other *Salmonella* cause D&V: p390 & p246.) *Incubation:* 3-21d. *Spread:* Faecal-oral (acid suppression from PPIs ↑risk). *Presentation:* Malaise, headache, high fever with relative bradycardia, cough, and constipation. CNS signs (coma, delirium, meningism, cerebellar signs, fits)[326] are serious. Diarrhoea is more common after the 1st week. Rose spots occur on the trunk of 40%, but may be difficult to see. Epistaxis, bruising, abdominal pain, and splenomegaly may occur. *Δ:* Can be made by isolation of *S. typhi* from blood, bone marrow or a specific anatomical lesion. Clinical symptoms or serology are suggestive but not definitive for diagnosis. Blood culture is the mainstay of the diagnosis, which is +ve in 1st 10d.[327] *Later:* urine/ stool cultures. Marrow culture has best yield. LFT↑. Widal test is unreliable (-ve in ~30% of culture-proven cases). DNA probes and PCR tests have been developed.
*R̃:* Fluid replacement and good nutrition + **ciprofloxacin** 500mg/12h PO for 10d. *Alternatives for ciprofloxacin resistance:* (common, eg in Asia)—**ceftriaxone** 2g IV/24h for 14d; or **azithromycin** 1g PO on day 1 with 500g PO on days 2-6.[328] *In severe disease*, give IV ciprofloxacin or IV cefotaxime for 10-14d. In encephalopathy ± shock, give dexamethasone 3mg/kg IV stat just before antibiotics, then 1mg/kg/6h for 48h.
*Complications:* Osteomyelitis (eg if sickle-cell); GI bleed/perforation; cholecystitis; myocarditis; pyelonephritis; meningitis; abscess; DVT. *Clearance:* 6 consecutive cultures of urine + faeces are -ve. 1% become chronic carriers; treat if a food handler, etc. Ciprofloxacin 500mg/12h PO for 6wks ± cholecystectomy.
*Prognosis:* If untreated, 10% die; if treated, 0.1% die. *Vaccine:* p377.

## Bacillary dysentery[ND]

**Shigella** causes abdominal pain and bloody diarrhoea ± sudden fever, headache, and occasionally neck stiffness. CSF is sterile. UK school epidemics are often mild (often *S. sonnei*), but imported dysentery may be severe (often *S. flexneri* or *S. dysenteriae*). *Incubation:* 1-7d. *Spread:* Faecal-oral. *Diagnosis:* Stool culture. *Treatment:* Fluids PO. Avoid antidiarrhoeal drugs. Drugs: ciprofloxacin 500mg/12h PO for 3-5d. Imported shigellosis is often resistant to several antimicrobials: sensitivity testing is important for all enteric fevers. There may be associated spondyloarthritis (p553).

## Cholera[ND] Deaths/yr: ≈100,000[329]

*Cholera loves filth.* Anything soiled, polluted or corrupt, where politics and tainted water mix, gives cholera life, spelling death to the poor and undernourished. Where there is no corruption there is no cholera: clean water with clean politics *abolishes* it.
*Cause:* *Vibrio cholerae* (Gram -ve curved or comma-shaped flagellated motile vibrating/swarming rod). Only types O1 and O139 cause disease, eg explosive outbreaks or pandemics that affect whole countries (eg Zimbabwe and Angola), then continents.
*Incubation:* A few hours to 5d. *Spread:* Faecal-oral. *Signs:* Profuse (eg 1L/h) watery ('rice water') stools, fever, vomiting, and rapid dehydration (the cause of death, with associated metabolic acidosis). *Δ:* Stool microscopy (±dark ground) & culture.
*R̃:* Strict barrier nursing. ▸▸Prompt oral rehydration with pre-prepared sachets drunk in large amounts (0.9% saline IVI if shocked; add 20mmol/L K+ until U&E known; not plain Ringer's lactate ∵ fatal K+↓). Oral rehydration with WHO formula (20g glucose/L) is not as good as cooked rice powder solution (50-80g/L) in reducing stool volume.[330] Its high osmolarity (310mmol/L *vs* 200mmol/L) is also unfavourable to water absorption. Oral *erythromycin* or *ciprofloxacin* 1g PO stat may ↓fluid loss.[331] Zinc supplements shorten the illness (15mg elemental Zn/12h, as acetate).
*Mortality:* 1-3%; up to 50% if unprepared (war, ecological disaster, slum areas).
*Prevention:* Education. Good hygiene/sewage disposal. More primary care. Fewer slums. Only drink boiled or treated water. Cook all food well; eat it hot. Avoid shellfish. Peel all vegetables. Heat-killed vaccine (serovar O1) gives limited protection and is no longer needed for international travel; newer vaccines are non-standard.[332] *Ineffective public health measures:* Quarantine; a *cordon sanitaire* to halt introduction of cholera by travellers, vaccination, and mass chemoprophylaxis.[333]

## Whose deaths really matter?

DNA analysis of pulp in the teeth of Athenians dying in the great plague of 430BC reveals that the cause was typhoid fever.[334] 30% of Athenians died, including Pericles, their leader. He gave us the Parthenon, juries, free theatre, and, in his own immortal oratory, the notion that it is better to die resisting than to live in submission.[335] This is definitely *not* the right approach to infectious diseases: Pericles should have promulgated a third way: neither victory nor submission, but, more subtly, *accommodation*, or something even more symbiotic.

For the next 23 centuries, typhoid fever carried on killing, teaching us nothing much, until noon on 23 April 1851, when a little-known girl was quietly expiring in Malvern. Her name was Annie Darwin, her father's, Charles. Annie was his favourite fun-loving daughter, and with her lingering enteric death Darwin gave up all belief in a just and moral universe. Thus unimpeded, his mind was able to frame and compellingly justify the most devastating answer to the oldest question: that we are here by accident, thanks to natural selection, the survival of the fittest, and the 'wasteful, blundering, low and horridly cruel works of nature'.[1]

The next significant enteric death was 3 short summers later in 1854 at 40 Broad St (fig 1, p664), in the Parish of St James, London, where a child became ill with diarrhoea, dying on 2 September. Her mother rinsed the soiled nappies into the house drains. These led close to the supply to the Broad St pump. Both the drain and the pump's well had faulty brickwork allowing the waters to mix. From this confluence sprung the discipline of Public Health, for many of the 500 or so ensuing late summer deaths from cholera clustered around this pump, as diagrammed by the local doctor, Dr John Snow. He used his now famous diagrams locating each death to motivate the Board of Guardians of St James's parish at its meeting of 7 September: "In consequence of what I said, the handle of the pump was removed the following day"[2][336]—so inaugurating the control of cholera. If Snow were alive today, he might be busy unplugging all our carbon-emitting power-stations (maybe as killing as cholera), but note that Snow worked through committees to save his countless lives, not by direct action.

These events illustrate two counter-intuitive truths: knowledge of the microscopic cause of a disease is not required for public health measures to succeed (*Vibrio cholerae* was as yet undiscovered)—and even the most parochial Church Council is capable of prompt and decisive action affecting the lives of millions, when informed by an intelligent doctor in command of the facts.

There is one metaphysical truth revealed by these enteric deaths, which would not have escaped Pericles had he only taken the trouble to become a medical student for long enough to realize that his overvalued ideal of heroism is often pointless.[3] Pericles never gave his condolences to parents who lost their sons in battle, because, he said, a hero's death was the finest thing that could befall a man. We meet many heroic deaths on our wards, but they seem oddly pointless in retrospect. This is why we owe the highest favour to Annie, whose unheroic death so transforms the inner landscapes of the mind. With Annie in mind, we can confidently relieve our patients of the notion that they must die fighting.

**1** A remark of Darwin's in 1856, before starting his *Origin of Species*, quoted in *Darwin* (Desmond & Moore, Penguin). This reminds us of Thomas Hobbes' (1588-1679) dictum: owing to scarcity of natural resources, there is constant war of all against all ('*bellum omnium contra omnes*'). Life in the state of nature is 'solitary, poor, nasty, brutish and short'. It was Thomas Hobbes who first brought Pericles to our attention through his great translations of Thucydides, the biographer of Pericles.

**2** Snow (a teetotaller, a vegetarian, and a virgin) is unfairly portrayed as secular saviour; he was really just the man on the spot who took logical decisions.[337]

**3** If you doubt that heroism is often pointless, visit the Somme where lies buried the old lie '*dulce et decorum est pro patria mori*'. Wilfred Owen (1893-1918) wrote in a letter to his mother: 'The famous Latin tag [Horace] means *It is sweet and meet to die for one's country*. Sweet! and decorous!...'[338]

Infectious diseases

▶In an endemic area, any individual should be regarded as having leprosy if they show **one** of the following signs: 1 skin lesion consistent with leprosy (fig 1) and with definite sensory loss, with or without thickened nerves; 2 positive skin smears.

Leprosy is a chronic disease caused by *Mycobacterium leprae*. It affects millions of people in the tropics and subtropics. Since the widespread use of dapsone, and WHO elimination campaigns, prevalence has fallen (from 0.5% to 0.4/10,000 in Uganda; from 11% to 4/10,000 in parts of India).[339] Incidence remains stable, at ~800,000 new cases/yr worldwide, many of whom are children. It mainly affects skin, peripheral nerves, mucosa of upper airways and the eyes. ~1-2 million people are disabled, visibly and irreversibly, from leprosy, and need care in the community in which they live.

**Diagnosis** is based on the clinical signs and symptoms, and laboratory and other investigations are rarely needed.[340] Skin lesions can be single or multiple, and usually manifest as hypopigmented anaesthetic macules, papules, or annular lesions (with raised erythematous rims). Erythema nodosum (fig 1, p565) occurs in 'lepromatous' disease, especially during the 1st year of treatment. Sensory loss is a typical feature of leprosy. The skin lesion may show loss of sensation to pin-prick and/or light touch. A thickened nerve is another feature of leprosy, and is often accompanied by other signs as a result of damage to the nerve (eg loss of sensation in the skin and weakness of muscles supplied by the affected nerve). Sometimes a thickened sensory nerve may be felt running into the skin lesion (eg ulnar nerve above the elbow, median nerve at the wrist, or the great auricular nerve running up behind the ear). In the absence of these signs, nerve thickening by itself, without sensory loss and/or muscle weakness is often not a reliable sign of leprosy. In a few cases, rod-shaped, red-stained leprosy bacilli, which are diagnostic of the disease, may be seen in the smears taken from the affected skin. *Eye lesions:* ▶*Refer promptly to an ophthalmologist.* The lower temperature of the anterior chamber favours corneal invasion (so secondary infection and cataract). Inflammatory signs: chronic iritis, scleritis, episcleritis. There may be reduced corneal sensation (V nerve palsy) and reduced blinking (VII nerve palsy) and lagophthalmos (difficulty in closing the eyes), ± ingrowing eyelashes (trichiasis).

**Classification**[341]*Paucibacillary* ('tuberculoid') *leprosy:* there is a vigorous immune response, with granulomata containing epithelioid cells and lymphocytes, but few or no demonstrable bacilli. Patients show negative smears at all sites. *Multibacillary* ('lepromatous') *leprosy:* immune response is ↓. There are foamy histiocytes full of bacilli, but few lymphocytes. Patients show +ve smears at any site. *Borderline:* Between these two poles. *Method of transmission:* the exact method is not known;[342] however, it seems to be transmitted by contact between cases of leprosy and healthy persons. More recently, the possibility of transmission by the respiratory route has been gaining ground. There are also other possibilities, such as transmission through insects, which cannot be completely ruled out.

 ℞[343] Tackle: ☻Poverty ☻Ignorance ☻Nutritional state ☻Shame and stigma, as well as the bacterium—otherwise transmission inevitably continues in endemic countries.[344] Ask a local expert about: •Resistance patterns, eg to dapsone, when ethionamide may (rarely) be needed •Using prednisolone for severe complications •Is surgery ± physiotherapy needed as well as drug therapy? In the UK, get advice from the Leprosy Opinion panel. *Paucibacillary leprosy:* Rifampicin: 600mg once a month, dapsone: 100mg/d. Duration: 6 months. *Multibacillary leprosy:* Rifampicin: 600mg once a month, dapsone: 100mg/d, clofazimine: 300mg once a month (supervised) and 50mg/d. Duration: 1yr. *Single skin lesion paucibacillary leprosy:* A stat dose of rifampicin 600mg + ofloxacin 400mg + minocycline 100mg.[345]

▶Beware sudden permanent *paralysis* from nerve inflammation caused by dying bacilli (± *orchitis, prostration, or death*); this 'lepra reaction' may be mollified by thalidomide (*NOT* if pregnant) or prednisolone. Liaise urgently with a leprologist. Supervised therapy may be problematic as many patients find it hard to attend (nomads, jungle-dwellers). WHO has proposed 'accompanied' multi-drug therapy where someone close to the patient takes responsibility for ensuring treatment.[339-344]

### What is more communicable than leprosy?

This page is dedicated to Joseph deVeuster (Father Damien) of Kalawao, Molokai, in Hawaii, who befriended sufferers of leprosy in a remote Pacific colony. Here the leprosy victims, arriving by ship, were sometimes told to jump overboard and swim for their lives, so frightened were the sailors of contagion that they dared not land. Those swimmers who made it found a friend who was both doctor and priest to them, whose self-imposed duty was to build their homes, their churches—and their coffins. Without any distinction of race or religion, he gave a voice to the voiceless, building a unique community where the joy of being together gave people new reasons for living.

It is said that after spilling boiling water painlessly on his foot, he diagnosed his own leprosy. After that, his sermons beginning "We lepers..." had added veracity.

He gave everything to leprosy—and leprosy took all it could from him, including, on 15 April 1889, his life.

We may look upon that water flowing over his foot not so much as a death sentence, but as one of those initiation ceremonies devised by ancient shamans who realized that it was by these close encounters with death that we augment our spirituality, and so are able to heal.

Joseph deVeuster also invalidates all our definitions of health (soundness in body and mind...total physical wellbeing, etc). More importantly, he demonstrates that optimism works and is more communicable than leprosy, proving that there is nothing that cannot be transcended.

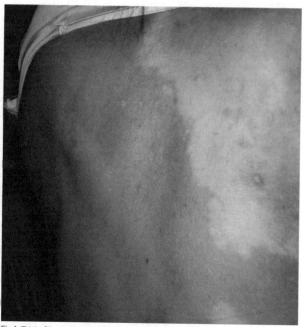

**Fig 1.** Think of leprosy in everyone with anaesthetic hypopigmented macules or plaques. Could this be vitiligo? No: vitiligo is more demarcated and depigmented (chalk white). See fig 4 on p565.
Courtesy of Prof Jayakar Thomas.

Infectious diseases

**Lyme disease**[347] is a tick-borne (fig 1) infection caused by *Borrelia burgdorferi*. *Signs:* ►≤75% remember the tick bite. The 1st sign is usually **erythema migrans**; a circular rash (*OHCS* p587 fig 3) occurring in ~80%, which begins at the site of a tick bite after 3-30d (p564). It gradually expands, reaching up to 30cm across. Its centre may clear as it enlarges (bull's-eye appearance). *Also:* fatigue, chills, fever, headache, muscle and joint pain, lymphadenopathy, myocarditis; heart block; meningitis; ataxia; amnesia; cranial nerve palsies; neuropathy; lymphocytic meningoradiculitis (Bannwarth's syndrome). *Diagnosis* is based on symptoms, physical findings, and a history of exposure to infected ticks. Lab tests are not needed in presence of erythema migrans.[348] *R:* Skin rash: doxycycline 100mg/12h PO (amoxicillin or penicillin V if <8yrs or pregnant) for 14-21d. Later complications: high-dose IV benzylpenicillin, ceftriaxone. *Prevention:* Keep limbs covered; use insect repellent; tick collars for pets; check skin often when in risky areas. Vaccination is available, eg if living in high-risk areas. Advice differs on prophylaxis after a tick bites. A single dose of doxycycline 200mg PO given within 72h of a bite is effective prophylaxis; in highly endemic areas, this may be worthwhile (eg if risk >1%). *Removing ticks:* Use fine (tick-removing) tweezers to grasp the tick very close to the skin. With a steady motion, pull the tick's body away; clean with soap and water. Don't worry if the tick's mouthparts remain in the skin—they won't transmit Lyme disease.[349] Skin complications: **acrodermatitis chronica atrophicans** (ACA; skin is as 'thin as cigarette paper'); **borrelia lymphocytoma** manifests, eg as a blue/red discolouration of the earlobe.

Fig 1. *Amblyomma americanum.*
© Prof S. Upton, Kansas Univ.

**Endemic treponematoses** *Yaws* is caused by *T. pertenue* (serologically indistinguishable from *T. pallidum*). It is a chronic granulomatous disease common in children in the rural Tropics. Spread: direct contact, via skin abrasions, promoted by poor hygiene. The primary lesion (an ulcerating papule) appears ~4wks after exposure. Scattered 2nd lesions then appear, eg in moist skin, but can be anywhere. These may become exuberant. Tertiary lesions are subcutaneous gummatous ulcerating granulomata, affecting skin and bone. CVS and CNS complications do not occur. *Pinta* (*T. carateum*) affects only skin; seen in Central and S America. *Endemic nonvenereal syphilis* (*bejel*; *T. pallidum*) is seen in Third World children, when it resembles yaws. In the developed world, *T. pallidum* causes *syphilis* (see BOX). Δ: Clinical. *R:* Procaine penicillin (p378).

**Weil's disease**ND is caused by *Leptospira interrogans* (eg serogroup *L. icterohaemorrhagiae*). Spread is typically by contact with infected rat urine, eg in slums or while swimming, canoeing or cycling through puddles. After an incubation of 2-20d there is abrupt fever, myalgia/myositis, cough, chest pain ± haemoptysis—then recovery, or jaundice, meningitis, uveitis, and renal failure. Δ: Blood culture +ve only up to day 4 of illness; serology. *R: Mild:* doxycycline, amoxicillin, or ampicillin. *Severe:* IV penicillin G. *Alternatives:* ampicillin, amoxicillin, erythromycin. Prophylaxis: doxycycline 200mg/wk may have a role—eg for water sports in dangerous places.

**Canicola fever** is an aseptic meningitis caused by *Leptospira canicola*.

**Relapsing fever**ND This is caused by *Borrelia recurrentis* (louse-borne) or *B. duttoni* (tick-borne). It typically occurs in pandemics following war or disaster, and may kill millions. *Incubation:* 4-18d. *Presentation:* Abrupt onset fever, rigors, and headache. A petechial rash (which may be faint or absent), jaundice, and tender hepatosplenomegaly may develop. Serious signs: myocarditis, hepatic failure, and DIC. Crises of very high fever and tachycardia occur; on abating, fatal hypotension from vasodilatation may occur. Relapses occur, but are milder. *Tests:* Organisms are seen on Leishman-stained thin or thick films. *R:* Doxycyline 100mg/12h PO. The Jarisch–Herxheimer reaction (p431) is fatal in 5%: meptazinol 100mg IV slowly is given as prophylaxis with the tetracycline, repeated ½h later (with the chill phase) and during the flush phase (if systolic BP <75mmHg). Delouse the patient and their clothes.[350] Doxycycline (p380) is useful prophylaxis in high-risk groups.

▶*Any anogenital ulcer or sore is syphilis until proven otherwise.* UK incidence: >2250 infections/yr.[351] Serious outbreaks exist in the UK and USA[352–354] as safe-sex messages are forgotten, ignored, or trounced (some clubs ban condoms on 'raw nights').[355] ~70% are in men who have sex with men (rates rising since 2001, esp if black or Hispanic, aged 15–19yrs).[356] Female prevalence (screening in London antenatal clinics): 0.44% (vs 0.34% for HIV & 1.1% for hepatitis B).[357]

*Treponema pallidum* (fig 1) enters during sex, via a graze, forming the very infectious hard ulcer (chancre) of *primary syphilis.* All 4 stages are due to an endarteritis obliterans. *Incubation:* 9–90d.

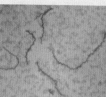

*Secondary syphilis:* 6 weeks to 6 months after infection: rash (trunk, face, palms, soles; may be scaly), malaise, lymphadenopathy, T°↑, tonsillitis, condylomata lata (flat papules around/beyond genitals),[358] oral snail-track ulcers, alopecia, hepatitis (in up to ⅓, esp. if HIV+ve too[359]), hepatosplenomegaly, uveitis, optic neuritis, meningism, glomerulonephritis ± periosteitis.

Fig 1. *T. pallidum.* ©Prof S Spilatro.

*Tertiary syphilis* follows ≥2yrs latency (when patients are non-infectious): there are *gummas* (granulomas in skin, mucosa, bone, joints, viscera, eg lung, testis).

*Quaternary Vascular:* Ascending aortic aneurysm/aortic regurgitation. Neurosyphilis (Δ: CSF analysis; consider if RPR titre ≥1:32) *(a) Meningovascular:* Cranial nerve palsies (eg vision↓), stroke *(b) General paresis of insane (GPI):* Dementia, psychoses/reversible dementia (fatal if untreated) *(c) Tabes dorsalis:* Ataxia, numb legs, chest & bridge of nose, lightning pains ("like a bolt from the blue"), gastric crises, reflex loss, plantars↑↑, Charcot's joints (p520). Argyll Robertson pupil (p79).

*Cardiolipin antibody:* Not treponeme-specific. Detectable in primary disease but wanes in late syphilis. Indicates active disease and becomes -ve after treatment. *False +ves* (with -ve treponemal antibody): pregnancy, immunization, pneumonia, malaria, SLE, TB, leprosy. Examples: Venereal Disease Research Laboratory slide test (VDRL), rapid plasma reagin (RPR), Wassermann reaction (WR).

*Treponeme-specific antibody:* Positive in 1° disease, remains so despite treatment. Examples: *T. pallidum* haemagglutination assay (TPHA), fluorescent treponemal antibody (FTA), *T. pallidum* immobilization test (TPI). Non-specific, also +ve in non-venereal yaws, bejel, or pinta. *ELISA:* Syphilis ELISA IgG and ELISA IgM.

*Other tests:* In 1° syphilis, treponemes may be seen by *dark ground microscopy* of chancre fluid; serology at this stage is often -ve. In 2° syphilis, treponemes are seen in the lesions and both types of antibody tests are positive. In late syphilis, organisms may no longer be seen, but both types of antibody test usually remain +ve (cardiolipin antibody tests may wane). In neurosyphilis, CSF antibody tests (particularly FTA and TPHA) are +ve. ▶*Look for other STIs.* If HIV+ve, serology may be negative during syphilis reactivation. PCR may help. Do contact tracing.

℞: Simplest regimen: 2–3 doses (1wk apart) of benzathine penicillin G 1.8g.[380] As this is only available in the UK on a named-patient basis (see *BNF*) an alternative is benzylpenicillin 0.6–1.2g/24h IM for ~28d (17d in early syphilis) + probenecid, eg 500mg/6h (to prevent penicillin loss in urine).[360]

Or doxycycline: early syphilis, 100mg/12h for 14d; late latent syphilis, 100mg/12h for 28d. Neurosyphilis, ceftriaxone (unlicensed) 2g/d IM for 14d. *If pregnant:* erythromycin 500mg/6h PO (*OTM* dose).

Beware *Jarisch-Herxheimer reaction:* T°↑, pulse↑, and vasodilatation hours after the 1st dose of antibiotic (? from sudden release of endotoxin). Commonest in 2° disease; most dangerous in 3°. Consider steroids. If HIV+ve, penicillin may not stop neurosyphilis; consult microbiologist. *Congenital syphilis: OHCS* p35.

Infectious diseases

219 virus species are known to infect humans. Yellow fever was the 1st to be discovered (in 1901). New species are added at a rate of ~3/year (with careful observation you may be able to make a name for yourself by discovering the 220th).

*Yellow fever:* An epidemic arbovirus disease spread by *Aedes* mosquitoes (Brazil, Bolivia, Peru, Central and West Africa). *Immunization:* p391. *Incubation:* 2–14d. *The patient:* In mild forms, fever, headache, nausea, albuminuria, myalgia, and relative bradycardia. If severe: 3 days of headache, myalgia, anorexia ± nausea, then abrupt fever, a brief remission, then prostration, jaundice (± fatty liver), haematemesis, other bleeding, oliguria. *Mortality:* <10% (day 5–10). Δ: ELISA. ℞: Symptomatic.

*Lassa fever*[ND], *Ebola virus*[ND], *Marburg virus*[ND], *dengue haemorrhagic fever* (DHF, BOX 1—this 'unofficial' haemorrhagic fever is the commonest arbovirus disease).[361] They start with sudden headache, pleuritic pain, backache, myalgia, conjunctivitis, prostration, dehydration, facial flushing (dengue), and T°↑. Bleeding soon supervenes. There may be resolution, or renal failure, encephalitis, coma, and death. ℞: Primarily symptomatic; ribavirin helps in Lassa fever if given early.[362] ►Use special infection control measures (Lassa, Ebola, Marburg); get expert help at once.

## Poliomyelitis[ND]

Polio is a highly contagious picornavirus (fig 1), though only a few patients develop any illness from the infection. *Spread:* Droplet or faecal-oral. *Incubation:* 7 days. *Signs: Flu prodrome* for 48h then a *pre-paralytic stage:* T°↑, pulse↑, headache, vomiting, neck stiffness, and unilateral tremor. In <50% this progresses to a *paralytic stage:* myalgia, LMN signs[1] ± respiratory failure. No sensory signs. *Tests:* CSF: WCC↑, polymorphs then lymphocytes, otherwise normal; paired sera (14 days apart); throat swab and stool culture identify virus. *Natural history:* <10% of those with paralysis die. There may be *delayed progression* of paralysis (*post-polio syndrome*, PPS). *Risk of severe paralysis* ↑ if: Adult; pregnant; muscle fatigue/trauma during incubation period. PPS causes fatigue, weakness, myalgia, and worsening function, not necessarily at sites originally affected (advise enough exercise to prevent wasting but not so much as to ↑weakness in already damaged muscles). No drug works.[363] *Vaccine:* p391.

## Rabies[ND]

50,000 deaths/yr world-wide

Rabies is a rhabdovirus spread by bites from an infected mammal, eg bats, dogs, cats, foxes, or raccoons (bites may go unnoticed).[364] There is slight risk from scratches, or licks to cuts, mouth or eyes. *The patient:* ~9–90 days' incubation, so give prophylaxis even several months after exposure. Prodrome: headache, malaise, odd behaviour, agitation, fever, and itch around the bite. Progresses to 'furious rabies', eg with water-provoked muscle spasms often accompanied by terror (hydrophobia). In 20%, 'dumb rabies' starts with flaccid paralysis in the bitten limb. *Deaths/yr:* 50,000.

*Advice in countries not declared rabies-free:* Avoid animal contact; get help if bitten. Wash all bites meticulously with soapy water (takes 20min and ↓incidence by ~65%).

*Pre-exposure prophylaxis* (vets, zoo-keepers, customs workers, bat handlers, travellers in rabies area for >1 month or at especial risk, or if access to post-exposure treatment is hard): give human diploid cell strain vaccine (1mL IM, deltoid) on days 0, 7, & 28, and again at 2–3yrs if still at risk. *Treatment if bitten where rabies is endemic* (if unvaccinated): wash as above. ►Seek help (*Health Protection Agency, tel.:* UK020 8200 6868). Watch the biting animal to see if it dies (it is possible that it may not die of rabies before the patient does)[365] *If previously immunized:* give vaccine (1mL IM) on days 0 & 3. *If previously unimmunized:* give vaccine on days 0, 3, 7, 14 & 30 + rabies immunoglobulin (RIg, 20U/kg on day 0; ½ IM & ½ infiltrated around wounds). HRIg is probably unnecessary > a week after vaccination has started, as an active antibody response has already begun. ►Never mix vaccine and antiserum or inject in the same limb.[366] Rabies is 'always' fatal once symptoms start (survival has occurred, with optimal CNS/cardiorespiratory support). Vaccinate attending staff. *Public health:* ☺Wherever rabies is a problem, put it on the national curriculum, along with dog-handling.[367] Philippines success story Vaccinate dogs; make houses bat-proof.[368]

## Dengue fever (DF) and dengue haemorrhagic fever (DHF)

*Incidence:* 50–100×10⁶/yr (DF); 250,000–500,000/yr get DHF. The global pandemic of this RNA flavivirus relates to poor vector control (eg of Asian tiger *Aedes* mosquitoes), urbanization[2] poor waste disposal, and migrations bringing new strains (DEN-2) that get more virulent in those who have had mild dengue. Global warming is extending the range of DF (eg to southern USA). English winters are now warm enough to support transmission.[369]

Infants typically have a simple febrile illness with a rash. Older children/adults have flushes (face, neck, chest) ± centrifugal maculopapular rash from day 3, or late confluent petechiae with round pale areas of normal skin ± headache, arthralgia, jaundice, hepatosplenomegaly, anuria. *Haemorrhagic signs:* (Unlikely if AST normal)[370] Petechiae, GI, gum or nose bleeds, haematuria, menorrhagia.

*Monitor:* BP; urine flow; WCC↓; platelets↓; PCV; +ve tourniquet test (>20 petechiae/inch²) + PCV↑ by 20% are telling signs (rapid endothelial plasma leak is the key pathophysiology of DHF). ΔΔ: Chikungunya[3] measles, leptospirosis, typhoid, malaria. *Exclusion:* If symptoms start >2wks after leaving a dengue area, or if fever lasts >2wks, dengue is 'ruled out'. R: Supportive. Prompt IV resuscitation, eg Ringer's lactate. ►►If shocked (mortality 40%) get help; it is traditional to try a bolus of 15mL/kg repeated every ½h until BP rises and urine flows at >30mL/h. Evidence is lacking.[371,372] *Mosquito control:* Problematic![4]

## Polio: a tantalizing exercise in prevention and (near) eradication

Eradication makes economic and humanitarian sense, even if it costs US\$billions.[373]
• Pre-1950s, polio distribution was worldwide. In 1952 CO₂ retention was found to be the cause of death. Mechanical ventilation began (≈the birth of ITU).[374]
• 12 April 1955: vaccination starts with Salk's inactivated vaccine.
• 1958: Sabin donated his 3 attenuated strains to Chumakov in Moscow, who produced the 3 vaccines, giving them to 15 million people in 1 year.
• 1960s: the 3 vaccines are mixed, to produce a single oral polio vaccine (OPV).
• 1988: Estimated 350,000 cases worldwide, occurring in 125 countries. The Global Polio Eradication Initiative, aiming to protect children worldwide through vaccination, is launched; the aim was eradication by the year 2000.
• 1991–4: transmission interrupted in the West. 80,000,000 vaccinated in 48h in China.
• 1994: WHO declares the Americas polio-free.
• 1997: 1 case of wild polio in all of Europe.
• 1999: Only 7090 cases worldwide.
• 2000: WHO declares Western Pacific polio-free.
• 2001: 483 cases in 10 endemic countries.
• 2002: WHO declares Europe polio-free.
• 2004: 6 polio-endemic countries remain.[375]
• 2006: Transmission re-established in: Nigeria, Sudan, Egypt, Central African Republic, Mali, Côte d'Ivoire, Somalia, Burkina Faso, Uttar Pradesh.[376, 377]
• 2008: 1655 cases in 17 countries.[378]

Fig 1. Poliovirus ©D Belnap (Utah Univ.) & J Hogle (Harvard).

• 2012: outbreak of circulating vaccine-derived poliovirus in Yemen & Mozambique.

Before 2005 most cases in the West were adult contacts of child vaccinees; these cases have stopped as live vaccine has been replaced by inactivated vaccine.

NB: Sabin viruses and their genetic revertants can cause chronic infection in immunodeficient people, who may shed neurovirulent virus in faeces for years. So programmes of oral vaccination must not continue one day longer than needed.

---

**1** *Non-viral causes of flaccid paralysis*: Borrelia; mycoplasma; diphtheria; botulism; heavy metals; transverse myelitis; polymyositis

**2** Southern UK, northern France, parts of Germany, Italy, Sicily, Balkan and Benelux countries are now at risk. Conversely, cities high in the Andes are dengue-free, as *Aedes* mosquitoes cannot survive high up.

**3** Haemorrhagic features in Chikungunya virus infections are rare; arthralgia, fever, myalgia and a rash are more common, eg in Indian Ocean islands.

**4** Mosquito control has shown limited success owing to: •Modern urban complexity •Increasing insecticide resistance •Labour-intensive and logistically demanding nature of the work •Entomological surveys having limited ability to predict future epidemics. Different approaches are now envisaged: 1 Use of transgenic mosquitoes or adult mosquitoes as vehicles of juvenile hormone transfer between resting and oviposition sites 2 Using mosquito microbiota or its symbionts to manipulate disease transmission.[79]

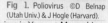

**Q fever** is caused by *Coxiella burnetii* (100 cases/yr in the UK). It is so named because it was first labelled 'query' fever in workers in an Australian abattoir.

*Epidemiology:* Occurs worldwide, and is usually rural, with reservoirs in cattle and sheep. The organism is resistant to drying and is usually inhaled from infected dust. It can be contracted from unpasteurized milk, directly from carcasses in abattoirs, sometimes by droplet spread, and rarely from tick bites.

*Clinical features:* Suspect Q fever in anyone with a PUO or atypical pneumonia. It may present with fever, myalgia, sweats, headache, cough, and hepatitis (± spleno-megaly).[280] If the disease becomes chronic, suspect endocarditis (typically 'culture-negative'). This usually affects the aortic valve, but clinical signs may be absent. It also causes miscarriages and CNS infection.

*Tests:* CXR may show consolidation, eg multilobar or slowly resolving. Liver function tests may be hepatitic and biopsy may show granulomata. Diagnosis is serological: indirect immunofluorescence assay (IFA) is the most dependable and widely used method. Increased IgG and IgA antibodies to phase I are often indicative of Q fever endocarditis.[381] Phase I antigens suggest chronic infection; phase II antigens suggest acute infection. PCR may be used on tissue samples. CSF tests may be needed.

*Treatment:* Get expert microbiological help. *Acute:* Doxycycline 100mg/12h PO for 2-3wks. Minocycline, clarithromycin, ciprofloxacin (in pregnancy) and co-trim-oxazole are used. *Q fever endocarditis:* Treatment is difficult, eg doxycycline plus hydroxychloroquine, eg 600mg/d PO for at least 18 months ± valve replacement.[381]

*Prevention:* Vaccination for those whose occupation places them at high risk.

**Bartonellosis** is caused by *Bartonella bacilliformis*, a Gram -ve, motile, bacillus-like organism which parasitizes RBCs. Spread is by sandflies in the Andes, Peru, Ecuador, Colombia, Thailand, and Niger. Transient immunosuppression leads to other infections (eg Salmonella). *Incubation:* 10-210d (mean = 60d).

*Signs:* Fever, rashes, lymphadenopathy, hepatosplenomegaly, jaundice, cerebellar syndromes, dermal nodules (verrucas), retinal haemorrhages, myocarditis, pericard-ial effusion, oedema, and, rarely, meningo-encephalomyelitis.

*Tests:* Giemsa-stained blood films. Blood culture (prolonged). Coombs' -ve haemo-lytic anaemia, and hypochromic, macrocytic red cells with a megaloblastic marrow. CSF pleocytosis. Serological tests are not widely available.

*Treatment:* Responds to **penicillin**, but ciprofloxacin (500mg/12h PO for 10d) is often used because of frequent association with salmonelloses. Steroids if CNS involved.

**Trench fever** is caused by *Bartonella quintana* inoculated from infected louse fae-ces, not only in soldiers, but also in the homeless, and in alcoholics.

*Clinical features:* Fever, headache, myalgia, dizziness, back pain, macular rash, eye pain, leg pain, splenomegaly, endocarditis (rare). In HIV-infected patients, the skin lesions may resemble Kaposi's sarcoma. It is not fatal; it may relapse.

*Tests:* Blood culture, serology, PCR. ℞: Doxycycline 100mg/12h PO for 15 days.

**Ehrlichiosis** is caused by *Ehrlichia chaffeensis*, an obligate intracytoplasmic Gram -ve organism, related to Rickettsia. It is spread by ticks. It causes fever, headache, anorexia, malaise, abdominal pain, epigastric pain, conjunctivitis, lymphadenopathy, jaundice, rash, confusion, and cervical lymphadenopathy.

*Tests:* Leucopenia, thrombocytopenia, AST↑.[282] Serology/PCR are diagnostic.

*Treatment:* May respond to **doxycycline** 100mg/12h PO for 7-14d.

## Typhus: the archetypal rickettsial disease

Rickettsiae are parasitic bacteria that are obligate intracellular parasites; they are bigger than viruses but smaller than classical bacteria. They are carried by host arthropods (figs 1–3) and invade human mononuclear cells, neutrophils, or blood vessel endothelium ('vasculotropic'). All the cataclysmic events of the last century (war, revolution, flood, famine, genocide, and overcrowding) have been helpful to lice. As a result, Rickettsiae (especially typhus) have killed untold millions.

**Pathology** Widespread vasculitis and endothelial proliferation may affect any organ and thrombotic occlusion may lead to gangrene.

**Signs** ▶*Think of typhus in all travellers or inhabitants of endemic areas who seem to have septicaemia, but have -ve blood cultures*:[50] Incubation: 2–23d. Infection may be mild/asymptomatic or severe/systemic, with sudden fever, frontal headache, confusion, and jaundice. With some species, an eschar (dark crusty ulcer at the site of a bite) is found. A rickettsial rash may be macular, papular, petechial, or haemorrhagic. Tests: haemolysis, neutrophilia, platelets↓, clotting↓, hepatitis, renal impairment. Patients die of shock, renal failure, DIC (p346), stroke, respiratory distress syndrome, cardiac arrest, and multi-organ dysfunction.

*Epidemic typhus (R. prowazeki):* Spread: human lice *Pediculus humanus* (fig 1; faeces are inhaled or pass through skin). It may recrudesce decades later (Brill-Zinsser disease). The rash is truncal, then peripheral (opposite to *R. rickettsii*).

*Rocky Mountain spotted fever (R. rickettsii)* is tick-borne (fig 2). Endemic in Rocky Mountains and south-eastern USA. The rash (seen in 90%) begins as macules on hands/feet, spreading and becoming petechial or haemorrhagic in 50%.

*Tick typhus (R. conorii;* Mediterranean spotted fever/boutonneuse, African tick bite fever, Marseilles fever, Indian/Israeli tick typhus) is the chief imported rickettsial disease in the UK (endemic in Africa, the Mediterranean, eg Croatia, and parts of Asia; sporadic in Laos, Korea,[etc]). Vector example: fig 3. The rash starts in the axillae, becoming purpuric as it spreads. *Other signs:* conjunctival suffusion; jaundice; deranged clotting; meningoencephalitis; cerebritis;[383] renal failure.

*Scrub typhus (Orientia tsutsugamushi)* Most common in SE Asia. Signs: Eschar from chigger bite (75%); hepatomegaly (65%); cough (60%); lymphadenopathy (46%);[50] tachypnoea (35%); constipation (25%); abdominal pain (20%); oedema (20%); splenomegaly (15%); vomiting (15%); rash (15%); petechiae (5%); sudden deafness.[384] CXR: bilateral infiltrations (85%).[385] Blood: LFT↑ (90%); platelets↓ (80%); neutrophilia (60%); lymphocytosis ± atypical lymphocytosis (5%). Complications: pneumonia ± pulmonary oedema, meningitis, and shock.

*Murine (endemic) typhus (R. typhi)* is spread by fleas from rats to humans. It is more prevalent in warm, coastal ports (eg Dalmatia, Laos, southern USA).[386]

*Rickettsialpox (R. akari)* Variegate rash: macular, papular, or vesicular.

*Mediterranean spotted fever (R. conorii )*: meningoencephalitis; cerebellitis.[387]

**Δ** Culture is difficult; traditional heterophil antibody Weil-Felix tests are insensitive and non-specific. A rise in antibody titre in paired sera is diagnostic. Latex agglutination, indirect immunofluorescence, ELISAs and PCR are available (may be done on the eschar).[388] An accurate, rapid dotblot immunoassay is available for scrub typhus. Skin biopsy may be diagnostic in Rocky Mountain spotted fever.

**℞** Doxycycline 100mg/12h PO/IV for 7d (or 48h after T°↔) or chloramphenicol 500mg/6h PO for 10–14d. Resistance, eg in Thailand. Azithromycin 500mg stat may work in tick and scrub typhus.[389] Extracorporeal membrane oxygenation may help.[390]

**Poor prognostic factors** Older age, male, black, G6PD deficiency.

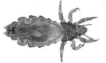

Fig 1. *Pediculus humanus:* endemic typhus vector.

Fig 2. *Dermacentor variabilis* is a vector for Rocky Mountain spotted fever.

Fig 3. Dog tick

Figs 1–3 © Prof S Upton, Kansas Univ.

*Giardia lamblia* (fig 1) is a flagellate protozoon that lives in the duodenum and jejunum. Spread: faecal-oral (↑ risk if, eg immunosuppression, travel, anal sex, achlorhydria, playgroups,[391] and swimming)—or from pets or birds. Drinking water may be contaminated.

*The patient* is often asymptomatic. Lassitude, bloating, flatulence, abdominal pain, loose stools ± explosive diarrhoea are typical. Malabsorption, weight loss, and lactose intolerance may occur.

*Δ:* •Stool microscopy for cysts and trophozoites may be -ve so repeat ≥ 3 times •Duodenal fluid aspirate analysis •Stool ELISA/PCR • Therapeutic trial. *ΔΔ:* Any cause of diarrhoea (p246), sprue (p280), coeliac.

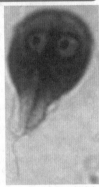

Fig 1. *Giardia:* the only diplomonadid to trouble us.

*R̟:* Scrupulous hygiene. **Tinidazole** 2g PO stat (avoid alcohol); if pregnant, **paromomycin** 500mg/6h PO for 7d. If this fails, check compliance and consider treating *all* the family. If diarrhoea persists, avoid milk as lactose intolerance may persist for 6wks.

*Entamoeba histolytica* (amoebiasis; figs 2-5) affects 50 million people worldwide; ~100,000 die annually.[392] Spread: faecal-oral (eg oral-anal sex).[393] Boil water and infected food to destroy cysts. Most symptoms are from involvement of the colon, but 1% present with potentially fatal invasive liver disease. Distinguishing invasive forms (*E. histolytica*) from a morphologically identical but *usually*[394] non-invasive *E. dispar* requires PCR *et al*.

**Amoebic dysentery**ND may occur some time after initial infection. Diarrhoea starts slowly, becoming profuse & bloody. An acute febrile prostrating illness can

Fig 2. *E. histolytica* cyst with an endosome inside each of its 4 nuclei.

occur but high fever, colic, and tenesmus are rare. May remit and relapse. *Δ:* Stool microscopy: trophozoites, blood, pus cells. Faecal antigen detection also helps. Serology indicates previous or current infection and may be unhelpful in acute infection. *ΔΔ: Bacillary dysentery* often starts more suddenly, is more dehydrating, and stools are more watery. *Acute ulcerative colitis* is more gradual and stools are bloodier. Other causes of bloody diarrhoea: p426 & p246.

**Amoebic colonic abscesses** may perforate causing peritonitis.

**Amoebomas** are inflammatory masses, eg in the caecum (a cause of RIF masses).

**Amoebic liver abscess** is often a single mass in the right lobe containing 'anchovy-sauce' pus. *Signs:* High swinging fever, sweats, RUQ pain/tenderness ± chest pain (eg if intrapleural rupture). WCC↑. LFT normal or ↑ (cholestatic). 50% have no history of amoebic dysentery. *Δ:* PCR; ultrasound/CT ± aspiration; don't rely on microscopy.

*R̟:* **Metronidazole** 800mg/8h PO for 5d for acute amoebic dysentery (active against vegetative amoebae), then **diloxanide furoate** 500mg/8h PO for 10d to destroy gut cysts (it's a luminal agent to prevent recurrence; SE rare); diloxanide is also best in chronic disease when *Entamoeba* cysts, not vegetative forms, are in stools. Amoebic liver abscess/severe infections: **tinidazole** 2g/24h for 5d ± ultrasound-guided aspiration (by an expert in theatre) if not improving within days, eg via catheter (not needle) if >10cm across.[395] Check INR/clotting pre-op. Give diloxanide post-metronidazole.

*Balantidium coli* is a big ciliate protozoan with a sausage-shaped nucleus. Explosive diarrhoea may occur when it gains access via water contaminated by pigs. Inhalation is a rarer way in (→haemoptysis). *R̟:* Oxytetracycline + metronidazole.[396]

**Other protozoa** *Cryptosporidium*, p390; *Microsporidium & Isospora*, p410 (with HIV).

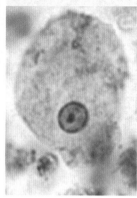

**Fig 3.** A trophozoite of *Entamoeba histo-lytica*.

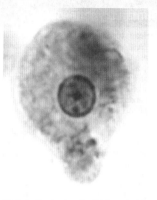

**Fig 4.** Another trophozoite of *Entamoeba histolytica*.

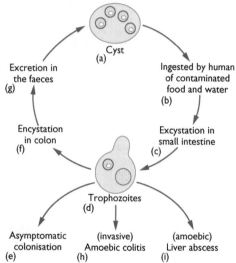

**Fig 5.** The lifecycle of *Entamoeba histolytica* is in 2 stages: cysts and trophozoites. Cysts (10-15μm across) typically contain 4 nuclei. During excystation in the gut lumen, nuclear division is followed by cytoplasmic division, giving rise to 8 trophozoites. Trophozoites (10-50μm across) contain one nucleus with a central karyosome; they live in the caecum and colon. ~90% of individuals infected with *E. histolytica* are asymptomatic. Re-encystation of the trophozoites occurs in the colon, and excretion of cysts in faeces perpetuates the lifecycle. Trophozoites may also invade colon epithelium, causing amoebic colitis in ~10%.

*E. histolytica* can spread haematogenously after breaching colon epithelium and can establish persistent extra-intestinal infection (eg amoebic liver abscess).

Figs 1–4 courtesy of Prof S Upton, Kansas University. Fig 5 is adapted with permission from *Expert Reviews in Molecular Medicine*, CUP, 1999; www-ermm.cbcu.cam.ac.uk/99000617h.htm.

Infectious diseases

### African trypanosomiasis (sleeping sickness)

In West and Central Africa, *Trypanosoma gambiense* (fig 1) causes a slow, wasting illness with long latency. In East Africa, *T. rhodesiense* causes a more rapidly progressive illness. Uganda is the only country where both species are endemic.[397] Trypanosome parasites, spread by tsetse flies, proliferate in blood, lymphatics, and CNS, causing progressive dysfunction, then death. Prevalence: ≤70,000 in the early 2000s, but active surveillance has now stopped in some areas and mortality is increasing (now probably ~10% vs 5% earlier)[397] despite great work done by Stamp Out Sleeping Sickness (SOS) interventions, WHO, the Gates Foundation, Aventis, and Médecins sans Frontières.[398] Wars and famines can cause upsurges.

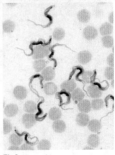
Fig 1. *T. gambiense.*
©S Upton, Kansas Univ.

*Staging:* A tender subcutaneous nodule *(chancre)* develops at the infection site, then...

*Stage I (haemolymphatic):* Non-specific fever, rash, rigors, headaches, hepatosplenomegaly, lymphadenopathy, and joint pains. Winterbottom's sign (posterior cervical nodes↓) is a reliable sign (esp. in *T. gambiense*). In *T. rhodesiense* infections, this stage may be particularly severe, with potentially fatal myocarditis.

*Stage II (meningoencephalitic):* Weeks (*T. rhodesiense*) or months (*T. gambiense*) after initial infection, convulsions, agitation, and confusion—and then apathy, depression, ataxia, dyskinesias, dementia, hypersomnolence, and coma occur.

*Diagnosis:* Microscopy shows trypomastigotes in blood film, lymph node aspirate, or CSF. Serology (see card agglutination text) is reliable in *T. gambiense* infections.

*Treatment:* ▶Seek expert help. Treat anaemia and other infections first; then: early (pre-CNS) phase: pentamidine isethionate 4mg/kg/d deep IM for 10d. SE: WCC↓, BP↓, Ca²⁺↓, GFR↓, platelets↓. Alternative: suramin; SE: proteinuria, GFR↓.

CNS disease: get help. MSF regimen:[Médecins sans Frontières] nifurtimox 5mg/kg/8h PO for 10d + eflornithine 200mg/kg/12h IVI in 250mL of 0.9% saline over 2h for 7d. SE: Hb↓, diarrhoea, fits, leucopenia, hair loss. ~8% relapse (risk↑ if CSF leucocytes >20×10⁹/L or ♂).[399]

### American trypanosomiasis

(Chagas' disease) is caused by *T. cruzi.* Spread: blood-sucking reduviids (triatomine bugs, fig 2) in Latin America and southern USA. ▶Emigration means that chronic Chagas disease could turn up today in your heart or GI clinic: keep alert! Acute disease mostly affects children. A red indurated nodule *(chagoma)* forms at the site of infection; it may scar. *Signs:* (mild/insidious over 2 months): T°↑, myalgia, rash, lymphadenopathy, hepatosplenomegaly ± unilateral conjunctivitis ± periorbital oedema *(Romaña's sign)* ± myocarditis/meningoencephalitis. Chronic disease occurs after a latency of 20yrs. Multi-organ invasion causes serious dilated cardiomyopathy (p146), mega-oesophagus (dysphagia, aspiration), mega-colon (abdominal distension, constipation) + CNS lesions, eg if HIV +ve.

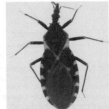
Fig 2. The blood-sucking vector (*Triatoma*) hides in thatch or cracks in walls (rural & urban). Transmission occurs if its faeces are rubbed into wounds or mouths (or via infected blood).
©S Upton, Kansas Univ.

Δ: (no gold standard): *Acute:* trypomastigotes seen in or grown from blood, CSF, or node aspirate. *Chronic:* serology (Chagas' IgG ELISA).

R: Unsatisfactory. Benznidazole (2.5-3.5mg/kg/12h PO for 60d) or nifurtimox 2mg/kg/6h PO pc for 120d in acute disease (toxic, and eliminate parasites in ≤50%). Chronic disease can only be treated symptomatically. Surgery may be needed.

*Prevention:* Better housing, spraying houses with insecticides.

# Leishmaniasis

*Leishmania* are protozoa (fig 1, inset, with 2 RBCs, from a spleen aspirate) that cause granulomata. They are spread by sandflies in Africa, India, Latin America, southern USA, Middle East/Mediterranean. Clinical effects reflect: 1 The ability of each species to induce or suppress the immune response, to metastasize, and to invade cartilage, and 2 the efficiency of our immune response. *L. major* is the most immunogenic and allergenic of cutaneous Old World *Leishmania* and causes most necrosis. *L. tropica* is less immunogenic and causes less inflamed, slow-healing sores with relapsing lesions and a tuberculoid histology.

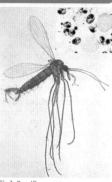

Fig 1. Sandfly. ©S Upton, Kansas Univ.

**Cutaneous leishmaniasis** (oriental sore) affects >300,000 people, eg in Africa, India and S. America; caused by *L. mexicana*, *L. major*, *L. tropica* or *L. amazonensis*.[400] Lesions develop at the bite site, beginning as an itchy papule; crusts fall off to leave an ulcer (*Chiclero's ulcer*). Most heal in ~2 (Old World disease) to 15 months, with scarring (disfiguring if extensive). *L. mexicana* may cause pinna destruction (*Chiclero's ear*). Δ: Microscopy and culture of aspiration from the base of the ulcer.[401] ℞: Topical paromomycin, or IM drugs if unhealed by 6 months or lesion >5cm across (or multiple). Get help. Pentavalent antimony, eg **meglumine antimoniate** (Glucantime) or **sodium stibogluconate** (Pentostam); 20mg/kg/d for 20d. Oral fluconazole or ketoconazole are alternatives.[402]

**Mucocutaneous leishmaniasis** (*L. brasiliensis*) occurs in S America. Primary skin lesions may spread to the mucosa of the nose, pharynx, palate, larynx, and upper lip and cause severe scarring. Nasopharyngeal lesions are called *espundia*. Δ: As parasites may be scanty, a Leishmanin skin test may be needed for distinguishing from leprosy, TB, syphilis, yaws, and cancer. Indirect fluorescent antibody tests and PCR are available. ℞: Sodium stibogluconate (below). Treatment is unsatisfactory once mucosae are involved, so treat all cutaneous lesions early.

**Visceral leishmaniasis (VL)** (kala-azar, means black sickness) is the 2nd most deadly parasitic disease in the world after malaria (50,000 deaths/year).[403] It occurs in Asia, Africa, S America and Mediterranean areas. Cause: *L. donovani*, *L. chagasi*, or *L. infantum* (or, rarely, 'visceralizing' of *L. tropica*).[404] Incubation: months to years. Protozoa spread via lymphatics from minor skin lesions and multiply in macrophages of the reticuloendothelial system (Leishman-Donovan bodies). There are 30 subclinical cases for every overt case. ♀:♂ >3:1. It can be HIV-associated. *Signs:* Dry, warty, hyperpigmented skin lesions; T°↑; sweats; burning feet; arthralgia; cough; epistaxis; abdo pain; splenomegaly (96%); hepatomegaly (63%); lymphadenopathy; emaciation; pancytopenia; hypergammaglobulinaemia.
Δ:[405] *Microscopic exam* of lymph nodes, bone marrow or spleen are confirmatory.
*Ab-detection:* Indirect fluorescence antibody (IFA), ELISA, western blot, direct agglutination test (DAT) and RK39-based immunochromatographic test (ICT). Serology limitations: 1 Ab levels are detectable for years after cure, so cannot diagnose VL relapse. 2 Tests are +ve in many with no history of VL. Serology may be -ve if HIV+ve.
*Ag-detection:* detects heat-stable Ag by latex agglutination. ℞: **Liposomal amphoterin B** (1st-line in Europe/USA), or **miltefosine** (1st effective oral drug for VL; 0.75–1.2mg/kg/12h PO for 28d). There are increasing cases of antimony-resistant strains of *L. donovani*, eg in India.[406,407]
*Prevention:* Sandfly control is not working well, eg in India, as indoor spraying (the basis of *P. argentipes* control) is poorly implemented.[408]
*Post kala-azar dermal leishmaniasis:* Years after successful ℞, lesions resemble leprosy.

Infectious diseases

Pathogenic fungi produce either toxins or allergic reactions. They are *superficial* (pityriasis versicolor), *cutaneous* (tinea/ringworm; intertrigo; restricted to keratinized skin, hair and nails), *subcutaneous* (mycetoma; madura foot or sporotrichosis; ℞ is complex and may need limb amputation)—or *systemic* (from the lung, spreading to many organs, eg histoplasmosis; blastomycosis; coccidioidomycosis; fungal meningitis).

**Superficial/cutaneous mycoses** *Candida* (figs 1 & 3). Dermatophytes (*Trichophyton, Microsporum, Dermatophyton*) cause tinea (ringworm). Δ: Skin scraping microscopy. ℞: Topical clotrimazole 1%. Continue for 14d after healing. If intractable, try itraconazole (100–200mg/24h PO for 7d if eGFR >80; SE: D&V; CCF), terbinafine (250mg/24h PO for 4wks) or griseofulvin (0.5–1g/24h; SE: agranulocytosis; SLE). *Malassezia furfur* causes pityriasis versicolor, a macular rash which appears brown on pale skin and pale on tanned skin. Δ: Microscopy of skin scrapings under Wood's light. ℞: Ketoconazole cream (2%) or selenium shampoo used as a lotion; leave on for 10min daily for 7d).

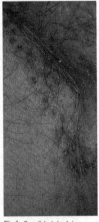

Fig 1. *Candida intertrigo*.

**Systemic mycoses** *Aspergillus fumigatus* may precipitate asthma, allergic bronchopulmonary aspergillosis (ABPA), or cause aspergilloma (p168) ± pneumonia and invasive aspergillosis if immunosuppressed. Voriconazole may be better than amphotericin B in invasive aspergillosis,[409] esp. in cerebral aspergillosis[410]

*Systemic candidiasis* occurs in the immunocompromised: consider this *whenever* they get a PUO, eg *Candida* UTI in DM or as a rare cause of prosthetic valve endocarditis. Do repeated blood cultures. If infection does not resolve when the predisposing factor (eg IV line) is removed, the treatment is fluconazole (400mg stat then 200mg/d PO, halved if eGFR <50) or an echinocandin (they are embryotoxic). Caspofungin 70mg/d IVI on day 1, then 50mg/d (70mg/d if >80kg) is an alternative.[411]

*Cryptococcus neoformans* causes meningitis or pneumonia. It is commonest in the immunocompromised, eg AIDS, sarcoid, Hodgkin's, or steroid ℞. The history may be long. Look for signs of ICP↑, eg confusion, papilloedema, cranial nerve lesions. Δ: Indian ink CSF stain; blood culture. Cryptococcal antigen is detected in CSF & blood by latex tests. ℞: It may be necessary to ↓CSF pressure by ~50% by removing CSF. *Non-AIDS meningitis:* Amphotericin B 0.7mg/kg/d IV + flucytosine 25mg/kg/6h PO for 2wks then fluconazole 200mg/d PO for 8wks. *AIDS meningitis:* As above, but continue fluconazole 400mg/d PO for 10wks, then 200mg/d PO until CD4 >200 for >6 months (or lifelong). *Non-CNS infections* (AIDS or non-AIDS): Do LP to rule out meningitis, then treat with fluconazole, itraconazole or flucytosine.[412] Prophylaxis with fluconazole 200mg/d PO is needed until CD4 >150 × 10⁶/L and cryptococcal antigen -ve (p410).

**New World and Africa fungi** causing deep infection: *Histoplasma* (fig 2), *Coccidioides immitis, Paracoccidioides brasiliensis* & *Blastomyces dermatitidis* may be asymptomatic or cause acute/chronic lung disease, or disseminated infection. Histoplasma pneumonitis: arthralgia, erythema nodosum (fig 1, p565), and multiforme (p565). Chronic disease causes upper-zone fibrosis ± CXR

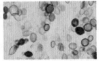

Fig 2. Histoplasma × 1000.

coin lesions. Δ: CXR, serology, culture, biopsy. ℞: *Histoplasmosis:* 1 week's methylprednisolone (0.5 mg/kg/d) + amphotericin B 0.7mg/kg/d IV, eg if HIV +ve & severe; liposomal form may be better (+less renal failure), then itraconazole 200mg/8–12h PO for 12wks. *Paracoccidioides:* Itraconazole 200mg/d PO for >26wks. *Blastomycosis:* Itraconazole.

**HIV: which systemic mycoses occur?** Cryptococcosis, histoplasmosis, blastomycosis, paracoccidioidomycosis, penicilliosis, aspergillosis, and coccidioidomycosis.[413]

Figures courtesy of A Huntley (figs 1, 5 & 8), Subhash Mohan (fig 2) & P-Y Guillaume (figs 3, 4, 6 & 7).

## Candida on ITU: colonization → invasion → dissemination

Not everyone with +ve yeast cultures needs treating: *Candida* is a common commensal on skin, pharynx, or vagina but in some contexts (MINIBOX) or if many sites are colonized (surgical drains, urine ± sputum), risk of invasion is high:[414] *Invasion* implies fungus in normally sterile tissues. *Dissemination* involves infection of remote organs via blood (eg endophthalmitis + fungi in lung or kidney). Options: amphotericin (p440); fluconazole; caspofungin if at risk (see MINIBOX; especially if your patient is deteriorating):[415]

| *Risk of dissemination ↑ if:* |
| --- |
| • Prolonged ventilation |
| • Broad-spectrum antibiotics |
| • Urinary catheters |
| • Immunosuppression |
| • Intravascular lines |
| • IV nutrition |

• A single well-taken +ve blood culture—if risk factors are present (above).
• Isolation of *Candida* from any sterile site except urine.
• Yeasts on microscopy on a sterile-site specimen, before cultures are known.
• Positive histology from normally sterile tissues in those at risk (above).
• Removal/change of IV lines is essential in patients with candidaemia.

►Consult an ID physician/microbiologist before starting systemic antifungals.

**Prevention when immunocompromised** Fluconazole 50–400mg/d after chemo/radiotherapy, started before onset of neutropenia, and continued for 1 week after WCC normalizes. It only protects against yeasts. NB: posaconazole is the only drug licensed for prophylaxis in this setting and is active against moulds and yeasts.

## Facts of life for budding mycologists (figs 1-8)[1]

To the uninitiated, fungi are like bacteria, but their chitin cell walls and their knack of mitosis puts them in their own kingdom. They are larger than bacteria (eg 8µm across), and mostly reproduce by budding of germ tubes (fig 4), not by fission. Yeasts occur as single cells or as clusters. Hyphae often occur in a mass of cells (called moulds). A hyphal cell with cross-walls is called a mycelium. Some yeasts are dimorphic: single cells at 37°C but forming structures called mycelia, containing fruiting bodies (hyphae), at room temperature.

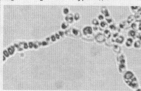

Fig 3. *Candida albicans*.

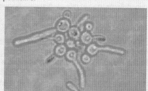

Fig 4. Germ tubes emerging from dimorphic *Candida albicans* blastospores.

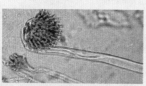

Fig 5. *Aspergillus niger*. If spores are inhaled, aspergillosis can occur (rare, p169):[416] If HIV +ve, bone or eye infection may occur.

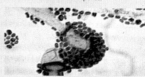

Fig 6. Mucor blastospores. Think of mucormycosis in diabetics with black pus in the nose ± proptosis/sinusitis or pneumonia. *R:* amphotericin B; posaconazole.

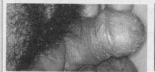

Fig 7. Candida of the glans.

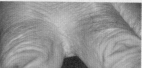

Fig 8. Web-space candida.

1 billion people are hosts to nematodes (± few hundred million[417]). Many live with us seemingly peacefully ▶but with significant loss in quality of life.[418] Ascariasis can cause GI obstruction, hookworms can stunt growth and cause anaemia. Mass use of albendazole 400mg/24h PO for 3d to school children or immigrants from endemic areas? Maybe. But don't think *"Drugs..."* 🙂think *"Education...hygiene".*[419]

*Necator americanus and Ankylostoma duodenale (hookworm)* occur in SE Asia, India, central/N Africa, and parts of Europe. Necator is also found in the Americas & sub-Saharan Africa. Many small worms attach to upper GI mucosa, causing chronic bleeding and iron-deficiency with devastating effects on children and mothers. Eggs are excreted in faeces and hatch in soil. Larvae penetrate feet, so starting new infections. Oral transmission of *Ankylostoma* occurs. *Δ:* Stool microscopy (fig 1). *R:* Mebendazole 100mg/12h for 3d.

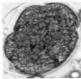
Fig 1. *Necator americanus* eggs (~70×38μm).

*Strongyloides stercoralis* is endemic in the sub-tropics. Transmitted via skin, it causes migrating urticaria on legs and trunk (*cutaneous larva migrans*) ± pneumonitis, enteritis/malabsorption (chronic diarrhoea/abdominal; pain). Worms may take bacteria into the blood, causing septicaemia ± meningitis. *Δ:* Stool microscopy, serology, or duodenal aspiration. *R:* Ivermectin 0.2mg/kg/24h PO for 48h. Hyperinfestation occurs in AIDS; consider albendazole 400mg/12h PO for 7-10d.

*Ascaris lumbricoides* looks like a garden worm (*Lumbricus*). It has 3 finely toothed lips. Transmission: faecal-oral. It migrates through liver & lungs, settling in small bowel. Often asymptomatic; GI obstruction/perforation is rare, as is migration to pancreatic ducts. If in bile ducts, cholangitis or pancreatitis can result. Worms may be >25cm long with a hooked end if ♂, fig 2. *Δ:* Stool microscopy (ova stain orange in bile); worms on barium x-rays; eosinophilia. *R:* Mebendazole (100mg/12h PO for 3d), albendazole (400mg PO once), ivermectin (150–200μg/kg PO once).

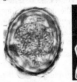
Fig 2. *Ascaris* eggs (45× 40μm) & ♂ worm (20cm).

*Enterobius vermicularis* Threadworms (fig 3; 9mm long) cause anal itch as they leave the gut to lay eggs on the perineum. Apply sticky tape there to identify eggs (~55×25μm) microscopically. *R:* Mebendazole 100mg PO stat. Repeat at 2wks if ≥2yrs, eg if re-infection. If aged <2yrs, try piperazine (see *BNF*). Treat the whole family. *Hygiene is more important than drugs* as adult worms die after 6wks. Continued symptoms means *reinfection*.

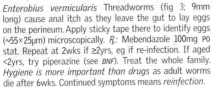
Fig 3. *Enterobius:* the folded worm is seen squirming in its egg. On the right is a ♀ worm.

*Trichuris trichiura* (whipworm) causes non-specific abdominal pain, dysentery, and sometimes rectal prolapse. *Δ:* Eggs in stool. *R:* Mebendazole 100mg/12h for 3d.

*Trichinella spiralis* (worldwide) Transmitted by under-cooked pork[etc] (bushpigs; warthogs), it migrates to muscle/CNS;[420] causing myalgia, fever, rash, fatigue, myocarditis, eyelid oedema ± T°↑. *Δ:* Eggs; MRI. *R:* Albendazole 400mg/24h PO for 3d.

*Toxocara canis* is the main cause of visceral[1] and ocular larval migrans (eye granulomas, retinal detachment, ophthalmitis, uveitis, squint, blindness)—also meningoencephalitis (rare). *Δ:* Fundoscopy, serology, histology. FBC: eosinophilia. *R:* Albendazole 400mg/12h PO for 5d. Severe lung, heart, or CNS disease may warrant steroids. In eye disease, visible larvae can be lasered. *Toxocara* is contracted by ingesting dirt, so de-worm pets often (exclude from play areas).

*Dracunculus medinensis* (Guinea worm) is the longest nematode (~70cm). Transmission: water containing tiny crustaceans (copepods).[421] *R:* Slow extraction of pre-emerging worms as they exit through the skin helped by metronidazole (±steroids). It is almost eradicated (except in Mali, south Sudan and Ethiopia).

1 Visceral larval migrans occurs when larvae migrate through a host's internal organs. We get it by ingesting parasite eggs, or by eating tissues from intermediate hosts containing larvae, eg *Ascaris* in raw beef. Signs vary with location, eg ↓appetite, T°↑, myalgia, big liver, asthma, cough, myeloradiculitis.[422]

## Filarial infection

This is common—prevalence of lymphatic filariasis: 120 million worldwide.

**1 Onchocerciasis** (caused by *Onchocerca volvulus*, transmitted by the black fly) is the world's second leading infectious cause of blindness.[423] It causes **river blindness** in 72% of some communities in Africa and S America (17 million worldwide). A nodule forms at the site of the bite, shedding microfilariae to distant skin sites which develop altered pigmentation, lichenification, loss of elasticity, and poor healing. Signs are mainly from localized host responses to moribund microfilariae. Eye signs: keratitis, uveitis, cataract, fixed pupil, fundal degeneration, or optic neuritis/atrophy. Lymphadenopathy & elephantiasis also occur.

*Diagnosis:* Visualization of microfilaria in eye or skin snips. Remove a fine shaving of clean, unanaesthetized skin with a scalpel. Put on slide with a drop of 0.9% saline and look for swimming larvae after 30min. ℞: *Ivermectin* 150μg/kg stat, repeat eg 6-monthly to suppress dermal and ocular microfilariae. If the eye is involved start *prednisolone* 1mg/kg/24h PO a few days before ivermectin (probably OK in pregnancy). Worm survival requires symbiosis with Wolbachia bacteria (susceptible to doxycycline 100mg/d PO for 6 weeks; give *before* ivermectin). Ivermectin resistance may be evolving.[424]

**2 Lymphatic filariasis** occurs in Asia, Africa, and S America and is transmitted by 5 genera of mosquito. Acute infection causes fever, lymphadenitis & chyluria.[1] *Wuchereria bancrofti* causes leg lymphoedema (elephantiasis) and hydroceles (may be huge). *Brugia malaya* causes elephantiasis below the elbow/knee. *Wuchereria* lifecycle: a mosquito bites an infected human→ingested microfilariae develop into larvae→larvae migrate to mosquito's mouth→biting of another human→access to bloodstream→adult filariae lodge in lymphatics.

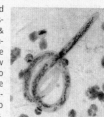

Fig 4. Blood smear of *W. bancrofti* (290×8.5μm).

Δ: Blood film (fig 4); or rapid immuno-chromatographic fingerprick field test. As lymphoedema may develop years after infection, tests may be -ve.

*Complications:* Immune hyperreactivity may cause tropical pulmonary eosinophilia (cough, wheeze, lung fibrosis, high eosinophil counts, IgE↑ and IgG↑). It is a major public health problem and is a WHO target for elimination by the year 2020 (starting with Nigeria, Samoa and Egypt). The current elimination strategy involves mass treatment with one yearly dose of 2 drugs for 5yrs: albendazole (400mg) + *either* ivermectin (200μg/kg) *or diethylcarbamazine* (see BNF).[425] Giving *diethylcarbamazine*-fortified salt to families for 1yr might help too.

*Prevention:* Avoiding mosquitoes + annual mass treatment of entire communities. Marvellous! Free drugs!! Elimination of a disease!!! Not quite...free drugs are often rejected for cultural reasons.[426] ✿Think again...ask a medical anthropologist.

**3 Loiasis (eye-worm)** Loa loa is a parasite that causes tropical eye worm—seen in tropical forests of Africa where it is transmitted by Tabanid flies of the genus *Chrysops*. It causes pruritus, urticaria, myalgia arthralgia, and mysterious wandering Calabar swellings.[2] The worm may migrate over the surface of the eye ("Something's wiggling in my eye, doctor"). This eerie trip causes intense conjunctivitis, which luckily heals OK if left alone (don't treat until the transmigration is over: on detecting your therapy the worm tends to panic).[427] Check for glomerulonephritis, eosinophilia, and encephalitis. Δ: Blood smears (often -ve, or show squirming microfilariae),[428] serology, or PCR. ℞: Diethylcarbamazine.

---

**1** Chyluria entails fistulae (eg pyelo-lymphatic) between lymphatic and urinary systems: hence milky lymph in urine (ΔΔ: filariasis, TB, trauma, neoplasia, congenital; it is also associated with nephrosis).[429]

**2** Calabar swellings occur anywhere (face, arms, legs, eg induced by local trauma). Oedema is preceded by local pain or itching lasting 1–2h. There then develops a 10–20cm non-erythematous, non-pitting swelling, resolving after 2 days to several weeks. Severe swellings can cause paraesthesiae or entrapment neuropathy. Recurrences are common at the same site (or elsewhere). Cause: unknown (?allergic responses to antigens released in the tracks of adult migrating parasites).[430]

Figs 1–4 ©Prof S Upton, Kansas Univ. Fig 3's eggs: ©JML.

***Taenia solium*** (pork tapeworm; fig 1) infection occurs by eating uncooked pork, or from drinking contaminated water.[1] *T. saginata* is from uncooked beef. Both cause vague abdominal symptoms and malabsorption. Contaminated food and water contain cysticerci which adhere to the gut and develop into adult worms. On swallowing the eggs of *T. solium* they may enter the circulation and disseminate widely, becoming cysticerci within the human host (cysticercosis; 50,000 deaths/yr worldwide and the cause of much chronic disability).[431] This tapeworm encysts in muscle, skin, heart, eye, and CNS, causing focal signs. *Subcutaneous cysticercosis* causes subcutaneous nodules (arms, legs, chest). *Ocular cysticercosis* causes conjunctivitis; uveitis; retinitis; choroidal atrophy; blindness.

*Neurocysticercosis* is the main cause of seizures in some places, eg Mexico, and is getting more prevalent, eg in the southern USA. Other signs: focal CNS signs, eg hemiplegia, foot drop, odd behaviour, mood or personality change, dementia (reversible if you are quick)[432]—or no symptoms. Cysticerci may cluster like bunches of grapes ('racemose' form) in the ventricles (causing hydrocephalus) and basal cisterns (causing

Fig 1. *Taenia solium* (note the two rows of hooks).

basal meningitis, cranial nerve lesions and ↑ICP). Spinal cysticerci may cause radicular or compressive symptoms (p470). Δ: •Stool microscopy of perianal swabs. •Serology: indirect haemagglutination test. •CSF: eosinophils in neurocysticercosis, and a CSF antigen test is available. •MRI locates cysts (CT may be normal). •SXR and x-ray of soft tissue: calcified cysts. •Detecting *T. solium* DNA in brain biopsy tissue.[433] R: Get help (*tel: 0151 705 3100*[UK]). Neurocysticercosis: **albendazole**, eg 7.5mg/kg/12h (max 400mg/12h) PO for 8–30d, or **praziquantel**. **Dexamethasone** ↓allergic responses to dying larvae (0.1mg/kg/d for 29d), but using steroids routinely is controversial. NB: if CSF ventricles are involved, you may need to shunt before starting drugs. Drugs may worsen the acute phase of cysticercotic encephalitis.[434]

*Hymenolepis nana; H. diminuta* (dwarf tapeworm; rarely symptomatic). R: Praziquantel 25mg/kg PO (1 dose; adults & children) or niclosamide 500mg/d for 3d.

*Diphyllobothrium latum* (fig 2) is a fish tapeworm (via uncooked fish, eg salmon, trout) causing similar symptoms to *T. solium* + tapeworm segments passed PR. It is a cause of vitamin B$_{12}$↓. R: Praziquantel 10mg/kg stat PO.

Fig 2. *D. latum.*

**Hydatid** Cystic hydatid disease is a zoonosis caused by eating eggs of the dog parasite, eg *Echinococcus granulosus* (fig 3), eg in rural sheep-farming regions. Hydatid is a worldwide public health problem (not confined to traditional rural areas in China, Russia, Japan, Alaska, Wales, Italy, India, Pakistan). In one Tunisian study, prevalence of cysts was: 16% in sheep, 9% in cattle, 6% in dromedaries (1-humped camels) and 3% in goats.[435]

Fig 3. Hydatid.

In humans, cysts may inhabit: *liver* (hepatomegaly, obstructive jaundice, cholangitis, PUO); *lung* (dyspnoea, chest pain, haemoptysis, anaphylaxis—alveolar hydatid is caused by *E. multilocularis*); *CNS* (space-occupying signs); *bone* (an interesting osteolytic cause of knee pain, cord compression, etc) or often silently in breast, kidney, adrenals, bladder, heart, psoas.

Δ: Plain x-ray, ultrasound, CT/MRI—cysts may look like tumours.[436] A good serological test has replaced the variably sensitive Casoni intradermal test.

R: Get help (including surgical). 1$^{st}$-choice: **albendazole** pre & post drainage (if >60kg, 400mg/12h; if <60kg, 7.5mg/kg/12h with food). Excise/drain symptomatic cysts (some favour hepatic resection).[437] Beware spilling cyst contents (causes anaphylaxis; give **praziquantel** here). PAIR approach: puncture→aspirate cyst→inject hypertonic saline → re-aspirate after 25min; continue albendazole for 30d to prevent recurrence.[438]

**1** While eating undercooked pork is the only way to acquire intestinal *T. solium*, any food contaminated by faeces from hosts infected with cysticerci can carry the eggs that may lead to development of cysticercosis. Even vegetarians are at risk. The lack of public awareness of this poses big problems.[439]

Figs 1-3 ©Prof S Upton, Kansas Univ.

**Schistosomiasis** (bilharzia) is caused by blood-dwelling schistosoma worms: *S. mansoni* (Africa and Americas), *S. japonicum* (S and East Asia→GI and hepatosplenic schistosomiasis), *S. haematobium* (~230 million people in Africa—bladder and vulva involved. Lesser species: *S. mekongi* (Mekong River; similar to *S. japonica*); *S. intercalatum*. Snails release cercariae that penetrate skin, eg during paddling, causing itchy papular rashes ('swimmer's itch'). Cercariae shed their tails to become schistosomules, migrating via lungs to liver where they grow. ~2wks later, there may be fever, urticaria, diarrhoea, cough, wheeze, and hepatosplenomegaly (Katayama fever). In 8wks flukes mature (14♂-20♀mm long), mate (fig 1), and migrate to resting habitats, eg bladder or mesenteric veins, releasing eggs, causing local granulomas and scars (important sites of

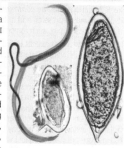

Fig 1. *S. mansoni* ♂/♀ mating; right: egg with sublateral spine (arrow).
Fig 2. *S. haematobium*; terminal spine.
Figs 1-3 ©S Upton, Kansas Univ.

HIV entry). Signs reflect our immune response to eggs (type IV hypersensitivity, eg for *S. mansoni*).

*Signs: S. mansoni:* abdominal pain; D&V; later, hepatic fibrosis, granulomatous inflammation, anaemia, and portal hypertension (variceal bleeding is common, but transformation into true cirrhosis has not been well documented). *S. japonicum*, often the most serious, occurs in SE Asia, tends to affect the bowel and liver, and may migrate to lung and CNS ('traveller's myelitis'). Urinary schistosomiasis (*S. haematobium*) occurs in Africa, the Middle East, and the Indian Ocean. Signs: frequency, dysuria, haematuria (± haematospermia), incontinence. Complications: hydronephrosis; renal failure; squamous cell cancer of the bladder. *Δ:* Eggs in urine (*S. haematobium*; fig 2, with 3 RBCs for scale) or faeces (*S. mansoni* and *japonicum*) or rectal biopsy (all types). AXR may show bladder calcification in chronic *S. haematobium* infection. Ultrasound (renal obstruction, hydronephrosis ± thick bladder wall). Ab to *S. mansoni*, *S. haematobium*, and *S. japonicum* adult worm microsomal Ag are specific for all 3 species (ELISA and immunoblot assays).[440] *R:* Praziquantel: 40mg/kg PO with food divided into 2 doses separated by 4-6h for *S. mansoni* and *S. haematobium*, or 20mg/kg/8h for 1d in *S. japonicum*. Sudden transitory abdominal pain ± bloody diarrhoea may occur shortly after. Oxamniquine is an alternative for *S. mansoni*.

*Fasciola hepatica* (liver fluke) is spread by sheep, water, and snails. It causes T°↑, abdominal pain, diarrhoea, weight↓, jaundice, hepatomegaly, liver fibrosis and eosinophilia. *Tests:* Stool microscopy, serology. *R:* Get help. Triclabendazole 10mg/kg PO, 1 dose, or bithionol 30mg/kg alternate days for 10-15 doses, max 2g/day IM.

*Opisthorchis* & *Clonorchis* (fig 3) are liver flukes common in SE Asia, where they cause cholangitis, cholecystitis & cholangiocarcinoma. *Risk factor:* Raw fish. *Tests:*[441] Stool microscopy; PCR. *R:* Praziquantel 25mg/kg/8h PO for 2d.

*Fasciolopsis buski* is a GI fluke 7cm long, causing ulcers/abscesses at sites of attachment. *R:* Praziquantel 25mg/kg/8h PO for 1d.

*Paragonimus westermani* (lung fluke) is got by eating raw freshwater crabs & crayfish. Flukes migrate through gut and diaphragm to invade lungs (hence cough, dyspnoea, haemoptysis, ± lung abscess/bronchiectasis). It occurs in the Far East, S America, and Congo; often mistaken for TB (similar signs and CXR). *Tests:* Ova in sputum. MRI/CT for lung/CNS lesions. *R:* Praziquantel 25mg/kg/8h for 2d.

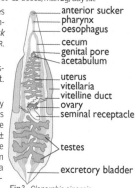

anterior sucker
pharynx
oesophagus
cecum
genital pore
acetabulum
uterus
vitellaria
vitelline duct
ovary
seminal receptacle
testes
excretory bladder

Fig 3. *Clonorchis sinensis*.

Infectious diseases

Exotic infections may be *community-acquired* or *nosocomial*, ie acquired in hospital. Immunosuppression and antibiotic overuse have caused an increase in exotic infections. Techniques such as PCR have identified more putative infective agents.

*A good gossip:* Don't expect to find the pertinent question in any textbook—eg:

1 "Have you delivered any infected babies in the last year?" You can impress/cure your obstetrician friends who don't know about baby-to-obstetrician brucellosis who tell you that "I'm so depressed about not being able to shake off this flu"[442]

2 "Are your carp well at present?" (*Mycobacterium marinum* skin infection).[443]

3 "Could that be a Hyalomma tick bite from when you rode your ostrich in last week's race?" (Crimean-Congo haemorrhagic fever, CCHF, p388; a bunyavirus→DIC/ARDS).

4 "Who has been licking your face recently?" (*Pasteurella multocida*).[444]

5 "Has your dog been on holiday this year?" (monkeypox from prairie dogs).

6 "Has your pet hedgehog lost weight?" (salmonella).[445]

7 "I expect you have a pet magpie causing your headache" (zoonotic transmission of *Cryptococcus neoformans* causing meningitis in an immunocompetent adult)[446]

8 "Did you have a stray pig living under your house when the monsoon started?" (pigs + standing water + mosquitoes ≈ Japanese encephalitis).

9 "Any contact with invasive snails?" Angiostrongyliasis→eosinophilic meningitis.[447]

10 "Do you sometimes wonder if your goat miscarried last year?" (brucellosis).[448]

11 "Were you over-enthusiastic at last month's Festival of Sacrifice?" (Turkish Kurban Bayrami) (*Erysipelothrix rhusiopathiae* endocarditis via swine erysipelas).

12 "Show me your pet lobster: he may be the cause of your bad hand", ask about: an erysipeloid infection from *Erysipelothrix*.[449] Pet lobsters have a grand pedigree: Gérard de Nerval (OHCS p397) used to take his pet lobster for walks, on a blue silk lead, beside the Seine (fig 1). A lobster, he said, is "serious-minded and quiet, doesn't scratch or bark like a dog, and knows all of the secrets of the deep." His lobster's mission was to combat the Philistinism chaining us all to mediocrity.[450]

Fig 1. "Is your pet lobster well?" (Gérard de Nerval).

When you suspect infection (T°↑, sweats, inflammation, D&V, WCC↑, or *any* unexplained symptom), ask about: •Foreign travel (recent and past) •Foreign bodies (hip prosthesis, heart valve) •Work or hobby or family exposure to infectious agents •Any bites/stings •Sexual exploits •Any necrotic tissue? •HIV risk or reason for immunosuppression (eg pregnancy; steroids) •Any pets, exotic or otherwise?

**Diagnosis** ♥*Listen to your patient.* Don't just think pathogens! You have two cultures to master: the host's and the pathogen's (culture blood, urine, stool, CSF; take swabs). *Prolonged immersion in both cultures may be needed.* Liaise early with infectious disease doctors & microbiologists. Imaging: CXR, ultrasound, CT/MRI. If the infection seems localized, consider surgical debridement ± drainage. Don't give up if culture is negative; tests may need repeating. Perhaps the organism is 'fastidious' in its nutritional requirement or requires longer incubation? Even if culture *is* achieved, it may be that the organism is non-pathogenic/commensal (ie part of the normal flora for that patient). If culture fails, look for antibodies or antigen in the serum or body fluids. It is generally agreed that a 4-fold rise in antibody titres in convalescence (compared with the acute sera 2-3wks before) *may* indicate recent infection. PCR is increasingly used for identification, but it is far from infallible, and contamination with DNA from the lab or elsewhere is a big problem.

℞ "What worked for you last time this happened?" Empirical therapy (p382) may be needed if the patient is ill—see opposite. Draining pus is as important as antibiotics. Ask about local diseases, antibiotic resistance and the need for isolation/contact tracing. *Doses:* Penicillins (p378); cephalosporins (p379); gentamicin[1 *et al*] (p380).

---

1 Prescribing by **surface area**, or **lean** body weight (LBW), eg for gentamicin, or **ideal** body weight (IBW):
body surface area = 0.20247 × Height (metres)$^{0.725}$ × weight (kg)$^{0.425}$      halls.md/ideal-weight/devine.htm
lean body weight   ♂ = (1.10 × weight in kg) − 128 (weight$^2$/(100 × height in metres)$^2$)
lean body weight   ♀ = (1.07 × weight in kg) − 148 (weight$^2$/(100 × height in metres)$^2$)
ideal body weight  ♂ = 50 + 2.3 for every inch over 5ft tall (♀ = 49 + 1.7 for each inch over 5ft)

Infectious diseases

| Exotic/unusual organism | Site or type of infection | Treatment example |
|---|---|---|
| | *IE=infective endocarditis*[1] | |
| *Acanthamoeba* | Corneal ulcers | Propamidine + neomycin |
| *Acinetobacter calcoaceticus* | UTI; CSF; lung; bone; conjunctiva | Meropenem or amikacin[461] |
| *Actinobacillus lignieresii* | CSF; IE; wounds; bone; lymph nodes | Ampicillin ± gentamicin |
| *Actinobacillus ureae* | Bronchus; CSF post-trauma; hepatitis | Ampicillin ± gentamicin |
| *Aerococcus viridans* | Empyema; UTI; CSF; bone; IE | Penicillin ± gentamicin |
| *Aeromonas hydrophila* | IE; CSF; cornea; bone; D&V; liver abscess | Ciprofloxacin |
| *Afipia broomeae* | Marrow; synovium | Imipenem or ceftriaxone |
| *Aggregatibacter actinomycetemcomitans* | IE; CNS; UTI; bone; thyroid; lung; peri-odontitis; abscesses | Penicillin ± gentamicin |
| *Alcaligenes* species | Dialysis peritonitis; ear; lung | Co-amoxiclav or ceftazidime |
| *Arachnia propionica* | Actinomycosis; tear ducts; CNS | Penicillin |
| *Arcanobacterium* | Throat; cellulitis; leg ulcer | Penicillin |
| *Babesia microti* (protozoa) | PUO ± haemolysis if old/splenectomy | Atovaquone + azithromycin |
| *Bacillus cereus* | Wounds; eye; ear; lung; UTI; IE | Vancomycin |
| *Bifidobacterium* | Vagina; UTI; IE; peritonitis; lung | Penicillin |
| *Bordetella bronchiseptica* | URTI; CSF (after animal contact) | Co-amoxiclav |
| *Burkholderia cepacia*, etc (formerly *pseudomonas*) | Wounds; feet; lungs; IE; CAPD; UTI ecthyma gangrenosa; peritonitis | Ciprofloxacin or meropenem |
| *Burkholderia pickettii* (formerly a pseudomonas) | CSF | Cefalosporin |
| *Burkholderia pseudomallei* (formerly *Pseudomonas pseudomallei*) | Melioidosis: self-reactivating septic-aemia + multi-organ, protean signs, eg in rice farmers, via water/soil in Papua, Thailand, Vietnam, Torres Straits | Ceftazidime (14d) + co-trimoxazole for 3 months |
| *Capnocytophaga* | Oral ulcer; stomatitis; arthritis | Ertapenem |
| *Cardiobacterium hominis* | IE (=infective endocarditis) | Ceftrixone for 4wks |
| *Chromobacterium violaceum* | Nodes; eye; bone; liver; pustules | Gentamicin, chloramphenicol |
| *Citrobacter koseri/diversus* | CSF; UTI; blood; cholecystitis | Imipenem |
| *Corynebacterium jeikeium* | IE; CSF; otitis; leg ulcer; lung | Vancomycin |
| *Corynebacterium pseudoTB* | Lymphadenitis | Ciprofloxacin |
| *Corynebacterium ulcerans* | Diphtheria-like ± CNS signs | Rifampicin + diphtheria antitoxin |
| *Cyclospora cayetanensis* | Diarrhoea (via raspberries) | Co-trimoxazole |
| *Edwardsiella tarda* | Cellulitis; abscesses; BP↓; dysentery via penetrating fish injuries | Cefuroxime + gentamicin |
| *Eikenella corrodens* | Sinus; ears; PE post-jugular vein phle-bitis (post-anginal sepsis) via bites | Penicillin ± gentamicin |
| *Erysipelothrix rhusiopathiae* | Erysipelas-like (*OHCS* p598); IE | Penicillin |
| *Eubacterium* | Wounds; gynaecologic sepsis; IE | Penicillin + cefoxitin |
| *Flavobacterium meningo-septicum* | Lungs; epidemic neonatal meningitis; post-op sepsis; contact lens keratitis | Piperacillin |
| *Flavobacterium multivorum* | Peritonitis (spontaneous); pneumonia in HIV | Ciprofloxacin |
| *Gemella haemolysans* | IE; meningitis after neurosurgery | Linezolid + chloramphenicol |
| *Helicobacter cinaedi* | Proctitis in homosexual men | Ciprofloxacin + rifampicin |
| *Kingella kingae* | Throat; larynx; eyelid; joint; skin | Penicillin ± cephalosporin |
| *Lactobacillus* | Teeth; chorioamnionitis; pyelitis | Penicillin or ampicillin |
| *Mobiluncus curtisii/mulieris* | Vagina | Clindamycin (topical) |
| *Moraxella osloensis* and *M. nonliquefaciens* | Conjunctiva; wound; vagina; UTI; CSF CNS; bone; haemorrhagic stomatitis | Co-amoxiclav |
| *Pasteurella multocida*[452, 453] (Gram-red) | Skin; bone; lung; CSF; UTI; pericarditis; epiglottitis. From cat or dog bites | β-lactam antibiotics |
| *P. pneumotrophica* | Wounds; joints; bone; CSF | Penicillin; cipro-/moxifloxacin |
| *Peptostreptococcus* | Bone/joint/discitis; wound; teeth; face | Clindamycin or metronidazole |
| *Plesiomonas shigelloides* | D&V; eye; sepsis—post fishbone injury | Ciprofloxacin |
| *Propionibacterium acnes* (see *OHCS* p600) | Face; wounds; CSF shunts; bone; IE; liver granuloma (botyromycosis) | Tetracycline or ceftriaxone |
| *Prototheca wickerhamii* & *zopfii=achlorophyllous algae* | Subcutaneous granuloma; plaques; bursitis; adenitis; nodules[454] | Amphotericin or ketoconazole |
| *Providencia stuartii* | UTI; purple urine bag syndrome | Ceftriaxone |
| *Pseudomonas maltophilia* | stenotrophomonas wounds; ear; eye; lung; UTI; IE | Co-trimoxazole or cefepime |
| *Pseudomonas putrefaciens* | CSF post CNS surgery/head trauma | Cefotaxime |
| *Rothia dentocariosa*[455] | Appendix abscess; infective emboli | Penicillin + gentamicin |
| *Serratia marcescens* (may be non-pathogenic)[456] | Wounds; burns; lung; UTI; liver; CSF; bone; IE; red diaper/nappy syndrome | Imipenem, ceftazidime, ciprofloxacin |
| *Sphingomonas paucimobilis* | Superficial leg ulcer; CSF; UTI | Ceftazidime |
| *Streptococcus bovis* | IE if colon cancer; do colonoscopy | Penicillin + gentamicin |
| *Vibrio vulnificus* | Wounds; muscle; uterus; fasciitis | Tetracycline + cephalosporin |

**1 Rare causes of endocarditis** often involve the *HACEK* organisms: *Haemophilus aphrophilus, Act-inobacillus, Cardiobacter, Eikenella,* and *Kingella.*

Source: *GAT Sandford.*

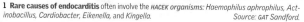

**Contents**

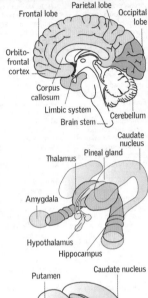

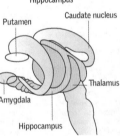

Fig 1. *Conflicting systems:* cerebral hemispheres and limbic system (last 2 images). 'We know...about how there isn't a unitary ego—how we're made up of conflicting, interacting systems.' A.S. Byatt *Possession*

Our bodies are not a bicycle with a single rider—more like a tandem with various processes in various saddles. The front(al) drivers may decide to bear right, but if the rear drivers now lean left we go awry, and our will seems mysteriously subverted. Those few doctors whose processes are in perpetual harmony are at a disadvantage here as they never understand what makes their patients good and bad.

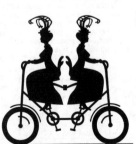

Fig 2. A body has more than one rider.

W e dedicate this page to those carers who find themselves responsible for a friend or relative who has a chronic neurological illness, such as stroke, Parkinson's disease, Alzheimer's disease, or motor neuron disease. As a thought experiment, try spending a morning imagining that you are such a carer, trying to expunge the smell of soiled sheets from your clothes, while awaiting a visit from a neighbour, who said he would 'sit with him' so you can catch the bus into town, and, like a guilty hedonist, play truant from your role as nurse for a few sanity-giving hours of normal life. You wait. No one comes. You stop bothering about the smell on your clothes, and turn towards your husband, about to say something, but when your eyes meet his, you realize he does not recognize you—and you keep your thoughts to yourself. Knuckles whiten as you grasp his collar to lift him forward on the commode, and you seem to hear a mocking voice over your shoulder saying: "... so I see we're getting angry with him today, are we?" The ceaseless round from mouth to anus, from bed to chair, from twilight to twilight, continues, *ad infinitum*.

It is all we can do to spend *2 minutes* on this thought experiment, let alone a morning—or the rest of our lives. We need to be aware of the strategies we adopt to avoid involvement with the naked truth of the shattered lives, which, like a tragic subplot, stand behind the farce of morning surgery or outpatients in which we hear ourselves forever saying in tones of plummy complacency: "And how are *you* today Mrs Salt—your husband, I know... marvellous how you manage. You are a real support to each other. Let me know if I can do anything." We pretend to be busy, we ensure that we *are* busy, we surround ourselves with students, uniforms, and a miasma of technical expertise—we surround ourselves with *anything* to ensure that there is no chink through which Mrs Salt can shine her rays of darkness. Poor Mrs Salt. Poor us—to be frightened of the dark, panicking at the thought that we might not have anything to offer, or that we might be called to offer up our equanimity as a sacrifice to Mrs Salt. How dare one little grain upset our carefully contrived universe?

Respite care, medical charities, meals on wheels, laundry services, physiotherapy, occupational therapy (OT), transport, day care centres, clubs for carers, visits from the doctor (which may cure the plummy complacency), district nurses or from a nurse-matron specializing in chronic diseases will go some way to mitigate Mrs Salt's problems. As ever, the way forward is by taking time to listen. Congratulate the carer, and acknowledge that they may be accomplishing more than what *3* full-time nurses working round the clock could achieve.

Carers' needs evolve. First there is uncertainty, and the need for help in handling this. Next comes the moment of diagnosis, with the numbness, denial, and anger that may follow. Then there may be an adjustment to reality, with frenzied searching for information and advice, or a careful titration by the carer of how much information he or she can handle.

Issues of driving, mobility, finance, sex, and employment are likely to occur throughout the illness, and advice will need to be constantly tailored to suit individual circumstances. But the best thing you can ever offer is the unwritten contract that, come what may, you will be there, available, often ineffectual, but incapable of being alienated by whatever the carer may disclose to you.

*Pages elsewhere with a neurological flavour:* CNS exam (p72–80); mental state (p82); tremor (p71); facial pain (p71); how to do an LP (p782).
Emergencies: headache (p794); coma (p800); GCS (p802); meningitis (p832); encephalitis (p834); cerebral abscess (p835); status epilepticus (p836); head injury/↑ICP (p838–840).

We thank Dr Thomas Hughes, our Specialist Reader, and Zuzana Sipkova, our Junior Reader, for their contribution to this chapter.

**Where is the lesion?** A helpful feature in determining if a focal lesion is present is lack of symmetry—eg one pupil dilated, or one upgoing plantar response. Also a spinal level (below) is a localizing sign (effects may be symmetrical below the lesion).

Localizing the lesion depends on recognizing characteristic patterns of cognitive, cranial nerve, motor, and sensory deficits that occur with lesions at different sites. *Where?* is a great question, but note that sometimes there is no single lesion, rather, a *general insult*, eg trauma, encephalitis, anoxia, poisoning, or post-ictal states—or *diffuse neurodegeneration* (may have specific local effects, eg amnesia).

*Patterns of motor loss:* Weakness can arise from lesions of the cortex, corona radiata, internal capsule, brainstem, cord, roots, plexi, peripheral nerves, neuromuscular junction, or muscle. Is the pattern upper or lower motor neuron (UMN or LMN; see BOXES)? *Cortical lesions* may cause an unexpected pattern of weakness of all movements of a hand or foot, with normal or even ↑tone—but ↑reflexes more proximally in the arm or leg will suggest a UMN rather than LMN lesion. *Internal capsule* (p474) and *corticospinal tract* lesions cause contralateral hemiparesis. If this occurs with epilepsy, ↓cognition, or homonymous hemianopia (p453), the lesion is in a cerebral hemisphere. A cranial nerve palsy (III–XII) contralateral to a hemiplegia implicates the brainstem on the side of the cranial nerve palsy. *Cord lesions* causing paraparesis (both legs) or quadriparesis/tetraplegia (all limbs) are suggested by finding a motor and reflex level (power is unaffected above the lesion, with LMN signs at the level of the lesion, and UMN signs *below* the lesion). *Peripheral neuropathies:* (p506) Most cause distal weakness, eg foot-drop; weak hand (in Guillain-Barré syndrome weakness is often *proximal* due to root involvement). Involvement of a single nerve (mononeuropathy) occurs with trauma or entrapment (carpal tunnel, p507); involvement of several nerves (mononeuritis multiplex) is seen, eg in DM or vasculitis.

*Sensory deficits: Distribution* of sensory loss and modality involved (pain, temperature, touch, vibration, joint-position sense) helps localize the lesion. Pain and T° sensations travel along small fibres in peripheral nerves and the *anterolateral (spinothalamic) tracts* in the cord and brainstem (p520), whereas joint-position and vibration sense travel in large fibres in peripheral nerves and the large *dorsal columns* of the cord. *Distal sensory loss* suggests a neuropathy and may involve all sensory modalities or be selective, depending on nerve fibre size involved. Individual nerve lesions are identified by their anatomical territories, which are usually more sharply defined than those of root lesions (dermatomes, p458), which often show considerable overlap. A *sensory level* is the hallmark (albeit a rather unreliable one) of a cord lesion—ie decreased sensation below the lesion (eg the legs) with normal sensation above this level (eg in abdomen, trunk, and arms). Hemi-cord lesions cause a Brown-Séquard picture (p710) with dorsal column loss on the side of the lesion and contralateral spinothalamic loss. *Dissociated sensory loss* may occur, eg in *cervical cord lesions*—loss of fine touch and proprioception without loss of pain and temperature (or vice-versa, eg syringomyelia, p520; or cord tumours). Lateral brainstem lesions show both dissociated and crossed sensory loss with pain and T° loss on the side of the face ipsilateral to the lesion, and contralateral arm and leg sensory loss. Lesions above the brainstem give a contralateral pattern of generalized sensory loss. In *cortical lesions*, sensory loss is confined to more subtle and discriminative sensory functions (2-point discrimination and stereognosis; p503).

**What is the lesion?** Are the cells diseased, dysfunctional, disconnected (anatomically, eg after a stroke, or functionally, as in autism[1])● or under- or over-excited (migraine; epilepsy)? Is there loss of a specific type of nerve cell, as in motor neuron disease or subacute combined degeneration of the cord (B₁₂↓, p328, fig 1 p471). Arteriopaths get strokes, tropical travellers get wormy lesions[etc etc].

**Why?** Do a general examination. Example: a man comes in with dysphasia: where?=dominant hemisphere; what?=infarct; why?=embolus from atrial fibrillation. After a few years of bedside neurology you will find your finger automatically fumbling under the bedclothes to reveal an irregularly irregular pulse long before the stuttering history is half complete. But beware putting 2 and 2 together *too* soon.

## UMN (upper motor neuron) lesions

These are caused by damage to motor pathways (corticospinal tracts) anywhere from motor nerve cells in the precentral gyrus of the frontal cortex, through the internal capsule, brainstem, and cord, to the synapse with the anterior horn cells in the cord. UMN weakness affects *muscle groups*, not individual muscles. *Weakness* is typically 'pyramidal'[1,2] in distribution, ie weakness involving arm extensors (shoulder abduction; elbow, wrist, and finger extension), the small muscles of the hand, and lower limb flexors (at hip and knee, and ankle dorsiflexors and everters). There is no muscle wasting; *loss of skilled fine finger movements* may be greater than expected from the overall grade of weakness (BOX). *Spasticity* develops in stronger muscles (arm flexors and leg extensors). It manifests as ↑tone that is *velocity-dependent* and *non-uniform*,[3] ie the faster you move the patient's muscle the greater the resistance, until it finally gives way in a clasp-knife manner. There is *hyperreflexia*: reflexes are brisk; *plantars are upgoing* (+ve Babinski sign) ± *clonus* (elicited by rapidly dorsiflexing the foot; ≤3 rhythmic, downward beats of the foot are normal; more suggest an UMN lesion) ± a positive *Hoffman's reflex:* brief flexion of thumb and index finger in a pincer movement following a flick to the pulp of the middle finger (it is a stretch reflex so the often-used way of flicking the finger towards the palm isn't ideal). Neck extension is said to increase sensitivity of this test. NB: UMN lesions can mimic LMN lesions in the first few hours before the spasticity and hyperreflexia develop.

## LMN (lower motor neuron) lesions

These are caused by damage anywhere from anterior horn cells in the cord, nerve roots, plexi, or peripheral nerves. The distribution of weakness corresponds to those muscles supplied by the involved cord segment, nerve root, part of plexus, or peripheral nerve. See p456. A combination of anatomical knowledge, good muscle testing technique, and experience is needed to distinguish, eg a radial nerve palsy from a C7 root lesion, or a common peroneal nerve palsy from an L5 root lesion (p456).[4] Affected muscles show *wasting ± fasciculation* (spontaneous involuntary twitching), and the limb feels soft and floppy, providing little resistance to passive stretch (*hypotonia/flaccidity*). *Reflexes are reduced* or absent, the *plantars remain flexor*. The chief differential is weakness from primary muscle disease—here there is symmetrical loss, reflexes are lost later than in neuropathies, and there is no sensory loss. Myasthenia gravis (p516) causes weakness worsening with use (fatiguability); there is little wasting, normal reflexes, and no sensory loss.
*Reflexes and spinal cord level:* p73. *Spinal roots for each muscle:* p456.
For *mixed LMN and UMN signs*, see p471 (MND, ↓B₁₂, taboparesis, etc).

## Muscle weakness grading (MRC classification)[4]

| | | | |
|---|---|---|---|
| **Grade 0** | No muscle contraction | **Grade 3** | Active movement against gravity |
| **Grade 1** | Flicker of contraction | **Grade 4** | Active movement against resistance |
| **Grade 2** | Some active movement | **Grade 5** | Normal power (allowing for age) |

Grade 4 covers a big range: 4−, 4, and 4+ denote movement against slight, moderate, and stronger resistance; avoid fudging descriptions—'strength 4/5 throughout' suggests a mild quadriparesis or myopathy. It is better to document 'poor effort' and the maximum grade for each muscle tested. ▶Distribution of weakness tells us more than grade of weakness (grade does help document improvement).

---

**1** The pyramidal (=corticospinal) tract starts at the pyramidal cells of Betz in area 4 and 6 of the motor cortex. It descends in the internal capsule to the medulla oblongata where fibres pass through the medullar pyramids (hence the name); here most decussate (uncrossed corticospinal fibres descend in the anterior funiculus as the anterior corticospinal tract). Lesions cause paresis and spasticity.¹

**2** 'Extrapyramidal' denotes CNS motor phenomena relating to the basal ganglia. Extrapyramidal lesions cause motor initiation and maintenance of movement—**negative symptoms** include bradykinesia/akinesia (slow/absent movement) and loss of postural reflexes. **Positive symptoms** include tremor, rigidity, involuntary movements (p472, eg chorea, athetosis, ballismus, and dystonia).

**3** Whereas with *rigidity*, ↑ tone is not velocity-dependent but constant throughout passive movement.

**4** The booklet *Aids to the Examination of the Peripheral Nervous System* is invaluable here. ISBN 0-7020-2512-7

Knowledge of the anatomy of the blood supply of the brain helps in diagnosing and managing cerebrovascular disease (p474–p482). Always try to identify the area of brain that correlates with a patient's symptoms and identify the affected artery.

**Blood supply** The brain is supplied by the internal carotid arteries (anteriorly) and the basilar artery (posteriorly, formed by the joining of the vertebral arteries, which supply the brainstem). These 3 vessels feed the anastomotic ring (circle of Willis) at the base of the brain. This arrangement may lessen the effects of occlusion of a feeder vessel proximal to the anastomosis by allowing supply from unaffected vessels. But the anatomy of the circle of Willis is variable and in many people it does not provide much protection from ischaemia due to carotid, vertebral, or basilar artery occlusion. Anastomotic supply from other vessels in the neck may mitigate occlusions of feeder vessels—occlusion of the internal carotid in the neck, for example, may not cause infarction if flow from the external carotid artery enters the circle of Willis via its anastomosis with the ophthalmic artery.

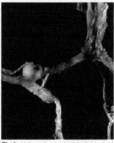

**Fig 1.** Where (and what) is the lesion? Answer: p482.  ©Dr D Hamoundi.

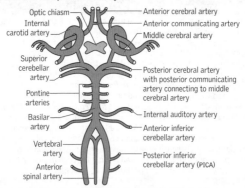

**Fig 2.** The circle of Willis at the base of the brain. See also fig 1 and fig 2, p483.

Labels (clockwise):
- Optic chiasm
- Internal carotid artery
- Superior cerebellar artery
- Pontine arteries
- Basilar artery
- Vertebral artery
- Anterior spinal artery
- Anterior cerebral artery
- Anterior communicating artery
- Middle cerebral artery
- Posterior cerebral artery with posterior communicating artery connecting to middle cerebral artery
- Internal auditory artery
- Anterior inferior cerebellar artery
- Posterior inferior cerebellar artery (PICA)

### ☙ Thomas Willis

Thomas Willis (1621–75) is one of those happy Oxford heroes who hold a bogus DM degree, awarded in 1646 for his Royalist sympathies while at Christ Church, the most loyally royal college in the University. He had a busy life inventing terms such as 'neurology' and 'reflex'. Not only has his name been given to his famous circle, but he was the first to describe myasthenia gravis, whooping cough, and the sweet taste of diabetic urine. He was the first person (few have followed him[3]) to know the course of the spinal accessory nerve. He is unusual among Oxford neurologists in that he developed the practice of giving his lunch away to the poor. He also espoused iatrochemistry: a theory of medicine according to which all morbid conditions of the body can be explained by disturbances in the fermentations and effervescences of its humours.

Dizzy-plus syndromes and arterial events: SCA →dizzy
AICA →dizzy and deaf
PICA →dizzy and dysphagic and dysphonic

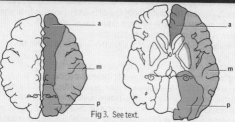

Fig 3. See text.

**Carotid artery** At worst, internal carotid artery occlusion causes total fatal infarction of the anterior two-thirds of its hemisphere and basal ganglia (lenticulostriate arteries). More often, the picture is like middle cerebral artery occlusion.

**Cerebral arteries** 3 pairs of arteries leave the circle of Willis to supply the cerebral hemispheres: the anterior, middle and posterior cerebral arteries. The anterior and middle cerebrals are branches of the internal carotid arteries; in 80%, the basilar artery divides into the 2 posterior cerebral arteries. Ischaemia from occlusion of any one of them may be lessened by retrograde supply from leptomeningeal vessels.

*Anterior cerebral artery:* (a in fig 3) Supplies the frontal and medial part of the cerebrum. Occlusion may cause a weak, numb contralateral leg ± similar, if milder, arm symptoms. The face is spared. Bilateral infarction can cause akinetic mutism from damage to the cingulate gyri (also a rare cause of paraplegia).

*Middle cerebral artery:* (m in fig 3) Supplies the lateral part of each hemisphere. Occlusion may cause contralateral hemiparesis, hemisensory loss (esp. face & arm), contralateral homonymous hemianopia due to involvement of the optic radiation, cognitive change including dysphasia with dominant hemisphere lesions, and visuo-spatial disturbance (eg cannot dress; gets lost) with non-dominant lesions.

*Posterior cerebral artery:* (p in fig 3; fig 4) Supplies the occipital lobe. Occlusion gives contralateral homonymous hemianopia (often with macula sparing).

**Vertebrobasilar circulation** Supplies the cerebellum, brainstem, occipital lobes; occlusion causes signs relating to any or all 3: hemianopia; cortical blindness; diplopia; vertigo; nystagmus; ataxia; dysarthria; dysphasia; hemi- or quadriplegia; unilateral or bilateral sensory symptoms; hiccups; coma. Infarctions of the brainstem can produce various syndromes, eg *lateral medullary syndrome*, in which occlusion of one vertebral artery or the posterior inferior cerebellar artery causes infarction of the lateral medulla and the inferior cerebellar surface (→vertigo, vomiting, dysphagia, nystagmus, ipsilateral ataxia, soft palate paralysis, ipsilateral Horner's syndrome, and a crossed pattern sensory loss—analgesia to pin-

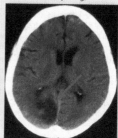

Fig 4. CT of stroke in posterior cerebral artery territory. ©J Trobe.

prick on ipsilateral face and contralateral trunk and limbs). *Locked-in syndrome* is caused by damage to the ventral pons due to pontine artery occlusion. Patients are unable to move, but retain full cognition and awareness, communicating, eg by blinking, electronic boards or special computers. ☯Right-to-die legislation may be invoked...as one sufferer blinked: "My life is dull, miserable, demeaning, undignified, and intolerable." Locked-in syndrome is different from other right-to-die conditions because patients need someone to do the act for them.◆※4

*Subclavian steal syndrome:* Subclavian artery stenosis proximal to the origin of the vertebral artery may cause blood to be *stolen* by retrograde flow down this vertebral artery down into the arm, causing brainstem ischaemia typically after use of the arm. Suspect if the BP in each arm differs by >20mmHg.

Neurology

The brain is a gland that secretes both thoughts and molecules: both products are modulated by neurotransmitter systems. Some target sites for drugs:

1 Precursor of the transmitter (eg levodopa).
2 Interference with the storage of transmitter in vesicles within the pre-synaptic neuron (eg tetrabenazine).
3 Binding to the post-synaptic receptor site (bromocriptine).
4 Binding to the receptor-modulating site (benzodiazepines).
5 Interference with the breakdown of neurotransmitter within the synaptic cleft (acetylcholinesterase inhibitors; monoamine oxidase inhibitors—MAOIs).
6 Reduce reuptake of transmitter from synaptic cleft into pre-synaptic cell (selective serotonin reuptake inhibitors—SSRIs, eg fluoxetine, or serotonin and noradrenaline reuptake inhibitors—SNRIs, eg mirtazapine).[1]
7 Binding to presynaptic autoreceptors. There are 3 kinds of autoreceptors: neurotransmitter release modulators, synthesis modulators, and impulse modulators. These offer sites for intervention. Augmenting antidepressant therapy with 5HT autoreceptor antagonists such as pindolol is possible.

The proven neurotransmitters include:

**Amino acids** Glutamate and aspartate act as excitatory transmitters on NMDA and non-NMDA receptors (BOX)—relevant in epilepsy and CNS ischaemia. $\gamma$-aminobutyric acid (GABA) is mostly inhibitory. *Drugs enhancing GABA activity:* Used in epilepsy and neuropathic pain (gabapentin, valproate); spasticity (baclofen, benzodiazepines).

**Peptides** Opioids and substance P.

**Histamine and purines** (such as ATP) Clinical relevance is not clear.

**Dopamine (DA)** *Drugs enhancing DA activity:* Used in Parkinson's; hyperprolactinaemia; acromegaly. SE: vomiting; BP↓; chorea; dystonia; hallucinations/psychosis. *Drugs that reduce DA activity:* Used in schizophrenia (OHCS p360, $D_2$ antagonists); chorea; tics; nausea; vertigo. SE: parkinsonism; dystonias; akathisia.

**Serotonin** (5-hydroxytryptamine; 5HT) There are many types of receptor, eg $5HT_{1-4}$. $5HT_1$ has 5 subtypes ($5HT_{1A-E}$). *Agonists:* Lithium$_{1A}$; sumatriptan$_{1D}$. *Partial agonists:* Buspirone$_{1A}$; LSD$_2$. *Antagonists:* Ondansetron$_3$, pizotifen$_{1\&2}$, methysergide$_{1\&2}$, clozapine$_{2C}$—known as low $D_2$-high 5HT$_2$, while risperidone is high $D_2$-high 5HT$_2$ (low $D_2$ means <60% $D_2$ occupancy at conventional sites; traditional antipsychotics are just high $D_2$, ie 60-80%). *Reuptake inhibitors:* Fluoxetine, sertraline, venlafaxine. Ecstasy increases nerve-terminal 5HT release.

**Adrenaline (epinephrine) and noradrenaline (norepinephrine)** 4 receptor types: $\alpha_1$, $\alpha_2$, $\beta_1$, $\beta_2$. Noradrenaline is more specific for $\alpha$-receptors but both transmitters affect all receptors. In the periphery, $\alpha$-receptor stimulation leads to arteriolar vasoconstriction and pupillary dilatation, $\beta_1$ stimulation leads to increase in pulse and myocardial contractility, and $\beta_2$ stimulation leads to bronchodilatation, uterine relaxation, and arteriolar vasodilatation.

*Drugs enhancing adrenergic activity:* Used in asthma ($\beta_2$); anaphylaxis (adrenaline); heart failure (dobutamine); depression (MAOIs and tricyclics; the latter may act by increasing synaptic norepinephrine in the CNS).[1]

*Drugs reducing adrenergic activity:* Used in angina, ↑BP, arrhythmias ($\beta_1$); anxiety, thyrotoxicosis ($\beta$); ↑BP from phaeochromocytoma, prostatism ($\alpha$).

**Acetylcholine** (Muscarinic and nicotinic receptors)

*Centrally acting anticholinergics:* Used in parkinsonism, dystonias, motion sickness. Central toxic effects (especially in the elderly): confusion, delusions.

*Peripherally acting antimuscarinics:* Used in asthma (ipratropium); incontinence; to dry secretions pre-op; to dilate pupils; to ↑ heart rate (atropine).

*Peripherally acting cholinergic agonists:* Used in glaucoma (pilocarpine); myasthenia (anticholinesterases). SE: sweating, hypersalivation, colic.

---

1 Noradrenaline may be more involved in the symptoms of anergia, fatigue and loss of drive in depression, and 5-HT may be more involved in the alteration in subjective mood and anxiety.

## Neurotransmitters and CNS drugs

Here we list drugs used to modify CNS transmitters. When prescribing bear in mind that: • The drug (or a metabolite) must be able to pass through the blood-brain barrier to have an effect. • The consequences of any sedative effects may be severe. • There will be short- and long-term side-effects (eg tardive dyskinesia with neuroleptic drugs). • Drugs may affect many neurotransmitters, increasing therapeutic scope (and uncertainty). • One neurotransmitter may have many effects, eg dopaminergic neurons go awry in Parkinson's disease, schizophrenia, and addiction to drugs and gambling, by affecting motor control, motivation, effort, reward,[1] analgesia, stress, learning, attention, and cognition.[9]

Don't just think about neurotransmitters! In migraine, for example, targets include calcitonin gene-related peptide (CGRP) antagonists, nitric oxide synthetase inhibitors, and ion channel antagonists, as well as 5-HT$_{1F}$ receptor agonists.[10]

| Drugs increasing activity (≈agonists) | Drugs decreasing activity (≈antagonists) |
|---|---|
| **Dopamine** | |
| Pergolide; apomorphine; amantadine | Benzisoxazoles (D$_2$), eg risperidone |
| Bromocriptine (D$_2$) | Haloperidol, chlorpromazine |
| Pramipexole;[1] ropinirole (D$_3$)^To do with mood, behaviour & rewards | Metoclopramide (D$_2$) |
| Selegiline (MAOI-B inhibitor) | |
| **Noradrenaline and adrenaline** (=norepinephrine and epinephrine) | |
| Salbutamol (β$_2$); adrenaline | Propranolol (β); bisoprolol, metoprolol (β$_1$) |
| ?Tricyclic antidepressants | Clonidine (α$_2$-agonist) |
| MAOIs | Phentolamine (α) |
| **Serotonin (5HT)** | |
| LSD and other hallucinogens | Pizotifen |
| Sumatriptan (5HT$_{1B \& 1D}$) | Benzisoxazoles (5HT$_2$), eg risperidone |
| Antidepressants, eg fluoxetine, trazodone | Olanzapine, clozapine (5HT$_{2A}$) |
| Buspirone, lithium | Mirtazapine, ondansetron (5HT$_3$) |
| **Acetylcholine** | |
| Carbachol | Atropine; scopolamine |
| Pilocarpine | Ipratropium |
| Anticholinesterases, eg donepezil, rivastigmine, pyridostigmine | Trihexyphenidyl (= Benzhexol) |
| | Orphenadrine; procyclidine |
| **GABA** (=gamma aminobutyric acid—an inhibitory neurotransmitter) | |
| Benzodiazepines (GABA$_A$) | Baclofen (GABA$_B$) |
| Valproate | |
| Gabapentin, pregabalin | Alcohol abuse:[2] *acute effects* block N-methyl-D-aspartate (NMDA) receptors; *with chronic use*, numbers of NMDA receptors rise, mediating alcohol craving |
| Barbiturates | |
| Acamprosate (used in alcohol addiction; taurine and GABA analogue)[11] | |
| **Glutamate**[2] (an excitatory amino acid) | |
| None | Lamotrigine (used in epilepsy) |
| | Topiramate (used in epilepsy)[2] |
| | Acamprosate (↓craving in alcoholics) |
| | Memantine (Alzheimer's, p492) |
| | Zonisamide (+ carbonic anhydrase activity, and modulates T-TYPE Ca$^{2+}$ channels) |

New drugs are often aimed at 2-3 neurotransmitters, eg *risperidone* (blocks D$_2$, 5HT$_2$, α$_1$ & α$_2$ receptors). The smoking-cessation drug *bupropion* (=amfebutamone) may act by ↑ dopamine in the mesolimbic system (mediates dependence) *and* via noradrenergic effects in the locus ceruleus (mediates symptoms of nicotine withdrawal).[12]

1 Use of D$_3$ receptor agonists in Parkinson's causes pathological behavioural patterns such as hypersexuality, pathological gambling or hobbying, and obsessive-compulsive disorders of impulse control in people having no history of these. These remit on stopping the drug. Expression of the D$_3$ receptor is richest in the limbic system, where it modulates emotional experience of novelty, reward, and risk assessment.[13]
2 Alcoholics have more glutamate binding sites, facilitating midbrain dopamine neurotransmission (pathways that, in the ventral tegmental area, mediate alcohol's rewarding effects). Topiramate and baclofen[14] facilitate GABA function, antagonizing glutamate at kainate receptors, and ↓craving in alcoholism.[15]

Neurology

## Upper limb

| Nerve root | Muscle | Test by asking the patient to: |
|---|---|---|
| C3, 4 | Trapezius | Shrug shoulder (via accessory nerve) |
| C5, 6, 7 | Serratus anterior | Push arm forward against resistance; look for scapula winging (p515) if weak |
| C5, 6 | Pectoralis major (P major) clavicular head | Adduct arm from above horizontal, and push it forward |
| C6, 7, 8 | P major sternocostal head | Adduct arm below horizontal |
| C5, 6 | Supraspinatus | Abduct arm the first 15° |
| C5, 6 | Infraspinatus | Externally rotate semi-flexed arm, elbow at side |
| C6, 7, 8 | Latissimus dorsi | Adduct arm from horizontal position |
| C5, 6 | Biceps | Flex supinated forearm |
| C5, 6 | Deltoid | Abduct arm between 15° and 90° |

**Radial nerve** (p506)

| | | |
|---|---|---|
| C6, 7, 8 | Triceps | Extend elbow against resistance |
| C5, 6 | Brachioradialis | Flex elbow with forearm half way between pronation and supination |
| C5, 6 | Extensor carpi radialis longus | Extend wrist to radial side |
| C6, 7 | Supinator | Arm by side, resist hand pronation |
| C7, 8 | Extensor digitorum | Keep fingers extended at MCP joint |
| C7, 8 | Extensor carpi ulnaris | Extend wrist to ulnar side |
| C7, 8 | Abductor pollicis longus | Abduct thumb at 90° to palm |
| C7, 8 | Extensor pollicis brevis | Extend thumb at MCP joint |
| C7, 8 | Extensor pollicis longus | Resist thumb flexion at IP joint |

**Median nerve** (p506)

| | | |
|---|---|---|
| C6, 7 | Pronator teres | Keep arm pronated against resistance |
| C6, 7 | Flexor carpi radialis | Flex wrist towards radial side |
| C7, 8, T1 | Flexor digitorum superficialis | Resist extension at PIP joint (with proximal phalanx fixed by the examiner) |
| C7, 8 | Flexor digitorum profundus I & II | Resist extension at index DIP joint of index finger |
| C7, 8, T1 | Flexor pollicis longus | Resist thumb extension at interphalangeal joint (fix proximal phalanx) |
| C8, T1 | Abductor pollicis brevis | Abduct thumb (nail at 90° to palm) |
| C8, T1 | Opponens pollicis | Thumb touches base of 5th fingertip (nail parallel to palm) |
| C8, T1 | 1st lumbrical/interosseus (median and ulnar nerves) | Extend PIP joint against resistance with MCP joint held hyperextended |

**Ulnar nerve** (p506)

| | | |
|---|---|---|
| C7, 8, T1 | Flexor carpi ulnaris | Flex wrist to ulnar side; observe tendon |
| C7, C8 | Flexor digitorum profundus III & IV | Resist extension of distal phalanx of 5th finger while you fix its middle phalanx |
| C8, T1 | Dorsal interossei | Finger abduction: cannot cross the middle over the index finger (tests index finger adduction too)[16] |
| C8, T1 | Palmar interossei | Finger adduction: pull apart a sheet of paper held between middle and ring finger DIP joints of both hands; the paper moves on the weaker side[117] |
| C8, T1 | Adductor pollicis | Adduct thumb (nail at 90° to palm) |
| C8, T1 | Abductor digiti minimi | Abduct little finger |
| C8, T1 | Flexor digiti minimi | Flex little finger at MCP joint |

**1** Also, metacarpophalangeal joint flexion may be more on the affected side as flexor tendons are recruited—the basis of Froment's paper sign. Wartenberg's sign is persistent little finger abduction.

## Lower limb

| Nerve root | Muscle | Test by asking the patient to: |
|---|---|---|
| **Femoral nerve** | | |
| L1, 2, 3 | Iliopsoas (also supplied via L1, 2, & 3 spinal nerves) | Flex hip against resistance with knee flexed and lower leg supported: patient lies on back |
| L2, 3, 4 | Quadriceps femoris | Extend at knee against resistance. Start with knee flexed |
| **Obturator nerve** | | |
| L2, 3, 4 | Hip adductors | Adduct leg against resistance |
| **Inferior gluteal nerve** | | |
| L5, S1, S2 | Gluteus maximus | Hip extension ('bury heel into the couch')—with knee in extension |
| **Superior gluteal nerve**[13] | | |
| L4, 5, S1 | Gluteus medius and minimus | Abduction and internal hip rotation with leg flexed at hip and knee |
| **Sciatic (and common peroneal\*) and sciatic (and tibial\*\*) nerves** | | |
| \*L4, 5 | Tibialis anterior | Dorsiflex ankle |
| \*L5, S1 | Extensor digitorum longus | Dorsiflex toes against resistance |
| \*L5, S1 | Extensor hallucis longus | Dorsiflex hallux against resistance |
| \*L5, S1 | Peroneus longus and brevis | Evert foot against resistance |
| \*L5, S1 | Extensor digitorum brevis | Dorsiflex proximal phalanges of toes |
| (\*)L5, S1, 2 | Hamstrings (short head of biceps femoris is from the common peroneal nerve) | Flex knee against resistance |
| \*\*L4, 5 | Tibialis posterior | Invert plantarflexed foot |
| \*\*S1, 2 | Gastrocnemius | Plantarflex ankle or stand on tiptoe |
| \*\*L5, S1, 2 | Flexor digitorum longus | Flex terminal joints of toes |
| \*\*S1, 2 | Small muscles of foot | Make the sole of the foot into a cup |

## Quick screening test for muscle power

| | | | | | |
|---|---|---|---|---|---|
| **Shoulder** | Abduction | C5 | **Hip** | Flexion | L1-L2 |
| | Adduction | C5-C7 | | Adduction | L2-3 |
| **Elbow** | Flexion | C5-C6 | | Extension | L5-S1 |
| | Extension | C7 | **Knee** | Flexion | L5-S1 |
| **Wrist** | Flexion | C7-8 | | Extension | L3-L4 |
| | Extension | C7 | **Ankle** | Dorsiflexion | L4 |
| **Fingers** | Flexion | C8 | | Eversion | L5-S1 |
| | Extension | C7 | | Plantarflexion | S1-S2 |
| | Abduction | T1 | **Toe** | Big toe extension | L5 |

Remember to test proximal muscle power: ask the patient to sit from lying, to pull you towards himself, and to rise from squatting (if reasonably fit).

▶Observe walking—easy to forget, even if the complaint is of difficulty walking!

▶Sources vary in ascribing particular nerve roots to muscles, and there is some biological variation in individuals. The above is a reasonable compromise, based on MRC/*Brain* guidelines: ISBN 0-7020-2512-7.
▶We don't react to nerve damage according to simple anatomy; eg ulnar neuropathy may initiate dystonic flexion or tremor of 4th and 5th digits by inducing a central motor disorder.[19]

**Neurology**

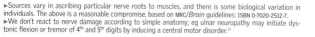

Neurology

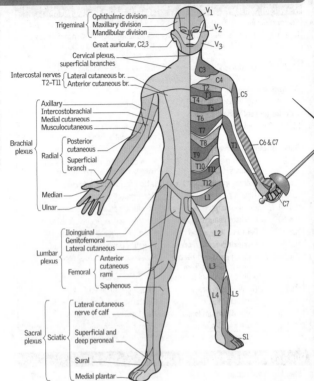

Fig 1. The white areas denote terra incognita, not because a neurologist's prick has never entered there, but because these 2011 evidence-based dermatomes reveal much more individual variation than originally thought, and no single best option can be given. Great: one less thing to remember! This is only 1 reason why knowing what we don't know is brilliant.

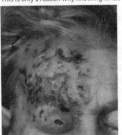

Fig 2. Pain in a dermatomal distribution suggests a problem with a cranial nerve or dorsal root ganglion (radiculopathy)—where the cell bodies of sensory fibres live.[10] What is the dermatome? What is the lesion? See p400 for the answer.

| Aim to keep a few key dermatomes up your sleeve (C5-T2) | |
|---|---|
| C3–4 | Clavicles |
| C6-7 | Lateral arm/forearm |
| T1 | Medial side of arm |
| C6 | Thumb |
| C7 | Middle finger |
| C8 | Little finger |
| T4 | Nipples |
| T10 | Umbilicus |
| L1 | Inguinal ligament |
| L2-3 | Anterior and inner leg |
| L5 | Medial side of big toe |
| L5, S1-2 | Posterior and outer leg |
| S1 | Lateral margin of foot and little toe |
| S2-4 | Perineum    Rough approximations! |

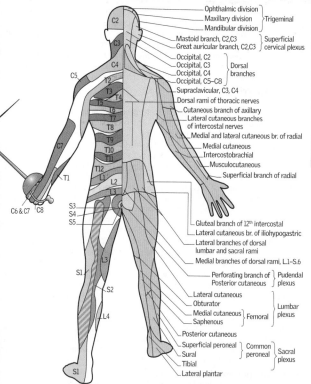

Ophthalmic division ⎫
Maxillary division ⎬ Trigeminal
Mandibular division ⎭
Mastoid branch, C2,C3 ⎫ Superficial
Great auricular branch, C2,C3 ⎬ cervical plexus
Occipital, C2 ⎫
Occipital, C3 ⎬ Dorsal
Occipital, C4 ⎪ branches
Occipital, C5–C8 ⎭
Supraclavicular, C3, C4
Dorsal rami of thoracic nerves
Cutaneous branch of axillary
Lateral cutaneous branches
of intercostal nerves
Medial and lateral cutaneous br. of radial
Medial cutaneous
Intercostobrachial
Musculocutaneous
Superficial branch of radial

Gluteal branch of 12th intercostal
Lateral cutaneous br. of iliohypogastric
Lateral branches of dorsal
lumbar and sacral rami
Medial branches of dorsal rami, L1–S.6
Perforating branch of ⎫ Pudendal
Posterior cutaneous ⎬ plexus
Lateral cutaneous
Obturator ⎫ Lumbar
Medial cutaneous ⎬ Femoral plexus
Saphenous ⎭
Posterior cutaneous
Superficial peroneal ⎫ Common
Sural ⎬ peroneal ⎫ Sacral
Tibial ⎪ ⎬ plexus
Lateral plantar ⎭ ⎭

**Fig 3.** Although this guy is crossing swords with his forward-looking self, don't think "Suicide pact" or "Delusion of doubles" (Capgras syndrome, *OHCS* p640): simply note that each sword points to the top dermatome (Vi) depicted in fig 2.

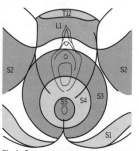

**Fig 4.** **3** views. In 2, the anterior ⅓ of the scrotum is L1; the posterior ⅔ is S3. The penis is S2/3 (L1 at its root).

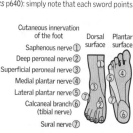

Cutaneous innervation
of the foot
Saphenous nerve ①
Deep peroneal nerve ②
Superficial peroneal nerve ③
Medial plantar nerve ④
Lateral plantar nerve ⑤
Calcaneal branch ⑥
(tibial nerve)
Sural nerve ⑦

Dorsal surface    Plantar surface

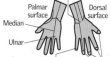

Superficial branch of radial
Palmar surface    Dorsal surface
Median
Ulnar
Dorsal cutaneous branch of ulnar    Median

**Fig 5.** Feet and hands.

Dermatome divisions after M Lee *et al* 2008 An evidence-based approach to human dermatomes. *Clin Anatomy* 21 363; John Wiley with permission. Artwork ©OUP

Every day, *thousands* visit their doctors complaining of headache. These consultations are rewarding as the chief skill is in interpreting the history—don't *take* it... let it *unfold*. ☺Let patients tell you about all the headache's associations, or even *who* their headache is. Tension headache is the most common cause of headache, for which stress relief may have more to offer than a neurologist, but some headaches are disabling and treatable (migraine, cluster headache), while others are sinister (space-occupying lesions, meningitis, subarachnoid haemorrhage).

### Acute single episode
- *With meningism:* If the headache is acute, severe, felt over most of the head and accompanied by neck stiffness (≈meningeal irritation) you must exclude:
  - meningitis (p832): fever, photophobia, stiff neck, purpuric rash, coma
  - encephalitis (p834): fever, odd behaviour, fits, or consciousness↓
  - subarachnoid haemorrhage (p482): *sudden*-onset, 'worst ever' headache, often occipital, stiff neck, focal signs, consciousness↓.

Admit immediately for urgent CT head. If CT –ve, do LP to look for signs of infection or blood products in the CSF.
- *Head injury:* Headache is common at the site of trauma but may be more generalized. It lasts ~2wks; often resistant to analgesia. Do CT to exclude subdural or extradural haemorrhage if drowsiness ± lucid interval, or focal signs (p486).
- *Venous sinus thrombosis:* (p484) Subacute or sudden headache, papilloedema.
- *Sinusitis* causes dull, constant ache over frontal or maxillary sinuses, with tenderness ± postnasal drip. Pain is worse on bending over. Ethmoid or sphenoid sinus pain is felt deep in the midline at the root of the nose. Common with coryza (p402). The pain lasts ~1-2 weeks. CT can confirm diagnosis but is rarely needed.
- *Tropical illness:* eg malaria: travel history, flu-like illness (p388); typhus (p435).
- *Low pressure headache:* From CSF leak (post LP or skull fracture).
- *Acute glaucoma:* Typically elderly, long-sighted people. Constant, aching pain develops rapidly around one eye, radiating to the forehead. *Symptoms:* Markedly reduced vision, visual haloes, nausea/vomiting. *Signs:* Red, congested eye (p563); cloudy cornea; dilated, non-responsive pupil, may be oval; ↓acuity. Attacks may be precipitated by dilating eye-drops, emotional upset or sitting in the dark, eg the cinema. ℞: Seek expert help at once. If delay in treatment of >1h is likely, start acetazolamide 500mg IV over several minutes.

### Recurrent acute attacks of headache
*Migraine:* p462. *Cluster headache:* BOX 1. *Trigeminal neuralgia:* BOX 2.
- *Recurrent (Mollaret's) meningitis:* Suspect if fever/meningism with each headache. Send CSF for herpes simplex PCR (HSV2). Is there access to subarachnoid spaces via a skull fracture, or a recurring cause of aseptic meningitis (SLE, Behçet's, sarcoid)?

### Headaches of subacute onset
- *Giant cell arteritis:* (p558). *Exclude in all >50yrs old with a headache that has lasted a few weeks.* Tender, thickened, pulseless temporal arteries; jaw claudication; ESR >40mm/h. Prompt diagnosis and steroids avoid blindness.

### Chronic headache
- *Tension headache:* The usual cause of bilateral, non-pulsatile headache ± scalp muscle tenderness, but without vomiting or sensitivity to head movement. Stress relief, eg massage or antidepressants, may be helpful.
- *Raised intracranial pressure:* Typically worse on waking, lying, bending forward, or coughing. Also vomiting, papilloedema, seizures, false localizing signs, or odd behaviour. Do imaging to exclude a space-occupying lesion, and consider idiopathic intracranial hypertension. LP *is contraindicated until after imaging.*
- *Medication overuse (analgesic rebound) headache:* Culprits are mixed analgesics (paracetamol+codeine/opiates), ergotamine and triptans. This is a common reason for episodic headache becoming chronic daily headache. Analgesia must be withdrawn—aspirin or naproxen may mollify the rebound headache. A preventive may help once off other drugs (eg tricyclics, valproate, gabapentin; p508). Limit use of over-the-counter analgesia (no more than 6 days per month).

## Cluster headache (AKA migrainous neuralgia)

Cluster headache may be the most disabling of the primary headache disorders. The cause (unknown) *may* be superficial temporal artery smooth muscle hyperreactivity to 5HT. There are hypothalamic grey matter abnormalities too. An autosomal dominant gene has a role. ♂:♀ ≥5:1; onset at any age; commoner in smokers.

**Symptoms** Rapid-onset of excruciating pain around one eye that may become watery and bloodshot with lid swelling, lacrimation, facial flushing, rhinorrhoea, miosis ± ptosis (20% of attacks). Pain is strictly unilateral and almost always affects the same side. It lasts 15–160min, occurs once or twice a day, and is often nocturnal. Clusters last 4–12wks and are followed by pain-free periods of months or even 1-2yrs before the next cluster. Sometimes it is chronic, not episodic.

**℞** "Keep calm ... carry oxygen". [21]
*Acute attack:* 100% O₂ for ~15min via non-rebreathable mask (not if COPD); [22] sumatriptan SC 6mg at onset (or zolmitriptan nasal spray 5mg).

*Preventives:* Level B evidence: suboccipital steroid injections (many SE); intranasal civamide (a synthetic isomer of capsaicin; SE nasal burning)—modestly effective but not available in the UK. [23] Level C: verapamil 360mg, lithium 900mg, and melatonin 10mg. [24,25] Methysergide may be effective but causes retroperitoneal fibrosis ∴ take a 1-month 'drug holiday' every 6 months (get expert advice).

**☁ The father in extremis** "I am careful not to wake the children as I make my way down the stairs. If they were to witness my nightly cluster ritual, they would never see me the same way again. Their father, fearless protector, diligent provider, crawling about in tears, beating his head on the hard wood floor. The pain is so intense I want to scream, but I never do. I go down 3 flights of stairs where I can't be heard, and drop to my knees. I place my hands on the back of my neck, and lock my fingers together. I bind my head between my arms and squeeze as hard as I can in an attempt to crush my skull. I begin to roll around, banging my head on the floor, pressing my left eye with full force of my palm. I search for the phone that has always been my weapon of choice for creating a diversion, and I beat my left temple with the hand piece. I create a rhythm as I strike my skull, cursing the demon with each blow...". [26]

## Trigeminal neuralgia

*Symptoms:* Paroxysms of intense, stabbing pain, lasting seconds, in the trigeminal nerve distribution. It is unilateral, typically affecting mandibular or maxillary divisions. The face screws up with pain (*hence tic douloureux*). *Triggers:* Washing affected area, shaving, eating, talking, dental prostheses. *Typical patient:* ♂ >50yrs old; in Asians ♀:♂ ≈ 2:1. *Secondary causes:* Compression of the trigeminal root by anomalous or aneurysmal intracranial vessels or a tumour, chronic meningeal inflammation, MS, zoster, skull base malformation (eg Chiari). MRI is necessary to exclude secondary causes (~14% of cases). [27] ℞: **Carbamazepine** (start at 100mg/12h PO; max 400mg/6h; **lamotrigine; phenytoin** 200–400mg/24h PO; or **gabapentin** (p508). If drugs fail, surgery may be necessary. This may be directed at the peripheral nerve, the trigeminal ganglion or the nerve root. *Microvascular decompression:* Anomalous vessels are separated from the trigeminal root. Stereotactic gamma knife surgery can work, but length of pain relief and the time to treatment response are limiting factors. *Facial pain ∆∆:* p71.

Neurology

Neurology

Migraine causes much misery, often because patients haven't teamed up with a doctor to master the art of prophylaxis.[28] Economic costs are enormous ($£ billions/yr).[29]
*Symptoms Classically:* •Visual or other aura (see below) lasting 15–30min followed within 1h by unilateral, throbbing headache. Or: •Isolated aura with no headache; •Episodic severe headaches without aura, often premenstrual, usually unilateral, with nausea, vomiting ± photophobia/phonophobia ('common migraine'). There may be allodynia—all stimuli produce pain: "I can't brush my hair, wear earrings or glasses, or shave, it's so painful". *Signs:* None. *Associations:* Obesity (weight loss may ↓ excess oestrogen/oestradiol production in adipose tissue—but benefit is unproven);[30] patent foramen ovale (some say catheter closure may help).[31] *Tests:* None if typical history. *Prodrome:* Precedes headache by hours/days: yawning, cravings, mood/sleep change. *Aura:* Precedes headache by minutes and may persist during it. • *Visual:* chaotic cascading, distorting, 'melting' and jumbling of lines, dots, or zigzags, scotomata or hemianopia; • *Somatosensory:* paraesthesiae spreading from fingers to face; • *Motor:* dysarthria and ataxia (basilar migraine), ophthalmoplegia, or hemiparesis; • *Speech:* (8% of auras) dysphasia or paraphasia, eg phoneme substitution.

**Criteria if no aura** ≥5 headaches lasting 4–72h + nausea/vomiting (or photo/phonophobia)+any 2 of: •Unilateral •Pulsating •Impairs (or worsened by) routine activity.

**Partial triggers** Seen in 50%: CHOCOLATE or: chocolate, hangovers, orgasms, cheese, oral contraceptives, lie-ins, alcohol, tumult, or exercise.

**Differential** Cluster or tension headache, cervical spondylosis, ↑BP, intracranial pathology, sinusitis/otitis media, caries. TIAs may mimic migraine aura. Migraine is rarely a sign of other pathology: don't look too hard for antiphospholipid syndrome, arteriovenous malformations, or microemboli (but in some they may be important).

**Treatment** NSAIDs (eg ketoprofen 100mg, dispersible aspirin 900mg/6h) are good as there is less chance of developing medication misuse headache (p460), and they have similar efficacy to oral 5HT agonists (triptans and ergot alkaloids).[32] Triptans[1] are generally better tolerated than ergots: in one QALY-based study, rizatriptan was better/cheaper than sumatriptan[2], which was better/cheaper than Cafergot® (below).[33] Triptans are CI if IHD, coronary spasm, uncontrolled ↑BP, recent lithium, SSRIs, or ergot use. Rare SE: arrhythmias or angina ± MI, even if no pre-existing risk. Ergotamine 1mg PO as headache starts, repeated at ⅓h, up to 3mg in a day, and 6mg in a week; or better, as a *Cafergot®* suppository (2mg ergotamine + 100mg caffeine up to 2 in 24h; then ≥4 days without). Emphasize dangers of ergotamine (gangrene, vascular damage). CI: the Pill (OHCS p300); peripheral vascular disease, IHD; pregnancy; breastfeeding; hemiplegic migraine; Raynaud's; liver or renal impairment; BP↑. 12-weekly botulinum toxin type A injections are a last resort in chronic migraine.[3] *Non-pharmacological therapies:* Warm or cold packs to the head, or rebreathing into paper bag (↑P₄CO₂) may help abort attacks.[34] Spinal manipulation,[35] riboflavin[36] and magnesium may have a role. ►Migraine often co-exists with other chronic conditions—and the combined negative impact is immense. **Rx** Don't treat each disease in isolation. Rather, attempt to restore a good relationship with the self—and the recovery of the purpose of life. This is the hardest and the most rewarding task. Can these structured holistic dialogues help? Yes, definitely,[37] so don't be daunted.

**Prevention** Remove triggers; ensure analgesic rebound headache is not complicating matters (p460). *Drugs,* eg if frequency ≥2 a month or not responding to drugs—1st-line: Propranolol 40–120mg/12h, amitriptyline 10–75mg nocte (SE: drowsiness, dry mouth, vision↓), topiramate 25–50mg/12h (SE: memory↓),[38] or Ca²⁺ channel blockers.[39] 2nd-line: Valproate, pizotifen (effective, but unacceptable weight gain in some), gabapentin, pregabalin, ACE-i, NSAIDs.[40] There is less evidence for levetiracetam, tiagabine and lamotrigine.[41] If one drug doesn't work after 3 months, try another; be guided by patient choice and SEs. Most (>65%) achieve ~50% ↓ in attack frequency.

---

**1** Triptans are 5HT₁ᵦ/₁ᴅ agonists, constricting cranial arteries. They also inhibit release of substance P, and pro-inflammatory neuropeptides, blocking transmission from the trigeminal nerve to 2nd-order neurons in the trigeminal nucleus caudalis;[c] hence use in any process that activates trigeminal fibres, including migraine, cluster headache and subarachnoid haemorrhage.

## What is going on in migraine?

The idea that migraine is a primary brain disorder resulting from altered modulation of normal sensory stimuli and trigeminal nerve dysfunction[43] is replacing the old idea that vascular events are primary (constriction during aura, with dilatation causing pain). MRIs during attacks show episodic cerebral oedema, dilatation of intracranial vessels, and ↓water diffusion not respecting vascular territories, so the primary event may be neurological.[44] PET (p752) implicates ↑hypothalamic activity; this matches food cravings and neuroendocrine data.[45] *Is migraine due to a hyperexcitable brain?* Magneto-encephalographic (MEG) studies have shown resting (interictal) hyperexcitability at least in the visual cortex, suggesting a failure of inhibitory circuits.[46] Cortical hyperexcitability may relate to imbalance between neuronal inhibition (mediated by GABA, p455) and excitation (via excitatory amino acids). Putative causes: ↓cerebral $Mg^{2+}$ levels, mitochondrial abnormalities, dysfunctions related to ↑nitric oxide, and $Ca^{2+}$ channelopathy.[47] ☺Don't neglect the social context of migraine. We might pat

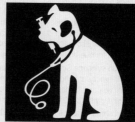

Fig 1. Migraine? Ask the dog.

ourselves on the back when we ask about family members and migraine, but we are missing the point if we don't ask about pets. In one study (n=1029)[48] most dog owners said their pet recognized their migraine before they did themselves, or during the early visual phases—and the dogs would typically show unusual attentiveness. It would be nice to think we are of more use to our patients than their dogs—but we mustn't get above our station.

## Migraine considerations in women

NICE 2012

Preventives (eg topirimate) may cause embryopathy, and interfere with the Pill. *Migraine, stroke, and the Pill (combined contraception):* Incidence of migraine + Pill-related ischaemic stroke is 8/100,000 if aged 20 (80/100,000 if 40). Only use low-dose Pills. Those with migraine+aura have ↑risk, precluding the Pill (but progesterone-only or non-hormonal contraception is OK). Risk is augmented by: •Smoking •Age >35yrs •BP↑ •Obesity (body mass index >30) •Diabetes mellitus •Hyperlipidaemia •Family history of arteriopathy when aged <45yrs. Warn women with migraine to stop Pills at once if they develop aura or worsening migraine; see OHCS p301. *If the problem is migraine without aura in the pill-free interval* consider: •Alternative contraception method or a pill with a lower dose of the same progestogen or lowest available dose of a different progestogen. •Tricycling: take the pill continuously for 3 packets (9 weeks) followed by a 7 day pill-free interval, so that the number of menstrual bleeds is reduced. •Oestrogen supplements (below) from 3 days before menses, continuing for 1wk.
*Perimenstrual migraine: Prophylaxis:* If no asthma, CCF, peptic ulcer, etc, NSAID (eg mefenamic acid) at onset of menses to last day of bleeding ± transdermal oestradiol 50–100μg patches 3 days before menses, continue for 1wk.
*Pregnancy:* Be optimistic: migraine often improves; if not, get help—evidence suggests that worsening migraine in pregnancy is associated with a greater risk of pre-eclampsia and cardiovascular complications.[49] *Prophylaxis:* stop, or use amitriptyline (most, esp. anti-convulsants, are teratogenic). *Anti-emetic:* cyclizine or promethazine. *Analgesia:* ibuprofen or aspirin may be used up to 30 weeks' gestation. If attacks persist in the 2nd and 3rd trimesters (uncommon) and paracetamol is insufficient, try partial agonist opioids.[50] Don't use aspirin if breastfeeding.

**2** Of the oral triptans, rizatriptan is said to have quick efficacy; rizatriptan and zolmitriptan are available as rapid-dissolving wafers. Imigran Recovery® may be bought 'over the counter'. Almotriptan is similar to oral sumatriptan, but ?fewer SEs;[51] 12.5mg is an effective, well-tolerated alternative if there is a poor response to sumatriptan 50mg. Rizatriptan interacts with propranolol (halve rizatriptan dose).
**3** Chronic migraine=headaches on >14 days a month. Consider botulinum toxin if no response to 3 prophylactic drugs—and only if medication overuse headache is not an issue. (NICE 2012)

Neurology

**History** It is vital to establish exactly what patients mean by 'blackout': loss of consciousness (LOC)?—a fall to the ground without loss of consciousness?—or clouding of vision, diplopia, or vertigo? ☺Take time with the patient *and* witnesses: let them tell you as much as possible without you prompting or leading them (see BOX).

**Vasovagal (neurocardiogenic) syncope** Due to reflex bradycardia ± peripheral vasodilatation provoked by emotion, pain, fear or standing too long. Onset is over seconds (*not* instantaneous), and is often preceded by nausea, pallor, sweating and closing in of visual fields (pre-syncope). *It cannot occur if lying down.* He falls to the ground, being unconscious for ~2min. Brief clonic jerking of the limbs may occur (reflex anoxic convulsion due to cerebral hypoperfusion), but there is no stiffening or tonic/clonic sequence. Urinary incontinence is uncommon (but can occur), and there is no tongue-biting. Recovery is rapid (but not as quick as with a dysrhythmia).

**Situation syncope** Syncopal symptoms are as described for vasovagal syncope.
• *Cough syncope:* Syncope after a paroxysm of coughing.
• *Effort syncope:* Syncope on exercise; cardiac origin, eg aortic stenosis, HCM.
• *Micturition syncope:* Syncope during or after micturition. Mostly men, at night.

**Carotid sinus syncope** Hypersensitive baroreceptors cause excessive reflex bradycardia ± vasodilatation on minimal stimulation (eg head-turning, shaving).

**Epilepsy** Attacks vary with the type of seizure (p494), but certain features are more suggestive of epilepsy: attacks when asleep or lying down; aura; identifiable triggers, eg TV; altered breathing; cyanosis; typical tonic-clonic movements; incontinence of urine; tongue-biting (ask about a sore tongue after the fit); prolonged post-ictal drowsiness, confusion, amnesia and transient focal paralysis (Todd's palsy).

**Stokes-Adams attacks** Transient arrhythmias (eg bradycardia due to complete heart block) causing ↓cardiac output and LOC. The patient falls to the ground (often with *no* warning except palpitations), pale, with a slow or absent pulse. Recovery is in seconds, the patient flushes, the pulse speeds up, and consciousness is regained. Injury is typical of these intermittent arrhythmias. As with vasovagal syncope, a few clonic jerks may occur if an attack is prolonged, due to cerebral hypoperfusion (reflex anoxic convulsion). Attacks may happen several times a day and in any posture.

**Drop attacks** Sudden weakness of the legs causes the patient, usually an older woman, to fall to the ground. There is no warning, no LOC and no confusion afterwards. The condition is benign, resolving spontaneously after a number of attacks. *Other causes:* hydrocephalus (these patients, however, may not be able to get up for hours); cataplexy—triggered by emotion (associated with narcolepsy, p714).

**Other causes** *Hypoglycaemia:* Tremor, hunger, and perspiration herald lightheadedness or LOC; rare in non-diabetics but see p206. *Orthostatic hypotension:* Unsteadiness or LOC on standing from lying in those with inadequate vasomotor reflexes: the elderly; autonomic neuropathy (p509); antihypertensive medication; overdiuresis; multisystem atrophy (MSA; p499). *Anxiety:* Hyperventilation, tremor, sweating, tachycardia, paraesthesiae, light-headedness, and no LOC suggest a panic attack. *Factitious blackouts:* pseudoseizures, Münchausen's (p720). *Choking:* If a large piece of food blocks the larynx, the patient may collapse, become cyanotic, and be unable to speak. Do the Heimlich manoeuvre immediately to eject the food.

**Examination** Cardiovascular, neurological. BP lying and standing.

**Investigation** ECG ± 24h ECG (arrhythmia, long QT, eg Romano-Ward, p90);[1] U&E, FBC, glucose; tilt-table tests; EEG; sleep EEG; echocardiogram; CT/MRI brain; HUT.[2] $P_aCO_2$↓ in attacks suggests hyperventilation as the cause.

▶*While the cause is being elucidated, advise against driving.*

---

**1** Consider elevating $V_1$–$V_3$ leads from 4th to the 2nd intercostal space to reveal saddle-shaped ST elevation, a telltale sign of **Brugada syndrome** (p709)—a SCN5A channelopathy predisposing to VT—and ameliorable by an implantable defibrillator.[52]

**2** Head-up tilt (HUT) tests distinguish vasodepressor from cardio-inhibitory syncope. HUT is +ve if symptoms are associated with a BP drop >30mmHg (vasodepressor; consider β-blockers to counter ↑sympathetic activity)—or bradycardia (cardio-inhibitory; consider pacing).[53]

## Taking a history of blackouts

*Ask a witness:*
• Does the patient lose awareness?
• Does the patient injure himself?
• Does the patient move? Are they stiff or floppy? (Not everything that twitches is epilepsy—a few clonic jerks may occur with syncope or arrhythmias, but are not preceded by a tonic phase. Ask for exact details of movements.)
• Is there incontinence? (More common in epilepsy, but can occur with syncope.)
• Is the complexion changed? (Cyanosis suggests epilepsy; white or red suggests arrhythmia, but may also occur in temporal lobe seizures.)
• Does the patient bite the side of his tongue? (Suggests epilepsy.)
• Any associated symptoms (palpitations, sweats, pallor, chest pain, dyspnoea)?
• How long does the attack last?
• If a 'drop attack', is the patient always sleepy? (Narcolepsy, p714.)

*Before the attack:*
• Is there any warning?—eg typical epileptic aura or cardiac pre-syncope.
• In what circumstances do attacks occur? (If watching TV, presume epilepsy).
• Can the patient prevent attacks?

*After the attack:*
• How much does the patient remember about the attack afterwards?
• Muscle ache afterwards suggests a tonic-clonic seizure.
• Is the patient confused or sleepy? (Suggests epilepsy.)

*Background to attacks:*
• When did they start?
• Are they getting more frequent?
• Is anyone else in the family getting them? Sudden arrhythmic death syndrome (SADS)[1] may leave no cardiac trace at post mortem, or there may be hereditary cardiomyopathy.

▶Witnesses often give conflicting accounts: the most reliable may not be the one with the most medical knowledge. He or she may know what you expect to hear, and furnish you with extra (imagined) material. Remember that only judges, historians and scientists are trained as impartial observers of phenomena, and even they are rarely completely objective.

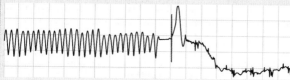

Fig 1. What is the cause of this patient's blackouts? Try to work out how they have been treated before reading footnote 1 opposite. What is the event illustrated here, and what happens just afterwards? Clue: ⬜DDMS (p126).
▶All with recurrent syncope (or falls) need cardiac assessment—urgently if associated with palpitations, arrhythmias, 3ʳᵈ-degree AV block, or prolonged QT interval (p725).¹ᵗ Also refer those with a relative who has had a sudden unexplained death (<40yrs old)—genetic counselling is vital: bshg.org.uk/genetic_centres/uk_genetic_centres.htm.

Neurology

Complaints of 'dizzy spells' are very common and are used by patients to describe many different sensations. The key to diagnosis is to find out exactly what the patient means by 'dizzy' and then decide whether or not this represents vertigo.

**Is this vertigo?** *Definition:* An illusion of movement, often rotatory, of the patient or his surroundings. In practice, simple 'spinning' is rare—the floor may tilt, sink, or rise, or "I veer sideways on walking as if pulled by a magnet". Vertigo is always[1] worsened by movement. *Associated symptoms:* Difficulty walking or standing (may even fall suddenly to the ground), relief on lying or sitting still; nausea, vomiting, pallor, sweating. Associated hearing loss or tinnitus implies labyrinth or VIII[th] nerve involvement. *What is not vertigo:* Faintness may be due to anxiety with associated palpitations, tremor, and sweating. *Light-headedness* may be due to anaemia, orthostatic hypotension, or effort in an emphysematous patient. But in all of these there is no illusion of movement or typical associated symptoms. *Lost awareness* during attacks should prompt thoughts of epilepsy or syncope, not vertigo.

**Causes** Look to the labyrinth, vestibular nerve, vestibular nuclei, or their central connections. Other structures are rarely involved (MINIBOX).

| Causes of vertigo |
|---|
| *Labyrinth & VIII[th] nerve* |
| • Ménière's disease |
| • Vestibular neuronitis (ie acute labyrinthitis) |
| • Benign positional vertigo (*OHCS* p554) |
| • Motion sickness |
| • Trauma |
| • Ototoxic drugs |
| • Zoster (ie Ramsay Hunt syndrome, p505) |
| • Tullio phenomenon[2] |
| *Brainstem, cerebellum, cerebello-pontine angle* (Look for nystagmus and cranial nerve lesions) |
| • MS; acoustic neuroma |
| • Stroke/TIA; haemorrhage |
| • Migraine |
| *Cerebral cortex* |
| • Vertiginous epilepsy |
| *Alcohol intoxication* |

*Benign positional vertigo* is due to canalolithiasis—debris in the semicircular canal, disturbed by head movement, resettles causing vertigo lasting a few seconds after the movement (often turning over in bed). Nystagmus on performing the Hallpike manoeuvre is diagnostic. Epley manoeuvres clear the debris from the semicircular canals (*OHCS* p555).

*Acute labyrinthitis (vestibular neuronitis):* Abrupt onset of severe vertigo, nausea, vomiting ± prostration. No deafness or tinnitus. Causes: virus; vascular lesion. Severe vertigo subsides in days, complete recovery takes 3–4wks. ℞: Reassure. Sedate.

*Ménière's disease:* Endolymphatic hydrops causes recurrent attacks of **vertigo** lasting >20min (± nausea/vomiting), fluctuating (± permanent) sensorineural **hearing loss**, and **tinnitus** (with a sense of aural fullness ± drop attacks (no loss of consciousness or vertigo, but falling to one side, ie Tumarkin otolithic catastrophes)). ℞: Acute attacks—bed rest and reassurance. An antihistamine (eg cinnarizine) is useful if prolonged, or buccal prochlorperazine if severe, for up to 7d. In very severe disease, consider endolymphatic sac surgery or ablation of the vestibular organ with gentamicin. *Prophylaxis:* low-Na⁺ diets or betahistine may be tried, but there is no evidence of efficacy.[65] Trimetazidine, thiazide diuretics and lithium are not recommended.

*Ototoxicity:* Aminoglycosides, loop diuretics or cisplatin can cause deafness±vertigo.

*Acoustic neuroma* (figs 1 & 2) is doubly misnamed: it is a Schwannoma (not neuroma) arising from the vestibular (not auditory) nerve. It often presents with unilateral hearing loss, with vertigo occurring later. With progression, ipsilateral V[th], VI[th], IX[th], & X[th] nerves may be affected (also ipsilateral cerebellar signs). Paradoxically, the VII[th] nerve is rarely involved pre-operatively. Signs of ↑ICP occur late, indicating a large tumour. They account for 80% of cerebello-pontine angle tumours (ΔΔ meningioma).[56] Commoner in ♀; also in neurofibromatosis (esp. NF2, p518). Not all need removing.

*Traumatic damage* involving the petrous temporal bone or the cerebello-pontine angle often affects the auditory nerve, causing vertigo, deafness and/or tinnitus.

*Herpes zoster:* Herpetic eruption of the external auditory meatus; facial palsy ± deafness, tinnitus, and vertigo (Ramsay Hunt syndrome, see p505).

[1] The single exception is *mal de debarquement*, in which vertiginous motion sickness persists long after alighting from, for example, the ship or train that triggered the motion sickness.

[2] Dizziness induced by sound, eg one's own voice or a musical instrument. Causes: superior canal dehiscence, perilymph fistula, Ménière's syndrome, post fenestration surgery, and vestibulofibrosis

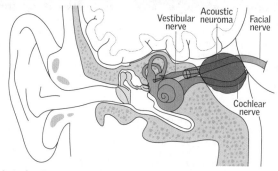

**Fig 1.** An acoustic neuroma (vestibular schwannoma) growing dangerously near the facial nerve. It helps to understand their natural history, since you may be able to save patients a difficult and dangerous operation. For each patient, growth rate is constant and predictable after a few years of serial MRIs: ~30% do not progress; ~50% grow slowly (1–2mm/yr); and ~20% grow > 2mm/yr. Malignancy is rare but not negligible, and every so often we all get tricked by these tumours. *Microsurgical removal* has ~1% operative mortality. Near-normal post-op facial movement, sensation and perhaps hearing is the aim, but damage to VII[th] nerve is common. Likelihood of surgical cure is > 95%.[57]

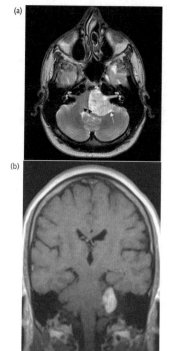

**Fig 2.** Large vestibular schwannoma. **(a)** Axial T2w and **(b)** Contrast enhanced coronal MRI.[58]
Reproduced from Manji *et al*, *Oxford Handbook of Neurology*, 2007,
with permission from OUP.

One reasonable bedside method to establish hearing loss is to whisper numbers increasingly loudly in one ear while blocking the other ear with a finger. Ask your patient to repeat the number. Make sure that failure is not from misunderstanding. The anatomy of the auditory apparatus is shown in fig 1.

**Tuning fork tests** No single test is diagnostic, but tuning fork tests do give useful information (also popular in exams). Use a 512Hz or 256Hz tuning fork, struck ⅓ from its free end on your patella to make it vibrate.

• *Rinne:* Hold a vibrating tuning fork so that the prongs and auditory canal lie on the same line, testing air conduction (AC). Then place the vibrating stem on the mastoid for bone conduction (BC). Ask "Which is louder?" *Rinne negative:* BC > AC. This occurs with conductive deafness >20dB, but also severe sensorineural hearing loss (SNHL)—ie a false -ve Rinne: the other cochlea picks up the sound by bone conduction. Using a Barany noise box to mask the other ear during the test prevents this. *Rinne positive:* AC > BC, indicating normality or SNHL. Remember 'SNAC-RIP': in sensorineural loss and normal ears, air conduction is better—Rinne is positive.

• *Weber:* With the vibrating tuning fork on the vertex, forehead or upper incisors(!), ask the patient which ear the sound is heard in. Sound localizes to the affected ear with conductive loss (>10dB loss), to the contralateral ear in SNHL, and to the midline if both ears are normal (or if bilateral sensorineural loss).

**Conductive deafness** *Causes:* wax (remove, eg by syringing with warm water after softening with olive oil drops), otosclerosis, otitis media, or glue ear (*OHCS* p546).

**Chronic sensorineural deafness** Often due to accumulated environmental noise toxicity, presbyacusis or inherited disorders. *Presbyacusis:* Loss of acuity for high-frequency sounds starts before 30yrs old. We do not usually notice it until hearing of speech is affected. Hearing is most affected in the presence of background noise. Hearing aids are the usual treatment.

**Sudden sensorineural deafness** ►Get an ENT opinion *today* (steroids may cure)! *Causes:* noise exposure; gentamicin/other toxin; mumps; acoustic neuroma; MS; stroke; vasculitis; TB. *Tests:* ESR, FBC, LFT, pANCA, viral titres and TB Elispot; evoked response audiometry; CXR; MRI; lymph node and nasopharyngeal biopsy for culture.

## Tinnitus (See also *OHCS* p552)

This ringing or buzzing in the ears is common, and may cause depression or insomnia. ►Investigate unilateral tinnitus fully to exclude an acoustic neuroma (p466).

**Causes** Focal hyper-excitability in the auditory cortex (postulated to be the cause of common tinnitus[59]), hearing loss (20%), wax, viral, presbyacusis, excess noise (eg gunfire), head injury, septic otitis media, post-stapedectomy, Ménière's, anaemia, ↑BP (in up to 16%, but it may not be causative).[60] *Drugs:* Aspirin (reversible), loop diuretics, aminoglycosides. *Psychological associations:* Redundancy, divorce, retirement. *Mean age at onset:* 40-50yrs. ♂:♀≈1:1. *Causes of pulsatile tinnitus:* Carotid artery stenosis or dissection[61] AV fistulae, and glomus jugulare tumours (*OHCS* p552). May be audible with stethoscope. Discuss imaging with a neuroradiologist.

**Management** ►Psychological support is very important (eg from a hearing therapist). Exclude serious causes; reassure that tinnitus does not mean madness or serious disease and that it often improves in time. Cognitive therapy helps, as does 'tinnitus coping training'. Patient support groups can help greatly.[62] Drugs are disappointing. Avoid tranquillizers, particularly if depressed (use tricyclic antidepressants here, eg amitriptyline[63] or nortriptyline).[64] Hypnotics at night may help. Carbamazepine rarely helps. If Ménière's disease is the cause, betahistine helps only a few. Masking may give relief. White noise (like an off-tuned radio) is given via a noise generator worn like a post-aural hearing aid. Hearing aids may help by amplifying desirable sounds. Cochlear nerve section can relieve disabling tinnitus in 25% (at the expense of deafness). Repetitive transcranial magnetic stimulation of the auditory cortex can help (a novel and non-standard therapy).[59]

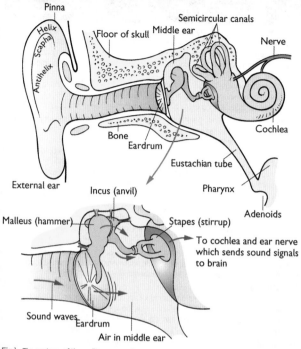

Fig 1. The anatomy of the auditory apparatus.

Neurology

►Cord compression typically presents with weak legs. There are many causes of weak legs (see BOX): addressing these 5 questions helps with diagnosis:

1 Was onset sudden? ►Sudden or progressive weakness is an emergency: get help to prevent permanent paralysis, faecal incontinence, and a neurogenic bladder).[1]
2 Are the legs flaccid or spastic (causes of UMN lesions, p451)?
3 Is there sensory loss?[1] A sensory level usually means spinal cord disease.
4 Is there loss of sphincter control (bowels, bladder)?
5 Any signs of infection, eg extradural abscess (tender spine, T°↑, WCC↑, ESR↑, CRP↑)?

*Symptoms:* Spinal or root pain[2] may precede leg weakness and sensory loss. Arm weakness is often less severe (suggests a cervical cord lesion). Bladder (and anal) sphincter involvement is late and manifests as hesitancy, frequency, and, later, as painless retention. *Signs:* Look for a motor, reflex, and sensory level, with normal findings above the level of the lesion, LMN signs at the level (especially in cervical cord compression, see p512), and UMN signs *below* the level (but remember tone and reflexes are usually reduced in *acute* cord compression; OHCS p768).

**Causes** ►Secondary malignancy (breast, lung, prostate, thyroid, kidney) in the spine is commonest. Rarer: infection (epidural abscess), cervical disc prolapse, haematoma (warfarin), intrinsic cord tumour, atlanto-axial subluxation, myeloma. Occasionally one can get caught out by causes that are not in the spine, eg bilateral frontal lobe infarcts, or a parasagittal meningioma (see BOX 1).

ΔΔ Transverse myelitis, MS, carcinomatous meningitis, cord vasculitis (PAN, syphilis), spinal artery thrombosis, trauma, dissecting aneurysm, Guillain-Barré (though not a cord pathology, but one of roots and peripheral nerves ∴ LMN; p716).

**Investigations** ►Do not delay imaging at any cost. Speed of imaging should parallel the rate of clinical progression. Spinal x-rays are unreliable; MRI is the definitive modality. Biopsy or surgical exploration may be needed to identify the nature of any mass. *Screening blood tests:* FBC, ESR, $B_{12}$, syphilis serology, U&E, LFT, PSA, serum electrophoresis. Do a CXR (primary lung malignancy, lung secondaries, TB).

**Treatment** ►If malignancy, give dexamethasone IV 4mg/6h while considering more specific therapy, eg radiotherapy or chemotherapy ± decompressive laminectomy; which is most appropriate depends on tumour type, quality of life, and likely prognosis. Epidural abscesses must be surgically decompressed and antibiotics given.

**Cauda equina and conus medullaris lesions** The big difference between these lesions and those high up in the cord is that leg weakness is flaccid and areflexic, not spastic and hyperreflexic. *Causes:* As above, plus congenital lumbar disc disease and lumbosacral nerve lesions. *Signs:* Conus medullaris lesions feature a mixed UMN/LMN leg weakness; early urinary retention and constipation; back pain; sacral sensory disturbance; and erectile dysfunction. Cauda equina lesions feature back pain and radicular pain down the legs; asymmetrical, atrophic, areflexic paralysis of the legs; sensory loss in a root distribution; and ↓sphincter tone; do PR.

*Paralysed patients need especial care* Avoid pressure sores by turning. Review weight-bearing areas often. Avoid thrombosis in paralysed limbs by frequent passive movement and pressure stockings ± low molecular weight heparin (p344). Bladder care is vital; catheterization is only one option. Do not control incontinence by decreasing fluid intake (OHCS p774). Bowel evacuation may be manual or aided by suppositories. Increasing dietary fibre intake may help. Exercise of unaffected or partially paralysed limbs is important to avoid unnecessary loss of function.

---

1 Get help *today* from a neurosurgeon or your spinal cord compression co-ordinator. Prevent DVTs and pressure sores. See p526.
2 *Nerve root sensations* may be sharp or dull (like angina if T3–T4 affected) or 'warm glows', or 'as if if bandages were wrapped round my leg' or rubbed with sandpaper, or sprayed with hot water. *Dorsal column damage* may cause hypersensitivity or vibratory feelings, as if on the deck of a ship under full power or the limbs may feel twice their normal size. *Spinothalamic symptoms* may be 'as if my bones burned and the flesh was torn away'.

## Other causes of leg weakness

*Unilateral foot drop:* DM, common peroneal nerve palsy, stroke, prolapsed disc, MS.

*Weak legs with no sensory loss:* MND, polio, parasagittal meningioma (an exception to the rule that weak legs mean cord or distal lesion).

*Chronic spastic paraparesis:* MS, cord tumour (astrocytoma, haemangioblastoma, ependymoma),[65] cord metastases,[66] MND, syringomyelia, subacute combined degeneration of the cord (fig 1), hereditary spastic paraparesis, taboparesis,[1] histiocytosis X, parasites (eg schistosomiasis; look for eosinophilia).[67]

*Chronic flaccid paraparesis:* Peripheral neuropathy, myopathy (rare; arms also involved).

*Absent knee jerks and extensor plantars:* Combined cervical and lumbar disc disease, conus medullaris lesions, or a 'MAST': MND (or myeloradiculitis[2]), Friedreich's ataxia, subacute combined degeneration of the cord (vit. B₁₂ deficiency; fig 1), taboparesis.[1]

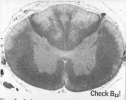

Check B₁₂!

Fig 1. Subacute combined degeneration of the cord, due to vit. B₁₂ deficiency (p329). Why 'combined'? Both lateral (motor) *and* dorsal (sensory, at the top of fig 1) columns lose myelin (at ~C5-T3), then axons. Eventually *all* the cord's rim is affected, if vit B₁₂ injections are delayed (p328). NB: if vit B₁₂ is normal, do copper studies (hypocupric myelopathy).

©Prof D Agamanolis.

## Gait disorders

(Even the best professionals have to employ extraordinary tactics just to *describe* gaits accurately,😔[3] never mind *diagnose* them accurately.)

*Spastic:* Stiff, circumduction of legs ± scuffing of the toe of the shoes.

*Extrapyramidal:* Flexed posture, shuffling feet, slow to start, postural instability. Example: Parkinson's disease.

*Apraxic:* Pathognomonic 'gluing-to-the-floor' on attempting walking or a wide-based unsteady gait with a tendency to fall, like a novice on an ice-rink. *Causes:* normal pressure hydrocephalus, multi-infarct states.

*Ataxic:* Wide-based; falls; cannot walk heel-to-toe. *Causes:* cerebellar lesions (eg MS, posterior fossa tumours, alcohol, phenytoin toxicity); proprioceptive sensory loss (eg sensory neuropathies, ↓B₁₂). Often worse in the dark, or with eyes closed.

*Myopathic:* Waddle (hip girdle weakness). Cannot climb steps or stand from sitting.

*Psychogenic:* Often a bizarre gait not conforming to any pattern of organic gait disturbance. Suspect if there is profound gait disturbance with inability even to stand, without any signs when examined on the couch (Paul Blocq's[68] 'astasia abasia'[4])—but this may occur with midline cerebellar lesions, normal pressure hydrocephalus, and rare tumours[69]—hence the adage that psychogenic disorders are only to be diagnosed by doctors over 40 in patients under 40. Video analysis reveals 6 'signs of psychogenicity', seen in 97% of patients in one study:[70]

- Fluctuations in response to suggestion or distraction.
- Excessive hesitation of locomotion incompatible with CNS disease.
- 'Psychogenic' building-up of sway amplitudes on Romberg test.
- Uneconomic postures wasting muscular energy.
- 'Walking on ice' gait, ie small cautious steps, with ankle joints fixed.
- Sudden buckling of the knees, usually without falls.

**Tests** Spinal x-rays; MRI; FBC; ESR; syphilis serology; serum B₁₂; U&E; LFT; PSA; serum electrophoresis; CXR; LP; EMG; muscle ± sural nerve biopsy.

1 Tertiary syphilis (p431): in tabes dorsalis the afferent pathways from muscle spindles are lost, with reduced tone and tendon reflexes (without weakness). Later, additional involvement of the pyramidal tracts causes taboparesis—a spastic paraparesis with the peculiar combination of extensor plantars (from the taboparesis) and absent tendon reflexes (from the tabes dorsalis).
2 Infections can inflame roots *and* cord (eg visceral larva migrans); hence the mixed picture.[71]
3 Unda her brella mid piddle med puddle she ninnygoes nannygoes nancing by. *James Joyce, Finnegans Wake*
4 Greek for no standing/no walking, eg the 'hysterical'● unwalking unwounded cadet.

Neurology

Movement disorders are clinically and pathologically heterogenous, and are characterized by impairment of the planning, control or execution of movement.[72,73] They may manifest with symptoms of ataxia, dystonia, gait problems (p471), parkinsonism, chorea, myoclonus, spasticity, dyskinesia, tics and tremor.

**Tremor** Note frequency, amplitude, and exacerbating factors (stress; fatigue).
• *Rest tremor:* abolished on voluntary movement. *Cause:* parkinsonism (p498).
• *Intention tremor:* irregular, large-amplitude, worse at the end of purposeful acts, eg finger-pointing or using a remote control. *Cause:* cerebellar damage (eg MS, stroke).
• *Postural tremor:* absent at rest, present on maintained posture (arms outstretched) and may persist (but is not worse) on movement. *Causes:* Benign essential tremor (autosomal dominant; improves with alcohol), thyrotoxicosis, anxiety, β-agonists.
• *Re-emergent tremor:* postural tremor developing after a delay of ~10sec (eg in Parkinson's).[74] Surgery/deep brain stimulation (DBS) helps some tremors.[75]

**Chorea, athetosis, and hemiballismus** *Chorea:*[1] Non-rhythmic, jerky, purposeless movements flitting from one place to another—eg facial grimacing, raising the shoulders, flexing/extending the fingers. *Causes:* Huntington's disease, Sydenham's chorea (choreoathetoid movements as a rare complication of strep infection). The anatomical basis of chorea is uncertain but it may be the pharmacological mirror image of Parkinson's disease (L-dopa worsens chorea). *Hemiballismus:* Large-amplitude, flinging hemichorea (affects proximal muscles) contralateral to a vascular lesion of the subthalamic nucleus (often elderly diabetics). Recovers spontaneously over months. *Athetosis:* Slow, sinuous, confluent, purposeless movements (esp. digits, hands, face, tongue), often difficult to distinguish from chorea. *Causes:* commonest is cerebral palsy (*OHCS* p214). Most other 'athetoid' patterns may now be better classed as dystonias. *Pseudoathetosis* is caused by severe proprioceptive loss.

**Tics** Brief, repeated, stereotyped movements which patients may suppress for a while. Tics are common in children (and usually resolve). In *Tourette's syndrome* (p714), motor and vocal tics occur. Consider psychological support, clonazepam or clonidine if tics are severe (haloperidol may help but risks tardive dyskinesia).

**Myoclonus** Sudden involuntary focal or general jerks arising from cord, brainstem or cerebral cortex, seen in metabolic problems (below), neurodegenerative disease (eg lysosomal storage enzyme defects), CJD (p710), and myoclonic epilepsies (infantile spasms). *Benign essential myoclonus:* Childhood onset with frequent generalized myoclonus, without progression. Often autosomal dominant. It may respond to valproate, clonazepam or piracetam. *Asterixis ('metabolic flap'):* Jerking (~1-2 jerks/sec) of outstretched hands, worse with wrists extended, from loss of extensor tone—ie incoordination between flexors and extensors (='negative myoclonus'). *Causes:* liver or kidney failure, ↓Na⁺, ↑CO₂, gabapentin, thalamic stroke (consider if unilateral).[76]

**Tardive syndromes** Tardive means 'delayed onset', in this case after chronic exposure to dopamine antagonists (eg antipsychotics, antiemetics). Tardive syndromes are a source of much distress and disability, and may be permanent, despite discontinuing all drugs. *Classification:*[77] • *Tardive dyskinesia* (orobuccolingual, truncal, or choreiform movements, eg vacuous chewing and grimacing movements); • *Tardive dystonia* (sustained, stereotyped muscle spasms of a twisting or turning character, eg retrocollis and back arching/opisthotonic posturing); • *Tardive akathisia* (unpleasant inner sense of restlessness or unease ± repetitive, purposeless movements (stereotypies, eg pacing)); • *Tardive myoclonus*; • *Tardive tourettism* (p714). • *Tardive tremor* (may respond to donepezil).[78] *Treating tardive dyskinesia:* Get help. Gradually withdraw neuroleptics and wait 3-6 months. If still a problem, consider **tetrabenazine** 12.5-50mg/8h PO.[79] Quetiapine, olanzapine and clozapine are examples of atypical antipsychotics that are less likely to cause tardive syndromes.

---

**1** Paracelsus used the term *chorea* to describe the jerking movements of medieval pilgrims travelling to the healing shrine of St Vitus—reflecting the ancient Greek round dance accompanied by singing (hence choreography). He recognized 3 types: chorea arising from the imagination (chorea imaginativa), or from sexual desire (chorea lasciva) or from corporeal causes (chorea naturalis).[80]

Dystonia describes prolonged muscle contractions causing abnormal posture or repetitive movements. Verbatim example of dystonic symptoms (writer's cramp, in this example): ☺"I cannot, for example, draw the instrument [pen, pencil] toward me in a circular motion, eg the left arc of a circle, or the letter O. If I force the move, the movements become jerky and I lose all smoothness in the character. The same thing will happen when eating and trying to use a fork...I end up moving my mouth to the fork...instead of moving my hand to my mouth—awkward."[81]

**Classification** can be by *age of onset*—childhood (<12yrs old), adolescent (13-20yrs) or adult (>20yrs); by *part of the body affected*; or by *cause* (there are many).

*Idiopathic generalized dystonia* is suggested by onset in childhood and often starts with dystonia in one leg, spreading to that side of the body over 5-10yrs. Autosomal dominant inheritance is common (genetics often show a deletion in DYT1). Treatment is challenging; exclude Wilson's disease and dopa-responsive dystonia (often better after sleep; needs an L-dopa trial). High-dose **trihyphenidyl** (=benzhexol, an anticholinergic) and **deep-brain stimulation** may help.[82]

*Focal dystonias* are confined to one part of the body, eg *spasmodic torticollis* (head pulled to one side), *blepharospasm* (involuntary contraction of orbicularis oculi, *OHCS* p460), *writer's cramp*. Focal dystonias in adults are typically idiopathic, and rarely generalize. They are worsened by stress. Patients may develop a *geste antagonistique* to try to resist the dystonic posturing (eg a touch of the finger to the jaw in spasmodic torticollis).[83] Injection of **botulinum toxin** into the overactive muscles (*OHCS* p460) is usually effective, but there may be SEs.

*Writer's cramp* (scrivener's palsy; graphospasm) When trying to write, the pen is driven into the paper and flow of movement is poor. ☺"I would look at [my fingers] and tell them to do one thing, and they'd do jagged things instead, I'd have full muscle control for everything, except putting a pen to a piece of paper."[84] Look for hand and forearm spasm, dystonic arm posture, focal tremor, myoclonus, and dominant-hand muscle hypertrophy.[85] *Association:* obsessive-compulsive disorder.[86] *EMG:* May correlate with physiological events; ↓reciprocal inhibition of wrist flexor motor neurons at rest, and ↑co-contraction of antagonist muscles of the forearm during voluntary activity.[87] *EEG:* Abnormal motor command (sensorimotor region β rhythm).[88] *R:* β-blockers and valproate often fail. Breath-holding or arm-cooling may work, as may botulinum toxin and EMG biofeedback.[85]

*Acute dystonia* (fig 1) may occur on starting many drugs, including neuroleptics and some antiemetics (eg metoclopramide, cyclizine). There is torticollis (head pulled back), trismus (oromandibular spasm), and/or oculogyric crisis (eyes drawn up). You may mistake this for tetanus or meningitis, but such reactions rapidly disappear after a dose of an anticholinergic, see p855.

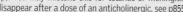

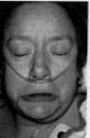 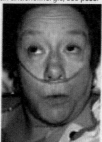 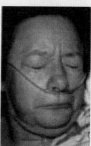

**Fig 1.** Oromandibular/oculogyric crisis in acute dystonia.
From *Mayo Clinic Proc* 2003; 78:1150-2. Used with permission.[89]

Strokes result from ischaemic infarction or bleeding into part of the brain, manifest by rapid onset (eg seconds-minutes) of focal CNS signs and symptoms. It is the major neurological disease of our time. *Mortality after 1st stroke:* 12% by day 56 (UK data; was 21% in 1999). *Incidence* is falling too (now 1/1000/yr, perhaps due to a more vigorous approach to risk factors in primary care, ie statin use and control of BP).[90]

**Causes** • Small vessel occlusion/cerebral microangiopathy[91] or thrombosis *in situ*
• Cardiac emboli (AF; endocarditis; MI—see BOX on p477)
• Atherothromboembolism (eg from carotids)
• CNS bleeds (BP↑, trauma, aneurysm rupture, anticoagulation, thrombolysis)

*Other causes:* (most important to consider in younger patients) Sudden BP drop by ≥40mmHg (boundary zone/'watershed'[1] stroke, eg in sepsis), carotid artery dissection (spontaneous, or from neck trauma or fibromuscular dysplasia), vasculitis, subarachnoid haemorrhage, venous sinus thrombosis (acute venous infarct, p484), antiphospholipid syndrome, thrombophilia, Fabry's disease (p712), CADASIL,[2] CARASIL (autosomal recessive).
►Do not hesitate to get a neurology, cardiology, or haematology opinion.

**Modifiable risk factors** BP↑, smoking, DM, heart disease (valvular, ischaemic, AF), peripheral vascular disease, past TIA, ↑PCV, carotid bruit, the Pill, ↑lipids, ↑alcohol use, ↑clotting (eg ↑plasma fibrinogen, ↓antithrombin III, p368), thomocysteine, syphilis.

**Signs** ►Sudden onset, maybe with further progression over hours (rarely days). In theory, focal signs relate to distribution of the affected artery (p452), but collaterals cloud the issue. *Pointers to bleeding (unreliable!):* Meningism, severe headache, and coma within hours. *Pointers to ischaemia:* Carotid bruit, AF, past TIA, IHD.
• *Cerebral infarcts:* (50%) Depending on site there may be contralateral sensory loss or hemiplegia—initially flaccid (floppy limb, falls like a dead weight when lifted), becoming spastic (UMN); dysphasia; homonymous hemianopia; visuo-spatial deficit.
• *Brainstem infarcts:* (25%) Wide range of effects, which include quadriplegia, disturbances of gaze and vision, locked-in syndrome (aware, but unable to respond).
• *Lacunar infarcts:* (25%) In basal ganglia,[3] internal capsule, thalamus, and pons. 5 syndromes: ataxic hemiparesis, pure motor, pure sensory, sensorimotor, and dysarthria/clumsy hand. Cognition/consciousness are intact except thalamic stroke.

**Action** (1st hr; see p476-7 for later) ►*Protect the airway* to avoid hypoxia/aspiration.
►►*Pulse, BP and ECG:* Is it an embolus from AF? NB: treating even very high BPs may harm (unless there is encephalopathy, or aortic dissection): even a 20% fall may compromise cerebral perfusion, as autoregulation is impaired. If on HRT, stop it.
►►*Blood glucose:* If low, see p844. Aim for 4-11 mmol/L. Sliding scale (p591) if DM.
►►*Urgent CT/MRI if:* Thrombolysis considered, cerebellar stroke (cerebellar haematomas may need urgent referral for evacuation),[92] unusual presentation (alternative diagnosis likely?—BOX), or high risk of haemorrhage (↓GCS, signs of ↑ICP, severe headache, meningism, progressive symptoms, known bleeding tendency or anticoagulated). Otherwise imaging can wait (aim <24h). Diffusion-weighted MRI is most sensitive for an acute infarct, but CT helps rule out primary haemorrhage.
►►*Thrombolysis:* Consider if onset of symptoms ≤4.5h ago; BOX.
►►*'Nil by mouth':* Only if swallowing attempts might lead to choking. Keep hydrated (eg IVI), but don't overhydrate (risk of cerebral oedema).
►►*Antiplatelet agents:* Once haemorrhagic stroke is excluded, give **aspirin 300mg**.
☼Communicate fully with your patient, the relatives, and carers over difficult decisions, eg deciding on the kindest/best level of intervention taking into account quality of life, coexisting conditions, and prognosis. Is there a living will? See p478.
*Take to a stroke unit with special nursing/physio* to save life,[93] and to motivate.

---

**1** In medical parlance a watershed is the zone between 2 vascular beds where supply is most tenuous.
**2** CADASIL=cerebral Autosomal Dominant Arteriopathy with subcortical Infarcts & Leucoencephalopathy. This NOTCH3 gene mutation (19q) is the main genetic cause of stroke. Presents from 40yrs with migraine, TIA, mood disorders, dementia ± pseudobulbar palsy. MRI: hypointensities on T1-weighted images; hyperintensities on T2+confluent white matter lesions. Skin,spleen,liver,muscle,aorta & glomeruli involved too.[94]
**3** Basal ganglia strokes may cause a grasp reflex (p503); also unilateral choreoathetosis.

## Differential diagnosis of stroke

- Head injury
- CNS lymphoma
- Mitochondrial cytopathies[1]
- Hypo/hyperglycaemia
- Pneumocephalus; air entry
- Herpes encephalitis
- Subdural haemorrhage
- via otitis or mastoid air cells
- HIV; HTLV-1; toxoplasmosis
- Intracranial tumours
- Wernicke's encephalopathy
- Abscesses (eg typhoid)
- Hemiplegic migraine
- Drug overdose (if coma)
- Mycotic aneurysm[95]
- Epilepsy (Todd's palsy)
- Hepatic encephalopathy
- *Coccidioides immitis*[96]
- NB: status epilepticus *can* cause CNS infarcts.[97]
- Acanthamoeba/naegleria[98]

## ▶▶ Thrombolysis in acute non-haemorrhagic stroke

See IST3 trial

If an expert team (neuroimaging and clinicians) is in place, *and* the patient is seen within ~4.5h[2,3] of the onset of symptoms, *and* no contraindication exists (see below), refer with *utmost urgency* for consideration of reperfusion with IV recombinant tissue plasminogen activator (tPA: alteplase—eg 0.9mg/kg over 1h). This reduces death and dependency (odds ratio 0.64) despite a small increase in intracranial haemorrhage (these are usually small and asymptomatic).[99] Recent use of antiplatelet agents does not appear to ↑ this risk.[99] Always do CT 24h post-lysis to identify bleeds (if +ve, register at SITS, www.acutestroke.org). <sup>Safe Implementation of Thrombolysis in Stroke (SITS) database</sup>

CI • Major infarct or haemorrhage on CT • Mild/non-disabling deficit • Recent birth, surgery, trauma, or artery or vein puncture at uncompressible site • Past CNS bleed • AVM or aneurysm • Severe liver disease, varices or portal hypertension • Seizures at presentation • Anticoagulants or INR >1.7 • Platelets <100 × 10⁹/L • BP >220/130. *The future:* Those with CI may be eligible for a flow-restoration device, eg the Solitaire, in large-vessel intracranial occlusive stroke (SWIFT and TREVO2 trials).[100]

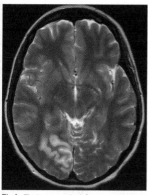
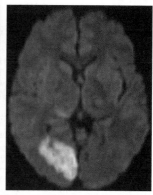

**Fig 1.** The image on the left is T2-weighted (p760); the more water present, the more white the appearance. In the right occipital lobe, the cerebral cortex is abnormal with high signal, most likely from oedema. If so, it is cytotoxic oedema from cell ischaemia and death, rather than vasogenic oedema from leaky capillaries that involves more of the white matter. The diagnosis could be an infarct (distribution is the right PCA territory), inflammation, or tumour. The diffusion-weighted image on the right shows limited (abnormal) diffusion in the region, indicating this is an infarct. ©Prof Peter Scally.

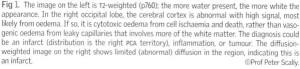

**1** Mitochondrial Encephalopathy with Lactic Acidosis & stroke-like episodes (MELAS). Episodes triggered by metabolic stress, with lactic acidosis ffl seizures. Due to a point mutation in mitochondrial DNA.
**2** Alteplase is licensed within 3h of onset of stroke, but ECASS3 and SITS studies show benefit up to 4.5h.[101,102] IST3 + meta-analyses suggest at up to 6h (also if >80yrs old).[103] ▶▶Best results are at <90min; *don't dawdle!*[104] Public health 'Brain Attack' awareness campaigns address this point: we should all know what the **FAST** acronym stands for: Facial weakness, Arm/leg weakness, or Speech difficulty = Time to act.
**3** Intra-arterial r-tPA has a role seen between 3 and 6h post symptom onset.[105]

**Primary prevention** *(ie before any stroke)* Control risk factors (p474): Look for and treat hypertension, DM, ↑lipids (p704; statins ↓risk by ~17%),[106] and cardiac disease (see BOX). Exercise helps (↑HDL, ↑glucose tolerance). Folate supplements[1] may also help somewhat (↓serum homocysteine).[107] *Help quit smoking:* ►p87. In middle-aged men (esp. if ↑BP), quitting ↓risk of stroke, with benefits seen in ≤5yrs (switching to pipes or cigars achieves little; former heavy smokers retain some excess risk). Use *lifelong anticoagulation* if rheumatic or prosthetic heart valves on left side, and consider in chronic non-rheumatic atrial fibrillation (AF), especially if there are other vascular risk factors (see BOX). For prevention post-TIA see p480.

**Secondary prevention** *(ie preventing further strokes)* Control risk factors (as *Primary prevention* above). Several large studies suggest considerable advantages from lowering blood pressure and cholesterol (even if not particularly raised). *Antiplatelet agents after stroke:* (assuming no primary haemorrhage on CT) Clopidogrel monotherapy is the best way to prevent CNS and heart events and is probably superior to aspirin plus slow-release dipyridamole. *Anticoagulation after stroke from AF:* Start warfarin if indicated (BOX), 2wks after the stroke (if clinically and radiologically small, from 7-10 days). Use antiplatelet therapy until anticoagulated; if anticoagulated already, replace with antiplatelet for 1wk. Warfarin CI: p344.

**Tests** (see p474 for imaging) Investigate promptly to identify risk factors for further strokes, but consider whether results will affect management. Look for:
- *Hypertension:* Look for retinopathy (p562), nephropathy, and a big heart on CXR. Raised BP is common in early stroke. In general, don't treat acutely.
- *Cardiac source of emboli:* (see also BOX) 24h ECG to look for atrial fibrillation (p124). CXR may show an enlarged left atrium. Echocardiogram may reveal mural thrombus due to AF or a hypokinetic segment of cardiac muscle post-MI. It may also show valvular lesions in infective endocarditis or rheumatic heart disease. Transoesophageal echo is more sensitive than transthoracic.
- *Carotid artery stenosis:* Do carotid Doppler ultrasound ± CT/MRI angiography. ≥70% stenosis is significant. Results of ECST-2 are awaited to see who benefits most from endarterectomy (earlier studies were in the pre-statin era). Endovascular carotid artery stenting is an alternative if not suitable for surgery, but safety and long-term benefits (in-stent re-stenosis) are problems.[108]
- *Hypoglycaemia, hyperglycaemia, dyslipidaemia* and *hyperhomocysteinaemia.*
- *Vasculitis:* ↑ESR, ANA +ve,[etc] (p558). VDRL to look for active, untreated syphilis (p431).
- *Prothrombotic states:* eg thrombophilia (p368), antiphospholipid syndrome (p556).
- *Hyperviscosity:* eg polycythaemia (p360), sickle-cell disease (p334).
- *Thrombocytopenia* and other bleeding disorders.
- *Genetic tests:* CADASIL (p474); Fabry's disease (x-linked, but some ♀ affected too).

**Prognosis** Good nursing (eg to prevent pressure ulcers—see fig 1) on a stroke unit, antiplatelet agents, and prompt intervention (eg after carotid Doppler imaging) are key. For those with a minor ischaemic stroke/TIA, urgent assessment and treatment saves lives (p480). *Overall mortality:* 60,000/yr; UK 20% at 1 month, then ≤10%/yr. *Full recovery:* ≤40%. Drowsiness≈poor prognosis. *Complications:* Aspiration pneumonia (keep 'nil by mouth' until assessed, p478); pressure sores (fig 1; turn regularly and keep dry—consider catheter); contractures; constipation; depression; "I'm a prisoner in my body"; stress in spouse (eg alcoholism), p449.

---

1 ↑Plasma homocysteine is associated more strongly with stroke risk than with cardiovascular risk. Folic acid lowers homocysteine and folic acid supplementation in grain food has been shown to be associated with a ↓stroke incidence in USA and Canada. Other studies show that any +ve effects on all-cause mortality of folic acid are likely to be small, at best (SEARCH, WENBIT, WAFACS, CHAOS-2, VISP, NORVIT, and HOPE-2 trials).[109-111]

## Cardiac causes of stroke

Cardioembolic causes are the source of stroke in >30% of patients in population studies. These may recur, unless you prevent them.

▶So examine the heart with as much attention as you examine the brain.

- *Non-valvular atrial fibrillation* is associated with an overall risk of stroke of 4.5%/yr. Age, prior stroke/TIA, diabetes and hypertension are additive risks. Ischaemic strokes in AF are often worse than ischaemic stroke with sinus rhythm. Warfarin (or dabigatran 150mg/12h PO, p125)[112] is effective for primary and secondary prevention of ischaemic stroke, reducing ↓risk by 68% (>80% if CHADS2 score[1] ≥2).[113] Aspirin alone may be OK if CHADS2 ≤1 (safer and needs no monitoring).[114] Explain risks and benefits of warfarin, and let the patient decide, giving a steer towards warfarin the higher CHADS2 is—if there are no contraindications (falls, poor compliance/concordance). If warfarin is chosen, aim for an INR of 2.5-3.5 (stroke risk doubles if INR ~1.7 vs 2). Adding aspirin to warfarin does not help. Warfarin can be stopped after ablation for AF if CHADS2 ≤3.[115]
- *External cardioversion* is complicated in 1-3% by peripheral emboli: pharmacological cardioversion may carry similar risks.
- *Prosthetic valves* risk major emboli; anticoagulate (INR 3.5-4.5, p345).
- *Acute myocardial infarct* with large left ventricular wall motion abnormalities on echocardiography predispose to left ventricular thrombus. Emboli arise in 10% of these patients in the next 6-12 months; risk is reduced by two-thirds by warfarin anticoagulation. Mural thrombus is best seen by echocardiography.
- *Paradoxical systemic emboli* via the venous circulation in those with patent foramen ovale, atrial and ventricular septal defects.
- *Cardiac surgery*, eg bypass graft, carries particular risk (0.9-5.2%).
- *Valve vegetations from SBE/IE* may embolize (p144). 20% of those with endocarditis present with CNS signs due to septic emboli from valves. ▶Is there fever or a murmur? Treat as endocarditis; ask a cardiologist's opinion.

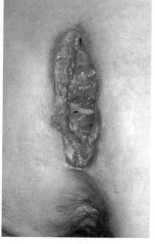

Fig 1. Sacral pressure ulcer after a stroke. Easy to prevent, given good nursing and nutrition—but so hard to treat, and so often a prelude to death. Lying still for too long also causes severe constipation and hypostatic pneumonia, eg in 9%.[116]

**1 The CHADS2 score** (see also CHA2DS2, p125)

| | |
|---|---|
| C Congestive heart failure | 1 |
| H Hypertension: blood pressure consistently above 140/90mmHg (or treated hypertension on medication) | 1 |
| A Age ≥75yrs | 1 |
| D Diabetes mellitus | 1 |
| S2 Prior stroke or TIA or thromboembolism | 2 |

Neurology

Enablement can focus on the specific disability or it can take a holistic approach and recognize that understanding an individual's past abilities is as important as knowing about present disabilities. *Summary of the Enablement Approach:*

&Give equal weight to assessing physical and cognitive function.

&Agree the tasks to be done. Which elements of each task is the person finding difficult? Don't be too helpful by taking over doing the whole task yourself.

&Assess risks involved in doing each task. How can these be reduced or avoided?

&Plan each small step. Agree realistic *relevant* goals, that can be achieved soon.

&Frequently review and reset specific goals.[117]

▶Each person is an individual and no two people will require the exact same support. 6 *points in the early management of stroke which bear on later plans:*

1 Watch the patient swallow a small volume of water; if signs of aspiration (a cough or voice change) make *nil by mouth* until formal assessment by a speech therapist. Use IV fluids, then semi-solids (eg jelly; avoid soups and crumbly food). Avoid early NG tube feeds (needed only in the few with established chronic swallowing problems). Speech therapists skilled in assessing swallowing difficulties are invaluable here.

2 Avoid falls and damaging patient's shoulders through careless lifting.

3 Ensure good bladder and bowel care through frequent toileting. Avoid early catheterization which may prevent return to continence.

4 Position to minimize spasticity (occurs in ~40%). Get prompt physiotherapy. Botulinum toxin injections are helpful for focal spasticity.[118]

5 Measure time taken to sit up, and to transfer from lying to sitting in a chair; this is a good way to monitor progress with physio/occupational therapy.[119]

6 In pseudo-emotionalism/emotional lability (sobbing unprovoked by sorrow, from failure of cortical inhibition of the limbic system), tricyclics or fluoxetine may help.

▶Involve the carer/spouse with all aspects of care-giving. Good rehab saves lives.

**Tests** Asking to point to a named part of the body tests perceptual function. Copying matchstick patterns tests spatial ability. Dressing or copying a clock face tests for *apraxia* (p80). Picking out and naming easy objects from a pile tests for agnosia (acuity OK, but cannot mime use; guesses are way-out, semantically, and phonetically). Screen for depression (low mood; inability to feel pleasure or to concentrate).

**Making physio fun** aids motivation, eg swimming (a hemiplegic arm may be supported on a special float), music and video games (↑recovery by aiding coordination).[120] The aim is to promote cerebral reorganization. To this end, constraint of the good arm has been found to be helpful (*constraint-induced movement therapy*).[121]

**End-of-life decisions** ▶If the patient's views are known, comply with them, except perhaps where doing so entails an illegal act, or one that clearly harms others.

&No person has authority to impose views on end-of-life decisions. You cannot tell a nurse to stop feeding someone, and expect her to obey you. Consensus is the only practical value. Try to get the opinion of more than one relative, and more than one shift of nurses (eg at changeover time). Let everyone have their say. You may learn new, important facts about your patient, which make decisions easier—or harder.

&If consensus is impossible, recourse to the Courts is one option: but remember that judges have no special skill in this area.

&Beware guidelines giving doctors special powers (such as the BMA guidelines).[122] Doctors may be the worst decision-makers as closeness to life and death may make them tolerant of ending life—eg if the bed could be used for 'something better'. Even if *not* the case, if society thinks this, then doctors are in an untenable position. We *do* have a role, though, in facilitating consensus, and documenting it.

Success is often impossible (there are too many grey areas), but if you can stumble from one ambiguity to another without being disheartened, then that is good enough. Your patients will respect your honesty.

## Assessing handicap, disability, and independence in daily life

*Handicap* entails inability to carry out social functions. 'A disadvantage for a given individual, resulting from an impairment or disability, that limits or prevents the fulfilment of a role.' Two people with the same *impairment* (eg paralysed arm) may have different *disabilities* (one can dress, the other cannot). Disabilities are likely to determine quality of future life. Treatment is often best aimed at reducing disability, not curing disease. For example, Velcro® fasteners in place of buttons may enable a person to dress.

A person with a severe hearing impairment may seem to you to have no disability if they can lip-read. But ask yourself (and your patients, when you get to know them) about the price they pay for rising above their disabilities. Lip-reading, for example, is exhausting, requiring 100% vigilance to make sense of transitory and incomplete visual clues.

### Barthel's index of activities of daily living

| | | |
|---|---|---|
| Bowels | 0 | Incontinent (or needs to be given enemas) |
| | 1 | Occasional accidents (once a week) |
| | 2 | Continent |
| Bladder | 0 | Incontinent, or catheter inserted but unable to manage it |
| | 1 | Occasional accidents (up to once per 24h) |
| | 2 | Continent (for more than 7 days) |
| Grooming | 0 | Needs help with personal care: face, hair, teeth, shaving |
| | 1 | Independent (implements provided) |
| Toilet use | 0 | Dependent |
| | 1 | Needs some help but can do some things alone |
| | 2 | Independent (on and off, wiping, dressing) |
| Feeding | 0 | Unable |
| | 1 | Needs help in cutting, spreading butter, etc. |
| | 2 | Independent (food provided within reach) |
| Transfer | 0 | Unable to get from bed to commode: the vital transfer to prevent the need for 24-hour nursing care |
| | 1 | Major help needed (physical, 1–2 people), can sit |
| | 2 | Minor help needed (verbal or physical) |
| | 3 | Independent |
| Mobility | 0 | Immobile |
| | 1 | Wheelchair-independent, including corners, etc. |
| | 2 | Walks with help of one person (verbal or physical) |
| | 3 | Independent |
| Dressing | 0 | Dependent |
| | 1 | Needs help but can do about half unaided |
| | 2 | Independent (including buttons, zips, laces, etc.) |
| Stairs | 0 | Unable |
| | 1 | Needs help (verbal, physical, carrying aid) |
| | 2 | Independent up and down |
| Bath/shower | 0 | Dependent |
| | 1 | Independent (must get in and out unaided and wash self) |

The aim is to establish the degree of independence from any help.

Mahoney FI, Barthel DW: Functional evaluation: the Barthel Index. *Maryland State Medical Journal.* 1965; 14:61–65. Used with permission.

**Barthel's paradox** The more we contemplate Barthel's eulogy of independence, the more we see it as a mirage reflecting a greater truth about human affairs: ►there is no such thing as independence[1]—only inter-dependence—and in fostering this interdependence lies our true vocation.

**1** No man is an Island, *intire of it selfe; every man is a peece of the Continent, a part of the maine; if a Clod bee washed away by the Sea, Europe is the lesse, as well as if a promontorie were, as well as if a Mannor of thy friends or of thine owne were. Any man's death diminishes me, because I am involved in mankinde; And therefore never send to know for whom the bell tolls: It tolls for thee.* John Donne 1572–1631; Meditation XVII.

What happens when we take up John Donne's offer of meditation? Some very interesting CNS events: brain activity slows, and blood is relocated to the anterior cingulate and dorsolateral prefrontal areas.[2]

The sudden onset of focal CNS phenomena due to temporary occlusion of part of the cerebral circulation, usually by emboli, is termed a TIA if symptoms last <24h (often much shorter). Incidence: 0.4/1000/yr. ▶▶15% of 1st strokes are preceded by TIAs; they are also harbingers of MI, so...*good management may avert disaster.*

**Signs of TIA** Attacks are single or many. Features of a TIA should always mimic those of a stroke in the same arterial territory (p453), and may be the same or different for each TIA. *Global* events (eg syncope, dizziness) are not typical of TIAs. Multiple highly stereotyped attacks suggest a critical intracranial stenosis (commonly the superior division of the MCA, p452). Emboli may also pass to the retinal artery, causing *amaurosis fugax* (one eye's vision is progressively lost "like a curtain descending over my field of view"). Limb-shaking TIAs may be mistaken for a focal motor seizure.

**Signs of causes** Carotid bruit (p38), but absence does not rule out a carotid source of emboli: tight stenoses often have *no* bruit;[124] BP↑; heart murmur from valve disease; atrial fibrillation. Fundoscopy during TIAs may show retinal artery emboli.

**Causes** (see also p474) *Atherothromboembolism* from the carotid is the chief cause. *Cardioembolism:* mural thrombus post-MI or in AF, valve disease, prosthetic valve. *Hyperviscosity:* (p366), eg polycythaemia, sickle-cell anaemia, WCC↑↑ (leukostasis; may need urgent chemotherapy), myeloma.[125] *Vasculitis* (eg cranial arteritis, PAN, SLE, syphilis, etc) is a rare cause, and perhaps shouldn't be classified as TIA.

**Differential** Hypoglycaemia, migraine aura (symptoms spread and intensify over minutes, often with visual scintillations), focal epilepsy (symptoms spread over seconds and often include twitching and jerking), hyperventilation, retinal bleeds. *Rare mimics of TIA:* Malignant hypertension, MS (paroxysmal dysarthria), intracranial tumours, peripheral neuropathy, phaeochromocytoma, somatization.

**Tests** Aim to find the cause and define vascular risk: FBC, ESR, U&Es, glucose, lipids, CXR, ECG, carotid Doppler ± angiography, CT or diffusion-weighted MRI (any existing infarcts? If bilateral, it suggests cardioembolism), echocardiogram (rarely shows cardiac cause if no suggestive signs).

**Treatment** ▶▶Time to intervention is crucial. Risk of stroke within 90 days of TIA is 2% in those treated within 72h of TIA, compared to 10% in those treated by 3wks.[126]
• *Control cardiovascular risk factors:* ↑BP (cautiously lower; aim for <140/85mmHg, p134); hyperlipidaemia (p704); DM (p198); help to stop smoking (p87 & OHCS p512).
• *Antiplatelet drugs:* **Clopidogrel** (75mg/d), a thienopyridine that inhibits platelet aggregation by modifying platelet ADP receptors, prevents further strokes and MIs, as does (to a lesser extent) aspirin 300mg/d (↓after 2wks 75mg/d). NB: dipyridamole MR 200mg/12h should be added to aspirin, where used. Dipyridamole ↑cAMP and ↓thromboxane A2.
• *Warfarin indications:* Cardiac emboli (eg AF, mitral stenosis, recent big septal MI).
• *Carotid endarterectomy* If ≥70% stenosis at the origin of the internal carotid artery and operative risk is good.[1][124][127] Surgery should be performed within 2 weeks of first presentation.[128] Operating on 50–70% stenoses may be valuable if the team's perioperative stroke and mortality rate <3%.[129] Intra-operative transcranial Doppler can monitor middle cerebral artery flow. Using patches may reduce chance of restenosis. Do not stop aspirin beforehand. Endovascular carotid artery stenting is an alternative if not suitable for surgery, but safety and long-term benefits (in-stent restenosis is common) remain under investigation.[108]

**Driving** Avoid for 1 month; patients in the UK should inform the DVLA only if multiple attacks in short period or residual deficit.

**Prognosis** The combined risk of stroke and MI is ~9%/yr; if carotid stenosis is ≥70% risk of stroke ↑ to 12% in 1st year and up to 10% subsequently. More frequent TIAs ↑ risk yet further. Mortality is ~3-fold that of a TIA-free matched population. In one Dutch study in 2005, 60% of patients were dead within 10 years of a TIA.[130]

---

**1** *Who risks death/CVA from endarterectomy?* ♀ sex, >75yrs old, systolic BP↑, contralateral artery occluded; stenosis of ipsilateral carotid syphon/external carotid; wide-territory TIAs (against just amaurosis fugax).

## ►► When should TIA lead to prompt or emergency referral?

An ABCD2 score[131] of ≥6 (see TABLE) strongly predicts a stroke (8.1% within 2 days, 35.5% in the next week). Patients with a score ≥4 should be assessed by a specialist within 24h, and all patients with a suspected TIA should be seen within 7 days.

| Age ≥60 yrs old | 1 point |
|---|---|
| Blood pressure ≥140/90 | 1 point |
| Clinical features | |
| Unilateral weakness | 2 points |
| Speech disturbance without weakness | 1 point |
| Duration of symptoms | |
| Symptoms lasting ≥1h | 2 points |
| Symptoms lasting 10–59min | 1 point |
| Diabetes | 1 point |

In assessing urgency, bear in mind Warlow's 2005 data: in stroke patients who had a preceding TIA, 17% occurred on the day of the stroke, 9% on the previous day, and 43% at some point during the 7 days before the stroke.[132] These sobering figures should remind us to rehearse routes for referral for emergency endarterectomy—at present this is typically performed >90 days post-TIA.[133]

Neurology

Neurology

Spontaneous bleeding into the subarachnoid space is often catastrophic. *Incidence:* 9/100,000/yr; typical age: 35–65. *Causes:* Rupture of saccular aneurysms (80%); arteriovenous malformations (AVM; 15%). No cause is found in <15%. *Risk factors:* Smoking, alcohol misuse, BP↑,[1] bleeding disorders, mycotic aneurysm (SBE), perhaps post-menopausal ↓ oestrogen (♀:♂≈3:2 if >45yrs old).[134] Close relatives have 3–5-fold ↑risk of SAH.[135]

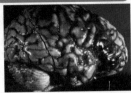

Fig 1. Middle cerebral artery SAH at the Sylvian fissure. ©Dr D Hamoudi

**Berry aneurysms** Common sites: junction of posterior communicating with the internal carotid or of the anterior communicating with the anterior cerebral artery or bifurcation of the middle cerebral artery (figs 1, 2 & fig 1, p452). 15% are multiple. Some are hereditary. *Associations:* Polycystic kidneys, coarctation of the aorta, Ehlers-Danlos syndrome (hypermobile joints with ↑skin elasticity, *OHCS* p642).

**Symptoms** Sudden (usually, but not always, within seconds)[136] devastating typically occipital headache—"I thought I'd been kicked in the head". Vomiting, collapse, seizures and coma often follow. Coma/drowsiness may last for days.

**Signs** Neck stiffness, Kernig's sign (takes 6h to develop), retinal, subhyaloid and vitreous bleeds (=Terson's syndrome; it carries a worse prognosis: mortality ↑×5).[137] Focal neurology at *presentation* may suggest site of aneurysm (eg pupil changes indicating a III^rd nerve palsy with a posterior communicating artery aneurysm) or intracerebral haematoma. Later deficits suggest complications (see below).[138]

**Differential** In primary care, only 25% of those with severe, sudden 'thunderclap' headache have SAH. In 50–60%, no cause is found; the remainder have meningitis, migraine, intracerebral bleeds, or cortical vein thrombosis (p484).

**Sentinel headache** SAH patients may earlier have experienced a sentinel headache, perhaps due to a small warning leak from the offending aneurysm (~6%), but recall-bias clouds the picture.[138] As surgery is more successful in the least symptomatic, be suspicious of any *sudden* headache especially with neck or back pain.[138]

**Tests** CT detects >90% of SAH within the 1^st 48h (fig 3).[139] LP if CT −ve and no contraindication >12h after headache onset. CSF in SAH is uniformly bloody early on, and becomes xanthochromic (yellow) after several hours due to breakdown products of Hb (bilirubin). Finding xanthochromia confirms SAH, showing that the LP was not a 'bloody tap' (don't rely on finding fewer CSF RBCs in each successive bottle).

**Management** ▶Refer all proven SAH to neurosurgery immediately.
- Re-examine CNS often; chart BP, pupils and GCS (p802). Repeat CT if deteriorating.
- Maintain cerebral perfusion by keeping well hydrated, and aim for <160mmHg.
- Nimodipine (60mg/4h PO for 3wks, or 1mg/h IVI) is a Ca²⁺ antagonist that reduces vasospasm and consequent morbidity from cerebral ischaemia.
- Endovascular coiling is preferred to surgical clipping where possible (7% ↑ in independent survival over 7yrs follow-up, but ↑ risk of rebleeding).[140] Do catheter or CT angiography to identify single *vs* multiple aneurysms *before* intervening. Intracranial stents and balloon remodelling enable treating wide-necked aneurysms. Microcatheters can now traverse tortuous vessels to treat previously unreachable lesions.[141] AV malformations and fistulae may also benefit from this.

**Complications** *Rebleeding* is the commonest cause of death, and occurs in 20%, often in the 1^st few days. *Cerebral ischaemia* due to vasospasm may cause a permanent CNS deficit, and is the commonest cause of morbidity. If this happens, surgery is not helpful at the time but may be so later. *Hydrocephalus*, due to blockage of arachnoid granulations, requires a ventricular or lumbar drain. *Hyponatraemia* is common but should not be managed with fluid restriction. Seek expert help.

---

1 For each 20mmHg rise in systolic BP, relative risks of ischaemic stroke, intracerebral haemorrhage, and subarachnoid haemorrhage are 1.8, 2.5, and 1.6 in ♂, and 1.6, 3.1, and 2.3 in ♀, respectively.[142]

## Mortality in subarachnoid haemorrhage

| Grade | Signs | Mortality: % |
|---|---|---|
| I | None | 0 |
| II | Neck stiffness and cranial nerve palsies | 11 |
| III | Drowsiness | 37 |
| IV | Drowsy with hemiplegia | 71 |
| V | Prolonged coma | 100 |

Almost all the mortality occurs in the 1st month. Of those who survive the 1st month, 90% survive a year or more.

### Unruptured aneurysms: 'the time-bomb in my head'

Bear in mind the old adage: 'if it ain't broke; don't fix it'—usually, risks of *preventive* intervention outweigh any benefits, except perhaps in young patients (more years at risk, and surgery is twice as hazardous if >45yrs old)[143] who have aneurysms >7mm in diameter, especially if located at the junction of the internal carotid and the posterior communicating cerebral artery, or at the rostral basilar artery bifurcation, and especially if there is uncontrolled hypertension or a past history of bleeds.[143] Data from the 2003 International Study of Unruptured Intracranial Aneurysms (ISUIA) show that relative risk of rupture for an aneurysm 7–12mm across is 3.3 compared with aneurysms <7mm across; if the diameter is >12mm, the relative risk is 17.[144]

Patients with a *previous SAH* have a raised risk for new aneurysm formation and enlargement of untreated aneurysms. Screening these patients might be beneficial, eg if multiple aneurysms, hypertension, or a history of smoking.[145]

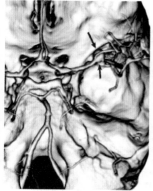

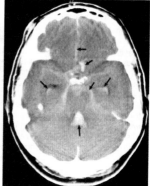

**Fig 2.** CT images can be manipulated to show only high-density structures such as bones and arteries containing contrast. Here is a middle cerebral artery aneurysm.

**Fig 3.** Blood from a ruptured aneurysm occupies the interhemispheric fissure (top arrow), a crescentic intracerebral area presumably near the aneurysm (2nd arrow), the basal cisterns, the lateral ventricles (temporal horns), and the 4th ventricle (bottom arrow).

We thank Prof. Peter Scally for these CT images and the commentaries on them.

Neurology

**Dural venous sinus thrombosis** Most commonly sagittal sinus thrombosis (figs 1 & 2; 47% of all IVT) or transverse sinus thrombosis (35%). Sagittal sinus thrombosis often coexists if other sinuses are thrombosed. Symptoms come on gradually over days or weeks. Thrombosis within a dural venous sinus may extend into the cortical veins and cause infarction within a venous territory (fig 3; see under *Cortical vein thrombosis* below for symptoms and signs).

- *Sagittal sinus:* Headache, vomiting, seizures, ↓vision, papilloedema.
- *Transverse sinus:* Headache ± mastoid pain, focal CNS signs, seizures, papilloedema.
- *Sigmoid sinus:* Cerebellar signs, lower cranial nerve palsies.
- *Inferior petrosal sinus:* Vᵗʰ and VIᵗʰ cranial nerve palsies, which, with temporal and retro-orbital pain, comprise Gradenigo's syndrome.[149]
- *Cavernous sinus:* Often due to spread from facial pustules or folliculitis, causing headache, chemosis, oedematous eyelids, proptosis, painful ophthalmoplegia, fever.[150]

**Cortical vein thrombosis (CVT)** Often causes venous infarcts, with stroke-like focal symptoms that develop over days. However, the associated headache may come on suddenly (thunderclap headache).[151] Seizures are common, unlike in arterial stroke, and focal (p494). It usually occurs with sinus thromboses.[152] Galen vein thrombosis is a rare cause of CVT and is usually associated with vascular malformation.[153] *Signs:* Encephalopathy, focal seizures, headache (including thunderclap headache), slowly evolving focal deficits (paresis, speech disorders, cognition↓, vision↓).

**Differential diagnosis** Subarachnoid haemorrhage (p482; thunderclap headaches also occur in dissection of a carotid or vertebral artery, and in benign thunderclap headache, triggered by Valsalva manoeuvre (eg cough, coitus)), meningitis, encephalitis, intracranial abscess, arterial infarction.

**Investigations** Exclude SAH if thunderclap headache (p482). Check there are no signs of meningitis (p832). *Imaging:* CT/MRI venography may show the absence of a sinus (fig 1), though an absent transverse sinus can be a normal variant. MRI T2-weighted gradient echo sequences can visualize thrombus directly (fig 2), and also identify haemorrhagic infarction.[154] CT may be normal early; then at ~1wk develops the delta sign, where a transversely cut sinus shows a contrast filling defect. *Lumbar puncture* (unless CI by MRI/CT): if raised opening CSF pressure, with persistent headache and SAH excluded, suspect cerebral vein thrombosis. CSF may be normal, or show RBCs and xanthochromia.

**Management** Seek expert help. Heparin improves outcome,[155] possibly even in those with haemorrhagic venous infarction. Fibrinolytics (eg streptokinase) have been used via selective catheterization.[156,157] Thrombophilia screen and ENT review to help identify the cause.

**Prognosis** Variable. Death is mainly due to transtentorial herniation from unilateral focal mass effects or diffuse oedema, and multiple parenchymal lesions. Independent predictors of death in one study were coma (odds ratio OR≈8.8), deep cortical vein thrombosis (OR≈8.5), posterior fossa lesion (OR≈6.5) right intracerebral haemorrhage (OR≈3.4), and mental disturbance (OR≈2.5). Evolving focal deficits are also associated with ↑ mortality.[158]

| Common causes |
|---|
| • Pregnancy/puerperium |
| • Oral contraceptives |
| • Head injury |
| • Dehydration |
| • Blood dyscrasias |
| • Intracranial malignancy (local invasion/pressure) |
| • Extracranial malignancy (hypercoagulability) |
| • Recent LP |

| Systemic causes |
|---|
| • Hyperthyroidism |
| • Nephrosis |
| • Ketoacidosis[146] |
| • Heart failure |
| • SLE |
| • Homocystinuria |
| • Hyperviscosity (p366) |
| • Crohn's or UC (p272-4) |
| • Behçet's disease (p708) |
| • Activated protein C resistance (p368) |
| • Antiphospholipid syn |
| • Klippel-Trénaunay syn |
| • Paroxysmal nocturnal haemoglobinuria |

| Infectious causes |
|---|
| • Meningitis; TB |
| • Cerebral abscess |
| • Septicaemia |
| • Fungal infections |
| • Otitis media |
| • Cerebral malaria |
| • HIV with nephrosis |

| Drug causes |
|---|
| • Androgens, eg oxymetholone[147] |
| • Antifibrinolytics, eg tranexamic acid |
| • Infliximab[148] |

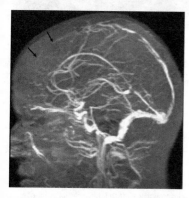

**Fig 1.** This magnetic resonance venogram (MRV) could look normal at first glance: the hardest thing to see in imaging is often that which is not there. Much of the superior sagittal sinus is not seen because it is filled with clot—a superior sagittal sinus thrombosis. The arrows point to where it should be seen. Posteriorly, the irregularity of the vessel indicates non-occlusive clot.

Image and commentary courtesy of Prof. P. Scally.

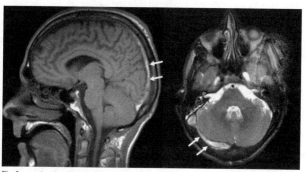

**Fig 2.** MRI showing thrombus (arrows) in the sagittal sinus (sagittal T1-weighted image, LEFT), and in the right transverse sinus (axial T2-weighted image, RIGHT). Often more than one sinus is involved.

Image courtesy of Dr David Werring.

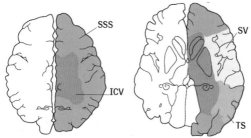

**Fig 3.** Venous territories (compare with arterial territories on p453). SSS—superior sagittal sinus; TS—transverse sinus; SV—Sylvian veins; ICV—internal cortical veins.

There is much greater variation in venous anatomy between individuals than there is in arterial anatomy, so this diagram is only a rough guide. The key point is to realize that infarction that crosses boundaries between arterial territories may be venous in origin.

Neurology

▶Consider this very treatable condition in all whose conscious level fluctuates, and also in those having an 'evolving stroke', especially if on anticoagulants. Bleeding is from bridging veins between cortex and venous sinuses (vulnerable to deceleration injury), resulting in accumulating haematoma between dura and arachnoid. This gradually raises ICP, shifting midline structures away from the side of the clot and, if untreated, eventual tentorial herniation and coning. Most subdurals are from trauma but the trauma is *often forgotten as it was so minor or so long ago* (up to 9 months).[159] It can also occur without trauma (eg ↓ICP;[1] dural metastases).[160] The elderly are most susceptible, as brain atrophy makes bridging veins vulnerable. *Other risk factors:* falls (epileptics, alcoholics); anticoagulation.

**Symptoms** Fluctuating level of consciousness (seen in 35%) ± insidious physical or intellectual slowing, sleepiness, headache, personality change, and unsteadiness.

**Signs** ↑ICP (p840); seizures. Localizing neurological symptoms (eg unequal pupils, hemiparesis) occur late and often long after the injury (mean=63 days).

**Imaging** (figs 1 & 2) CT/MRI shows clot ± midline shift (but beware bilateral isodense clots). Look for crescent-shaped collection of blood over 1 hemisphere. The sickle-shape differentiates subdural blood from extradural haemorrhage.

**ΔΔ** Stroke, dementia, CNS masses (eg tumours, abscess, neurocysticercosis).[161]

**Treatment** Irrigation/evacuation, eg via burr twist drill and burr hole craniostomy, can be considered 1st-line; craniotomy is 2nd-line,[162] if the clot has organized.[163] Address causes of the trauma (eg falls due cataract or arrhythmia; abuse).

## Extradural (epidural) haemorrhage

▶*Suspect this if, after head injury, conscious level falls or is slow to improve, or there is a lucid interval.* Extradural bleeds are often due to a fractured temporal or parietal bone causing laceration of the middle meningeal artery and vein, typically after trauma to a temple just lateral to the eye. Any tear in a dural venous sinus will also result in an extradural bleed. Blood accumulates between bone and dura.

**The patient** Beware deteriorating consciousness after any head injury that initially produced no loss of consciousness or after initial drowsiness post injury seems to have resolved. This **lucid interval** pattern is typical of extradural bleeds (ΔΔ: epilepsy,[164] carotid dissection,[165] and carbon monoxide poisoning).[166] It may last a few hours to a few days before a bleed declares itself by ↓GCS from rising ICP. Increasingly severe headache, vomiting, confusion, and fits follow, ± hemiparesis with brisk reflexes and an upgoing plantar. If bleeding continues, the ipsilateral pupil dilates, coma deepens, bilateral limb weakness develops, and breathing becomes deep and irregular (brainstem compression). Death follows a period of coma and is due to respiratory arrest. Bradycardia and raised blood pressure are late signs.

**Tests** CT (fig 3) shows a haematoma (often biconvex/lens-shaped; the blood forms a more rounded shape compared with the sickle-shaped subdural haematoma as the tough dural attachments to the skull keep it more localized). Skull x-ray may be normal or show fracture lines crossing the course of the middle meningeal vessels. Skull fracture after trauma greatly increases risk of an extradural haemorrhage, and should lead to prompt CT. ▶*Lumbar puncture is contraindicated.*

**Management** ▶▶Stabilize and transfer urgently (with skilled medical and nursing escorts) to a neurosurgical unit for clot evacuation ± ligation of the bleeding vessel. Care of the airway in an unconscious patient and measures to ↓ICP often require intubation and ventilation (+ mannitol IVI, p841).

**Prognosis** Excellent if diagnosis and operation early. Poor if coma, pupil abnormalities, or decerebrate rigidity are present pre-op.

---

1 *Intracranial hypotension* (↓ICP) is due to CSF leaks, amenable to epidural blood patches over the leak.[167] Suspect if headaches are worse on standing.[168] *Causes:* arachnoid diverticula/dural ectasia (eg in Marfan's syndrome); after lumbar puncture or epidural anaesthesia; dehydration; hyperpnoea (↑tidal volume). *MRI:* engorged venous sinuses, meningeal enhancement, and subdural fluid.

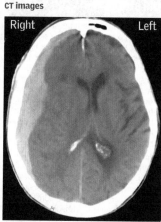

**Fig 1.** This image explains the cause as well as the pathology. On the patient's left, cerebral sulci are prominent and prior to this adverse event would have been even larger. The brain had shrunk within the skull as a result of atherosclerosis, and poor perfusion, leaving large subarachnoid spaces. A simple, quick rotation of the head is enough to tear a bridging vein, causing this *acute subdural haematoma*.

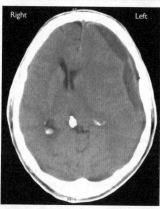

**Fig 2.** This fluid collection is of low attenuation compared to the brain, except for a small area of increased attenuation. It is an *acute on chronic (mixed-density) subdural haematoma*. But there is more! Look at the shift of midline structures across under the falx cerebri—subfalcine herniation. It is not just caused by the subdural. The left hemisphere is swollen as a result of the compression of the bridging veins in the subdural space, shifting the ventricles and calcified pineal across to the right.

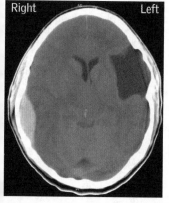

**Fig 3.** The blood (high attenuation, fusiform or biconvex collection) on the right side is limited anteriorly by the coronal suture and posteriorly by the lambdoid suture. This is therefore an *extradural haematoma*. The low attenuation CSF density collection on the left is causing scalloping of the overlying bone. It is in the typical location of an arachnoid cyst; an incidental finding of a congenital abnormality.

We thank Professor Peter Scally for the images and commentary.

20% of elderly patients on medical and surgical wards have some form of delirium:[1] consider *any* acute fluctuating baffling behaviour change as possible delirium. Look for organic causes (UTI, pneumonia, MI). The 8 signs of DELIRIUM are:

*Disordered thinking:* slow, irrational, rambling, jumbled up, incoherent ideas.
*Euphoric, fearful, depressed or angry:* Labile mood, eg anxious then torpid.
*Language impaired:* Speech is reduced or gabbling, repetitive, and disruptive.
*Illusions/delusions/hallucinations:* Tactile or visual (auditory suggests psychosis).
*Reversal of sleep-awake cycle:* May be drowsy by day and hypervigilant at night.
*Inattention:* Focusing, sustaining, or shifting attention is poor; no real dialogue.
*Unaware/disorientated:* Doesn't know it's evening, or his own name, or location.
*Memory deficits:* Often marked. (Later he may be amnesic for the episode.)
*Summary:* Globally impaired cognition and impaired awareness/consciousness.

**Illustration from Conrad's** *Heart of Darkness* 'The wastes of his weary brain were haunted by shadowy images now—images of wealth and fame...Sometimes he was contemptibly childish. He desired to have kings meet him at railway-stations on his return from some ghastly Nowhere ..."Close the shutter", said Kurtz suddenly "I can't bear to look at this." I did so. There was a silence. "Oh, but I will wring your heart yet!" he cried at the invisible wilderness.'[169] Impaired consciousness is difficult to describe (which is why we have to resort to Conrad—the master of multilayered descriptions). When you talk to the patient you have the sense that he is not with you, but away with the fairies—inaccessible and lost.

**Causes** (Pain and other psychological states are important co-factors.)
• Systemic infection: pneumonia, UTI, malaria, wounds, IV lines.
• Intracranial infection: encephalitis, meningitis.
• Drugs: opiates, anticonvulsants, levodopa, sedatives, recreational, post-GA.
• Alcohol withdrawal (2-5d post-admission; ↑LFTs, ↑MCV; history of alcohol abuse). Also drug withdrawal. See p282 for management of alcohol withdrawal.
• Metabolic: uraemia, liver failure, Na⁺ or glucose ↑↓, Hb↓, malnutrition (beri-beri, p278).
• Hypoxia: respiratory or cardiac failure.
• Vascular: stroke, myocardial infarction.
• Head injury, ↑ICP, space-occupying lesions (eg tumour, subdural haematoma).
• Epilepsy: non-convulsive status epilepticus (see BOX 2), post-ictal states.
• Nutritional: thiamine, nicotinic acid, or B₁₂ deficiency.

**Differential** If agitated, is it **anxiety**? Check conscious level. If delusions or hallucinations, is it a **primary mental illness** (eg schizophrenia), but this is rare on the wards (esp. if no past history) and delirium is very common in ill patients.

**Tests** Consider FBC, U&E, LFT, blood glucose, ABG, septic screen (urine dipstick, CXR, blood cultures); also ECG, malaria films, LP, EEG, CT/MRI.

**Management** After identifying and treating the underlying cause, aim to:
• Reduce distress and prevent accidents; encourage family to sit with the patient.
• Nurse in a *moderately lit*, quiet room, ideally with the *same* staff in attendance (minimizes confusion) where the patient can be watched closely. Improve orientation to time and place—**hunt down hearing aids/glasses**, give repeated reassurance.
• Do not use physical restraints—and remove catheters and other impedimenta.
• Augment self-care. Discourage passive dependency and inappropriate napping.
• Use the 3M non-drug cures for agitation: music, massage, and muscle relaxation.
• Minimize medication (especially sedatives); but if disruptive, some sedation may be wanted, eg haloperidol 0.5-2mg, or chlorpromazine 50-100mg, PO if they will take it, IM if not (p11). Wait 20min to judge effect—further doses can be given if needed. NB: Avoid chlorpromazine in the elderly and in alcohol withdrawal (p282).

►Be aware that delirium may persist beyond the duration of the original illness by several weeks in the elderly. Do not assume this must be dementia—provide support and reassess 1-2 months later.

---

**1** Delirium, from the latin *de* (from) and *lira* (ridge between furrows), meaning 'out of one's furrow'.

## 48

## Tests of consciousness, and an explanation of dissociative states

Consciousness results wherever four entities co-exist: perception, memory, emotion, and orientation in space and time. Remorse, for example, is a blend of these constructs. If a black box exhibited remorse no further test would be needed to establish its consciousness. Patients are often black boxes to us: we are never *sure* what is going on inside. How do we find out? Dialogue is the first method. Patients with clouding of consciousness often engage in dialogue, but we get the feeling that they are not quite with us. A conversation may suggest clouding of consciousness—until the moment when the patient makes an ironic remark, banishing the need for formal tests of consciousness.

If a patient knows where he is, the time of day, and his memory is OK, we think there is no problem with consciousness—and move on to more mundane issues. This is a pity because changes in consciousness are often subtle—and we need to ask others who know the patient well if there has been any change. So elucidating changes in consciousness depends on triangulation between 3 interacting centres of consciousness—our own, the patient's, and a third party. These issues are exemplified in the next boxes, where we illustrate the concept of derealization. Here, it is enough to say that *depersonalization* and *derealization* are part of the *dissociative states* (one example of a disorder of consciousness). Dissociation is a mechanism that separates streams of memories or thoughts from 'now' consciousness. These fragments may resurface and pursue a life of their own. *Causes:* migraine, epilepsy, head injury, stress, and prolonged sleeplessness (which is why all doctors instinctively understand this odd syndrome).

## Non-convulsive status epilepticus as a cause of confusion

Non-convulsive status epilepticus is under-diagnosed, and may manifest as confusion, impaired cognition/memory, odd behaviour, and dreamy derealization[170] (the external world appears unfamiliar and unreal—its objects, anchored neither in space nor time, float as in a more or less lucid dream). Other features: aggression, psychosis ± abnormalities of eye movement, eyelid myoclonus, and odd postures. It may occur in the context of classic convulsive seizures (eg prolonged 'post-ictal' state) or ischaemic brain injury (especially haemorrhagic).[171] Other causes/associations: drugs (eg antidepressants), infections (arboviruses; HIV; syphilis), neoplasia, dementia, sudden ↑↓$Ca^{2+}$,[172] renal failure (eg with cephalosporin therapy or peritoneal dialysis). *Diagnosis:* EEG evidence of rhythmical discharges (eg prolonged 3-per-second spike-wave complexes). Subsequent MRI may show focal oedema (eg in the hippocampus). ℞: lorazepam 2mg IV as 1st-line. Valproate IV may be indicated (this requires specialist evaluation).

## Ganser syndrome—an example of dissociative symptoms

There are absurd or approximate answers to questions (*paralogias*)—wrong but suggesting that the answers are unconsciously known but have been passed by or half-ignored by the current (dissociated) stream of consciousness. There are also: clouding of consciousness (or hypervigilance); somatic conversion symptoms (eg inexplicable paralysis—formerly known as hysterical symptoms); hallucinations; and amnesia, regarding the episode. *Causes/associations:* head injury, Munchausen's syndrome, solitary confinement, very stressful events.[173]

When asked to spell WORLD backwards, one Ganser patient replied 'EBOLG'. When asked to recall the words 'honesty', 'window', and 'lace', he replied 'modesty', 'house', and 'shoes'.[174] *NB:* ▸ictal and post-ictal states may present with similarly impaired consciousness, perceptual abnormalities, and odd behaviour.

Dementia is a syndrome encompassing progressive deficits in several cognitive domains. The initial presentation is usually of memory loss over months or years (►if over days think infection or stroke; if over weeks think depression). In later stages, non-cognitive symptoms such as agitation, aggression or apathy may complicate care, which becomes increasingly difficult requiring specialist input.

**Prevalence** Rare if <5yrs of age; 5–10% if >65yrs; 20% if >80yrs; 70% if >100yrs.

**Diagnosis** The key is a good history both from the patient and someone who knows them well (eg spouse, relatives, or friends). Ask about the *timeline* of the progression of their impaired cognition/memory, what was noticed first and what particular aspects of it they have most difficulty with (autobiographical, political,[1] etc). Ask also about how it affects their *activities of daily living*, and their ability to cope with tasks such as *financial affairs* and *medications*—some may cope well with significant impairment, others may be disproportionately affected. Examples from the spouse or relative will be helpful. There may also be agitation, aggression, wandering, hallucinations, slow repetitious speech, apathy, mood disturbance (NB: depression is common in dementia, but can also cause cognitive impairment). *Cognitive testing:* use a validated dementia screen such as the AMTS (p70), TYM (p85), or similar, plus short tests of verbal recall (eg HVLT, which is more sensitive in mild impairment) and executive function (eg CLOX).[175] *Mental state examination* may reveal anxiety, depression or hallucinations. *Physical examination* may identify a physical cause of the cognitive impairment, risk factors (esp. for vascular dementia), or parkinsonism.

**Investigations** FBC, ESR, U&E, $Ca^{2+}$, LFT, TSH, autoantibodies, $B_{12}$/folate (treat low-normals, p328); syphilis serology.[176] CT/MRI (for vascular damage, haemorrhage or structural pathology). Consider also: EEG, CSF, functional imaging (FDG, PET, SPECT).[177] Metabolic, genetic, and HIV tests if indicated.

**Commonest causes** *Alzheimer's disease (AD)* See p492.

*Vascular dementia:* ~25% of all dementias. It represents the cumulative effects of many small strokes, thus sudden onset and stepwise deterioration is characteristic (but often hard to recognize). Look for evidence of vascular pathology (BP↑, past strokes, focal CNS signs).

*Lewy body dementia:* The 3rd commonest cause (15–25%) after Alzheimer's and vascular causes, typically with fluctuating cognitive impairment, detailed visual hallucinations (eg small animals or children) and later, parkinsonism (p498). Histology is characterized by Lewy bodies[2] in brainstem and neocortex.

| Ameliorable causes |
|---|
| • $T_4$↓; $B_{12}$/folate↓ |
| • Thiamine↓ (eg alcohol) |
| • Syphilis |
| • Tumours (meningioma) |
| • Subdural haematoma |
| • Parkinson's (p498) |
| • CNS cysticercosis (p444) |
| • HIV (± cryptococcosis) |
| • Normal pressure hydrocephalus (dilated ventricles *without* enlarged cerebral sulci. *Signs:* gait apraxia, incontinence, dementia; CSF shunts help) |
| • Whipple's disease (p730) |
| • Pellagra (p278) |

*Fronto-temporal (Pick's[3]) dementia:* Frontal & temporal atrophy without Alzheimer histology (p493); genes on chromosome 9 are important, as in MND (p510). *Signs:* Executive impairment; behavioural/personality change; early preservation of episodic memory and spatial orientation; disinhibition (not *always* bad[4]); hyperorality, stereotyped behaviour, and emotional unconcern.

*Other causes:* Alcohol/drug abuse; repeated head trauma; pellagra (p278), Whipple's disease (p730); Huntington's (p716); CJD (p710); Parkinson's (p498); HIV; cryptococcosis (p440); familial autosomal dominant Alzheimer's; CADASIL (p474).

---

1 Autobiographical and political memory are held in different areas: S Black 2004 *Neuropsychologia* 42 25.
2 Lewy bodies are eosinophilic intracytoplasmic neuronal inclusion bodies; there is overlap between Lewy body dementia, Alzheimer's and Parkinson's (PD), making treatment hard as L-dopa can precipitate delusions, and antipsychotic drugs worsen PD. Rivastigmine may help all 3.[178]
3 Pick's dementia is a term now reserved for fronto-temporal dementia with Pick inclusion bodies.
4 ☺An artist who had been constrained by over-adherence to one school of art had a fascinating blossoming of creativity and emotional insight with the arrival of fronto-temporal dementia.[178] Similarly, the unique writing style of 19th century critic and author John Ruskin is thought to be a consequence of CADASIL. This poses the question of what counts as a disease. If you can answer this question unequivocally perhaps you are over-endowed, fronto-temporally? Let some ambiguity in!

## 49

### The positive features of dementia (Auntie Kathleen's syndrome)

Positive features include wandering, aggression, flight of ideas, and logorrhoea:

"Not for her a listless, dull-eyed wordless decline; with her it is all rush, gabble, celerity. She had always been a talker, but now her dementia unleashes torrents of speech...one train of thought switching to another without signal or pause, rattling across points and through junctions at a rate no listener can follow... Following the sense is like trying to track a particular ripple in a pelting torrent of talk."

Alan Bennett *Untold Stories*, 87

### Practical issues in managing dementia

• Patients with dementia become increasingly dependent and develop increasingly complex needs as the disease progresses. Most will at some stage experience behavioural or psychological symptoms, which can be particularly distressing for the carer. ►See *Living with neurological disease*, p449. Issues to consider are:
• *A care coordinator* (via Social Services or the local Old Age Community Mental Healthcare Team) is vital to coordinate the various teams and services that may at various times become necessary, and to arrange the *special help* that is available for those caring for demented relatives at home, eg in the UK:
    • Laundry services for soiled linen
    • Car badge giving priority parking
    • Carers' groups for mutual support
    • Help from occupational therapist, district nurses, and community psychiatric nurses
    • Attendance allowance
    • Respite care in hospital
    • Day care/lunch clubs
    • Council tax rebate (forms from local council office)
• *Capacity:* Can the patient make decisions regarding medical or financial affairs? Wherever possible, allow the patient to guide decisions. If currently capacitous suggest making an advanced directive or appointing a Lasting Power of Attorney.
• *Develop routines:* Routines learned early on are retained until late in the disease, helping patients to maintain their independence for longer. Habitually keeping house keys in the same place, for example, will help to avoid losing them by forgetting their whereabouts later on.
• *Plan ahead:* Relocation to a new house or to a care home can be very disruptive for a patient with dementia. Discuss this with the patient and their family. If the family are keen to help but live far away, consider moving earlier rather than later, when a new environment will be harder to become accustomed to. Equally, regular respite visits to the same care home may make a final move there easier at a later date.
• *Day services* can be invaluable for stimulating patients and providing regular, much-needed breaks for carers. Multisensory stimulation, massage, music,[180] animal therapy and aromatherapy[181] can help mood, aggression, anxiety, and speech.[182] Structured conversation and exercise also help.[183]
• *Who will care for the carers?* Carer stress is inevitable, causing ↑morbidity and mortality. Support groups, telephone helplines, respite care and your unswerving loyalty can all ease the burden; eg UK Alzheimer's Disease Society: 0845 300 0336.
• *Challenging behaviour:* First rule out pain and infection as the cause of the worsening behaviour. Then, if non-pharmacological therapies fail, consider trazodone (50-300mg at night) or lorazepam (0.5-1mg/12-24h PO). If the agitation is severe, get help: antipsychotics such as quetiapine, risperidone and olanzapine may improve positive symptoms, but cognition, verbal fluency, and longevity may be worsened.[184] Haloperidol (0.5-4mg) can be useful in the short term.
    ►Avoid using antipsychotics for agitation in Lewy body dementia (↑↑risk of SE). There is some evidence that acetylcholinesterase inhibitors may help (see p493).
• *Depression* is common. Try an SSRI (eg citalopram 10-20mg OD) or, if severe, mirtazapine (15-45mg at night if eGFR >40). Cognitive behavioural therapy can help with social withdrawal and catastrophic thinking.
• *Avoid drugs that impair cognition* (eg neuroleptics, sedatives, tricyclics, pII).

Neurology

This leading cause of dementia is *the* big neuropsychiatric disorder of our times, dominating the care of the elderly and the lives of their families who give up work, friends, and ways of life to support relatives through the long final years. Their lives can be tormented—"*I am chained to a corpse*" (p449)—or transformed, depending on how gently patients exit into their "*worlds of preoccupied emptiness*". *Onset* may be from 40yrs (earlier in Down's syndrome, in which AD is inevitable).

**Presentation** See p490 for diagnosing dementias (any type). Suspect Alzheimer's in adults with enduring,[1] progressive and global cognitive impairment (unlike other dementias which may affect certain domains but not others): visuo-spatial skill (gets lost), memory, verbal abilities and executive function (planning) are all affected (use neuropsychometric testing to identify affected domains; see p490), and there is anosognosia—a lack of insight into the problems engendered by the disease, eg missed appointments, misunderstood conversations or plots of films, and mishandling of money and clerical work.[185] Later there may be irritability; mood disturbance (depression or euphoria); behavioural change (eg aggression, wandering, disinhibition); psychosis (hallucinations or delusions); agnosia (may not recognize self in the mirror). There is no standard natural history. Cognitive impairment is progressive, but non-cognitive symptoms may come and go over months. Towards the end, often but not invariably, patients become sedentary, taking little interest in anything.

**Cause** Modest concordance between monozygotic and dizygotic twins suggests that environmental and genetic factors both play a role. Accumulation of β-amyloid peptide, a degradation product of amyloid precursor protein, results in progressive neuronal damage, neurofibrillary tangles, ↑numbers of amyloid plaques, and loss of the neurotransmitter *acetylcholine* (fig 1). Defective clearance of β-amyloid plaques by macrophages appears to relate to altered macrophage gene expression.[2] Neuronal loss is selective—the hippocampus, amygdala, temporal neocortex and subcortical nuclei (eg nucleus basalis of Meynert) are most vulnerable (p448).[186] Vascular effects are also important—95% of AD patients show evidence of vascular dementia.

**Risk factors** 1st-degree relative with AD; Down's syndrome; homozygosity for apolipoprotein e (ApoE) e4 allele; PICALM, CL1 & CLU mutations;[187] vascular risk factors (↑BP, diabetes, dyslipidaemia, ↑homocysteine, AF); ↓physical/cognitive activity; depression; loneliness (risk↑×2; simply living alone is not a risk factor). Evidence on alcohol is inconsistent: ≥2 drinks/day accelerated onset of AD by 5yrs in one study; others report that red wine is protective; ≥20 cigarettes/day accelerates onset by 2.3yrs.● Delaying onset by 5yrs would ↓ prevalence by ~50%.[188]

**Management** ▶See p491 for a general approach to management in dementia. • Refer to a specialist memory service. • Acetylcholinesterase inhibitors (BOX). • BP control (complex interaction between vasculopathy and AD)[3] • Ginkgo biloba (EGb 761® 240mg/d) may improve wellbeing of patients *and* carers;[189,190] data on other antioxidants are mixed. Huperzine A (traditional Chinese Qian Ceng Ta) is promising.

*Prevention in the context of AD's time-course:* Changes in CSF amyloid-β are seen ~25yrs before onset of unequivocal symptoms (USy) and its deposition is detected 15yrs before USy. CSF tau protein & brain atrophy are also detected 15yrs before USy.[191] Cerebral hypometabolism and impaired episodic memory occur 10yrs before USy. Global cognitive impairment occurs 5yrs before USy. Prevention will probably be most effective before any of this starts. Polyunsaturated fatty acid (PUFA), folic acid and B vitamins (BOX) may have a role here.[192] NB: there is no simple relationship between brain structure, neurofibrillary tangles, and function.[193] *Mean survival:* 7 yrs from USy.

---

1 'Enduring' doesn't mean unfluctuating: cognition comes and goes, allowing poetic insights, as in Iris Murdoch's poignant self-diagnosis: "I am sailing into the dark".
2 This is partly correctable by bisdemethoxycurcumin, found in the turmeric component of curries;[194] just one reason why AD may be less prevalent in India: 0.5% *vs* 1.7% in USA.[195,196]
3 In heart failure there is a 2-fold risk of AD; excess risk halves with antihypertensive use.[197] Doppler middle cerebral artery monitoring for 1h finds that small emboli occur in 40% in AD *vs* 15% in controls.[198]

## Pharmacological treatment of cognitive decline

*Acetylcholinesterase inhibitors:* Evidence that acetylcholinesterase inhibitors are modestly effective in treating Alzheimer's is good.[199] There is also limited evidence for their efficacy in the dementia of Parkinson's disease[200] and rivastigmine may improve behavioural symptoms in Lewy body dementia.[201] They appear to help the laying down of new memories more than accessing old ones,[202] and delay the need for institutional care, but not its duration.[203] They are currently available in the UK only through specialist memory services, for patients whose MMSE lies between 10 and 20. However, one cannot say "Stop these drugs as he has only scored x on the MMSE" (notoriously variable from day to day) if the wife says "but he's brighter, more motivated".[204] ►Be aware that using QALYs (p10) relentlessly can make us cruel; sentiment (the alternative to QALYs) may make us useless, but it is better to be useless than cruel. The Scottish Intercollegiate Guidelines Network (SIGN) states that all AD patients could benefit from acetylcholinesterase inhibitors, although this did not take into account a cost-benefit analysis.

- **Donepezil:**[1] initially 5mg PO, eg doubled after 1 month.
- **Rivastigmine:**[2] 1.5mg/12h initially, ↑ to 3-6mg/12h. Patches are also available.
- **Galantamine:** initially 4mg/12h, ↑ to 8-12mg/12h PO. Originally isolated from daffodils. *SE:* D&V, cramps, incontinence, headache, dizziness, insomnia, LFT↑; rarely, but importantly, heart block/arrhythmias, hallucinations, peptic ulcers.

►The cholinergic effects of acetylcholinesterase inhibitors may exacerbate peptic ulcer disease and heart block. Always ask about dyspepsia and cardiac symptoms, and do an ECG before starting treatment.

*Antiglutamatergic treatment:* Randomized trials show that **memantine** (an NMDA antagonist, see p455) is reasonably effective in late stage disease. *Dose:* 5mg/24h initially, ↑ by 5mg/d weekly to 10mg/12h. *SE:* hallucinations, confusion, hypertonia, hypersexuality.

*Targetting β amyloid* has proved disappointing, except for an equivocal effect of solanezumab—mild AD patients may get up to a 42% reduction in decline in cognition after 18 months treatment (but the *EXPEDITION 2* study was negative).[205]

*Folic acid and B vitamins:* 0.8mg folic acid, 0.5mg vit $B_{12}$ + 20mg vit $B_6$/day PO decreases mild cognitive impairment (MCI) if baseline homocysteine >11μmol/l. B vitamins also ↓rates of MRI brain atrophy in MCI (Celeste de Jager's VITACOG trials).[206]

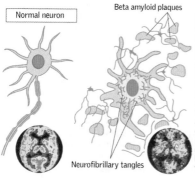

Normal neuron

Beta amyloid plaques

Neurofibrillary tangles

Fig 1. Alzheimer's has 2 hallmarks: senile plaques and neurofibrillary tangles. 30yrs ago their proteins were identified, precipitating an avalanche of molecular research and promises of new drugs. So why is progress so slow? Do we need a paradigm shift from the reductionism that defines amyloid and tau hypotheses—to recognition that AD is a manifestation of cellular adaptation, eg a defence against oxidative injury? If AD pathology is a host response rather than a manifestation of protein injury, it is unlikely to be the best target for drugs.

**1** Pre-treatment orbitofrontal signs (agitation, disinhibition, odd motor activity) may predict good response to donepezil.[207]
**2** Pre-treatment hallucinations predict a response to rivastigmine.[208]

*Epilepsy* is a recurrent tendency to spontaneous, intermittent, abnormal electrical activity in part of the brain, manifesting as *seizures*.[1] These may take many forms, but for each individual patient they tend to be stereotyped. *Convulsions* are the motor signs of electrical discharges. Many of us would have seizures in abnormal metabolic circumstances—eg Na+↓, hypoxia (eg reflex anoxic seizures in faints): we would not normally be said to have epilepsy. The prevalence of active epilepsy is ~1%.

**Elements of a seizure** A *prodrome* lasting hours or days may rarely precede the seizure. It is not part of the seizure itself: the patient or others notice a change in mood or behaviour. An *aura* is part of the seizure of which the patient is aware, and may precede its other manifestations. The aura may be a strange feeling in the gut, or an experience such as *déjà vu* (disturbing sense of familiarity), or strange smells or flashing lights. It implies a partial (focal) seizure, often, but not necessarily, from the temporal lobe. *Post-ictally* there may be headache, confusion, myalgia, and a sore tongue; or temporary weakness after a focal seizure in motor cortex (Todd's palsy, p726), or dysphasia following a focal seizure in the temporal lobe.

**Causes** ⅔ are idiopathic (often familial). *Structural:* Cortical scarring (eg head injury years before onset), developmental (eg dysembryoplastic neuroepithelial tumour or cortical dysgenesis), space-occupying lesion, stroke, hippocampal sclerosis (eg after a febrile convulsion), vascular malformations. *Others:* Tuberous sclerosis, sarcoidosis, SLE, PAN. *Non-epileptic causes of seizures:* Trauma, stroke, haemorrhage, ↑ICP; alcohol or benzodiazepine withdrawal; *metabolic disturbance* (hypoxia, Na+↑↓, Ca²⁺↓, glucose↑↓, uraemia); liver disease; infection (eg meningitis, encephalitis, syphilis, cysticercosis, HIV; T°↑; drugs (tricyclics, cocaine, tramadol, theophylline); pseudoseizures (p496).

**Diagnosis** There are three key questions to consider:

1 *Are these really seizures?* A detailed description from a witness of 'the fit' is vital (but ask yourself: "Are they reliable?") In the heat of the moment many witnesses report twitching when none took place. Tongue-biting and a slow recovery are very suggestive. Not everything that twitches is epilepsy—reflex anoxic convulsions due to syncope are particularly difficult. Try hard not to diagnose epilepsy in error—therapy has significant side-effects, and the diagnosis is stigmatizing and has implications for employment, insurance, and driving. See p464 for ΔΔ.

2 *What type of seizure is it*—partial or generalized? The attack's *onset* is the key concern here. If the seizure begins with focal features, it is a partial seizure, however rapidly it then generalizes. See BOX.

3 *Any triggers?* Eg alcohol, stress, fevers, certain sounds, flickering lights/TV, contrasting patterns, reading/writing? Does he recognize warning events (eg twitches) so he can abort the fit before it generalizes? TV-induced fits rarely need drugs.

*In assessing a first-ever seizure*, consider also:

• *Is it really the first?* Ask the family and patient about past funny turns/odd behaviour. Déjà vu and odd episodic feelings of fear may well be relevant.

• *Was the seizure provoked?* (see 'Non-epileptic causes' above) Provoked 1st seizures are less likely to recur (3-10%, unless the cause is irreversible, eg an infarct or glioma); if it was unprovoked, recurrence rates are 30-50%.[209] NB: provocations are different to triggers: most people would have a seizure given sufficient provocation, but most people do not have seizures however many triggers they are exposed to, so triggered seizures suggest epilepsy. Triggered attacks tend to recur.

• Prompt investigation, eg with admission for 24h for bloods, drugs screen, LP (if safe), EEG—p496 CT/MRI± enhancement (or else infective causes, eg TB, may be missed).[210] Admit to substantiate ideas of pseudoseizures, or for recurrent seizures.

**☼Counselling** After any 'fit', advise about dangers (eg swimming, driving, heights) until the diagnosis is known; then give *individualized* counselling on employment, sport, insurance and ►conception (OHCS p29). Avoid driving until seizure-free for >1yr; if in the UK, say "you must contact DVLA" (p153). Document this.

---

1 ↑Membrane excitation (epileptogenicity) may be related to disorders of synaptic transmission, K⁺ channelopathies, or α-subunit mutations (eg SCN2A; SCN1A) of voltage-gated Na⁺ channel.

## Seizure classification[211]

**Partial seizures** Focal onset, with features referable to a part of one hemisphere (see BOX). Often seen with underlying structural disease.
• *Simple partial seizure:* Awareness is unimpaired, with focal motor, sensory (olfactory, visual, etc), autonomic or psychic symptoms. No post-ictal symptoms.
• *Complex partial seizures:* Awareness is impaired. May have a simple partial onset (=aura), or impaired awareness at onset. Most commonly arise from the temporal lobe. Post-ictal confusion is common with seizures arising from the temporal lobe, whereas recovery is rapid after seizures in the frontal lobe.
• *Partial seizure with secondary generalization:* In ⅔ of patients with partial seizures, the electrical disturbance, which starts focally (as either a simple or complex partial seizure), spreads widely, causing a secondary generalized seizure, which is typically convulsive.

**Primary generalized seizures** Simultaneous onset of electrical discharge throughout cortex, with no localizing features referable to only one hemisphere.
• *Absence seizures:* Brief (≤10s) pauses, eg suddenly stops talking in mid-sentence, then carries on where left off. Presents in childhood.
• *Tonic-clonic seizures:* Loss of consciousness. Limbs stiffen (tonic), then jerk (clonic). May have one without the other. Post-ictal confusion and drowsiness.
• *Myoclonic seizures:* Sudden jerk of a limb, face or trunk. The patient may be thrown suddenly to the ground, or have a violently disobedient limb: one patient described it as *'my flying-saucer epilepsy'*, as crockery which happened to be in the hand would take off.
• *Atonic (akinetic) seizures:* Sudden loss of muscle tone causing a fall, no LOC.
• *Infantile spasms:* (OHCS p206) Commonly associated with tuberous sclerosis.

NB: the classification of *epileptic syndromes* is separate to the classification of seizures, and is based on seizure type, age of onset, EEG findings and other features such as family history. Seizure classifications based on semiology also exist.[212]

## Localizing features of partial (focal) seizures

**Temporal lobe** •Automatisms—complex motor phenomena, but with impaired awareness and no recollection afterwards, varying from primitive oral (lip smacking, chewing, swallowing) or manual (fumbling, fiddling, grabbing) movements, to complex actions (singing, kissing, driving a car and violent acts);[213] •Abdominal rising sensation or pain (± ictal vomiting; or rarely episodic fevers[214] or D&V[215]); •Dysphasia (ictal or post-ictal); •Memory phenomena—*déjà vu* (when everything seems strangely familiar), or *jamais vu* (everything seems strangely unfamiliar); •Hippocampal involvement may cause emotional disturbance, eg sudden terror, panic, anger or elation, and derealization (out-of-body experiences)[216], which in combination may manifest as excessive religiosity;[1][217] •Uncal involvement may cause hallucinations of smell or taste and a dreamlike state,[218] and seizures in auditory cortex may cause complex auditory hallucinations, eg music or conversations, or palinacousis[219]; •Delusional behaviour; •Finally, you may find yourself not believing your patient's bizarre story—eg "Canned music at Tesco's always makes me cry and then pass out, unless I wear an earplug in one ear"[220] or "I get orgasms when I brush my teeth" (right temporal lobe hyper- and hypoperfusion, respectively)[221]

**Frontal lobe** •Motor features such as posturing, versive movements of the head and eyes,[222] or peddling movements of the legs •Jacksonian march (a spreading focal motor seizure with retained awareness, often starting with the face or a thumb) •Motor arrest •Subtle behavioural disturbances (often diagnosed as psychogenic) •Dysphasia or speech arrest •Post-ictal Todd's palsy (p726).

**Parietal lobe** •Sensory disturbances—tingling, numbness, pain (rare) •Motor symptoms (due to spread to the pre-central gyrus).

**Occipital lobe** •Visual phenomena such as spots, lines, flashes.

1 The temporolimbic system tags certain stimuli as derealized, crucially important, harmonious, and/or joyous or ecstatic, making us prone to describe these experiences within religious frameworks.[223]

Neurology

Don't just think about drugs! We get better results if we take time to teach patients about their brain and its functioning, and to explain how their feelings, thinking, and behaviour can help living with epilepsy, and, perhaps,•☜ partly to control seizures. Relaxation training or aura interruption (eg smelling a pleasant smell if the aura is a certain bad smell)[224,225] may abort emotion-triggered seizures (p494). *Andrews-Reiter hypotheses 22b*

▶*Involve patients in all decisions.* Concordance depends on communication and doctor-patient negotiation (p3). Living with *active* epilepsy creates many problems (eg inability to drive or operate machinery, drug side-effects) and fears (eg of sudden death). Neurologists may have little time to explore these issues, while GPs may have no special interest in epilepsy. Enlist the help of an **epilepsy nurse specialist**, who can provide telephone advice and annual reviews to monitor drug efficacy and side-effects, to address employment, leisure, and reproductive issues, and, after a few seizure-free years, to consider drug withdrawal.

**Drugs** We do not advise drugs after one fit, unless risk of recurrence is high (eg structural brain lesion, focal CNS deficit, or unequivocal epileptiform EEG). After a 2nd fit, discuss options with the patient; drugs are probably indicated (provided a specialist has confirmed the diagnosis). If only 1 fit every 2yrs, he or she may accept the risk (if there is no need to drive or operate machinery) rather than have to take drugs every day. Drug choice depends on seizure type and epilepsy syndrome, other medications and co-morbidities, plans for pregnancy, and patient preference:

• *Generalized tonic-clonic seizures:* Sodium valproate or lamotrigine (often better tolerated,[227] and less teratogenic) are 1st-line, then carbamazepine or topiramate. Others: levetiracetam, oxcarbazepine, clobazam.
• *Absence seizures:* Sodium valproate, lamotrigine or ethosuximide.[228]
• *Tonic, atonic and myoclonic seizures:* As for generalized tonic-clonic seizures, but avoiding carbamazepine and oxcarbazepine, which may worsen seizures.
• *Partial seizures ± secondary generalization:* Carbamazepine is 1st-line, then sodium valproate, lamotrigine, oxcarbazepine or topiramate. Others: levetiracetam, gabapentin, tiagabine, phenytoin, clobazam.

Treat with *one* drug and with *one* doctor in charge only. Slowly build up doses over 2-3 months (see BOX 1) until seizures are controlled, side-effects are bad, or maximum dosage is reached. If ineffective or not tolerated, switch to the next most appropriate drug. To switch drugs, introduce the new drug (see BOX 1), and only withdraw the 1st drug once established on the 2nd. Dual therapy is necessary in <10% of patients—consider if all appropriate drugs have been tried singly at the optimum dose.

**EEG** An EEG cannot exclude or refute epilepsy; it forms part of the context for diagnosis, so don't do one if simple syncope is the likely diagnosis (often false +ve). In 1st unprovoked fits, unequivocal epileptiform activity on EEG helps assess risk of recurrence.[229] Only do *emergency* EEGs if non-convulsive status is the problem (p489). Other tests: MRI (structural lesions, p494). Drug levels (is he taking the tablets?). Magnetoencephalography (MEG), PET, cognitive assessment, and ictal SPECT may help localize the epileptogenic focus when evaluating for epilepsy surgery.

**Non-epileptic attack disorder** *(pseudo- or psychogenic seizures)* These are not infrequent: suspect this if there are uncontrollable symptoms, no learning disabilities, and CNS exam, CT, MRI, and EEG are normal.[203] It may coexist with true epilepsy.

**If drugs don't work...** If a single epileptogenic focus can be identified (see above) such as hippocampal sclerosis or a small low-grade tumour, **neurosurgical resection** offers up to 70% chance of seizure freedom, depending on the location of the focus, with the risk of causing focal neurological deficits such as memory impairment, dysphasia or hemianopia.[230] An alternative is **vagal nerve stimulation**, which can reduce seizure frequency and severity in ~33%.

**When it all goes wrong** Sudden unexpected death in epilepsy (SUDEP) is more common in uncontrolled epilepsy, and may be related to nocturnal seizure-associated apnoea or asystole.[231] Those with epilepsy have a mortality rate 3-fold that of controls. >700 epilepsy-related deaths are recorded/yr in the UK; up to 17% are SUDEPs. For help with families of those with SUDEP, contact *Epilepsy Bereaved* UK 01235 772852.

## Anti-epileptic drugs (AED): doses and side-effects (see formulary for details)

*Carbamazepine:* (as slow-release) Initially 100mg/12h, increase by 200mg/d every 2wks up to max 1000mg/12h. SE: leucopenia, diplopia, blurred vision, impaired balance, drowsiness, mild generalized erythematous rash, SIADH (rare; see p687).

*Lamotrigine:* As monotherapy, initially 25mg/d, ↑ by 50mg/d every 2wks up to 100mg/12h (max 250mg/12h). ►Halve monotherapy dose if on valproate; double if on carbamazepine or phenytoin (max 350mg/12h). SE: maculopapular rash—occurs in 10% (but 1/1000 develop *Stevens-Johnson syndrome* or *toxic epidermal necrolysis*) typically in 1$^{st}$ 8wks, esp if on valproate; warn patients to see a doctor at once if rash or flu symptoms develop; also associated with hypersensitivity, ↑LFTs and disseminated intravascular coagulopathy). Other SEs: diplopia, blurred vision, photosensitivity (SLE-like), tremor, agitation, vomiting, aplastic anaemia.

*Levetiracetam:* If >16yrs, initially 250mg/24h, increase by 250mg/12h every 2wks up to max 1.5g/12h (if eGFR >80). Psychiatric side-effects are common, eg depression, agitation. Other SEs: D&V, dyspepsia, drowsiness, diplopia, blood dyscrasias.

*Phenytoin:* Effective and well-tried, but no longer 1$^{st}$-line for generalized or partial epilepsy due to toxicity (nystagmus, diplopia, tremor, dysarthria, ataxia) and SEs (↓intellect, depression, coarse facial features, acne, gum hypertrophy, polyneuropathy, blood dyscrasias). Dosage is difficult—do blood levels (p766).

*Sodium valproate:* Initially 300mg/12h, increase by 100mg/12h every 3 days up to max 30mg/kg (or 2.5g) daily. Nausea is very common (take with food).

*Vigabatrin:* Only used in infantile spasms (due to a high incidence of visual field defects).

►Carbamazepine, phenytoin and barbiturates are liver enzyme inducing.

| Valproate side-effects |
|---|
| Appetite↑, weight gain |
| Liver failure (watch LFT esp. during 1$^{st}$ 6 months) |
| Pancreatitis |
| Reversible hair loss (grows back curly) |
| Oedema |
| Ataxia |
| Teratogenicity, tremor, thrombocytopenia |
| Encephalopathy (due to hyperammonaemia) |

## Women with epilepsy

- *Teratogenicity of AEDs:* Women of child-bearing age should take folic acid 5mg/d. Valproate in particular should be avoided (use lamotrigine).
- *Pre-conception counselling* is vital (5% risk of fetal abnormality, OHCS p29).
- *Breastfeeding:* most AEDs except carbamazepine and valproate are present in breast milk. Lamotrigine is not thought to be harmful to infants.
- *The Pill:* Non-enzyme-inducing AEDs have no effect on the Pill. With other AEDs ≥50μg of oestrogen may be needed (Norinyl-1®; ↓pill-free days from 7 to 4; use condoms too) or Depo-Provera® (10-weekly IM). Progesterone-only pills are also affected. Coils are OK for emergency contraception, or levonorgestrel 3mg PO stat.

## Stopping anticonvulsants

►*Discuss risks and benefits with patients. Informed choices are vital.* Most patients are seizure-free within a few years of starting drugs. More than 50% remain so when drugs are withdrawn. After assessing risks and benefits for the individual patient (eg the need to drive), withdrawal may be tried, if the patient meets these criteria: normal CNS examination, normal IQ, normal EEG prior to withdrawal, seizure-free for >2yrs, and no juvenile myoclonic epilepsy. In one study (n =459), over 5yrs 52% remained seizure-free, compared with 67% who continued their medication.[203] However, in another study, resuming medication did not return the patient to his/her status quo, and not all seizures could be controlled (risk factors: cognitive deficits and partial epilepsy).[232] One way to withdraw drugs in adults is to decrease the dose by 10% every 2–4wks (for carbamazepine, lamotrigine, phenytoin, valproate, and vigabatrin) and by 10% every 4–8wks for phenobarbital, benzodiazepines, and ethosuximide.[233]

Neurology

James Parkinson (1755-1824) described this cardinal triad:
1 *Tremor:* Worse at rest; often 'pill-rolling' of thumb over fingers. 4-6 cycles/sec (slower than cerebellar tremor). Distinguish from 'essential tremor', which is a symptomatic postural and action tremor of the upper limbs and head.
2 *Rigidity/↑tone:* Rigidity + tremor gives 'cogwheel rigidity', felt by the examiner during rapid pronation/supination.
3 *Bradykinesia/hypokinesia:* Slow to initiate movement and slow, low-amplitude excursions in repetitive actions, eg ↓blink rate, monotonous hypophonic speech, micrographia. Gait: ↓arm-swing, festination (shuffling steps with flexed trunk, as if chasing one's centre of gravity, fig 1), freezing at obstacles or doors. Expressionless face (hypomimesis).

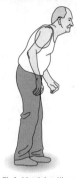

Fig 1. *March à petit pas.*

**Cause** Idiopathic PD[1], or drugs (neuroleptics, metoclopramide, prochlorperazine)[et al]. Rarely: trauma/boxing; encephalopathy post 'flu; manganese or copper toxicity (Wilson's disease); HIV (HAART helps, p413); Parkinson's-plus syndromes: see BOX.

## Idiopathic Parkinson's disease (PD)

**Presentation** Bradykinesia/hypokinesia + one or more of: tremor at rest (one side worse), postural instability ± muscular rigidity. Other signs (MINIBOX) may be subtle, eg poor decoding of the emotional content of speech (prosody),[234] poor executive functioning, and REM sleep disorders. Poor *simultaneous* motor and cognitive functions can lead to freezing while walking[235] (a devastating symptom) *Typical age at onset:* 65yrs. *Prevalence:* 0.6% at 60-64yrs; 3.5% at 85-89yrs (Europe).

| *Non-motor features:* |
|---|
| Sense of smell reduced |
| Constipation |
| Visual hallucinations |
| Frequency/urgency |
| Dribbling of saliva |
| Depression & dementia |

**Pathology** Mitochondrial DNA dysfunction causes degeneration of dopaminergic neurons in the substantia nigra pars compacta (associated with Lewy bodies), hence ↓striatal dopamine levels.[236]

**Rx** ►Take time! Sit down over a cup of tea[2] to clarify how PD, though incurable and progressive, *is* amenable to palliation. ►Explain how you will assemble a multidisciplinary team (GP, neurologist, PD nurse, social worker, carers, physio- & occupational therapist) to boost quality of life. Assess disability & cognition objectively and regularly, eg via UPDRS.[Unified PD rating scale] ►Postural exercises, eg Chinese qigong, help both.[237] Weight lifting has also been 'validated' as superior to simple fitness programs (N=48). ►Do all you can to make your patient happy talking about their symptoms: letting their dentist or barber know that their shaking is no big deal will then be easier.
• **Drugs** (BOX 1); a key decision is when to start levodopa. ►*Personalize your care plan.* Discuss pros & cons with your patient, eg end-of-dose wearing off and dopamine-induced dyskinesias (develops over 5-10yrs). In view of these, starting late may be wise, eg when >70yrs or when PD seriously interferes with life. NICE recommends referring to a neurologist *before* drugs are used. Dopamine agonists and MAO-B inhibitors may allow delay in starting levodopa, or allow lower doses of levodopa.
• **Neuropsychiatric complications**, such as depression, dementia and psychosis, are common and may reflect disease progression or drug SEs. Try SSRIs for depression. Distinguish drug-induced psychosis (consider reducing DA-agonist doses) from disease progression (try atypical antipsychotics, eg quetiapine, olanzapine).
• **Respite care** is much valued by carers in advanced disease.
• **Deep brain stimulation** (DBS) may help those who are partly dopamine-responsive.[240]
• **Surgical ablation** of overactive basal ganglia circuits (eg subthalamic nuclei).

1 Mutations in FbXo7 may be important in disrupting mitophagy, the process CNS cells use to eliminate faulty mitochondria. PINK1 and Parkin also play a role.
2 Tea might be just the thing: no therapy has proven neuroprotection in PD, but polyphenols in green tea and turmeric (*Curcuma longa*) are strong candidates.[238,239]

## Medical therapy in Parkinson's disease

*Levodopa* is used combined with a dopa-decarboxylase inhibitor such as **Madopar®** (co-beneldopa) or **Sinemet®** (co-careldopa). 'Modified-release' has little benefit over normal preparations; dispersible tablets have rapid bioavailability and may help 'jump-start' patients in the morning, or during sudden 'off' freezing. SEs: nausea and vomiting can be helped by domperidone; taking the pills with a non-protein snack may help too (protein ↓ effectiveness). Efficacy reduces with time, requiring larger and more frequent dosing, with worsening SE. In the long term, dyskinesias, painful dystonias, and response fluctuations such as unpredictable 'off' freezing and pronounced end-of-dose reduced response are common problems (~50% at 6yrs). Non-motor SE: psychosis; visual hallucinations.

*Dopamine agonists (DA):* **Ropinirole** and **pramipexole** (D3, p455) monotherapy can delay starting L-dopa in early stages of PD, and allow lower doses of L-dopa as PD progresses. **Rotigotine** transdermal patches are available as mono- or additive. SEs: drowsiness, nausea, hallucinations, compulsive behaviour (gambling, hypersexuality, p455). Ergot-derived DA-agonists (bromocriptine, pergolide, cabergoline) can cause heart valvulopathy and serosal fibrosis, and are late not favoured.[241] **Amantadine** (weak DA) is used for drug-induced dyskinesias in late PD.

*Apomorphine* is a potent DA agonist used with continuous SC infusion to even out end-of-dose effects, or as a rescue-pen for sudden 'off' freezing. SE: injection-site ulcers.

*Anticholinergics* (eg benzhexol, orphenadrine) help tremor, but cause confusion in the elderly. SE: dry mouth, dizziness, vision↓, urinary retention, pulse↑, anxiety, confusion, excitement, hallucinations, insomnia, memory↓.[242]

*MAO-B inhibitors* (eg rasagiline, selegiline) are an alternative to dopamine agonists in early PD. SEs include postural hypotension and atrial fibrillation.

*COMT inhibitors* (eg entacapone, tolcapone) may lessen the 'off' time in those with end-of-dose wearing off. Tolcapone has better efficacy, but may cause severe hepatic complications and requires close monitoring of LFT.[203]

*The future:* Non-dopaminergic receptors in the basal ganglia are giving new options: *istradefylline*, an adenosine A$_{2A}$ receptor blocker, potentiates responses to low-dose L-dopa and reduces 'off' time,[243] and *endocannabinoid receptors* have been successfully targeted in PD mouse models.[244] Animal studies also hint at a possible neuroprotective and neuroregenerative role for glial cell line-derived neurotrophic factor (GDNF), by using gene therapy to increase local GDNF levels.[245] Neural stem cell transplantation remains unproven.[246]

*Neurology*

## Is a Parkinson's-plus syndrome present? 5 **VIVID** red flags to unfurl...

🏳 Early postural instability and **v**ertical gaze palsy ± falls; rigidity of trunk > in limbs; symmetrical onset; speech and swallowing problems; little tremor→*progressive supranuclear palsy*: (PSP, Steele-Richardson-Olszewski syndrome).

🏳 Early autonomic features, eg **i**mpotence/incontinence, postural ↓BP; cerebellar + pyramidal signs; rigidity > tremor→*multiple system atrophy* (MSA; Shy-Drager).

🏳 Fluctuating cognition with **v**isual hallucinations and early dementia→*Lewy body dementia* (p490).

🏳 Akinetic rigidity **i**nvolving one limb; cortical sensory loss (eg astereognosis); apraxia (even autonomous interfering activity by affected limb—the 'alien limb' phenomenon)→*cortico-basal degeneration* (CBD).

🏳 Pyramidal signs (legs), eg in **d**iabetic/hypertensive patient who falls[247] or has gait problems, eg ataxia (*no* festination)→*vascular parkinsonism* (2-5% of 'PD').

**Cause** Discrete plaques of demyelination occur at multiple CNS sites, from T-cell-mediated immune response (trigger is unknown, but see vit. D, below). Demyelination heals poorly, causing *relapsing and remitting* symptoms. Prolonged demyelination causes axonal loss and clinically *progressive* symptoms. *Prevalence:* commoner in temperate areas (England ≥42:100,000; SE Scotland 200:100,000;[248] rarer in Black Africa/Asia). Lifetime UK risk 1:1000. Adult migrants take their risk with them; children acquire the risk of where they settle. *Mean age of onset:* 30yrs. ♀:♂ ≥3:1.[249]

Early exposure to sunlight/vit. D is important, and vit. D status relates to prevention of MS, and fewer symptoms and fewer new lesions on MRI in established MS.[250, 251]

**Presentation** Usually monosymptomatic: unilateral optic neuritis (pain on eye movement and rapid ↓ central vision); numbness or tingling in the limbs; leg weakness; brainstem or cerebellar symptoms (eg diplopia, ataxia). Other signs: see BOX. Symptoms may worsen with heat (eg hot bath) or exercise. Rarely polysymptomatic. *Progression:* Early on, relapses (which can be stress induced)[252] may be followed by remission and full recovery. With time, remissions are incomplete, so disability accumulates. Steady progression of disability from the outset also occurs, while some patients experience no progressive disablement at all. *Poor prognostic signs:* Older ♂; motor signs at onset; many relapses early on; many MRI lesions; axonal loss.

**Diagnosis** This is clinical, as no test is pathognomonic. It requires *lesions disseminated in time and space*, unattributable to other causes; thus after a 1st episode further evidence is needed. ►Early diagnosis and treatment reduce relapse rates and disability. A careful history may reveal past episodes, eg brief unexplained visual loss, and detailed examination may show more than 1 lesion. *MRI* is sensitive but not specific for plaque detection (*McDonald criteria*, see BOX 2).

~90% presenting with an MS-like 1st episode and consistent MRI lesions go on to develop MS.[253] MRI may also exclude other causes, eg cord compression. *CSF:* Oligoclonal bands of IgG on electrophoresis that are not present in serum suggest CNS inflammation. Delayed visual, auditory, and somatosensory *evoked potentials*. NMO-IgG antibodies are highly specific for Devic's syndrome.[1] MOG and MBP antibodies in those with a single MS-like clinical lesion can predict time to conversion to definite MS.[254]

**℞** Encourage a happy, stress-free life if possible.[255 RCT N=121] Minimize disability (disabled living foundation). If poor diet or ↓sun exposure, give vit. D to achieve serum 25(OH)D levels of ≥50nmol/L.

*Steroids:* Methylprednisolone, eg ½-1g/24h IV/PO for ≤3d shortens acute relapses; use sparingly (≤ twice/yr; steroid SE, p371). It doesn't alter overall prognosis.

*Interferons (IFN-1β & IFN-1α):* ↓ relapses by 30% in active relapsing-remitting MS;[257] and ↓lesion accumulation on MRI.[258, 259] Their power to delay disability is modest at best, as is their role in progressive MS. SE: flu symptoms, depression, anxiety. NB: new gadolinium-enhancing lesions on IFN correlate with severe disability 15yrs later.[259]

*Monoclonal antibodies:* Alemtuzumab acts against T cells in relapsing-remitting MS. 2 trials show it's better than INF.[260] SE: infections, while the immune system reconstitutes itself; autoimmune disease (thyroid, skin, kidney). Natalizumab acts against VLA-4 receptors that allow immune cells to cross the blood-brain barrier. It ↓ relapses in relapsing-remitting MS by 68% and ↓MRI lesions by 92%. SE: progressive leucoencephalopathy; antibody-mediated resistance.

*Non-immunosuppressives:* Glatiramer; mitoxantrone (doxorubicin analogue; helps in secondary progressive MS; safety is an issue).

*Other drugs:* Azathioprine may be as good as interferons for relapsing-remitting MS and is 20× cheaper.[261] NB: there are no good drugs for primary progressive MS.[262]

*Palliation: Spasticity:* Baclofen 5-25mg/8h PO; diazepam 5mg/8-24h PO (addictive); dantrolene 25mg/24h (max 100mg/6h); tizanidine 2mg/24h PO, ↑ every 4d in steps of 1mg/12h (max 9mg/6h). Endocannabinoid system modulation (Sativex®) has a role.[263]
*Tremor:* Botulinum toxin type A injections improve arm tremor and functioning.[264]
*Urgency/frequency:* If post-micturition residual urine >100mL, teach intermittent self-catheterization; if <100mL, try tolterodine.

## 50

## Clinical features (and some personal/social consequences) of MS

> "I'm not worried about losing my life; but I am worried about losing my demeanour, my mind, my interaction with life... ."
> J Hinkleton

| Sensory: | •Dysaesthesia[2]<br>•Pins and needles<br>•Vibration sense↓<br>•Trigeminal neuralgia | GI: Swallowing disorders; constipation.<br><br>Eye: Diplopia; hemianopia; optic neuritis;[3] visual phenomena (eg on exercise);[4] bilateral internuclear ophthalmoplegia (p78); pupil defects.[5,6] |
|---|---|---|
| Motor: | •Spastic weakness<br>•Myelitis[1] | Cerebellum: Trunk and limb ataxia; intention tremor; scanning (ie monotonous) speech; falls. |
| Sexual/GU:<br>(don't be too shy to ask!) | •Erectile dysfunction<br>•Anorgasmia; urine retention; incontinence | Cognitive/visuospatial decline: ►A big cause of unemployment, accidents/isolation;[265] amnesia; mood ↑ or ↓ (avoid ECT); ↓executive functioning. |

**NB:** T°↑, malaise, nausea, vomiting, positional vertigo, seizures, aphasia, meningism, bilateral optic neuritis, CSF leucocytosis and ↑ CSF protein are rare in MS, and may suggest non-MS recurrent demyelinating disease, eg vasculitis or sarcoidosis.[266]

**Neurology**

## McDonald criteria for diagnosing MS (2010)[267]

►MS remains a clinical diagnosis! These criteria may give too much weight to MRI.[268]

| Clinical presentation | Additional data needed |
|---|---|
| 2 or more attacks (relapses) with 2 or more objective clinical lesions | None; clinical evidence will do; imaging evidence desirable; must conform to MS |
| 2 or more attacks with 1 objective clinical lesion | Typical disseminated lesions on MRI or +ve CSF and ≥2 MRI lesions consistent with MS or 2nd attack at a new site |
| 1 attack with 2 or more objective clinical lesions | Dissemination in time:<br>•MRI or 2nd clinical attack |
| 1 attack with 1 objective clinical lesion (monosymptomatic presentation) | Dissemination in space: •MRI or +ve CSF if ≥2 MRI lesions consistent with MS •and dissemination in time (by MRI or a 2nd clinical attack) |
| Insidious neurological progression suggestive of MS (primary progressive MS) | +ve CSF and dissemination in space, ie:<br>•MRI evidence of ≥9 T2 brain lesions;<br>or 2 or more cord lesions;<br>or 4-8 brain and 1 cord lesion; or +ve visual evoked potential (VEP) with 4-8 MRI lesions;<br>or +ve VEP + <4 brain lesions +1 cord lesion and dissemination in time seen on MRI;<br>or continued progression for ≥1yr |

*Attacks* must last >1h, eg weakness, etc (see above), with >30d between attacks.

*MRI abnormality:* 3 out of 4:
• Gadolinium-enhancing or ≥9 T2 hyperintense lesions if no Gd-enhancing lesions
• 1 or more infratentorial lesions •1 or more juxtacortical lesions
• ≥3 periventricular lesions (1 spinal cord lesion = 1 brain lesion)

*CSF:* Oligoclonal IgG bands in CSF (and not serum) or ↑IgG index.

*Evoked potentials: (EP)* This counts if delayed but well-preserved waveform.

*What provides MRI evidence of dissemination in time?* A Gd-enhancing lesion demonstrated in a scan done at least 3 months following onset of clinical attack at a site different from attack, or if no Gd-enhancing lesions at a 3-month scan, follow-up scan after another 3 months showing Gd-lesion or new T2 lesion.[269]

*Six MS eponyms:* Loss of motor, sensory, autonomic, reflex, and sphincter function below the level of a lesion indicates transverse myelitis. Longitudinal myelitis also occurs. Devic's syndrome[1] (neuromyelitis optica—NMO) is an MS variant with transverse myelitis, optic atrophy and NMO-IgG antibodies (p712).

In Lhermitte's sign[2], neck flexion causes 'electric shocks' in trunk/limbs. Also +ve in cervical spondylosis, cord tumours and subacute combined degeneration of the cord ($B_{12}$↓). Along with dysaesthetic pain, trigeminal neuralgia, and painful tonic MS spasms, it comprises the MS-related central pain disorders.[270]

*Optic neuritis symptoms:* •Acuity↓/temporary blindness ± complex visual hallucinations of rays, ie Charles Bonnet syndrome[3] (rare) • Uthhoff's phenomenon[4] (↓vision on exercise, hot meals, hot baths); •Phosphenes (flashes) on eye movement • Pulfrich effect[5] (unequal eye latencies, causing disorientation in traffic as straight trajectories seem curved and distances are misjudged on looking sideways).[271]

*Efferent, afferent* or *relative afferent pupillary defects* (p79). An **Argyle Robertson-type pupil**[5] is rarer (p79; ΔΔ: syphilis, DM, MS or sarcoidosis—lesion in or near the **Edinger-Westphal nucleus**[6]).[272]

**Neurology**

**Signs** •↑*ICP* (see p840): Headache worse on waking, lying down, bending forward, or with coughing (p460); vomiting; papilloedema (only in 50% of tumours); ↓GCS.
- *Seizures:* Seen in ≤50%. Exclude SOL in all adult-onset seizures, especially if focal, or with a localizing aura or post-ictal weakness (Todd's palsy, p726).
- *Evolving focal neurology:* See BOX for localizing signs. ↑ICP causes *false localizing signs:* VIᵗʰ nerve palsy is commonest (p76) due to its long intracranial course.
- *Subtle personality change:* Irritability, lack of application to tasks, lack of initiative, socially inappropriate behaviour.

**Causes** Tumour (primary or metastatic, below), aneurysm, abscess (25% multiple); chronic subdural haematoma, granuloma (p187, eg tuberculoma), cyst (eg cysticercosis). *Tumours:* 30% are metastatic (eg breast, lung, melanoma). *Primaries:* astrocytoma, glioblastoma multiforme (opinion remains divided over association with mobile phone use),²⁷⁴,²⁷⁵ oligodendroglioma, ependymoma. Also meningioma (♀:♂≈2:1), primary CNS lymphoma (eg as non-infectious manifestation of HIV), and cerebellar haemangioblastoma.

**Differential diagnosis** Stroke, head injury, venous sinus thrombosis, vasculitis (p558; eg SLE, syphilis, PAN, giant cell arteritis), MS, encephalitis, post-ictal (Todd's palsy, p726), metabolic, or U&E disturbance. Also colloid cyst of the 3ʳᵈ ventricle and idiopathic intracranial hypertension.

**Tests** CT ± MRI (good for posterior fossa masses). Consider biopsy. Avoid LP before imaging (risks *coning*, ie cerebellar tonsils herniate through the foramen magnum).

**Tumour management** *Benign:* Removal if possible but some may be inaccessible. *Malignant:* Excision of gliomas is hard as resection margins are rarely clear, but surgery does give a tissue diagnosis, it debulks pre-radiotherapy, and makes a cavity for inserting carmustine wafers²⁷⁶ (may cause serious cerebral oedema).²⁷⁷ If a tumour is inaccessible but causing hydrocephalus, a ventriculo-peritoneal shunt can help. Chemo-radiotherapy is used post-op for gliomas or metastases, and as sole therapy if surgery is impossible. Oligodendroglioma with 1p/19q deletions is especially sensitive. In glioblastoma, temozolomide (a new alkylating agent) ↑survival²⁷⁸ (benefit is mainly if tumours have methylated methylguanine methyltransferase gene promoters and are thus unable to repair chemotherapy-induced DNA damage).²⁷⁹ Seizure prophylaxis (eg phenytoin) is important, but often fails. Treat headache (eg codeine 60mg/4h PO). *Cerebral oedema:* Dexamethasone 4mg/8h PO; mannitol if ↑ICP acutely (p841). Plan meticulous palliative treatment (p536).

**Prognosis** Poor but improving (<50% survival at 5yrs) for CNS primaries; 40% 20yr survival for cerebellar haemangioblastoma; benign tumours are curable by excision.

**Third ventricle colloid cysts** These congenital cysts declare themselves in adult life with amnesia, headache (often positional), obtundation (blunted consciousness), incontinence, dim vision, bilateral paraesthesiae, weak legs, and drop attacks. *R:* Excision or ventriculo-peritoneal shunting.

## Idiopathic intracranial hypertension (=pseudotumour cerebri)

Think of this in those presenting as if with a mass (headache, ↑ICP and papilloedema)—*when none is found.* Typical patients are obese women with narrowed visual fields, blurred vision ± diplopia, VIᵗʰ nerve palsy, and an enlarged blind spot, if papilloedema is present (it usually is). Consciousness and cognition are preserved.

*Cause:* Often unknown, or secondary to venous sinus thrombosis, or drugs, eg tetracycline, minocycline, nitrofurantoin, vitamin A, isotretinoin, danazol, and somatropin.

*R:* Weight loss, acetazolamide, loop diuretics, and prednisolone (start at ~40mg/24h PO; more SE than diuretics) *may* reverse papilloedema.²⁸⁰ Consider optic nerve sheath fenestration or lumbar-peritoneal shunt if drugs fail and visual loss worsens.²⁸¹

*Prognosis:* Often self-limiting. Permanent significant visual loss in 10% (ie not so benign). CSF shunting or optic nerve sheath fenestration can help vision.²⁸²

►Ask first *where* the mass is, then *what it is*. Localizing features of SOLs can be thought of as dividing into *negative symptoms* (deficits caused by direct pressure or tumour invasion) and *positive symptoms* (due to localized seizure activity caused by irritation of the brain parenchyma). Both depend on the function of the area of the brain affected. Negative symptoms are listed below. See p495 for positive (seizure) symptoms. Frontal lobe, midline, and non-dominant temporal lobe masses present late.

**Temporal lobe** •Dysphasia (p80); •Contralateral homonymous hemianopia (or upper quadrantanopia if only Meyer's loop affected); •Amnesia; •Many odd or seemingly inexplicable phenomena, p495.

**Frontal lobe** •Hemiparesis; •Personality change (indecent, indolent, indiscreet, facetious, tendency to pun; see also orbitofrontal syndrome below); •Release phenomena such as the grasp reflex (fingers drawn across palm are grasped), significant only if unilateral; •Broca's dysphasia (p80), or more subtle difficulty with initiating and planning speech with intact repetition and no anomia—but loss of coherence; •Unilateral anosmia (loss of smell); •General lack of drive or initiative; •Concrete thinking; •Perseveration (unable to switch from one line of thinking to another); •Executive dysfunction (unable to plan tasks); •↓verbal fluency, eg unable to list words beginning with the letter 'A' or 'F' (normal is ~15 words in 1 min).[283]

*Orbitofrontal[1] syndrome* (fig 1, p448): Lack of empathy; over-eating; disinhibition; impulsive behaviour; ↓social skills; over-familiar; unconscious imitation of postures (eg when you put your feet on the desk, or sit on the floor); 'utilization behaviour' (whatever is provided is used, eg hand the patient spectacles, and he puts them on, hand him another pair, and this goes on his nose too, ditto for a 3rd pair).

**Parietal lobe** •Hemisensory loss; •↓2-point discrimination; •Astereognosis (unable to recognize an object by touch alone); •Sensory inattention; •Dysphasia (p80); •Gerstmann's syndrome (p714).

**Occipital lobe** •Contralateral visual field defects; •Palinopsia;[2] •Polyopia (seeing multiple images).

**Cerebellum** Remember DASHING: dysdiadochokinesis (impaired *rapidly alternating* movements, p73) and dysmetria (past-pointing); ataxia (limb/truncal);[3] slurred speech (dysarthria); hypotonia; intention tremor; nystagmus; gait abnormality.

**Cerebellopontine angle** (eg acoustic neuroma/vestibular Schwannoma; p466) Causes ipsilateral deafness, nystagmus, ↓corneal reflex, facial weakness (rare), ipsilateral cerebellar signs (above), papilloedema, VIth nerve palsy (p77).

**Corpus callosum** (a rare site for lesions) Severe rapid intellectual deterioration with focal signs of adjacent lobes and signs of loss of communication between lobes (eg left hand unable to carry out verbal commands).

**Midbrain** (eg pineal tumours or midbrain infarction) Failure of up or down gaze; light/near dissociated pupil responses (p79), with convergence globe-retracting nystagmus[284] from co-contraction of opposing horizontal muscles, on attempted up-gaze.[285] Elicited by looking at a down-moving target.[285] video link

Neurology

---

1 The orbitofrontal cortex (fig 1, p448) and right amygdala[286] appreciate beauty (and sexual allure). The poets were nearly right that *Beauty is in the eye of the beholder*: it is ~1cm *above* the orbit.[287]
2 Palinopsia: persisting or recurring images, once the stimulus has left the field of view, from the Greek word *palin* meaning 'again'.
3 If truncal ataxia is worse on eye closure, blame the dorsal columns, not the cerebellum.

Bell's palsy is partly a diagnosis of exclusion (~30% of facial palsies have a defined cause, see MINIBOX, but features distinguishing it from other causes are: abrupt onset (eg overnight or after a nap) with complete unilateral facial weakness at 24-72h; ipsilateral numbness or pain around the ear; ‡taste (ageusia); hypersensitivity to sounds (ie hyperacusis from stapedius palsy).[291] Other pathologies may be indicated by bilateral symptoms,[1] UMN signs, other cranial neuropathies (eg V or XII, but also seen in 8% of idiopathic cases),[292] limb weakness, and rashes.

**Incidence** 15–40/100,000/yr (~1 patient/2yrs/GP).[293]
♂≈♀. Risk ↑ in pregnancy (×3) and in diabetes (×5).

**Other symptoms of VII[th] palsy (from any cause)**
•Unilateral sagging of the mouth, which is drawn upwards on the normal side on smiling, causing a grimace •Drooling of saliva •Food trapped between gum and cheek •Speech difficulty •Failure of eye closure may cause a watery or dry eye, ectropion (sagging and turning-out of the lower lid), injury from foreign bodies, or conjunctivitis.

**Signs** Ask him to wrinkle his forehead and close his eyes forcefully (under bilateral cortical control so spared in UMN lesion). Whistling/blowing out the cheeks tests buccinator (*buccina* is Latin for trumpet).

**Tests** *Blood:* ESR; glucose; ↑*Borrelia* antibodies in Lyme disease (indistinguishable clinically from Bell's);[294] ↑VZV antibodies in Ramsay Hunt syndrome (BOX).[295] *MRI:* Space-occupying lesions; stroke; MS; *CSF* (rarely done) for infections. *Nerve conduction tests* at 2wks predict slow recovery by showing axon degeneration but don't influence treatment, so not routinely done.

| Causes of VII[th] nerve palsy |
| --- |
| Bell's palsy (70% of cases) |
| Ramsay Hunt syn. (BOX) |
| Lyme disease (*Borrelia* sp.) |
| Meningitis (eg fungal) |
| TB; viruses (HIV, polio) |
| Mycoplasma (rare) |
| **Brainstem lesions** |
| Stroke, tumour, MS |
| **Cerebello-pontine angle** |
| Acoustic neuroma (p466) |
| Meningioma |
| **Systemic disease** |
| Diabetes mellitus |
| Sarcoidosis[288] |
| Guillain-Barré (often bilateral) |
| **ENT and other causes** |
| Orofacial granulomatosis |
| Parotid tumours |
| Otitis media or cholesteatoma |
| Trauma to skull base |
| Diving (barotrauma + temporal bone pneumocoele)[289] |
| Intracranial hypotension[290] |

**Prognosis** *Incomplete paralysis* without axonal degeneration usually recovers completely within a few weeks. Of those with *complete paralysis* ~80% make a full spontaneous recovery, but ~15% have axonal degeneration (~50% in pregnancy) in which case recovery is delayed, starting after ~3 months, and may be complicated by aberrant reconnections: *synkinesis*, eg eye blinking causes synchronous upturning of the mouth; misconnection of parasympathetic fibres (red in fig 1) can produce *crocodile tears* (gusto-lacrimal reflex) when eating stimulates unilateral lacrimation, not salivation (intra-lacrimal gland botulinum toxin may help).[296]

**Management** If given within 72h of onset, prednisolone (eg 60mg/d PO for 5d, tailing by 10mg/d) speeds recovery, with 95% making a full recovery),[297,298 NNT=8] perhaps by reducing axonal oedema and thus damage. Antivirals (eg aciclovir) don't help; although some 'Bell's cases' are thought to be associated with HSV-1, no-one has shown actively replicating virus.[299] There are little data to guide treatment if presenting after 72h of onset, but corticosteroids are widely used (but remember: high doses can cause psychosis and hyperglycaemia)[300]. No advice on the use of steroids is universally agreed in pregnancy.[301] Protect the eye: •Dark glasses and artificial tears (eg hypromellose) if evidence of drying •Encourage regular eyelid closure by pulling down the lid by hand •Use tape to close the eyes at night. *Surgery:* If eye closure remains a long-term problem (lagophthalmos), a lid loading procedure (eg with gold) to the upper lid may help.[302] If ectropion is severe, lateral tarsorrhaphy (partial lid-to-lid suturing) can help; if no recovery in 1yr, plastic surgery to help lid closure and to straighten the drooping face can be tried. Botulinum toxin can augment facial symmetry,[303] and hence self-esteem (beauty is symmetry according to Greek ideals—and *Vogue*).[304] There is low quality evidence that tailored facial exercises can improve facial function with moderate and chronic paralysis and ↓sequelae in acute cases.[305]

---

**1** Common causes of bilateral facial weakness: Lyme disease, Guillain-Barré syndrome, leukaemia, sarcoidosis, EBV, trauma and myasthenia gravis.

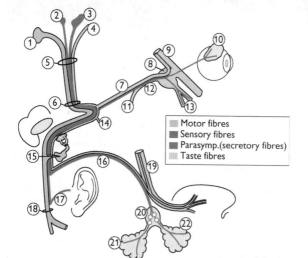

1 Facial nerve nucleus, deep in reticular formation of lower pons
2 Spinal nucleus of v
3 Superior salivary nuc.
4 Solitary tract
5 Porus acusticus internus
6 Meatal foramen
7 Large petrosal nerve
8 Sphenopalatine ganglion
9 Superior maxillary nerve
10 Lacrimal gland
11 Large deep petrosal nerve
12 Vidian nerve
13 Nose/palate gland nerves
14 Small petrosal nerve at geniculate ganglion[306]
15 Stapedial nerve
16 Chorda tympani
17 Auricular branch
18 Stylomastoid foramen
19 Lingual nerve—visceral motor[VII] and taste[VII] and general sensory to tongue ($v^3$)[307]
20 Submandibular ganglion (and gland, 21)
22 Sublingual gland

**Fig 1.** Facial nerve branches. The motor part moves the muscles of the face, scalp, and ears—also buccinator (puffs out the cheeks), platysma, stapedius, and the posterior belly of the digastric. It also contains the sympathetic motor fibres (vasodilator) of the submaxillary and sublingual glands (via the chorda tympani nerve). The sensory part contains the fibres of taste for the anterior ⅔ of the tongue and a few somatic sensory fibres from the middle ear region.

After Baylor College of Med. bcm.edu/oto/studs/face.html.

### Rare facial nerve eponyms (and why neurology is so easy)

**Ramsay Hunt syndrome** Described by James Ramsay Hunt in 1907,[308] this occurs when latent varicella zoster virus (p400) reactivates in the geniculate ganglion of the VII[th] cranial nerve. *Symptoms:* Painful vesicular rash on the auditory canal—*herpes zoster oticus* ± on drum, pinna, tongue palate or iris (→hyphema, ie blood under the cornea)[309] with ipsilateral facial palsy, loss of taste, vertigo, tinnitus, deafness, dry mouth & eyes. The rash may be too subtle for ordinary mortals to see—*herpes sine herpete*, ie herpes without herpes (neurology is easy, honestly... there's nothing to it). *Incidence:* ~5/100,000 (higher if >60yrs). *Δ:* Clinical, as antiviral treatment is thought to be most effective within the 1ˢᵗ 72h, while the virus is replicating. *R:* Antivirals (eg *aciclovir* 800mg PO 5× daily for 7d; if ₑGFR low, see p834)[310]+ *prednisolone*, as for Bell's palsy (according to a small retrospective analysis;[311] no definitive RCTs). *Prognosis:* If treated within 72h, ~75% recover well; if not, ~⅓ make a good recovery, ⅓ a reasonable recovery, and ⅓ a poor recovery.

**Foville's syndrome** Pontine lesion giving VII palsy, ipsilateral horizontal gaze palsy + contralateral hemiparesis, hemisensory loss & internuclear ophthalmoplegia.

**Millard-Gubler syndrome** Occlusion of basilar artery branches in the pons gives lateral rectus palsy (VI), ipsilateral facial paralysis and contralateral hemiplegia.

These are lesions of individual peripheral or cranial nerves. Causes are usually local, such as trauma,[1] or entrapment (eg tumour), except for carpal tunnel syndrome (BOX 1). The term *mononeuritis multiplex* is used if 2 or more peripheral nerves are affected, when causes tend to be systemic ('WARDS PLC'): Wegener's, aIDS/amyloid, rheumatoid, diabetes mellitus, sarcoidosis, pAN, leprosy, carcinomatosis). Electromyography (EMG) helps define the anatomic site of lesions.

**Median nerve C6-T1** The median nerve is the nerve of precision grip—muscles involved are easier to remember if you use your 'LOAF' (2 lumbricals, opponens pollicis, abductor pollicis brevis, and flexor pollicis brevis)[312] *At the wrist:* (eg lacerations, carpal tunnel syndrome, BOX 1) weakness of abductor pollicis brevis and sensory loss over the radial 3½ fingers and palm. *Anterior interosseous nerve lesions:* (eg trauma) weakness of flexion of the distal phalanx of the thumb and index finger. *Proximal lesions* (eg compression at the elbow) may show combined defects.

**Ulnar nerve C7-T1** Vulnerable to elbow trauma. *Signs:* Weakness/wasting of medial (ulnar side) wrist flexors, interossei (cannot cross the fingers in the good luck sign) and medial two lumbricals (claw hand); hypothenar eminence wasting (∴ weak little finger abduction); sensory loss over medial (ulnar) 1½ fingers and ulnar side of the hand. Flexion of 4th & 5th DIP joints is weak. With lesions at the wrist (digitorum profundus intact), claw hand is more marked. *Treatment:* BOX 2.

**Radial nerve C5-T1** This nerve opens the fist. It may be damaged by compression against the humerus. *Signs:* Test for wrist and finger drop with elbow flexed and arm pronated; sensory loss is variable—the dorsal aspect of the root of the thumb (the anatomical snuff box) is most reliably affected. Muscles involved: ('BEST') brachioradialis; extensors; supinator; triceps.[313]

**Brachial plexus** Pain/paraesthesiae and weakness in the affected arm in a variable distribution. *Causes:* trauma, radiotherapy (eg for breast carcinoma), prolonged wearing of a heavy rucksack, cervical rib, neuralgic amyotrophy,[2] thoracic outlet compression (also affects vasculature).

**Phrenic nerve C3-5** <sup>C3,4,5 keeps the diaphragm alive</sup> Consider phrenic nerve palsy if orthopnoea with raised hemidiaphragm on CXR. *Causes:* Lung cancer, myeloma, thymoma, cervical spondylosis/trauma, thoracic surgery, C3-5 zoster, HIV, Lyme disease, TB, paraneoplastic syndromes, muscular dystrophy, big left atrium, phrenic nucleus lesion, eg MS.

**Lateral cutaneous nerve of the thigh L2-L3** *Meralgia paraesthetica* is anterolateral burning thigh pain from entrapment under the inguinal ligament.

**Sciatic nerve L4-S3** Damaged by pelvic tumours or fractures to pelvis or femur. Lesions affect the hamstrings and all muscles below the knee (foot drop), with loss of sensation below the knee laterally.

**Common peroneal nerve L4-S1** Originates from sciatic nerve just above knee. Often damaged as it winds round the fibular head (trauma, sitting cross-legged). *Signs:* Foot drop, weak ankle dorsiflexion/eversion, and sensory loss over dorsum of foot.

**Tibial nerve L4-S3** Originates from the sciatic nerve just above the knee. Lesions lead to an inability to stand on tiptoe (plantarflexion), invert the foot, or flex the toes, with sensory loss over the sole.

---

1 Hereditary neuropathy with liability to pressure palsies is an autosomal dominant hereditary neuropathy presenting as recurrent isolated or multiple neuropathies. Onset is during teenage years.
2 Neuralgic amyotrophy (Parsonage-Turner syndrome) is a poorly understood inflammatory condition affecting the brachial plexus on one side only. Sudden onset severe pain, followed over hours by profound weakness, resolving completely over several days. It may rarely involve the phrenic or lower cranial nerves.

## Carpal tunnel syndrome: the commonest mononeuropathy

**The median nerve** and 9 tendons compete for space within the wrist. Compression is common, especially in women who have narrower wrists but similar-sized tendons to men. For similar reasons, the tibial nerve may be compressed: the tarsal tunnel syndrome, causing unilateral burning sole pain, eg on walking or standing.

**The patient:** Aching pain in the hand and arm (especially at night), and paraesthesiae in thumb, index, and middle fingers, all relieved by dangling the hand over the edge of the bed and shaking it (remember 'wake and shake'). There may be sensory loss and weakness of abductor pollicis brevis ± wasting of the thenar eminence. Light touch, 2-point discrimination, and sweating may be impaired.

**Famous median traps:** Myxoedema; enforced flexion (eg in a Colles' splint); diabetic neuropathy; idiopathic; acromegaly; neoplasms (eg myeloma); benign tumours (lipomas, ganglia); rheumatoid arthritis; amyloidosis; pregnancy/premenstrual oedema; sarcoidosis.

**Tests:** Neurophysiology helps by confirming the lesion's site and severity (and likelihood of improvement after surgery). Maximal wrist flexion for 1 min (*Phalen's test*) may elicit symptoms (unreliable!). Tapping over the nerve at the wrist induces tingling (*Tinel's test*; also rather non-specific).

**Treatment:** Splinting, local steroid injection (OHCS p710) ± decompression surgery; many alternative therapies are tried: meta-analyses are doubtful.[1]

Neurology

## Managing ulnar mononeuropathies from entrapments

**The ulnar nerve** asks for trouble in at least 5 places at the elbow, starting proximally at the arcade of Struthers (a musculofascial band ~8cm proximal to the medial epicondyle), and ending distally where it exits the flexor carpi ulnaris muscle in the forearm.[314] Most often, compression occurs at the *epicondylar groove* or at the point where the nerve passes between the 2 heads of flexor carpi ulnaris (true *cubital tunnel syndrome*). Trauma can easily damage the nerve against its bony confines (the medial condyle of the humerus—the 'funny bone'). Normally, stretch and compression forces on the ulnar nerve at the elbow are moderated by its ability to glide in its groove. When normal excursion is restricted, irritation ensues. This may cause a vicious cycle of perineural scarring, consequent loss of excursion, and progressive symptoms—without antecedent trauma. Compressive ulnar neuropathies at the wrist (*Guyon's canal*—between the pisiform and hamate bones) are less common, but they can also result in disability.

**Treatment** centres on rest and avoiding pressure on the nerve, but if symptoms continue, night-time soft elbow splinting (to prevent flexion to >60°)[315] is warranted, eg for 6 months.[316] A splint for the hand may help prevent permanent clawing of the fingers. For chronic neuropathy associated with weakness, or if splinting fails, a variety of *surgical procedures* have been tried. For moderately severe neuropathies, decompressions *in situ* may help, but often fail. Medial epicondylectomies are effective in ≤50% (but many will recur). Subcutaneous nerve re-routing (transposition) may be tried. Intramuscular and submuscular transpositions are more complicated, but the latter may be preferable.[317]

1 *Cochrane meta-analysis of 21 carpal tunnel trials:* 7 (but not 2) weeks' ultrasound can help. Compared to placebo, diuretics and NSAIDs gave no benefit. Vit B₆ did not help (N = 50). Those adopting the namaste (prayer) posture in yoga may obviate need for surgery: the forced wrist extension helps (N = 53). Trials of ergonomic keyboards give equivocal results for pain and function. Trials of magnet therapy, laser acupuncture, and exercise showed no benefit. Chiropractic care can increase distress.

Neurology

Polyneuropathies are disorders of peripheral or cranial nerves, whose distribution is usually symmetrical and widespread, often with distal weakness and sensory loss ('glove and stocking'). They are classified by course (*acute* or *chronic*), by function (*sensory, motor, autonomic, mixed*), or by pathology (*demyelination, axonal degeneration,* or *both*). For example, Guillain-Barré syndrome (p716) is an acute, predominantly motor, demyelinating neuropathy, whereas chronic alcohol abuse leads to a chronic, initially sensory then mixed, axonal neuropathy.

| **Mostly motor** | **Mostly sensory** |
|---|---|
| Guillain-Barré syndrome (p716) | Diabetes mellitus |
| Lead poisoning | Renal failure |
| Charcot-Marie-Tooth syndrome[1] | Leprosy |

**Diagnosis** The history is vital: be clear about the time course, the precise nature of the symptoms, and any preceding or associated events (eg D&V before Guillain-Barré syndrome; weight↓ in cancer; arthralgia from a connective tissue disease. Ask about travel, alcohol and drug use, sexual infections, and family history. If there is palpable nerve thickening think of leprosy or Charcot-Marie-Tooth. Examine other systems for clues to the cause, eg alcoholic liver disease.

*Sensory neuropathy:* Numbness; pins & needles, "feels funny" or "burning"; affects extremities 1st ('glove and stocking' distribution—map out each modality, p450). There may be difficulty handling small objects such as buttons. Signs of trauma (eg finger burns) or joint deformation may indicate sensory loss. Diabetic and alcoholic neuropathies are typically painful.

*Motor neuropathy:* Often progressive (may be rapid); weak or clumsy hands; difficulty in walking (falls; stumbling); difficulty in breathing (vital capacity↓). Signs: LMN lesion: wasting and weakness most marked in the distal muscles of hands and feet (foot or wrist drop). Reflexes are reduced or absent.

*Cranial nerves:* Swallowing/speaking difficulty; diplopia. *Autonomic system:* BOX 1.

**Tests** FBC, ESR, glucose, U&E, LFT, TSH, B₁₂, electrophoresis, ANA & ANCA (p555), CXR, urinalysis, and consider an LP ± specific genetic tests for inherited neuropathies (eg for PMP22 in Charcot-Marie-Tooth),³¹⁸ lead level, antiganglioside antibodies. Nerve conduction studies help distinguish demyelinating from axonal causes.

**Management** Treat the cause. Involve physio & OT (p449). Foot care and shoe choice are important in sensory neuropathies to minimize trauma. Splinting joints helps prevent contractures in prolonged paralysis. In Guillain-Barré and CIDP² IV immunoglobulin helps.³¹⁹ For vasculitic causes, steroids/immunosuppressants may help. Treat neuropathic pain with amitriptyline or nortriptyline (10-25mg at night; may not work in HIV neuropathy).³²⁰ If this fails, try gabapentin³ or pregabalin.³²¹

### Causes

**Metabolic**
Diabetes mellitus
Renal failure
Hypothyroidism
Hypoglycaemia
Mitochondrial disorders

**Vasculitides** (p558)
Polyarteritis nodosa
Rheumatoid arthritis
Wegener's• granulomatosis

**Malignancy**
Paraneoplastic syndromes
Polycythaemia rubra vera

**Inflammatory**
Guillain-Barré syndrome
Sarcoidosis; CIDP²

**Infections** Leprosy
HIV, syphilis
Lyme disease (p430)

**Nutritional**
↓ vit B₁, B₁₂ (eg EtOH abuse)
↓ vit E, folate
↑ vit B₆ (if >100mg/d)

**Inherited syndromes**
Charcot-Marie-Tooth (p710)
Refsum's syndrome (p724)
Porphyria (p706)
Leucodystrophy

**Toxins** Lead, arsenic

**Drugs** Vincristine
Alcohol Cisplatin
Isoniazid Nitrofurantoin
Phenytoin Metronidazole

**Others**
Paraproteinaemias
Amyloidosis (p364)

---

1 The *presentation* of Charcot-Marie-Tooth is typically motor, although the sensory deficit is present on examination, because the sensory loss is so gradual & long-standing that it feels 'normal' to the patient.
2 Chronic inflammatory demyelinating polyradiculoneuropathy (CIDP) autoimmune demyelination of peripheral nerves (distal onset of weakness/sensory loss in limbs + nerve enlargement + CSF protein↑).
3 300mg on day 1, 300mg/12h on day 2, 300mg/8h on day 3, then ↑ according to response in steps of 100mg/8h; max 600mg/8h if eGFR >80. SE: diarrhoea, dry mouth, dyspepsia, vomiting, oedema, dizziness.

## Autonomic neuropathy

Sympathetic and Parasympathetic neuropathies may be isolated or part of a generalized sensorimotor peripheral neuropathy.

*Causes:* DM, amyloidosis, Guillain–Barré and Sjögren's syndrome, HIV, leprosy, SLE,[322] toxic, genetic (eg porphyria), or paraneoplastic, eg paraneoplastic encephalo-myeloneuropathies and Lambert-Eaton myasthenic syndrome (LEMS, p516).

*Signs:* Postural hypotension[s] (faints on standing, eating, or hot bath), erectile dysfunction[p]/ejaculatory failure[s] (remember 'point & shoot'), sweating↓[s], constipation, nocturnal diarrhoea, urine retention[p], Horner's[s] (p716), Holmes–Adie pupil[p] (p79)[323]

**Autonomic function tests** • *Postural drop* of ≥20/10mmHg is abnormal. $R$: p39.
• *ECG:* A variation of <10bpm with respiration is abnormal.
• *Cystometry:* Bladder pressure studies.
• *Pupils:* Instil 0.1% epinephrine (dilates if post-ganglionic sympathetic denervation, not if normal); 2.5% cocaine (dilates if normal; not if sympathetic denervation); 2.5% methacholine (constricts if parasympathetic lesion)—rarely used.
• *Paraneoplastic antibodies:* Anti-Hu, anti-Yo, anti-Ri, antiamphiphysin, anti-CV2, anti-Ma2). *Other ab:* Antiganglionic acetylcholine receptor antibody presence shows that the cause may be autoimmune autonomic ganglionopathy.[324]

**Primary autonomic failure** Occurs alone (autoimmune autonomic ganglionopathy), as part of multisystem atrophy (MSA, p499), or with Parkinson's disease, typically in a middle-aged/elderly man. Onset: insidious; symptoms as above.

MND is a cluster of major degenerative diseases characterized by selective loss of neurons in motor cortex, cranial nerve nuclei, and anterior horn cells. Upper and lower motor neurons are affected but there is *no* sensory loss or sphincter disturbance, thus distinguishing MND from MS and polyneuropathies. MND never affects eye movements, distinguishing it from myasthenia (p516). Events at the ALS-FTD locus (amyotrophic lateral sclerosis-frontotemporal dementia locus on 9p21) explain 87% of familial ALS (eg autosomal-dominant D90A SOD1 mutation).[325] 4 clinical patterns:

1 *ALS/amyotrophic lateral sclerosis* (archetypal MND; 50%) Loss of motor neurons in motor cortex *and* the anterior horn of the cord, so weakness + UMN signs (eg upgoing plantars) + LMN wasting/fasciculation (p451). Worse prognosis if: bulbar onset, ↑age; ↓FVC. The split hand sign:[326] the thumb's side of the hand seems cast adrift owing to excessive wasting around it—there is much less hypothenar wasting.

2 *Progressive bulbar palsy* (10%) Only affects cranial nerves IX–XII. Signs: BOX 1.

3 *Progressive muscular atrophy* (10%) Anterior horn cell lesion only, thus no UMN signs. Affects distal muscle groups before proximal. Better prognosis than ALS.

4 *Primary lateral sclerosis* Loss of Betz cells in motor cortex, thus mainly UMN signs + marked spastic leg weakness and pseudobulbar palsy. No cognitive decline.

▶Think of MND in those >40yrs with stumbling spastic gait, foot-drop ± proximal myopathy, weak grip (door-handles don't turn) and shoulder abduction (hair-washing is hard), or aspiration pneumonia. Look for UMN signs: spasticity, brisk reflexes; ↑plantars; and LMN signs: wasting, fasciculation of tongue, abdomen, back, thigh. Is speech or swallowing affected (bulbar signs)? Fasciculation is not enough to diagnose an LMN lesion: look for weakness too. Frontotemporal dementia occurs in ~25%.

**Diagnostic criteria** See BOX 2. There is no diagnostic test. Brain/cord MRI helps exclude structural causes, LP helps exclude inflammatory ones, and neurophysiology can detect subclinical denervation and help exclude mimicking motor neuropathies.[1]

**Prevalence** 6/100,000. ♂:♀ ≈ 3 : 2. Median UK age at onset: 60yrs. Often fatal in 2–4yrs.

**Treatment** Due to MND's implacable course, its rarity, and its frightening nature, a multidisciplinary approach is best:[327] neurologist, palliative nurse,[328] hospice, physio, OT, speech therapist, dietician, social services—all orchestrated by the GP. Death by choking is rare, so warmly reassure that a dignified end is the rule. MNDassociation.org UK tel. 08457 626262

*Antiglutamatergic drugs:* Riluzole (BOX) prolongs life by ~3 months; it is costly. *Caution:* LFT↑ (do 3-monthly). SE: vomiting, pulse↑, somnolence, headache, vertigo, LFT↑.

*Drooling:* Propantheline 15–30mg/8h; amitriptyline 25–50mg/8h (doctors think this is quite effective, but patients disagree: and example of our wishful thinking; BOX).

*Dysphagia:* Blend food; would he or she like a nasogastric tube, or percutaneous catheter gastrostomy?—or would this prolong death? *Spasticity:* See MS (p500).

*Joint pains and distress:* Analgesic ladder—NSAIDs, etc, then opioids (p539).

*Respiratory failure (± aspiration pneumonia and sleep apnoea):* Non-invasive ventilation (NIV) at home in selected patients may give valuable palliation.

**✿Ethical problems: beyond autonomy** Patients with MND may be ventilated (eg NIV), and then decide they want NIV withdrawn.[329] This may be fatal, making decisions difficult for everyone. Ethicists tend to speak in black-and-white prose: "Do whatever promotes autonomy", and this is the *raison d'être* of assisted-suicide organizations such as Dignitas (increasingly popular, worldwide, even if illegal). Sometimes nature contrives something more ambiguous and poetic, in which rationality and rage[330] uncertainty and the forked emotions of hope and despair produce a heady internal world which the ethicist can never quite catch or tame; if this internal world is one of perpetual change and oscillation of the will, ideas of autonomy become incoherent. Rather than aiming to apply Kantian universal rules (p15), our role may be more to offer a well-placed hug to signal metaphysical complicity, and to stand beside our patients, come what may.

---

1 If no UMN signs and distal arm muscles are affected in the distribution of individual nerves, suspect multifocal motor neuropathy with conduction block (diagnose on nerve conduction studies; ℞: IV Ig). Gynaecomastia, atrophic testes ± infertility suggests Kennedy syndrome (bulbospinal muscular atrophy).

## Bulbar and corticobulbar ('pseudobulbar') palsy

**Bulbar palsy** denotes diseases of the nuclei of cranial nerves IX–XII in the medulla. *Signs* are of an *LMN lesion* of the tongue and muscles of talking and swallowing: flaccid, fasciculating tongue (like a sack of worms); jaw jerk is normal or absent, speech is quiet, hoarse, or nasal. *Causes:* MND, Guillain-Barré, polio, myasthenia gravis, syringobulbia (p520), brainstem tumours, central pontine myelinolysis (p686).

**Corticobulbar palsy** *UMN lesion* of muscles of swallowing and talking due to bilateral lesions above the mid-pons, eg corticobulbar tracts (MS, MND, stroke, central pontine myelinolysis). It is commoner than bulbar palsy. *Signs:* Slow tongue movements, with slow deliberate speech; ↑jaw jerk; ↑pharyngeal and palatal reflexes; pseudobulbar affect (PBA)—weeping unprovoked by sorrow or mood-incongruent giggling (emotional incontinence *without* mood change is also seen in MS, Wilson's, and Parkinson's disease, dementia, nitrous oxide use, and head injury)[331] In some countries, dextromethorphan + quinidine is licensed for PBA.

## Revised El Escorial diagnostic criteria for ALS

**Definite** Lower + upper motor neuron signs in 3 regions.
**Probable** Lower + upper motor neuron signs in 2 regions.
**Probably with lab support** Lower + upper motor neuron signs in 1 region, or upper motor neuron signs in ≥1 region + EMG shows acute denervation in ≥2 limbs.
**Possible** Lower + upper motor neuron signs in 1 region.
**Suspected** Upper or lower motor neuron signs only—in 1 or more regions.

## Following in the footprints of free radicals

Autopsies show that changes to proteins and DNA that are signs or 'footprints' of free-radical damage are more pronounced in MND brains than in controls[332] Also, cultured fibroblasts from MND brains show ↑sensitivity to oxidative insults (pesticides may have a role).[333] But these findings don't explain 2 key MND phenomena: *Why is there a predilection for motor neurons?* One answer may be the sheer length and complex cytoarchitecture of motor cells, with their 1 metre axons and high levels of neurofilament proteins, and low levels of $Ca^{2+}$-buffering proteins (thought to be protective). We note that motor cells with the shortest axons (to the extraocular muscles) are unaffected in MND; this is not true of the tongue, which only requires slightly longer axons. Also, it isn't *only* motor neurons that are affected: specific aphasias and dementias are part of the MND picture too.[334] *Why do some MND brains have excess levels of glutamate?* (Glutamate is the chief excitatory neurotransmitter.) This is thought to be from ↓ activity of the excitatory amino acid transporter (EAAT2), which mops up glutamate—hence the notion that MND is an 'excitotoxic' phenomenon. Motor cells have high levels of Cu/Zn superoxide dismutase (thought to protect normal motor cells from glutamate toxicity/oxidative stress). But a high level may itself be damaging, given certain genetic or acquired vulnerabilities.[335] Transgenic mice exhibiting high levels of superoxide dismutase do indeed develop an MND phenotype.

These ideas are speculative,[336] but help understanding and criticism of future therapies. Riluzole is an $Na^+$-channel blocker inhibiting glutamate release. Neurotrophic factors can protect motor neurons in animal studies, but clinical trials have proved disappointing. CI: hepatic or renal problems. Effects of free-radical manipulation can be unpredictable. The antioxidant vitamin E protects transgenic mice from developing an MND-like picture, and in at least one human trial high intake of polyunsaturated fatty acids and vitamin E associated with a 50% decreased risk of developing ALS (these nutrients appear to act synergistically).[337]

Apoptosis is a hallmark of MND,[338] and overexpression of proteins inhibiting cell death via apoptosis (Bcl-2) in transgenic mice can slow MND degeneration.

## PatientsLikeMe.com

Patient-organized sites such as these have now got so big that reliable(ish) data can be obtained about what works for MND symptoms[et al.339] There are intriguing disparities between what doctors and patients think works. We think we know everything about symptoms: sites like these show how we lead ourselves astray.

Cervical spondylosis with compression of the cord (myelopathy) and nerve roots is the leading cause of progressive spastic quadriparesis with sensory loss below the neck.[340] Most people with cervical spondylosis have no impairment, however—just degeneration of the annulus fibrosus of cervical intervertebral discs ± osteophytes, which narrow the spinal canal and intervertebral foramina. As the neck flexes and extends, the cord is damaged as it is dragged over these protruding bony spurs anteriorly and indented by a thickened ligamentum flavum posteriorly.

**Signs** Limited, painful neck movement ± crepitus—be careful! Neck flexion may produce tingling down the spine—a positive Lhermitte's symptom. This does not help decide if cord or roots (or both) are involved.

*Root compression (radiculopathy):* Pain/'electrical' sensations in arms or fingers at the level of the compression (TABLE), with dull reflexes, dynatomal[1] sensory disturbance (numbness, tingling, ↓pain & T°), LMN weakness and eventual wasting of muscles innervated by the affected root. Below the level of the affected root (examine the legs) there may be UMN signs suggesting cord compression: spasticity, weakness, brisk reflexes, and upgoing plantars. Position & vibration sense may be lost. Is there a sensory level?

| Complaints may be of: |
| --- |
| • Neck stiffness (but common in anyone >50yrs old) |
| • Crepitus on moving neck |
| • Stabbing or dull arm pain (brachialgia) |
| • Forearm/wrist pain |
| *Signs of cord compression:* |
| • Spastic leg weakness (often 1 leg > other) |
| • Weak, clumsy hands |
| • Numbness in hands |
| • 'Heavy' legs |
| • Foot-drop/poor walking |
| • Incontinence, hesitancy & urgency are often late[341] |

**Dynatomes**[1] *C3 and C4* symptoms are neck pain or trapezius pain.
*C5* pain occurs in the shoulder and radiates down the front of the arm to below the elbow. There is overlap in the pain of *C6* radiculopathy and carpal tunnel syndrome (p507)—CTS causes pain worse on wrist flexion+while abductor pollicis brevis+thenar atrophy; in contrast, C6 root innervates elbow flexors and wrist extensors. Spurling's manoeuvre[2] may exacerbate C6 radicular pain (but not CTS).
*C7* pain radiates down the dorsal arm, via the elbow and into the 3rd finger.
*C8* symptoms go down the inferior medial aspect of the arm in 4th & 5th digits and are often confused with the pain of ulnar neuropathy (but here there is splitting of sensory symptoms in either the 3rd or 4th digit).[342]

**Tests** MRI to localize the lesion (fig 1). An AP compression ratio ≥30% usually induces histopathological changes in the cord (cadaver studies). Time to walk 30m helps monitor progress (valid & cheap)[340]

ΔΔ MS; nerve root neurofibroma; subacute combined degeneration of the cord (↓B₁₂); compression by bone or cord tumours; intramedullary spinal sarcoidosis.[343]

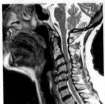

Fig 1. A T2-weighted MRI (∴ CSF looks bright). The cord is compressed between osteophytes anteriorly and the ligamentum flavum posteriorly.

**Management** A firm neck collar restricts anterior-posterior movement of the neck so may relieve pain, but patients dislike them. Don't dismiss those with chronic root pain in the arm as suffering simply from 'wear and tear' spondylosis. Be optimistic: they may improve over months; if not, they *may* benefit greatly from surgical root decompression (laminectomy, fig 2, or laminoplasty, fig 3) if there is significant MRI abnormality,[344] and especially if the history is short and the neurological deficit is progressing. As a rule of thumb, opt for conservative treatment if the spinal transverse area is >70mm², the patient is elderly, and motor conduction time is normal.[345] If surgery *is* done, progression is usually halted and leg weakness may improve. Operative risk is less than with anterior spinal fusion (needs bone grafts with more complications but no extra benefit).[346] Transforaminal steroid injection is gaining popularity on the rationale that nerve root inflammation causes radicular pain. Pain reduction is reported.

**Rare complications** Diaphragm paralysis,[347] spinal artery syndrome mimicking angina (from spinal artery compression; pain & T° are lost before vibration sense).[348]

| Typical motor and sensory deficits from individual root involvement (c5-8) | |
|---|---|
| **C5 (C4/C5 disc)** | Weak deltoid & supraspinatus; ↓supinator jerks; numb elbow. |
| **C6 (C5/C6 disc)** | Weak biceps & brachioradialis; ↓biceps jerks; numb thumb & index finger. |
| **C7 (C6/C7 disc)** | Weak triceps & finger extension; ↓triceps jerks; numb middle finger. |
| **C8 (C7/T1 disc)** | Weak finger flexors & small muscles of the hand; numb 5ᵗʰ & ring finger. |

►*Worrying symptoms:* Night pain, weight↓, fever.

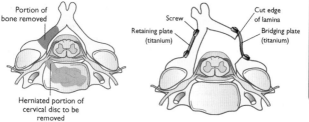

**Fig 2.** Laminectomy.

**Fig 3.** Laminoplasty (screws and plates).

*Laminectomy or laminoplasty?* Laminectomy and laminoplasty improve gait, strength, sensation, pain, and degree of myelopathy, to a roughly equal extent, but in one study of 44 consecutive patients, laminoplasty was associated with more pain reduction and fewer late complications (but there was more neck stiffness).[349] At appropriate level, the ligamentum flavum (overlies the dura) is incised and cut away with part of adjacent laminae, as necessary to expose the extradural space.[350]

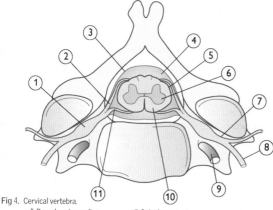

**Fig 4.** Cervical vertebra.

| | |
|---|---|
| 1 Dorsal root ganglion | 7 Spinal nerve |
| 2 Dorsal root | 8 Ventral ramus |
| 3 Dura mater | 9 Vertebral artery in the transverse foramen |
| 4 Subarachnoid space | 10 White matter |
| 5 Pia mater | 11 Ventral spinal nerve |
| 6 Grey matter | |

Fig 1 ©Prof P Scally; figs 2-4 after Dr C Carpenter.

**1** A dynatome is the area of pain or pins and needles caused by a trapped nerve root. It differs from a dermatome or myotome because it relates to complex referred pain mechanisms, not nerve root function (which is what radiculopathy relates to). Dynatomes don't map neatly to dermatomes or myotomes, so according to Slipman, we should try not use dynotomes *in isolation* to blame individual nerve roots.[351]
**2** Reproduction of the patient's symptoms when the examiner moves the patient's head.

Neurology

**Myopathy or neuropathy?** In favour of myopathy: •Gradual onset of symmetric *proximal* weakness—difficulty combing hair and climbing stairs (NB: weakness is also *distal* in myotonic dystrophy); •Dystrophies usually affect specific muscle groups (ie selective weakness on first presentation); •Preserved tendon reflexes.

A neuropathy is more likely if there are paraesthesiae, bladder problems or distal weakness. **Rapid onset** suggests a neuropathy or a toxic, drug, or metabolic myopathy. **Excess fatigability** (↑weakness with exercise) suggests myasthenia (p516). Spontaneous **pain** at rest and local tenderness occurs in inflammatory myopathies. Pain on exercise suggests ischaemia or metabolic myopathy (eg McArdle's disease). **Oddly firm** muscles (due to infiltrations with fat or connective tissue) suggest pseudohypertrophic muscular dystrophies (eg Duchenne's). **Lumps** are commonly caused by haematoma, herniation of muscle through fascia, and tendon rupture. Muscle tumours are rare. **Fasciculation** suggests anterior horn cell or root disease. Look for evidence of systemic disease. *Tests:* ESR, CK, AST and LDH may be raised. Do EMG and tests relevant to systemic causes (eg TSH↑↓, p208). Many genetic disorders of muscle are detectable by DNA analysis: use muscle biopsy only if genetic tests are non-diagnostic.

**Muscular dystrophies** are a group of genetic diseases with progressive degeneration and weakness of specific muscle groups. The primary abnormality may be in the muscle membrane. Secondary effects are marked variation in size of individual fibres and deposition of fat and connective tissue. The commonest is Duchenne's muscular dystrophy (3/1000 male live births; sex-linked recessive—30% from spontaneous mutation). The Duchenne gene is on the short arm of X (xp665), and its product, dystrophin, is non-functional. It presents at ~4yrs old with clumsy walking, then difficulty in standing, and respiratory failure. Pseudohypertrophy is seen, especially in the calves. Serum creatine kinase ↑ >40-fold. There is no specific treatment. Some survive beyond 20yrs. Home ventilation improves prognosis. Genetic counselling is vital. Becker's muscular dystrophy (~0.3/1000 ♂ births) results from a Duchenne gene mutation that produces partially functioning dystrophin. It presents with similar but milder symptoms, at a later age than Duchenne's, and with a better prognosis. Facioscapulohumeral muscular dystrophy (Landouzy-Dejerine) is almost as common as Duchenne's. *Inheritance:* Autosomal dominant (locus 4q35). Onset is ~12-14yrs old, with inability to puff out the cheeks and difficulty raising the arms above the head (eg changing light-bulbs). *Signs:* Weakness of face ('ironed out' expression), shoulders, and upper arms (often asymmetric with deltoids spared), foot-drop, scapular winging (fig 1),[352] scoliosis, anterior axillary folds,[353] and horizontal clavicles.[354] ≤20% need a wheelchair by 40yrs old.

**Myotonic disorders** cause tonic muscle spasm (myotonia). *Histology:* long chains of central nuclei within muscle fibres. The chief one is dystrophia myotonica (DM1), an autosomal dominant Cl⁻ channelopathy.[355] *Typical onset:* 25yr-old with distal-onset weakness (hand/foot drop), weak sternomastoids and myotonia. Facial weakness and muscle wasting give a long, haggard appearance. *Also:* cataracts, male frontal baldness, diabetes, testis/ovary atrophy, cardiomyopathy, and ↓cognition. Most patients die in middle age of intercurrent illness. Mexiletine, phenytoin and acetazolamide may help. Genetic counselling is important. Myotonia caused by Na⁺ **channelopathy:** paramyotonia congenita, adynamia episodica hereditaria.

**Acquired myopathies of late onset** are often part of systemic disease—eg hyperthyroidism, malignancy, Cushing's, hypo- and hypercalcaemia.

**Inflammatory myopathies** Inclusion body myositis is the chief example if aged >50yrs. Aggregates of Alzheimer tau proteins suggest a 'peripheral tauopathy'.[356] *Signs:* weakness starts with quads, finger flexors or pharyngeal muscles. Ventral extremity muscle groups are more affected than dorsal or girdle groups. Wheelchair dependency is <3%. *Histology:* ringed vacuoles + intranuclear inclusions. *R:* nothing is consistently effective. For polymyositis and dermatomyositis, see p554.

**Drug causes** Alcohol; statins; steroids; chloroquine; zidovudine; vincristine; cocaine.

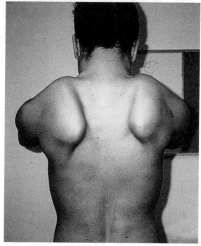

**Fig 1.** Winging of both scapulae in facioscapulohumeral muscular dystrophy. Winging is due to weakness of thoracoscapular muscles.

Reproduced from Donaghy, *Brain's Diseases of the Nervous System*, 12th edition, with permission from Oxford University Press.

MG is an autoimmune disease mediated by antibodies to nicotinic acetylcholine receptors (AChR), interfering with the neuromuscular transmission via depletion of working post-synaptic receptor sites (fig 1). Both B and T cells are implicated.[357,358]

**Presentation** Increasing muscular fatigue. Muscle groups affected, in order: extraocular; bulbar (swallowing, chewing); face; neck; limb girdle; trunk. Look for: ptosis, diplopia, myasthenic snarl on smiling, 'peek sign'.[1] On counting to 50, the voice fades (dysphonia is a rare presentation). *Tendon reflexes* are normal. Weakness is worsened by: pregnancy, K⁺↓, infection, over-treatment, change of climate, emotion, exercise, gentamicin, opiates, tetracycline, quinine, procainamide, β-blockers.

**Associations** If under 50yrs, MG is commoner in women, associated with other autoimmune diseases and thymic hyperplasia. Over 50, it is commoner in men, and associated with thymic atrophy or thymic tumour, rheumatoid arthritis, and SLE.

**Tests** •*Antibodies:* Anti-AChR antibodies ↑ in 90% (70% in ocular-confined MG); if seronegative look for MuSK antibodies (muscle specific tyrosine kinase; ♀:♂≈15:2).[359] •*Neurophysiology:* Decremental muscle response to repetitive nerve stimulation ± ↑single-fibre jitter. •*Imaging:* CT of thymus.[360] •*Other:* ptosis improves by >2mm after ice application to the (shut) affected lid for >2min—a neat, non-invasive test.[361] The Tensilon® test may not give clear answers and has dangers, so is less used.

**Treatment** *Symptom control* Anticholinesterase, eg pyridostigmine (60-120mg PO up to 6×daily; max 1.2g/d). Cholinergic SE: salivation↑, lacrimation, sweats, vomiting, miosis. Other SE: diarrhoea, colic (controllable with propantheline 15mg/8h).

*Immunosuppression:* Treat relapses with prednisolone—start at 5mg on alternate days, ↑ by 5mg/wk up to 1mg/kg on each treatment day. ↓dose on remission (may take months). Give osteoporosis prophylaxis. SE: weakness (hence low starting dose). Steroids may be combined with azathioprine 2.5mg/kg/day (do FBC and LFT weekly for 8wks, then 12-weekly) or weekly methotrexate.[362] IV methylprednisolone has a role.

*Thymectomy:* Consider if onset before 50yrs old and disease is not easily controlled by anticholinesterases. Expect remission in 25% and worthwhile benefit in a further 50%. Thymectomy is also necessary for thymomas to prevent local invasion (but MG symptoms are often unaffected). Some give IV immunoglobulin (IV Ig) 0.4g/kg daily for 5 days pre-op.[363]

**Myasthenic crisis** Weakness of the respiratory muscles during a relapse can be life-threatening. ►Monitor forced vital capacity. Ventilatory support is unlikely to be needed if vital capacity >20mL/kg.[364] Treat with plasmapheresis or IV Ig[365] and identify and treat the trigger for the relapse (eg infection, medications).

**Prognosis** Relapsing or slow progression. If thymoma, 5yr survival is 68%.[366]

**Other causes of muscle fatigability** Polymyositis; SLE; Takayasu's arteritis (fatigability of the extremities); botulism (see BOX). For other myopathies, see p514.

## Lambert-Eaton myasthenic syndrome (LEMS, *ALSO* ELMS)

LEMS can be paraneoplastic (from small-cell lung cancer) or autoimmune.[2] Unlike true MG there is: •Gait difficulty before eye signs; •Autonomic involvement (dry mouth, constipation, impotence); •Hyporeflexia and weakness, which improve after exercise; •Less response to edrophonium; •Antibody to the pre-synaptic membrane's voltage-gated Ca²⁺ channels (see fig 2; anti-P/Q type VGCC antibodies are +ve in 85%).[367] •Electrical post-tetanic potentiation with >60% ↑ in post-exercise facilitation of abductor digiti quinti.[368] *R:* 3,4-diaminopyridine or IV immunoglobulin (get specialist help).[369] ►Do regular CXR/high-resolution CT as symptoms may precede the cancer by >4yrs.

---

1 After brief opposition to gentle sustained lid closure, the lids separate ('peek') to show white sclerae.[370]
2 64% of those with non-tumour LEMS have a family member with autoimmune thyroid disease or DM.[371]

1 Before transmission can occur, neurotransmitter must be packed into synaptic vesicles. At the neuromuscular junction (NMJ) this is acetylcholine (ACh). Each vesicle contains ~8000 ACh molecules.

2 When an action potential arrives at the pre-synaptic terminal, depolarization opens voltage-gated $Ca^{2+}$ channels (VGCC). In **Lambert-Eaton** syndrome anti-P/Q type VGCC antibodies disrupt this stage of synaptic transmission.

3 Influx of $Ca^{2+}$ through the VGCCs triggers fusion of synaptic vesicles with the pre-synaptic membrane (a process that **botulinum toxin** interferes with), and neurotransmitter is released from the vesicles into the synaptic cleft.

4 Transmitter molecules cross the synaptic cleft by diffusion and bind to receptors on the post-synaptic membrane, causing depolarization of the post-synaptic membrane (the end-plate potential). This change in the post-synaptic membrane triggers muscle contraction at the NMJ, or onward transmission of the action potential in neurons. In **myasthenia gravis**, antibodies block the post-synaptic ACh receptors, preventing the end-plate potential from becoming large enough to trigger muscle contraction—and muscle weakness ensues.

5 Transmitter action is terminated by enzyme-induced degradation of transmitter (eg acetylcholinesterase), uptake into the pre-synaptic terminal or glial cells, or by diffusion away from synapse.[372] Anticholinesterase treatments for myasthenia gravis, such as **pyridostigmine**, reduce the rate of degradation of ACh, increasing the chance that it will trigger an end-plate potential.

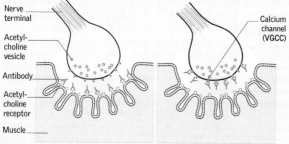

Nerve terminal

Acetyl-choline vesicle

Antibody

Acetyl-choline receptor

Muscle

Calcium channel (VGCC)

Fig 1. Myasthenia gravis features *post-synaptic* acetylcholine receptor antibodies. Tendon reflexes are normal because the synapses do not have time to become fatigued with such a brief muscle contraction. Ocular palsies are common (it's not exactly clear why).

Fig 2. Lambert-Eaton syndrome features **pre-synaptic** $Ca^{2+}$-channel antibodies. Diplopia and involvement of the muscles of respiration are rare. Depressed tendon reflexes are common, because less transmitter is released, but reflexes may ↑ after maximum voluntary contraction due to a build of transmitter in the synaptic cleft (post-tetanic potentiation). Dysfunction of the autonomic nervous system is also common.

Neurology

### Type 1 neurofibromatosis (NF1, von Recklinghausen's disease)

Autosomal dominant inheritance (gene locus 17q11.2). Expression of NF1 is variable, even within a family. *Prevalence:* 1 in 2500, ♀:♂≈1:1; no racial predilection.

*Signs:* Café-au-lait spots: flat, coffee-coloured patches of skin seen in 1st year of life (clearest in UV light), increasing in size and number with age. Adults have ≥6, >15mm across. They do *not* predispose to skin cancer. **Freckling:** typically in skin-folds (axillae, groin, neck base, and submammary area♀), and usually present by age 10. **Dermal neurofibromas:** small, violaceous nodules, gelatinous in texture, which appear at puberty, and may become papillomatous. They are not painful but may itch. Numbers increase with age. **Nodular neurofibromas** arise from nerve trunks. Firm and clearly demarcated, they can give rise to paraesthesiae if pressed. Lisch nodules (fig 1) are tiny harmless regular brown/ translucent mounds (hamartomas) on the iris (use a slit lamp)≤2mm in diameter. They develop by 6yrs old in 90%. Also short stature and macrocephaly.

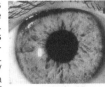
Fig 1. Multiple brown Lisch nodules on the iris. ©Jon Miles.

*Complications:* Occur in 30%. Mild learning disability is common. *Local effects of neurofibromas:* Nerve root compression (weakness, pain, paraesthesiae);[373] GI—bleeds, obstruction; bone—cystic lesions, scoliosis, pseudarthrosis. BP↑ (6%) from renal artery stenosis or phaeochromocytoma. Plexiform neurofibromas (large, subcutaneous swellings). *Malignancy* (5% patients with NF1): optic glioma, sarcomatous change in a neurofibroma. Epilepsy risk ↑ (slight). *Rare association:* carcinoid syndrome (p278).[374]

*Management:* Multidisciplinary team with geneticist, neurologist, surgeon, and physiotherapist,[373] orchestrated by a GP. Yearly measurement of BP and cutaneous survey. Dermal neurofibromas are unsightly, and catch on clothing; if troublesome, excise, but removing all lesions is unrealistic. Genetic counselling is vital (OHCS p154).

### Type 2 neurofibromatosis (NF2)

Autosomal dominant inheritance, though 50% are *de novo*, with mosaicism in some (NF2 gene locus is 22q11). Rarer than NF1 with a prevalence of only 1 in 35,000.

*Signs:* Café-au-lait spots are fewer than in NF1. **Bilateral vestibular Schwannomas** (= acoustic neuromas; p466) are characteristic, becoming symptomatic by ~20yrs old when sensorineural hearing loss is the 1st sign. There may be tinnitus and vertigo. The rate of tumour growth is unpredictable and variable. The tumours are benign but cause problems by pressing on local structures and by ↑ICP. They may be absent in mosaic NF2. **Juvenile posterior subcapsular lenticular opacity** (a form of cataract) occurs before other manifestations and can be useful in screening those at risk.

*Complications:* Tender Schwannomas of cranial and peripheral nerves, and spinal nerve roots. Meningiomas (45% in NF2, often multiple). Glial tumours are less common. Consider NF2 in any young person presenting with one of these tumours in isolation.

*Management:* Hearing tests yearly from puberty in affected families, with MRI brain if abnormality is detected. A normal MRI in the late teens is helpful in assessing risk to any offspring. A clear scan at 30yrs (unless a family history of late onset) indicates that the gene has not been inherited. Treatment of vestibular Schwannomas is neurosurgical and complicated by hearing loss/deterioration and facial palsy. Mean survival from diagnosis is ~15yrs,[375] but with best practice should be better.[376]

**Schwannomatosis** Multiple tender cutaneous Schwannomas without the bilateral vestibular Schwannomas that are characteristic of NF2. Indistinguishable from mosaic NF2, where vestibular Schwannomas are also absent, except by genetic analysis of tumour biopsies.[377] There is typically a large tumour load, assessable only by whole-body MRI. INI1 gene mutations with autosomal dominant inheritance and spontaneous NF2 mutations have both been described.[378] Life expectancy is normal.

## Diagnostic criteria for neurofibromatosis

*NF1 (von Recklinghausen's disease)*

Diagnosis is made if 2 of the following are found:
1 ≥6 *café-au-lait* macules >5mm (pre-pubertal) or >15mm (post-pubertal)
2 ≥2 neurofibromas of any type or 1 plexiform
3 Freckling in the axillary or inguinal regions
4 Optic glioma
5 ≥2 Lisch nodules
6 Distinctive osseous lesion typical of NF1, eg sphenoid dysplasia
7 First-degree relative with NF1 according to the above criteria

*Differential:* McCune–Albright syndrome (*OHCS* p649), multiple lentigines,[1] urticaria pigmentosa (*OHCS* p610).

*NF2*

Diagnosis is made if either of the following are found:
1 Bilateral vestibular Schwannomas seen on MRI or CT
2 First-degree relative with NF2, and either:
    a) Unilateral vestibular Schwannoma; or
    b) One of the following:
       • Neurofibroma
       • Meningioma
       • Glioma
       • Schwannoma
       • Juvenile cataract (NF2 type)

*Differential:* NF1, Schwannomatosis.

*Causes of café-au-lait spots:* Normal (eg up to 5); NF1 (melanocyte density↑ vs 'normal' café-au-lait spots); NF2; rare syndromes: Gaucher's; McCune–Albright; Russel–Silver; tuberous sclerosis; Wiskott–Aldrich.

Neurology

1 May be part of LEOPARD syndrome: autosomal dominant Lentigines, ECG anomalies, Ocular hypertelorism (eyes wide-spaced), Pulmonary stenosis, Anomalies of genital organs, Retarded growth, Deafness.

Syrinx was one of those versatile virgins of Arcadia who, on being pursued by Pan beside the River Ladon, turned herself into a reed, from which Pan made his pipes, so giving her name to various tubular structures, eg syringe, and syrinx, which is a tubular or slit-like cavity in or close to the central canal of the cervical cord. It may extend up or down. *Mean age of onset:* 30yrs. *Incidence:* 8/100,000/yr. Symptoms may be static for years, but then worsen fast—eg on coughing or sneezing, as ↑ pressure causes extension, eg into the brainstem (*syringobulbia*).[379]

**Causes** *Typically*, blocked CSF circulation (without 4th ventricular communication), with ↓flow from basal posterior fossa to caudal space, eg Arnold–Chiari malformation (cerebellum herniates through foramen magnum); basal arachnoiditis (after infection, irradiation, subarachnoid haemorrhage); basilar impression/invagination;[1] masses (cysts, rheumatoid pannus, encephalocoele, tumours). *Less commonly*, a syrinx may develop after myelitis, cord trauma or rupture of an AV malformation, or within spinal tumours (ependymoma or haemangioblastoma) due to fluid secreted from neoplastic cells or haemorrhage.

**Cardinal signs:** Dissociated sensory loss (absent pain and T° sensation, with preserved light touch, vibration, and joint-position sense) due to pressure from the syrinx on the decussating anterolateral pathway (fig 1) in a root distribution reflecting the location of the syrinx (eg over typical cervical syrinx then sensory loss is over trunk and arms); wasting/weakness of hands ± claw-hand (then arms→shoulders→respiratory muscles). Anterior horn cells are also vulnerable.

*Other signs:* Horner's syndrome; UMN leg signs; body asymmetry, limb hemi-hypertrophy, or unilateral odo- or chiromegaly (enlarged hand or foot), perhaps from release of trophic factors via anterior horn cells; *Syringobulbia* (brainstem involvement): nystagmus, tongue atrophy, dysphagia, pharyngeal/palatal weakness, Vth nerve sensory loss. *Charcot's (neuropathic) joints:* Increased range of movement (from lost joint proprioception), destroys the joint, which becomes swollen and mobile (see fig 2, p205).[380] Causes: tabes dorsalis (eg knee), diabetic neuropathy, paraplegia (eg hips),[381] syringomyelia (shoulder, wrist),[382] leprosy, spinal osteolysis/cord atrophy (systemic sclerosis).[382]

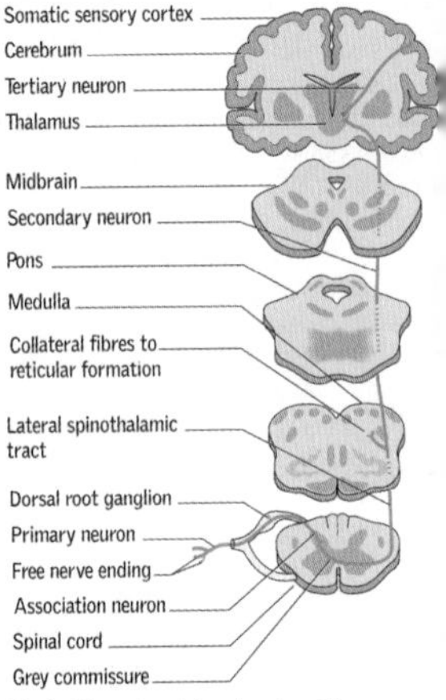

**MRI imaging** How big is the syrinx? Any base-of-brain (Chiari) malformation?

**Surgery** Don't wait for gross deterioration to occur. Decompression at the foramen magnum may be tried in Chiari malformations, to promote free flow of CSF, and so prevent syrinx dilatation. Surgery may relieve pain, and slow progression.[384]

Fig 1. The anterolateral system.[383]

Labels (top to bottom): Somatic sensory cortex; Cerebrum; Tertiary neuron; Thalamus; Midbrain; Secondary neuron; Pons; Medulla; Collateral fibres to reticular formation; Lateral spinothalamic tract; Dorsal root ganglion; Primary neuron; Free nerve ending; Association neuron; Spinal cord; Grey commissure

## Retroviruses and neurology

**HIV/AIDS** is part of the differential diagnosis of meningitis (eg fungal/TB), intracranial mass lesions (toxoplasmosis), dementia, encephalomyelitis, cord problems,[385] and peripheral nerve problems, eg mononeuritis multiplex and Guillain–Barré syndrome.

**Tropical spastic paraplegia/HTLV-1 myelopathy** is a slowly progressing spastic paraplegia, with paraesthesiae, sensory loss, and disorders of micturition.

1 The top of the odontoid process (part of C2) migrates upwards (congenitally, or in rheumatoid arthritis or osteogenesis imperfecta) causing foramen stenosis ± medulla oblongata compression. Consider basilar invagination if the odontoid tip is ≥4mm above McGregor's line (drawn from the upper surface of the posterior edge of the hard palate to the most caudal point of the occipital curve).

## ☼ Models of brain functioning

A superficial reading of the foregoing pages might lead one to the conclusion that the structure of the adult brain is fixed, and that a circumscribed lesion will cause reproducible, predictable results (if we remember our neuroanatomy correctly). Furthermore, if a certain phenomenon appears when part of the brain (say area A) is stimulated, and is lost when the same part of the brain is injured, we happily conclude that area A is the centre for laughter, fear, or whatever the phenomenon is. A lesion here, and you will stop laughing for ever, we might think. An area on the hard disk of our mind has been scratched. The grey cells do not regenerate themselves, so the brain carries on as before with this one defect. The more we look at the brain, the more wrong this model becomes.

If our brains were like a computer, the more tasks we did at the same time, the slower we would do any one task. In fact, our performance can *improve*, the more simultaneous tasks we take on. This is why music helps some of us concentrate. Experiments using functional MRI show that listening to polyphonic music recruits memory circuits, promotes attention, and aids semantic processing, target detection, and some forms of imagery.[388]

Another way in which our brains are not like a computer is that we are born with certain predispositions and expectations. Our hard disk was never blank. Just as the skin on the feet of new-born babies is thicker than other areas, as if feet were made with a prior knowledge of walking or somehow expecting walking, so our brains are made expecting a world of stimuli, which need making sense of by reframing sequential events in terms of cause and effect. We cannot help unconsciously imposing cause and effect relationships on events which are purely sequential. This unconscious reframing no doubt has survival value.

The model we have of brain function is important because it influences our attitude to our patients. If we are stuck with a neuroanatomical model, we will be rather pessimistic and guarded in our assessment of how patients may recover after neurological events. If we use a model that is more holistic and reality-based, such as the Piaget-type model in which the brain is seen as intrinsically unstable and continually re-creating itself, we will grant our patients more possibilities.[387] Our model of the brain must encompass its ability to set goals for itself, and to be self-actuating.[388] Unstructured optimism is unwarranted, but structured optimism is to some extent a self-fulfilling prognosis. For many medical conditions, the more optimistic we are, and the more we involve our patients in their own care and its planning, the faster and better they will recover.[389] If we combine this with the observed fact that those with an optimistic turn of mind are less likely to suffer stroke,[390] we can reach the conclusion that emotional wellbeing predicts subsequent functional independence and survival. When this hypothesis is tested directly in a prospective way, the effect of emotional wellbeing is found to be direct and strong and independent of other factors such as functional status, sociodemographic variables, chronic conditions, body mass index, etc.[391]

So the conclusion is that the brain has an unknown amount of inherent plasticity, and an unknown potential for healing after injury—uninjured areas may take on new functions, and injured parts may function in new ways.[1] The great challenge of neurology is to work to maximize this potential of recovery and re-creation. This demands knowledge of your patient, as well as knowledge of neuroanatomy and neurophysiology. The point is that there is no predefined limit to what is possible.

◀ In early frontotemporal dementia, artistic creativity may blossom—suggesting that language is not required for, and may even inhibit, certain types of visual creativity. See p490.

**Contents**

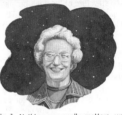

Fig 1. Nothing ever really matters, we might think, on gazing into the heavens, and spotting a few exploding galaxies or dying suns. But if we lead a more or less insignificant life we might rather like to matter. Dame Cicely Saunders (who combined nursing, social work and medicine, as well as founding the first hospice) matters to us because she never stopped telling her patients *"You matter because you are you. You matter to the last moment of your life."* Was she right? We are better doctors if we believe her.

Consciously and continually strive to make your patients feel that they matter. Then you will realize that you matter too—and the exploding galaxies and dying suns will, for a moment, be eclipsed.

*Relevant pages in other chapters:* Active management of death (p7); immuno-suppressive drugs (p370); pain (p576); dying at home (*OHCS* p498).

## ☼ Communicating about cancer

Communication forms the first step in understanding, treating, or coming to terms with cancer. A range of overwhelming feelings can surface on receiving this diagnosis, including shock, numbness, denial, panic, anger and resignation ("I knew all along..."). Some doctors instinctively turn away from 'undisciplined squads of emotions' and try to stop them taking over consultations. A more positive approach is to try to use these to benefit and motivate your patient, through listening to and addressing their worst fears. ►*Include your patient in all decision-making processes.* Many patients (not just the young and well informed) will appreciate this, and the giving of information and the sharing of decisions is known to reduce treatment morbidity. So, even when this is physically exhausting (the same ground may need covering many times) it is definitely worth spending this time. A huge amount is forgotten or fails to register initially, so videos and written information are important. Be sure to question, in an open way, about use of alternative therapies, which can indicate psychosocial distress and is frequently a sign of undisclosed worry of recurrence.[1] Ask about this and through good communication and the promotion of autonomy, your patient's fear-driven wish to try dangerous or untried therapies may be trumped by a spirit of rational optimism.

*We thank Professor Max Watson, our Specialist Reader, and James Sewell, our Junior Reader, for their contribution to this chapter.*

## ☼ Looking after people with cancer

No rules guarantee success, but getting to know your patient, making an agreed management plan, and seeking out the right expert for each stage of treatment *all* need to be central activities in oncology. The patient will bring worries from all aspects of their family, work and social life. Communication is central to resolving these issues and the personal attributes of the doctor as a physician are key. Remember, it is never too early to start palliative care (*with* other treatments) and that *quality of life* is of the utmost importance.

**Psychological support** Meta-analyses have suggested that psychological support can ↓pain² & improve outcome measures such as survival.³ Examples include:
• *Allowing negative feelings*, eg fear or anger (anger can anaesthetize pain).
• *Counselling*, eg with a breast cancer nurse in preparation for mastectomy.
• *Biofeedback and relaxation therapy* can ↓ side-effects of chemotherapy.⁴
• *Cognitive behavioural therapy* reduces psychological morbidity associated with cancer treatments. See OHCS p370.
• *Group therapy* (OHCS p376) reduces pain, mood disturbance and the frequency of maladaptive coping strategies.

**Streamlining care pathways** Care pathways map journeys in a health system: symptoms felt→unknown psychic processes↓→GP appointment→referral→hospital appointment→consultant clinic→imaging→initial treatment (surgery, etc). Each arrow represents a possibly fatal delay. 48h access to GPs, GP referral under a '2-week rule' (hospital must see within 2wks, inevitably making other equally or more deserving patients wait longer) and e-booking (like on-line airline reservations) are unreliable ways of speeding up the crucial arrow pointing to initial treatment.⁵ The only way to do this is to increase capacity (beds, nurses, doctors, equipment, theatres).

### Hints for breaking bad news⁶

1 Set the environment up carefully. Choose a quiet place where you will not be disturbed. Make sure family are present if wanted. Be sure of your facts.
2 Find out what the patient already knows or surmises (often a great deal). This may change rapidly, and different perceptions may all be relevant.
3 Ascertain how much the person wants to know. You can be surprisingly direct. "If anything were amiss, would you want to know all the details?"
4 Give some warning—"There is some bad news for us to address". Offer small amounts of information at a time, as this can soften the impact.
5 Share information about diagnosis and treatments. Specifically list supporting people (eg nurses) and institutions (eg hospices). Break information down into manageable chunks and check understanding for each. Ask "Is there anything else you want me to explain?" Don't hesitate to go over the same ground repeatedly. Allow denial: don't force the pace, give them time.
6 'Cancer' has negative connotations for many people. Address this, and explain that ~50% of cancers are cured in the developed world.⁷
7 Listen to any concerns raised; encourage the airing of feelings and empathize.
8 Prognosis questions are often hardest to answer, doctors are usually too optimistic.⁸ Encourage an appropriate level of hope, refer to an expert.
9 Summarize, make a plan and offer availability. Record details of the conversation in the notes (including the language used).
10 Follow through. ►Leave the patient with the strong impression that come what may, you are with them, and that this unwritten contract will not be broken.

Don't imagine that a single blueprint will always work. Use whatever the patient gives you—closely observe both verbal and non-verbal cues.⁹ Practise in low-key interactions with patients, so that when great difficulties arise you have a better chance of helping. Humans are very complex, and we all frequently fail—don't be put off: keep trying, and recap with colleagues afterwards, so you keep learning.

1 Why is there so much variation in cancer 5-yr survival rates? In breast cancer, 5-yr survival is 82% in England, 88% in Australia and 89% in Sweden. One reason is NHS inefficiency; another is cultural. If an English woman feels a lump she may say "I haven't got time to be ill," or "Let's see if it goes away," or "If this is how I'm going to die, so be it," but others may say "I'd better get this sorted *now*."¹⁰

Oncology and palliative care

Genetic changes drive the pathogenesis of cancer. These changes occur most commonly as acquired events, but they may be inherited as germline mutations causing a cancer predisposition syndrome.

**Familial breast/ovarian cancer** Around 5-10% of breast cancers are due to mutation in BRCA1 (17q) or BRCA2 (13q). Both genes function as tumour suppressors (see BOX 2). Carrying a BRCA1 mutation confers a 65% lifetime risk of developing breast cancer and a 40% risk of developing ovarian cancer. For BRCA2 the risk of breast cancer is 45% (6% in affected males) and 11% for ovarian cancer. In BRCA1 there is also a 40-60% risk of developing a second breast cancer.[11] Incidence of mutations varies among populations. In families with ≥4 cases of breast cancer collected by the Breast Cancer Linkage Consortium, the disease was linked to BRCA1 in 52% of families and BRCA2 in 32%. Individuals from families in which a mutation has not been detected can be given risk estimation based on the number of individuals affected and age of onset of cancer.

*Treatment* is essentially that for non-hereditary disease (p604). It is less clear how to manage asymptomatic carriers or prevent second breast cancers. Annual MRI surveillance is more sensitive than mammography in detecting cancer in women <50 years.[12] It should be offered to all BRCA1/2 carriers aged 30-50, and to those aged 30-39 with >8% 10 year risk, or >20% if aged 40-49.[13] Bilateral prophylactic mastectomy in BRCA1/2 reduces risk of breast cancer by ~90%[14] and may be offered in conjunction with oophorectomy. No drug has been fully assessed for prevention in high-risk patients. *Tamoxifen* is associated with a reduction of contralateral breast cancer in BRCA1/2 carriers but has unacceptable side-effects. The aromatase inhibitor *exemestane* is effective in reducing breast cancer in non-BRCA postmenopausal women.[15] Trials of letrozole for prevention in BRCA patients are ongoing.[16] There is optimism for a new class of agents known as *poly(ADP)-ribose polymerase* (PARP) inhibitors.

**Familial prostate cancer** ~5% of those with prostate cancer have a family history: the genetic basis is multifactorial. Risk is modestly elevated for male carriers of BRCA1 and BRCA2 mutations, although the molecular basis of this remains to be elucidated. Mutations in BRCA1/BRCA2 or in the genes on chromosomes 1 and X do not account for all family clusters of prostate cancer and so it is clear that other genes must be involved. In one twin study, 42% of the risk was found to be genetic.[17]

**Familial colorectal cancer** ~20% of those with colorectal cancer have a family history of the disease. An individual's relative risk (RR) of colorectal cancer is related to the degree of family history—refer to a genetic clinic if: • Two affected 1st-degree relatives aged <70 (RR×5); • One affected 1st-degree relative aged <45yrs at diagnosis (RR×3); • 3 close relatives affected with average age at onset <60yrs (RR×2); • Familial adenomatous polyposis (below); • Potential family history of HNPCC (below).

*Familial adenomatous polyposis* is due to germline mutations in the APC gene (5q). Offspring are at 50% risk of being a gene carrier, and gene penetrance approaches 100% for colorectal cancer by 50yrs old. Once diagnosed, total colectomy prevents the inevitable development of carcinoma.

*Peutz-Jeghers syndrome* (p722) has a 10-20% lifetime risk of colorectal cancer, and is due to germline mutations in STK11, a serine threonine kinase (locus: 19p14).

*Hereditary non-polyposis colorectal cancer* (HNPCC) entails familial aggregation of colorectal cancer (HNPCC 1) ± cancer of uterus, ovary, stomach, renal pelvis, small gut, or pancreas (HNPCC 2) with mutations in 1 of 5 DNA mismatch repair genes. Suspect a family history if ≥3 affected relatives (one 1st-degree), from 2 successive generations, of whom one was affected <50yrs old. Inheritance is autosomal dominant (incomplete penetrance). Genetic testing may be indicated. Lifetime risk of colorectal cancer for relatives who carry a mutation is 60%, and women with a mutation have a 40% lifetime risk of endometrial cancer. There is no consensus on prophylactic surgery/most centres use colonoscopic surveillance.

## Characteristics of cancer cells

It is proposed that six alterations in cell physiology collectively dictate malignant growth: 1 Autonomy from growth signals; 2 Insensitivity to growth inhibitory signals; 3 Evasion of programmed cell death (apoptosis); 4 Unlimited replication potential; 5 Recruitment and proliferation of blood vessels (angiogenesis); 6 Invasion and metastasis. Each of these new capabilities represents the successful breach of an inherent anticancer defence mechanism.[18]

## Oncogenes and tumour suppressor genes[19]

Mutations in normal genes involved in pathways associated with cell growth, differentiation, and death contribute to carcinogenesis. These mutations may result in a 'gain of function' (oncogenes) or 'loss of function' (tumour suppressor genes).

**Oncogenes** are mutated genes that increase activity in the absence of a relevant signal. For example, *ras* is a protein involved in signal transduction as part of a tiered cascade of molecular interactions. It is mutated in ~30% of human cancers. Oncogenes behave in a dominant manner, therefore mutation to one allele results in continuous unchecked activation. Oncogene mutations occur most often as somatic events in sporadic tumours, or during the progression to malignancy in those with a predisposition gene. They are rarely inherited.

**Tumour suppressor genes** act as inhibitors of cellular growth. Suppression of pro-malignant processes are therefore lost in mutated genes. Unlike oncogenes, mutations to both alleles must occur before cellular effects are evident—usually as separate somatic events, but in the case of predisposition genes, the first 'hit' is inherited and the second may occur somatically. Thus the same gene can be involved in both inherited and sporadic tumours and explains why tumours occur at an earlier age and more than once in familial cancers. *p53* is a tumour suppressor gene mutated in ~50% of human cancers. Loss of function results in increased mutation, angiogenesis and tumour growth.

## Multistep carcinogenesis

Most cancers arise from multiple mutations. This is perhaps best represented in the stepwise accumulation of cellular mutations in the pathogenesis of colorectal cancer, where virtually all carcinomas develop from adenomatous polyps (fig 1). It is thought to be the accumulation of mutations rather than the order that is critical to developing colorectal cancer.

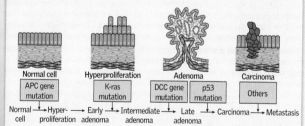

Fig 1. Stepwise cellular mutations and contributing genes in the development of colorectal cancer.[20]

**Other familial cancer syndromes:** Von Hippel-Lindau (kidney, CNS) (p726); Carney complex (p215); MEN1 (pituitary, pancreas, thyroid; p215); MEN2 (p215); Neurofibromatosis type 1 (CNS—rare; p518); Neurofibromatosis type 2 (common—meningiomas, auditory neuromas; p518).

▶A patient who becomes acutely unwell can often be made more comfortable with simple measures, but some problems require specific treatment.

**Febrile neutropenic patients** ▶▶ Immediate treatment saves lives. See p346.

**Spinal cord compression** (see also p470) Urgent and efficient treatment is required to preserve neurological function. A high index of suspicion is essential (BOX). *Causes:* Typically extradural metastases. *Other causes:* extension of tumour from a vertebral body, direct extension of the tumour, or crush fracture. *Signs and symptoms:* Back pain, weakness or sensory loss with a root distribution (or a sensory level), bowel and bladder dysfunction. Have a low threshold for investigating patients with known cancer, who present with new or worsening back pain (especially thoracic or cervical) and any deterioration in mobility or sensation. *Investigations:* Urgent MRI of the whole spine. *Management: Dexamethasone* 16mg/24h PO. Palliative radiotherapy is the commonest treatment. Selected patients should have decompressive surgery.[21] Discuss with a neurosurgeon and clinical oncologist immediately.

**Superior vena cava (SVC) obstruction with airway compromise** SVC obstruction is not an emergency unless there is tracheal compression *with airway compromise:* otherwise there is usually time to plan optimal treatment, which is preferable to rushing into therapy that may not be beneficial.[22] *Causes:* Malignancy accounts for >90% of SVC obstruction, ¾ of which are from lung cancer. *Rare causes:* mediastinal enlargement (eg germ cell tumour), thymus malignancy, mediastinal lymphadenopathy (eg lymphoma), thrombotic disorders (eg Behçet's or nephrotic syndromes), thrombus around an IV central line, hamartoma. *Signs and symptoms:* Dyspnoea, orthopnoea, plethora/cyanosis, swollen face and arm, cough, headache and engorged veins. *Pemberton's test:* Lifting the arms over the head for >1min causes facial plethora/cyanosis, JVP↑ (non-pulsatile), and inspiratory stridor. *Investigations:* Urgent contrast enhanced CT. *Management:* Get a tissue diagnosis if the cause is unknown (eg biopsy of peripheral lymph node; bronchoscopy may be hazardous). Give oral *dexamethasone* 8–16mg/24h. Consider balloon *venoplasty* and SVC stenting as this provides the most rapid relief of symptoms[23] (eg prior to radical or palliative chemo- or radiotherapy, depending on tumour type).

**Malignancy associated hypercalcaemia** Affects 10–20% of patients with cancer, and 40% of those with myeloma. It is a very poor prognostic sign with 75% of patients dead within 3 months of starting hypocalcaemic treatment. *Causes:* Lytic bone mets, myeloma, production of osteoclast activating factor or PTH-like hormones by the tumour. *Symptoms:* Lethargy, anorexia, nausea, polydipsia, polyuria, constipation, dehydration, confusion, weakness. Most obvious with corrected serum $Ca^{2+}$ >3mmol/L (but >2.6mmol/L may be enough in some patients). *Acute management* involves rehydration followed by IV bisphosphonate (or calcitonin if resistant) ▶ See p691 for treatment of *acute hypercalcaemia*. Maintenance therapy with IV bisphosphonates is often required. The best treatment is control of underlying malignancy.

**Raised intracranial pressure** (see also p840). Due to either a primary CNS tumour or metastatic disease. *Signs and symptoms:* Headache (often worse in the morning, when coughing or bending over), nausea, vomiting, papilloedema, fits, focal neurological signs. *Investigations:* Urgent CT/MRI is important to diagnose an expanding mass, cystic degeneration, haemorrhage within a tumour, cerebral oedema, or hydrocephalus due to tumour or blocked shunt, since the management of these scenarios can be very different. *Treatment: Dexamethasone* 8–16mg/24h PO, radiotherapy, and surgery as appropriate depending on cause. *Mannitol* may be tried for symptom relief for cerebral oedema (not evidence-based).[24]

**Tumour lysis syndrome** Rapid cell death on starting chemotherapy for rapidly proliferating leukaemia, lymphoma, myeloma, and some germ cell tumours can result in a rise in serum urate, $K^+$, and phosphate, precipitating renal failure. Prevention is key, with good hydration and *allopurinol* started 24h before chemotherapy (300mg/12h PO if good renal function; if creatinine >100μmol/L give 100mg on alternate days).[25] Haemodialysis may be needed in renal failure. A more potent uricolytic agent is *rasburicase* (recombinant urate oxidase) 200μg/kg/d IVI for 5–7d.[26]

### When you suspect cord compression from metastases...[27]

▶Get advice today—eg from a neurosurgeon, or, where appointed, from your *metastatic spinal cord compression co-ordinator*. He or she will want to know:
- Why you think it is urgent—eg back pain disturbing sleep (p544), radicular pain, local spinal tenderness with weak legs, sphincter disturbance, or a sensory level.
- Has a tissue diagnosis of cancer been made?
- Is the patient too frail for specialist treatment?
- How is the compression progressing? If paraplegic for >24h, you may be too late.
- How long is the patient likely to live? Is it >3 months? *Urgent radiotherapy* may have a role. If longer, *spinal reconstruction* with a bone graft may be appropriate. *Vertebral body reinforcement* is one option for pain. *Laminectomy* alone should only be done for isolated epidural tumours or neural arch metastases.
- What is the fluid status (over-hydration is a danger)?
- Has DVT prophylaxis been considered (p580)?
- Have bisphosphonates (p696) been started? (Needed in all those with vertebral involvement from myeloma or breast cancer—they help pain and stability.)
- Has the option of palliative radiotherapy been considered?

### Cancer staging

Staging systems are used to describe the extent to which a cancer has spread when first diagnosed. This is vital to determine the most appropriate treatment and to assess prognosis. It also provides a common language for doctors to communicate. Note that the stage of a cancer does not change, even if the cancer progresses or recurs. Most solid organ cancers are staged using the TNM system[1], which is based on the extent of tumour (T), the extent of spread to lymph nodes (N), and the presence of metastases (M). Each cancer using the TNM system has its own classification—some use additional values and more detailed subcategories to those listed below:

| | | | |
|---|---|---|---|
| Tx | Primary tumour cannot be assessed | Nx | Nodes cannot be assessed |
| T0 | No evidence of primary tumour | N0 | No node involvement |
| $T_{is}$ | Carcinoma *in situ* | N1-3 | Regional node metastases |
| T1-4 | Size and/or extent of primary tumour | M0 | No distant spread |
| | (1=small tumour with minimal invasion; 4=large tumour with extensive invasion) | M1 | Distant metastases |

A number of prefixes may also be used: c refers to clinical stage (based on information gained prior to surgery, eg from imaging or biopsy); p is the stage given after pathological examination; y refers to assessment of stage after neoadjuvant therapy; r is used if a tumour is re-staged after a disease-free interval; a indicates stage determined at autopsy.

A colorectal cancer staged as pT2 pN1b M0 describes a tumour staged after pathological examination that invades the muscularis propria of the bowel and has metastases in 2-3 regional lymph nodes, with no evidence of distant metastases. For specific TNM staging see p171 (lung cancer); p604 (breast cancer); p621 (oesophageal cancer); p649 (bladder cancer). Some cancers may also have alternative staging systems such as Duke's classification for colorectal cancer (p619) or the FIGO system used in gynaecological malignancies.

The TNM stage may be combined to assign an overall 'Stage'. In some cancers this may also require non-anatomical factors, such as the histological Gleason score in prostate cancer (p647), or the presence of serum tumour markers in testicular cancer. Stage 0 refers to carcinoma *in situ*; Stages I-III describe local, locally advanced and regional disease; Stage IV indicates distant metastatic disease.

---

**1** The TNM system was developed and is maintained by the American Joint Committee on Cancer (AJCC) and the International Union Against Cancer (UICC). Gynaecological malignancies use both the TNM and FIGO classifications for staging. Haematological malignancies and CNS tumours do not use the TNM system.

Cancer affects 30% of the population; 20% die from it. Management requires a multidisciplinary team, and communication is vital. Most patients wish to have some part in decision-making at the various stages of their treatment, and to be informed of their options. The majority will undergo a variety of therapies during the treatment of their cancer and your job may be to orchestrate these. ►*Include the patient in the decision-making process* (p522).

**Surgery** Has a number of roles: •Surgical biopsy may be required to provide tissue for histological diagnosis. •Staging may be undertaken laparoscopically. •Surgery is often performed with curative intent and is the mainstay of treatment (and principal hope of cure) in most patients with solid tumours. It may be the only treatment required in early GI tumours, soft tissue sarcomas, and gynaecological tumours, but best results are often achieved when used in combination with radiotherapy or chemotherapy. •Palliative surgery may be required in advanced disease, eg surgical debulking of large tumours or stabilization of pathological fractures. •Occasionally surgery may be used prophylactically, eg in BRCA/FAP (p524).

**Radiotherapy** Uses ionizing radiation to kill tumour cells. See p530.

**Chemotherapy** Cytotoxics should be given under expert guidance by people trained in their administration. Drugs are given with a variety of intents, often in combination: *Neoadjuvant*—to shrink tumours prior to surgery and thus reduce the need for major surgery (eg mastectomy). There is also a rationale that considers early control of micro-metastasis. *Primary therapy*—as the sole treatment, eg for haematological malignancies. *Adjuvant*—to reduce the chance of relapse after primary surgery in, eg breast and bowel cancers. *Palliative*—to provide relief from symptomatic metastatic disease and possibly to prolong survival.

*Important classes of drugs include:*
• *Alkylating agents:* Antiproliferative drugs that bind via alkyl groups to DNA, eg cyclophosphamide, chlorambucil, busulfan.
• *Antimetabolites:* Interfere with normal cellular metabolism of nucleic acids, eg methotrexate, 5-fluorouracil.
• *Vinca alkaloids:* 'Spindle poisons' which target mechanisms of cell division, eg vincristine, vinblastine.
• *Antitumour antibiotics:* Vary in action (depending on type), eg dactinomycin, doxorubicin, mitomycin.
• *Monoclonal antibodies:* Inhibit a specific targeted process, such as angiogenesis, (eg bevacizumab for renal cell carcinoma), or epidermal growth factor receptors (eg panitumumab and cetuximab). NB: over-expression of epidermal growth factor receptors correlates with poor prognosis in many cancers.
• *Others:* eg etoposide, taxanes, platinum compounds.

*Side-effects* depend on the types of drugs used, and include:
• *Vomiting:* A source of much anxiety and should be prevented before the $1^{st}$ dose, thus avoiding anticipatory vomiting: eg metoclopramide 10-20mg/8h, ondansetron 4-8mg/8h can be effective. See p241, BOX.
• *Alopecia:* Can have a profound impact on self esteem and quality of life.
• *Neutropenia:* Most commonly seen 10-14d after chemotherapy (but can occur within 7d for taxanes). ►►Neutropenic sepsis requires immediate attention (p346).

*Principles of combination chemotherapy:*
Combination therapy has important advantages over single-agent use. It increases tumour cell kill, leading to improved overall response. It offers a broader range of drug activiy against resistant tumour cells and it prevents or slows the development of new drug-resistant cells. Each drug should have: •Single-agent activity in that tumour type (preferentially including drugs that induce complete remission) •A different mechanism of activity—ideally with additive or synergystic cytotoxic effect •Non-overlapping toxicitiy—to maximize the benefit of full therapeutic doses •Action on a different part of the cell cycle •Different mechanisms of resistance.[28]

## Planning or avoiding surgery in patients with cancer

Ambitious surgery may be futile if a cancer has already metastasized—knowing when to halt further intervention is essential. A key process in planning the right procedure is to interest a radiologist in your problem. This may require more than scrawling a brief request on an x-ray form. The range of imaging available is constantly changing, so discussing the request in person with a radiologist may help direct the use of the most appropriate modality to answer your question.[29]

*CT:* Extensive application in many cancers.

*MRI:* Used for precise staging in areas occult to CT (eg marrow, CNS). See p748.

*Bone scan:* Used for staging/follow-up of prostate, breast, and lung cancer.

*Sestamibi scan:* Used for localizing active disease in breast cancer and thyroid (eg if not iodine-avid). Like bone scans, it uses technetium ($^{99m}$Tc).

*Thallium scan:* Used to localize viable tissue, eg in brain tumours.

*Gallium scan:* Used for staging and follow-up in lymphoma.

*Octreotide scan:* Used to demonstrate cancers with somatostatin receptors (eg pancreas, medullary thyroid, neuroblastoma, and carcinoid tumours).

*Monoclonal antibodies:* $^{99m}$Tc-labelled tumour antibodies are used in staging by detecting tumour antigen, eg in lung, colon, and prostate cancer.

*FDG PET:* 2-[$^{18}$F] fluoro-2-deoxy-D-glucose positron emission tomography detects high rates of aerobic metabolism, eg in lung, colon, breast, and testis.

*MIBG scan ($^{131}$I):* Used to localize noradrenaline production, eg phaeochromocytoma. MIBG = meta-iodobenzylguanidine.

## Extravasation of chemotherapeutic agents

Do not use an IV line for cytotoxic drugs if there is any doubt about its patency. Extravasation of vesicant agents can cause severe tissue necrosis. ►Suspect if there is pain, burning or swelling at the infusion site.

*Management:*[30] Stop the infusion and disconnect the drip. Attempt to aspirate any residual drug from the cannula before removing. Take advice and follow local policies if available (many cancer wards have 'extravasation kits'). Follow any drug-specific managment recommendations. Apply a cold pack (if extravasation of a DNA binding drug) to vasoconstrict and minimize drug spread, or a heat pack (if non-DNA binding drug) to vasodilate and increase drug distribution/absorption. Local injection of corticosteroids is controversial and their effectiveness is not proven. Topical steroids may help reduce non-specific inflammation. Evidence surrounding the use of antidotes is conflicting.[1][31] Liaise early with a plastic surgeon, eg to discuss flush-out. Elevate the arm, mark the affected area and review regularly. Give analgesia if required. Consider reporting to the National Extravastion Scheme.[32]

## Beau's lines

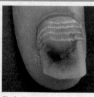

Beau's lines (fig 1) are horizontal depressions in the nail plate that run parallel to the moon-shaped portion of the nail bed. They result from a sudden interruption of nail keratin synthesis and may be due to local infection or trauma, systemic illness or from medication (see p32). Each line in this photo coincided with a round of chemotherapy for breast cancer. The patient was triumphant at having survived it all (just).

Fig 1. Beau's lines.

1 Some recommend (on scant evidence) topical dimethylsulfoxide (DMSO) and cooling after extravasation of anthracyclines or mitomycin, locally injected hyaluronidase if vinca alkaloids involved, and locally injected sodium thiosulfate (sodium hyposulfite) if chlormethine (mechlorethamine; mustine). NB all uses unlicensed.

Radiotherapy is used in >50% of cancer patients. It uses ionizing radiation to produce free radicals which damage DNA. Normal cells are better at repairing this damage than cancer cells, so are able to recover before the next dose (or fraction) of treatment.

**Radical treatment** is given with curative intent. The total doses given range from 40-70 gray (Gy) in 15-35 daily fractions. Some regimens involve giving several smaller fractions a day with a gap of 6-8h. Combined chemoradiation is used in some sites, eg anus and oesophagus, to increase response rates.

**Palliation** aims to relieve symptoms—it may not impact on survival time. Doses are 8-30Gy, given in 1, 2, 5, or 10 fractions. Bone pain, haemoptysis, cough, dyspnoea, and bleeding are helped in >50% of patients. *"Will this patient benefit from radiotherapy?"* is a frequently asked question.[33,34] When in doubt, ask an expert (or two). Remember it may take 3 weeks before radiotherapy begins to produce a therapeutic effect.

**Early reactions** occur within 8 weeks of treatment.
• *Tiredness:* Common after radical treatments. It can last weeks to months.
• *Skin reactions:* These vary from erythema to dry desquamation to moist desquamation to ulceration. On completing treatment, use moisturizers.
• *Mucositis:* All patients receiving head and neck treatment should have a dental check-up before therapy. Avoid smoking, alcohol, and spicy foods. Antiseptic mouthwashes may help. Aspirin gargle and other soluble analgesics are helpful. Treat oral thrush, eg with *Nystatin* oral solution (1mL swill and swallow every 6h) ± fluconazole 50mg/24h PO.
• *Nausea and vomiting:* Occur when stomach, liver, or brain treated. Try *metoclopramide* (dopamine antagonist) 10-20mg/8h PO, or *domperidone* (blocks the central chemoreceptor trigger zone) 10-20mg/8h PO. If unsuccessful, try a serotonin (5HT₃) antagonist, eg *ondansetron* 4-8mg/8h PO/IV. See p241, BOX 3.
• *Diarrhoea:* Usually after abdominal or pelvic treatments. Maintain good hydration. Avoid high-fibre bulking agents; try loperamide 2mg PO after each loose stool (max 16mg/24h).
• *Dysphagia:* Following thoracic treatments.
• *Cystitis:* After pelvic treatments. Drink plenty of fluids. Use NSAIDs.
• *Bone marrow suppression:* More likely after chemotherapy unless large areas are being irradiated. Usually reversible.

**Late reactions** occur months or years after treatment.
• *CNS: Somnolence,* 6-12wks after brain radiotherapy. Treat with steroids. *Spinal cord myelopathy*—progressive weakness. MRI is needed to exclude cord compression. *Brachial plexopathy*—numb, weak, and painful arm after axillary radiotherapy. Reduced IQ can occur in children receiving brain irradiation if <6yrs old.
• *Lung: Pneumonitis* may occur 6-12wks after thoracic treatment, eg with dry cough ± dyspnoea. Treat with *prednisolone* 40mg OD, reducing over 6wks.
• *GI: Xerostomia*—reduced saliva. Treat with *pilocarpine* 5mg/8h PO or artificial saliva with meals (OHCS p579). Care must be taken with all future dental care as healing is reduced. *Benign strictures*—of oesophagus or bowel. Treat with dilatation. *Fistulae* need surgery. *Radiation proctitis* may be a problem after prostate irradiation. NB: those having radiotherapy for rectal cancer seem to have a *lower* than expected incidence of prostate cancer in the next decade (risk ↓ by 72%).[35]
• *GU: Urinary frequency:* small fibrosed bladder after pelvic treatments. *Fertility:* pelvic radiotherapy (and cytotoxics) may ↓ fertility, so consider ova or sperm storage. This is a complex area: get expert help. See BOX 2. In premature female menopause or reduced testosterone, replace hormones. *Vaginal stenosis* and *dyspareunia*. *Erectile dysfunction* can occur several years after pelvic radiotherapy.
• *Others: Panhypopituitarism* following radical treatment involving pituitary fossa. Children need hormones checking regularly as growth hormone may be required. *Hypothyroidism*—neck treatments, eg for Hodgkin's lymphoma. *Secondary cancers*, eg sarcomas, usually wait 10 or more years before appearing, as do *Cataracts*.

## Methods of delivering radiotherapy

*Conventional external beam radiotherapy* (EBRT) is the most common form of treatment and delivers beams of ionizing radiation to the patient from an external linear accelerator.

*Stereotactic radiotherapy* is a highly accurate form of EBRT used to target small lesions with great precision—most frequently in treating intracranial conditions. It is often referred to by the manufacturer's name, eg *Gamma Knife®, Truebeam®*.

*Brachytherapy* involves a radiation source being placed within or close to a tumour, allowing high local radiation dose to a small tumour. Implants may be placed within a cavity (eg uterus) or interstitially (eg prostate or breast).

*Radioisotope therapy* uses tumour-seeking radionuclides to target specific tissues. For example, $^{131}$I (radioiodine) to ablate remaining thyroid tissue after thyroidectomy for thyroid cancer. MIBG (p529) is used to treat neural crest tumours.

## ☼ Fertility issues in cancer patients

Plan with patients *before* treatment and get expert help.

Chemotherapy and radiotherapy often damage germ cell spermatogonia (causing impaired spermatogenesis or male sterility), and may hasten oocyte depletion (premature menopause). GNRH agonists, eg goserelin, used concurrently during chemotherapy may help to preserve ovarian function.[36] As treatments become more effective and survival improves, there are more survivors in the reproductive years for whom parenting is a top priority.[37] There is nothing like the hope of creating new life to sustain patients through the difficult times of radio- and chemotherapy, so make sure this hope is well founded.[38]

*Semen cryopreservation* from men and older boys with cancer must be offered before therapy. With modern fertility treatment (*OHCS* p293), even poor quality samples can yield successful pregnancies.[39] Another option is use of sperm from cryopreserved testicular tissue followed up with intracytoplasmic sperm injection (ICSI). If your patient is a man some years after cancer therapy who is unable to have children, refer him to a specialist. ▶*Do not write him off as infertile*—testicular sperm extraction (TESE) with ICSI can yield normal pregnancies.[40]

*Cryopreservation of embryos* and *ovarian tissue banking* are harder options in women.[41] Cryopreservation requires ovarian stimulation and oocyte collection, which may result in unacceptable delays to treatment. Harvesting and storing ovarian cortical tissue from girls and young women before potentially gonadotoxic therapy is only available in some centres.[42]

For ethical issues see *OHCS* p293.

Oncology and palliative care

Diagnosis of cancer on clinical grounds alone can be difficult; however, a variety of clinical scenarios and symptoms should alert you to the possible presence of malignancy and prompt urgent referral to the appropriate specialist. The list below is by no means exhaustive but covers the commonest presentations.

**Lung** •Immediate admission if there are signs of superior vena caval obstruction (p526) or stridor; •Urgently (within 2 weeks) if persistent haemoptysis (smokers or non-smokers over 40); •Suggestive CXR (pleural effusion, slowly resolving consolidation); •Normal CXR but high suspicion; •History of asbestos exposure and recent chest pain or dyspnoea; •Unexplained systemic symptoms with suspicious CXR. ►*High-risk groups:* ex- and current smokers, COPD (p176), asbestos exposure (p192), previous cancer.

**Upper gastrointestinal** •Urgent referral should be regardless of *H. pylori* status if there is *dyspepsia* plus any one of chronic GI bleeding, dysphagia, progressive unintentional weight loss, persistent vomiting, iron-deficiency anaemia, epigastric mass, or suspicious barium meal result. *Also:* •Isolated dysphagia; •Unexplained upper abdominal pain and weight loss, with or without back pain; •Upper abdominal mass without dyspepsia; •Obstructive jaundice; •Consider referral in vomiting or iron deficiency anaemia with weight loss, or in dyspepsia with Barrett's oesophagus, dysplasia, atrophic gastritis or old (>20yrs ago) peptic ulcer surgery. ►*For endoscopy:* those over 55 with persistent unexplained recent onset dyspepsia.

**Lower gastrointestinal** If there are equivocal symptoms and you are not anxious, it is reasonable to watch and wait. Do PR examination and FBC in all. •Over 40 with PR bleeding *and* bowel habit change (more loose/frequent >6 weeks); •Any age with a right lower abdominal mass likely to be bowel; •Palpable rectal mass; •Men or non-menstruating women with unexplained iron-deficiency anaemia and Hb less than 11 or 10 respectively. ►*High-risk groups:* Ulcerative colitis; it is unproven whether a family history of colon cancer assists decisions in symptomatic patients (p524).

**Breast** •Discrete, hard lump with fixation; •Over 30 with a discrete lump persisting after a period or presenting post-menopause; •Under 30 with an enlarging lump, fixed and hard lump, or family history; •Previous breast cancer with a new lump or suspicious symptoms; •Unilateral eczematous skin or nipple change unresponsive to topical treatment; •Recent nipple distortion; •Spontaneous bloody unilateral nipple discharge; •Men over 50 with a unilateral firm subareolar mass; •Consider referral if under 30 with a lump or persistent breast pain.

**Gynaecology** •Examination suggestive of cervical cancer (don't wait for a smear test); •Postmenopausal bleeding in non-HRT patients or those on HRT after 6 weeks cessation; •Vulval lump or bleeding; •Consider in persistent intermenstrual bleeding. ►*Ultrasound:* any abdominal or pelvic mass not GI or urological in origin. Do pelvic and abdominal examinations, with speculum as appropriate.

**Urology** •Hard irregular prostate (refer with PSA result); •Normal prostate but raised PSA (p534) and urinary symptoms; •Painless macroscopic haematuria at any age; •Over 40 with persistent or recurrent UTI and haematuria; •Over 50 with unexplained microscopic haematuria; •Any abdominal mass arising from the urinary tract; •Swelling or mass in the body of the testis; •Ulceration or mass in the penis.

**Central nervous system** •New onset cranial nerve palsy or unilateral sensorineural deafness (p468); •Recent-onset headaches with features of raised intracranial pressure (eg vomiting, drowsiness, posture-related headache, pulse-synchronous tinnitus; p468) or other CNS symptoms; •A new and different unexplained headache of progressive severity; •Recent-onset seizures; •Consider in rapid progression of subacute focal deficit, unexplained cognitive impairment, or personality change with features indicative of a tumour.

*Haematological* p346; *Thyroid* p602; *Skin* p598.

## Is the energy we expend in speeding up referrals paying off?

Possibly not. There is evidence that reducing breast cancer waits from a few months to a few weeks is helpful—but there is little evidence that a few weeks here or there make any difference in colon and other cancers.[44] There is (as yet) no evidence to suggest that the '2-week wait' for suspected cancers in the UK has improved survival.[45] One concern with referral guidelines is the poor predictive value of symptoms for cancer, another is the suggestion that guidelines are abused (although one study found GP compliance to be over 90%).[46] The number of patients referred urgently has increased; however, patients not meeting urgent criteria may present with suspicious signs—yet they will not be seen urgently because other cases are forced to jump the queue. As a result, routine waiting times have increased and an increasing proportion of cancers are being diagnosed in routine patients.[47] This is just one example of the aphorism that *all targets distort clinical priorities*.

Studies of how well dermatology cancer guidelines work conclude that the best way forward is by education regarding recognition of benign conditions.[48] It also seems likely that dialogue between local consultants and referring GPs is a key factor—although this dialogue has become harder and less coherent with the 'choose and book' referral system.

On the good side, establishing clear referral responsibilities forces everyone to look at what they are doing—and this has facilitated many care pathways.

## Multidisciplinary cancer meetings

These essential meetings aim to improve quality of life for cancer sufferers by standardizing and optimizing screening, early detection and treatment of cancer.[49] At any meeting you should be able to spot:

• Paired surgeons and physicians (eg upper GI surgeon and gastroenterologist)
• Radiologists
• Oncologists
• Histopathologists
• Palliative care physicians
• Specialist care nurses
• Meeting administrators

This expert forum aims to provide the most up-to-date and relevant options for treatment individualized for each patient. However, despite everyone's best efforts, there can still remain an inherent uncertainty as to what is exactly the best treatment for the patient—something which in the end may only be known to the patient him- or herself when given the options.

Oncology and palliative care

Tumour markers are specific molecules (usually glycoproteins) that may be found in higher concentrations in the serum and other tissues in patients with certain cancers (see TABLE p535). ▶They are rarely sufficiently specific to be diagnostic and do not replace biopsy for establishing a diagnosis. Many tumour markers are raised in several cancers and may also be raised in benign conditions. Normal levels do not exclude malignancy or disease recurrence.

The main value of tumour markers is in monitoring the course of an illness, determining the effectiveness of treatment and in detecting cancer recurrence. Screening of asymptomatic populations to detect early cancer has yet to consistently demonstrate a survival benefit (trials for PSA are conflicting and for CA 125 ongoing).

Measuring ≥1 tumour marker is unlikely to aid diagnosis (except if suspecting a germ cell tumour). Therefore opportunistic requests for panels of tumour markers in patients with non-specific symptoms is not helpful. It may cause the patient additional stress and anxiety, result in inappropriate and costly investigations, and could delay correct diagnosis. Similarly unhelpful is testing PSA in women or CA 125 in men. An audit in 1 UK hospital found that 17% of requests for CA 125 (the marker of ovarian cancer) were for men.[51]

### Prostate specific antigen (PSA)

As well as being a marker of prostate cancer, PSA is (unfortunately) raised in benign prostatic hyperplasia. See p647 for advising men who ask for a PSA test. 25% of large benign prostates give PSA up to 10 ng/mL. PSA may also be raised if:
• BMI <25 (↑BMI associated with ↓PSA concentrations ?2° haemodilution)[52] • Black Africans • Taller men • Recent ejaculation (avoid for 24h prior to measurement) • Recent rectal examination (usually insignificant●[※]) • Prostatitis • UTI (PSA levels may not return to baseline for some months after a UTI).[53] Plasma reference interval is age specific; the age specific cut-off for PSA measurements recommended by the Prostate Cancer Risk Management Programme are shown below left[1]. Refer urgently if age-specific PSA is raised. The proportion of patients with a raised PSA and benign hypertrophy or carcinoma is shown below right.

| Age (yrs) | PSA cut-off values ng/mL |
|-----------|--------------------------|
| 50–59     | ≥3.0                     |
| 60–69     | ≥4.0                     |
| 70 and over | ≥5.0                   |

| | PSA ng/mL | |
|---|-----------|---|
| Benign prostatic hyperplasia | <4 in 91% | PSA will be ~50% lower after 6 months on 5α reductase inhibitors (see p644) |
| | 4–10 in 8% | |
| | >10 in 1% | |
| Prostate carcinoma | <4 in 15% | |
| | 4–10 in 20% | |
| | >10 in 65% | |

The above is a guide; reference ranges and populations vary. More specific assays, such as free PSA/total PSA index and PSA density, are also available, which may partly solve these problems. It is shown to illustrate the common problem of interpreting a PSA of ~8—and as a warning against casual requests for PSAs in the (vain) hope of simple answers. NB: PSA should be 'undetectable' after radical prostatectomy—refer to a urologist if >0.04ng/mL.

**1** Note there are no age specific reference ranges for men over 80 years. Nearly all will have a focus of cancer, which only needs to be diagnosed if likely to need palliative treatment.

### Paraneoplastic syndromes

*Antineuronal antibody associated paraneoplastic syndromes* are rare, fascinating non-metastatic manifestations of malignancy mediated by hormones, cytokines or antibodies. They are triggered by an altered immune system response to a neoplasm and their importance is that they often pre-date symptoms associated with the cancer itself. They are worth knowing about: if you do, you will occasionally save a life by making a rather clever double diagnosis, eg of an odd eyelid rash (dermatomyositis p554) and of its associated cancer (eg colon cancer); examples are given in *OHCS* p589.

| Tumour marker | Relevant cancer | Use | Associated cancers | Associated benign conditions |
|---|---|---|---|---|
| | | | Other cancers and benign conditions in which the same tumour marker may be raised (not comprehensive) | |
| Alpha-fetoprotein (αFP) | Germ cell/testicular Hepatocellular | Diagnosis, prognosis, monitoring treatment & detecting recurrence | Colorectal; gastric; hepatobiliary; lung | Cirrhosis; pregnancy; neural tube defects |
| Calcitonin | Medullary thyroid | Diagnosis, monitoring treatment & detecting recurrence | None known | C-cell hyperplasia |
| Cancer antigen (CA) 125 | Ovarian | Diagnosis, prognosis, monitoring treatment & detecting recurrence | Breast; cervical; endometrial; hepatocellular; lung; non-Hodgkin's lymphoma; pancreatic; medullary thyroid carcinoma; peritoneal; uterine | *Many:* Liver disease; cystic fibrosis; pancreatitis; urinary retention; diabetes; heart failure; pregnancy; SLE; sarcoid; RA; diverticulitis; IBS; endometriosis; fibroids |
| CA 19-9 | Pancreatic | Diagnosis, prognosis, monitoring treatment & detecting recurrence | Colorectal; gastric; hepatocellular; oesophageal; ovarian | Acute cholangitis; cholestasis; pancreatitis; diabetes; IBS; jaundice |
| CA15-3 | Breast | Monitoring treatment & detecting recurrence | Hepatocellular; pancreatic | Cirrhosis; benign breast disease; in normal health |
| Carcinoembryonic antigen (CEA) | Colorectal | Prognosis, monitoring treatment & detecting recurrence | Breast; gastric; lung; mesothelioma; oesophageal; pancreatic | Smoking; chronic liver disease; chronic kidney disease; diverticulitis; jaundice |
| Human chorionic gonadotrophin (β-HCG) | Germ cell/testicular Gestational trophoblastic | Diagnosis, prognosis, monitoring treatment & detecting recurrence | Lung | Pregnancy |
| Paraproteins | B cell proliferative disorders (eg myeloma) | Diagnosis, monitoring treatment & detecting recurrence | None known | None known |
| Thyroglobulin | Thyroid (follicular/papillary) | Monitoring treatment & detecting recurrence | None known | None known |

Adapted from 'Serum tumour markers: how to order and interpret them', Sturgeon C M, Lai L C, Duffy M J, 2012, with permission from BMJ Publishing Ltd.

Oncology and palliative care

Palliative care is the medicine of palliating (relieving) symptoms. Though this most often applies in the later stages of a malignancy, it does not necessarily have to—something that doctors and patients all too often forget.

℞ Take time to find out exactly what is troubling a patient and approach problems holistically. Remember, each person comes with a set of emotions, preconceptions and a family already attached. Most hospitals now have a dedicated palliative care team for help and advice. See also p7.

**Pain** See p538.

**Nausea and vomiting** Causes include chemotherapy, constipation, GI obstruction, drugs, severe pain, cough, oral thrush, infection and uraemia. *Management:* Aim to treat reversible causes, eg with laxatives, fluconazole, analgesia or antibiotics; consider stopping, reducing or changing drugs or route. Consider the likely cause and base anti-emetic choice on mechanism of nausea and site of drug action (see p241). Give orally if possible, but remember alternative routes (IV/SC/IM/PR). Patients starting strong opioids should be prescribed a regular antiemetic for first week, then PRN. A third of patients will need more than one medication.[54] Consider non-pharmacological methods, eg relaxation. *Oral agents: Cyclizine* 50mg/8h (antihistamine; anticholinergic; central action); *domperidone* 10–20mg/8h (peripheral antidopaminergic, no acute dystonic SEs); *metoclopramide* 10mg/8h (blocks central chemoreceptor trigger zone, *and* peripheral prokinetic effects, good in gastric stasis); *haloperidol* 0.5–1.5mg/12h (dopamine antagonist, effective in drug- or metabolic-induced nausea); *ondansetron* 4–8mg/8h (serotonin antagonist, good for chemo/radiotherapy-related nausea); *levomepromazine* 3–12.5mg/12h (broad spectrum, but can sedate).[55]

**Constipation** Very common SE with opiates, and better prevented than treated. May also be due to $\uparrow Ca^{2+}$ or dehydration. Use *bisacodyl* 5mg at night, or combine a stimulant with a softener (co-danthramer 5–10mL nocte). *Macrogols* 2–4 sachets/12h are useful in resistance. Try glycerol suppositories or an enema if oral therapy fails.

**Breathlessness** Consider fans, air supply, and *supplementary $O_2$. Morphine* reduces respiratory drive, and thus relieves the sensation of breathlessness. Use of relaxation techniques and benzodiazepines can be useful. Look for pleural or pericardial effusion. Consider thoracocentesis ± pleurodesis for a significant pleural effusion. If there is a malignant pericardial effusion, a number of options exist including pericardiocentesis (p787), pleuropericardial windows, and external beam radiotherapy.[56]

**Mouthcare** Treat any candida infection or other underlying cause. Simple measures such as chewing ice chips, pineapple chunks (release proteolytic enzymes) or gum should be tried. Good oral hygiene with mouth washes, chorhexidine and saliva substitutes, such as *Biotene Oralbalance®* gel, can help.

**Pruritus** (itching) See p26.

**Venepuncture problems** Repeated venepuncture with the attendant risk of painful extravasation and phlebitis may be avoided by insertion of a single or multilumen skin-tunnelled catheter (eg a Hickman line) into a major central vein (eg subclavian or internal jugular) using a strict aseptic technique. Patients can look after their own lines at home, and give their own drugs. Problems include: infection, blockage (flush with 0.9% saline or dilute heparin, eg every week), axillary, subclavian, or superior vena cava thrombosis/obstruction, and line slippage.

**The last days and weeks of life** Once a decision has been made that a patient is entering the very final days of their illness, comfort should be the main concern. Think about stopping observations, unnecessary blood tests and medications (such as those for long-term prophylaxis). Prescribe 'as required' subcutaneous end of life drugs before they are needed (see BOX 2). Start a syringe driver if any of these are being given regularly. Ensure that a 'do not attempt resuscitation' order has been made and clearly documented (usually by a senior doctor). Personalised end-of-life care plans should be made, which focus on control of symptoms, comfort and cessation of unnecessary interventions. Consider whether transfer to a hospice may be appropriate. If going home is a priority, it can be arranged at very short notice.

## Syringe drivers

Syringe drivers allow a continuous subcutaneous infusion of drugs when the oral route is no longer feasible and avoids repeated cannulation attempts. Several drugs can be administered subcutaneously to palliate a number of symptoms:

| Indication | Drug | Subcutaneous dose | Comment |
|---|---|---|---|
| Pain | Diamorphine | Start 10–20mg/24h<br>If converting from oral morphine divide total 24h dose by 3 (see p539). | If using regular breakthrough doses, ↑ daily dose by total breakthrough dose required. |
| Agitation | Midazolam | 20–100mg/24h | |
| Nausea and vomiting | Cyclizine | 150mg/24h | |
| | Haloperidol | 1.5–10mg/24h | |
| Respiratory secretions | Hyoscine hydrobromide[1] | 0.6–2.4mg/24h | |
| | Glycopyrronium | 0.6–1.2mg/24h | |
| Bowel colic | Hyoscine butylbromide[1] | 20–120mg/24h | |

## 'As required' end of life medication

Prescribe the following PRN subcutaneous medications for all dying patients *before* they are needed, in anticipation of any symptoms. Also write them up for any patients on syringe drivers who may require breakthrough doses.

| Indication | Drug | Subcutaneous dose | Comment |
|---|---|---|---|
| Pain | Diamorphine | 2.5–5mg/3–4h | Breakthrough dose = 1/6th of total 24h dose. |
| Agitation | Midazolam | 2.5mg–5mg/4h | |
| Nausea and vomiting | Haloperidol | 1–2.5mg/8h | |
| Respiratory secretions | Hyoscine hydrobromide[1] | 0.4mg/8h | |

## Other agents that may help relieve symptoms

**Other agents and procedures to know about** (alphabetically listed)
- Colestyramine 4g/6h PO (1h after other drugs) may help itch with jaundice.
- Dexamethasone 8mg IV stat relieves symptoms of SVC or bronchial obstruction, and lymphangitis carcinomatosa. 4mg/24h PO may stimulate appetite, reduce ↑ICP headache, or induce (in some patients) a satisfactory sense of euphoria (short-term benefits must be balanced against side-effects).
- Fluconazole 50mg/24h PO for candida.
- Haloperidol 0.5–5mg/24h PO helps agitation, hallucinations, and vomiting.
- Hyoscine hydrobromide 0.4–0.6mg/8h SC or 0.3mg sublingual: vomiting from upper GI obstruction or noisy bronchial rattles.
- Metronidazole 400mg/8h PO mitigates anaerobic odours from tumours; so do charcoal dressings (Actisorb®).
- Naproxen 250mg/8h with food: fevers caused by malignancy or bone pain from metastases (consider splinting joints if this fails).
- Nerve blocks may lastingly relieve pleural or other resistant pains.
- Sodium chloride nebulizers 5mL as needed, can aid persistent cough.
- Spironolactone 100mg/12h PO + bumetanide 1mg/24h PO for ascites associated with portal hypertension (but not for ascites caused by abdominal malignancy, ie where serum-ascites albumin gradient <11g/L).

---

1 Do not confuse the vastly different doses for hyoscine hydrobromide and hyoscine butylbromide!

**Pain** is one of the most feared sequelae of a terminal diagnosis and yet is largely preventable. Studies show that cancer pain is particularly poorly managed in most settings,[57] especially in the elderly. No patient should live or die with unrelieved pain; aim to prevent or eliminate it.

**Assessment** Don't assume a cause—take a detailed history and examine to understand the aetiology. Evaluate severity, nature, functional deficit and psychological state—depression occurs in up to 25% of cancer patients.[58] Pain from nerve infiltration or local pressure damage may respond better to amitriptyline or gabapentin than to opioids.

**Management** Explain and plan rehabilitation goals. Aim to modify the pathological process when possible, eg radiotherapy, hormones, chemotherapy, surgery. Effective analgesia is possible in 70–90% of patients[59] by adhering to 5 simple guidelines:

1 *By the mouth*—give orally wherever possible.
2 *By the clock*—give at fixed intervals to give continuous relief.
3 *By the ladder*—following the WHO stepwise approach (BOX).
4 *For the individual*—there are no standard doses for opiates, needs vary.
5 *With attention to detail*—inform, set times carefully, warn of side-effects.

Use the WHO ladder (BOX) until pain is relieved. Monitor the response carefully—review of results and side-effects is crucial to good care. Start regular laxatives and anti-emetics with strong opiates. *Paracetamol* PO/PR/IV at step 1 may have an opiate-sparing effect, and should be continued at steps 2 and 3.[60]

**Morphine** Start with oral solution 5–10mg/4h PO with an equal breakthrough dose as often as required. A double dose at bedtime can enable a good night's sleep. Patient needs will vary greatly and there is no maximum dose; aim to control symptoms with minimum side-effects. If not effective, increase doses in 30–50% increments (5mg→10mg→20mg→30mg→45mg). Change to modified release preparations (eg *MST Continus®* 12h) once daily needs are known by totalling 24h use and dividing by 2. Prescribe 1/6ᵗʰ of the total daily dose as oral solution for breakthrough pain. Side-effects (common) are drowsiness, nausea/vomiting, constipation and dry mouth. Hallucinations and myoclonic jerks are signs of toxicity and should prompt dose review. ►*If the oral route is unavailable try morphine/diamorphine* IV/SC (see BOX for conversions). If difficulty tolerating morphine/diamorphine, try *oxycodone* PO/IV/SC/ PR, starting at an equivalent dose. It is as effective as morphine and is a useful 2ⁿᵈ-line opioid with a different range of receptor activity.[61] *OxyNorm®* is the oral liquid form. There are also *fentanyl* transdermal patches which should usually be started under specialist supervision (after opioid dose requirements have been established). Remove after 72h, and place a new patch at a different site. 45mg oral morphine/24h is approximately equivalent to a 12mcg/h fentanyl patch.

*Suppositories* for pain: try *oxycodone* 30mg PR (eg 30mg/8h ≈ 30mg morphine).

*Syringe drivers* See BOX on p537.

*Unfounded fears:* Patients often shrink from using morphine analgesia, usually as a result of common misconceptions—that it is addictive, for the dying, signifying 'The End'. It is important to address and allay these fears. Addiction is not a problem in the palliative care setting, neither is respiratory depression with correct titration—pain stimulates the respiratory centre. Reassure the patient that it is simply a good painkiller, used in many situations. There is evidence it has no effect on life expectancy.[62] See BOX for dose escalation required to ensure total sedation.

*Prescribing morphine and other controlled drugs:* Include the total quantity in both words and figures, and include the formulation (tablets, capsules, oral liquid, etc). On charts rewrite medications in full if doses change and always give the amount in milligrams, especially when using liquid preparations.

**Morphine-resistant pain** Consider methadone or ketamine, and adjuvants such as NSAIDs, steroids, muscle relaxants or anxiolytics + seek expert help. If *neuropathic pain* is suspected, try *amitriptyline* (10–25mg ON) or *pregabalin* (25–300mg/12h). *Depression* is common, and can amplify pain, so consider starting an SSRI.

## The WHO analgesic ladder[63]

(See p576 for NNT)

| Rung 1 | Non-opioid | Paracetamol; NSAIDs |
|---|---|---|
| Rung 2 | Weak opioid | Codeine; dihydrocodeine; tramadol |
| Rung 3 | Strong opioid | Morphine; diamorphine; hydromorphone; oxycodone; fentanyl; buprenorphine (± adjuvant analgesics) |

Unlike other ladders this ladder is not used to fetch something out of reach—adequate pain relief should be attainable to all. If one drug fails to relieve pain, move up—do not try other drugs at the same level. In new, severe pain, rung 2 may be omitted.[64]

## Opiate dose equivalents[65]

| | 24h dose (mg) | 4h dose (mg) | Relative potency to oral morphine |
|---|---|---|---|
| Morphine PO | 30 | 5 | 1× |
| Morphine IV | 15 | 2.5 | 2× |
| Morphine SC | 15 | 2.5 | 2× |
| Diamorphine IV | 12 | 2 | 3× |
| Diamorphine SC | 12 | 2 | 3× |
| Oxycodone PO | 15 | 2.5 | 2× |
| Oxycodone SC | 12 | 2 | 3× |
| Oxycodone SC | 7.5–15 | 1.25–2.5 | 3× |
| Alfentanil SC[1] | 1 | — | 30× |

To convert oral codeine, dihydrocodeine, or tramadol to oral morphine, divide the total daily dose by about 10.

Conversions are not exact; these tables are intended as a rough guide. The potency figures in particular can vary widely. If in doubt, use a dose below your estimate.

## ☼ Total sedation

The active management of death may need geometric increments in drug doses to avoid suffering.[2] If a patient is dying and prefers total sedation, opiate doses may need to be doubled every 12h (or increased by 5–50% every few hours if on a syringe driver).[66] Don't be frightened to use big or very big doses if smaller doses are not working. It's whatever is needed and this is very variable:

• *Parenteral morphine:* 2.5–100mg/1–4h SC. If many breakthrough doses are needed, increase background analgesia by ≥50%.[67] In one study, 91% needed 5–299mg of morphine/day, 7% needed 300–599mg/day, and 2% needed ≥600mg of morphine/day.[68,69] Morphine doses SC via a syringe driver range from 0.5–300mg/h.[70] If 10mg/h is not working, give a bolus of 10mg, and then increase the rate by ≥50% (15mg/h). If distress continues, re-bolus with 15mg, and ↑rate to 22mg/h and so on until full comfort is achieved.[71] It often helps to add midazolam 0.8–8mg/h;[72,73] NB: validated protocols for dose escalation are lacking.[74]

• *Modified-release morphine sulfate:* 10–260mg/12h.[66,75,76] *Oxycodone* is an alternative, eg *OxyContin®*. In one study, the mean daily *OxyContin®* dose was ~80mg/d. 20% need at least 3 times as much.[77]

• *Transdermal fentanyl patches* are useful once dose requirements are known.[78]

---

1 Alfentanil can be used in patients with marked renal failure—discuss with the palliative care team first

2 Document that this is the patient's wishes, each dose increase is proportionate and plans have been discussed with an experienced colleague; take into account GMC guidance.

## Contents

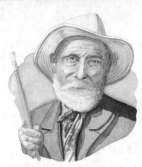

Fig 1. The painter Pierre-Auguste Renoir (1841-1919) suffered from severe rheumatoid arthritis which caused crippling hand deformity. In later life, he painted with a brush fixed between his index and middle fingers. In this way, and despite shoulder ankylosis, he completed some of his greatest works of impressionist art. Through his work he communicated the joy he took from his subjects. "Why shouldn't art be pretty?" he said, "There are enough unpleasant things in the world".

Try to encourage those who are struggling to overcome the adversities of physical disease by engaging them in positive activities that are within their reach (or from which they can adapt). This may allow them to break through the barriers hindering them—whether perceived or real.

We like to see our rheumatology patients before destructive changes take place. Rheumatic disease can present an array of symptoms—the skill of the rheumatologist is to stand back and see the whole. This involves not only making a diagnosis, but also understanding the relationship between patient and disease. The swan is famously mute, and serene, just as our most afflicted patients can appear so serene, bearing the arthritic agony of daily life. But when you see painted fingernails at the end of swan-neck fingers, remember the great effort the swan must make to take flight.

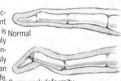

Normal

Swan-neck deformity
Fig 2. Swan-neck finger deformity.

*Relevant pages elsewhere:* Cervical spondylosis (p512); Charcot's joints (p520); osteoporosis (p696); Behçet's disease (p708); Sjögren's syndrome (p724); Wegener's granulomatosis (p728). *Orthopaedics:* OHCS chapter 11.

*We thank Professor Kevin Davies, our Specialist Reader, and William Hunt, our Junior Reader, for their contribution to this chapter.*

# Some points to note in a rheumatological history

In the assessment of an arthritic presentation, pay particular attention to the distribution of joint involvement (including spine) and the presence of symmetry. Also look for disruption of joint anatomy, limitation of movement (by pain or contracture), joint effusions and peri-articular involvement (see p542 for a fuller assessment). Ask about, and examine for, *extra-articular features:* skin and nail (see p32) involvement (include scalp, hairline, umbilicus, genitalia, and natal cleft—psoriasis can easily be missed); eye signs (see p562); lungs (eg fibrosis)(see p188); kidneys (see p314); heart; GI (eg mouth ulcers, diarrhoea); GU (eg urethritis, genital ulcers); and CNS.

## 3 screening questions for musculo-skeletal disease:
1 Are you free of any pain or stiffness in your joints, muscles or back?
2 Can you dress yourself without too much difficulty?
3 Can you manage walking up and down stairs?

If *yes* to all 3, serious inflammatory muscle/joint disease is unlikely.

*Presenting symptoms:*
- Pattern of involved joints
- Symmetry (or not)
- Morning stiffness >30min (eg RA)
- Pain, swelling, loss of function, erythema, warmth

*Extra-articular features:*
- Rashes, photosensitivity (eg SLE)
- Raynaud's (SLE; CREST; polymyositis and dermatomyositis)
- Dry eyes or mouth (Sjögren's)
- Red eyes, iritis (eg AS)
- Diarrhoea/urethritis (Reiter's•)
- Nodules or nodes (eg RA; TB; gout)
- Mouth/genital ulcers (eg Behçet's)
- Weight loss (eg malignancy, any systemic inflammatory disease)

*Related diseases:*
- Crohn's/UC (in ankylosing spondylitis), gonorrhoea, psoriasis

*Current and past drugs:*
- NSAIDs, DMARDs (p549)
- Biological agents (eg TNFα inhibitors)

*Family history:*
- Arthritis, psoriasis, autoimmune disease

*Social history:*
- Age
- Occupation
- Sexual history
- Ethnicity (eg SLE is commoner in African-Caribbeans and Asians)
- Ability to function, eg dressing, grooming, writing, walking
- Domestic situation, social support, home adaptations
- Smoking (may worsen RA)

## Patterns of presentation of arthritis

| Monoarthritis | Oligoarthritis (≤5 joints) | Polyarthritis (>5 joints involved) | |
|---|---|---|---|
| | | **Symmetrical:** | **Asymmetrical:** |
| Septic arthritis | Crystal arthritis | Rheumatoid arthritis | Reactive arthritis |
| Crystal arthritis (gout, CPPD) | Psoriatic arthritis | | |
| | Reactive arthritis, eg *Yersinia, Salmonella, Campylobacter* | Osteoarthritis | Psoriatic arthritis |
| Osteoarthritis | | Viruses (eg hepatitis A, B & C; mumps) | |
| Trauma, eg haemarthrosis | | | |
| | Ankylosing spondylitis Osteoarthritis | Systemic conditions[1] (can be either) | |

▶▶Exclude septic arthritis in any acutely inflamed joint, as it can destroy a joint in under 24h (p546). Inflammation may be less overt if immunocompromised (eg from the many immunosuppressive drugs used in rheumatological conditions) or if there is underlying joint disease. Joint aspiration (p543) is the key investigation, and if you are unable to do it, find someone who can.

1 Connective tissue disease (eg SLE and relapsing polychondritis), sarcoidosis, malignancy (eg leukaemia), endocarditis, haemochromatosis, sickle-cell anaemia, familial Mediterranean fever, Behçet's.

*Rheumatology*

This aims to screen for rheumatological conditions primarily affecting mobility (as a consequence of underlying joint disease). It is based on the GALS locomotor screen (**G**ait, **A**rms, **L**egs, **S**pine).[1]

**Essence** 'Look, feel and move' (active and passive). If a *joint looks normal* to you, *feels normal* to the patient, and has *full range of movement*, it usually is normal. Make sure the patient is comfortable, and obtain their consent before examination. The GALS screening examination should be done in light underwear.

*Spine: Observe from behind:* Is muscle bulk normal (buttocks, shoulders)? Is the spine straight? Are paraspinal muscles symmetrical? Any swellings/deformities? *Observe from the side:* Is cervical and lumbar lordosis normal? Any kyphosis? "Touch your toes, please": Is lumbar spine flexion normal, eg Schober's test?[1] *Observe from in front:* "*Tilt your head*" (without moving the shoulders)—tests lateral neck flexion. Palpate for typical fibromyalgia tender points (see p560).

*Arms:* "*Try putting your hands behind your head*"—tests functional shoulder movement. "*Arms out straight*"—tests elbow extension and forearm supination/pronation. Examine the hands: (See p32). Any deformity, wasting, or swellings? *Squeeze across 2nd–5th metacarpophalangeal joints.* Pain may denote joint or tendon synovitis. "*Put your index finger on your thumb*"—tests pincer grip. Assess dexterity, eg fastening a button or picking up a coin.

*Legs: Observe legs:* Normal quadriceps bulk? Any swelling or deformity? *With patient lying supine:* Any leg length discrepancy? *Internally/externally rotate each hip in flexion. Passively flex knee and hip to the full extent.* Is movement limited? Any crepitus? *Find any knee effusion* using the patella tap test. If there is fluid, consider aspirating and testing for crystals or infection. *With patient standing:* Observe feet: Any deformity? Are arches high or flat? Any callosities? These may indicate an abnormal gait of some chronicity. *Squeeze across metatarsophalangeal joints:* see above. Also: although not in the GALS system, *palpate the heel and Achilles tendon* to identify plantar fasciitis and Achilles tendonitis often associated with seronegative rheumatological conditions. *Examine the patient's shoes* for signs of uneven wear.

*Gait: Observe walking:* Is the gait smooth? Good arm swing? Stride length OK? Normal heel strike and toe off? Can they turn quickly?

| The GALS system for quickly recording your findings | | |
|---|---|---|
| **G** (Gait) | ✓ | |
| | *Appearance:* | *Movement:* |
| **A** (Arms) | ✓ | ✓ |
| **L** (Legs) | ✓ | ✓ |
| **S** (Spine) | ✓ | ✓ |
| ✓ means normal. If not normal, then put a cross with a note to explain what the exact problem is. | | |

**Range of joint movement** is noted in degrees, with anatomical position being the neutral position—eg elbow flexion 0°-150° normally, but with fixed flexion and limited movement, range may be reduced to 30°-90°. A valgus deformity deviates laterally (away from the mid-line, fig 1); a varus deformity points towards the mid-line.

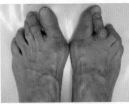

Fig 1. Bilateral hallux valgus.
Reproduced from *British Medical Journal*, 'Hallux valgus',
R Choa, R Sharp, K R Mahtani, 2010,
with permission from BMJ Publishing Group Ltd.

1 Schober's test: make a mark on the lumbar spine at the level of the posterior iliac spine. Measure out a line from 5cm below to 10cm above the mark. Ask to bend forward as far as they can. If the line does not lengthen by at least 5cm in flexion, there is reduced lumbar flexion, eg in ankylosing spondylitis.

### Some important rheumatological investigations

**Joint aspiration** is the most important investigation in any monoarthritic presentation (see also *OHCS* p708). Send synovial fluid for urgent white cell count, Gram stain, polarized light microscopy (for crystals, p550). The risk of inducing septic arthritis, using sterile precautions, is <1:10,000.[2] Look for blood[1], pus, and crystals (gout or CPPD crystal arthropathy; p550). ►Do not attempt joint aspiration through inflamed and potentially infected skin (eg through a psoriatic plaque).

#### Synovial fluid in health and disease

|  | Appearance | Viscosity | WBC/mm³ | Neutrophils |
|---|---|---|---|---|
| *Normal* | Clear, colourless | ↔ | ≤200 | None |
| *Osteoarthritis* | Clear, straw | ↑ | ≤1000 | ≤50% |
| *Haemorrhagic*[1] | Bloody, xanthochromic | Varies | ≤10,000 | ≤50% |
| *Acutely inflamed:* |  |  |  |  |
| • RA | Turbid, yellow | ↓ | 1–50,000 | Varies |
| • *Crystal* | Turbid, yellow | ↓ | 5–50,000 | ~80% |
| *Septic* | Turbid, yellow | ↓ | 10–100,000 | >90% |

**Blood tests** FBC, ESR, urate, U&E, CRP. Blood culture for septic arthritis. Consider rheumatoid factor, anti-CCP, ANA, other autoantibodies (p555), and HLA B27 (p552) —as guided by presentation. Consider causes of reactive arthritis (p552), eg viral serology, urine chlamydia PCR, hepatitis and HIV serology if risk factors are present.

**Radiology** Look for erosions, calcification, widening or loss of joint space, changes in underlying bone of affected joints (eg periarticular osteopenia, sclerotic areas, osteophytes). Characteristic x-ray features for various arthritides are shown in figs 1–3. Irregularity of the lower half of the sacroiliac joints is seen in spondyloarthritis. Ultrasound and MRI are more sensitive in identifying effusions, synovitis, enthesitis and infection than plain radiographs—discuss further investigations with a radiologist. Do a CXR for RA, vasculitis, TB and sarcoid.

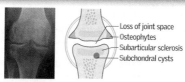

Loss of joint space
Osteophytes
Subarticular sclerosis
Subchondral cysts

Fig 1. x-ray features of osteoarthritis.

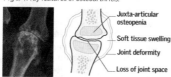

Juxta-articular osteopenia
Soft tissue swelling
Joint deformity
Loss of joint space

Fig 2. x-ray features of rheumatoid arthritis (MCPJ).

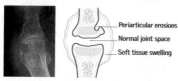

Periarticular erosions
Normal joint space
Soft tissue swelling

Fig 3. x-ray features of gout (1st MTPJ).

x-ray figs 1–3 courtesy of Dr DC Howlett.

1 Eg trauma, tumour or haemophilia.

Back pain is very common, and often self-limiting, but *be alert to sinister causes*, ie malignancy, infection or inflammatory causes. See below for red-flag symptoms, and BOX opposite for neurosurgical emergencies.

| Red flags for sinister causes of back pain³ | |
|---|---|
| ►Aged <20yrs or >55yrs old | ►Thoracic back pain |
| ►Acute onset in elderly people | ►Morning stiffness |
| ►Constant or progressive pain | ►Bilateral or alternating leg pain |
| ►Nocturnal pain | ►Neurological disturbance (incl sciatica) |
| ►Worse pain on being supine | ►Sphincter disturbance |
| ►Fever, night sweats, weight loss | ►Current or recent infection |
| ►History of malignancy | ►Immunosuppression, eg steroids/HIV |
| ►Abdominal mass | ►Leg claudication or exercise-related leg weakness/numbness (spinal stenosis) |

**Examination**

1 With the patient standing, gauge the extent and smoothness of lumbar forward/ lateral flexion and extension (see p542).
2 *Clinical tests for sacroiliitis:* direct pressure, lateral compression, sacroiliac stretch test (pain on adduction of the hip, with the hip and knee flexed).
3 Neurological deficits (see BOX 1): test lower limb sensation, power, and deep tendon and plantar reflexes. Digital rectal examination for perianal tone and sensation.
4 Examine for nerve root pain: this is distributed in relevant dermatomes, and is worsened by coughing or bending forward. *Straight leg test* (L4, L5, S1): positive if raising the leg with the knee extended causes pain below the knee, which increases on foot dorsiflexion (Lasègue's sign). It suggests irritation to the sciatic nerve. The main cause is lumbar disc prolapse. Also *femoral stretch test* (L4 and above): pain in front of thigh on lifting the hip into extension with the patient lying face downwards and the knee flexed.
5 Signs of generalized disease—eg malignancy. Examine other systems (eg abdomen) as pain may be referred.

**Causes** Age determines the most likely causes:

| 15–30yrs: | Prolapsed disc, trauma, fractures, ankylosing spondylitis (AS; p552), spondylolisthesis (a forward shift of one vertebra over another, which is congenital or due to trauma), pregnancy. |
|---|---|
| 30–50yrs: | Degenerative spinal disease, prolapsed disc, malignancy (primary or secondary from lung, breast, prostate, thyroid or kidney ca). |
| >50yrs: | Degenerative, osteoporotic vertebral collapse, Paget's (see p699), malignancy, myeloma (see p362), spinal stenosis. |

*Rarer:* Cauda equina tumours, psoas abscess, spinal infection (eg discitis, usually staphylococcal but also *Proteus, E. coli, S. typhi* and TB—there are often no systemic signs).

**Investigations** Arrange relevant tests if you suspect a specific cause, or if red flag symptoms: FBC, ESR and CRP (myeloma, infection, tumour), U&E, ALP (Paget's), serum/urine electrophoresis (myeloma), PSA. *x-rays* can exclude bony abnormality but are generally not indicated. *MRI* is the image of choice and can detect disc prolapse, cord compression (fig 1), cancer, infection or inflammation (eg sacroiliitis).

**Management** ►►Urgent neurosurgical referral if any neurological deficit (see BOX 1). ℞ Keep the diagnosis under review. For non-specific back pain, focus on **education** and **self-management**. Advise patients to continue with normal activites and be active. Manage pain to allow this—regular paracetamol ± NSAIDs ± codeine. Consider low dose amitriptyline if these fail (do not use SSRIs for treating pain). Offer **physiotherapy, acupuncture** or an **exercise programme** if not improving.⁴ Address **psychosocial issues**, which may predispose to developing chronic pain and disability (see p561). Surgical options may be considered in selected patients with intractable symptoms who fail to respond to other measures.

## Neurosurgical emergencies (see also p470)

►*Acute cauda equina compression:* Alternating or bilateral root pain in legs, saddle anaesthesia (perianal), loss of anal tone on PR, bladder ± bowel incontinence.
►*Acute cord compression:* Bilateral pain, LMN signs (p451) at level of compression, UMN and sensory loss below, sphincter disturbance.
►*Immediate urgent treatment* prevents irreversible loss, eg laminectomy for disc protrusions, radiotherapy for tumours, decompression for abscesses.
►*Causes* (same for both): bony metastasis (look for missing pedicle on x-ray), large disc protrusion, myeloma, cord or paraspinal tumour, TB (p398), abscess.

## Nerve root lesions

| Nerve root | Pain | Weakness | Reflex affected |
|---|---|---|---|
| L2 | Across upper thigh | Hip flexion and adduction | Nil |
| L3 | Across lower thigh | Hip adduction, knee extension | Knee jerk |
| L4 | Across knee to medial malleolus | Knee extension, foot inversion and dorsiflexion | Knee jerk |
| L5 | Lateral shin to dorsum of foot and great toe | Hip extension and abduction<br>Knee flexion<br>Foot and great toe dorsiflexion | Great toe jerk |
| S1 | Posterior calf to lateral foot and little toe | Knee flexion<br>Foot and toe plantar flexion<br>Foot eversion | Ankle jerk |

Rheumatology

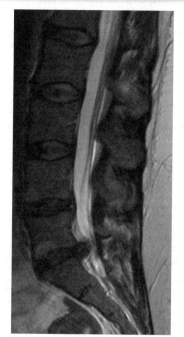

Fig 1. Sagittal T2-weighted MRI of the lumbar spine showing a herniated L5–S1 disc.

Courtesy of Norwich Radiology Department.

Osteoarthritis (OA) is the commonest joint condition. ♀:♂≈3:1, onset typically >50yrs. It is usually primary (generalized), but may be secondary to joint disease or other conditions (eg haemochromatosis, obesity, occupational).

**Signs and symptoms** *Localized disease* (usually knee or hip): pain on movement and crepitus; background pain at rest; joint gelling—stiffness after rest up to ~30min; joint instability. *Generalized disease* (primary OA): with Heberden's nodes ('nodal OA', seen mainly in post-menopausal ♀), commonly affected joints are the DIP joints, thumb carpo-metacarpal joints and the knees. There may be joint tenderness, derangement and bony swelling (Heberden's nodes at DIP, Bouchard's nodes at PIP), ↓range of movement and mild synovitis. Assess effect of symptoms on occupation, family duties, hobbies and lifestyle expectations.

**Tests** Plain radiographs show: **L**oss of joint space, **O**steophytes, **S**ubarticular sclerosis and **S**ubchondral cysts (fig 1 p543). CRP may be slightly elevated.[5]

**Management**[6] *Core treatments:* Exercise to improve local muscle strength and general aerobic fitness (irrespective of age, severity or comorbidity). Weight loss if overweight. *Analgesia:* Regular paracetamol ± topical NSAIDs. If ineffective use codeine or short-term oral NSAID (+PPI)—see BOX. Topical capsaicin (derived from chillies) may help. Intra-articular steroid injections temporarily relieve pain in severe symptoms. Intra-articular hyaluronic acid injections (viscosupplementation) are as effective as NSAIDs or steroid injection, but are much more expensive.[7] Glucosamine and chondroitin products are not recommended. *Non-pharmacological:* Use a multi-disciplinary approach, including physiotherapists and occupational therapists. Try heat or cold packs at the site of pain, walking aids, stretching/manipulation or TENS. *Surgery:* Joint replacement (hips, or knees) is the best way to deal with severe OA that has a substantial impact on quality of life.

## Septic arthritis

▶▶Consider septic arthritis in any acutely inflamed joint, as it can destroy a joint in under 24h. Inflammation may be less overt if immunocompromised (eg from medication) or if there is underlying joint disease. The knee is affected in >50% cases.

**Risk factors** Pre-existing joint disease (especially rheumatoid arthritis); diabetes mellitus, immunosuppression, chronic renal failure, recent joint surgery, prosthetic joints (where infection is particularly difficult to treat), IV drug abuse, age >80yrs.[8]

**Investigations** Urgent joint aspiration for synovial fluid microscopy and culture is the key investigation (p543), as plain radiographs and CRP may be normal. The main differential diagnoses are the crystal arthropathies (p550). Blood cultures may be helpful for guiding antibiotic choice later.

*Ask yourself* "How did the organism get there?" Is there immunosuppression, or another focus of infection, eg from indwelling IV lines, infected skin, or pneumonia (present in up to 50% of those with pneumococcal arthritis)?[9]

**Treatment** If in doubt start empirical IV antibiotics (after aspiration) until sensitivities are known. Common causative organisms are *Staph. aureus*, streptococci, *Neisseria gonococcus* and Gram -ve bacilli. Follow local guidelines for antibiotic choice. Consider **flucloxacillin** 1g/6h IV (*clindamycin* if penicillin allergic); **vancomycin** 1g/12h IV if MRSA (or history of MRSA); or **cefotaxime** 1g/8h IV if gonococcal or Gram -ve organisms suspected.[10] If HIV +ve, look for atypical mycobacteria and fungi. Antibiotics are required for a prolonged period but there is no consensus on which route or for how long they should be continued (eg ~2 weeks IV, then 2-4 weeks PO)—ask a microbiologist.[11] Ask for orthopaedic advice for consideration of arthrocentesis, lavage and debridement, especially if there is a prosthetic joint involved.[12] This may be done arthroscopically (eg for knee) or open under GA (eg for hip; this allows for biopsy—helpful in TB). Splint for ≤48h, give adequate analgesia and consider physiotherapy.

Around 60% of patients will respond to any NSAID, but there is considerable variation in response and tolerance—if one isn't effective, try another. If taken regularly, NSAIDs have both analgesic and anti-inflammatory effect, but the full anti-inflammatory effect may take up to 3 weeks.[10] NSAIDs cause ~1000 deaths/yr in the UK[12] so only use after risk:benefit analysis individualized for each patient, including indication, dose, proposed duration of use, and comorbidity. Follow local recommendations and national guidelines where available.

**NSAID SEs** The main serious side-effects are GI bleeding (►gastrointestinal damage may occur without dyspeptic symptoms) and renal impairment. NSAIDs are contraindicated in severe heart failure. SEs increase with: prolonged use, ↑age, polypharmacy, history of peptic ulcers and renal impairment (review before *and after* starting therapy). Avoid giving NSAIDs to patients on aspirin and do not use in active GI ulceration. Ibuprofen has the lowest GI risk.

**Inform your patients** Many patients prescribed NSAIDs do not need them all the time, so say "Take the lowest possible dose for the shortest possible time". *Bleeding is more common in those who know less about their drugs.*[13] Explain:
- Drugs are to relieve symptoms: on good days, don't take any. In rheumatoid arthritis, cod liver oil (eg 10g/d) reduces reliance on NSAIDs by 30%.[14]
- Abdominal pain may be a sign of impending GI problems: stop the tablets, and come back for more advice if symptoms continue.
- Report black stools ± faints at once.
- Don't supplement prescribed NSAIDs with ones bought over the counter (eg ibuprofen): mixing NSAIDs can increase risks 20-fold.
- Smoking and alcohol increase NSAID risk.[15]

**Cardiovascular side-effects:**[16] Consider cardiovascular risk when prescribing any NSAID—all are associated with a small increased risk of MI and stroke (independent of cardiovascular risk factor or duration of use). Specifically implicated are celecoxib (any dose), diclofenac (>150mg/24h) and ibuprofen (>1200mg/24h). Naproxen appears to be least harmful.[16]

**When should COX-2 selective NSAIDs be tried?** Not often—COX-2 selective NSAIDs are associated with a lower risk of serious upper GI SEs but are not as safe as we had hoped. Commonly used COX-2 drugs include celecoxib and etoricoxib. Meta-analyses of cardiovascular risk for celecoxib are inconsistent, but appear similar to other conventional NSAIDs (above); for etoricoxib there is increased risk when compared to naproxen or ibuprofen.[13] Perhaps use COX-2 selective NSAIDs *only* when an NSAID is essential *and* there is past peptic ulceration (but risk is not eliminated, and bleeds that do occur may be very serious) *if an* ordinary NSAID with PPI (eg omeprazole) is problematic *or* >65yrs old (not on aspirin) *or* needing high-dose NSAID over a long time. If at very high risk of GI bleed, ideally avoid altogether, or combine a COX-2 (eg celecoxib 200mg/12h; avoid if eGFR <30) with a PPI.[17]

Rheumatology

Rheumatology

RA is a chronic systemic inflammatory disease, characterized by a symmetrical, deforming, peripheral polyarthritis. *Epidemiology:* Prevalence is ~1% (↑ in smokers). ♀:♂ >2:1. Peak onset: $5^{th}$–$6^{th}$ decade. HLA DR4/DR1 linked (associated with ↑ severity).

**Presentation** *Typically:* symmetrical swollen, painful, and stiff small joints of hands and feet, worse in the morning. This can fluctuate and larger joints may become involved. *Less common presentations:* •Sudden onset, widespread arthritis; •Recurring mono/polyarthritis of various joints (*palindromic RA*);[1] •Persistent monoarthritis (often knee, shoulder or hip); •Systemic illness with extra-articular symptoms, eg fatigue, fever, weight loss, pericarditis and pleurisy, but initially few joint problems (commoner in ♂); •Polymyalgic onset—vague limb girdle aches; •Recurrent soft tissue problems (eg frozen shoulder, carpal tunnel syndrome, de Quervain's tenosynovitis).

**Signs** *Early* (inflammation, no joint damage): swollen MCP, PIP, wrist, or MTP joints (often symmetrical). Look for tenosynovitis or bursitis. *Later* (joint damage, deformity): ulnar deviation of the fingers and dorsal wrist subluxation. Boutonnière and swan-neck deformities of fingers (fig 1 on p540) or Z-deformity of thumbs occur. Hand extensor tendons may rupture. Foot changes are similar. Larger joints can be involved. Atlanto-axial joint subluxation may threaten the spinal cord (rare).

**Extra-articular** Nodules—elbows & lungs; lymphadenopathy; vasculitis; fibrosing alveolitis, obliterative bronchiolitis; pleural & pericardial effusion; Raynaud's; carpal tunnel syndrome; peripheral neuropathy; splenomegaly (seen in 5%; only 1% have Felty's syndrome: RA + splenomegaly + neutropenia, see p712); episcleritis, scleritis, scleromalacia, keratoconjunctivitis sicca (p562); osteoporosis; amyloidosis (p364).

**Investigations** Rheumatoid factor (RhF) is positive in ~70% (p555). A high titre is associated with severe disease, erosions and extra-articular disease. Anticyclic citrullinated peptide antibodies (ACPA/anti-CCP) are highly specific (~98%) for RA. There is often anaemia of chronic disease. Inflammation causes ↑platelets, ↑ESR, ↑CRP. *X-rays* show soft tissue swelling, juxta-articular osteopenia and ↓joint space. Later there may be bony erosions, subluxation or complete carpal destruction (see fig 2 on p543). Ultrasound and MRI can identify synovitis more accurately, and have greater sensitivity in detecting bone erosions than conventional x-rays.[18]

**Diagnostic criteria** see BOX 1.

**Management** ►Refer early to a rheumatologist (before irreversible destruction).
• Disease activity is measured using the DAS28.[2] Aim to reduce score to <3.
• Early use of DMARDs and **biological agents** improves long-term outcomes (see BOX).
• **Steroids** rapidly reduce symptoms and inflammation. Avoid starting unless appropriately experienced. They are useful for treating acute exacerbations ('flares'), eg IM depot *methylprednisolone* 80–120mg. Intra-articular steroids have a rapid but short-term effect (*OHCS* p708–711). Oral steroids (eg *prednisolone* 7.5mg/d) may control difficult symptoms, but side-effects preclude routine long-term use.
• NSAIDs (see p547) are good for symptom relief, but have no effect on disease progression. Paracetamol and weak opiates are rarely effective.
• Offer specialist physio- and occupational therapy, eg for aids and splints.
• Surgery may relieve pain, improve function and reduce deformity.
• There is ↑ risk of cardiovascular and cerebrovascular disease, as atherosclerosis is accelerated in RA.[19] Manage risk factors (p87). Smoking also ↑ symptoms of RA.

☺ Patients want to live as unencumbered by the disease as possible. Depressive symptoms and pain are better predictors of quality of life than disease markers or radiological damage. Assess impact on relationships, work and hobbies. Psychological interventions (eg relaxation, cognitive coping skills) may help. There is little evidence for the long-term efficacy of complementary therapies but don't prejudice patients who may decide to try.

**1** In rheumatological palindromes, arthritis lasting hours or days runs to and fro, visiting and revisiting 3 or more sites, typically knees, wrists, and MCP joints. It may presage RA, SLE, Whipple's, or Behçet's disease. Remissions are (initially) complete, leaving no radiological mark.
**2** 28-joint Disease Activity Score—assesses tenderness and swelling at 28 joints (MCPs, PIPs, wrists, elbows, shoulders, knees), ESR and patient's self-reported symptom severity.

| **Criteria for diagnosing RA[20]** | | | |
|---|---|---|---|
| *Who should be tested?* Those with ≥1 joint with definite swelling which is not better explained by another disease. Add total A–D score. Scores ≥6/10 are diagnostic. | | | |
| **A** | *Joint involvement* (swelling or tenderness ± imaging evidence) | | |
| | 1 large joint =0 | 2–10 large joints =1 | 1–3 small* joints[†] =2 |
| | 4–10 small* joints[†] =3 | > 10 joints (at least 1 small joint) =5 | |
| **B** | *Serology* (at least 1 test result needed) | | |
| | Negative RF *and* negative anti-CCP =0 | Low +ve RF *or* low +ve anti-CCP =2 | |
| | High +ve RF *or* high +ve anti-CCP =3 | | |
| **C** | *Acute phase reactants* (at least 1 test result needed) | | |
| | Normal CRP and normal ESR =0 | Abnormal CRP or abnormal ESR =1 | |
| **D** | *Duration of symptoms* | | |
| | <6 weeks =0 | ≥6 weeks =1 | |

*= MCPJ, PIPJ, 2–5th MTPJ, wrists and thumb IPJ; †= with or without involvement of large joints.

## Influencing biological events in RA

The chief biological event is inflammation. Over-produced cytokines and cellular processes erode cartilage and bone, and produce the systemic effects seen in RA.

**Disease-modifying antirheumatic drugs** (DMARDs) are 1st-line for treating RA and should ideally be started within 3 months of persistent symptoms. They can take 6–12 weeks for symptomatic benefit. Best results are often achieved with a combination of methotrexate, sulfasalazine and hydroxychloroquine.[21] Other DMARDs include leflunomide and IM gold (now rarely used). The role of penicillamine, azathioprine and ciclosporin is less clear.

▶*Immunosuppression* is a potentially fatal SE of treatment (especially in combination with methotrexate) which can result in pancytopenia, ↑susceptibility to infection and neutropenic sepsis (p346). Regular FBC monitoring is required.[22]

*Other SE:* •Methotrexate—pneumonitis (get urgent respiratory help), oral ulcers, hepatotoxicity •Sulfasalazine—rash, ↓sperm count, oral ulcers •Leflunomide—teratogenicity (♂ and ♀), oral ulcers, ↑BP, hepatotoxicity •Hydroxychloroquine—irreversible retinopathy (request annual ophthalmology review).[23]

**Biological agents and NICE guidance:** There are 4 approaches, which should be initiated under specialist supervision:

1 *TNFα inhibitors*, eg Infliximab (p275), etanercept, adalimumab, certolizumab-pegol and golimumab. All are approved by NICE (usually in combination with methotrexate) as 1st-line biological agents for active RA after failure to respond to 2 DMARDs and with a DAS28 >5.1.[24,25,26] Where methotrexate is contraindicated, adalimumab and etanercept can be used as monotherapy. Clinical response can be striking, with improved function and health outcomes, although some patients may have inadequate or unsustained response.[24]

2 *B cell depletion*, eg Rituximab, used in combination with methotrexate and approved by NICE for severe active RA where DMARDs and a TNFα blocker have failed.[28]

3 *IL-1 and IL-6 inhibition*, eg Tocilizumab (IL-6 receptor blocker), approved by NICE in combination with methotrexate for patients where both a TNFα blocker and rituximab have failed (or are contraindicated).[29] Anakinra (IL-1 receptor inhibitor) is not recommended. Cochrane review shows less clinical improvement in comparison to other agents.[30]

4 *Disruption of T cell function*, eg Abatacept—used infrequently for patients with severe active RA who have not responded to DMARDs, a TNFα blocker or rituximab.[31]

**SEs of biological agents:** Serious infection, including reactivation of TB (∴ screen and consider prophylaxis) and hepatitis B; worsening heart failure; hypersensitivity; injection-site reactions and blood disorders. Neutralizing antibodies may ↓ efficacy with infliximab and adalimumab; ANA and reversible SLE-type illness may evolve. Long-term safety is unknown (no clear evidence for ↑ risk of cancer).

Rheumatology

Gout typically presents with an acute monoarthropathy with severe joint inflammation (fig 1). >50% occur at the metatarsophalangeal joint of the big toe (podagra). Other common joints are the ankle, foot, small joints of the hand, wrist, elbow or knee. It can be polyarticular. It is caused by deposition of monosodium urate crystals in and near joints, precipitated, for example, by trauma, surgery, starvation, infection or diuretics. It is associated with raised plasma urate. In the long term, urate deposits (= tophi, eg in pinna, tendons, joints; see fig 2) and renal disease (stones, interstitial nephritis) may occur. *Prevalence:* ~1%. ♂:♀ ≈ 4:1.

**Differential diagnoses** Exclude septic arthritis in any acute monoarthropathy (p546). Then consider haemarthrosis, CPPD (below) and palindromic RA (p548).

**Causes** Hereditary, ↑dietary purines, alcohol excess, diuretics, leukaemia, cytotoxics (tumour lysis). *Associations:* Cardiovascular disease, hypertension, diabetes mellitus and chronic renal failure (see p694).[32] Gout is a marker for these, therefore seek out and treat if needed.

**Investigations** Polarized light microscopy of synovial fluid shows *negatively birefringent* urate crystals (fig 3). Serum urate is usually raised but may be normal.[33] Radiographs show only soft-tissue swelling in the early stages. Later, well-defined 'punched out' erosions are seen in juxta-articular bone (see fig 3 on p543). There is no sclerotic reaction, and joint spaces are preserved until late.

**Treatment of acute gout**[34] Use high-dose NSAID or coxib (eg *etoricoxib* 120mg/24h PO).[35] Symptoms should subside in 3–5d. If CI (eg peptic ulcer; heart failure; anticoagulation), *colchicine* (0.5mg/6–12h PO) is effective but slower to work (note new BNF guidelines of max 6mg per course). **NB:** in renal impairment, NSAIDs and colchicine are problematic. Steroids (oral, IM or intra-articular) may also be used.[36] Rest and elevate the affected joint. Ice packs and 'bed cages' can be effective.

**Prevention** Lose weight. Avoid prolonged fasts, alcohol excess, purine-rich meats and low-dose aspirin (↑serum urate). *Prophylaxis:* Start if >1 attack in 12 months, tophi or renal stones. The aim is to ↓ attacks and prevent damage caused by crystal deposition. Use *allopurinol* and titrate from 100mg/24h, increasing every 2 weeks until plasma urate <0.3mmol/L (max 300mg/8h). SE: rash, fever, WCC↓. Introduction of allopurinol may trigger an attack so wait until 3 weeks after an acute episode, and cover with regular NSAID (for up to 6 weeks) or colchicine (0.5mg/12h PO for up to 6 months). Avoid stopping allopurinol in acute attacks once established on treatment. *Febuxostat* (80mg/24h) is an alternative if allopurinol is CI or not tolerated. It ↓ uric acid by inhibiting xanthine oxidase (SE: ↑ LFTs) and is more effective at reducing serum urate than allopurinol (although the number of acute attacks is the same).[37] Uricosuric drugs ↑ urate excretion. They are rarely used in patients who under-excrete uric acid or who are resistant to other treatment (eg sulfinpyrazine).

## Calcium pyrophosphate deposition (CPPD)

CPPD is an umbrella term used to describe different patterns of disease including:[38]
- *Acute CPP crystal arthritis* (previously **pseudogout**) like gout it causes an acute monoarthropathy typically of larger joints in elderly patients. It is usually spontaneous and self-limiting, but can be provoked by illness, surgery or trauma.
- *Chronic CPPD* inflammatory RA-like (symmetrical) polyarthritis and synovitis.
- *Osteoarthritis with CPPD* chronic polyarticular osteoarthritis with superimposed acute CPP attacks.

**Risk factors** Old age, hyperparathyroidism (see p214), haemochromatosis (see p262), hypophosphataemia (see p693).

**Tests** Polarized light microscopy of synovial fluid shows weakly positively birefringent crystals (fig 4). It is associated with soft tissue calcium deposition on x-ray.

**Management** Acute attacks: cool packs, rest, aspiration and intra-articular steroids. NSAIDs (+PPI) ± *colchicine* 0.5–1.0mg/24h (used with caution) may prevent acute attacks. Methotrexate and hydroxychloroquine have a role in chronic CPPD.[39]

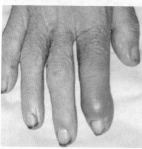

Fig 1. Acute monoarthritis in gout.

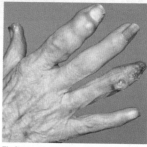

Fig 2. Ulcerated tophi in gout.

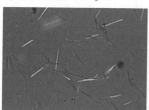

Fig 3. Needle-shaped monosodium urate crystals found in gout, displaying negative birefringence under polarized light.

Reproduced from Warrell *et al*, *Oxford Textbook of Medicine*, 2010, with permission from Oxford University Press.

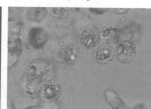

Fig 4. Rhomboid-shaped calcium pyrophosphate dihydrate crystals in Pseudogout, showing Positive birefringence in polarized light.

Image courtesy of Prof. Eliseo Pascual, Sección de Reumatología, Hospital General Universitario de Alicante.

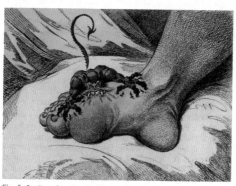

Fig 5. Don't underestimate the severity of pain caused by gout—as illustrated by satirical artist and gout sufferer James Gillray (1756–1815).

Rheumatology

**1 Ankylosing spondylitis (AS)** is a chronic inflammatory disease of the spine and sacroiliac joints, of unknown aetiology. *Prevalence:* 0.25-1%. *Men present earlier:* ♂:♀ ≈ 6:1 at 16yrs old, and ~2:1 at 30yrs old. ~90% are HLA B27 +ve (see BOX 2).

*Symptoms and signs:* The typical patient is a man <30yrs old with gradual onset of low back pain, worse at night, with spinal morning stiffness relieved by exercise. Pain radiates from sacroiliac joints to hips/buttocks, and usually improves towards the end of the day. There is progressive loss of spinal movement (all directions)—hence ↓thoracic expansion. See p542-4 for tests of spine flexion and sacroiliitis. The disease course is variable; a few progress to kyphosis, neck hyperextension (question-mark posture; fig 1), and spino-cranial ankylosis. Other features include **enthesitis** (see BOX 1), especially Achilles tendonitis, plantar fasciitis, at the tibial and ischial tuberosities, and at the iliac crests. Anterior mechanical chest pain due to costochondritis and fatigue may feature. **Acute iritis** occurs in ~⅓ of patients and may lead to blindness if untreated (but may also have occurred many years before, so enquire directly). AS is also associated with osteoporosis (up to 60%), aortic valve incompetence (<3%) and pulmonary apical fibrosis.

*Tests:* Diagnosis is clinical, supported by imaging (MRI is most sensitive and better at detecting early disease).[40] Sacroiliitis is the earliest x-ray feature, but may appear late: look for irregularities, erosions, or sclerosis affecting the lower half of the sacroiliac joints, especially the iliac side. Vertebral syndesmophytes are characteristic (often T11-L1 initially): bony proliferations due to enthesitis between ligaments and vertebrae. These fuse with the vertebral body above, causing ankylosis. In later stages, calcification of ligaments with ankylosis lead to a 'bamboo spine' appearance. *Also:* FBC (normocytic anaemia), ↑ESR, ↑CRP, HLA B27+ve (not diagnostic).

*Management:* Exercise, not rest, for backache, including intense exercise regimens to maintain posture and mobility—ideally with a physiotherapist specializing in AS. NSAIDs (eg ibuprofen or naproxen, if no CI—see p547) usually relieve symptoms within 48h, and they may slow radiographic progression.[41] TNFα blockers etanercept, adalimumab and golimumab are indicated in severe active AS if NSAIDs fail (p549).[42] Local steroid injections provide temporary relief. Surgery includes hip replacement to improve pain and mobility if the hips are involved, and rarely spinal osteotomy. There is increased risk of osteoporotic spinal fractures (consider bisphosphonates).

*Prognosis:* There is not always a clear relationship between the activity of arthritis and severity of underlying inflammation (as for all the spondyloarthritides). Prognosis is worse if ESR >30; onset <16yrs; early hip involvement or poor response to NSAIDs.[43]

**2 Enteric arthropathy** *Associations:* Inflammatory bowel disease, GI bypass, coeliac and Whipple's disease (p730). Arthropathy often improves with the treatment of bowel symptoms (beware NSAIDs). Use DMARDs for resistant cases.

**3 Psoriatic arthritis** (OHCS p594) Occurs in 10-40% with psoriasis and can present before skin changes. Patterns are: •Symmetrical polyarthritis (like RA); •DIP joints; •Asymmetrical oligoarthritis; •Spinal (similar to AS); •Psoriatic arthritis mutilans (rare, ~3%, severe deformity). *Radiology:* Erosive changes, with 'pencil-in-cup' deformity in severe cases. Nail changes in 80%, synovitis (dactylitis—see BOX 1), acneiform rashes and palmo-plantar pustulosis. *Management:* NSAIDs, sulfasalazine, methotrexate and ciclosporin. Anti-TNF agents are also effective.

**4 Reactive arthritis** A *sterile* arthritis, typically affecting the lower limb ~1-4 weeks after urethritis (p416; *Chlamydia* or *Ureaplasma* sp.), or dysentery (*Campylobacter, Salmonella, Shigella,* or *Yersinia* sp.). It may be chronic or relapsing. *Also there may be* iritis, keratoderma blennorrhagica (brown, raised plaques on soles and palms), circinate balanitis (painless penile ulceration secondary to *Chlamydia*), mouth ulcers and enthesitis. *Reiter's* syndrome[44] is a triad of urethritis, arthritis, and conjunctivitis. *Tests:* ESR & CRP↑. Culture stool if diarrhoea. Infectious serology. Sexual health review. X-ray may show enthesitis with periosteal reaction. *Management:* There is no specific cure. Splint affected joints acutely; treat with NSAIDs or local steroid injections. Consider sulfasalazine or methotrexate if symptoms >6 months. Treating the original infection may make little difference to the arthritis.

## Shared features of the spondyloarthropathies

The spondyloarthropathies show much overlap, with several features in common:
1 Seronegativity (= rheumatoid factor -ve).
2 HLA B27 association—see BOX below.
3 'Axial arthritis': pathology in spine (spondylo-) and sacroiliac joints.
4 Asymmetrical large-joint oligoarthritis (ie <5 joints) or monoarthritis.
5 Enthesitis: inflammation of the site of insertion of tendon or ligament into bone, eg plantar fasciitis, Achilles tendonitis, costochondritis.
6 Dactylitis: inflammation of an entire digit ('sausage digit'), due to soft tissue oedema, and tenosynovial and joint inflammation.
7 Extra-articular manifestations: eg iritis (anterior uveitis), psoriaform rashes, oral ulcers, aortic valve incompetence, inflammatory bowel disease.

NB Behçet's syndrome (p708) can also present with uveitis, skin lesions and arthritis and is not always associated with gross oral or genital ulcerations.

## HLA-B27 disease associations[45]

The HLA system plays a key role in immunity and self-recognition. More than one hundred HLA B27 disease associations have been made, yet the actual role of HLA B27 in triggering an inflammatory response is not fully understood. ~5% of the UK population are HLA B27 positive—most do not have any disease. The chance of an HLA B27 positive person developing spondyloarthritis or eye disease is 1 in 4. Common associations include:

*Ankylosing spondylitis:* 88% of all those with AS are HLA B27 positive.
*Acute anterior uveitis:* 50–60% are HLA B27 positive.
*Reactive arthritis:* 60–85% are HLA B27 positive.
*Enteric arthropathy:* 50–60% are HLA B27 positive.
*Psoriatic arthritis:* 60–70% are HLA B27 positive.

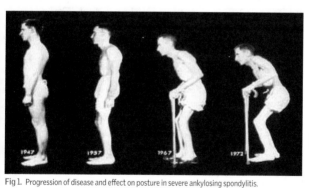

Fig 1. Progression of disease and effect on posture in severe ankylosing spondylitis.
Reproduced from *American Journal of Medicine* 1976:60:279-85 with permission from Elsevier.

*Rheumatology*

Included under this heading are SLE (p556), systemic sclerosis, primary Sjögren's syndrome (p724), idiopathic inflammatory myopathies (myositis—see below), mixed connective tissue disease, relapsing polychondritis, and Behçet's disease (p708). They overlap with each other, affect many organ systems, and often require immunosuppressive therapies (p370). Consider as a differential in unwell patients with multi-organ involvement, especially if there is no infection.

**Systemic sclerosis** features scleroderma (skin fibrosis) and vascular disease:

•*Limited cutaneous systemic sclerosis:* (formerly CREST syndrome) Calcinosis (subcutaneous tissues), Raynaud's, oesophageal and gut dysmotility, Sclerodactyly (swollen tight digits), and Telangiectasia. Skin involvement is 'limited' to the face, hands and feet. It is associated with anticentromere antibodies in 70–80%. Pulmonary hypertension is often present subclinically, and can become rapidly life-threatening, so should be looked for (℞: sildenafil, bosentan).

•*Diffuse cutaneous systemic sclerosis:* 'Diffuse' skin involvement (whole body in severe cases) and early organ fibrosis: lung, cardiac, GI and renal (p314). Antitopoisomerase-1 [Scl70] antibodies in 40% and anti-RNA polymerase in 20%. Prognosis is often poor. Control BP meticulously. Perform annual echocardiogram & spirometry.

*Management:* Currently no cure. Immunosuppressive regimens, including IV cyclophosphamide, are used for organ involvement or progressive skin disease. Trials of antifibrotic tyrosine kinase inhibitors are ongoing.[46] Monitor BP and renal function. Regular ACE-i or A2RBs ↓ risk of renal crisis (p314). *Raynaud's phenomenon:* (see p722).

**Mixed connective tissue disease** combines features of systemic sclerosis, SLE and polymyositis. Debate continues as to whether this is a distinct disease.[47, 48]

**Relapsing polychondritis** attacks cartilage, affecting the pinna (floppy ears), nasal septum, larynx (hence stridor) and joints. *Associations:* aortic valve disease, polyarthritis and vasculitis. 30% have underlying rheumatic or autoimmune disease. Diagnosis is clinical. ℞: Steroids and immunosuppressives.

## Polymyositis and dermatomyositis

These rare conditions are characterized by insidious onset of progressive symmetrical proximal muscle weakness and autoimmune-mediated *striated* muscle inflammation (myositis), associated with myalgia ± arthralgia. Muscle weakness may also cause dysphagia, dysphonia (ie poor phonation, *not* dysphasia), or respiratory weakness. The myositis (esp. in dermatomyositis) may be a paraneoplastic phenomenon, commonly from lung, pancreatic, ovarian or bowel malignancy.

**Dermatomyositis** features myositis plus skin signs: •Macular rash (*shawl sign* is +ve if over back & shoulders); •Lilac-purple (*heliotrope*) rash on eyelids often with oedema (fig 8, p565); •Nailfold erythema (*dilated capillary loops*); •*Gottron's papules:* Roughened red papules over the knuckles, also seen on elbows and knees (pathognomonic if CK↑ + muscle weakness); •Subcutaneous calcifications.

**Extra-muscular signs** in both conditions include fever, arthralgia, Raynaud's, interstitial lung fibrosis and myocardial involvement (myocarditis, arrhythmias).

**Tests** Muscle enzymes (ALT, AST, LDH, CK & aldolase) ↑ in plasma; electromyography (EMG) shows characteristic fibrillation potentials; muscle biopsy confirms the diagnosis (and excludes mimicking conditions). MRI shows muscle oedema in acute myositis. *Autoantibody associations:* anti-Mi2, anti-Jo1—associated with a syndrome of acute onset and interstitial lung fibrosis that should be treated aggressively.

**Differential diagnoses** Carcinomatous myopathy, inclusion-body myositis, muscular dystrophy, PMR, endocrine/metabolic myopathy (eg steroids), rhabdomyolysis, infection (eg HIV), drugs (penicillamine, colchicine, statins or chloroquine).

**Management** Screen systematically for malignancy. Start *prednisolone* (eg 1mg/kg/d PO). Immunosuppressives (p370) and cytotoxics are used early in resistant cases, eg azathioprine, methotrexate, cyclophosphamide or ciclosporin. Hydroxychloroquine or topical tacrolimus may help with skin disease.

## Plasma autoantibodies (Abs): disease associations

▶ Always interpret in the context of clinical findings:

*Rheumatological* Rheumatoid factor (RhF) positive in:

| | | | |
|---|---|---|---|
| Sjögren's syndrome | ≤100% | Mixed connective tissue disease | 50% |
| Felty's syndrome | ≤100% | SLE | ≤40% |
| RA | 70% | Systemic sclerosis | 30% |
| Infection (SBE/IE; hepatitis) | ≤50% | Normal | 2-10% |

Anticyclic citrullinated peptide Ab (anti-CCP):[1] Rheumatoid arthritis (~96% specificity)

Antinuclear antibody (ANA) positive by immunofluorescence in:

| | | | |
|---|---|---|---|
| SLE | >95% | Systemic sclerosis | 96% |
| Autoimmune hepatitis | 75% | RA | 30% |
| Sjögren's syndrome | 68% | Normal | 0-2% |

ANA titres are expressed according to dilutions at which antibodies can be detected, ie 1:160 means antibodies can still be detected after the serum has been diluted 160 times. Titres of 1:40 or 1:80 may not be significant. The pattern of staining may indicate the disease (although these are not specific):

- *Homogeneous* SLE
- *Speckled* Mixed CT disease
- *Nucleolar* Systemic sclerosis
- *Centromere* Limited systemic sclerosis

Anti-double-stranded DNA (dsDNA): SLE (60% sensitivity, but highly specific).

Antihistone Ab: Drug-induced SLE (~100%).

Antiphospholipid Ab (eg anti-cardiolipin Ab): antiphospholipid syndrome, SLE.

Anticentromere Ab: limited systemic sclerosis.

Anti-extractable nuclear antigen (ENA) antibodies (usually with +ve ANA):

- Anti-Ro (SSA) — SLE, Sjögren's syndrome, systemic sclerosis. Associated with congenital heart block.
- Anti-La (SSB) — Sjögren's syndrome, SLE (15%).
- Anti-Sm — SLE (20-30%).
- Anti-RNP — SLE, mixed connective tissue disease.
- Anti Jo-1; Anti-Mi-2 — Polymyositis, dermatomyositis.
- Anti-Scl70 — Diffuse systemic sclerosis.

*Gastrointestinal* (for liver autoantibodies, see p268).

Antimitochondrial Ab (AMA): Primary biliary cirrhosis (>95%), autoimmune hepatitis (30%), idiopathic cirrhosis (25-30%).

Anti-smooth muscle Ab (SMA): Autoimmune hepatitis (70%), primary biliary cirrhosis (50%), idiopathic cirrhosis (25-30%).

Gastric parietal cell Ab: Pernicious anaemia (>90%), atrophic gastritis (40%), 'normal' (10%).

Intrinsic factor Ab: Pernicious anaemia (50%).

α-gliadin Ab, antitissue transglutaminase, anti-endomysial Ab: Coeliac disease.

*Endocrine* Thyroid peroxidase Ab: Hashimoto's thyroiditis (~87%), Graves' (>50%). Islet cell Ab (ICA), glutamic acid decarboxylase (GAD) Ab: Type 1 diabetes mellitus (75%).

*Renal* Glomerular basement membrane Ab (anti-GBM): Goodpasture's disease (100%). Antineutrophil cytoplasmic Ab (ANCA):

- Cytoplasmic (c-ANCA), specific for serine proteinase-3 (PR3 +ve). Granulomatosis with polyangiitis (Wegener's•) (90%); also microscopic polyangiitis (30%), polyarteritis nodosa (11%).
- Perinuclear (p-ANCA), specific for myeloperoxidase (MPO +ve). Microscopic polyangiitis (45%), Churg-Strauss, some pulmonary-renal vasculitides (Goodpasture's syndrome).

Unlike immune-complex vasculitis, in ANCA-associated vasculitis no complement consumption or immune complex deposition occurs (ie pauci-immune vasculitis).[49]

ANCA may also be +ve in UC/Crohn's, sclerosing cholangitis, autoimmune hepatitis, Felty's, RA, SLE, or drugs (eg antithyroid, allopurinol, ciprofloxacin).

*Neurological* Acetylcholine receptor Ab: Myasthenia gravis (90%)(see p516).

Anti-voltage-gated K⁺-channel Ab: Limbic encephalitis.

Anti-voltage-gated $Ca^{2+}$-channel Ab: Lambert-Eaton syndrome (see p516).

Anti-aquaporin 4: Neuromyelitis optica (Devic's disease, p712).

---

1 Most centres now use anti-CCP antibodies for the initial workup of suspected RA.

Rheumatology

SLE is a multisystemic autoimmune disease in which autoantibodies are made against a variety of autoantigens (eg ANA). Immunopathology results in polyclonal B-cell secretion of pathogenic autoantibodies causing tissue damage via multiple mechanisms including immune complex formation and deposition, complement activation and other direct effects. *Prevalence:* ~0.2%. ♀:♂≈9:1, typically women of child-bearing age. Commoner in African-Caribbeans, Asians, and if HLA B8, DR2 or DR3 +ve. ~10% of relatives may be affected. It may be triggered by EBV (p401).[50]

**Clinical features** It is a remitting and relapsing illness of variable presentation and course, typically presenting with non-specific constitutional symptoms of malaise, fatigue, myalgia and fever. See BOX opposite for specific features. Other features include lymphadenopathy, weight loss, alopecia, nail-fold infarcts, non-infective endocarditis (Libman-Sacks syndrome), Raynaud's (30%; see p722), migraine (40%), stroke, and retinal exudates.

**Immunology** >95% are ANA +ve. A high anti-double-stranded DNA (dsDNA) antibody titre is highly specific, but only +ve in ~60% of cases. ENA (p555) may be +ve in 20-30% (anti-Ro, anti-La, anti-Sm, anti-RNP); 40% are RhF +ve; antiphospholipid antibodies (anticardiolipin or lupus anticoagulant) may also be +ve. SLE may be associated with other autoimmune conditions: Sjögren's (15-20%), autoimmune thyroid disease (5-10%).

**Diagnosis** see BOX. *Monitoring activity 3 best tests:* 1 Anti-dsDNA antibody titres. 2 Complement: C3↓, C4↓ (denotes consumption of complement, hence C3 and C4↓, and C3d and C4d↑, their degradation products). 3 ESR. *Also:* BP, urine for casts or protein (lupus nephritis, below), FBC, U&E, LFTs, CRP (usually normal) ►*think of SLE whenever someone has a multisystem disorder and ↑ESR but CRP normal.* If ↑CRP, think instead of infection, serositis or arthritis. Skin or renal biopsies may be diagnostic.

**Drug-induced lupus** Causes (>50 drugs) include isoniazid, hydralazine (if >50mg/24h in slow acetylators), procainamide, quinidine, chlorpromazine, minocycline, phenytoin. It is associated with antihistone antibodies in ~100%. Skin and lung signs prevail (renal and CNS are rarely affected). The disease remits if the drug is stopped. Sulfonamides or the oral contraceptive pill may worsen idiopathic SLE.

**Management** should be through specialist SLE and lupus nephritis clinics.
- ►►*Severe flares:* Acute SLE (eg haemolytic anaemia, nephritis, severe pericarditis or CNS disease) requires urgent IV **cyclophosphamide + high-dose prednisolone.**
- *Cutaneous symptoms:* treat rashes with topical steroids. Prevent rashes with high-factor sunblock creams. Sun exposure may also trigger acute systemic flares.
- *Maintenance:* use NSAIDs and **hydroxychloroquine** (see p549 for SE) for joint and skin symptoms. *Low-dose steroids* may be of value in chronic disease. Azathioprine, methotrexate and mycophenolate are used as steroid-sparing agents.
- *Lupus nephritis:* (p314) May require more intensive immunosuppression with steroids and **cyclophosphamide** or **mycophenolate.** NB: immunosuppressed patients are prone to infection (especially atypicals). BP control is vital: ACE-i, α-blockers (eg doxazosin) or Ca²⁺-channel blockers (eg nifedipine). Renal replacement therapy (p298) may be needed if disease progresses; nephritis recurs in ~50% post-transplant, but is a rare cause of graft failure.[51]
- *B-cell depletion:* Trials of rituximab (p356) have been disappointing.[52] Belimumab has shown significant clinical benefit and is licensed in the US.[53] Trials with epratuzumab are ongoing.[54]
- *Future treatments:* Interferon-α, interleukin-6 inhibition,[55] and T-cell targets are currently being evaluated.

**Prognosis** is ~80% survival at 15 years.[50] There is an increased long-term risk of cardiovascular disease and osteoporosis.

**Antiphospholipid syndrome** can be associated with SLE (20-30%). More often it occurs as a primary disease. Antiphospholipid antibodies (anticardiolipin & lupus anticoagulant) cause CLOTS: Coagulation defect, Livedo reticularis (p559), Obstetric (recurrent miscarriage), Thrombocytopenia (↓platelets). There is a thrombotic tendency, affecting the cerebral, renal and other vessels. ℞: Low-dose aspirin, or warfarin if recurrent thromboses (aim INR of 2-3).[56] Seek advice in pregnancy.

## Revised criteria (serial or simultaneous) for diagnosing SLE[57, 58]

A favourite differential diagnosis, SLE mimics other illnesses, with wide variation in symptoms that may come and go unpredictably. Diagnose SLE in an appropriate clinical setting if ≥4 out of 11 criteria are present:

1 *Malar rash (butterfly rash):* Fixed erythema, flat or raised, over the malar eminences, tending to spare the nasolabial folds (fig 1). Occurs in up to 50%.

2 *Discoidrash:* Erythematous raised patches with adherent keratotic scales and follicular plugging ± atrophic scarring (fig 2). Think of it as a 3-stage rash affecting ears, cheeks, scalp, forehead, and chest: erythema→pigmented hyperkeratotic oedematous papules→atrophic depressed lesions.

3 *Photosensitivity:* On exposed skin representing unusual reaction to light. Exposure to sun may also cause disease to flare, so sunblocks are advised.

4 *Oral ulcers:* Oral or nasopharyngeal ulceration, usually painless.

5 *Non-erosive arthritis:* Involving ≥2 peripheral joints (tenderness, swelling, or effusion). Joint involvement is seen in 90% of patients, and may present similarly to RA. A reversible deforming arthropathy may occur due to capsular laxity (Jaccoud's arthropathy). Aseptic bone necrosis may also occur.

6 *Serositis:* (a) **Pleuritis** (presents as pleuritic pain or dyspnoea due to pleural effusion—80% have lung function abnormalities) OR (b) **Pericarditis** (chest pain, ECG, pericardial rub or signs of pericardial effusion).

7 *Renal disorder:* (a) **Persistent proteinuria** >0.5g/d (or >3+ on urinalysis) OR (b) **Cellular casts**—may be red cell, granular, or mixed. See p314.

8 *CNS disorder:* (a) **Seizures**, in the absence of causative drugs or metabolic imbalance, eg uraemia, ketoacidosis, or electrolyte imbalance, OR (b) **Psychosis** in the absence of causative drugs/metabolic derangements, as above.

9 *Haematological disorder:* (a) **Haemolytic anaemia** with reticulocytosis (p330), OR (b) **Leukopenia** <4×10⁹/L on ≥2 occasions, OR (c) **Lymphopenia** <1.5 × 10⁹/L on ≥2 occasions, OR (d) **Thrombocytopenia** <100×10⁹/L, in the absence of a drug effect.

10 *Immunological disorder:* Presence of (a) **Anti-dsDNA** antibody, (b) **Anti-Sm** antibody, OR (c) **Antiphospholipid** antibody +ve based on:
   • An abnormal serum level of IgG or IgM anticardiolipin antibodies,
   • Positive result for lupus anticoagulant using a standard method, or
   • False +ve syphilis serology: If +ve for >6 months and confirmed by -ve *Treponema pallidum* immobilization and fluorescent treponemal antibody absorption tests.[42] (The phospholipid reagents used to test for syphilis can cause false positive results in patients with antiphospholipid antibodies.)

11 *Antinuclear antibody (ANA):* +ve in >95%.

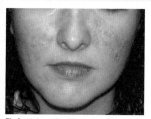

**Fig 1.** Malar rash, with sparing of the nasolabial folds.

Courtesy of David F Fiorentino, MD, PhD; by kind permission of *Skin & Aging*.

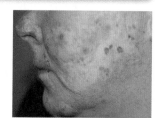

**Fig 2.** Discoid rash.

Courtesy of Amy McMichael, MD; by kind permission of *Skin & Aging*.

Vasculitis is defined as an inflammatory disorder of blood vessel walls, causing destruction (aneurysm/rupture) or stenosis. It can affect the vessels of any organ, and presentation depends on which organs are involved. It may be a primary condition or secondary to other diseases, eg SLE, RA, hepatitis B & C, HIV. It is categorized according to the main size of blood vessel affected:

- *Large:* Giant cell arteritis, Takayasu's arteritis (see p726).
- *Medium:* Polyarteritis nodosa, Kawasaki disease (OHCS p646).
- *Small:* • ANCA +ve vasculitis has a predilection for respiratory tract and kidneys. It includes p-ANCA associated microscopic polyangiitis, glomerulonephritis and Churg-Strauss syndrome (p710) and c-ANCA associated Wegener's granulomatosis (p728).
- ANCA –ve vasculitis includes Henoch-Schönlein purpura (p716), Goodpasture's syndrome (p714) and cryoglobulinaemia.

*Symptoms:* Different vasculitides preferentially affect different organs, causing different patterns of symptoms (see BOX 1), but the presentation may often be of only overwhelming fatigue with ↑ESR/CRP. ▶▶*Consider vasculitis in any unidentified multisystem disorder.* If presentation does not fit clinically or serologically into a specific category consider malignancy-associated vasculitis. A severe vasculitis flare is a medical emergency. If suspected, seek urgent help, as organ damage may occur rapidly (eg critical renal failure <24h).

*Tests:* ESR/CRP↑. ANCA may be +ve. ↑Creatinine if renal failure. Urine: proteinuria, haematuria, casts on microscopy. Angiography ± biopsy may be diagnostic.

*Management:* Large-vessel vasculitis: steroids in most cases. Medium/small: standard therapy is steroids and IV *cyclophosphamide* (15mg/kg).[59] Azathioprine may be useful as steroid-sparing maintenance treatment.

## Giant cell arteritis (GCA)[60] = cranial or temporal arteritis

It is common in the elderly—consider Takayasu's if under 55yrs (p726). It is associated with PMR in 50% (see BOX 2). *Symptoms:* Headache, temporal artery and scalp tenderness (eg when combing hair), jaw claudication, amaurosis fugax, or sudden blindness, typically in one eye. Extracranial symptoms may include dyspnoea, morning stiffness, and unequal or weak pulses.[61] ▶▶If you suspect GCA, do ESR and start *prednisolone* 60mg/d PO *immediately*. The risk is irreversible bilateral visual loss, which can occur suddenly if not treated (some advocate IV methylprednisolone for 3d if visual symptoms—ask an ophthalmologist). *Tests:* ESR & CRP↑↑, platelets↑, alk phos↑, Hb↓. Get a temporal artery biopsy within 7 days of starting steroids. Skip lesions occur, so don't be put off by a negative biopsy (up to 10%). *Prognosis:* Typically a 2-year course, then complete remission. Reduce prednisolone once symptoms have resolved and ↓ESR; ↑dose if symptoms recur. The main cause of death and morbidity in GCA is long-term steroid treatment so consider risks and benefits! Give gastric and bone protection (PPI & bisphosphonate).

## Polyarteritis nodosa (PAN)

PAN is a necrotizing vasculitis that causes aneurysms and thrombosis in medium-sized arteries, leading to infarction in affected organs (fig 2), with severe systemic symptoms. ♂:♀≈2:1. It may be associated with hepatitis B, and is rare in the UK. *Symptoms:* Typically systemic features, plus predominantly skin (rash and 'punched out' ulcers), renal (main cause of death, though glomerulonephritis is not seen), cardiac, GI and GU involvement. See BOX. Coronary aneurysms occur in Kawasaki disease (childhood PAN variant, OHCS p646). *Tests:* Often WCC↑, mild eosinophilia (in 30%), anaemia, ESR↑, CRP↑, ANCA –ve. Renal or mesenteric angiography, or renal biopsy can be diagnostic. *Treatment:* Control BP meticulously. Refer to experts. Most respond to corticosteroids and cyclophosphamide. Hepatitis B should be treated with an antiviral (p407) after initial treatment with steroids.[62]

## Microscopic polyangiitis

A necrotizing vasculitis affecting small- and medium-sized vessels. *Symptoms:* Rapidly progressive glomerulonephritis usually features; pulmonary haemorrhage occurs in up to 30%; other features are rare. *Tests:* pANCA (MPO) +ve (p555). *Treatment:* As for PAN.

## Features of vasculitis

The presentation of vasculitis will depend on the organs affected:

*Systemic:* fever, malaise, weight loss, arthralgia, myalgia.
*Skin:* purpura, ulcers, livedo reticularis (fig 1), nailbed infarcts, digital gangrene.
*Eyes:* episcleritis, scleritis, visual loss.
*ENT:* epistaxis, nasal crusting, stridor, deafness.
*Pulmonary:* haemoptysis and dyspnoea (due to pulmonary haemorrhage).
*Cardiac:* Angina or MI (due to coronary arteritis), heart failure and pericarditis.
*GI:* Pain or perforation (infarcted viscus), malabsorption (chronic ischaemia).
*Renal:* Hypertension, haematuria, proteinuria, casts, and renal failure (renal cortical infarcts; glomerulonephritis in ANCA +ve vasculitis).
*Neurological:* Stroke, fits, chorea, psychosis, confusion, impaired cognition, altered mood. Arteritis of the vasa nervorum (arterial supply to peripheral nerves) may cause mononeuritis multiplex or a sensorimotor polyneuropathy.[63]
*GU:* Orchitis—testicular pain or tenderness.

## Polymyalgia rheumatica (PMR) [64]

PMR is not a true vasculitis and its pathogenesis is unknown. PMR and GCA share the same demographic characteristics and, although separate conditions, the two frequently occur together.

*Features:* Age >50yrs; subacute onset (<2 weeks) of bilateral aching, tenderness and morning stiffness in shoulders and proximal limb muscles ± mild polyarthritis, tenosynovitis, and carpal tunnel syndrome (10%). Weakness is not a feature. There may be associated fatigue, fever, weight↓, anorexia and depression.

*Investigations:* CRP ↑, ESR typically >40 (but may be normal); ALP is ↑ in 30%. Note creatinine kinase levels are normal (helping to distinguish from myositis/myopathies).

*Differential diagnoses:* Recent onset RA, polymyositis, hypothyroidism, primary muscle disease, occult malignancy or infection, osteoarthritis (especially cervical spondylosis, shoulder OA), neck lesions, bilateral subacromial impingement (OHCS p664), spinal stenosis (OHCS p674).

*Management: Prednisolone* 15mg/d PO. Expect a dramatic response within 1 week and consider an alternative diagnosis if not. ↓dose slowly, eg by 1mg/month (according to symptoms and ESR). Investigate apparent 'flares' during withdrawal—recurrent symptoms may be attributable to another condition (above). Most need steroids for ≥2yrs, so give gastric and bone protection. NSAIDs are not effective and trials with steroid-sparing agents have been inconsistent. Inform patients to seek urgent review if symptoms of GCA develop.

Rheumatology

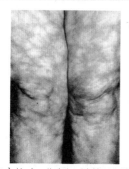

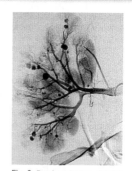

Fig 1. Livedo reticularis: pink-blue mottling caused by capillary dilatation and stasis in skin venules. Causes: physiological, eg cold, or vasculitis.

Fig 2. Renal angiogram showing multiple aneurysms in PAN.
Courtesy of Dr William Herring.

Rheumatology

Fibromyalgia and chronic fatigue syndrome are part of a diffuse group of overlapping syndromes, sharing similar demographic and clinical characteristics, in which chronic symptoms of fatigue and widespread pain feature prominently. Their existence as discrete entities is controversial, especially in the absence of clear pathology, and some find such dysfunctional diagnoses frustrating. However, a correct diagnosis enables the doctor to give appropriate counselling and advise appropriate therapies, and allows the patient to begin to accept and deal with their symptoms.

## Fibromyalgia

Fibromyalgia comprises up to 10% of new referrals to the rheumatology clinic.[65] *Prevalence:* 0.5-4%. ♀:♂≈10:1. *Risk factors:* BOX. Also female sex, middle age, low household income, divorced, low educational status. *Associations:* Other somatic syndromes such as chronic fatigue syndrome, irritable bowel syndrome (p276) and chronic headaches syndromes (see *OHCS* p528). Also found in ~25% of patients with RA, AS and SLE.

*Features:* Diagnosis depends on pain that is *chronic* (>3months) and widespread (involves left and right sides, above and below the waist, and the axial skeleton) in the absence of inflammation; and the presence of pain on palpation of at least 11/18 'tender points'—left- and right-sided: •Suboccipital muscle insertions; •Anterior aspects of the inter-transverse spaces at C5-C7; •Midpoint of the upper border of trapezius; •Origin of supraspinatus near the medial border of the scapular spine; •Costochondral junction of 2nd rib; •2cm distal from lateral humeral epicondyle; •Upper outer gluteal quadrant; •Posterior to the greater trochanter; •Knee, at medial fat pad proximal to joint line. Patients may have more tender points than those listed, but these are the most consistent and helpful diagnostically.[66] Healthy individuals may also have tender points, but it is their widespread and severe nature that indicates fibromyalgia. *Additional features:* morning stiffness (~80-90%), fatigue (~80-90%, often severe), poor concentration, low mood and sleep disturbance (~70%).

*Investigations:* are all normal. Over-investigation can consolidate illness behaviour; however, other causes of pain and/or fatigue must be excluded (eg RA, PMR see p559, vasculitis see p558, hypothyroidism see p212, myeloma see p362).

*R℞:* The manner in which management is discussed is almost as important as the management itself, which should focus on **education** of the patient *and their family* and on developing coping strategies. Such a diagnosis may be a relief or a disappointment to the patient. *Explain* that fibromyalgia is a relapsing and remitting condition, with no easy cures, and that they will continue to have good and bad days. *Reassure* them that there is no serious underlying pathology, that their joints are not being damaged, and that no further tests are necessary, but be sympathetic to the fact that they may have been seeking a physical cause for their symptoms. Discuss psychosocial issues (see BOX). Cognitive-behavioural therapy (CBT) aims to help patients develop coping strategies and set achievable goals.[67] Pacing of activity is vital to avoid over-exertion and consequent pain and fatigue. Long-term graded exercise programmes improve functional capacity.[68,69] *Pharmacotherapy:* Pain in fibromyalgia rarely responds to NSAIDs and steroids as there is no inflammation (if it does respond, reconsider your diagnosis!). Low-dose tricyclic antidepressants (eg *amitriptyline* 10-20mg at night) and *pregabalin* (150-300mg/12h PO) may improve pain (especially combined with tramadol), sleep and morning stiffness, but effects may not be apparent for up to a month.[70,71] High-dose SNRIs, eg venlafaxine, may also be effective (unlicensed use). SSRIs appear to be less useful.

## Chronic fatigue syndrome (aka myalgic encephalomyelitis)[72]

Chronic fatigue syndrome is defined as persistent disabling fatigue lasting >6 months, affecting mental and physical function, present >50% of the time, plus ≥4 of: myalgia (~80%), polyarthralgia, ↓ memory, unrefreshing sleep, fatigue after exertion >24h, persistent sore throat, tender cervical/axillary lymph nodes. Management principles are similar to fibromyalgia above and include graded exercise and CBT. No pharmacological agents have yet been proved effective for chronic fatigue syndrome (see also *OHCS* p528).

## Yellow flags[73]

☼ Psychosocial risk factors for developing persisting chronic pain and long-term disability have been termed 'yellow flags'. These include:

► Belief that pain and activity are harmful.
► Sickness behaviours such as extended rest.
► Social withdrawal.
► Emotional problems such as low mood, anxiety or stress.
► Problems or dissatisfaction at work.
► Problems with claims for compensation or time off work.
► Overprotective family or lack of support.
► Inappropriate expectations of treatment, eg low active participation in treatment.

Rheumatology

### ☼ An existential approach to difficult symptoms

We all at some stage come across a patient with difficult symptoms and an ex-asperating lack of pathology to explain them. Investigations are all normal, and medications do not seem to work. It is tempting to dismiss such patients as malin-gerers, but often this conclusion comes from the clinician approaching the problem from the wrong angle. The patient has symptoms that are real and disabling to them, and that will not improve without help. Perhaps a more pragmatic approach is to take advice from the Danish philosopher Kierkegaard who wrote to a friend in 1835, *'What I really lack is to be clear in my mind what I am to do, not what I am to know ... The thing is to understand myself ... to find a truth which is true for me.'* Listen to the patient and accept their story. Then help them to focus on what they can *do* to improve their situation, and to move away from dwelling on finding a physical answer to their symptoms.

### ☼ Is fibromyalgia a real disease?

The current hypothesis is that fibromyalgia is caused by aberrant peripheral and central pain processing. Two key features of the condition are *allodynia* (pain in response to a non-painful stimulus) and *hyperaesthesia* (exaggerated perception of pain in response to a mildly painful stimulus), examined for by palpation of tender points. Research is beginning to suggest that certain antidepressants can relieve pain and other symptoms, and especially those that have both serotonergic and noradrenergic activity (tricyclics and venlafaxine). Those acting on serotonergic receptors only are less effective. There is also some evidence to support the use of alternative therapies such as acupuncture and spa therapies, which have been postulated to act through similar spinal pain-modulatory pathways.[74] Thus far, trials have involved relatively small numbers of patients or short time periods, and lack the power to draw strong conclusions. However, it is interesting to note that the CSF of patients with fibromyalgia appears to have increased levels of substance P, while levels of noradrenaline and serotonin metabolites are decreased. All three are neurotransmitters involved in descending pain-modulatory pathways in the spinal cord.[75,76] Evidence from PET imaging suggests that patients with fibromyalgia may have an abnormal central dopamine response to pain.[77] The critical question is: Is this cause or effect?

*The eye is host to many diseases: the more you look, the more you'll see, and the more you'll enjoy, not least because the eye is as beautiful as its signs are legion.*

**Granulomatous disorders** Syphilis, TB, sarcoidosis, leprosy, brucellosis, and toxoplasmosis may inflame either the front chamber (anterior uveitis/iritis) or back chamber (posterior uveitis/choroiditis). Refer to an ophthalmologist.

**Systemic inflammatory diseases** may manifest as iritis in ankylosing spondylitis and Reiter's•; *conjunctivitis* in Reiter's; *scleritis* or *episcleritis* in RA, vasculitis and SLE. Scleritis in RA and Wegener's• may damage the eye. Refer urgently if eye pain. Giant cell arteritis causes optic nerve ischaemia presenting as sudden blindness.

**Keratoconjunctivitis sicca** is a reduction in tear formation, tested by the Schirmer filter paper test (<5mm in 5min). It causes a gritty feeling in the eyes, and a dry mouth (xerostomia from ↓ saliva production). It is found on its own (Sjögren's syndrome), or with other diseases, eg SLE, RA, sarcoidosis. ℞: artificial tears/saliva (eg Tears Naturale®, hypromellose drops, Saliveze® oral spray).

**Hypertensive retinopathy** ↑BP accelerates atherosclerosis in retinal vessels. Hardened arteries are shiny ('silver wiring'; fig 1) and 'nip' veins where they cross (AV nipping; fig 2). Narrowed arterioles may become blocked, causing localized retinal infarction, seen as cotton-wool spots. Leaks from these in severe hypertension manifest as hard exudates or macular oedema. Papilloedema (fig 3) or flame haemorrhages suggest accelerated hypertension (p132) requiring urgent treatment.

**Vascular occlusion** *Emboli* passing through the retinal vasculature may cause *retinal artery occlusion* (global or segmental retinal pallor) or *amaurosis fugax* (p480). Roth spots (small retinal infarcts, fig 1 on p386) occur in infective endocarditis. In dermatomyositis, there is orbital oedema with retinopathy showing cotton-wool spots (micro-infarcts). *Retinal vein occlusion* is caused by ↑BP, age, or hyperviscosity (p366). Suspect in any acute fall in acuity. If it is the central vein, the fundus is like a stormy sunset (those angry red clouds are haemorrhages). In branch vein occlusion, changes are confined to a wedge of retina. Get expert help.

**Haematological disorders** *Retinal haemorrhages* occur in leukaemia; commashaped *conjunctival haemorrhages* and retinal new vessel formation may occur in sickle-cell disease. *Optic atrophy* is seen in pernicious anaemia (and also MS).

**Metabolic disease** Diabetes mellitus: p202. Hyperthyroid exophthalmos: p211. Lens opacities are seen in hypoparathyroidism. Conjunctival and corneal calcification can occur in hypercalcaemia. In gout, conjunctival urate deposits may cause sore eyes.

**Systemic infections** Septicaemia may seed to the vitreous causing endophthalmitis. Syphilis can cause iritis (+ pigmented retinopathy if congenital). Systemic fungal infections may affect the eye, eg in the immunocompromised or in IV drug users, requiring intra-vitreal antibiotics. **AIDS and HIV:** CMV retinitis (pizza-pie fundus—a mixture of cotton-wool spots, infiltrates and haemorrhages, p405) may be asymptomatic but can cause sudden visual loss. If present, it implies AIDS (CD4 count <100 × 10⁶/L; p410). Cotton-wool spots on their own indicate HIV retinopathy and may occur in early disease. Kaposi's sarcoma may affect the lids (non-tender purple nodule) or conjunctiva (red fleshy mass).

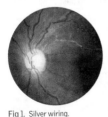

Fig 1. Silver wiring.   Fig 2. AV nipping.   Fig 3. Papilloedema.

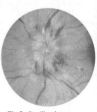

Figs 1-3 ©Prof Jonathan Trobe.

## Differential diagnosis of a red eye

| | Symptoms | Visual acuity | Cornea | Pupil | Other features |
|---|---|---|---|---|---|
| Acute angle closure glaucoma | severe ache, haloes, vomiting | ↓↓ | hazy | unreactive, semi-dilated | Typically hypermetropic (long sighted), elderly &/or East Asian |
| Bacterial corneal ulcer | sharp pain, photophobia | normal or ↓ | white spot, stains with fluorescein | normal | Often contact lens wearers. May have purulent discharge |
| Acute anterior uveitis (iritis) | sharp pain, photophobia | normal or ↓ | normal or hazy | normal - or unreactive, irregular & small | Typically young/ middle aged. Often recurrent. May be associated with ankylosing spondylitis, IBD, JIA, psoriatic arthritis, Reiters, sarcoid |
| Scleritis | severe ache (may wake patient at night) | usually normal | normal | normal | Often bilateral. Eyeball tender to touch Often associated with rheumatoid arthritis, sarcoid, lupus, Wegeners |
| Conjunctivitis | gritty or sticky | normal | normal | normal | Usually bilateral Discharge: purulent (bacterial); watery (viral); mucoid (allergic) |

With thanks to Dr Jim McHugh for contributing this table.

**Rheumatology**

**Erythema nodosum** (fig 1) Painful, blue-red, raised lesions on shins (± thighs/arms). *Causes:* sarcoidosis, drugs (sulfonamides, the Pill, dapsone), streptococcal infection. *Less common:* Crohn's/UC, BCG vaccination, leptospirosis, *Mycobacterium* (TB, leprosy), *Yersinia* or various viruses and fungi. Cause unknown in 30–50%.

**Erythema multiforme** (see *OHCS* p588) (fig 3) 'Target' lesions: symmetrical ± central blister, on palms/soles, limbs, and elsewhere. *Stevens-Johnson syndrome* (p724): a rare, severe variant with fever and mucosal involvement (mouth, genital, and eye ulcers), associated with a hypersensitivity reaction to drugs (NSAIDs, sulfonamides, anti-convulsants, allopurinol) or infections (herpes, *Mycoplasma*, orf—). Also seen in collagen disorders. 50% of cases are idiopathic. Get expert help in severe disease.

**Erythema migrans** (fig 7) Presents as a small papule at the site of a tick bite which develops into a spreading large erythematous ring, with central fading. It lasts from 48h to 3 months and there may be multiple lesions in disseminated disease. *Cause:* The rash is pathognomonic of Lyme disease and occurs in ~80% of cases (p430).

**Erythema marginatum** Pink coalescent rings on trunk which come and go. It is seen in rheumatic fever (or rarely other causes, eg drugs). See fig 1, p137.

**Pyoderma gangrenosum** (fig 2) Recurring nodulo-pustular ulcers, ~10cm wide, with tender red/blue overhanging necrotic edge, purulent surface, and healing with cribriform scars on leg, abdomen, or face. *Associations:* UC/Crohn's, autoimmune hepatitis, Wegener's•, myeloma, neoplasia. ♀>♂. *Treatment:* Get help. Oral steroids ± ciclosporin should be 1st-line therapy.[78]

**Vitiligo** (fig 4) *Vitellus* is Latin for *spotted calf:* typically white patches ± hyperpigmented borders. Sunlight makes them itch. *Associations:* autoimmune disorders; premature ovarian failure. Treat by camouflage cosmetics and sunscreens (± steroid creams ± dermabrasion). UK Vitiligo Society: 0800 018 2631.

## Specific diseases and their skin manifestations

**Crohn's** Perianal/vulval/oral ulcers; erythema nodosum; pyoderma gangrenosum.

**Dermatomyositis** Gottron's papules (rough red papules on the knuckles/extensor surfaces); shawl sign; heliotrope rash on eyelids (fig 8). It may be associated with lung, bowel, ovarian or pancreatic malignancy (p554).

**Diabetes mellitus** Ulcers, *necrobiosis lipoidica* (shiny yellowish area on shin ± telangiectasia; fig 5), *granuloma annulare* (*OHCS* p586), *acanthosis nigricans* (pigmented, rough thickening of axillary, neck or groin skin with warty lesions; fig 6).

**Gluten-sensitive enteropathy (coeliac disease)** *Dermatitis herpetiformis*—itchy blisters, in groups on knees, elbows, and scalp. The itch (which can drive patients to suicide) responds to *dapsone* 25–200mg/24h PO within 48h—and this may be used as a diagnostic test. The maintenance dose may be as little as 50mg/wk. A gluten-free diet should be adhered to, but in 30% dapsone will need to be continued. SE (dose-related): haemolysis (CI: anaemia, G6PD-deficiency), hepatitis, agranulocytosis (monitor FBC and LFTs). There is a ↑ risk of small bowel lymphoma with coeliac disease *and* dermatitis herpetiformis—so surveillance is needed.

**Hyperthyroidism** *Pretibial myxoedema*—red oedematous swellings above lateral malleoli, progressing to thickened oedema of legs and feet, *thyroid acropachy*—clubbing + subperiosteal new bone in phalanges. *Other endocrinopathies:* p197.

**Liver disease** Palmar erythema; spider naevi; gynaecomastia; decrease in pubic hair; jaundice; bruising; scratch marks.

**Malabsorption** Dry pigmented skin, easy bruising, hair loss, leuconychia.

**Neoplasia** *Acanthosis nigricans:* (see above under diabetes and fig 6) associated with gastric cancer. *Dermatomyositis*—see above. *Thrombophlebitis migrans:* Successive crops of tender nodules affecting blood vessels throughout the body, associated with pancreatic cancer (especially body and tail). Acquired ichthyosis: Dry scaly skin associated with lymphoma. *Skin metastases:* Especially melanoma, and colonic, lung, breast, laryngeal/oral, or ovarian malignancy.

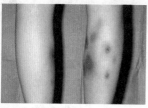

Fig 1. Erythema nodosum.

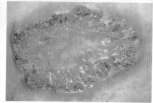

Fig 2. Pyoderma gangrenosum.

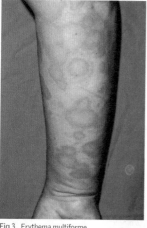

Fig 3. Erythema multiforme.

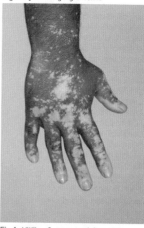

Fig 4. Vitiligo. Compare with fig 1, p429.

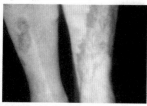

Fig 5. Necrobiosis lipoidica.

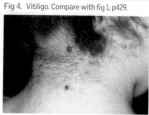

Fig 6. Acanthosis nigricans.

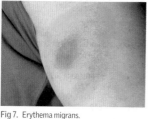

Fig 7. Erythema migrans.

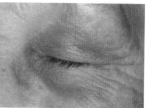

Fig 8. Heliotrope rash.

Fig 2 Reproduced from *BMJ* 2006; 333:181, with permission from BMJ Publishing Ltd; Fig 5 reproduced from Warrel *et al*, *Oxford Textbook of Medicine*, 2010, with permission from Oxford University Press; Fig 6 reproduced from Lewis-Jones, *Oxford Specialist Handbook of Paediatric Dermatology*, 2010, with permission from Oxford University Press; Fig 7 courtesy of CDC/James Gathany; Fig 8 courtesy of Nick Taylor, East Sussex Hospitals Trust.

**Contents**
Language of surgery 567

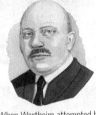

Fig 1. When Wertheim attempted his radical hysterectomy for cervical cancer, the first dozen women died. Undeterred, he continued. Thousands of women owe their lives to his skill—and to the sacrifice of those 12 dead women (see p595 for more).

*See also in other chapters:* Gastroenterology (p234), Radiology (p732), UTI (p288); haematuria (p286); prostatism (p65); gynaecological urology (*OHCS* p306); IV fluids (p680).

We thank our Specialist Readers for this chapter: Mr Mohamed Elkalaawy (General and GI surgery); Professor Thomas Lennard (Breast and endocrine surgery); Mr David Chadwick (Urology); Mr George Peach (Vascular surgery); Mr Graham Cox (Head and neck surgery); Mr Mark Malak (Urogynaecology). We also thank our Junior Reader, Eleanor Zimmermann.

## The language of surgery

1 Right upper quadrant (RUQ) or hypochondrium
2 Epigastrium
3 Left upper quadrant (LUQ) or hypochondrium
4 Right flank (merges posteriorly with right loin, p57)
5 Periumbilical or central area
6 Left flank (merges posteriorly with left loin, p57)
7 Right iliac fossa (RIF)
8 Suprapubic area
9 Left iliac fossa (LIF)

Fig 1. Abdominal areas.

 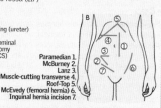

1. Kocher
2. Midline
3. Muscle splitting (ureter)
4. Pfannenstiel
5. Thoraco-abdominal (oesophagectomy) 9th or 10th ICS)

Paramedian 1.
McBurney 2.
Lanz 3.
Muscle-cutting transverse 4.
Roof-Top 5.
McEvedy (femoral hernia) 6.
Inguinal hernia incision 7.

Fig 2. Incisions.

| | |
|---|---|
| -ectomy | Cutting something out. |
| -gram | A radiological image. |
| -pexy | Anchoring of a structure to keep it in position. |
| -plasty | Surgical refashioning in order to regain good function/cosmesis. |
| -scopy | Procedure with instrumentation for looking into the body. |
| -stomy | An artificial union between a conduit and the outside or another conduit. |
| -tomy | Cutting something open to the outside world. |
| -tripsy | Fragmentation of an object. |

| | | | |
|---|---|---|---|
| angio- | Tube or vessel | lith- | Stone |
| appendic- | Appendix | mast- | Breast |
| chole- | Relating to gall/bile | meso- | Mesentery |
| colp- | Vagina | nephr- | Kidney |
| cyst- | Bladder | orchid- | Testicle |
| -doch- | Ducts | oophor- | Ovary |
| enter- | Small bowel | phren- | Diaphragm |
| eschar- | Dead tissue, eg from burn | pyloro- | Pyloric sphincter |
| gastr- | Stomach | pyel- | Renal pelvis |
| hepat- | Liver | proct- | Anal canal |
| hyster- | Uterus | salping- | Fallopian tube |
| lapar- | Abdomen | splen- | Spleen |

| | |
|---|---|
| **abscess** | A cavity containing pus. Remember: *if there is pus about, let it out.* |
| **cyst** | Fluid-filled cavity lined by epi/endothelium. |
| **fistula** | An abnormal connection between two epithelial surfaces. Fistulae often close spontaneously, but will not in the presence of malignant tissue, distal obstruction, foreign bodies, chronic inflammation, and the formation of a muco-cutaneous junction (eg stoma). |
| **hernia** | The protrusion of a viscus/part of a viscus through a defect of the wall of its containing cavity into an abnormal position. |
| **ileus** | Used in this book as a term for adynamic bowel. |
| **colic** | Intermittent pain from over-contraction/obstruction of a hollow viscus. |
| **sinus** | A blind-ending tract, typically lined by epithelial or granulation tissue, which opens to an epithelial surface. |
| **stent** | An artificial tube placed in a biological tube to keep it open. |
| **stoma** | (p584) An artificial union between conduits and the outside. |
| **ulcer** | (p662) Interruption in the continuity of an epi/endothelial surface. |
| **volvulus** | (p613) Twisting of a structure around itself. Common GI sites include the sigmoid colon and caecum, and more rarely the stomach. |

| | | | | | |
|---|---|---|---|---|---|
| epi- | Upon | pan- | Whole | peri- | Around |
| end- | Inside | para- | Alongside | sub- | Beneath |
| mega- | Enlarged | per- | Going through | trans- | Across |

Surgery

**Aims** ►To provide diagnostic and prognostic information. To ensure the patient understands the nature, aims, and expected outcome of surgery. To allay anxiety and pain:
- Ensure that the right patient gets the right surgery. Have the symptoms and signs changed? If so, inform the surgeon.
- Get informed consent (p570).
- Assess/balance risks of anaesthesia, and maximize fitness. Comorbidities? Drugs? Smoker? Optimizing oxygenation **before** major surgery improves outcome.[1]
- Check proposed anaesthesia/analgesia with anaesthetist.

**Pre-op checks** Assess cardiorespiratory system, exercise tolerance, existing illnesses, drugs, and allergies. Is the neck unstable (eg arthritis complicating intubation)? Assess past history of: MI[1], diabetes, asthma, hypertension, rheumatic fever, epilepsy, jaundice. Assess any specific risks, eg is the patient pregnant? Is the neck/jaw immobile and teeth stable (intubation risk)? Has there been previous anaesthesia? Were there any complications (eg nausea, DVT)? ►The World Health Organization 'Surgical Safety Checklist'[2] should be completed for every patient undergoing a surgical procedure. ►Is DVT/PE prophylaxis needed (p580)? ►Special tests, eg sickle cell, see BOX 1. ►If for 'unilateral' surgery, mark the correct arm/leg/kidney.

**Family history** May be relevant, eg in malignant hyperpyrexia (p574); dystrophia myotonica (p514); porphyria; cholinesterase problems; sickle-cell disease.

**Drugs** Any drug/plaster/antiseptic allergies? ►Inform the anaesthetist about **all** drugs even if 'over-the-counter'. ►Steroids: see p592; diabetes: see p590.
- *Antibiotics: Tetracycline* and *neomycin* may ↑neuromuscular blockade.
- *Anticoagulants:* ►Tell the surgeon. Avoid epidural, spinal, and regional blocks. *Aspirin* should probably be continued unless there is a major risk of bleeding. Discuss stopping *clopidogrel* therapy with the cardiologists/neurologists.
- *Anticonvulsants:* Give as usual pre-op. Post-op, give drugs IV (or by NGT) until able to take orally. *Valproate:* give usual dose IV. *Phenytoin:* give IV slowly (<50mg/min, on cardiac monitor). IM *phenytoin* absorption is unreliable.
- *β-blockers:* Continue up to and including the day of surgery as this precludes a labile cardiovascular response.
- *Contraceptive pill:* See BNF. Stop 4wks before major/leg surgery; ensure alternative contraception is used. Restart 2wks after surgery, provided patient is mobile.
- *Digoxin:* Continue up to and including morning of surgery. Check for toxicity (ECG; plasma level); do plasma K+ and Ca2+ (*suxamethonium* can ↑K+ and lead to ventricular arrhythmias in the fully digitalized).
- *Diuretics:* Beware hypokalaemia, dehydration. Do U&E (and bicarbonate).
- *Eye-drops:* β-blockers get systemically absorbed.
- *HRT:* As with contraceptive pill there may be an increased risk of DVT/PE.
- *Levodopa:* Possible arrhythmias when patient under GA.
- *Lithium:* Get expert help; it may potentiate neuromuscular blockade and cause arrhythmias. See OHCS p354.
- *MAOIs:* Get expert help as interactions may cause hypotensive/hypertensive crises.
- *Thyroid medication:* see p593.
- *Tricyclics:* These enhance *adrenaline* (epinephrine) and arrhythmias.

**Preparation** ►Starve patient; NBM ≥2h pre-op for clear fluids and ≥6h for solids.[3]
- Is any bowel or skin preparation needed, or prophylactic antibiotics (p572)?
- Start DVT prophylaxis as indicated, eg graduated compression stockings (not if there is peripheral arterial disease); low molecular weight heparin (LMWH, p344): eg *enoxaparin* 20mg/d SC, increased to 40mg/d in major-risk surgery or *heparin* 5000U SC 2h pre-op, then every 8-12h SC for 7d or until ambulant.
- Write up the pre-meds (p574); book any pre-, intra-, or post-operative x-rays or frozen sections. Book post-operative physiotherapy.
- If needed, catheterize (p776) and insert a Ryle's tube (p773) before induction. These can reduce organ bulk, making it easier to operate in the abdomen.

**1** If within the last 6 months, the perioperative risk of re-infarction (up to 40%) makes most elective surgery too risky. Echo and stress testing (+ exercise ECG or MUGA scan, p755) should be done.

## Pre-operative examination and tests—see NICE guidelines[4]

►Careful planning prevents peri-operative death.[1] A good thought exercise is to imagine yourself at the next surgical *Mortality Meeting* and ask "If I were looking back at the pre-op period, knowing that this patient had died, would I still consider that surgery was indicated?" The UK National Confidential Enquiry into Perioperative Deaths (NCEPOD) found that 'too many' operations are performed on high-risk patients.[5]

It is the anaesthetist's duty to assess suitability for anaesthesia. The ward doctor assists with a good history and examination, and can also reassure, inform, and get informed written consent (p570; ideally this should be from the surgeon).

Be alert to chronic lung disease, BP↑, arrhythmias, and murmurs.

**Tests** ►Be guided by the history and examination, and local/NICE protocols.

- **U&E, FBC, and finger-prick blood glucose in most patients.** If Hb <100g/L tell anaesthetist. Investigate/treat as appropriate. U&E are particularly important if the patient is starved, diabetic, on diuretics, a burns patient, has hepatic or renal disease, has an ileus, or is parenterally fed.
- **Crossmatch:** Blood type is identified and units are allocated to the patient. *Group and save (G&S):* Blood type is identified and held, pending crossmatch (if required). Contact your lab to discuss requirements—this decreases wastage and allows increased efficiency of blood stocks.
- **Specific blood tests:** LFT in jaundice, malignancy, or alcohol abuse. Amylase in acute abdominal pain. Blood glucose if diabetic (p590). Drug levels as appropriate (eg *digoxin, lithium*). Clotting studies in liver or renal disease, DIC (p346), massive blood loss, or if on *valproate, warfarin,* or *heparin.* HIV, HBsAg in high-risk patients, after counselling. Sickle test in those from Africa, West Indies, or Mediterranean—and if origins are in malarial areas (including most of India). Thyroid function tests in those with thyroid disease.
- **CXR** if known cardiorespiratory disease, pathology or symptoms, possible lung metastases, or >65yrs old. Remember to check the film prior to surgery.
- **ECG** if >55yrs old or poor exercise tolerance, or history of myocardial ischaemia, hypertension, rheumatic fever, or other heart disease.
- **Echocardiogram** may be performed if there is a suspicion of poor LV function.
- **Pulmonary function tests** in known pulmonary disease/obesity.
- **Lateral cervical spine x-ray** (flexion and extension views) if history of rheumatoid arthritis/ankylosing spondylitis/Down's syndrome, to warn of difficult intubations.
- **MRSA screen:** Screen and decolonize nasal carriers according to local policy (eg nasal mupirocin ointment). Colonization is **not** a contraindication to surgery. Place patients last on the list to minimize transmission to others and cover with appropriate antibiotic prophylaxis, eg vancomycin or teicoplanin.

### Pre-op checklist

- Blood tests (inc. G & S or crossmatch)
- IV cannula
- ECG + CXR
- Drug chart:
  regular medications
  analgesia/anti-emetic
  antibiotics
  **LMWH/heparin**
- Compression stockings
- Consent
- Marked site/side
- Anaesthetist informed
- Theatres informed
- Infection risk? (eg MRSA/HIV/HBV/HCV)
- NBM since when?

...not all will be required. WHO Surgical Safety checklists ensure pre-op preparation, intraoperative monitoring and post-operative review[2]

*Surgery*

---

## American Society of Anesthesiologists (ASA) classification

| | |
|---|---|
| Class I | Normally healthy patient |
| Class II | Mild systemic disease |
| Class III | Severe systemic disease that limits activity but is not incapacitating |
| Class IV | Incapacitating systemic disease which poses a constant threat to life |
| Class V | Moribund: not expected to survive 24h even with operation |

You will see a space for an ASA number on most anaesthetic charts. It is a health index at the time of surgery. The suffix E is used in emergencies, eg ASA 2E.

---

**1** Risk of mortality from elective surgery is currently about 1:100,000 to 1:150,000.

Surgery

*In which of the following situations would you seek 'informed written consent' from a patient?* 1 Feeling for a pulse. 2 Taking blood. 3 Inserting a central line. 4 Removing a section of small bowel during a laparotomy for division of adhesions. 5 Orchidectomy after a failed operation for testicular torsion.

English law states that *any* intervention or treatment needs consent—ie all of the above—yet, for different reasons, we know that, for some, informed formal consent is not regularly sought! In fact, **written** consent itself is not required by law, but it does constitute 'good medical practice' in the best interests of the patient and practitioner. Sometimes actions and words can imply valid consent, eg by simply entering into conversation or holding out an arm. In these situations your actions and their consequences are understood by the patient as a product of their knowledge, previous interactions with doctors and learning through experience.[1] However, if the consequences are not clear and the patient has capacity to give consent (see below), you should seek informed written consent as a record of your conversation.[6]

### For consent to be valid

- It can be given any time before the intervention/treatment is initiated. Earlier is better as this will give the patient time to think about the risks, benefits and alternatives—he may even bring forward questions on issues that you had not considered relevant. Think of consent as an ongoing process throughout the patient's time with you, not just the moment of signing the form.
- The proposed treatment or test must be clearly understood by the patient, taking into account the benefits, risks (including complication rates if known), additional procedures, alternative courses of action and their consequences.
- It must be given **voluntarily**. This can be difficult to evaluate—eg when live organ donation is being considered—see BOX for other difficult situations.
- The doctor who is providing treatment or undertaking the test needs to ensure that the patient has given valid consent. The act of seeking consent is ultimately the responsibility of the doctor looking after the patient, though the task may be delegated to another health professional, as long as they are suitably trained and qualified. Sometimes you may have to be certified to get consent.
- The patient must have the **capacity** (can understand, retain, and weigh the necessary information) to give consent. Assessment of capacity must be time- and decision-specific.

### When taking consent

- Think about whether you are the right person to be obtaining consent.
- Use words the patient understands and avoid jargon and abbreviations.
- Ensure that he believes your facts and can retain 'pros' and 'cons' long enough to inform his decision. Fact sheets/diagrams for individual operations help.
- Make sure his choice is free from pressure from others, and explain that after he has signed the form he is free to choose not to have the proposed treatment (ie withdraw consent) at any time. Some patients may view the consent form as a contract from which they cannot *renege*.
- If the patient is illiterate, a witnessed mark does endorse valid consent. Similarly, if the patient is willing but physically unable to sign the consent form, then an entry into the medical notes stating so is valid.
- Remember to discuss further procedures that may become necessary during the proposed treatment. This avoids waking up to a nasty surprise (eg a missing testicle as in scenario 5 above).
- If you suspect the patient is not capable of giving consent then a formal assessment needs to be documented in the medical notes.

Consent is complex, but remember that it exists for the benefit of the patient **and** the doctor, giving you an opportunity to revisit expectations and involve the patient in his own care.

---

**1** In agreeing to a blood test, the patient understands that it may be an uncomfortable experience, but he also knows that the results of the test may help you in making a diagnosis and hopefully restore him to full health. But grey areas exist everywhere: when he extends his arm towards you, does he know that you could accidentally injure an artery or nerve, with all the complications that follow—does he need to know...?

## Special circumstances for consent...and who to ask

There are some areas of treatment or investigation for which it may be advisable to seek specialist advice if it is not part of your regular practice:

- Photography of a patient.
- Innovative or novel treatment.
- Living organ donation.
- Storage, use, or removal of human tissue (for any length of time), as regulated under the Human Tissue Act 2004.

| Who to ask if you are unsure? |
| --- |
| • Your team's senior/consultant |
| • Your employing organization |
| • Legal defence organization |
| • National medical association |
| • Local research ethics committee |

- The storage, loss, or use of gametes, as regulated under the Human Fertilisation and Embryology Act 1990.
- The use of patient records or tissue in research or teaching.
- In the presence of an advanced directive or living will expressly refusing a particular treatment, investigation or action.
- Consent if <16yrs (consent form 3 in NHS).[7] In the UK, those >16yrs can give valid consent. Those <16yrs can give consent for a medical decision provided they understand what it involves—the concept of *Gillick* competence.[8] It is still good practice to involve the parents in the decision, if the child is willing. If <18yrs and refusing life-saving surgery, talk to the parents and your senior; the law is unclear. You may need to contact the duty judge in the High Court.
- Consent in the incapacitated (NHS consent form 4).[7] No-one (parents, relatives, or even members of a healthcare team) is able to give consent on behalf of an adult in England, and the High Court may be required to give a ruling on the matters of lawfulness of a proposed procedure. Proceeding in a patient's best interest is decided by the clinician overseeing their care, although it is always good practice to involve family in the proposed course of treatment.

## The right to refuse treatment

*Theirs not to make reply,*
*Theirs not to reason why,*
*Theirs but to do and die.*     Alfred, Lord Tennyson from *The Charge of the Light Brigade*, 1854

The rights of a patient are something of an antithesis to this military macabre of Tennyson, and it is our responsibility to respect the legal and ethical rights of those we treat. We do this not only for the sake of the individual, but also for the sake of an enduring trust between the patient and doctor, remembering that is the patient's right to refuse treatment (if a fully competent adult) even when this may result in death of the patient, or even the death of an unborn child, whatever the stage of pregnancy. The only exception is in circumstances outlined by the Mental Health Act 2007 (amends Mental Health Act 1983 and Mental Capacity Act 2005).

### 5 Principles of capacity:

1 Assumption of capacity (unless it is established a person lacks capacity).
2 A person is not to be treated as unable to make a decision unless all practicable steps to help him to do so have been taken without success.
3 A person is not to be treated as unable to make a decision merely because he makes an unwise decision.
4 An act done, or decision made for or on behalf of a person who lacks capacity must be done, or made, in his best interests.
5 Before the act is done or the decision is made, regard must be paid as to whether the purpose for which it is needed can be effectively achieved in a way that is less restrictive of the person's rights and freedom of action.

Futher reading: *Consent: patients and doctors making decisions together.* General Medical Council (2008).
*Reference guide to consent for examination or treatment.* Department of Health (2009).

Surgery

Prophylactic antibiotics are given to counter the risk of wound infection (see TABLE), which occurs in ~20% of elective GI surgery (up to 60% in emergency surgery). Antibiotics are also given if infection elsewhere, although unlikely, would have severe consequences (eg when prostheses are involved). A single dose given before surgery has been shown to be just as good as more prolonged regimens in biliary and colorectal surgery.[9,10] Additional doses may be given if high-risk/prolonged procedures, or if major blood loss. ►Wound infections are not necessarily trivial since sepsis may lead to haemorrhage, wound dehiscence, and initiate a fatal chain of events, so take measures to minimize the risk of wound infection:

• Time administration correctly (eg IV prophylaxis should be given 30min prior to surgery to maximize skin concentration; metronidazole PR is given 2h before).
• Use antibiotics which will kill anaerobes and coliforms.
• Consider use of peri-operative supplemental oxygen. This is a practical method of reducing the incidence of surgical wound infections.[11]
• Practise strictly sterile surgical technique. (Ask for a hand with scrubbing up if you are not sure—theatre staff will be more than pleased to help!)

**Antibiotic regimens** Check for local preferences. BNF examples include:[12]
• *Appendicectomy; colorectal resections and open biliary surgery:* A single dose of IV cefuroxime 1.5g + metronidazole 500mg *or* gentamicin 1.5mg/kg + metronidazole 500mg *or* co-amoxiclav 1.2g alone.
• *Oesophageal or gastric surgery:* 1 dose of IV gentamicin *or* cefuroxime *or* co-amoxiclav (doses above).
• *Vascular surgery:* 1 dose of IV cefuroxime *or* flucloxacillin 1-2g + gentamicin. Add metronidazole if risk of anaerobes (eg amputations, gangrene or diabetes).
• *MRSA:* For high-risk patients add teicoplanin or vancomycin to the above.

## Bowel preparation in colorectal surgery

Vigorous pre-operative bowel cleansing had been thought to reduce the risk of anastomotic leakage and septic complications, but meta-analyses have shown no benefit to patients from mechanical bowel cleansing before open colonic surgery—its omission is now widely recommended.[13,14] There is also no evidence for the use of enemas prior to rectal surgery. Mechanical bowel preparation may be used selectively in rectal surgery, but an awareness of the associated complications is essential:
• Liquefying bowel contents which are spilled during surgery • Perforation
• Electrolyte loss leading to hyponatraemia and seizures[14] • Dehydration
• A higher rate of post-operative anastomotic leakage[15]
►If in doubt, check with the surgeon to see if preparation is required.

Bowel preparation prior to colonoscopy does provide obvious benefit for visualizing the lumen.[16] Check your hospital's preferred regimen. *Example:* 1 sachet of *Picolax®* (10mg sodium picosulfate + magnesium citrate) at 8AM; another 6-8h later on the day before endoscopy. SE: dehydration and electrolyte disturbances.

## Sutures

Sutures (stitches) are central to the art of surgery. In their broadest sense they are absorbable or non-absorbable, synthetic or natural, and their structure may be divided into monofilament, twisted, or braided. See TABLE (BOX). Monofilament sutures are quite slippery but minimize infection and produce less reaction. Braided sutures have plaited strands and provide secure knots, but they may allow infection to occur between their strands. Twisted sutures have 2 twisted strands and similar qualities to braided sutures. 3-0 or 4-0 (smaller) are the best sizes for skin closure.

Timing of suture removal depends on site and the general health of the patient. Face and neck sutures may be removed after 5d (earlier in children), scalp and back of neck after 5d, abdominal incisions and proximal limbs (including clips) after ~10d, distal extremities after 14d. In patients with poor wound healing, eg steroids, malignancy, infection, cachexia (p29), the elderly, or smokers, sutures may need ~14d.

## Classification of surgical procedures and wound infection risk

| Category | Description | Infection risk |
|---|---|---|
| Clean | Incising uninfected skin without opening a viscus | <2% |
| Clean-contaminated | Intra-operative breach of a viscus (but not colon) | 8–10% |
| Contaminated | Breach of a viscus + spillage or opening of colon | 12–20% |
| Dirty | The site is already contaminated with pus or faeces, or from exogenous contagion, eg trauma | 25% |

Table after *MRCS Core Modules: Essential Revision Notes*, S. Andrews, Pastest

Surgery

## Surgical drains in the post-operative period (OHClinSurg p80)

The decision when to insert and remove drains may seem to be one of the great surgical enigmas—but there are basically 3 types to get a grip of:

1 Most are inserted to drain the area of surgery and are often put under suction or -ve pressure (Redivac® uses a 'high vacuum'). These are removed when they stop draining. They protect against collection, haematoma and seroma formation (in breast surgery this can cause overlying skin necrosis).

2 The second type of drain is used to protect sites where leakage may occur in the post-operative period, such as bowel anastomoses. These form a tract and are removed after about 1 week.

3 The third type (eg Bellovac®) collects red blood cells from the site of the operation, which can then be autotransfused within 6h, protecting from the hazards of allotransfusion—it is used commonly in orthopaedics.

'Shortening a drain' means withdrawing it (eg by 2cm/d) to allow the tract to seal, bit by bit. Evidence suggests that certain types of drain are not effective and may even lead to more complications, such as when used to protect colorectal anastomoses.[17] ►Check the individual surgeon's wishes before altering a drain.

## Some commonly encountered suture materials (OHClinSurg p84)

The perfect suture material is monofilament, strong, easy to handle, holds knots well, has predictable absorption and causes minimal tissue reaction. Unfortunately no single suture fits the bill for every occasion, and so suture selection (including size) depends on the job in hand:

**Absorbable**

| Name | Material | Construction | Use |
|---|---|---|---|
| Monocryl® | Poliglecaprone | Monofilament | Subcuticular skin closure |
| PDS® | Polydioxanone | Monofilament | Closing abdominal wall |
| Vicryl® | Polyglactin | Braided multifilament | Tying pedicles; bowel anastomosis; subcutaneous closure |
| Dexon® | Polyglycolic acid | Braided multifilament | Very similar to vicryl® |

**Non-absorbable**

| Name | Material | Construction | Use |
|---|---|---|---|
| Ethilon® | Polyamide | Monofilament | Closing skin wounds |
| Prolene® | Polypropylene | Monofilament | Arterial anastomosis |
| Mersilk®N | Silk | Braided multifilament | Securing drains |
| Metal | Eg steel | Clips or monofilament | Skin wound/sternotomy closure |

N = natural; other natural materials (eg cotton and catgut) are rarely used these days.

Surgery

Before anaesthesia, explain to the patient what will happen and where they will wake up, otherwise the recovery room or ITU will be frightening. Explain that they may feel ill on waking. The premedication aims to allay anxiety and to make the anaesthesia itself easier to conduct (see BOX 1). Typical regimens might include:

- *Anxiolytics:* Benzodiazepines, eg *lorazepam* 2mg PO; *temazepam* 10-20mg PO. In children, use oral premeds as first choice eg *midazolam* 0.5mg/kg (tastes bitter so often put in paracetamol suspension).
- *Analgesics:* See p576. Pre-emptive analgesia is not often used and effects are hard to determine. The aim is to dampen pain signals before they arrive. In children or anxious adults, local anaesthetic cream may be used on a few sites before inserting an IVI (►the anaesthetist may prefer to site the cannula themselves!)
- *Anti-emetics:* Post-operative nausea and vomiting is experienced by ~25% of all patients. 5HT₃ antagonists (eg *ondansetron* 4mg IV/IM) are the most effective agents; others, eg *metoclopramide* 10mg/8h IV/IM/PO, are also used—see p241.
- *Antacids:* Ranitidine 50mg IV or *omeprazole* 40mg PO/IV in patients at particular risk of aspiration.
- *Antisialogues: Glycopyrronium* (200-400µg in adults, 4-8µg/kg in children; given IV/IM 30-60min before induction) is sometimes used to decrease secretions that may cause respiratory obstruction in smaller airways.
- *Antibiotics:* See p572.

Give oral premedication 2h before surgery (1h if IM route used).

### Side-effects of anaesthetic agents

- *Hyoscine, atropine:* Anticholinergic ∴ tachycardia, urinary retention, glaucoma, sedation (especially in the elderly).
- *Opioids:* Respiratory depression, cough reflex↓, nausea and vomiting, constipation.
- *Thiopental:* (induction agent) laryngospasm.
- *Propofol:* (induction agent) respiratory depression, cardiac depression, pain on injection.
- *Volatile agents, eg isoflurane:* Nausea and vomiting, cardiac depression, respiratory depression, vasodilatation, hepatotoxicity (see *BNF*).

### The complications of anaesthesia are due to loss of:

- *Pain sensation:* Urinary retention, diathermy burns, pressure necrosis, local nerve injuries (eg radial nerve palsy from arm hanging over the table edge).
- *Consciousness:* Cannot communicate 'wrong leg/kidney'. NB: in some patients (eg 0.15%) *retained* consciousness is the problem. Awareness under GA sounds like a contradiction in terms, but remember that anaesthesia is a process rather than an event. Such awareness can lead to ill-defined, delayed neuroses and post-traumatic stress disorder (*OHCS* p347).[18]
- *Muscle power:* Corneal abrasion (∴ tape the eyes closed), no respiration, no cough (leads to pneumonia and atelectasis—partial lung collapse causing shunting ± impaired gas exchange: it starts minutes after induction, and may be related to the use of 100% O₂, supine position, surgery, age and to loss of power).

**Local/regional anaesthesia** If unfit/unwilling to undergo general anaesthesia, local nerve blocks (eg brachial plexus) or spinal blocks (contraindication: anticoagulation, local infection) using long-acting local anaesthetics such as *bupivacaine* may be indicated. See TABLE for doses and toxicity effects.

**Drugs complicating anaesthesia** ►Inform anaesthetist. See p568 for lists of specific drugs, and actions to take.

**Malignant hyperpyrexia** This is a rare complication, precipitated by any volatile agent, eg *halothane*, or *suxamethonium*. It exhibits autosomal dominant inheritance. There is a rapid rise in temperature (>1°C every 30min); masseter spasm may be an early sign. Complications include hypoxaemia, hypercarbia, hyperkalaemia, metabolic acidosis, and arrhythmias. ►Get expert help immediately. Prompt treatment with *dantrolene*[1] (skeletal muscle relaxant), active cooling and ITU care can reduce mortality significantly.

1 Give 1mg/kg every 5min IV—up to 10mg/kg in total (*OHCS* p628).

## Principles and practical conduct of anaesthesia (fig 1)

```
                Hypnosis              Analgesia



                    Muscle relaxation
```

Fig 1. ▶The general principles of anaesthesia centre on the triad of hypnosis, analgesia, and muscle relaxation.

The conduct of anaesthesia typically involves:
* *Induction:* Either intravenous (eg *propofol* 1.5-2.5mg/kg IV at a rate of 20-40mg every 10s; *thiopental* is an alternative) or, if airway obstruction or difficult IV access, gaseous (eg *sevoflurane* or *nitrous oxide*, mixed in $O_2$).
* *Airway control:* Either using a facemask, an oropharyngeal (Guedel) airway or by intubation. The latter usually requires muscle relaxation with a depolarizing/ non-depolarizing neuromuscular blocker (*OHCS* p622).
* *Maintenance of anaesthesia:* Either a volatile agent added to $N_2O/O_2$ mixture, or high-dose opiates with mechanical ventilation, or IV infusion anaesthesia (eg *propofol* 4-12mg/kg/h IVI).
* *Recovery:* Change inspired gases to 100% oxygen only, then discontinue any anaesthetic infusions and reverse muscle paralysis. Extubate once spontaneously breathing, place patient in recovery position and give oxygen by facemask.
* For further details, see the *Anaesthesia* chapter in *OHCS* (p612).

## Local anaesthetic toxicity and maximum doses

After a few minutes' conversation with an anaesthetist at work, it becomes apparent that they are masters of the drug dose by weight! It is important to remember the maximum doses for local anaesthetics, not least because we use them so frequently, but because the effects of overdose can be lethal.

Local anaesthetic toxicity starts with peri-oral tingling and paraesthesiae, progressing to drowsiness, seizures, coma and cardiorespiratory arrest. If suspected (the patient feels 'funny' and develops early signs) then stop administration immediately and commence ABC resuscitation as required.

Handy to remember (though it can be worked out with a pen, paper and SI units) is that a 1% concentration is equivalent to 10mg/mL. Local anaesthetics are also basic, and so do not work well in acidic environments, eg abscesses.

| % conc$^n$ | Lidocaine conc$^n$ (mg/mL) | Approx. allowable volume (mL/kg) | Approx. allowable volume for 70kg adult (mL) |
|---|---|---|---|
| 0.25% | 2.5 | 1.12 | ≤80 |
| 0.5% | 5 | 0.56 | ≤40 |
| 1% | 10 | 0.28 | ≤20 |
| 2% | 20 | 0.14 | ≤10 |

Humans are the most exquisite devices ever made for experiencing pain: the richer our inner lives, the greater the varieties of pain there are for us to feel, and the more resources we have for dealing with pain. If we can connect with patients' inner lives we may make a real difference. Never forget how painful pain is, nor how fear magnifies pain. Try not to let these sensations, so often interposed between your patient and his recovery, be invisible to you as he bravely puts up with them.

**Guidelines for success** (see also analgesic ladder, p538–539) Review and chart each pain carefully and individually.
- Identify and treat the underlying pathology wherever possible.
- Give **regular** doses rather than on an 'as-required' basis.
- Choose the best route: PO, PR, IM, epidural, SC, inhalation, or IV.
- Explanation and reassurance contribute greatly to analgesia.
- Allow the patient to be in charge. This promotes wellbeing, and does not lead to overuse. Patient-controlled continuous IV morphine delivery systems are useful.
- Liaise with the Acute Pain Service, if possible.

**Non-narcotic (simple) analgesia** *Paracetamol* 0.5–1.0g/4h PO (up to 4g daily; 15mg/kg/4h IV over 15min in children <50kg; up to 60mg/kg/d). Caution in liver impairment. NSAIDs, eg *ibuprofen* 400mg/8h PO (see BNFc for dosing in children) or *diclofenac* 50mg/8h PO, or 100mg PR, or 75mg IM stat; these are good for musculoskeletal pain and renal or biliary colic. CI: peptic ulcer, clotting disorders, anticoagulants. Cautions: asthma, renal or hepatic impairment, heart failure, IHD, pregnancy and the elderly. Aspirin is contraindicated in children due to the risk of Reye's syndrome (*OHCS* p652).

**Opioid drugs for severe pain** *Morphine* (eg 10–15mg/2–4h IV/IM) or *diamorphine* (5–10mg/2–4h PO, SC, or slow IV, but you may need much more) are best. NB: these are 'controlled' drugs. For palliative care, see p538. *Side-effects of opioids:* These include nausea (so give with an anti-emetic, p241), respiratory depression, constipation, cough suppression, urinary retention, BP↓, and sedation (do not use in hepatic failure or head injury). Dependency is rarely a problem. *Naloxone* (eg 100–200μg IV, followed by 100μg increments, eg every 2min until responsive) may be needed to reverse the effects of excess opioids (p854).

**How effective are standard analgesics?** Pain is subjective, but its measurement by patients is surprisingly consistent and reproducible. The TABLE below gives 'number needed to treat' (NNT, p669), ie the number of patients who need to receive the drug for one to achieve at least 50% pain relief over 4–6h (the range is 95% confidence intervals).

| Codeine⁶⁰ᵐᵍ | 11–48 | Paracetamol¹⁰⁰⁰ᵐᵍ | 3–4 |
|---|---|---|---|
| Tramadol⁵⁰ᵐᵍ | 6–13 | Paracetamol¹⁰⁰⁰ᵐᵍ/codeine⁶⁰ᵐᵍ | 2–3 |
| Aspirin⁶⁵⁰ᵐᵍ/codeine⁶⁰ᵐᵍ | 4–7 | Diclofenac⁵⁰ᵐᵍ or ibuprofen⁴⁰⁰ᵐᵍ | 2–3 |

**Epidural analgesia** Opioids and anaesthetics are given into the epidural space by infusion or as boluses. Ask the advice of the Pain Service. SEs are thought to be less, as the drug is more localized: watch for respiratory depression and local anaesthetic-induced autonomic blockade (BP↓).

**Adjuvant treatments** Eg radiotherapy for bone cancer pain; anticonvulsants, antidepressants, *gabapentin* or steroids for neuropathic pain, antispasmodics, eg *hyoscine butylbromide*[1] (Buscopan® 10–20mg/8h PO/IM/IV) for intestinal, renal tract colic. If brief pain relief is needed (eg for changing dressings or exploring wounds), try inhaled *nitrous oxide* (with 50% O₂—as Entonox®) with an 'on-demand' valve. Transcutaneous electrical nerve stimulation (TENS), local heat, local or regional anaesthesia, and neurosurgical procedures (eg excision of neuroma) may be tried but can prove disappointing. Treat conditions that exacerbate pain (eg constipation, depression, anxiety).

---

1 Not to be confused with *hyoscine hydrobromide*; used for drying secretions and in motion sickness.

## Why is controlling post-operative pain so important?

- **Psychological reasons:** Pain control is a humanitarian undertaking.
- **Social reasons:** Pain relief makes surgery less feared.
- **Biological reasons:** There is evidence for the following sequence: pain → autonomic activation → increased adrenergic activity → arteriolar vasoconstriction → reduced wound perfusion → decreased tissue oxygenation → delayed wound healing → serious or mortal consequences.

Surgery

**Pyrexia** Mild pyrexia in the 1st 48h is often from atelectasis (needs prompt physio, not antibiotics), tissue damage/necrosis or even from blood transfusions, but still have a low threshold for infection screen. See MINIBOX for where to look for infection—also check the legs for DVT (causes ↑°T). Send blood for FBC, U&E, CRP, and cultures (±LFT). Dipstick the urine. Consider MSU, CXR, and abdominal ultrasound/CT depending on clinical findings.

> **Looking for infection:**
> Check for signs of:
> • Peritonism
> • Chest infection
> • UTI
> • Wound infection
> • Cannula site erythema
> • Meningism
> • Endocarditis

**Confusion** may manifest as agitation, disorientation, and attempts to leave hospital, especially at night. Gently reassure the patient in well-lit surroundings. See p488 for a full work-up. Common causes are:
• Hypoxia (pneumonia, atelectasis, LVF, PE) • Infection (see above)
• Drugs (opiates, sedatives, and many others) • Alcohol withdrawal (p282)
• Urinary retention • Liver/renal failure
• MI or stroke

Occasionally, sedation is necessary to examine the patient; consider *lorazepam* 1mg PO/IM (antidote: *flumazenil*) or *haloperidol* 0.5-2mg IM. Reassure relatives that post-op confusion is common (seen in up to 40%) and reversible.

**Dyspnoea or hypoxia** Any previous lung disease? Sit patient up and give O₂, monitor peripheral O₂ sats by pulse oximetry (p156). Examine for evidence of: •Pneumonia, pulmonary collapse or aspiration •LVF (MI; fluid overload) •Pulmonary embolism (p182) •Pneumothorax (p182; due to CVP line, intercostal block or mechanical ventilation). *Tests* FBC; ABG; CXR; ECG. Manage according to findings.

**BP↓** If severe, tilt bed head-down and give O₂. Check pulse and BP yourself; compare it with pre-op values. Post-op ↓BP is often from hypovolaemia resulting from inadequate fluid input, so check fluid chart and replace losses. Monitor urine output (may need catheterization). A CVP line can help monitor fluid resuscitation (normal is 0-5cm H₂O relative to sternal angle). Hypovolaemia may also be caused by haemorrhage so review wounds and abdomen. If unstable, return to theatre for haemostasis. Beware cardiogenic and neurogenic causes and look for evidence of MI or PE. Consider sepsis and anaphylaxis. *Management:* p804.

**BP↑** may be from pain, urinary retention, idiopathic hypertension (eg missed medication) or inotropic drugs. Oral cardiac medications (including antihypertensives) should be continued throughout the perioperative period even if NBM. Treat the cause, consider increasing the regular medication, or if not absorbing orally try 50mg *labetalol* IV over 1min (see p134).

**Urine output↓ (oliguria)** Aim for output of >30mL/h in adults (or >0.5mL/kg/h). Anuria often means a blocked or malsited catheter (see p777) rather than AKI and never, we hope, an impending lawsuit from both ureters tied. Flush or replace catheter. **Oliguria** is usually due to too little replacement of lost fluid. Treat by increasing fluid input. ►Acute renal failure may follow shock, drugs, transfusion, pancreatitis or trauma (see p292 for pre-renal/intrinsic/post-renal causes and management of AKI).

• Review fluid chart and examine for signs of volume depletion.
• Urinary retention is also common, so examine for a palpable bladder.
• Establish normovolaemia (a CVP line may help here); you may need 1L/h IVI for 2-3h. A 'fluid challenge' of 250-500mL over 30min may also help.
• Catheterize bladder (for accurate monitoring)—see p776; check U&E.
• If intrinsic renal failure is suspected, stop any nephrotoxic drugs (eg NSAIDs, ACE-i) and refer to a nephrologist early.

**Nausea/vomiting** Any mechanical obstruction, ileus, or emetic drugs (opiates, digoxin, anaesthetics)? Consider AXR, NGT, and an anti-emetic (►not *metoclopramide* because of its prokinetic property). See p241 for choice of anti-emetics.

**↓Na⁺** What was the pre-op level? Over-administration of IV fluids may exacerbate the situation. Correct slowly (p686). SIADH (p687) can be precipitated by perioperative pain, nausea, and opioids as well as chest infection.

## Post-operative bleeding

**Primary haemorrhage:** Continuous bleeding, starting during surgery. Replace blood loss. If severe, return to theatre for adequate haemostasis. Treat shock vigorously (p804).

**Reactive haemorrhage:** Haemostasis appears secure until BP rises and bleeding starts. Replace blood and re-explore wound.

**Secondary haemorrhage** (caused by infection) occurs 1-2 weeks post-op.

## Talking about post-op complications...

When asked to give your thoughts on the complications of an operation—maybe with an examiner or a patient—a good starting point is to divide them up accordingly (and for each of the following stratify as immediate, early and late):
• *From the anaesthetic:* (p574) eg respiratory depression from induction agents.
• *From surgery in general:* (see p578 and BOX 1) eg wound infection, haemorrhage, neurovascular damage, DVT/PE.
• *From the specific procedure:* eg saphenous nerve damage in stripping of the long varicose vein.

Tailor the discussion towards the individual who, eg if an arteriopath, may have a significant risk of cardiac ischaemia during hypotensive episodes whilst under the anaesthetic. For some other post-op complications, see:
• Pain (p576) • DVT (p580 and figs 1-4) • Pulmonary embolus (p182; massive, p828)
• Wound dehiscence (p582) • Complications in post-gastric surgery (p624)
• Other complications of specific operations (p582).

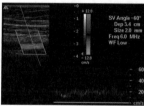

Fig 1. A normal duplex ultrasound (sagittal view) of the superficial femoral vein with a normal Doppler trace. Compression ultrasound (fig 2) is the best image in suspected DVT.

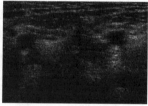

Fig 2. Transverse ultrasound of the superficial femoral vein and artery with (right) and without (left) compression. Collapse of the vein (deeper to the artery) on compression means absence of thrombus.

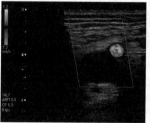

Fig 3. Ultrasound showing evidence of an acute thrombus within a dilated superficial femoral vein. This will not always show an intraluminal echo (compare with fig 4) and so confirm its presence by lack of compression of the vein with the ultrasound probe.

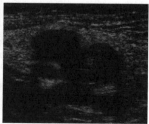

Fig 4. Ultrasound showing a transverse view of the femoral artery and vein. Here, the lumen of the femoral vein (deeper and medial to the artery) is occluded by thrombus, giving a hyperechoic signal compared to the arterial lumen.

Figs 1-4 courtesy of Norwich Radiology Dept.

Surgery

DVTs occur in 25–50% of surgical patients, and many non-surgical patients. All hospital inpatients should be assessed for DVT/PE risk and offered prophylaxis if appropriate (according to local guidelines).[19] 65% of below-knee DVTs are asymptomatic; these rarely embolize to the lung.

**Risk factors** Age↑, pregnancy, synthetic oestrogen, trauma, surgery (especially pelvic/orthopaedic), past DVT, cancer, obesity, immobility, thrombophilia (p368).

**Signs** •Calf warmth/tenderness/swelling/erythema •Mild fever •Pitting oedema.

**ΔΔ:** Cellulitis; ruptured Baker's cyst. Both may coexist with a DVT.

**Tests** D-dimer is sensitive but not specific for DVT (also ↑ in infection, pregnancy, malignancy, and post-op).[20] A -ve result, combined with a low pretest clinical probability score (see BOX 1), is sufficient to exclude DVT.[21] If D-dimer↑, or the patient has a high/intermediate pretest clinical probability score, do *ultrasound* (fig 3, p579).[22] If this is -ve, a repeat USS may be performed at 1wk to catch early but propagating DVTs. Think of a DVT as a symptom that needs to be investigated: Do *thrombophilia tests* (p368) **before** commencing anticoagulant therapy if there are no predisposing factors, in recurrent DVT, or if there is a family history of DVT. Look for *underlying malignancy:* Urine dip; FBC, LFT, $Ca^{2+}$; CXR ± CT abdomen/pelvis (& mammography in ♀) if >40yrs.[23]

**Prevention** •Stop the Pill 4wks pre-op. •Mobilize early. •Low molecular weight heparin (LMWH, eg *enoxaparin* 20mg/24h SC, ↑ to 40mg for high-risk patients, p369, starting 12h pre-op). •Graduated compression stockings ('thromboembolic deterrent (TED) stockings'; CI: ischaemia) and intermittent pneumatic compression devices reduce DVT risk by ⅔rds in surgical patients.[24] •*Fondaparinux* (a factor Xa inhibitor) reduces risk of DVT over LMWH without increasing the risk of bleeding.[25]

**Treatment** LMWH (eg *enoxaparin* 1.5mg/kg/24h SC) or *fondaparinux*. LMWH is superior to *unfractionated heparin* (which may be needed in renal failure or if ↑risk of bleeding; dose guided by APTT, p344). Cancer patients should receive LMWH for 6 months (then review).[23] In others, start *warfarin* simultaneously with LMWH (warfarin is prothrombotic for the first 48h). Stop heparin when INR is 2–3; treat for 3 months if post-op (6 months if no cause is found; lifelong in recurrent DVT or thrombophilia). *Inferior vena caval filters* may be used in active bleeding, or when anticoagulants fail, to minimize risk of pulmonary embolus. *Post-phlebitic change* can be seen in 10–30%. Graduated compression stockings help prevent long-term complications of DVT (pain, swelling and skin changes).[26] Thrombolytic therapy (to reduce damage to venous valves) may reduce complications but risks major bleeding.[27]

## Swollen legs
See also p29; treatment—see BOX 2

**Bilateral oedema** implies systemic disease with ↑venous pressure (eg right heart failure) or ↓intravascular oncotic pressure (any cause of ↓albumin, so test the urine for protein). It is **dependent** (distributed by gravity), which is why legs are affected early, but severe oedema extends above the legs. In the bed-bound, fluid moves to the new dependent area, causing a sacral pad. The exception is the local increase in venous pressure occurring in IVC obstruction: the swelling neither extends above the legs nor redistributes. *Causes:* •Right heart failure (p128); •Albumin ↓ (p700, eg renal or liver failure); •Venous insufficiency: acute, eg prolonged sitting, or chronic, with haemosiderin-pigmented, itchy, eczematous skin ± ulcers; •Vasodilators, eg *nifedipine, amlodipine.* •Pelvic mass (p57, p606); •Pregnancy—if BP↑ + proteinuria, diagnose pre-eclampsia (OHCS p48): find an obstetrician urgently. In all the above, both legs need not be affected to the same extent.

**Unilateral oedema:** Pain ± redness implies DVT or inflammation, eg cellulitis or insect bites (any blisters?). Bone or muscle may be to blame, eg tumours; necrotizing fasciitis (p662); trauma (check for sensation, pulses and severe pain esp. on passive movement: ►a compartment syndrome with ischaemic necrosis needs prompt fasciotomy). Impaired mobility suggests trauma, arthritis, or a Baker's cyst (p708).
**Non-pitting oedema** is oedema you cannot indent: see p29.

## Pretest clinical probability scoring for DVT: the Wells score[28]

In patients with symptoms in both legs, the more symptomatic leg is used.

| Clinical features | Score |
|---|---|
| Active cancer (treatment within last 6 months or palliative) | 1 point |
| Paralysis, paresis, or recent plaster immobilization of leg | 1 point |
| Recently bedridden for >3d or majory surgery in last 12wks | 1 point |
| Local tenderness along distribution of deep venous system | 1 point |
| Entire leg swollen | 1 point |
| Calf swelling >3cm compared with asymptomatic leg (measured 10cm below tibial tuberosity) | 1 point |
| Pitting oedema (greater in the symptomatic leg) | 1 point |
| Collateral superficial veins (non-varicose) | 1 point |
| Previously documented DVT | 1 point |
| Alternative diagnosis at least as likely as DVT | −2 points |

**Wells score:** ≤*1 point = DVT unlikely:* Perform D-dimer. If negative, DVT excluded. If positive, proceed to USS (if USS negative, DVT excluded; if positive, treat as DVT). ≥*2 points = DVT likely:* Do D-dimer and USS. If both negative, DVT excluded. If USS positive, treat as DVT. If D-dimer positive and USS negative, repeat USS in 1 week.

Reproduced from *CMAJ* 2006, Scarvelis D, Wells PS: Diagnosis and treatment of deep-vein thrombosis, Oct 24;175(9):1087–92. Vol 350, used with permission.

## 9 questions to ask those with swollen legs

| 1 Is it **both** legs? | 2 Is she pregnant? | 3 Is she mobile? |
|---|---|---|
| 4 Any trauma? | 5 Any pitting (p29)? | 6 Past diseases/on drugs? |
| 7 Any pain? | 8 Any skin changes? | 9 Any oedema elsewhere? |

**Tests** ►Look for proteinuria (+hypoalbuminaemia (≈nephrotic syndrome)). Is there CCF (echocardiogram)?

**Treatment of leg oedema** Treat the cause. Giving diuretics to everyone is not an answer. Ameliorate dependent oedema by elevating the legs (ankles higher than hips—do not just use footstools); raise the foot of the bed. Graduated support stockings may help (CI: ischaemia).[29]

## Air travel and DVT

In 1954, Homans reported an association between air travel and venous thrombo-embolism. Factors such as dehydration, immobilization, decreased oxygen tension, and prolonged pressure on the popliteal veins resulting from long periods in air-craft seats have all been suggested to be contributory factors. While the evidence linking air travel to an increased risk of DVT is still largely circumstantial, the following facts may help answer questions from your patients, family, and friends:

- The risk of developing a DVT from a long-distance flight has been estimated at 1 in 10,000 to 1 in 40,000 for the general population.
- The incidence of DVT in **high-risk** groups has been shown to be 4-6% for flights >10h. Travellers with ≥1 risk factor should consider compression stockings and/or a single dose of prophylactic LMWH for flights >6h.[30]
- There is ↑risk of pulmonary embolus associated with long-distance air travel.[31]
- Compression stockings may decrease the risk of DVT, though they may also cause superficial thrombophlebitis.[28,1]
- There is no evidence to support the use of prophylactic *aspirin*.[32]
- Measures to minimize risk of DVT include leg exercises, increased water intake, and refraining from alcohol or caffeine during the flight.

**Laparotomy** In the elderly, or the malnourished, the wound may break down from a few days to a few weeks post-op, eg if infection or haematoma is present, or this is major surgery in a patient already compromised, eg by cancer, or this is a 2ⁿᵈ laparotomy. The warning sign of wound dehiscence (incidence ≈3.5%) is a pink serous discharge. Always assume that the defect involves the whole of the wound. Serious wound dehiscence may lead to a 'burst abdomen' with evisceration of bowel (mortality 15-30%). If you are on the ward when this happens, put the guts back into the abdomen, place a sterile dressing over the wound, give IV antibiotics (eg cefuroxime + metronidazole; see local guidelines) and call your senior. Allay anxiety, give parenteral pain control, set up an IVI, and return patient to theatre. *Incisional hernia* is a common problem (20%), repairable by mesh insertion.[33]

**Biliary surgery** After exploration of the common bile duct (CBD), a T-tube is usually left in the bile duct draining freely to the exterior. A T-tube cholangiogram is done at 8-10d, and if there are no retained stones the tube may be pulled out. Retained stones may be removed by ERCP (p756), further surgery, or instillation of stone-dissolving agents (via T-tube). If there is distal obstruction in the CBD, fistula formation may occur with a chronic leakage of bile. Other complications of biliary surgery are CBD stricture; cholangitis; bleeding into the biliary tree (haemobilia) which may lead to biliary colic, jaundice, and haematemesis; pancreatitis; bile leak causing biliary peritonitis. If jaundiced, it is important to maintain a good urine output, monitor coagulation and consider antibiotics. There is a danger of hepatorenal syndrome (p259).

**Thyroid surgery** (See also p602) Recurrent (± superior) laryngeal nerve palsy (→hoarseness) can occur permanently in 0.5% and transiently in 1.5%[34]—warn the patient that their voice will be different for a few days post-op because of intubation and local oedema. (NB: pre-operative fibreoptic laryngoscopy should be performed to exclude pre-existing vocal cord dysfunction); hypoparathyroidism (p214), causing hypocalcaemia (p692) that is permanent in 2.5%; hypothyroidism in the long term; thyroid storm (p844); tracheal obstruction due to haematoma in the wound: ▶▶relieve by immediate removal of stitches or clips using the cutter/remover that should remain at the beside; may require urgent surgery.

**Mastectomy** Arm lymphoedema in up to 20% of those undergoing axillary node sampling or dissection.[35] The risk of lymphoedema increases with the level of axillary dissection: risk is lower with Level 1 dissection (remains inferior to *pec. minor* compared to Level 3 dissection (goes superior to *pec. minor*, rarely done); skin necrosis.

**Arterial surgery** Bleeding; thrombosis; embolism; graft infection; MI; AV fistula formation. *Complications of aortic surgery:* Gut ischaemia; renal failure; respiratory distress; aorto-enteric fistula; trauma to ureters or anterior spinal artery (leading to paraplegia); ischaemic events from distal trash from dislodged thrombus.

**Colonic surgery** Sepsis; ileus; fistulae; anastomotic leak (11% for radical rectal surgery);[36] obstruction from adhesions (BOX); haemorrhage; trauma to ureters or spleen.

**Small bowel surgery** Short gut syndrome (best defined functionally, though anatomically ≤250cm in the adult) may result from substantial resections of small bowel. Diarrhoea and malabsorption (particularly of fats) lead to a number of metabolic abnormalities including deficiency in vitamins A, D, E, K, and B₁₂, hyperoxaluria (causing renal stones), and bile salt depletion (causing gallstones).[37] The management of short bowel syndrome is complex and aims to correct these metabolic abnormalities.[38]

**Tracheostomy** Stenosis; mediastinitis; surgical emphysema.

**Splenectomy** (p367) Acute gastric dilatation (a serious consequence of not using a NGT, or to check that the one in place is working); thrombocytosis; sepsis. ▶Lifetime sepsis risk is partly preventable with pre-op vaccines—ie *Haemophilus* type B, meningococcal, and pneumococcal (p391 & p160) and prophylactic penicillin.

**Genitourinary surgery** Septicaemia (from instrumentation in the presence of infected urine)—consider a stat dose of *gentamicin*; urinoma—rupture of a ureter or renal pelvis leading to a mass of extravasated urine.

**Gastrectomy** See p624. **Prostatectomy** p645. **Haemorrhoidectomy** p634.

## Adhesions—legacy of the laparotomy, bane of the surgeon

When re-operating on the abdomen, the struggle against adhesions tests the farthest and darkest boundaries of patience of the abdominal surgeon and the assistant. The skill and persistence required to gently and atraumatically tease apart these fibrous bands that restrict access and vision makes any progression, no matter how slight, cause for subdued celebration. Perseverance is the name of this game.

Surgical division of adhesions is known as *adhesiolysis*. Any surgical procedure that breaches the abdominal or pelvic cavities can predispose to the formation of adhesions, which are found in up to 90% of those with previous abdominal surgery; this is why we do not rush to operate on small bowel obstruction: the operation predisposes to yet more adhesions. Handling of the serosal surface of the bowel causes inflammation, which over weeks to years can lead to the formation of fibrous bands that tether the bowel to itself or adjacent structures—though adhesions can also form secondary to infection, radiation injury and inflammatory processes such as Crohn's disease. Their main sequelae are intestinal obstruction (the cause in ~60% of cases—see p612) and chronic abdominal or pelvic pain. Studies have shown that adhesiolysis may help relieve chronic pain, though for a small proportion of patients the pain never improves or even worsens after directed intervention.[39]

As far as prevention is concerned, the best approach is to avoid operating, though there is evidence to suggest that laparoscopy compared with laparotomy reduces the rate of local adhesions.[40] Insertion of synthetic films (eg hyaluronic acid/carboxymethyl membrane) to prevent adhesions to the anterior abdominal wall reduces incidence, extent and severity of adhesions, but not incidence of obstruction or operative re-intervention.[41]

Surgery

*Surgery*

A stoma (Greek=*mouth*) is an artificial union between a conduit and the outside world—eg a colostomy, in which faeces are made to pass through an opening in the abdominal wall when a loop of colon is brought out onto the skin. NB A stoma can also be made between 2 internal conduits (eg a choledochojejunostomy).

**Colostomies** May be temporary or permanent. Pre-op, confirm that the patient is unsuited to one of the newer colostomy-avoiding operations (see below). Are they suitable for a laparoscopic operation?[242]

- *Loop colostomy:* A loop of colon is exteriorized and partially divided, forming 2 stomas that are joined together (the proximal end passes stool, the distal end passes mucus, see fig 1). A rod under the loop prevents retraction and may be removed after 7d. A loop colostomy is often temporary and performed to protect a distal anastamosis, eg after anterior resection.
- *End colostomy:* The bowel is divided and the proximal end brought out as a stoma; the distal end may be: 1 resected, eg abdominoperineal (AP) resection (inspect the perineum for absent anus when examining a stoma); 2 closed and left in the abdomen (Hartmann's procedure); 3 exteriorized, forming a 'mucous fistula'.
- *Paul-Mikulicz colostomy:* A double-barrelled colostomy in which the colon is divided completely (eg to excise a section of bowel). Each end is exteriorized as two separate stomas.

*Output:* Colostomies ideally pass 1-2 formed motions/day into an adherent plastic pouch. Some may be managed with irrigation, thus avoiding a pouch.
*Incidence:* 21,000 stomas/yr[UK] (>50% are permanent).[43] Most manage their stomas well. The cost for appliances is ~£1300/yr. If there is a skin reaction to the adhesive or pouch, a change of device may be all that is needed. Contact the stoma nurse.

**Ileostomies** protrude from the skin and emit frequent fluid motions which contain active enzymes (so the skin needs protecting), see fig 2. End ileostomy usually follows total proctocolectomy, typically for UC; loop ileostomies can also be formed.

**Defunctioning stomas** (eg loop colostomy or ileostomy) are used to relieve distal obstruction or to protect distal anastomoses. Although they do not reduce leakage rates, they probably minimize the severity of leakage when it does occur.[44]

**The alternatives to colostomy** *Low/ultralow anterior resection:* All or part of the rectum is excised and the proximal colon anastamosed to the top of the anal canal (the lower the level of anastamosis, the higher the risk of complication). *Ileoanal pouch formation:* The colon and rectum are removed and a pouch of ileum is joined to the upper anal canal. The 'J' pouch results in less frequent bowel movements and less incontinence compared with straight anastamosis.[45] *Total anorectal reconstruction:* An electrically stimulated sphincter is created using gracilis muscle, or an artificial mechanical sphincter implanted after, eg AP excision of the rectum. *Transanal endoscopic microsurgery:* Allows excision of small tumours within the rectum. Sphincter-saving operations for rectal cancer near the anal verge are not associated with increased recurrence rate compared with AP resection.[46]

 The physical and psychological aspects of stoma care must not be undervalued. Be alert to any vicious cycle in which a skin reaction leads to leakage and precipitates a fear of going out, or a fear of eating. This in turn may lead to poor skin nutrition and further skin reactions, resulting in further leakage and depression. These cycles can be circumvented by the *stoma nurse*, who is the expert in fitting secure, odourless devices.[47] Ensure patients are in contact before and after surgery—their advice is more useful than any doctor's in explaining what is going to happen, what the stoma will be like, and in troubleshooting post-op problems. ▶Early direct self-referral prevents problems. Without input from the stoma nurse, a patient may reject his colostomy, never attend to it, or even become suicidal.

**Urostomies** are fashioned after total cystectomy, bringing urine from the ureters to the abdominal wall via an *ileal conduit* that is usually incontinent. Formation of a catheterizable valvular mechanism may retain continence. Advances in urological surgery have seen an increase in continence-saving procedures such as orthotopic neobladder reconstruction, with good long-term continence rates.[48]

## Complications of stomas

▶Liaise early with the stoma nurse, starting pre-operatively.

*Early:*
- Haemorrhage at stoma site
- Stoma ischaemia—colour progresses from dusky grey to black
- High output (can lead to K⁺↓)—consider *loperamide ± codeine* to thicken output
- Obstruction secondary to adhesions (see p583)
- Stoma retraction

*Delayed:*
- Obstruction (failure at operation to close lateral space around stoma)
- Dermatitis around stoma site (worse with ileostomy)
- Stoma prolapse
- Stomal intussusception
- Stenosis
- Parastomal hernia (risk increases with time).[49] NB Prophylactic mesh insertion at the time of stoma formation reduces this risk[50]
- Fistulae
- Psychological problems

## Choosing a stoma site

When choosing the site for a stoma, avoid:
- Bony prominences (eg anterior superior iliac spine, costal margins)
- The umbilicus
- Old wounds/scars—there may be adhesions beneath
- Skin folds and creases
- The waistline
- The site should be assessed pre-operatively by the stoma nurse, with the patient both lying and standing

Colostomies are most often placed in the left iliac fossa (fig 3) whereas a stoma in the right iliac fossa is more likely to be an ileostomy/ileal conduit.

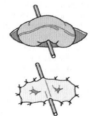

**Fig 1.** A loop colostomy with double-barrelled stoma and supporting ostomy rod.

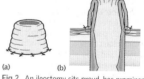

(a)    (b)

**Fig 2.** An ileostomy sits proud, has prominent mucosal folds, and is often right-sided.

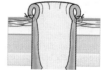

**Fig 3.** A colostomy sits flush with the skin and is typically sited in the left iliac fossa.

Surgery

▶Over 25% of hospital inpatients may be malnourished. Hospitals can become so focused on curing disease that they ignore the foundations of good health—malnourished patients recover more slowly and experience more complications.[1]

### Why are so many hospital patients malnourished?

1 Increased nutritional requirements (eg sepsis, burns, surgery)
2 Increased nutritional losses (eg malabsorption, output from stoma)
3 Decreased intake (eg dysphagia, nausea, sedation, coma)
4 Effect of treatment (eg nausea, diarrhoea)
5 Enforced starvation (eg prolonged periods nil by mouth)
6 Missing meals through being whisked off, eg for investigations
7 Difficulty with feeding (eg lost dentures; no one available to assist)
8 Unappetizing food

### Identifying the malnourished patient

• *History:* Recent weight↓ (>20%, accounting for fluid balance); recent reduced intake; diet change (eg recent change in consistency of food); nausea, vomiting, pain, diarrhoea which might have led to reduced intake.
• *Examination:* State of hydration (p680): dehydration can go hand-in-hand with malnutrition, and overhydration can mask malnutrition. Evidence of malnutrition: skin hanging off muscles (eg over biceps); no fat between fold of skin; hair rough and wiry; pressure sores; sores at corner of mouth. Calculate body mass index (p236); BMI <20kg/m² suggests malnourishment. Anthropomorphic indices, eg mid arm circumference, skin fold measures and grip strength are also useful.
• *Investigations:* Generally unhelpful. Low albumin suggestive, but is affected by many things other than nutrition. Albumin ↑ can be helpful in monitoring recovery.

**Prevention of malnutrition** Assess nutrition state and weight on admission, and, eg weekly thereafter. Identify those at risk (see above). Ensure that meals are uninterrupted, when possible. Provide appetizing food to the patient when they want to eat it. If the patient requires nutritional support, seek help from a dietician.

**Enteral nutrition** (ie nutrition given into gastrointestinal tract) If at all possible, give nutrition by mouth. An all-fluid diet can meet requirements (but get advice from dietician). If danger of choking or aspiration (eg after stroke), consider semi-solid diet before abandoning food by mouth. Early post-op enteral nutrition has been shown to benefit patients (eg after GI surgery) and may reduce complications.[51]

*Tube feeding:* Liquid nutrition via a tube, eg placed endoscopically, radiologically, or surgically (directly into stomach, ie gastrostomy). Use nutritionally complete, commercially prepared feeds. **Polymeric** feeds consist of undigested proteins, starches and long chain fatty acids (eg Nutrison standard®, Osmolite®). Normally contain ~1kCal/mL and 4-6g protein per 100mL. Most people's requirements are met with 2L/24h. **Elemental** feeds consist of individual amino acids, oligo- and monosaccharides needing minimal digestion. Also **disease-specific** feeds, eg in liver cirrhosis with hepatic encephalopathy branched-chain amino acid-enriched formulae, should be used.[52] Advice from dietician is essential. Nausea and vomiting less problematic if feed continuous, but may have disadvantages compared with intermittent nutrition.

### Guidelines for success

• Use fine-bore (9 Fr) nasogastric feeding tube when possible.
• Check position of nasogastric tube (pH testing) or nasoduodenal tube (x-ray) before starting feeding.
• Build up feeds gradually to avoid diarrhoea and distension.
• Weigh weekly, check blood glucose and plasma electrolytes (including phosphate, zinc, and magnesium, if previously malnourished).
• Treat underlying conditions vigorously, eg sepsis may impede +ve nitrogen balance.
▶Close liaison with a dietician is essential.

---

**1** For an in-depth guide to nutrition see *Manual of Dietetic Practice, 4e*, Briony Thomas, Blackwell.

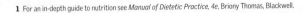

## Nil by mouth (NBM) before theatre

If in doubt about what is acceptable oral intake prior to induction for general anaesthesia (eg for GI surgery), it is best to liaise with the anaesthetist concerned. However, guidelines have been published by many colleges and societies to outline what is safe in the perioperative period:
- For **adult elective surgery** in healthy patients without GI comorbidity
  - Water or clear fluids (eg black tea/coffee) are allowed up to 2h beforehand
  - All other intake up to 6h beforehand[3]
- In **emergency surgery**, ≥6h NBM prior to theatre is best.

## Daily energy and nutritional requirements

| Substance | Requirement (/kg/d) | Notes |
|---|---|---|
| Energy | 20–40kCal | Normal adult requirements will be 2000–2500kCal/d; even catabolic patients rarely require >2500kCal/d. Very high calorie diets (eg >4000kCal/d) can lead to a fatty liver. |
| | 84–168kJ | Multiply kCal by a factor of 4.2. |
| Nitrogen | 0.2–0.4g | 6.25g of enteral protein gives 1g of nitrogen. Considering nitrogen balance is important because although catabolism is inevitable, replenishment is vital. |
| Protein | 0.5g | Contains 5kCal/g. |
| Fat | 3g | Contains 10kCal/g. |
| Carbohydrate | 2g | Contains 4kCal/g. |
| Water | 30–35mL | +500mL/d for each °C of pyrexia. |
| Na/K/Cl | 1.0mmol each | Electrolytes need to be considered, even if not on IVI. |

Do not undertake parenteral feeding lightly: it has risks. Specialist advice is vital. It should only be considered if the patient is likely to become malnourished without it—this normally means that the gastrointestinal tract is not functioning (eg bowel obstruction), and is unlikely to function for at least 7d. Parenteral feeding may supplement other forms of nutrition (eg in short bowel syndrome or active Crohn's disease, when nutrition cannot be sufficiently absorbed in the gut) or it can be used alone (total parenteral nutrition—TPN). ►Even if there is GI disease, studies show that enteral nutrition is safer, cheaper, and at least as efficacious as parenteral nutrition in the perioperative period.[1 53]

**Administration** Nutrition is normally given through a central venous line as this usually lasts longer than if given into a peripheral vein. A peripherally inserted central catheter (PICC line) is another option, though they can be trickier to insert and may have a higher rate of thrombophlebitis.[54] Insert under strict sterile conditions and check position on x-ray—figs 1 and 2.

**Requirements** There are many different regimens for parenteral feeding. Most provide 2000kCal and 10-14g nitrogen in 2-3L; this usually meets a patient's daily requirements (see TABLE, p587). ~50% of calories are provided by fat and ~50% by carbohydrate. Regimens comprise vitamins, minerals, trace elements, and electrolytes; these will normally be included by the pharmacist.

**Complications**
- *Sepsis:* (Eg *Staphylococcus epidermidis* and *Staphylococcus aureus*; *Candida*; *Pseudomonas*; infective endocarditis.) Look for spiking pyrexia and examine wound at tube insertion point. Take line **and** peripheral cultures. If central venous line-related sepsis is suspected, the safest course of action is always to remove the line. Do not attempt to salvage a line when *S. aureus* or *Candida* infection has been identified. Antimicrobial-impregnated central lines decrease the incidence of line-related infections.[55]
- *Thrombosis:* Central vein thrombosis may occur, resulting in pulmonary embolus or superior vena caval obstruction (p526). Heparin in the nutrient solution may be useful for prophylaxis in high-risk patients, though there is little clear-cut evidence in adult studies.
- *Metabolic imbalance:* Electrolyte abnormalities—see BOX; deranged plasma glucose; hyperlipidaemia; deficiency syndromes (TABLE, p281); acid-base disturbance (eg hypercapnia from excessive $CO_2$ production).
- *Mechanical:* Pneumothorax; embolism of IV line tip.

**Guidelines for success**
- ►Liaise closely with line insertion team, nutrition team and pharmacist.
- Meticulous sterility. Do not use central venous lines for uses other than nutrition. Remove the line if you suspect infection. Culture its tip.
- Review fluid balance at least twice daily, and requirements for energy and electrolytes daily.
- Check weight, fluid balance, and urine glucose daily throughout period of parenteral nutrition. Check plasma glucose, creatinine and electrolytes (including calcium and phosphate), and FBC daily until stable and then 3 times a week. Check LFT and lipid clearance three times a week until stable and then weekly. Check zinc and magnesium weekly throughout.
- Do not rush. Achieve the maintenance regimen in small steps.
- Treat underlying conditions vigorously—eg sepsis may impede +ve nitrogen balance.

---

**1** Enteral feeding promotes integrity of the gut mucosal barrier, thus preventing bacterial and endotoxin translocation across the gut wall, which can lead to multiple organ dysfunction syndrome (MODS) and perpetuation of a systemic inflammatory response—even when the gut is not the primary source of pathology.

## Refeeding syndrome

▶This is a life-threatening metabolic complication of refeeding via any route after a prolonged period of starvation.[56] As the body turns to fat and protein metabolism in the starved state, there is a drop in the level of circulating insulin (because of the paucity of dietary carbohydrates). The catabolic state also depletes intracellular stores of phosphate, although serum levels may remain normal (0.85-1.45mmol/L). When refeeding begins, the level of insulin rises in response to the carbohydrate load, and one of the consequences is to increase cellular uptake of phosphate.

**At risk with:**
- Malignancy
- Anorexia nervosa
- Alcoholism
- GI surgery
- Starvation

A hypophosphataemic state (<0.50mmol/L) normally develops within 4d and is mostly responsible for the features of 'refeeding syndrome', which include: rhabdomyolysis; red and white cell dysfunction; respiratory insufficiency; arrhythmias; cardiogenic shock; seizures; sudden death.

**Prevention** requires at-risk patients to be identified, assessed and monitored closely during refeeding (glucose, lipids, sodium, potassium, phosphate, calcium, magnesium, and zinc). Close involvement of a nutritionist is required.

**Treatment** is of the complicating features and includes parenteral phosphate administration (eg 18mmol/d) in addition to oral supplementation.[57]

## The venous system at the thoracic outlet

When trying to judge the position of a central venous line tip on CXR (see figs 2 and 3) it helps to know the anatomical landmarks of the venous system. The subclavian veins join the internal jugular veins behind the sternoclavicular joints to form the brachiocephalic veins. These come together behind the right 1st sternocostal joint to form the superior vena cava (SVC), which runs from this point to the right 3rd sternocostal joint. The right atrium starts here.

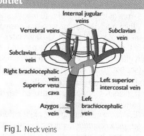

Fig 1. Neck veins

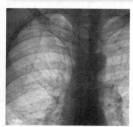

Fig 2. Right arm PICC (peripherally inserted central catheter) still with a wire in the lumen. This is a radiograph at the time of insertion to determine if placement is correct. The tip lies in the SVC—ie good positioning for long-term antibiotic therapy. The tip of a Hickman line, for cytotoxic administration, is better in the right atrium, to avoid possible irritation of the SVC and consequent thrombosis or stenosis.

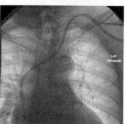

Fig 3. CXR showing placement of a dual lumen haemodialysis catheter. It is tunnelled through the subcutaneous tissues, enters the left internal jugular vein, and travels through the left brachiocephalic vein and SVC to enter the right atrium. The tip lies best in the SVC or right atrium, any further and it might damage the tricuspid valve.

Both images were acquired in the angiography room, where radio-opaque material appears black (it is easier to see contrast media against a white background).

Both images courtesy of Prof Peter Scally.

Surgery

Over 10% of surgical patients will have diabetes. This group face a greater risk of post-operative infection and cardiac complications.[59,60] Tight glycaemic control is therefore essential and improves outcome. Aim to achieve an $Hb_{A1c}$ of <69mmol/mol prior to elective surgery. Patients are often well informed about their diabetes—involve them fully in managing their diabetic care. Check your hospital's policy for managing diabetic patients who will be NBM before surgery. Below is a general guide.[61]

### Insulin-treated diabetes mellitus
• Try to place the patient first on the list in order to minimize the fasting period.
• Give all usual insulin the night before surgery.
• Long-acting (basal) insulin is usually continued at normal times (eg **Glargine**; **Detemir**), even when patients are on a variable rate intravenous insulin infusion (VRIII—previously known as a 'sliding scale' (see BOX 1).
• If on AM list, ensure no subcutaneous rapid-acting (bolus) or mixed insulin is given on the morning of surgery. If PM list, give the normal morning bolus insulin, or half the mixed insulin dose.
• If eating and drinking post-operatively, resume the usual insulin with evening meal. If AM list (or early PM) and eating a late lunch, give half the morning insulin dose with this meal. If not eating until evening, a VRIII may be needed if the capillary glucose readings are high.
• Omit all rapid-acting and mixed insulin whilst the patient is on a VRIII.
• It not eating or drinking post-op, start a VRIII 2 hours prior to surgery. Aim for serum glucose levels of 6-10mmol/L and check finger-prick glucose every 2 hours. When ready to eat, give normal dose of rapid acting or mixed insulin with the 1st meal and stop the VRIII 30-60min later.
• IV fluid is required whilst the patient is on a VRIII: see BOX 1.
• A glucose-potassium-insulin (GKI) infusion can be used as an alternative to a VRIII (see BOX 2), although it is no longer used as standard in the UK.

### Tablet-treated diabetes mellitus
• If diabetes is poorly controlled (eg fasting glucose >10mmol/L), treat as for patients on insulin (above).
• Give usual medications the night before surgery, except long-acting sulfonylureas (eg **glibenclamide**) which can cause prolonged hypoglycaemia when fasting and may need to be substituted 2-3 days pre-operatively. Discuss with the diabetes team.
• If eating and drinking post-operatively: On AM list, omit morning medication and take any missed drugs with lunch, after surgery. If PM list, take normal medications with breakfast, omit midday doses and take any missed drugs with a late lunch. The dose of these may need reducing, depending on dietary intake.
• If not eating or drinking post-op, start a VRIII 2 hours prior to surgery. Once eating and drinking, oral hypoglycaemics can be restarted.
• Some patients may need a phase of subcutaneous insulin following major surgery—refer to the diabetes team if serum glucose levels are persistently raised.
• *Metformin and iodine IV contrast:* Metformin can be continued after IV contrast in patients with normal serum creatinine and/or eGFR >60mL/min.[62] To minimize the risk of nephrotoxicity, if serum creatinine is raised or eGFR <60mL/min, stop metformin for 48h after contrast and check renal function has returned to baseline before restarting.

**Diet-controlled diabetes** There are usually no issues and patients should be treated as if not diabetic (and do not need to be first on the list). Check capillary blood glucose perioperatively. Avoid 5% glucose IV as this increases blood glucose levels.

**Perioperative morbidity and mortality** Diabetes mellitus is classed as in intermediate risk factor for increased perioperative cardiovascular risk by the American Heart Association, so screen for the presence of asymptomatic cardiac and renal disease (p569) and be aware of possible 'silent' myocardial ischaemia.[63] Long-term post-op survival has been found to be poorer for patients with diabetes; however, perioperative cardiovascular morbidity and mortality were only increased in the presence of congestive heart failure and haemodialysis—ie **not** diabetes alone.[64]

### How to write up a variable rate intravenous insulin infusion (VRIII)

*Variable rate intravenous insulin infusion (VRIII)* is more accurate a term than the previously used 'sliding scale'. Prescribe 50 units of short-acting insulin (eg *Actrapid®*) in 50mL of 0.9% saline to infuse at the rate shown in the TABLE below (according to blood glucose levels). NB: this is a guide only—infusions may vary between institutions and no one infusion rate is suitable for all patients. [65]

| Capillary blood glucose (mmol/L) | IV soluble insulin (rate of infusion) |
| --- | --- |
| <4.0 | 0.5 units/h (0.0 if long-acting insulin continued) |
| 4.1-7.0 | 1 unit/h |
| 7.1-9.0 | 2 units/h |
| 9.1-11.0 | 3 units/h |
| 11.1-14.0 | 4 units/h |
| 14.1-17.0 | 5 units/h |
| 17.1-20 | 6 units/h |
| >20 | 6 units/h; request urgent diabetic review |

Fluids should be prescribed to run with the VRIII (through the same cannula via a non-return valve). Ideally use 0.45% sodium chloride with 5% glucose *and* either 0.15% potassium chloride (KCI) (=20mmol/L) or 0.3% KCI (=40mmol/L). This provides a constant supply of substrate, but it is not widely available.

Alternatively, use 10% glucose + KCI. This has a lower risk of hypoglycaemia and hyponatraemia than 5% glucose. If capillary glucose >15mmol/L when starting the VRIII use 0.9% saline until <15mmol/L, then use 10% glucose.

Fluid should infuse at 83-125mL/h (ie 1L over 8-12 hours). Omit potassium if there is renal impairment or hyperkalaemia and slow the rate of infusion in heart failure.

### GKI infusions (glucose, K⁺ and insulin)

Although no longer commonly used in the UK, GKI infusions avoid the risks associated with running IV glucose and IV insulin through separate lines. If one cannula becomes blocked, the patient may become hypo- or hyperglycaemic. Even if glucose and insulin are given through the same cannula via a 3-way converter, this may also become blocked. The syringe driver may retrogradely fill the infusion set with insulin and when the cannula is subsequently resited and the infusion restarted, the patient will receive a large accumulated dose of insulin. This has caused lethal hypoglycaemia. In a GKI infusion, a 500mL bag of 10% glucose ± KCI is given over 6h, with a short-acting insulin (eg *Actrapid®*) added according to blood glucose: [66]

| Blood glucose (mmol/L) | Insulin dose (units/bag) | Serum K⁺ (mmol/L) | KCI to be added (mmol/bag) |
| --- | --- | --- | --- |
| <4 | None | <3 | 20 |
| 4-6 | 5 | 3-5 | 10 |
| 6-10 | 10 | >5 | None |
| 10-20 | 15 | | |
| >20 | 20 | | |

- Check blood glucose every 2h. If levels too high or low, start a new 500mL bag of glucose with the correct insulin dose (aim for 7-10mmol/L).
- GKI infusions are not suitable in poorly controlled diabetes or patients who are very unwell (where close serum glucose monitoring is required).
- If the patient is fluid restricted use 250mL of 20% glucose with the same insulin dose as above. If the patient is hyponatraemic then a concomitant infusion of 0.9% saline should be considered.
- Check U&E daily.
- NB: regimens vary and sometimes more insulin will be required. See *BNF* section 6.1.

Surgery

Operating in patients with obstructive jaundice is best avoided, especially with the availability of ERCP. There is increased risk of perioperative infection, bleeding and renal failure. Prevention of these is key:

**Coagulopathy** Vitamin K is reduced in obstruction as it requires bile in order to be absorbed. If no history of chronic liver disease, give parenteral vitamin K (consider even if clotting is normal). FFP may be required in liver disease or active bleeding.[67]

**Sepsis** Susceptibility to infection is due (in part) to •Increased bacterial translocation •Bacterial colonization of the biliary tree and •Reduced neutrophil function. Patients with cholangitis should be given antibiotics. Antibiotic prophylaxis for ERCP is not recommended unless biliary decompression fails, or there is a history of biliary disorders; liver transplantation; presence of a pancreatic pseudocyst; or neutropenia, in which case give oral *ciprofloxacin* or IV *gentamicin*.[68]

**Renal failure** Patients with obstructive jaundice are prone to developing renal failure post surgery, possibly due to absorption of endotoxin from the intestines (normally limited by the detergent effect of bile). This causes increased renal vasoconstriction and acute tubular necrosis (see hepatorenal syndrome, p259). Limited evidence suggests the use of lactulose or bile salts pre-op may help.[69] Prevention centres around adequate cardiac output achieved by maintenance of blood volume through IV fluids.[70] Ensure plenty of IV fluids pre- and post-operatively to maintain good urine output. Monitor urine output every 2 hours. Consider central line, inotropes and furosemide if urine output is poor despite adequate hydration. Measure U&E daily. Give 20mmol of K⁺ per litre of fluid after 24h post-op if urine output good.

## Surgery in those on steroids

Patients on steroids may not be able to mount an appropriate adrenal response to meet the stress of surgery due to suppression of the hypothalamic-pituitary-adrenal (HPA) axis. Extra corticosteroid cover may be required, depending on the type of surgery. Consider cover for any patient taking >5mg/d of *prednisolone* (or equivalent) for more than 2 weeks or any patient who has had their long-term steroid reduced in the last 2-4 weeks. There is also potential for HPA suppression in patients taking long-term high-dose inhaled or topical corticosteroids. A guide to supplementation is below.[71] Patients should take their normal morning steroid dose.
• *Minor procedures under local anaesthetic:* No supplementation required.
• *Moderate procedures:* (Eg joint replacement) Give 50mg *hydrocortisone* before induction and 25mg every 8h for 24h. Resume normal dose thereafter.
• *Major surgery:* Give 100mg *hydrocortisone* before induction and 50mg every 8h for 24h. After 24h, halve this dose each day until the level of maintenance.
Patients with primary adrenal insufficiency will need extra cover—discuss with an endocrinologist. The major risk with adrenal insufficiency is hypotension, so if this is encountered without an obvious cause, consider a stat dose of hydrocortisone. ►See p846 for treatment of Addisonian crisis and BNF section 6.3 for steroid dose equivalents.

## Surgery in those on anticoagulants

►Inform the surgeon and anaesthetist. *Minor surgery* can be undertaken without stopping *warfarin* (if INR <3.5 it may be safe to proceed).[72] In *major surgery*, drugs may be stopped for 2-5d pre-op. Risks and benefits are individual to each patient, so exact rules are impossible. Discuss these issues when arranging consent. *Vitamin K* ± FFP or *Beriplex®* may be needed for emergency reversal of INR. One elective option is conversion to *heparin* (stop 6h prior to surgery, and monitor APTT perioperatively): unfractionated heparin's short $t\frac{1}{2}$ allows swift reversal with *protamine* (p344).[73] When re-warfarinizing, continue heparin until the INR is therapeutic, as warfarin is prothrombotic in the early stages.

Stopping antiplatelet drugs is a complex business and best discussed with a cardiologist or neurologist. Premature discontinuation of *clopidogrel* in patients with drug-eluting stents can lead to stent thrombosis. The bleeding effects of *aspirin* are reversed 5d after stopping—check with local policy to see if cessation is required.[74]

## Thyroid disease and surgery[75]

Surgery can play a significant role in the management of thyroid disease. Operations include partial lobectomy or lobectomy (for isolated nodules); and thyroidectomy (for thyroid cancers, multinodular goitre or Graves' disease). See also p602.

• *Pre-operative management:*
  • The cause of hyperthyroidsim or swelling should be fully investigated prior to any surgery.
  • Check serum $Ca^{2+}$ (and PTH if abnormal).
  • Arrange laryngoscopy to visualize vocal cords (risk of recurrent laryngeal nerve injury).
  • Treat hyperthyroidism pre-operatively with antithyroid drugs until the patient is euthyroid (p210), eg **carbimazole** up to 20mg/12h PO or **propylthiouracil** 200mg/12h PO. **Potassium iodide** also has a role.
  • **Propranolol** up to 80mg/8h PO can be used to control tachycardia or tremor associated with hyperthyroidism (continue for 5d post-op).

• *Complications of thyroid surgery:* See p582.

▶▶**Thyrotoxic storm** is a rare but potentially fatal consequence of thyroid surgery (mortality 50%). See p845.

The terms 'keyhole surgery' or 'minimal access surgery' may be preferred, because these procedures can be as invasive as any laparotomy, having just the same set of side-effects—plus some new ones. It is the size of the incision and the use of laparoscopes that marks out this branch of surgery. Laparoscopy was developed within gynaecology and is now in widespread use for diagnostic purposes and surgical procedures such as appendicectomy, fundoplication, splenectomy, adrenalectomy, hernia repair, colectomy, prostatectomy and nephrectomy. Minimally invasive surgery is also used for thyroidectomy and parathyroidectomy.

As a rule of thumb, whatever can be done by laparotomy can also be done with the laparoscope. This does not mean that it should be done, but if the patient feels better sooner, has less post-operative pain, can return to work earlier, and has fewer complications, then these specific techniques will gain ascendency. Consider the benefits specific to laparoscopic inguinal hernia repair: post-operative pain is reduced, as is long-term chronic pain. Patients can return to normal activities (including work) sooner and there are fewer wound-related infections and haematomas, as well as a smaller scar. Rates of recurrence are similar to open hernia repair.[76] Laparoscopic repair may also allow diagnosis and repair of a previously undiagnosed contralateral hernia at the same operation. The complications of laparoscopic repair include accidental damage to other intra-abdominal organs and the risk of conversion to open procedure (~5%).[77] In laparoscopic surgery for colorectal cancer, long-term results show no difference in rate of complications or cancer recurrence between open and laparoscopic surgery.[78] Laparoscopic surgery may also have the benefit of a less suppressive effect on the immune system.[79] NB It is worth noting that advantages do not always include time—laparoscopic surgery may take longer than open procedures and set-up costs may be more than for conventional surgery.

### Problems with minimal access surgery:

#### For the surgeon
The 2-dimensional visual representation and different surgical approach alters the normal appearance of familiar anatomy. Palpation is impossible and it may be harder to locate colonic lesions prior to resection. As a result, pre-operative imaging may need to be more extensive. A fundamental problem is that of skill: not just that a new skill has to be learned and taught but that old skills may become attenuated. New surgeons may not achieve optimal skill in either open or laparoscopic surgery if they try to do both.

#### For patients and GPs
• *Post-operative complications:* What may be easily managed on a well-run surgical ward (eg haemorrhage) may be a challenge for a GP and terrify the patient, who may be all alone after early discharge.
• *Loss of tell-tale scars:* Afterwards there may only be a few abdominal wounds, so future carers have to guess at what has been done. The answer here is to communicate carefully with the patient, so that they know what has been done—see BOX 2.

#### For hospitals
Just because minimal access surgery is often cost-effective, it does not follow that hospitals can afford the procedures. Instruments are continuously being refined, and quickly become obsolete—so that many are now produced in disposable single-use form. Because of budgeting boundaries, hospitals cannot use the cash saved, by early return to work or by freeing-up bed space, to pay for capital equipment and extra theatre time that may be required.

See also: *OHClinSurg* p46.

## Who is not suitable for day-case surgery?

Perioperative care has evolved from the inpatient setting, with better results for the patient.[1] Many operations are performed as day-cases. Theoretically any procedure is suitable, provided the time under general anaesthetic does not exceed ~1h. The use of regional anaesthesia helps to avoid the SE of nausea and disorientation that may accompany a general anaesthetic, thus facilitating discharge.

To avoid putting the patient at unnecessary risk, it is important to identify those who are **not** suitable for day-case surgery:
- Severe dementia •Severe learning difficulties •Living alone (and no helpers)
- Children if supervision difficult—changes in expectation, delays and pain relief can be problematic[80] •BMI >32 (p237) •ASA category ≥III (p569) thus potentially unstable comorbidities—discuss with the anaesthetist as category III may be suitable with appropriate optimization •Infection at the site of the operation.

**Exclusions from local regional anaesthesia:** Poor communication (if co-operation required during anaesthetic procedure), severe claustrophobia.

## Discharge checklist for use after day-case surgery ('Leap-frog')

**L**ucid, not vomiting, and cough reflex established.
**E**asy breathing; easy urination.
**A**mbulant without fainting.
**P**ain relief + post-op drugs dispensed and given. Does the patient understand doses?
**F**ollow-up arranged (if required).
**R**hythm, pulse & BP checked: is trend satisfactory? Check no postural drop.
**O**peration site checked and explained to patient.
**G**P letter sent with patient or carer—the GP *must* know what has happened.

## ☼ Exposing patients to our learning curves? The jury is still out...

All surgeons get better over time (for a while), as they perform new techniques with increasing ease and confidence. When Wertheim did his first hysterectomies, his first dozen patients died—but then one survived. He assumed it was a good operation, and pressed ahead. He was a brave man, and thousands of women owe their lives to him. But had he tried to do this today, he would have been stopped. The UK's General Medical Council (GMC) and other august bodies tell us that we must protect the public by reporting doctors whose patients have low survival rates. The reason for this is partly ethical, and partly to preserve self-regulation.

We have the toughest codes of practice and disciplinary procedures of any group of workers. It is assumed that doctors are loyal to each other out of self-interest, and that this loyalty is bad. This has never been tested formally, and is not evidence-based. We can imagine two clinical worlds: one of constant 'reportings' and recriminatory audits, and another of trust and team-work. Both are imperfect, but we should not assume that the first world would be better for our patients.

When patients are sick with fear, they do not, perhaps, want to know everything. We may tell to protect ourselves. We may **not** tell to protect ourselves. Perhaps what we should do is, in our hearts, appeal to those 12 dead women-of-Wertheim—a jury as infallible as sacrificial—and try to hear their reply. And to those who complain that in doing so we are playing God, it is possible to reply with some humility that, whatever it is, it does not seem like play.

*"It is amazing what little harm doctors do when one considers all the opportunities they have"* M. Twain.

1 Advantages: shorter waiting lists, fewer infections, fewer days off work, and ↑patient satisfaction.[11]

▶Examine the regional lymph nodes as well as the lump. If the lump is a node, examine its area of drainage. Always examine the circulation & nerve supply distal to any lump.

**History** How long has it been there? Does it hurt? Any other symptoms, eg itch? Any other lumps? Is it getting bigger? Ever been abroad? Otherwise well?

**Physical exam** Remember the 6 S's: site, size, shape, smoothness (consistency), surface (contour/edge/colour), and surroundings. *Other questions:* Does it transilluminate (see below)? Is it fixed/tethered to skin or underlying structures (see BOX)? Is it fluctuant/compressible? Temperature? Tender? Pulsatile (US duplex may help)?

**Transilluminable lumps** After eliminating as much external light as possible, place a bright, thin 'pen' torch on the lump, from behind (or at least to the side), so the light is shining through the lump towards your eye. If the lump glows red it is said to transilluminate—a fluid-filled lump such as a hydrocele is a good example.

**Lipomas** These benign fatty lumps, occurring wherever fat can expand (ie **not** scalp or palms), have smooth, imprecise margins, a hint of fluctuance, and are not fixed to skin or deeper structures. Symptoms are only caused via pressure. Malignant change very rare (suspect if rapid growth/hardening/vascularization). Multiple scattered lipomas, which may be painful, occur in Dercum's disease, typically in postmenopausal women.[82]

**Sebaceous cysts** Refer to either *epidermal* (fig 1) or *pilar cysts* (they are not of sebaceous origin and contain keratin, not sebum). They appear as firm, round, mobile subcutaenous nodules of varying size. Look for the characteristic central punctum. Infection is quite common, and foul pus exits through the punctum. They are common on the scalp, face, neck and trunk. *Treatment:* Excision of cyst and contents.

**Lymph nodes** Causes of enlargement: *Infection:* Glandular fever; brucellosis; TB; HIV; toxoplasmosis; actinomycosis; syphilis. *Infiltration:* Malignancy (carcinoma, lymphoma); sarcoidosis.

**Cutaneous abscesses** Staphylococci are the most common organisms. Haemolytic streptococci only common in hand infections. *Proteus* is a common cause of nonstaphylococcal axillary abscesses. Below the waist faecal organisms are common (aerobes & anaerobes). *Treatment:* Incise and drain. *Boils (furuncles)* are abscesses involving a hair follicle and associated glands. A *carbuncle* is an area of subcutaneous necrosis which discharges itself on to the surface through multiple sinuses. Think of *hidradenitis suppurativa* if recurrent inguinal or axillary abscesses.

**Rheumatoid nodules** (fig 2) are collagenous granulomas which appear in established rheumatoid arthritis on the extensor aspects of joints—especially the elbows (fig 2).

**Ganglia** Degenerative cysts from an adjacent joint or synovial sheath commonly seen on the dorsum of the wrist or hand and dorsum of the foot. May transilluminate. 50% disappear spontaneously. Aspiration may be effective, especially when combined with instillation of steroid and *hyaluronidase*.[83] For the rest, treatment of choice is excision rather than the traditional blow from your bible (the *Oxford Textbook of Surgery*!). See fig 3.

**Fibromas** These may occur anywhere in the body, but most commonly under the skin. These whitish, benign tumours contain collagen, fibroblasts, and fibrocytes.

**Dermoid cysts** Contain dermal structures and are found at the junction of embryonic cutaneous boundaries, eg in the midline or lateral to the eye.

**Malignant tumours of connective tissue** Fibrosarcomas, liposarcomas, leiomyosarcomas (smooth muscle), and rhabdomyosarcomas (striated muscle). These are staged using modified TNM system including tumour grade. Needle-core (Trucut®) biopsies of large tumours precede excision. Any lesion suspected of being a sarcoma should not be simply enucleated. ▶Refer to a specialist.

**Neurofibromas** See p518.

**Keloids** Caused by irregular hypertrophy of vascularized collagen forming raised edges at sites of previous scars that extend outside the scar (fig 4). Common in dark skin. Treatment can be difficult. Intralesional steroid injections are a mainstay.

## In or under the skin?

| Intradermal | Subcutaneous |
|---|---|
| • Sebaceous cyst | • Lipoma |
| • Abscess | • Ganglion |
| • Dermoid cyst | • Neuroma |
| • Granuloma | • Lymph node |

If a lump is intradermal, you cannot draw the skin over it, while if the lump is subcutaneous you should be able to manipulate it independently from the skin.

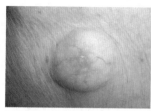

**Fig 1.** Epidermal cyst.
Courtesy of DermNetNZ, the web pages of the New Zealand Dermatological Society Inc. www.dermnetnz.org.

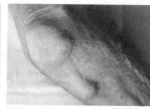

**Fig 2.** Rheumatoid nodule.
Courtesy of DermNetNZ, the web pages of the New Zealand Dermatological Society Inc. www.dermnetnz.org.

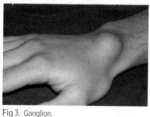

**Fig 3.** Ganglion.
Courtesy of John M Erikson, MD, Raleigh Hand Centre.

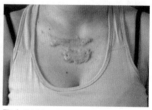

**Fig 4.** Keloid scar.
Courtesy of East Sussex Hospitals Trust.

**Malignant tumours**

1 *Malignant melanoma* ♀:♂ ≈ 1.3:1. UK incidence: ≥10:100,000/yr (up ≥200% in last 20yrs). Commonly affects younger patients ∴ early diagnosis is vital. Short periods of intense UV exposure is a major cause, particularly in the early years. May occur in pre-existing moles. If smooth, well-demarcated and regular, it is unlikely to be a melanoma but diagnosis can be tricky so ►if in doubt, refer. Refer if there are ≥3 points on the Glasgow scale, or with 1 point if suspicious.[84] See fig 1.

| Major (2 pts each) | Minor (1 pt each) | Less helpful signs |
|---|---|---|
| • Change in size | • Inflammation, crusting, or bleeding | • Asymmetry |
| • Change in shape | • Sensory change | • Irregular colour |
| • Change in colour | • Diameter >7mm (unless growth is in the vertical plane: beware) | • Elevation |
| | | • Irregular border |

**Superficial spreading melanomas** (70%) grow slowly, metastasize later and have better prognosis than **nodular melanomas** (10-15%) which invade deeply and metastasize early. Nodular lesions may be amelanotic in ~5%. *Others:* **Acral melanomas** occur on palms, soles and subungual areas (there is equal frequency amongst black patients and white patients); **Lentigo maligna melanoma** evolves from pre-existing lentigo maligna. Breslow thickness (depth in mm), tumour stage and presence of ulceration are important prognostic factors.[85] *℞:* Urgent excision can be curative. Chemotherapy gives a response in 10-30% with metastatic disease (*OHCS* p592).

2 *Squamous cell cancer* Usually presents as an ulcerated lesion, with hard, raised edges, on sun-exposed sites. May begin in solar keratoses (below), or be found on the lips of smokers or in long-standing ulcers (=Marjolin's ulcer). Metastasis to lymph nodes is rare, local destruction may be extensive. *℞:* Excision + radiotherapy to treat recurrence/affected nodes. See fig 2. NB: the condition may be confused with a keratoacanthoma—a fast-growing, benign, self-limiting papule plugged with keratin.

3 *Basal cell carcinoma* (aka **rodent ulcer**) **Nodular:** Typically a pearly nodule with rolled telangiectatic edge, on the face or a sun-exposed site. May have a central ulcer. See fig 3. Metastases are very rare. It slowly causes local destruction if left untreated. **Superficial:** Lesions appear as red scaly plaques with a raised smooth edge, often on the trunk or shoulders. *Cause:* (most frequently) UV exposure. *℞:* Excision; cryotherapy; for superficial BCCs topical flurouracil or imiquimod (see below).

**Pre-malignant tumours**

1 *Solar (actinic) keratoses* appear on sun-exposed skin as crumbly, yellow-white crusts. Malignant change to squamous cell carcinoma may occur after several years. *Treatment:* Cryotherapy; 5% *fluorouracil* cream or 5% *imiquimod*—these work by causing: erythema → vesiculation → erosion → ulceration → necrosis → healing epithelialization, leaving healthy skin unharmed. Warn patients of the expected inflammatory reaction. See *BNF* for dosing regimens. Alternatively try diclofenac gel (3%; Solaraze®, use thinly twice-daily for ≤90d).

2 *Bowen's disease* Slow-growing red/brown scaly plaque, eg on lower legs. *Histology:* Full-thickness dysplasia (carcinoma *in situ*). It infrequently progresses to squamous cell cancer. Penile Bowen's disease is called Queyrat's erythroplasia. *Treatment:* Cryotherapy, topical *fluorouracil* (see above) or photodynamic therapy.

3 *See also* Kaposi's sarcoma (p716); Paget's disease of the breast (p722).

**Others** •*Secondary carcinoma* Most common metastases to skin are from breast, kidney, or lung. Usually a firm nodule, most often on the scalp. See also acanthosis nigricans (p564) •*Mycosis fungoides* Cutaneous T-cell lymphoma usually confined to skin. Causes itchy, red plaques (Sézary syndrome-variant also associated with erythroderma) •*Leucoplakia* This appears as white patches (which may fissure) on oral or genital mucosa (where it may itch). Frank carcinomatous change may occur •*Leprosy* Suspect in any anaesthetic hypopigmented lesion (p428) •*Syphilis* Any genital ulcer is syphilis until proved otherwise. Secondary syphilis: papular rash—including, unusually, on the palms[1] (p431).

1 *Other palm rashes:* Stevens-Johnson syn.; hand, foot & mouth dis.; palmar erythema; palmoplantar pustulosis.

| **ABCDE** criteria for diagnosis of melanoma |
| :-- |
| **A**symmetry<br>**B**order—irregular<br>**C**olour—non-uniform<br>**D**iameter >7mm<br>**E**levation |

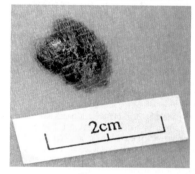

Fig 1. Melanoma.

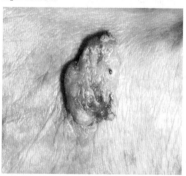

Fig 2. Squamous cell cancer.

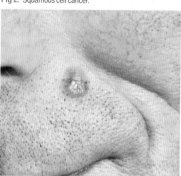

Fig 3. Basal cell carcinoma (BCC).

Surgery

▶ Don't biopsy lumps until tumours within the head and neck have been excluded by an ENT surgeon. Culture all biopsied lymph nodes for TB.

**Diagnosis** First, ask how long the lump has been present. If <3wks, self-limiting infection is the likely cause and extensive investigation is unwise. Next ask yourself where the lump is. Is it intradermal—eg sebaceous cyst with a central punctum (p596)? Is it a lipoma (p596)? If the lump is not intradermal, and is not of recent onset, you are about to start a diagnostic hunt over complicated terrain. 85% of neck swellings are lymph nodes (examine areas which they serve). Consider TB, viruses such as HIV or EBV (infectious mononucleosis), any chronic infection or, if >20yrs, consider lymphoma (hepatosplenomegaly?) or metastases (eg from GI or bronchial or head and neck neoplasia[1]), 8% are goitres (p602), and other diagnoses account for 7%.

**Tests** Ultrasound shows lump consistency: cystic, solid, complex, vascular. CT defines masses in relation to their anatomical neighbours. Do virology and Mantoux test. CXR may show malignancy or, in sarcoid, reveal bilateral hilar lymphadenopathy. Consider fine-needle aspiration (FNA).

**Midline lumps:** •If patient is <20yrs old, likely diagnosis is *dermoid cyst* (p596). •If it moves up on tongue protrusion and is below the hyoid, likely to be a *thyroglossal cyst*, a fluid-filled sac resulting from incomplete closure of the thyroid's migration path. ℞: surgery; they are the commonest congenital cervical cystic lump. •If >20yrs old, it is probably a *thyroid isthmus* mass. •If it is bony hard, the diagnosis may be a *chondroma* (benign cartilaginous tumour).

**Submandibular triangle:** (Bordered by the mental process, mandible, and the line between the two angles of the mandible.) •If <20yrs, self-limiting lymphadenopathy is likely. If >20yrs, exclude *malignant lymphadenopathy* (eg firm and non-tender). ▶ Is TB likely? •If it is not a node, think of submandibular *salivary stone*, *sialadenitis*, or *tumour* (see BOX for *Salivary gland pathology*).

**Anterior triangle:** (Between midline, anterior border of sternocleidomastoid, and the line between the two angles of the mandible.) •*Branchial cysts* emerge under the anterior border of sternocleidomastoid where the upper third meets the middle third (age <20yrs). Due to non-disappearance of the cervical sinus (where 2nd branchial arch grows down over 3rd and 4th). Lined by squamous epithelium, their fluid contains cholesterol crystals. Treat by excision. There may be communication with the pharynx in the form of a fistula •If lump in the supero-posterior area of the anterior triangle, is it a *parotid tumour* (more likely if >40yrs)? •*Laryngoceles* are an uncommon cause of anterior triangle lumps. They are painless and may be made worse by blowing. These cysts are classified as external, internal, or mixed, and may be associated with laryngeal cancer. If pulsatile may be: •*Carotid artery aneurysm*, •*Tortuous carotid artery*, or •*Carotid body tumours* (chemodectoma). These are very rare, move from side to side but not up and down, and splay out the carotid bifurcation. They are usually firm and occasionally soft and pulsatile. They do not usually cause bruits. They may be bilateral, familial, and malignant (5%). Suspect in any mass just anterior to the upper third of sternomastoid. Diagnose by duplex USS (splaying at the carotid bifurcation) or digital computer angiography. ℞: Extirpation by vascular surgeon.

**Posterior triangle:** (Behind sternocleidomastoid, in front of trapezius, above clavicle.) •*Cervical ribs* may intrude into this area. These are enlarged costal elements from C7 vertebra. The majority are asymptomatic but can cause Raynaud's syndrome by compressing subclavian artery and neurological symptoms (eg wasting of 1st dorsal interosseous) from pressure on lower trunk of the brachial plexus. •*Pharyngeal pouches* can protrude into the posterior triangle on swallowing (usually left-sided). •*Cystic hygromas* (usually infants) arise from jugular lymph sac. These macrocystic lymphatic malformations transilluminate brightly. Treat by surgery or hypertonic saline sclerosant injection. Recurrence can be troublesome. •*Pancoast's tumour* (see p722). •*Subclavian artery aneurysm* will be pulsatile.

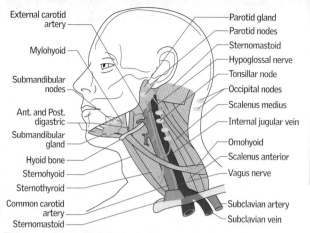

Fig 1. Important structures in the head and neck.

Labels — External carotid artery, Mylohyoid, Submandibular nodes, Ant. and Post. digastric, Submandibular gland, Hyoid bone, Sternohyoid, Sternothyroid, Common carotid artery, Sternomastoid; Parotid gland, Parotid nodes, Sternomastoid, Hypoglossal nerve, Tonsillar node, Occipital nodes, Scalenus medius, Internal jugular vein, Omohyoid, Scalenus anterior, Vagus nerve, Subclavian artery, Subclavian vein.

## Salivary gland pathology

There are 3 pairs of major salivary glands: parotid, submandibular, and sublingual (there are many minor glands). *History:* Lumps; swelling related to food; pain. *Examination:* Note external swelling; look for secretions; bimanual palpation for stones. Examine VII$^{th}$ nerve and regional lymph nodes. *Cytology:* This may be ascertained by FNA.

*Acute swelling* Think of mumps and HIV. *Recurrent unilateral pain and swelling* is likely to be from a stone. 80% are submandibular. The classical story is of pain and swelling on eating—with a red, tender, swollen, but uninfected gland. The stone may be seen on plain x-ray or by sialography (fig 2). Distal stones are removed via the mouth but deeper stones may require excision of the gland. *Chronic bilateral symptoms* may coexist with dry eyes and mouth and autoimmune disease, eg hypothyroidism, Mikulicz's or Sjögren's syndrome (p720 & p724)—also bulimia. *Fixed swelling* may be from a tumour/ALL (fig 5, p349), sarcoid, amyloid, Wegener's syndrome, or be idiopathic.

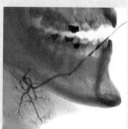

Fig 2. Normal sialogram of the submandibular gland. Wharton's (submandibular) duct opens into the mouth near the frenulum of the tongue.

**Salivary gland tumours** '80% are in the parotid, 80% of these are pleomorphic adenomas, 80% of these are in the superficial lobe.' Deflection of the ear outwards is a classic sign. ►Remove any salivary gland swelling for assessment if present for >1 month. VII$^{th}$ nerve palsy means malignancy.

| Benign or malignant | Malignant | Malignant |
|---|---|---|
| Cystadenolymphoma | Mucoepidermoid | Squamous or adeno ca |
| Pleomorphic adenoma | Acinic cell | Adenoid cystic ca |

Pleomorphic adenomas often present in middle age and grow slowly. Remove by superficial parotidectomy. Adenolymphomas (Warthin's tumour): usually older men; soft; treat by enucleation. Carcinomas: rapid growth; hard fixed mass; pain; facial palsy. Treatment: surgery + radiotherapy.

601

Surgery

If the thyroid is enlarged (=goitre), ask yourself: 1 Is the thyroid diffusely enlarged or nodular? 2 Is the patient euthyroid, thyrotoxic (p210), or hypothyroid (p212)?

**Diffuse goitre:** *Causes:* Endemic (iodine deficiency); congenital; secondary to goitrogens (substances that ↓ iodine uptake); acute thyroiditis (de Quervain's); physiological (pregnancy/puberty); autoimmune (Graves' disease; Hashimoto's thyroiditis).

**Nodular goitre:** •*Multinodular goitre (MNG):* The most common goitre in the UK. 50% who present with a single nodule actually have MNG. Patients are usually euthyroid, but may become hyperthyroid ('toxic'). MNG may be retro- or substernal. Hypothyroidism and malignancy within MNG are rare. Plummer's disease is hyperthyroidism with a single toxic nodule (uncommon). •*Fibrotic goitre:* Eg Riedel's thyroiditis. •*Solitary thyroid nodule:* See MINIBOX; ~10% are malignant.

**Investigations** •Do T₃, T₄ and TSH •Thyroid autoantibodies (p208, eg if Hashimoto's/Graves suspected) •CXR with thoracic inlet view (tracheal goitres and metastases?) •USS (solid, cystic, complex or part of a group of lumps) •Radionuclide scans may show malignant lesions as hypofunctioning or 'cold', whereas a hyperfunctioning 'hot' lesion suggests adenoma •FNA (fine-needle aspiration) and cytology on the fluid. ►No clinical/lab test good enough to tell for sure if follicular neoplasms found on FNA are benign, so refer for surgery.[86]

| Single thyroid nodule |
| --- |
| • Cyst |
| • Adenoma |
| • Malignancy |
| • Discrete nodule in multinodular goitre |

**What should you do if high-resolution ultrasound shows impalpable nodules?**
Such thyroid nodules can usually be observed provided they are:
• <1cm across (which accounts for most; ultrasound can detect lumps <2mm; such 'incidentalomas' occur in 46% of routine autopsies) and are asymptomatic.
• There is no past history of thyroid cancer or radiation.
• No family history of medullary cancer (if present, do USS-guided FNA).

**Thyroid cancer**[87]
1 *Papillary:* (60%). Often in younger patients. Spread: lymph nodes & lung (jugulo-digastric node metastasis is the so-called lateral aberrant thyroid). R̩: total thyroidectomy to remove non-obvious tumour ± node excision ± radioiodine (¹³¹I) to ablate residual cells. Give thyroxine to suppress TSH. Prognosis: better if young & ♀.

2 *Follicular:* (≤25%). Occur in middle-age & spreads early via blood (bone, lungs). Well-differentiated. R̩: total thyroidectomy + T₄ suppression + radioiodine ablation.

3 *Medullary:* (5%). Sporadic (80%) or part of MEN syndrome (p215). May produce calcitonin which can be used as a tumour marker. They do not concentrate iodine. ►Perform a phaeochromocytoma screen pre-op. R̩: thyroidectomy + node clearance. External beam radiotherapy should be considered to prevent regional recurrence.

4 *Lymphoma:* (5%). ♀:♂≈3:1. May present with stridor or dysphagia. Do full staging pre-treatment (chemoradiotherapy). Assess histology for mucosa-associated lymphoid tissue (MALT) origin (associated with a good prognosis).

5 *Anaplastic:* Rare. ♀:♂≈3:1. Elderly, poor response to any treatment. In the absence of unresectable disease, excision + radiotherapy may be tried.

**Thyroid surgery** *Indications:* Pressure symptoms, relapse hyperthyroidism after >1 failed course of drug treatment, carcinoma, cosmetic reasons, symptomatic patients planning pregnancy. Render euthyroid pre-op with antithyroid drugs (but stop 10 days prior to surgery as these increase vascularity). Check vocal cords by indirect laryngoscopy pre- and post-op.

**Complications:** See also p582. *Early:* Recurrent laryngeal nerve palsy; haemorrhage ►►if compresses airway, instantly remove sutures for evacuation of clot; hypoparathyroidism (check plasma Ca²⁺ daily; there is commonly a transient drop in serum concentration); ►►thyroid storm (symptoms of severe hyperthyroidism—see p844). *Late:* Hypothyroidism; recurrent hyperthyroidism.

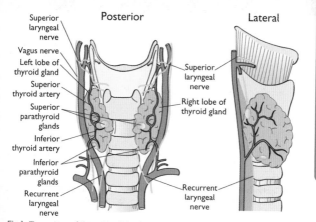

Posterior

Lateral

Superior laryngeal nerve

Vagus nerve

Left lobe of thyroid gland

Superior thyroid artery

Superior parathyroid glands

Inferior thyroid artery

Inferior parathyroid glands

Recurrent laryngeal nerve

Superior laryngeal nerve

Right lobe of thyroid gland

Recurrent laryngeal nerve

Surgery

**Fig 1.** The anatomy of the region of the thyroid gland. The important structures that must be considered when operating on the thyroid gland include:
- Recurrent laryngeal nerve
- Superior laryngeal nerve
- Parathyroid glands
- Trachea
- Common carotid artery
- Internal jugular vein (not depicted—see fig 3).

Uptake ratio is 6 : 1

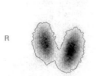
R          L

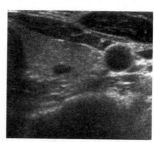

**Fig 2.** Radionuclide study of the thyroid showing changes consistent with Graves' disease (see also *hot and cold nodules* (p209) and *nuclear medicine*, p752). There is increased uptake of the radionuclide trace diffusely throughout both lobes of the gland (uptake ratio =6:1).

Image courtesy of Norwich Radiology Department.

**Fig 3.** Transverse ultrasound of the left lobe of the thyroid showing a small low-reflectivity cyst within higher-reflectivity thyroid tissue. Note the proximity to the gland of the common carotid artery and internal jugular vein (the latter compressed slightly by pressure from the probe), both seen beneath the body of sterno-cleidomastoid muscle.

Image courtesy of Norwich Radiology Department.

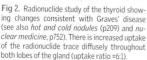

Surgery

**Epidemiology** Affects 1 in 9 ♀; ~40,000 new cases per year in UK (incidence increasing). Rare in men (~1% of all breast cancers).

**Risk factors** Risk is related to family history, age and uninterrupted oestrogen exposure, hence: nulliparity; 1st pregnancy >30yrs old, early menarche; late menopause; HRT; obesity; BRCA genes (p524); not breastfeeding; past breast cancer (metachronous rate ≈2%, synchronous rate ≈1%).

**Pathology** Non-invasive ductal carcinoma-*in-situ* (DCIS) is premalignant and seen as microcalcification on mammography (unifocal or widespread). Non-invasive lobular CIS is rarer and tends to be multifocal. Invasive ductal carcinoma is most common (~70%) whereas invasive lobular carcinoma accounts for 10-15% of breast cancers. Medullary cancers (~5%) tend to affect younger patients while colloid/mucoid (~2%) tend to affect the elderly. Others: papillary, tubular, adenoid-cystic and Paget's (p722). 60-70% of breast cancers are oestrogen receptor +ve, conveying better prognosis. ~30% over-express HER2 (growth factor receptor gene) associated with aggressive disease and poorer prognosis.

**Investigations** (See p66 for history & examination.) ▶All lumps should undergo *'triple' assessment:* Clinical examination + histology/cytology + mammography/ultrasound; see fig 1.

**Staging**: *Stage 1:* Confined to breast, mobile *Stage 2:* Growth confined to breast, mobile, lymph nodes in ipsilateral axilla *Stage 3:* Tumour fixed to muscle (but not chest wall), ipsilateral lymph nodes matted and may be fixed, skin involvement larger than tumour *Stage 4:* Complete fixation of tumour to chest wall, distant metastases. Also TNM staging: (p527) T1<2cm, T2 2-5cm, T3 >5cm, T4 Fixity to chest wall or *peau d'orange*; N1 Mobile ipsilateral nodes; N2 Fixed nodes; M1 Distant metastases.

**Treating stage 1-2 cancer** •*Surgery:* Removal of tumour by wide local excision (WLE) or mastectomy ± breast reconstruction + axillary node sampling/surgical clearance or sentinel node biopsy (BOX). •*Radiotherapy:* Recommended for all patients with invasive cancer after WLE. Risk of recurrence decreases from 30% to <10% at 10yrs and increases overall survival.[88] Axillary radiotherapy used if lymph node +ve on sampling and surgical clearance not performed (↑ risk of lymphoedema and brachial plexopathy). SE: pneumonitis, pericarditis and rib fractures. •*Chemotherapy:* Adjuvant chemotherapy improves survival & reduces recurrence in most groups of women (consider in all except excellent prognosis patients), eg epirubicin + 'CMF' (cyclophosphamide + methotrexate + 5-FU). Neoadjuvant chemotherapy has shown no difference in survival but may facilitate breast-conserving surgery. •*Endocrine agents:* Aim to ↓oestrogen activity and are used in oestrogen receptor (ER) or progesterone receptor (PR) +ve disease. The ER blocker *tamoxifen* is widely used, eg 20mg/d PO for 5yrs post-op (may rarely cause uterine cancer so warn to report vaginal bleeding).[89] Aromatase inhibitors (eg *anastrozole*) targeting peripheral oestrogen synthesis are also used (may be better tolerated). They are only used if post-menopausal. If pre-menopausal and an ER+ve tumour, ovarian ablation (via surgery or radiotherapy) or GnRH analogues (eg *goserelin*) ↓recurrence and ↑survival. •*Support:* Breastcare nurses •*Reconstruction options:* eg tissue expanders/implants, latissimus dorsi flap, TRAM (transverse rectus abdominis myocutaneous) flap.

**Treating distant disease** (Stage 3-4) Long-term survival is possible and median survival is >2yrs. Staging investigations should include CXR, bone scan, liver USS, CT/ MRI or PET-CT (p752) + LFTs and Ca²⁺. Radiotherapy (p530) to painful bony lesions (*bisphosphonates*, p696, may ↓pain and fracture risk). *Tamoxifen* is often used in ER+ve; if relapse after initial success, consider chemotherapy. *Trastuzumab* should be given for HER2 +ve tumours, in combination with chemotherapy. CNS surgery for solitary (or easily accessible) metastases may be possible; if not—radiotherapy. Get specialist help for arm lymphoedema (try decongestive methods first).[NICE]

**Preventing deaths** •Promote awareness •*Screening:* 2-view mammography every 3yrs for women aged 47-73 in UK has ↓breast cancer deaths by 30% in women >50yrs.

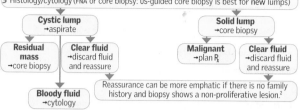

Fig 1. Triple assessment and investigation of a breast lump.

## Sentinel node biopsy

Decreases needless axillary clearances in lymph node -ve patients.[90]
• Patent blue dye and/or radiocolloid injected into periareolar area or tumour.
• A gamma probe/visual inspection is used to identify the sentinel node.
• The sentinel node is biopsied and sent for histology ± immunohistochemistry.
Trials suggest sentinel node identified in 90% of patients. False-negative rates are 9-14% (drop to <5% as surgeons become more experienced).

## Prognostic factors in breast cancer

Tumour size, grade, lymph node status, ER/PR status, presence of vascular invasion all help assess prognosis. Nottingham Prognostic Index (NPI) is widely used to predict survival and risk of relapse, and to help select appropriate adjuvant systemic therapy:[3] NPI = *0.2 × tumour size (cm) + histological grade + nodal status*.
If treated with surgery alone, 10yr survival rates are: NPI <2.4: 95%; NPI 2.4-3.4: 85%; NPI 3.4-4.4: 70%; NPI 4.4-5.4: 50%; NPI >5.4: 20%.

## Benign breast disease[91]

*Fibroadenoma:* Usually presents <30yrs but can occur up to menopause. Benign overgrowth of collagenous mesenchyme of one breast lobule. Firm, smooth, mobile lump. Painless. May be multiple. ⅓ regress, ⅓ stay the same, ⅓ get bigger. R: Observation and reassurance, but if in doubt refer for USS (usually conclusive) ± FNA. Surgical excision if large.

*Breast cysts:* Common >35yrs, esp. perimenopausal. Benign, fluid-filled rounded lump. Not fixed to surrounding tissue. Occasionally painful. R: Diagnosis confirmed on aspiration (perform only if trained).

*Infective mastitis/breast abscesses:* Infection of mammary duct often associated with lactation (usually *S. aureus*). Abscess presents as painful hot swelling of breast segment. R: Antibiotics. Open incision or percutaneous drainage if abscess.

*Duct ectasia:* Typically around menopause. Ducts become blocked and secretions stagnate. Present with nipple discharge (green/brown/bloody) ± nipple retraction ± lump. Refer for confirmation of diagnosis. Usually no R needed.

*Fat necrosis:* Fibrosis and calcification after injury to breast tissue. Scarring results in a firm lump. Refer for triple assessment. No R once diagnosis confirmed.

1 US is more accurate at detecting invasive breast cancer, though mammography remains most accurate at detecting ductal carcinoma *in situ* (DCIS). MRI is used in the assessment of multifocal/bilateral disease and patients with cosmetic implants who are identified as high risk.
2 There is a relatively ↑risk of malignancy if there is atypical hyperplasia or a proliferative lesion.[92]
3 Nodal status is scored 1-3: 1 = node -ve; 2 = 1-3 nodes +ve; 3 = >3 nodes +ve for breast cancer. Histological grade is also scored 1-3.

As with any mass (see p596), determine size, site, shape, and surface. Find out if it is pulsatile and if it is mobile. Examine supraclavicular and inguinal nodes. Is the lump ballotable (like bobbing an apple up and down in water)?

**Right iliac fossa masses:**

| | | |
|---|---|---|
| • Appendix mass/abscess | • Intussusception | • Transplanted kidney |
| • Caecal carcinoma | • TB mass | • Kidney malformation |
| • Crohn's disease | • Amoebic abscess | • Tumour in an |
| • Pelvic mass (see below) | • Actinomycosis (p421) | undescended testis |

**Abdominal distension** Flatus, fat, fluid, faeces, or fetus (p57)? Fluid may be outside the gut (ascites) or sequestered in bowel (obstruction; ileus). To demonstrate ascites elicit signs of a fluid thrill and/or shifting dullness (p60).

| Causes of ascites: | | Ascites with portal hypertension: | |
|---|---|---|---|
| • Malignancy* | • CCF; pericarditis | • Cirrhosis | • Portal nodes |
| • Infections*—esp TB | • Pancreatitis* | • Budd-Chiari syndrome* (p710) | |
| • ↓Albumin (eg nephrosis) | • Myxoedema | • IVC or portal vein thrombosis | |

*Tests:* Aspirate ascitic fluid (paracentesis, p778-779) for cytology, culture, and protein level (≥30g/L in diseases marked*); ultrasound.

**Left upper quadrant mass** Is it spleen, stomach, kidney, colon, pancreas, or a rare cause (eg neurofibroma)? Pancreatic cysts may be true (congenital; cystadenomas; retention cysts of chronic pancreatitis; cystic fibrosis) or pseudocysts (fluid in lesser sac from acute pancreatitis).

**Splenomegaly** Causes are often said to be infective, haematological, neoplastic, etc, but grouping by associated feature is more useful clinically:

| Splenomegaly with fever | With lymphadenopathy | With purpura |
|---|---|---|
| • Infection[HS] (malaria, SBE/IE hepatitis,[HS] EBV,[HS] TB, CMV, HIV) | • Glandular fever[HS] | • Septicaemia; typhus |
| • Sarcoid; malignancy[HS] | • Leukaemias; lymphoma | • DIC; amyloid[HS] |
| | • Sjögren's syndrome | • Meningococcaemia |
| **With arthritis** | **With ascites** | **With a murmur** |
| • Sjögren's syndrome | • Carcinoma | • SBE/IE |
| • Rheumatoid arthritis; SLE | • Portal hypertension[HS] | • Rheumatic fever |
| • Infection, eg Lyme (p430) | | • Hypereosinophilia |
| • Vasculitis/Behçet's (p558) | | • Amyloid[HS] (p364) |
| **With anaemia** | **With weight↓ + CNS signs** | **Massive splenomegaly** |
| • Sickle-cell;[HS] thalassaemia[HS] | • Cancer; lymphoma | • Malaria (hyper-reactivity after chronic exposure) |
| • Leishmaniasis;[HS] leukaemia[HS] | • TB; arsenic poisoning | • Myelofibrosis; CML[HS] |
| • Pernicious anaemia (p328) | • Paraproteinaemia[HS] | • Gaucher's syndrome[HS] |
| • POEMS syn. (p212) | | • Leishmaniasis |

HS=causes of hepatosplenomegaly.

**Smooth hepatomegaly** Hepatitis, CCF, sarcoidosis, early alcoholic cirrhosis (a small liver is typical later; tricuspid incompetence (→ pulsatile liver).

**Craggy hepatomegaly** Secondaries or 1° hepatoma. (Nodular cirrhosis typically causes a small, shrunken liver, not an enlarged craggy one.)

**Pelvic masses** *Is it truly pelvic?*—Yes, if by palpation you cannot get 'below it'.

**Investigating lumps** There is much to be said for performing an early CT to save time and money compared with leaving the test to be the last in a long chain. If unavailable, *ultrasound* is the first test (transvaginal approach may be useful). *Others:* IVU; liver and spleen radioisotope scans; Mantoux test (p398). Routine tests: FBC (with film); ESR; U&E; LFT; proteins; Ca²⁺; CXR; AXR; biopsy—a tissue diagnosis may be made using a fine needle guided by ultrasound or CT control. MRI also has a role.

| Pelvic masses |
|---|
| • Fibroids |
| • Fetus |
| • Bladder |
| • Ovarian cysts or malignancies |

Surgery

## ☺ The first successful laparotomy...

In 1809 an American surgeon by the name of Ephraim McDowell performed an astonishing operation: the first successful elective laparotomy for an abdominal tumour. It was an ovariotomy for an ovarian mass in a 44-year-old who, prior to physical examination by McDowell, was believed to be gravid. Not only was this feat performed in the age before anaesthesia and antisepsis, but it was also performed on a table in the front room of McDowell's Kentucky home, at that time on the frontier of the West in the United States. His account of the operation makes fascinating reading.[93] Whilst the strength of his diagnostic convictions combined with his speed and skill at operating is to be admired (the operation took 25 minutes), there is an even more laudable part played in this story. The patient, Mrs Jane Todd-Crawford, was fully willing to be involved with what can only be described as experimental surgery in the face of uncertainty. She defied pain simply by reciting psalms and hymns, and was back at home within 4 weeks with no complications. We would be well served in remembering the commitment of Mrs Todd-Crawford as most exceptional. In the rush and hurry of our daily tasks perhaps it is all to easy to forget that the undertaking of surgery today may be no less fear-provoking for patients than it was 200 years ago.

Surgery

Someone who becomes acutely ill and in whom symptoms and signs are chiefly related to the abdomen has an acute abdomen. Prompt laparotomy is sometimes essential: repeated examination is the key to making the decision.

## Clinical syndromes that usually require laparotomy

**1** *Rupture of an organ* (Spleen, aorta, ectopic pregnancy) Shock is a leading sign—see TABLE for assessment of blood loss. Abdominal swelling may be seen. Any history of trauma: blunt trauma → spleen; penetrating trauma → liver. Delayed rupture of the spleen may occur weeks after trauma. Peritonism may be mild.

**2** *Peritonitis* (Perforation of peptic ulcer/duodenal ulcer, diverticulum, appendix, bowel, or gallbladder) Signs: prostration, shock, lying still, +ve cough test (p62), tenderness (± rebound/percussion pain, p62), board-like abdominal rigidity, guarding, and no bowel sounds. Erect CXR may show gas under the diaphragm (fig 2). NB: acute pancreatitis (p638) causes these signs, but does **not** require a laparotomy so don't be caught out and ►*always check serum amylase*.

## Syndromes that may not require a laparotomy

*Local peritonitis:* Eg diverticulitis, cholecystitis, salpingitis, and appendicitis (the latter will need surgery). If abscess formation is suspected (swelling, swinging fever, and WCC↑) do ultrasound or CT. Drainage can be percutaneous (ultrasound or CT-guided), or by laparotomy. Local peritoneal inflammation can cause localized ileus with a 'sentinel loop' of intraluminal gas visible on plain AXR (p743).

*Colic* is a regularly waxing and waning pain, caused by muscular spasm in a hollow viscus, eg gut, ureter, salpinx, uterus, bile duct, or gallbladder (in the latter, pain is often dull and constant). Colic, unlike peritonitis, causes restlessness and the patient may well be pacing around when you go to see him!

## Obstruction of the bowel See p612.

**Tests** U&E; FBC; amylase; LFT; CRP; ABG (is there mesenteric ischaemia?); urinalysis. Erect CXR (fig 2), AXR may show Rigler's sign (p742). Laparoscopy may avert open surgery. CT can be helpful provided it is readily available and causes no delay (p746-747); USS may identify perforation or free fluid immediately, but appropriate performer training is important.

**Pre-op** ►Don't rush to theatre. Anaesthesia compounds shock, so resuscitate properly first (p805) unless blood being lost faster than can be replaced, eg ruptured ectopic pregnancy, (OHCS p262), aneurysm leak (p656), trauma.

> | *Plan: Bed rest—then:* |
> | :--- |
> | • Treat shock (p804) |
> | • Crossmatch/group and save |
> | • Blood culture |
> | • Antibiotics[1] |
> | • Relieve pain (p576) |
> | • IVI (0.9% saline) |
> | • Plain abdominal film |
> | • CXR if peritonitic or >50yrs |
> | • ECG if >50yrs |
> | • Consent |
> | • NBM |

**The medical acute abdomen** Irritable bowel syndrome (p276) is the chief cause, so always ask about episodes of pain associated with loose stools, relieved by defecation, bloating, and urgency (but **not** blood—this may be UC). Other causes:

| | | |
| :--- | :--- | :--- |
| ►►Myocardial infarction | Pneumonia (p160) | Sickle-cell crisis (p335) |
| Gastroenteritis or UTI | Thyroid storm (p844) | Phaeochromocytoma (p846) |
| Diabetes mellitus/DKA (p198) | Zoster (p400) | Malaria (p394) |
| Bornholm disease (p376) | Tuberculosis (p398) | Typhoid fever (p426) |
| Pneumococcal peritonitis | Porphyria (p706) | Cholera (p426) |
| Henoch-Schönlein (p716) | Narcotic addiction | *Yersinia enterocolitica* (p422) |
| Tabes dorsalis (p431) | PAN (p558) | Lead colic |

**Hidden diagnoses** ►►Mesenteric ischaemia (p622), ►►acute pancreatitis (p638) and ►►a leaking AAA (p656) are the *Unterseeboote* of the acute abdomen—unsuspected, undetectable unless carefully looked for, and underestimatedly deadly. They may have non-specific symptoms and signs that are surprisingly mild, so always think of them when assessing the acute abdomen and hopefully you will 'spot' them! ►Finally: *always exclude pregnancy* (± ectopic?) in females.

---

1 Give antibiotics if peritonitic, eg **cefuroxime** 1.5g/8h IV + **metronidazole** 500mg/8h IV/PR.

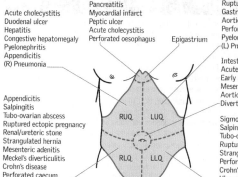

| | Pancreatitis | | Ruptured spleen |
| Acute cholecystitis | Myocardial infarct | | Gastric ulcer |
| Duodenal ulcer | Peptic ulcer | | Aortic aneurysm |
| Hepatitis | Acute cholecystitis | | Perforated colon |
| Congestive hepatomegaly | Perforated oesophagus | Epigastrium | Pyelonephritis |
| Pyelonephritis | | | (L) Pneumonia |
| Appendicitis | | | |
| (R) Pneumonia | | | Intestinal obstruction |

Acute cholecystitis
Duodenal ulcer
Hepatitis
Congestive hepatomegaly
Pyelonephritis
Appendicitis
(R) Pneumonia

Pancreatitis
Myocardial infarct
Peptic ulcer
Acute cholecystitis
Perforated oesophagus

Epigastrium

Ruptured spleen
Gastric ulcer
Aortic aneurysm
Perforated colon
Pyelonephritis
(L) Pneumonia

Intestinal obstruction
Acute pancreatitis
Early appendicitis
Mesenteric thrombosis
Aortic aneurysm
Diverticulitis

Appendicitis
Salpingitis
Tubo-ovarian abscess
Ruptured ectopic pregnancy
Renal/ureteric stone
Strangulated hernia
Mesenteric adenitis
Meckel's diverticulitis
Crohn's disease
Perforated caecum
Psoas abscess

RUQ   LUQ

RLQ   LLQ

Sigmoid diverticulitis
Salpingitis
Tubo-ovarian abscess
Ruptured ectopic pregnancy
Strangulated hernia
Perforated colon
Crohn's disease
Ulcerative colitis
Renal/ureteric stones

Fig 1. Causes of abdominal pain.

Surgery

## Assessing hypovolaemia from blood loss

The most likely cause of shock in a surgical patient is hypovolaemia (but don't forget the other causes—p804). The chief physiological parameters for assessing shock assess target organ perfusion rather than the direct measurement of BP and pulse, which may be 'normal' in one individual and yet totally abnormal for another. The most perfused organs in a normal state are the kidney, brain, and skin, so check **urine output**, GCS and **capillary refill** (CR). ▸▸ *The best quick test is:* "do you feel dizzy if you sit up?"

Of course, BP, pulse, and respirations are still **vital** signs, but the message here is: ▸▸treat suspected shock rather than wait for BP to fall. When there is any blood loss (eg a trauma situation), assess the status of the following:

| Parameter | Class I | Class II | Class III | Class IV |
|---|---|---|---|---|
| Blood loss | <750mL | 750-1500mL | 1500-2000mL | >2000mL |
| | <15% | 15-30% | 30-40% | >40% |
| Pulse | <100bpm | >100bpm | >120bpm | >140bpm |
| BP | ↔ | ↔ | ↓ | ↓ |
| Pulse pressure | ↔ or ↑ | ↓ | ↓ | ↓ |
| Respirations | 14-20/min | 20-30/min | 30-40/min | >35/min |
| Urine output | >30mL/h | 20-30mL/h | 5-15mL/h | Negligible |
| Mental state | Slightly anxious | Anxious | Confused → | →Lethargic |
| Fluid to give | Crystalloid | Crystalloid | Crystalloid + blood | |

Assumes a body mass of 70kg and a circulating blood volume of 5L.

Reproduced with permission from American Col. of Surgeons' Committee on Trauma, Advanced Trauma Life Support® for Doctors (ATLS®) Student Manual 7e, Chicago: Am Coll Surg, 2004.

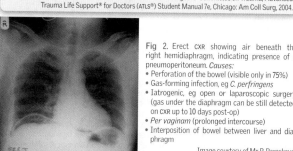

Fig 2. Erect CXR showing air beneath the right hemidiaphragm, indicating presence of a pneumoperitoneum. *Causes:*
• Perforation of the bowel (visible only in 75%)
• Gas-forming infection, eg *C. perfringens*
• Iatrogenic, eg open or laparoscopic surgery (gas under the diaphragm can be still detected on CXR up to 10 days post-op)
• Per vaginam (prolonged intercourse)
• Interposition of bowel between liver and diaphragm

Image courtesy of Mr P. Paraskeva.

Surgery

**Incidence** Most common surgical emergency (lifetime incidence = 6%). Can occur at any age, though highest incidence is between 10-20yrs. It is rare before age 2 because the appendix is cone shaped with a larger lumen.

**Pathogenesis** Gut organisms invade the appendix wall after lumen obstruction by lymphoid hyperplasia, faecolith, or filarial worms. This leads to oedema, ischaemic necrosis and perforation. There may be impaired ability to prevent invasion, brought about by improved hygiene & less exposure to pathogens (the 'hygiene hypothesis').

**Symptoms** Classically periumbilical pain that moves to the RIF (see MINIBOX). Anorexia is an important feature; vomiting is rarely prominent—pain normally precedes vomiting in the surgical abdomen. Constipation is usual. Diarrhoea may occur.

**Special tests** Rovsing's sign (pain > in RIF than LIF when the LIF is pressed). Psoas sign (pain on extending hip if retrocaecal appendix). Cope sign (pain on flexion and internal rotation of right hip if appendix in close relation to obturator internus).

**Investigations** Blood tests may reveal neutrophil leucocytosis and elevated CRP. USS may help,[94] but the appendix is not always visualized.[95] CT has high diagnostic accuracy and is useful if diagnosis is unclear: it reduces -ve appendicectomy rate, but may cause fatal delay.[96]

**Variations in the clinical picture**
- Inflammation in a retrocecal/retroperitoneal appendix (2.5%) may cause flank[97] or RUQ pain;[98] its only sign may be ↑tenderness on the right on PR.
- The child with vague abdominal pain who will not eat their favourite food.
- The shocked, confused octogenarian who is not in pain.
- Appendicitis occurs in ~1/1000 pregnancies. It is not commoner, but mortality is higher, especially from 20wks' gestation. Perforation is commoner, and increases fetal mortality. Pain is often less well localized (may be RUQ), & signs of peritonism less obvious.

| **General signs** |
|---|
| • Tachycardia |
| • Fever 37.5-38.5°C |
| • Furred tongue |
| • Lying still |
| • Coughing hurts (p62) |
| • Foetor ± flushing |
| • Shallow breaths |

| **Signs in the RIF** |
|---|
| • Guarding (p62) |
| • Rebound + percussion tenderness (p62) |
| • PR painful on right (sign of low-lying pelvic appendix) |

**Hints**
- If a child is anxious, use their hand to press their tummy—see also p629 for tips.
- Check for recent viral illnesses and lymphadenopathy—mesenteric adenitis?
- Don't **start** palpating in the RIF (makes it difficult to elicit pain elsewhere).
- Expect diagnosis to be wrong half the time. If diagnosis is uncertain re-examine often. A normal appendix is removed in up to 20% of patients.[99]

**Treatment** Prompt *appendicectomy. Antibiotics:* Metronidazole 500mg/8h + cefuroxime 1.5g/8h, 1 to 3 doses IV starting 1h pre-op, reduces wound infections. Give a longer course if perforated. *Laparoscopy:* Has diagnostic and therapeutic advantages (when done by an experienced surgeon), especially in women and the obese. It is not recommended in cases of suspected gangrenous perforation as the rate of abscess formation may be higher.[100]

| **ΔΔ** |
|---|
| • Ectopic (▶▶do a pregnancy test!) |
| • UTI (test urine!) |
| • Mesenteric adenitis |
| • Cystitis |
| • Cholecystitis |
| • Diverticulitis |
| • Salpingitis/PID |
| • Dysmenorrhoea |
| • Crohn's disease |
| • Perforated ulcer |
| • Food poisoning |
| • Meckel's diverticulum |

**Complications**
- *Perforation* is commoner if a faecolith is present[101] and in young children, as the diagnosis is more often delayed.[102] Perforation does not cause infertility in girls.[103]
- *Appendix mass* may result when an inflamed appendix becomes covered with omentum. US/CT may help with diagnosis.—Some advocate early surgery. Alternatively, initial conservative management—NBM and antibiotics. If the mass resolves, some perform an interval (ie delayed) appendicectomy. Exclude a colonic tumour (laparotomy or colonoscopy), which can present as early as the 4th decade.
- *Appendix abscess* May result if an appendix mass fails to resolve but enlarges and the patient gets more unwell. Treatment usually involves drainage (surgical or percutaneous under US/CT-guidance). Antibiotics alone may bring resolution.

## Explaining the pattern of abdominal pain in appendicitis

Internal organs and the visceral peritoneum have no somatic innervation, so the brain attributes the visceral (splanchnic) signals to a physical location whose dermatome corresponds to the same entry level in the spinal cord. Importantly, there is no laterality to the visceral unmyelinated c-fibre pain signals, which enter the cord bilaterally and at multiple levels. Division of the gut according to embryological origin is the important determinant here:

| Gut | Division points | Somatic referral | Arterial supply |
|---|---|---|---|
| Fore | Proximal to 2nd part of duodenum | Epigastrium | Coeliac axis |
| Mid | Above to ⅔ along transverse colon | Periumbilical | Superior mesenteric |
| Hind | Distal to above | Suprapubic | Inferior mesenteric |

Early inflammation irritates the structure and walls of the appendix, so a colicky pain is referred to the mid-abdomen—classically periumbilical. As the inflammation progresses and irritates the parietal peritoneum (especially on examination!) the somatic, lateralized pain settles at McBurney's point, ⅔ of the way along from the umbilicus to the right anterior superior iliac spine.

These principles also help us understand patterns of *referred pain*. In pneumonia, the T9 dermatome is shared by the lung and the abdomen. Also, irritation of the underside of the diaphragm (sensory innervation is from above through the phrenic nerve, C3-5) by an inflamed gallbladder or a subphrenic abscess refers pain to the right shoulder: dermatomes C3-5.

*Surgery*

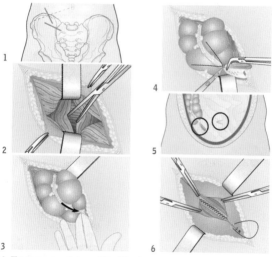

Fig 1. The open appendectomy. **1** Traditional approach is Gridiron incision over McBurney's point, at 90° to line from umbilicus to the anterior superior iliac spine. Lanz incision is more horizontal in Langer's lines (skin creases) and gives a better scar. **2** Divide subcutaneous fat and superficial/Scarpa's fascia. Fibres of external oblique, internal oblique and transversus abdominus divided with muscle splitting incision. **3** Incise pre-peritoneal fat and peritoneum to reveal caecum. Deliver caecum through incision. Appendix located at convergence of taenia coli. **4** Mesoappendix (blood vessels and mesentery) and appendix divided, ligated and excised (stump may be inverted). **5** In case of a normal-looking appendix, excise (may be histologically if not macroscopically inflamed); look for Meckel's diverticulum. **6** Wash, close in layers, dress wound.

**Features of obstruction** Vomiting, nausea and anorexia. Fermentation of the intestinal contents in established obstruction causes 'faeculent' vomiting ('faecal' vomiting is found when there is a colonic fistula with the proximal gut). Colic occurs early (may be absent in long-standing complete obstruction). **Constipation** need not be absolute (ie no faeces or flatus passed) if obstruction is high,

| Cardinal features of intestinal obstruction |
|---|
| • Vomiting |
| • Colicky pain |
| • Constipation |
| • Distension |

though in distal obstruction nothing will be passed. Abdominal distension is more marked as the obstruction progresses. There are active, 'tinkling' bowel sounds.

**The key decisions:**

1 *Is it obstruction of the small or large bowel?* In small bowel obstruction, vomiting occurs earlier, distension is less, and pain is higher in the abdomen. The AXR plays a key role in diagnosis—see p742. In small bowel obstruction, AXR shows central gas shadows with *valvulae conniventes* that completely cross the lumen and no gas in the large bowel. In large bowel obstruction, pain is more constant; AXR shows peripheral gas shadows proximal to the blockage (eg in caecum) but not in the rectum, unless you have done a PR examination ►which is always essential! Large bowel *haustra* do not cross all the lumen's width. If the ileocaecal valve is competent (ie doesn't allow reflux) pain may be felt over a distended caecum (see below).

| Causes: small bowel |
|---|
| • Adhesions (p567) |
| • Hernias (p614) |

| Causes: large bowel |
|---|
| • Colon ca (p618) |
| • Constipation (p248) |
| • Diverticular stricture |
| • Volvulus |
|   • Sigmoid (see BOX) |
|   • Caecal |

| Rarer causes |
|---|
| • Crohn's stricture |
| • Gallstone ileus (p636) |
| • Intussusception (p628) |
| • TB (developing world) |
| • Foreign body |

2 *Is there an ileus or mechanical obstruction?* Ileus is functional obstruction from reduced bowel motility (see box + p742). There is no pain and bowel sounds are absent.

3 *Is the obstructed bowel simple/closed loop/strangulated?* **Simple:** One obstructing point and no vascular compromise. **Closed loop:** Obstruction at two points (eg sigmoid volvulus, distension with competent ileocaecal valve) forming a loop of grossly distended bowel at risk of perforation (tenderness and perforation usually at caecum where the bowel is thinnest and widest; >12cm requires urgent decompression). **Strangulated:** Blood supply is compromised and the patient is more ill than you would expect. There is sharper, more constant and *localized* pain. Peritonism is the cardinal sign. There may be fever + WCC↑ with other signs of mesenteric ischaemia (p622).

**Management**

• *General principles:* Cause, site, speed of onset, and completeness of obstruction determine definitive therapy: strangulation and large bowel obstruction require surgery; ileus and incomplete small bowel obstruction can be managed conservatively, at least initially.

• *Immediate action:* ►'Drip and suck'—NGT and IV fluids to rehydrate and correct electrolyte imbalance (p680). Being NBM does not give adequate rest for the bowel because it can produce up to 9L of fluid/d. Also: analgesia, blood tests (inc. amylase, FBC, U&E), AXR, erect CXR, catheterize to monitor fluid status.

• *Further imaging:* Consider early CT if clinical and radiographic findings are inconclusive: it finds the cause and level of obstruction. It may show dilated, fluid-filled bowel and a transition zone at the site of obstruction (figs 1 & 2). There is a case for investigating the cause of large bowel obstruction by colonoscopy in some instances of suspected mechanical obstruction, though there is a danger of inducing perforation. Oral Gastrografin® can help identify partial small bowel obstruction (if contrast solution present in the colon within 24h it predicts conservative resolution).[104] It may also have mild therapeutic action against mechanical obstruction.

• *Surgery:* ►Strangulation needs emergency surgery, as does 'closed loop obstruction'. Stents may be used for obstructing large bowel malignancies either in palliation or as a bridge to surgery in acute obstruction (p618). Small bowel obstruction secondary to adhesions should rarely lead to surgery—see BOX, p583.

## Paralytic ileus or pseudo-obstruction?

**Paralytic ileus** is adynamic bowel due to the absence of normal peristaltic contractions. Contributing factors include abdominal surgery, pancreatitis (or any localized peritonitis), spinal injury, hypokalaemia, hyponatraemia, uraemia, peritoneal sepsis and drugs (eg tricyclic antidepressants).

**Pseudo-obstruction** is like mechanical GI obstruction but with no cause for obstruction found. **Acute** colonic pseudo-obstruction is called Ogilvie's syndrome (p720), and clinical features are similar to that of mechanical obstruction.[105] Predisposing factors: puerperium; pelvic surgery; trauma; cardiorespiratory disorders. *Treatment: Neostigmine* or colonoscopic decompression are sometimes useful. In **chronic** pseudo-obstruction weight loss from malabsorption is a problem.[106]

## Sigmoid volvulus

Sigmoid volvulus occurs when the bowel twists on its mesentery, which can produce severe, rapid, strangulated obstruction. There is a characteristic AXR with an 'inverted U' loop of bowel that looks a bit like a coffee bean. It tends to occur in the elderly, constipated and comorbid patient, and is often managed by sigmoidoscopy and insertion of a flatus tube. Sigmoid colectomy is sometimes required.
►If not treated successfully, it can progress to perforation and fatal peritonitis.

## Volvulus of the stomach

Gastric volvulus is rare. Rotation is typically 180° left to right, about a line joining the relatively fixed pylorus and oesophagus. This creates a closed loop obstruction that can result in incarceration and strangulation. The classical triad of gastro-oesophageal obstruction may occur: vomiting (then retching), pain, and failed attempts to pass an NG tube. Regurgitation of saliva also occurs. Dysphagia and noisy gastric peristalsis (relieved by lying down) may occur in chronic volvulus.

**Risk factors** *Congenital:* Paraoesophageal hernia; congenital bands; bowel malformations; pyloric stenosis. *Acquired:* Gastric/oesophageal surgery.

**Tests** Look for gastric dilatation and a double fluid level on erect films.

**Treatment** If acutely unwell arrange prompt resuscitation and laparotomy. Laparoscopic management is possible.[107]

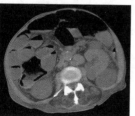

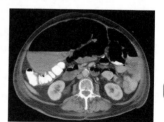

**Fig 1.** Unenhanced axial CT of the abdomen showing multiple loops of dilated, fluid-filled small bowel in a patient with small bowel obstruction.

Both images courtesy of Norwich Radiology Dept.

**Fig 2.** Axial CT of the abdomen post-oral contrast showing dilated loops of fluid and air-filled large bowel (contrast medium is in the small bowel). The cause or level of obstruction is not clear.

Surgery

**Definition** *The protrusion of a viscus or part of a viscus through a defect of the walls of its containing cavity into an abnormal position. Terminology:* Hernias involving bowel are said to be **irreducible** if they cannot be pushed back into the right place. This does not mean that they are either necessarily obstructed or strangulated. **Incarceration** implies that the contents of the hernial sac are stuck inside by adhesions. Gastrointestinal hernias are **obstructed** if bowel contents cannot pass through them—the classical features of intestinal obstruction soon appear (p612). They are **strangulated** if ischaemia occurs—the patient becomes toxic and requires urgent surgery. Care must be taken when attempting reduction (see p616 for the technique) as it is possible to perform reduction *en masse*, pushing the strangulated bowel and hernial sac back into the abdominal cavity, but giving the initial appearance of successful reduction.

**Inguinal hernia** The commonest type (far more common in men), described on p616.

**Femoral hernia** Bowel enters the femoral canal, presenting as a mass in the upper medial thigh or above the inguinal ligament where it points down the leg, unlike an inguinal hernia which points to the groin. They occur more often in women especially in middle age and the elderly. They are likely to be irreducible and to strangulate due to the rigidity of the canal's borders. *Anatomy:* The neck of the hernia is felt **inferior and lateral to the pubic tubercle** (inguinal hernias are superior and medial to this point). The boundaries of the femoral canal are **anteriorly** the inguinal ligament; **medially** the lacunar ligament (and pubic bone); **laterally** the femoral vein (and iliopsoas); and **posteriorly** the pectineal ligament and pectineus. The canal contains fat and Cloquet's node. *Differential diagnosis:*[108] (see also p653) 1 Inguinal hernia 2 Saphena varix 3 An enlarged Cloquet's node (p619) 4 Lipoma 5 Femoral aneurysm 6 Psoas abscess. *Treatment:* Surgical repair is recommended. (*Herniotomy* is ligation and excision of the sac, *herniorrhaphy* is repair of the hernial defect.)

**Paraumbilical hernias** occur just above or below the umbilicus. Risk factors are obesity and ascites. Omentum or bowel herniates through the defect. Surgery involves repair of the rectus sheath (Mayo repair).

**Epigastric hernias** pass through linea alba above the umbilicus.

**Incisional hernias** follow breakdown of muscle closure after surgery (11-20%). If obese, repair is not easy. Mesh repair has ↓recurrence but ↑infection over sutures.[109]

**Spigelian hernias** occur through the linea semilunaris at the lateral edge of the rectus sheath, below and lateral to the umbilicus.

**Lumbar hernias** occur through the inferior or superior lumbar triangles in the posterior abdominal wall.

**Richter's hernias** involve bowel wall only—not the whole lumen.

**Maydl's hernias** involve a herniating 'double loop' of bowel. The strangulated portion may reside as a single loop **inside** the abdominal cavity.

**Littre's hernias** are hernial sacs containing strangulated Meckel's diverticulum.

**Obturator hernias** occur through the obturator canal. Typically there is pain along the medial side of the thigh in a thin woman.

**Sciatic hernias** pass through the lesser sciatic foramen (a way through various pelvic ligaments). GI obstruction+a gluteal mass suggests this rare possibility.[110]

**Sliding hernias** contain a partially extraperitoneal structure (eg caecum on the right, sigmoid colon on the left). The sac does not completely surround the contents.

**Other examples of hernias:**
- Of the nucleus pulposus into the spinal canal (slipped disc).
- Of the uncus and hippocampal gyrus through the tentorium (tentorial hernia) in space-occupying lesions.
- Of brainstem and cerebellum through the foramen magnum (Arnold-Chiari, p708).
- Of the stomach through the diaphragm (hiatus hernia, p245).
- Of the terminal (intravesical) portion of the ureter into the bladder. This is a *uret erocele* and results from stenosis of the ureteral meatus.

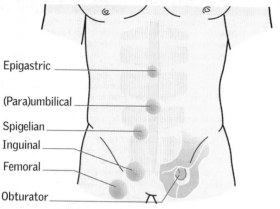

Fig 1. Some examples of hernias.

- Epigastric
- (Para)umbilical
- Spigelian
- Inguinal
- Femoral
- Obturator

## Abdominal wall defects in children

*(see OHCS, p130)*

**Gastroschisis** occurs with protrusion of the abdominal contents through a defect in the anterior abdominal wall to the right of the umbilicus. The protruding bowel is covered by a thin 'peel'. Prompt surgical repair is performed after cautious fluid resuscitation.[111] Concomitant congenital abnormalities are rare, but there is a 4% incidence of congenital heart defects.[112]

**Exomphalos** (also called *omphalocele*)[1] is associated with other congenital abnormalities, such as anencephaly, cardiac defects, hydrocephalus and spina bifida. In this condition the abdominal contents are found outside the abdomen, covered in a three-layer membrane consisting of peritoneum, Wharton's jelly and amnion. Surgical repair is less urgent than in gastroschisis because the bowel is protected by these membranes. The challenge of surgery is to fit the contents back into the relatively small abdominal cavity without compromising venous return and lung ventilation.

**Inguinal hernias** *Indirect* occur in ~4% of all male infants (due to patent *processus vaginalis*)—prematurity is a risk factor. They are uncommon in female infants and, if found, should prompt thoughts of testicular feminization. If the patent *processus vaginalis* contains peritoneal fluid only, then it is a *communicating hydrocele*. Surgical repair is required for both. Reinforcement of the posterior wall (eg with a mesh) is not needed as the internal ring has not been chronically dilated.

**True umbilical hernias** (3% of live births) are a result of a persistent defect in the transversalis fascia—the umbilical ring, through which the umbilical vessels passed to reach the fetus (more common in African-Caribbeans, trisomy 21 and congenital hypothyroidism). Surgical repair is rarely needed in children (3 in 1000) as most resolve by the age of 3.

The *omphalos* is the centre-stone at the Temple of Apollo in Delphi, centre of the ancient world—hence its umbilical association. Here Apollo persuaded Pan (the god of wild places, music, and syrinxes, p520) to reveal the art of prophesy, without which we would be without our most mysterious tool: *prognosis*.

**Indirect** hernias pass through the internal inguinal ring and, if large, out through the external ring. **Direct** hernias push their way *directly* forward through the posterior wall of the inguinal canal, into a defect in the abdominal wall (Hesselbach's triangle; medial to the inferior epigastric vessels and lateral to the rectus abdominus). *Predisposing conditions:* males ($\male$:$\female$≈8:1), chronic cough, constipation, urinary obstruction, heavy lifting, ascites, past abdominal surgery (eg damage to the iliohypogastric nerve during appendicectomy). There are 2 landmarks to identify: *The deep (internal) ring* may be defined as being the mid-point of the inguinal ligament, ~1½cm above the femoral pulse (which crosses the mid-inguinal point). *The superficial (external) ring* is a split in the external oblique aponeurosis just superior and medial to the pubic tubercle (the bony prominence forming the medial attachment of the inguinal ligament). Relations of the inguinal canal are:

- *Floor:* Inguinal ligament and lacunar ligament medially.
- *Roof:* Fibres of transversalis, internal oblique.
- *Anterior:* External oblique aponeurosis + internal oblique for the lateral ⅓.
- *Posterior:* Laterally, transversalis fascia; medially, conjoint tendon.

**Examination** Look for previous scars; feel the other side (more common on the right); examine the external genitalia. Then ask: •Is the lump visible? If so, ask the patient to reduce it—if he cannot, make sure that it is not a scrotal lump. Ask him to cough. Appears **above and medial to the pubic tubercle.** •If no lump is visible, feel for a cough impulse. •Repeat the examination with the patient standing. *Distinguishing direct from indirect hernias:* This is loved by examiners but is of little clinical use—not least because repair is the same for both (see below). The best way is to reduce the hernia and occlude the deep (internal) ring with two fingers. Ask the patient to cough or stand—if the hernia is restrained, it is indirect; if not, it is direct. The 'gold standard' for determining the type of inguinal hernia is at surgery: direct hernias arise medial to the inferior epigastric vessels; indirect hernias are lateral.

| Indirect hernias: | Direct hernias: | Femoral hernias: |
|---|---|---|
| • Common (80%) | • Less common (20%) | • More frequent in females |
| • Can strangulate | • Reduce easily | • Frequently irreducible |
| | • Rarely strangulate | • Frequently strangulate |

**Irreducible hernias** You may be called because a long-standing hernia is now irreducible and painful. It is always worth trying to reduce these yourself to prevent strangulation and necrosis (demanding prompt laparotomy). Learn how to do this from an expert, ie one of your patients who has been reducing his hernia for years. Then you will know how to act correctly when the emergency presents. Notice that such patients use the flat of the hand, directing the hernia from below, up towards the contralateral shoulder. Sometimes, as the hernia obstructs, reduction requires perseverance, which may be rewarded by a gurgle from the retreating bowel and a kiss from the attending spouse who had thought that surgery was inevitable.

**Repairs** Advise to diet (if over-weight) and stop smoking pre-op. Warn that hernia may recur. Mesh techniques (eg Lichtenstein repair) have replaced older methods. In mesh repairs, a polypropylene mesh reinforces the posterior wall. Recurrence rate is less than with other methods (eg <2% vs 10%). (CI: strangulated hernias contamination with pus/bowel contents.) Local anaesthetic techniques and day case 'ambulatory' surgery may halve the price of surgery. This is important because this is one of the most common operations (>100,000 per year in the UK). *Laparoscopic repair* gives similar recurrence rates.[113] Methods include *transabdominal pre-peritoneal* (TAPP) in which the peritoneum is entered and the hernia repaired, and *totally extraperitoneal* (TEP), which decreases the risk of visceral injury. For benefit of laparoscopic surgery see p594.

*Return to work:* We used to advise 4 weeks' rest and convalescence over 10 weeks but with new mesh or laparoscopic repairs, if comfortable, return to manual work (and driving) after ≤2 weeks is OK if all is well; explain this pre-operatively.

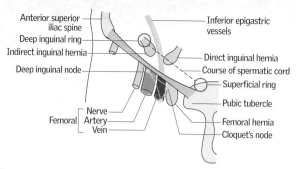

Fig 1. Anatomy of the inguinal canal.

### The contents of the inguinal canal in the male

• The external spermatic fascia (from external oblique), cremasteric fascia (from internal oblique and transverses abdominus) and internal spermatic fascia (from transversalis fascia) covering the cord.
• The spermatic cord:
   • Vas deferens, obliterated processus vaginalis, and lymphatics
   • Arteries to the vas, cremaster, and testis
   • The pampiniform plexus and the venous equivalent of the above
   • The genital branch of the genitofemoral nerve and sympathetic nerves
• The ilioinguinal nerve, which enters the inguinal canal via the anterior wall and runs anteriorly to the cord.

NB: in the female the round ligament of the uterus is in place of the male structures. A hydrocele of the canal of Nuck is the female equivalent of a hydrocele of the cord.

Surgery

This is the 3rd most common cancer and 2nd most common cause of UK cancer deaths (16,000 deaths/yr). Usually adenocarcinoma. 86% of presentations are in those >60yrs old.[114] Lifetime UK incidence: ♂ = 1:15; ♀ = 1:19.

**Predisposing factors** Neoplastic polyps (see below, & p525); IBD (UC and Crohn's); genetic predisposition (<8%), eg FAP and HNPCC (see p524); diet (low-fibre; ↑red and processed meat); ↑alcohol[115]; smoking[116]●; previous cancer. *Prevention:* Aspirin ≥75mg/d reduces incidence and mortality—it is thought to inhibit polyp growth. Benefit ↑ with duration of use and is greatest for proximal lesions. Widespread chemoprevention is not currently recommended due to gastrointestinal SEs.[117]

**Presentation** depends on site: *Left-sided:* Bleeding/mucus PR; altered bowel habit or obstruction (25%); tenesmus; mass PR (60%). *Right:* Weight↓; Hb↓; abdominal pain; obstruction less likely. *Either:* Abdominal mass; perforation; haemorrhage; fistula. See p532 for a guide to urgent referral criteria. See fig 1 for distribution.

**Tests** FBC (microcytic anaemia); faecal occult blood (FOB, see BOX); sigmoidoscopy; barium enema or colonoscopy (figs 2 & 3, p257), which can be done 'virtually' by CT (fig 1, p757); LFT, CT/MRI; liver USS. CEA (p535) may be used to monitor disease and effectiveness of treatment. If family history of FAP, refer for DNA test once >15yrs old.

**Spread** Local, lymphatic, by blood (liver, lung, bone) or transcoelomic. The TNM system (Tumour, Node, Metastases; p527) is most commonly used to stage disease and is largely replacing Dukes' classification (BOX).

**Surgery** aims to cure and may ↑survival times by up to 50% (eg in TME[1]). ●**Right hemicolectomy** for caecal, ascending or proximal transverse colon tumours. ●**Left hemicolectomy** for tumours in distal transverse or descending colon. ●**Sigmoid colectomy** for sigmoid tumours. ●**Anterior resection** for low sigmoid or high rectal tumours. Anastomosis is achieved at the 1st operation—stapling devices work well.[118] ●**Abdomino-perineal (AP) resection** for tumours low in the rectum (≤8cm from anus): permanent colostomy and removal of rectum and anus (but see p584 for total anorectal reconstruction). ●**Hartmann's procedure** in emergency bowel obstruction or perforation or palliation. ●**Transanal endoscopic microsurgery** allows local excision through a wide proctoscope in those unfit for major surgery. *Laparoscopic surgery* has revolutionized surgery for colon cancer. It is as safe as open surgery and there is no difference in overall survival or disease recurrence.[119] *Endoscopic stenting* should be considered for palliation in malignant obstruction and as a bridge to surgery in acute obstruction. Stenting ↓ need for colostomy, has less complications than emergency surgery, shortens intensive care and total hospital stays, and prevents unnecessary operations.[120] Surgery with liver resection may be curative if single-lobe hepatic metastases and no extrahepatic spread.[121]

**Radiotherapy** is mostly used in palliation for colonic cancer. It is occasionally used pre-op in rectal cancer to allow resection. Post-op radiotherapy is only used in patients with rectal tumours at high risk of local recurrence.

**Chemotherapy** Adjuvant chemotherapy reduces Dukes' C mortality by ~25%.[122] In Dukes' B there is absolute survival benefit of 3-5%.[123] The FOLFOX regimen has become standard (*5-FU, folinic acid* and *oxaliplatin*). Chemotherapy is also used in palliation of metastatic disease. *Biological therapies Bevacizumab* (anti-VEG antibody) improves survival when added to combination therapy in advanced disease.[124] *Cetuximab* and *Panitumumab* (anti-EGFR agents) improve response rate and survival in KRAS wild-type metastatic colorectal cancer.[125]

**Prognosis** Overall 5yr survival is ~50% but is dependent on age and stage (see BOX 1). Post-op anastomotic leakage is shown to ↓survival rates in otherwise potentially curative surgery.[126]

**Polyps** are lumps that appear above the mucosa. 1 *Inflammatory:* Ulcerative colitis, Crohn's, lymphoid hyperplasia. 2 *Hamartomatous:* Juvenile polyps, Peutz-Jeghers (p722). 3 *Neoplastic:* Tubular or villous adenomas: malignant potential, esp. if >2cm. Polyps should be biopsied and removed if they show malignant change. Most can be reached by flexible colonoscope; diathermy can avoid morbidity of colectomy.

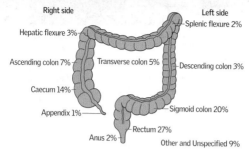

**Fig 1.** Distribution of colorectal carcinomas. These are averages: black females tend to have more proximal neoplasms. White men tend to have more distal neoplasms.

Surgery

## Dukes' classification for the staging of colorectal cancer

| Stage | Description | Treated 5yr survival rate[127] |
|-------|-------------|-------------------------------|
| A | Limited to muscularis mucosae | 93% |
| B | Extension through muscularis mucosae | 77% |
| C | Involvement of regional lymph nodes | 48% |
| D | Distant metastases | 6.6% |

See also TNM staging p527.

## UK screening for colorectal cancer

The NHS Bowel Cancer Screening Programme[128] (introduced in 2006) offers screening every 2 years to all men and women aged 60-75 by using Faecal Occult Blood (FOB) home testing kits. FOB screening reduces the relative risk of death from colorectal cancer by 16%.[129,130] The 11% increase in incidence rates since 2006 for people aged 60-69 is almost certainly due to the screening programme.[114]

Home test kits are used to sample 3 separate bowel motions and are returned for analysis. Approximately 2% of tests are positive and these patients are offered an appointment with a specialist nurse, plus further investigation (usually colonoscopy). The positive predictive value (p674) is 5-15%. There can be problems with 'acceptability' of home testing and also of high false positive rates (up to 10%).

In addition to this, the NHS is introducing a 'one-off' screening flexible sigmoidoscopy to all people in their 55th year. Trial results have shown the incidence of colorectal cancer in the intervention (screening) group is reduced by 33% and mortality from colorectal cancer is reduced by 43%. Number needed to screen to prevent one diagnosis (=191); or death (=489).[131]

TME = total mesorectal excision. It entails sharp dissection to yield an intact mesorectal envelope.[132]

Incidence of adenocarcinoma at the gastro-oesoph-ageal junction is increasing in the West, though incidence of distal and body gastric carcinoma has fallen sharply. It remains a tumour notable for its gloomy prognosis and non-specific presentation.

| **Associations** |
| --- |
| • Pernicious anaemia |
| • Blood group A |
| • *H. pylori* (p242) |
| • Atrophic gastritis |
| • Adenomatous polyps |
| • Lower social class |
| • Smoking |
| • Diet (high nitrate, high salt, pickling, low vitamin C) |
| • Nitrosamine exposure |

**Incidence** 23/100,000/yr in the UK, but there are unexplained wide geographical variations; it is especially common in Japan, as well as Eastern Europe, China, and South America. $\sigma$:$\varphi\approx2$:1.

**Pathology** Borrmann classification: i) Polypoid ii) Excavating iii) Ulcerating and raised iv) Diffusely infiltrative. Some are confined to mucosa and submucosa— 'early' gastric carcinoma.

**Presentation** *Symptoms:* Often non-specific. Dyspepsia (p59; for >1 month and age ≥50yrs demands investigation), weight ↓, vomiting, dysphagia, anaemia. *Signs* suggesting incurable disease: epigastric mass, hepatomegaly; jaundice, ascites (p606); large left supraclavicular (Virchow's) node (=Troisier's sign); acanthosis nigricans (p564). Most patients in the West present with locally advanced (inoperable) or metastatic disease. *Spread* is local, lymphatic, blood-borne, and transcoelomic, eg to ovaries (Krukenberg tumour).

**Tests** Gastroscopy + multiple ulcer edge biopsies. ▶*Aim to biopsy all gastric ulcers as even malignant ulcers may appear to heal on drug treatment.* Endoscopic ultrasound (EUS) can evaluate depth of invasion; CT/MRI helps staging. Staging laparoscopy is recommended for locally advanced tumours. Cytology of peritoneal washings can help identify peritoneal metastases.[133]

**Treatment** See p624 for a description of surgical resections. Partial gastrectomy may suffice for distal tumours. If more proximal, total gastrectomy may be needed. Combination chemotherapy (eg *epirubicin, cisplatin* and *5-fluorouracil*) appears to increase survival in advanced disease.[134] If given perioperatively in operable disease it improves survival compared to surgery alone.[135] Endoscopic mucosal resection is used for early tumours confined to the mucosa.[136] Surgical palliation is often needed for obstruction, pain, or haemorrhage. In locally advanced and metastatic disease chemotherapy increases quality of life and survival.[137] Targeted therapies are likely to have an increasing role, eg *trastuzumab* for HER-2 positive tumours.

**5yr survival** <10% overall, but nearly 20% for patients undergoing radical surgery. The prognosis is much better for 'early' gastric carcinoma.

## Carcinoma of the oesophagus *(OHOncol p334)*

**Incidence** Australia <5/100,000/yr; UK <9; Brittany >50; Iran >100. **Risk factors** Diet, alcohol excess, smoking, achalasia, Plummer-Vinson syn. (p240), obesity, diet ↓ in vit A&C, nitrosamine exposure, reflux oesophagitis ± Barrett's oesophagus (p708). $\sigma$:$\varphi\approx5$:1.

**Site** 20% occur in the upper part, 50% in the middle, and 30% in the lower part. They may be squamous cell (proximal) or adenocarcinomas (distal; incidence rising.

**Presentation** Dysphagia; weight↓; retrosternal chest pain. *Signs from the upper third of the oesophagus:* Hoarseness; cough (may be paroxysmal if aspiration pneumonia). *ΔΔ:* See Dysphagia, p240.

**Tests** Oesophagoscopy with biopsy is the investigation of choice ± EUS, CT/MRI for staging (fig 1), or laparoscopy if significant infra-diaphragmatic component. *Staging:* See TABLE.

**Treatment** Survival rates are poor with or without treatment. If localized T1-T2 disease, radical curative oesophagectomy may be tried. Pre-op chemotherapy (*cisplatin + 5-FU*) for localized disease may improve survival, but causes some morbidity.[138] Surgery alone may be preferable.[139] If surgery is not indicated, then chemoradiotherapy may be better than radiotherapy alone.[140] Palliation in advanced disease aims to restore swallowing with chemo/radiotherapy, stenting, and laser use.

## TNM staging in oesophageal cancer

(See also p527)

Spread of oesophageal cancer is direct, by submucosal infiltration and local spread—or to nodes, or, later, via the blood.

| | | | |
|---|---|---|---|
| **T$_{is}$** | Carcinoma *in situ* | **Nx** | Nodes cannot be assessed |
| **T1** | Invading lamina propria/submucosa | **N0** | No node spread |
| **T2** | Invading muscularis propria | **N1** | Regional node metastases |
| **T3** | Invading adventitia | **M0** | No distant spread |
| **T4** | Invasion of adjacent structures | **M1** | Distant metastasis |

## Oesophageal rupture

**Causes** •*Iatrogenic*, eg endoscopy/biopsy/dilatation (accounts for 85–90% of perforations) •*Trauma*, eg penetrating injury/ingestion of foreign body •*Carcinoma* •*Boerhaave syndrome*—rupture due to violent vomiting •*Corrosive ingestion*.

**Clinical features** Odynophagia, tachypnoea, dyspnoea, fever, shock, surgical emphysema (a crackling sensation felt on palpating the skin over the chest or neck caused by air tracking from the lungs; ∆∆: pneumothorax).

**℞** Iatrogenic perforations are less prone to mediastinitis and sepsis and may be managed conservatively with NG tube, PPI and antibiotics. Others require resuscitation, PPI, antibiotics, antifungals and surgery (debridement of mediastinum and placement of T-tube for drainage and formation of a controlled oesophagocutaneous fistula).

## Bile duct and gallbladder cancers[14]

All are rare, have an overall poor prognosis and are difficult to diagnose. They account for ~3% of all GI cancers worldwide, but there is geographical variation (↑ in north-east Thailand, Japan, Korea and Eastern Europe). Most are adenocarcinomas. Primary sclerosing cholangitis (p266) is the commonest predisposing factor in the West. *Presentation:* Varies according to location and may include obstructive jaundice, pruritus, abdominal pain, weight loss and anorexia. *Investigations:* USS, CT, and ERCP. MRI has a role for determining extent of invasion in bile duct cancers.

**Treatment**
- *Bile duct cancer:* Surgical resection is the only potentially curative treatment yet ~80% present with inoperable disease. Palliation includes biliary stenting and chemotherapy.
- *Gallbladder cancer:* Again, radical surgery is the only chance of cure. 25% of patients with a porcelain gallbaldder have cancer—prophylactic surgery should be considered. Palliative treatment of inoperable disease includes bilary stenting and chemotherapy.

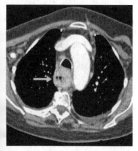

Fig 1. Axial CT of the chest after IV contrast medium showing concentric thickening of the oesophagus (arrow); the diagnosis here is oesophageal carcinoma. Loss of the fatty plane around the oesophagus suggests local invasion. Anterior to the oesophagus is the trachea and next to it is the arch of the aorta.

Image courtesy of Dr Stephen Golding.

Surgery

There are 3 main types of bowel ischaemia. ►AF with abdominal pain should always prompt thoughts of mesenteric ischaemia.

**1 Acute mesenteric ischaemia**[142] almost always involves the small bowel and may follow superior mesenteric artery (SMA) thrombosis or embolism, mesenteric vein thrombosis, or non-occlusive disease (see MINIBOX). Arterial thrombosis is becoming the commonest cause of acute ischaemia as embolism becomes rarer. Venous thrombosis is more common in younger patients with hypercoagulable states and tends to affect smaller lengths of bowel. Non-occlusive ischaemia occurs in low-flow states and usually reflects poor cardiac output, though there may be other factors such as recent cardiac surgery or renal failure.[143]

| *Acute ischaemia* |
|---|
| • Arterial |
|    • Thrombotic[(35%)] |
|    • Embolic[(35%)] |
| • Non-occlusive (20%) |
| • Venous (5%) |
| • Other |
|    • Trauma |
|    • Vasculitis (p558) |
|    • Radiotherapy |
|    • Strangulation, eg volvulus or hernia |
| *Chronic ischaemia* |
| Usually a combination of a low-flow state with atheroma. |

*Presentation* is a classical clinical triad: ►Acute severe abdominal pain; no abdominal signs; rapid hypovolaemia→shock. Pain tends to be constant, central, or around the RIF. The degree of illness is often far out of proportion with clinical signs.

*Tests:* There may be Hbt (due to plasma loss), WCCt, modestly raised plasma amylase, and a persistent metabolic acidosis. Early on, the abdominal x-ray shows a 'gasless' abdomen. Arteriography helps but many diagnoses are only made on finding a nasty necrotic bowel at laparotomy. CT/MR angiography provides a non-invasive alternative to simple arteriography.[144] Measurement of mucosal oxygen tension and MR oximetric measurements of superior mesenteric vein flow are emerging as diagnostic tools.[145]

*Treatment:* The main life-threatening complications secondary to acute mesenteric ischaemia are **1** septic peritonitis and **2** progression of a systemic inflammatory response syndrome (SIRS) into a multi-organ dysfunction syndrome (MODS), mediated by bacterial translocation across the dying gut wall. Resuscitation with fluid, antibiotics (*gentamicin + metronidazole*, p381) and, usually, *heparin* are required. If arteriography is done, thrombolytics may be infused locally via the catheter. At surgery dead bowel must be removed. Revascularization may be attempted on potentially viable bowel but it is a difficult process and often needs a 2nd laparotomy.

*Prognosis:* Poor for arterial thrombosis and non-occlusive disease (<40% survive), though not so bad for venous and embolic ischaemia.[146]

**2 Chronic mesenteric ischaemia** (AKA intestinal angina). The triad of severe, colicky post-prandial abdominal pain ('gut claudication'), ↓weight (eating hurts) and an upper abdominal bruit may be present ± PR bleeding, malabsoprtion and N&V. There is often a history of vascular disease (95% due to diffuse atherosclerotic disease in all 3 mesenteric arteries). It is rare and difficult to diagnose. *Tests:* CT angiography and contrast enhanced MR angiography are replacing traditional angiography.[147,148] Doppler USS may be useful. *Treatment:* Once diagnosis is confirmed, surgery should be considered due to the ongoing risk of acute infarction. Percutaneous transluminal angioplasty and stent insertion is replacing open revascularization.[149] It is associated with less post-operative morbidity and mortality, but has higher restenosis rates.[150]

**3 Chronic colonic ischaemia** (AKA ischaemic colitis) usually follows low flow in the inferior mesenteric artery (IMA) territory and ranges from mild ischaemia to gangrenous colitis. *Presentation:* Lower left-sided abdominal pain ± bloody diarrhoea. *Tests:* CT may be helpful but colonoscopy and biopsy is 'gold-standard'. Barium enema shows characteristic 'thumb printing' of submucosal swelling. *Treatment:* Usually conservative with fluid replacement and antibiotics. Most recover but strictures are common. Gangrenous ischaemic colitis (presenting with peritonitis and hypovolaemic shock) requires prompt resuscitation followed by resection of the affected bowel and stoma formation. Mortality is high.

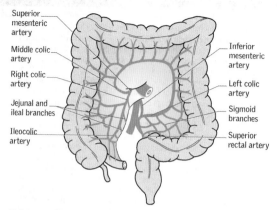

## 62

Superior mesenteric artery

Middle colic artery

Right colic artery

Jejunal and ileal branches

Ileocolic artery

Inferior mesenteric artery

Left colic artery

Sigmoid branches

Superior rectal artery

Fig 1. The arterial supply to the colon.

▶Indications for gastric surgery include gastric cancer (p620) and peptic ulcers, though medical therapy (p242) has made elective surgery for the latter rare.

**Operations for benign gastric ulceration** Pyloric ulcers may be considered similarly to duodenal ulceration (p626). Away from the pylorus, elective surgery is rarely needed as ulcers respond well to medical treatment, stopping smoking, and avoidance of NSAIDs. In patients who are unable to tolerate medical treatment, a laparoscopic highly selective vagotomy (HSV) can be done (p626). ▶▶*Emergency surgery* may be needed for haemorrhage or perforation. Haemorrhage is usually treated by under-running the bleeding ulcer base or excision of the ulcer. If the former is done, then a biopsy should be taken to exclude malignancy. Perforation is usually managed by excision of the hole for histology, then closure.

**Operations for duodenal ulceration** See p626.

**Gastric carcinoma** Localized disease may be treated by curative gastrectomy, either $D_1$ resection (excision of tumour and perigastric nodes) or $D_2$ resection (basically a $D_1$ resection extended to include nodes around the coeliac axis). $D_2$ resections should be performed in specialist centres.[151] Laparoscopic surgery is as effective and safe as open surgery.[152] A hand may be introduced into the peritoneal cavity (via a larger incision) for assistance (=laparoscopically assisted digital gastrectomy).

**Surgery** *Billroth I:* Partial gastrectomy with simple gastroduodenal re-anastomosis.

*Billroth II (aka Polya) gastrectomy* (fig 1) Partial gastrectomy with gastrojejunal anastamosis. The duodenal stump is oversewn (leaving a blind afferent loop), and anastomosis is achieved by a longitudinal incision into the proximal jejunum.

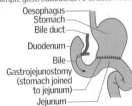

Oesophagus
Stomach
Bile duct
Duodenum
Bile
Gastrojejunostomy (stomach joined to jejunum)
Jejunum

**Fig 1.** Billroth II.

*Roux-en-Y* (fig 2) Following total or subtotal gastrectomy, the proximal duodenal stump is oversewn, the proximal jejunum is divided from the distal duodenum and connects with the oesophagus (or proximal stomach after subtotal gastrectomy) whilst the distal duodenum is connected to the distal jejunum.

**Physical complications of gastrectomy and peptic ulcer surgery**
• *Recurrent ulceration:* Symptoms are similar to those experienced pre-operatively but complications are more common and response to medical treatment is poor. Further surgery is difficult.
• *Abdominal fullness:* Feeling of early satiety (± discomfort and distension) improving with time. Advise to take small, frequent meals.
• *Afferent loop syndrome:* Post-gastrectomy (eg Billroth II), the afferent loop may fill with bile after a meal, causing upper abdominal pain and bilious vomiting. This is difficult to treat—but often improves with time.
• *Diarrhoea:* May be disabling after vagotomy. *Codeine phosphate* may help.
• *Gastric tumour:* A rare complication of any surgery which ↓acid production.
• *Amylase:* If with abdominal pain, this may indicate afferent loop obstruction after Billroth II surgery and requires emergency surgery.[153]

**Metabolic complications**
• *Dumping syndrome:*[154] Fainting and sweating after eating due to food of high osmotic potential being dumped in the jejunum, causing oligaemia from rapid fluid shifts. 'Late dumping' is due to rebound hypoglycaemia and occurs 1-3h after meals. Both tend to improve with time but may be helped by eating less sugar, and more guar and pectin (slows glucose absorption). *Acarbose* (p200) may also help to reduce the early hyperglycaemic stimulus to insulin secretion.[155]
• *Weight loss:* Often due to poor calorie intake.
• *Bacterial overgrowth ± malabsorption* (blind loop syndrome) may occur.
• *Anaemia:* Usually from lack of iron, hypochlorhydria and stomach resection. $B_{12}$ levels are frequently low but megaloblastic anaemia is rare.
• *Osteomalacia:* There may be pseudofractures which look like metastases.

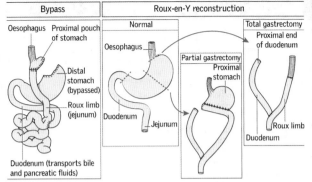

Fig 2. The Roux-en-Y reconstruction and gastric bypass

## Complications of peptic ulcer surgery

| | Partial gastrec-tomy | Vagotomy & pyloroplasty | Highly selective vagotomy |
|---|---|---|---|
| Recurrence | 2% | 7% | >7% |
| Dumping | 20% | 14% | 6% |
| Diarrhoea | 1% | 4% | <1% |
| Metabolic | ++++ | ++ | 0 |

(These values are approximate and depend on the skill of the surgeon.)

### Theodor Billroth

Theodor Billroth was a surgeon of German-Austrian origin, whose name lives on as a set of operations on the stomach. He was a pioneer of abdominal surgery and the use of aseptic techniques, performing the first Billroth I procedure in 1881 for the resection of a pyloric gastric carcinoma. Among the many of his remarkable achievements is included the first laryngectomy. He was also a talented musician (a close friend of Brahms) and a dedicated educator with something of a realist's view of the world:

*"The pleasure of a physician is little, the gratitude of patients is rare, and even rarer is material reward, but these things will never deter the student who feels the call within him."*     Theodor Billroth (1829-94) [56, 57]

Surgery

Peptic ulcers usually present as epigastric pain and dyspepsia (p242). There is no reliable method of distinguishing clinically between gastric and duodenal ulcers. Although management of both is usually medical in the first instance (eg with *H. pylori* eradication, p242); surgery is usually only required for complications such as *haemorrhage*, *perforation*, and *pyloric stenosis*, though may be considered for the few patients who are not responsive to, or tolerant of, medical therapy.

Several types of operation have been tried, but whenever surgery is considered, one must consider efficacy, side-seffects, and mortality.

**1 Elective surgery**
- *Highly selective vagotomy:* May be useful in patients unable to tolerate medical treatment. The vagus supply is denervated only where it supplies the lower oesophagus and stomach. The nerve of Latarget to the pylorus is left intact; thus, gastric emptying is unaffected. The results of surgery are greatly dependent on the skill of the surgeon.
- *Vagotomy and pyloroplasty:* This operation is now almost obsolete, and is only performed in exceptional circumstances.
- *Gastrectomy* (p624) is rarely required (eg Zollinger-Ellison syndrome, p730).

**2 Emergency surgery** may be required for the following complications:
- *Haemorrhage* may be controlled endoscopically by **adrenaline** injection, diathermy, laser coagulation, or heat probe. Surgery should be considered for severe haemorrhage or rebleeding, especially in the elderly—see p254 for indications. In theatre, the bleeding ulcer base is underrun or oversewn.
- *Perforation* Most patients undergo surgery, though some advocate an initial conservative approach in patients without generalized peritonitis (NBM, NG tube, IV antibiotics—this can prevent surgery in up to 50% of such cases). If emergency surgery is required, laparoscopic repair is as good (and may be better) than open repair.[158] *H. pylori* eradication should be commenced post-op (p242).
- *Pyloric stenosis* Adult pyloric stenosis is a late complication of duodenal ulcers due to scarring (and has nothing to do with congenital hypertrophic pyloric stenosis, p629). Patients complain of vomiting large amounts of food some hours after meals. *Treatment:* Endoscopic balloon dilatation, followed by maximal acid suppression (p242), may be tried in the first instance (NB: 5% risk of perforation). If this is unsuccessful, a drainage procedure (eg gastro-enterostomy or pyloroplasty) ± highly selective vagotomy may be performed, often laparoscopically. The operation should be done on the next available list, after correction of the metabolic defect—a hypochloraemic, hypokalaemic metabolic alkalosis.

## Fundoplication for gastro-oesophageal reflux

Laparoscopic fundoplication is the surgical procedure of choice when symtoms of GORD are retractable and refractory to medical therapy **and** there is severe reflux (confirmed by pH-monitoring)—see p244. Symptoms may be complicated by a hiatus hernia, which is repaired during the procedure.

**Surgery** The defect in the diaphragm is repaired by tightening the crura. Reflux is prevented by wrapping the gastric fundus around the lower oesophageal sphincter—see fig 1. There are various types of procedure, eg Nissen (360° wrap), Toupet (270° posterior wrap), Watson (anterior hemifundoplication).

Laparoscopic surgery is at least as effective at controlling reflux as open surgery but with a lower mortality and morbidity. Wound infections and respiratory complications are also more common in open surgery, though the incidence of dysphagia is similar for the two procedures—but see p594.

**Complications** Dysphagia (if the wrap is too tight), 'gas-bloat syndrome' (inability to belch/vomit) and new onset diarrhoea.[159]

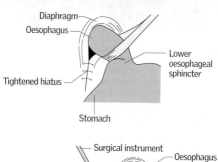

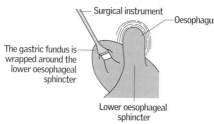

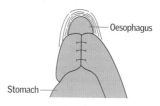

Fig 1. Laparoscopic Nissen fundoplication.

Fifty years ago obesity was considered a contraindication to elective surgery; however, obesity in itself may not be a risk factor for most complications.[160] In fact mild obesity confers an advantage to patients undergoing general and vascular surgery, with reduced complications and mortality compared to 'normal' weight patients.[161,162] Incidence of complications after elective surgery does not differ significantly between obese and non-obese patients, except for ↑ wound infection in obese patients.[160] Some studies have found obesity to increase complication risks (but not mortality) in cardiac surgery[163] and spinal surgery.[164] However, the practice of forcing patients to lose weight prior to elective surgery may be inappropriate if there are no clinical justifications.

**Surgical management of severe obesity** Severe obesity is increasing in prevalence worldwide and is associated with type 2 diabetes mellitus (T2DM); hypertension; ischaemic heart disease; sleep apnoea; osteoarthritis; and depression. Bariatric surgery has become very successful at weight reduction, symptom improvement,[165] and improving quality of life.[166] Surgery increases life expectancy by around 3 years[167] (but may not prolong survival in high-risk men).[168]

*Indications* According to NICE guidelines, weight-loss surgery in adults should be considered if *all* the following criteria are met:

1 BMI ≥40 or ≥35 with significant comorbidities that could improve with ↓weight.
2 Failure of non-surgical management to achieve and maintain clinically beneficial weight loss for 6 months.
3 Fitness for surgery and anaesthesia.
4 As part of an integrated programme that provides guidance on diet, physical activity, and psychosocial concerns, as well as lifelong medical monitoring.
5 The patient must be well-informed and motivated.

NB: if BMI ≥50 surgery is recommended as first-line treatment.

**Comparison with medical therapy** The *Swedish Obese Subjects Trial* compared conventional medical treatment (either diet, lifestyle or nothing) to surgery (including banding, gastroplasty and bypass). At 2 years surgical patients had a mean 23% weight loss (16% at 10 years). The medical group saw weight increase by 0.1% at 2 years and 1.6% at 10 years. The surgical group had higher recovery from comorbidities and improved quality of life.[169]

**Procedures** There are 2 main mechanisms causing weight loss: 1 Restriction of calorie intake by reducing stomach capacity 2 Malabsorption of nutrients by reducing the length of functional small bowel. NB: This also affects the levels of circulating gut peptides (eg PYY and GLP-1), which are thought to play a role in the mechanism of satiety and weight loss. The 2 most popular procedures are:

- *Laparoscopic adjustable gastric banding (LAGB):* This restrictive technique creates a pre-stomach pouch by placing a silicone band around the top of the stomach, which serves as a new smaller stomach. The band can be adjusted to alter the degree of restriction by addition or removal of saline through a subcutaneous port (see fig 1). One prospective study showed mean excess weight loss at 1 year of 45.7%.[170] LAGB is associated with improvements or recovery of T2DM, hypertension, asthma, joint pain, and depression, as well as improved quality of life.[171] Weight loss is slower and less than with gastric bypass but there is lower mortality and fewer complications. Long-term outcomes are yet to be firmly established. *Complications:* Pouch enlargement, band slip, band erosion and port infection/breakage.[172]

- *Roux-en-Y gastric bypass* (fig 2, p625): A portion of the jejunum is attached to a small stomach pouch to allow food to bypass the distal stomach, duodenum, and proximal jejunum. It can be performed laparoscopically and works by both restriction and malabsorption. Mean excess weight loss at 5 years is 62.8%.[173] Current evidence demonstrates greater weight loss, greater resolution of comorbidities and lower reoperation rates compared to LAGB.[174] *Complications:* Micronutrient deficiency (requires vitamin supplementation and lifelong follow-up with annual blood and micronutrient level tests), dumping syndrome, wound infection, hernias, malabsorption, diarrhoea, and a mortality of ~0.5% (at experienced centres).

# Some paediatric surgical emergencies

**Congenital hypertrophic pyloric stenosis** ►See *OHCS* p172. Usually presents in first 3-8wks as projectile vomiting (4 in 1000 live births). ♂:♀≈4:1. The baby is malnourished and always hungry. *Diagnosis:* palpate the olive-shaped pyloric mass in the RUQ during a feed. Visible gastric peristalsis starts in the LUQ. The baby can be severely alkalotic and depleted of water and ions from vomiting. Needs correcting **before** surgery. USS may be useful in assessment. Pass NGT (p773). *Treatment:* Ramstedt's pyloromyotomy (involves incision of muscle down to mucosa).

**Intussusception** See *OHCS*, p172. Small bowel telescopes, as if swallowing itself by invagination. *Presentation:* Any age (usually 5-12 months). **Episodic** intermittent inconsolable crying, with drawing the legs up (colic)±bilious vomiting± blood PR (like redcurrant jam or cranberry sauce).[175] A sausage-shaped abdominal mass may be felt. May become shocked and moribund. *Tests/Management:* Least invasive approach is USS with reduction by air enema or pneumatic reduction under radiographic control. If reduction fails, surgery is needed. Prompt treatment may avoid necrosis. *Pre-op care:* ►►Resuscitate, crossmatch blood, pass NGT. NB: children >4yrs present differently: rectal bleeding less common, more likely to have a long history (>3wks) and some sort of contributing pathology, eg Henoch-Schönlein purpura, cystic fibrosis, Peutz-Jeghers' syndrome or tumours, eg lymphomas—where obstructive symptoms caused by intussusception are the chief mode of presentation. Recurrence rate: ~5%.

**Midgut malrotation** See *OHCS* p130. During embryonic development, the midgut undergoes 270° anticlockwise rotation. If malrotated the gut is prone to undergo volvulus upon its abnormally pedicled mesentery. Usually presents in neonatal period with dark green bilious vomiting, distension, and rectal bleeding. Can be asymptomatic for years before acute presentation. *Treatment:* ►►Resuscitation, then surgery (involves broadening the mesentery and replacing bowel in a non-rotated position).

## Tips on examining the abdomen in children

Examining the abdomen of a child or infant can prove extremely difficult and requires patience, practice and opportunism. So:
- An age-directed approach will help develop your relationship with the child.
- Remember that the parents will be closely involved in what you do.
- Play specialists may be able to provide distraction.
- The abdomen may need to be examined with the child sitting in mum's lap.
- There is no hope of eliciting any signs whilst the child is crying and tensing his tummy—everyone will be better off if you return when the child has settled!
- Examining for rebound tenderness in young children is probably of little use for us and definitely uncomfortable for them.
- You should always examine the scrotum and inguinal regions in young boys to exclude the possibility of testicular torsion or a strangulated hernia.
- Performing a PR examination, if required, is best left to a specialist.
- Unless you have a magical way with children, don't be surprised to get the cold shoulder once in a while!

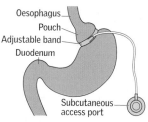

Fig 1. Adjustable gastric band.

A GI **diverticulum** is an outpouching of the gut wall, usually at sites of entry of perforating arteries. **Diverticulosis** means that diverticula are present, and **diverticular disease** implies they are symptomatic. **Diverticulitis** refers to inflammation of a diverticulum. Diverticulum can be aquired or congenital and may occur elsewhere, but the most important are acquired colonic diverticula, to which this page refers.

**Pathology** Most occur in the sigmoid colon with 95% of complications at this site, but right-sided and massive single diverticula can occur. Lack of dietary fibre is thought to lead to high intraluminal pressures which force the mucosa to herniate through the muscle layers of the gut at weak points adjacent to penetrating vessels. 30% of Westerners have diverticulosis by age 60. The majority are asymptomatic.

**Diagnosis** Diverticulae are a common incidental finding at colonoscopy (fig 6, p257), which should be performed if there is any suspicion of malignancy. Barium enema can clarify the diagnosis in patients with abdominal pain and altered bowel habit. CT abdomen is best to confirm acute diverticulitis and can identfy extent of disease and any complications.[178] Enema or colonoscopy risk perforation in the acute setting. Abdominal x-ray may identify obstruction, free air (perforation), or vesical fistulae.

**Complications of diverticulosis** There may be altered bowel habit ± left-sided colic relieved by defecation; nausea and flatulence. A high-fibre diet (wholemeal bread, fruit and vegetables) may be tried. Antispasmodics, eg *mebeverine* 135mg/8h PO, may help. Surgical resection is occasionally resorted to. Other complications:

**Diverticulitis**—with features above + pyrexia, WCC↑, CRP/ESR↑, a tender colon ± localized or generalized peritonism. ℞: analgesia, NBM, IV fluids, antibiotics, CT-guided percutaneous drainage (if abscess). ▶Beware diverticulitis in immunocompromised patients (eg on steroids) who often have few symptoms and may present late.

▶▶*Perforation* There is ileus, peritonitis ± shock. Mortality: 40%. Manage as for an acute abdomen. At laparotomy a Hartmann's procedure may be performed (temporary colostomy + partial colectomy). Primary anastomosis is possible and avoids repeat surgery to close the colostomy. This has comparable mortality to Hartmann's in patients with perforation (although selection bias limits sound conclusions).[177] Emergency laparoscopic management is an emerging alternative.[178]

• *Haemorrhage* is usually sudden and painless. It is a common cause of big rectal bleeds. ▶See BOX 2. Bleeding usually stops with bed rest. Transfusion may be needed. Embolization or colonic resection may be necessary after locating bleeding points by angiography or colonoscopy (here diathermy ± local *adrenaline* injections may obviate the need for surgery).

• *Fistulae* Enterocolic, colovaginal, or colovesical (pneumaturia ± intractable UTIs). Treatment is surgical, eg colonic resection.

• *Abscesses*, eg with swinging fever, leucocytosis, and localizing signs, eg boggy rectal mass (pelvic abscess—drain rectally). If no localizing signs, remember the aphorism: *pus somewhere, pus nowhere = pus under the diaphragm*. A subphrenic abscess is a horrible way to die, so do an urgent ultrasound. Antibiotics ± ultrasound/CT-guided drainage may be needed.

• *Post-infective strictures* may form in the sigmoid colon.

## Angiodysplasia

Angiodysplasia refers to submucosal arteriovenous malformations that typically present as fresh PR bleeding in the elderly. The underlying cause is unknown. *Pathology:* 70–90% of lesions occur in right colon, though angiodysplasia can affect anywhere in the GI tract. *Diagnosis:* PR examination, colonoscopy (fig 5, p257) may exclude competing diagnoses; [99mTc] radionuclide-labelled red-cell imaging (p752) is useful in identifying lesions during active bleeding (if >0.1mL/min). Mesenteric angiography is very helpful in diagnosing angiodysplasia (shows early filling at the lesion site, then extravasation), and allows therapeutic embolization during bleeding—it detects bleeding >1mL/min. CT angiography offers a non-invasive alternative. *Treatment options:* Embolization, endoscopic laser electrocoagulation, resection.

## Managing diverticulitis[179]

### Initial management

- Mild attacks can be treated at home with bowel rest (fluids only) ± antibiotics.[180]
- If oral fluids cannot be tolerated or pain cannot be controlled, admit to hospital for analgesia, NBM and IV fluids. IV antibiotics in uncomplicated diverticulitis are routinely given, but do not speed recovery or prevent comlications/recurrence.[181] Seek advice and follow local guidelines where available. Most attacks settle but complications include abscess formation (necessitating percutaneous CT-guided drainage), or perforation—see p630 for management.
- **Imaging** Erect CXR + USS can detect perforation, free fluid, and collections, though CT with contrast is more accurate, especially in complicated disease. If a contrast enema is performed, then water-soluble contrast should be used (see p762). ▶In an acute attack colonoscopy should not be done.[182]

**Surgery** The need for surgery is reflected by the degree of infective complications:

| | | |
|---|---|---|
| Stage 1 | Periolic or mesenteric abscess | Surgery rarely needed |
| Stage 2 | Walled off or pelvic abscess | May resolve without surgery |
| Stage 3 | Generalized purulent peritonitis | Surgery required |
| Stage 4 | Generalized faecal peritonitis | Surgery required |

- Elective resection after an acute episode is rarely recommended as most patients who develop complications present at the first episode. Indications for elective surgery include stenosis, fistule or recurrent bleeding.[183]
- For emergency colonic resection see p630.

## Rectal bleeding—an acute management plan

The causes of rectal bleeding are covered elsewhere (MINIBOX). Here let's make an acute management plan for this common surgical event:

▶▶ **ABC** resuscitation, if necessary.

▶▶ **History and examination**

▶▶ **Blood tests:** FBC, U&E, LFT, clotting, amylase (always thinking of pancreatitis), CRP, group and save—await Hb result before crossmatching unless unstable and bleeding.

▶▶ **Imaging** May only need plain AXR, but if there are signs of perforation (eg sepsis, peritonism) or if there is cardiorespiratory comorbidity, then request an erect CXR. See *angiodysplasia*, p630, for more imaging options.

> **Typical causes**
> - Diverticulitis, p630
> - Colorectal cancer, p618
> - Haemorrhoids, p634
> - Crohn's, UC, p272-275
> - Perianal disease, p632
> - Angiodysplasia, p630
> - Rarities—trauma, also:
>   - ischaemic colitis, p622
>   - radiation proctitis
>   - aorto-enteric fistula

▶▶ **Fluid management** Insert 2 cannulae (≥18G) into the antecubital fossae. Insert a urinary catheter if there is a suspicion of haemodynamic compromise—there is no absolute indication, but remember that you are weighing up the risks and benefits. Give crystalloid as replacement and maintenance IVI. Blood transfusion is rarely needed in the acute setting.

▶▶ **Antibiotics** may occasionally be required if there is evidence of sepsis or perforation, eg *cefuroxime* 1.5g/8h IV + *metronidazole* 500mg/8h IV.

▶▶ **PPI** Consider *omeprazole* 40mg/d IV as ~15% are from upper GI causes (p252-4).

▶▶ **Keep bedbound** The patient may feel the need to get out of bed to pass stool, but this could be another large bleed, resulting in collapse if they try to walk. ▶Don't allow them to mobilize and inform the nursing staff of this.

▶▶ **Start a stool chart** to monitor volume and frequency of motions. Send a sample for MC&S (x3 if known to have compromising comorbidity such as IBD).

▶▶ **Diet** Keep on clear fluids so that they can have something, yet the colon will be clear for colonoscopy (which is of little value until bleeding has stopped).

▶▶ **Surgery** The main indication for this is unremitting, massive bleeding.

Surgery

**Pruritus ani** Itch occurs if the anus is moist/soiled; fissures, incontinence, poor hygiene, tight pants, threadworm, fistula, dermatoses, lichen sclerosis, anxiety, contact dermatitis (perfumed goods). Cause is often unknown. $R$: Careful hygiene, anaesthetic cream, moist wipe post-defecation, no spicy food, no steroid/antibiotic cream. Capsaicin may help.[184]

**Fissure-in-ano** Painful tear in the squamous lining of the lower anal canal—often, if chronic, with a 'sentinel pile' or mucosal tag at the external aspect. 90% are posterior (anterior ones follow parturition). ♂>♀. *Causes:* Most are due to hard faeces. Spasm may constrict the inferior rectal artery, causing ischaemia, making healing difficult and perpetuating the problem.[185,186,187] Rare causes (multiple ± lateral): syphilis; herpes; trauma; Crohn's; anal cancer; psoriasis. Groin nodes suggest a complicating factor (eg immunosuppression/HIV). $R$: 5% *lidocaine* ointment + GTN ointment (0.2-0.4%) or topical *diltiazem* (2%)[188]; ↑dietary fibre, fluids ± stool softener and hygiene advice. *Botulinum toxin* injection (2ⁿᵈ line) and topical diltiazem (2%) are at least as effective as GTN with fewer side-effects.[189] If conservative measures fail, surgical options include *lateral partial internal sphincterotomy*.[190]

**Fistula-in-ano** A track communicates between the skin and anal canal/rectum. Blockage of deep intramuscular gland ducts is thought to predispose to the formation of abscesses, which discharge to form the fistula. *Goodsall's rule* determines the path of the fistula track: if anterior, the track is in a straight line (radial); if posterior, the internal opening is always at the 6 o'clock position. *Causes:* perianal sepsis, abscesses (see below), Crohn's disease, TB, diverticular disease, rectal carcinoma, immunocompromise. *Tests:* MRI;[191] endoanal US scan.[192] $R$: Fistulotomy + excision. High fistulae (involving continence muscles of anus) require 'seton suture' tightened over time to maintain continence; low fistulae are 'laid open' to heal by secondary intention—division of sphincters poses no risk to continence.

**Anorectal abscesses** usually caused by gut organisms (rarely staphs or TB). ♂:♀≈8:1. Perianal (~45%), ischiorectal (≤30%), intersphincteric (>20%), supralevator (~5%). $R$: Incise & drain under GA. *Associations:* DM, Crohn's, malignancy, fistulae.

**Perianal haematoma** (AKA thrombosed external pile—see p635). Strictly, it is actually a clotted venous saccule. It appears as a 2-4mm 'dark blueberry' under the skin at the anal margin. It may be evacuated under LA or left to resolve spontaneously.

**Pilonidal sinus** Obstruction of natal cleft hair follicles ~6cm above the anus. Ingrowing of hair excites a foreign body reaction and may cause secondary tracks to open laterally ± abscesses, with foul-smelling discharge. (Barbers get these between fingers.) ♂:♀≈10:1. Obese Caucasians and those from Asia, the Middle East, and Mediterranean at ↑risk. $R$: Excision of the sinus tract ± primary closure. Consider pre-op *antibiotics*. Complex tracks can be laid open and packed individually, or skin flaps can be used to cover the defect.[193] Offer hygiene and hair removal advice.

**Rectal prolapse** The mucosa (partial/type 1), or all layers (complete/type 2—more common), may protrude through the anus. Incontinence in 75%. It is due to a lax sphincter, prolonged straining, and related to chronic neurological and psychological disorders. $R$ *Abdominal approach*: fix rectum to sacrum (rectopexy) ± mesh insertion ± rectosigmoidectomy. Laparoscopic rectopexy is as effective as open repair.[194] *Perineal approach*: Delorme's procedure (resect close to dentate line and suture mucosal boundaries), anal encirclement with a Thiersch wire.[195]

**Perianal warts** Condylomata acuminata (viral warts) are treated with *podophyllotoxin* or *imiquimod* or cryotherapy/surgical excision. Giant condylomata acuminata of Bushke & Loewenstein may evolve into verrucous cancers (low-grade, non-metastasizing). Condylomata lata secondary to syphilis is treated with penicillin.

**Proctalgia fugax** Idiopathic, intense, brief, stabbing/crampy rectal pain, often worse at night. The mainstay of treatment is reassurance. Inhaled *salbutamol* or topical GTN (0.2-0.4%) or topical *diltiazem* (2%) may help.[196]

**Anal ulcers** are rare. Consider Crohn's disease, anal cancer, TB, and syphilis.

**Skin tags** seldom cause trouble but are easily excised.

## Examination of the rectum and anus

►It is necessary to have a chaperone present for the examination. Explain what you are about to do. Make sure curtains are pulled. Have the patient lie on their left side, with knees brought up towards the chest. Use gloves and lubricant. Part the buttocks and **inspect the anus:** •A gaping anus suggests a neuropathy or megarectum •Symmetry (a tender unilateral bulge suggests an abscess) •Prolapsed piles •A subanodermal clot may peep out •Prolapsed rectum (descent of >3cm when asked to strain, as if to pass a motion) •Anodermatitis (from frequent soiling). The anocutaneous reflex tests sensory and motor innervation—on lightly stroking the anal skin, does the external sphincter briefly contract?

Press your index finger against the side of the anus. Ask the patient to breathe deeply and insert your finger slowly. Feel for masses (haemorrhoids are not palpable) or impacted stool. Twist your arm so that the pad of your finger is feeling anteriorly. Feel for the cervix or prostate. Note consistency, size, and symmetry of the prostate. If there is faecal incontinence or concern about the spinal cord, ask the patient to squeeze your finger and note the tone. This is best done with your finger pad facing posteriorly. Note stool or blood on the glove and test for occult blood.

Wipe the anus. Consider proctoscopy (for the anus) or sigmoidoscopy (which mainly inspects the rectum).

## Anal cancer

**Incidence:** 300/yr.[uk] *Risk↑:* Syphilis, anal warts (HPV 16, 6, 11, 18, 31 & 33 implicated), anoreceptive homosexuals (often young). *Histology:* Squamous cell (85%); rarely basaloid, melanoma, or adenocarcinoma. Anal margin tumours are usually well-differentiated, keratinizing lesions with a good prognosis. Anal canal tumours arise above dentate line, are poorly differentiated and non-keratinizing with a poorer prognosis. *Spread:* Tumours above the dentate line spread to pelvic lymph nodes; those below spread to the inguinal nodes. *The patient* may present with bleeding, pain, bowel habit change, pruritus ani, masses, stricture. *ΔΔ:* Perianal warts; leucoplakia; lichen sclerosis; Bowen's disease; Crohn's disease. *Treatment:* Chemo-irradiation (radiotherapy + 5-fluorouracil + mitomycin/cisplatin) is usually preferred to anorectal excision & colostomy; 75% retain normal anal function.[197]

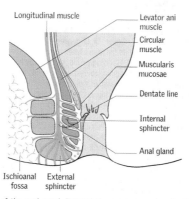

**Fig 1.** Anatomy of the anal canal. Perianal abscesses present as tender, inflamed, localized swellings at the anal verge. Ischiorectal abscesses are also tender but cause a diffuse, indurated swelling in the ischioanal fossa area. You will find your patient waiting anxiously for you, pacing about, or on the edge of their chair: avoiding all pressure is imperative. NB: Above the dentate line = visceral nerve innervation; below = somatic innervation (very sensitive to pain).

**Definition** Haemorrhoids are disrupted and dilated anal cushions. The anus is lined mainly by discontinuous masses of spongy vascular tissue—the anal cushions, which contribute to anal closure. Viewed from the lithotomy position, the 3 anal cushions are at 3, 7, and 11 o'clock (where the 3 major arteries that feed the vascular plexuses enter the anal canal). They are attached by smooth muscle and elastic tissue, but are prone to displacement and disruption, either singly or together. The effects of gravity (our erect posture), increased anal tone (?stress), and the effects of straining at stool may make them become both bulky and loose, and so to protrude to form piles (Latin *pila*, meaning a ball). They are vulnerable to trauma (eg from hard stools) and bleed readily from the capillaries of the underlying lamina propria, hence their other name, haemorrhoids (≈*running blood* in Greek). Because loss is from capillaries, it is bright red. NB: piles are **not** varicose veins.

As there are no sensory fibres above the dentate line (squamomucosal junction), piles are not painful unless they thrombose when they protrude and are gripped by the anal sphincter, blocking venous return.

**Differential diagnosis** Perianal haematoma; anal fissure; abscess; tumour; proctalgia fugax. ▶Never ascribe rectal bleeding to piles without adequate examination or investigation.

**Causes** Constipation with prolonged straining is a key factor. In many the bowel habit may be normal. Congestion from a pelvic tumour, pregnancy, CCF, or portal hypertension are important in only a minority of cases.

**Pathogenesis** There is a vicious circle: vascular cushions protrude through a tight anus, become more congested and hypertrophy to protrude again more readily. These protrusions may then strangulate. See TABLE for classification.

**Symptoms** Bright red rectal bleeding, often coating stools, on the tissue, or dripping into the pan after defecation. There may be mucous discharge and pruritus ani. Severe anaemia may occur. Symptoms such as weight loss, tenesmus and change in bowel habit should prompt thoughts of other pathology. ▶In all rectal bleeding do:
• An abdominal examination to rule out other diseases.
• PR exam: prolapsing piles are obvious. Internal haemorrhoids are not palpable.
• Proctoscopy to see the internal haemorrhoids.
• Sigmoidoscopy to identify rectal pathology higher up (you can get no higher up than the rectosigmoid junction).

**Treatment**[198] **1** *Medical:* (for 1$^{st}$-degree haemorrhoids) ↑fluid and fibre is key ± topical analgesics & stool softener. Topical steroids for short periods only.
**2** *Non-operative:* (for 2$^{nd}$ & 3$^{rd}$ degree, or 1$^{st}$ degree if medical therapy has failed). The best treatment is unknown as meta-analyses differ: •*Rubber band ligation:* A cheap treatment, but needs skill. Banding produces an ulcer to anchor the mucosa (SE: bleeding, infection; pain). It has the lowest recurrence rate. •*Sclerosants:* (for 1$^{st}$- or 2$^{nd}$-degree piles) 2mL of 5% *phenol* in almond/arachis oil is injected into the pile above the dentate line. Recurrence is higher (SE: impotence; prostatitis). •*Infra-red coagulation:* Applied to localized areas of piles, it works by coagulating vessels and tethering mucosa to subcutaneous tissue. It is as successful as banding and is less painful.[199] •*Cryotherapy* (freezing) has a high complication rate and is not recommended. In all but 4$^{th}$-degree piles, these measures may obviate the need for surgery.
**3** *Surgery:* •*Excisional haemorrhoidectomy* is the most effective treatment (excision of piles ± ligation of vascular pedicles, as day-case surgery, needing ~2wks off work). Scalpel, electrocautery or laser may be used. •*Stapled haemorrhoidopexy* (AKA *procedure for prolapsing haemorrhoids*) may result in less pain, a shorter hospital stay and quicker return to normal activity than conventional surgery.[200] It is used when there is a large internal component, but has a higher recurrence and prolapse rate than excisional surgery.[201] *Surgical complications:* Constipation; infection; stricture; bleeding.

**Prolapsed, thrombosed piles** are treated with analgesia, ice packs and stool softeners. Pain usually resolves in 2-3 weeks. Some advocate early surgery.

**Classification of haemorrhoids**

| | |
|---|---|
| **1st degree** | Remain in the rectum |
| **2nd degree** | Prolapse through the anus on defecation but spontaneously reduce |
| **3rd degree** | As for 2nd-degree but require digital reduction |
| **4th degree** | Remain persistently prolapsed |

External
haemorrhoid

Internal
haemorrhoid

Mixed
haemorrhoid

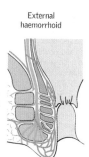
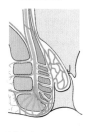
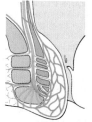

Origin below dentate
line (external rectal
plexus)

Origin above dentate
line (internal rectal
plexus)

Origin above and below
dentate line (internal and
external rectal plexus)

Fig 1. Internal and external haemorrhoids.

Bile contains cholesterol, bile pigments (from broken down Hb), and phospholipids. If the concentrations vary, different stones may form.[202] *Pigment stones:* (<10%) Small, friable, and irregular. *Causes:* haemolysis. *Cholesterol stones:* Large, often solitary. *Causes:* ♀, age, obesity (Admirand's triangle: ↑risk of stone if ↓lecithin, ↓bile salts, ↑cholesterol). *Mixed stones:* Faceted (calcium salts, pigment, and cholesterol). *Gallstone prevalence:* 8% of those over 40yrs. 90% remain asymptomatic. Risk factors for stones becoming symptomatic: smoking; parity.

**Acute cholecystitis** follows stone or sludge impaction in the neck of the gallbladder (GB), which may cause continuous epigastric or RUQ pain (referred to the right shoulder—see p611), vomiting, fever, local peritonism, or a GB mass. The main difference from biliary colic is the inflammatory component (local peritonism, fever, WCC↑). If the stone moves to the common bile duct (CBD), obstructive jaundice and cholangitis may occur—see BOX for complications. **Murphy's sign:** Lay 2 fingers over the RUQ; ask patient to breathe in. This causes pain & arrest of inspiration as an inflamed GB impinges on your fingers. It is only +ve if the same test in the LUQ does not cause pain. A phlegmon (RUQ mass of inflamed adherent omentum and bowel) may be palpable. *Tests:* WCC↑, ultrasound—a thick-walled, shrunken GB (also seen in chronic disease), pericholecystic fluid, stones, CBD (dilated if >6mm), HIDA cholescintigraphy (useful if diagnosis uncertain after US). Plain AXR only shows ~10% of gallstones; it may identify a 'porcelain' GB (~15% association with cancer).[203] *Treatment:* NBM, pain relief, IVI, and, eg cefuroxime 1.5g/8h IV. Laparoscopic cholecystectomy (either acute or delayed, see BOX 3) is the treatment of choice for all patients fit for GA. Open surgery is required if there is GB perforation. If elderly or high risk/unsuitable for surgery, consider percutaneous cholecystostomy; cholecystectomy can still be done later. Cholecystostomy is also the preferred treatment for acalculous cholecystitis.[204]

**Chronic cholecystitis** Chronic inflammation ± colic. 'Flatulent dyspepsia': vague abdominal discomfort, distension, nausea, flatulence, and fat intolerance (fat stimulates cholecystokinin release and GB contraction). US to image stones and assess CBD diameter. MRCP (p757) is used to find CBD stones. ℞: Cholecystectomy. If US shows a dilated CBD with stones, ERCP (p756) + sphincterotomy before surgery. If symptoms persist post-surgery consider hiatus hernia/IBS/peptic ulcer/relapsing pancreatitis/tumour.

**Biliary colic** Gallstones are symptomatic with cystic duct obstruction or if passed into the CBD. RUQ pain (radiates → back) ± jaundice. ℞: Analgesia (see p638), rehydrate, NBM. Elective laparoscopic cholecystectomy (see BOX 3). ΔΔ: The above may overlap as part of a spectrum of gallstone disease. Urinalysis, CXR, and ECG help exclude other diseases.

## Other presentations

- *Obstructive jaundice with CBD stones* (see p250)—if LFT worsening, ERCP with sphincterotomy ± biliary trawl, then cholecystectomy may be needed, or open surgery with CBD exploration. If CBD stones are suspected pre-operatively, they should be identified by MRCP (p762).
- *Cholangitis* (bile duct infection) causing RUQ pain, jaundice, and rigors (Charcot's triad, BOX). Treat with, eg cefuroxime 1.5g/8h IV and metronidazole 500mg/8h IV/PR.
- *Gallstone ileus:* A stone erodes through the GB into the duodenum; it may then obstruct the terminal ileum. AXR shows: air in CBD (= pneumobilia), small bowel fluid levels, and a stone. Duodenal obstruction is rarer (Bouveret's syndrome).[205]
- *Pancreatitis* (p638).
- *Mucocoele/empyema:* Obstructed GB fills with mucus (secreted by GB wall)/pus.
- *Silent stones:* Do elective surgery on those with sickle cell, immunosuppression (debatably diabetes) as well as all calcified/porcelain GBs.[206,207]
- *Mirizzi's syndrome:* A stone in the GB presses on the bile duct causing jaundice.[208]
- *Gallbladder perforation:* Rare because of dual blood supply (hepatic artery via cystic artery, and from small branches of the hepatic artery in the GB fossa).
- *Other:* Causes of cholecystitis and biliary symptoms other than gallstones are rare. Consider infection (typhoid, cryptosporidiosis and brucellosis); cholecystokinin release; parenteral nutrition; anatomical abnormality; polyarteritis nodosa (p558).

## Complications of gallstones

**In the gallbladder & cystic duct:**
- Biliary colic
- Acute and chronic cholecystitis
- Mucocoele
- Empyema
- Carcinoma
- Mirizzi's syndrome

**In the bile ducts:**
- Obstructive jaundice
- Cholangitis
- Pancreatitis

**In the gut:**
- Gallstone ileus

## Biliary colic, cholecystitis or cholangitis?

|  | RUQ pain | Fever / ↑wcc | Jaundice |
|---|---|---|---|
| **Biliary colic** | ✓ | ✗ | ✗ |
| **Acute cholecystitis** | ✓ | ✓ | ✗ |
| **Cholangitis** | ✓ | ✓ | ✓ |

## Early or delayed cholecystectomy?

**For acute cholecystitis** Laparoscopic cholecystectomy for acute cholecystitis has traditionally been performed 6–12wks after the acute episode due to anticipated increased mortality and conversion to open procedure. However, early laparoscopic cholecystectomy is becoming the treatment of choice. It is as safe as delayed surgery, there is no difference in the rate of conversion to open surgery or bile duct injury and early surgery shortens the length of hospital stay.[209] If surgery is delayed, repeat episodes of cholecystitis occur in 18% and may be associated with more complications.[210]

**For biliary colic** Patients with biliary colic due to gallstones waiting for an elective laparoscopic cholecystectomy may develop life-threatening complications, such as acute pancreatitis (p638) during the waiting period. Cochrane review of one high bias trial found early laparoscopic cholecystectomy (within 24 hours of an acute episode) decreased potential complications that may develop during the wait for elective surgery.[211]

## ☼ Is it possible to perform double-blind RCTs in surgery?

A double-blinded randomized controlled trial (RCT) looked at the differences between open and laparoscopic cholecystectomy.[212] This raises issues on both the place and validity of double-blinded RCTs in surgery.

Overcoming established treatments always has difficulties. When faced with either surgery or non-operative management, everyone's preference would be to avoid surgery especially if there is ambivalence about which treatment is superior. The negative influence of the learning curve for a new treatment must be considered and this may take time to overcome (p595). Furthermore, controlling the bias introduced by interperformer and patient variance is not least because each patient is different. There are also inherent difficulties in double-blinding surgical treatment: 'sham' surgery remains a contentious issue.[213] ✿☙

This unpredictable disease (mortality ~12%) is managed on surgical wards, but because surgery is often not involved, it's easy to think that there's no acute problem. There is: Self-perpetuating pancreatic inflammation by enzyme-mediated autodigestion; Oedema and fluid shifts causing hypovolaemia, as extracellular fluid is trapped in the gut, peritoneum, and retroperitoneum (worsened by vomiting). Progression may be rapid from mild oedema to necrotizing pancreatitis. ~50% of cases that advance to necrosis are further complicated by infection. Pancreatitis is mild in 80% of cases; 20% develop severe complicated and life-threatening disease.[214] For causes see MINIBOX.

| Causes 'GET SMASHED' |
|---|
| Gallstones[38%] |
| Ethanol[35%] |
| Trauma[1.5%] |
| Steroids |
| Mumps |
| Autoimmune (PAN) |
| Scorpion venom |
| Hyperlipidaemia, hypothermia, hypercalcaemia |
| ERCP[5%] and emboli |
| Drugs |
| Also pregnancy and neoplasia or no cause found[10-30%] |

**Symptoms** Gradual or sudden severe **epigastric** or **central abdominal pain** (radiates to back, sitting forward may relieve); vomiting prominent.

**Signs** may be mild in serious disease! Tachycardia, fever, jaundice, shock, ileus, rigid abdomen ± local/general tenderness, periumbilical bruising (**Cullen's sign**) or flanks (**Grey Turner's sign**) from blood vessel autodigestion and retroperitoneal haemorrhage.

**Tests** Raised serum *amylase* (>1000u/mL or around 3-fold upper limit of normal). The degree of elevation is not related to severity of disease. ►Amylase may be normal even in severe pancreatitis (levels starts to fall within the 1st 24-48h). Cholecystitis, mesenteric infarction, and GI perforation can cause lesser rises (usually). It is excreted renally so renal failure will ↑ levels. Serum *lipase* is more sensitive and specific for pancreatitis.[215] *ABG* to monitor oxygenation and acid-base status. *AXR*: No psoas shadow (retroperitoneal fluid↑), 'sentinel loop' of proximal jejunum from ileus (solitary air-filled dilatation). *Erect CXR* helps exclude other causes (eg perforation). *CT* is the standard choice of imaging to assess severity and for complications—*MRI* may be even better.[216] *US* (if gallstones + AST↑). *ERCP* if LFTs worsen. *CRP* >150mg/L at 36h after admission is a predictor of severe pancreatitis.

**Management** Severity assessment is essential (see BOX).
- Nil by mouth, likely to need NG tube (decrease pancreatic stimulation). Set up IVI and give lots of 0.9% saline, to counter third-space sequestration, until vital signs are satisfactory and urine flow stays at >30mL/h. Insert a urinary catheter and consider CVP monitoring. Think about nutrition early on (p586).
- Analgesia: *pethidine* 75-100mg/4h IM, or *morphine* (may cause Oddi's sphincter to contract more,[217] but it is a better analgesic and not contraindicated).[218]
- Hourly pulse, BP, and urine output; daily FBC, U&E, Ca²⁺, glucose, amylase, ABG.
- If worsening: ITU, O₂ if $P_aO_2$↓. In suspected abscess formation or pancreatic necrosis (on CT), consider parenteral nutrition ± laparotomy & debridement ('necrosectomy'). Antibiotics may help in specific severe disease, eg *imipenem* if >30% necrosis.[219] There is no consensus on prophylactic use if necrosis is present.[220]
- ERCP + gallstone removal may be needed if there is progressive jaundice.
- Repeat imaging (usually CT) is performed in order to monitor progress.

ΔΔ Any acute abdomen (p608), myocardial infarct. **Prognosis** See BOX.

**Early complications** Shock, ARDS (p178), renal failure (►give lots of fluid!), DIC, sepsis, Ca²⁺↓, glucose↑ (transient; 5% need insulin).

**Late complications** (>1wk) *Pancreatic necrosis* and *pseudocyst* (fluid in lesser sac, fig 1), with fever, a mass ± persistent ↑amylase/LFT; may resolve or need drainage. *Abscesses* need draining. *Bleeding* from elastase eroding a major vessel (eg splenic artery); embolization may be life-saving. *Thrombosis* may occur in the splenic/gastroduodenal arteries, or colic branches of the SMA, causing bowel necrosis. *Fistulae* normally close spontaneously. If purely pancreatic they do not irritate the skin. Some patients suffer *recurrent oedematous pancreatitis* so often that near-total pancreatectomy is contemplated. ►It can all be a miserable course.

## Modified Glasgow criteria for predicting severity of pancreatitis

▶3 or more positive factors detected within 48h of onset suggest severe pancreatitis, and should prompt transfer to ITU/HDU. Mnemonic: PANCREAS.[221]

| | |
|---|---|
| $P_aO_2$ | <8kPa |
| Age | >55yrs |
| Neutrophilia | WBC >15 x 10⁹/L |
| Calcium | <2mmol/L |
| Renal function | Urea >16mmol/L |
| Enzymes | LDH >600iu/L; AST >200iu/L |
| Albumin | <32g/L (serum) |
| Sugar | blood glucose >10mmol/L |

Courtesy of Mr Etienne Moore FRCS.

Moore EM. A useful mnemonic for severity stratification in acute pancreatitis. *Ann R Coll Surg Engl* 2000; 82: 16-17. © The Royal College of Surgeons of England. Reproduced with permission.

These criteria have been validated for pancreatitis caused by gallstones and alcohol; Ranson's criteria are valid for alcohol-induced pancreatitis, and can only be fully applied after 48h, which does have its disadvantages. Other criteria for assessing severity include the Acute Physiology and Chronic Health Examination (APACHE)-II, and the Bedside Index for Severity in Acute Pancreatitis (BISAP).

*Other methods of severity assessment:* Severity can also be assessed with the help of CT (Computed Tomography Severity Index).[1] CRP can be a helpful marker.[222]

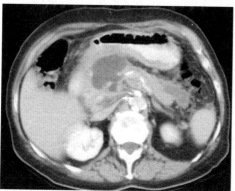

**Fig 1.** Axial CT of the abdomen (with IV and PO contrast media) showing a pancreatic pseudocyst occupying the lesser sac of the abdomen posterior to the stomach. It is called a 'pseudocyst' because it is not a true cyst, rather a collection of fluid in the lesser sac (ie not lined by epi/endothelium). It develops at ≥6wks. The cyst fluid is of low attenuation compared with the stomach contents because it has not been enhanced by the contrast media.

Image courtesy of Dr Stephen Golding.

Surgery

1 For a useful exposition on imaging in pancreatitis see www.emedicine.com/radio/topic521.htm.

Renal stones (calculi) consist of crystal aggregates. Stones form in collecting ducts and may be deposited anywhere from the renal pelvis to the urethra, though classically at 1 Pelviureteric junction 2 Pelvic brim 3 Vesicoureteric junction.

**Prevalence** Common: lifetime incidence up to 15%. *Peak age:* 20-40yr. ♂:♀≈3:1.

**Types** •Calcium oxalate (75%) •Magnesium ammonium phosphate (struvite/triple phosphate; 15%) •Also: urate (5%), hydroxyapatite (5%), brushite, cystine (1%), mixed.

**Presentation** Asymptomatic or: 1 *Renal colic:* excruciating ureteric spasms 'loin to groin' (or genitals/inner thigh), with nausea/vomiting. Often cannot lie still (differentiates from peritonitis). *Renal obstruction* felt in the loin, between rib 12 and lateral edge of lumbar muscles (like intercostal nerve irritation pain; the latter is not colicky, and is worsened by specific movements/pressure on a trigger spot). *Obstruction of mid-ureter* may mimic appendicitis/diverticulitis. *Obstruction of lower ureter* may lead to symptoms of bladder irritability and pain in scrotum, penile tip, or labia majora.[223] *Obstruction in bladder or urethra* causes pelvic pain, dysuria, strangury (desire but inability to void[224]) ± interrupted flow. 2 UTI can co-exist (↑risk if voiding impaired); *pyelonephritis* (fever, rigors, loin pain, nausea, vomiting), *pyonephrosis* (infected hydronephrosis) 3 Haematuria 4 Proteinuria 5 Sterile pyuria 6 Anuria.

**Examination** Usually no tenderness on palpation. May be renal angle tenderness especially to percussion if there is retroperitoneal inflammation.

**Tests** FBC, U&E, $Ca^{2+}$, $PO_4^{3-}$, glucose, bicarbonate, urate. *Urine dipstick:* Usually +ve for blood (90%). MSU: MC&S. *Further tests for cause:* Urine pH; 24h urine for: calcium, oxalate, urate, citrate, sodium, creatinine; stone biochemistry (sieve urine & send stone).

*Imaging:* Spiral non-contrast CT is superior to and has largely replaced IVU for imaging stones (99% visible) + helps exclude differential causes of an acute abdomen. ►A ruptured abdominal aortic aneurysm may present similarly. 80% of stones are visible on KUB XR (kidneys+ureters+bladder). Look along ureters for calcification over the transverse processes of the vertebral bodies. IVU: radio-opaque contrast injected and serial films taken until contrast seen down to level of obstruction. Cannot be interpreted without a plain control. Abnormal findings: failure of contrast to flow to bladder, dense nephrogram (contrast unable to flow from kidney), clubbed/blunted renal calyces (back pressure), filling defects in the bladder. (CI: contrast allergy, severe asthma, pregnancy, metformin.) USS to look for hydronephrosis or hydroureter.

**R:** *Initially:* Analgesia, eg *diclofenac* 75mg IV/IM, or 100mg PR.[225] (If CI: opioids) + IV fluids if unable to tolerate PO; antibiotics (eg *cefuroxime* 1.5g/8h IV, or *gentamicin*) if infection. *Stones <5mm in lower ureter:* ~90-95% pass spontaneously. ↑fluid intake. *Stones >5mm/pain not resolving:* Medical expulsive therapy: *nifedipine* 10mg/8h PO[226] or α-blockers (*tamsulosin* 0.4mg/d[227]) promote expulsion and reduce analgesia requirements:[228] ►start at presentation.[229] Most pass within 48h (>80% after ~30d). If not, try extracorporeal shockwave lithotripsy (ESWL) (if <1cm) or ureteroscopy using a basket.[230] ESWL: US waves shatter stone. SE: renal injury, may also cause ↑BP and DM.[231] Percutaneous nephrolithotomy (PCNL): keyhole surgery to remove stones, when large, multiple, or complex.[232] Open surgery is rare.

►*Indications for urgent intervention (delay kills glomeruli):* Presence of infection *and* obstruction—a percutaneous nephrostomy or ureteric stent may be needed to relieve obstruction (p642); urosepsis; intractable pain or vomiting; impending ARF; obstruction in a solitary kidney; bilateral obstructing stones.[232]

**Prevention** *General:* Drink plenty. *Normal* dietary $Ca^{2+}$ intake (low $Ca^{2+}$ diets increase oxalate excretion). *Specifically:* •*Calcium stones:* in hypercalciuria, a thiazide diuretic is used to ↓$Ca^{2+}$ excretion •*Oxalate:* ↓oxalate intake; pyridoxine may be used (p312) •*Struvite:* treat infection promptly •*Urate:* allopurinol (100-300mg/24h PO). Urine alkalinization may also help, as urate is more soluble at pH>6 (eg with potassium citrate or sodium bicarbonate) •*Cystine:* vigorous hydration to keep urine output >3L/d and urinary alkalinization (as above). D-penicillamine is used to chelate cystine, given with pyridoxine to prevent vitamin $B_6$ deficiency.

*What is its composition?*

| Type | Causative factors | Appearance on XR |
|---|---|---|
| Calcium oxalate (fig 1) | Metabolic or idiopathic | Spiky, radio-opaque |
| Calcium phosphate | Metabolic or idiopathic | Smooth, may be large, radio-opaque |
| Magnesium ammonium phosphate (fig 2) | UTI (proteus causes alkaline urine and calcium precipitation and ammonium salt formation) | Large, horny, 'staghorn' radio-opaque |
| Urate (p694) | Hyperuricaemia | Smooth, brown, radiolucent |
| Cystine (fig 3) | Renal tubular defect | Yellow, crystalline, semi-opaque |

*Why has he or she got this stone now?*
- *Diet:* Chocolate, tea, rhubarb, strawberries, nuts and spinach all ↑oxalate levels.
- *Season:* Variations in calcium and oxalate levels are thought to be mediated by vitamin D synthesis via sunlight on skin.
- *Work:* Can he/she drink freely at work? Is there dehydration?
- *Medications:* Precipitating drugs include: diuretics, antacids, acetazolamide, corticosteroids, theophylline, aspirin, allopurinol, vitamin C and D, indinavir.

*Are there any predisposing factors?* For example:
- *Recurrent UTIs* (in magnesium ammonium phosphate calculi).
- *Metabolic abnormalities:*
  - Hypercalciuria/hypercalcaemia (p690): hyperparathyroidism, neoplasia, sarcoidosis, hyperthyroidism, Addison's, Cushing's, lithium, vitamin D excess.
  - Hyperuricosuria/↑plasma urate: on its own, or with gout.
  - Hyperoxaluria (p312).
  - Cystinuria (p312).
  - Renal tubular acidosis (p310).
- *Urinary tract abnormalities:* eg pelviureteric junction obstruction, hydronephrosis (renal pelvis or calyces), calyceal diverticulum, horseshoe kidney, ureterocele, vesicoureteric reflux, ureteral stricture, medullary sponge kidney.[1]
- *Foreign bodies:* eg stents, catheters.

*Is there a family history?* ↑risk of stones × 3-fold. Specific diseases include x-linked nephrolithiasis and Dent's disease (proteinuria, hypercalciuria and nephrocalcinosis).

▶*Is there infection above the stone?* eg fever, loin tender, pyuria? This needs urgent intervention.

**Fig 1.** Calcium oxalate monohydrate.

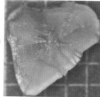

**Fig 2.** Struvite stone.

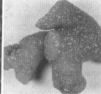

**Fig 3.** Cystine stone.

Figs 1-3 courtesy of Dr Glen Austin.

---

**1** Medullary sponge kidney is a typically asymptomatic developmental anomaly of the kidney mostly seen in adult females, where there is dilatation of the collecting ducts, which if severe leads to a sponge-like appearance of the renal medulla. *Complications/associations:* UTIs, nephrolithiasis, haematuria and hypercalciuria, hyperparathyroidism (if present, look for genetic markers of MEN type 2A, see p215).[233]

Surgery

▶*Urinary tract obstruction is common and should be considered in any patient with impaired renal function.* Damage can be permanent if the obstruction is not treated promptly. Obstruction may occur anywhere from the renal calyces to the urethral meatus, and may be *partial* or *complete*, *unilateral* or *bilateral*. Obstructing lesions are *luminal* (stones, blood clot, sloughed papilla, tumour: renal, ureteric, or bladder), *mural* (eg congenital or acquired stricture, neuromuscular dysfunction, schistosomiasis), or *extra-mural* (abdominal or pelvic mass/tumour, retroperitoneal fibrosis, or iatrogenic—eg post surgery). Unilateral obstruction may be clinically silent (normal urine output and U&E) if the other kidney is functioning. ▶Bilateral obstruction or obstruction with infection requires urgent treatment. See box p645.

**Clinical features**

• *Acute upper tract obstruction:* Loin pain radiating to the groin. There may be superimposed infection ± loin tenderness, or an enlarged kidney.

• *Chronic upper tract obstruction:* Flank pain, renal failure, superimposed infection. Polyuria may occur owing to impaired urinary concentration.

• *Acute lower tract obstruction:* Acute urinary retention typically presents with severe suprapubic pain, often preceded by symptoms of bladder outflow obstruction (as below). Clinically: distended, palpable bladder, dull to percussion.

• *Chronic lower tract obstruction: Symptoms:* urinary frequency, hesitancy, poor stream, terminal dribbling, overflow incontinence. *Signs:* distended, palpable bladder ± large prostate on PR. Complications: UTI, urinary retention.

**Tests** *Blood:* U&E, creatinine. *Urine:* MC&S. *Ultrasound* (p758) is the imaging modality of choice. If there is hydronephrosis or hydroureter (distension of the renal pelvis and calyces or ureter), arrange a CT scan. This will determine the level of obstuction. NB: in ~5% of cases of obstruction, no distension is seen on ultrasound. *Radionuclide imaging* enables functional assessment of the kidneys. MRI also has a role.

**Treatment** *Upper tract obstruction:* Nephrostomy or ureteric stent. NB: stents may cause significant discomfort and patients should be warned of this. α-blockers help reduce stent-related pain (↓ureteric spasm).[234] Pyeloplasty, to widen the PUJ, may be performed for idiopathic PUJ obstruction.

*Lower tract obstruction:* Insert a urethral or suprapubic catheter (p776). Treat the underlying cause if possible. Beware of a large diuresis after relief of obstruction; a temporary salt-losing nephropathy may occur resulting in the loss of several litres of fluid a day. Monitor weight, fluid balance, and U&E closely.

## Periaortitis (retroperitoneal fibrosis[et al])

Causes include idiopathic retroperitoneal fibrosis (RPF), inflammatory aneurysms of the abdominal aorta, and perianeurysmal RPF. Idiopathic RPF is an autoimmune disorder, where there is B-cell and CD4(+) T-cell associated vasculitis. This results in fibrinoid necrosis of the vasa vasorum, affecting the aorta and small and medium retroperitoneal vessels. The ureters get embedded in dense, fibrous tissue resulting in progressive bilateral ureteric obstruction. Secondary causes of RPF include malignancy, typically lymphoma.

**Associations** Drugs (eg β-blockers, bromocriptine, methysergide, methyldopa), autoimmune disease (eg thyroiditis, SLE, ANCA+ve vasculitis), smoking, asbestos.

**Typical patient** Middle-aged ♂ with vague loin, back or abdominal pain, BP↑.

**Tests** *Blood:* ↑urea and creatinine; ↑ESR; ↑CRP; anaemia. *Ultrasound:* dilated ureters (hydronephrosis). Then *CT/MRI:* periaortic mass (biopsy under imaging guidance is used to rule out malignancy).

**Treatment** Retrograde stent placement to relieve obstruction (removed after 12 months) ± ureterolysis (dissection of the ureters from the retroperitoneal tissue), and immunosuppression with low-dose steroids has good long-term results.[235]

## Problems of ureteric stenting (depend on site)

| Common | Rare |
|---|---|
| Stent-related pain | Obstruction |
| Trigonal irritation | Kinking |
| Haematuria | Ureteric rupture |
| Fever | Stent misplacement |
| Infection | Stent migration (especially if made of silicone) |
| Tissue inflammation | Tissue hyperplasia |
| Encrustation | Forgotton stents |
| Biofilm formation | |

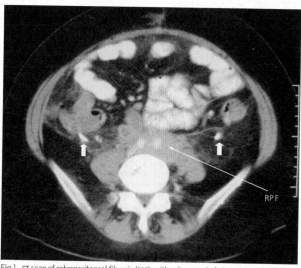

RPF

Fig 1. CT scan of retroperitoneal fibrosis (RPF), with subsequent obstruction and dilatation of the ureters (thick arrows). *Oxford Textbook of Nephrology*, 2465, OUP.

Surgery

Retention means not emptying the bladder (due to **obstruction** or **↓detrusor power**).

- **Acute retention** Bladder usually tender, containing ~600mL *Causes:* prostatic obstruction (usual cause in ♂), urethral strictures, anticholinergics, 'holding', alcohol, constipation, post-op (pain/inflammation/anaesthetics), infection (p292), neurological (cauda equina syndrome), carcinoma. *Examine:* Abdomen, DRE of prostate, perineal sensation (cauda equina compression). *Tests:* MSU, U&E, FBC, and prostate-specific antigen (PSA, p534).[1] Renal ultrasound if renal impairment. *Tricks to aid voiding:* Analgesia, privacy on hospital wards, ambulation, standing to void, voiding to the sound of running taps—or in a hot bath. *If the tricks fail:* Catheterize (p776) and start an α-blocker (eg *tamsulosin* 400μg/d PO). If in clot retention the patient will require a 3-way catheter and bladder washout. If >1L residual check U&E and monitor for post-obstructive diuresis (see BOX). After 2-3 days, trial without catheter (TWOC, p777) may work (esp. if <75yrs old and <1L drained or retention was triggered by a passing event, eg GA). α-blockers double the chance of successful voiding. *Prevention: Finasteride* (5mg/d PO) ↓ prostate size and retention risk. *Tamsulosin* (400μg/d PO) ↓ risk of recatheterization after acute retention.[236]

- **Chronic retention** More insidious and may be painless. Bladder capacity may be >1.5L. *Presentation:* Overflow incontinence, acute on chronic retention, lower abdominal mass, UTI, or renal failure (eg bilateral obstructive uropathy—see BOX). *Causes:* Prostatic enlargement is common, pelvic malignancy; rectal surgery; DM; CNS disease, eg transverse myelitis/MS; zoster (S2-S4). ►Only catheterize patient if there is pain, urinary infection, or renal impairment. Institute definitive treatment promptly. Intermittent self-catheterization is sometimes required (p777). **Catheters** p776. **Prostate carcinoma** p646.

**Benign prostatic hyperplasia (BPH)** is common (24% if aged 40-64; 40% if older). *Pathology:* Benign nodular or diffuse proliferation of musculofibrous and glandular layers of the prostate. Inner (transitional) zone enlarges in contrast to peripheral layer expansion seen in prostate carcinoma. *Features: Lower urinary tract symptoms* (LUTS) = nocturia, frequency, urgency, post-micturition dribbling, poor stream/flow, hesitancy, overflow incontinence, haematuria, bladder stones, UTI. *Management:* Assess severity of symptoms and impact on life. PR exam. *Tests:* MSU; U&E; ultrasound (large residual volume, hydronephrosis—fig 1). 'Rule out' cancer: PSA,[1] transrectal USS ± biopsy. Then consider:

- *Lifestyle:* Avoid caffeine, alcohol (to ↓urgency/nocturia). Relax when voiding. Void twice in a row to aid emptying. Control urgency by practising ↑distraction methods (eg breathing exercises). Train the bladder by 'holding on' to ↑time between voiding.
- *Drugs* are useful in mild disease, and while awaiting surgery. •α-**blockers** are 1ˢᵗ line (eg *tamsulosin* 400μg/d PO; also *alfuzosin, doxazosin, terazosin*). ↓smooth muscle tone (prostate and bladder). SE: drowsiness; depression; dizziness; BP↓; dry mouth; ejaculatory failure; extra-pyramidal signs; nasal congestion; weight↑.
- •5α-**reductase inhibitors:** can be added, or used alone, eg *finasteride* 5mg/d PO (↓testosterone's conversion to dihydrotestosterone).[2] Excreted in semen, so warn to use condoms; females should avoid handling. SE: impotence; ↓libido. Effects on prostate size are limited and slow. • There is no evidence for phytotherapy.[237]
- *Surgery:*
  - *Transurethral resection of prostate* (TURP) ≤14% become impotent (see BOX). Crossmatch 2u. Beware bleeding, clot retention and TUR syndrome: absorption of washout causing hyponatraemia and fits. ~20% need redoing within 10yrs.
  - *Transurethral incision of the prostate* (TUIP) involves less destruction than TURP,[238] and less risk to sexual function, but gives similar benefit.[239] It achieves this by relieving pressure on the urethra. It is perhaps the best surgical option for those with small glands <30g—ie ~50% of those operated on in some areas.
  - *Retropubic prostatectomy* is an open operation (if prostate very large).
  - *Transurethral laser-induced prostatectomy* (TULIP) may be as good as TURP.

---

**1** Do venepuncture for PSA before PR, as PR can ↑total PSA by ~1ng/mL (free PSA ↑by 10%).[240] It's difficult to know if acute retention raises PSA, but relieving obstruction does cause it to drop.[241]

**2** *Finasteride* can prevent retention but has odd effects on risk of prostate cancer. The PCPT trial showed ↓risk of indolent cancers, but ↑risk of Gleason >7 (p647).[242]

## Advice for patients concerning transurethral prostatectomy (TURP)

Pre-op consent issues may centre on risks of the procedure, eg:
- Haematuria/haemorrhage
- Haematospermia
- Hypothermia
- Urethral trauma/stricture
- Post TURP syndrome (T°↓; Na⁺↓)²⁴³
- Infection; prostatitis
- Erectile dysfunction ~10%
- Incontinence ≤10%
- Clot retention near strictures
- Retrograde ejaculation (common)

**Post-operative advice**
- Avoid driving for 2 weeks after the operation.
- Avoid sex for 2 weeks after surgery. Then get back to normal. The amount ejaculated may be reduced (as it flows backwards into the bladder—harmless, but may cloud the urine). It means you may be infertile. Erections may be a problem after TURP, but do not expect this: in some men, erections improve. Rarely, orgasmic sensations are reduced.
- Expect to pass blood in the urine for the first 2 weeks. A small amount of blood colours the urine bright red. Do not be alarmed.
- At first you may need to urinate more frequently than before. Do not be despondent. In 6 weeks things should be much better—but the operation cannot be guaranteed to work (8% fail, and lasting incontinence is a problem in 6%; 12% may need repeat TURPs within 8yrs, compared with 1.8% of men undergoing open prostatectomy).
- If feverish, or if urination hurts, take a sample of urine to your doctor.

## Obstructive uropathy

In chronic urinary retention, an episode of **acute** retention may go unnoticed for days and, because of their background symptoms, may only present when overflow incontinence becomes a nuisance—pain is not necessarily a feature.

After diagnosing acute on chronic retention and placing a catheter, the bladder residual can be as much as 1.5L of urine. Don't be surprised to be called by the biochemistry lab to be told that the serum creatinine is 1500μmol/L! The good news is that renal function usually returns to baseline after a few days (there may be mild background impairment). Ask for an urgent renal US (fig 1) and consider the following in the acute plan to ensure a safe course:

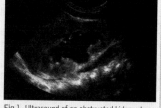

Fig 1. Ultrasound of an obstructed kidney showing hydronephrosis. Note dilatation of renal pelvis and ureter, and clubbed calyces.

Image courtesy of Norwich Radiology Department.

- **Hyperkalaemia** See p849.
- **Metabolic acidosis** On ABG there is likely to be a respiratory compensated metabolic acidosis. Concerns should prompt discussion with a renal specialist (a good idea anyway), in case haemodialysis is required (p292).
- **Post-obstructive diuresis** In the acute phase after relief of the obstruction, the kidneys produce a lot of urine—as much as a litre in the first hour. It is vital to provide resuscitation fluids and match input with output.
▶Fluid depletion rather than overload is the danger here.
- **Sodium- and bicarbonate-losing nephropathy** As the kidney undergoes diuresis, Na⁺ and bicarbonate are lost in the urine in large quantities. Replace 'in for out' (as above) with isotonic 1.26% sodium bicarbonate solution—this should be available from ITU. Some advocate using 0.9% saline, though the chloride load may exacerbate acidosis. Withhold any nephrotoxic drugs.
- **Infection** Treat infection, bearing in mind that the WCC↑ and CRP↑ may be part of the stress response. Send a sample of urine for MC&S.

Surgery

**Renal cell carcinoma** (aka RCC, hypernephroma, Grawitz tumour) arises from proximal renal tubular epithelium. *Epidemiology:* Accounts for 90% of renal cancers; mean age 55yrs. ♂:♀≈2:1. 15% of haemodialysis patients develop RCC. *Features:* 50% found incidentally. Haematuria, loin pain, abdominal mass, anorexia, malaise, weight loss, PUO—often in isolation. Rarely, invasion of left renal vein compresses left testicular vein causing a varicocele. Spread may be direct (renal vein), via lymph, or haematogenous (bone, liver, lung). 25% have metastases at presentation. *Tests:* BP: ↑from renin secretion. Blood: FBC (polycythaemia from erythropoietin secretion); ESR; U&E, ALP (bony mets?). Urine: RBCs; cytology. Imaging: US (p758); CT/MRI; IVU (filling defect ± calcification); CXR ('cannon ball' metastases). ℞: Radical nephrectomy (nephron-sparing surgery is good for T1 tumours + preserves renal function).[245] RCC is (in general) radio & chemo resistant. In those with unresectable or metastatic disease, some will have a good response to biological therapies, especially angiogenesis-targeted agents: *sunitinib, bevacizumab* and *sorafenib*. As 1st-line treatment for patients with multiple poor-risk factors, *temsirolimus* (inhibits mTOR) improves survival compared with interferon.[246] Interferon-α and interleukin-2 were formerly used on their own.[247] The *Mayo prognostic risk score (SSIGN)* was developed to predict survival and uses information on tumour **s**tage, **si**ze, **g**rade and **n**ecrosis.[248] *Prognosis:* 10yr survival ranges from 96.5% (scores 0–1) to 19.2% (scores ≥ 10).[249]

**Transitional cell carcinoma (TCC)** may arise in the bladder (50%), ureter, or renal pelvis. *Epidemiology:* Age >40yrs; ♂:♀≈4:1. *Risk factors:* p648. *Presentation:* Painless haematuria; frequency; urgency; dysuria; urinary tract obstruction. *Diagnosis:* Urine cytology; IVU; cystoscopy + biopsy; CT/MRI. ℞: See Bladder tumours, p648. *Prognosis:* Varies with clinical stage/histological grade: 10–80% 5yr survival.

**Wilms' tumour** (nephroblastoma) is a childhood tumour of primitive renal tubules and mesenchymal cells. *Prevalence:* 1:100,000—the chief abdominal malignancy in children. It presents with an abdominal mass and haematuria. ℞: OHCS p133.

**Prostate cancer** The commonest male malignancy. *Incidence:* ↑with age: 80% in men >80yrs (autopsy studies). *Associations:* +ve family history (×2–3 ↑risk, p524), ↑testosterone. Most are adenocarcinomas arising in peripheral prostate. Spread may be local (seminal vesicles, bladder, rectum) via lymph, or haematogenously (sclerotic bony lesions). *Symptoms:* Asymptomatic or nocturia, hesitancy, poor stream, terminal dribbling, or obstruction. Weight↓ ± bone pain suggests mets. *DRE exam of prostate:* May show hard, irregular prostate. *Diagnosis:* ↑PSA (normal in 30% of small cancers); transrectal USS & biopsy; x-rays; bone scan; CT/MRI. *Staging:* MRI. If contrast-enhancing magnetic nanoparticles used, sensitivity for detecting affected nodes rises from 35% to 90%.[250] *Treatment:* **Disease confined to prostate:**[251] Options depend on prognosis (BOX), patient preference and comorbidities. •*Radical prostatectomy* if <70yrs gives excellent disease-free survival (laparoscopic surgery is as good). The role of adjuvant hormonal therapy is being explored. •*Radical radiotherapy* (± neoadjuvant & adjuvant hormonal therapy) is an alternative curative option that compares favourably with surgery (no RCTs). It may be delivered as external beam or brachytherapy. •*Hormone therapy alone* temporarily delays tumour progression but refractory disease eventually develops. Consider in elderly unfit patients with high-risk disease. •*Active surveillance*—particularly if >70yrs and low-risk. **Metastatic disease:** •*Hormonal drugs* may give benefit for 1–2yrs. LHRH agonists, eg 12-weekly *goserelin* (10.8mg SC as Zoladex LA®) first stimulate, then inhibit pituitary gonadotrophin. NB: risks tumour 'flare' when first used—start anti-androgen, eg *cyproterone acetate*, in susceptible patients. The LHRH antagonist *degarelix* is also used in advanced disease. *Symptomatic ℞:* Analgesia; treat hypercalcaemia; radiotherapy for bone mets/spinal cord compression. *Prognosis:* 10% die in 6 months, 10% live >10yrs. *Screening:* DRE of prostate; transrectal USS; PSA (see BOX).

**Penile cancer** *Epidemiology:* rare in UK, more common in Far East and Africa, very rare in circumcised. Related to chronic irritation, viruses, smegma. *Presentation:* chronic fungating ulcer, bloody/purulent discharge, 50% spread to lymph at presentation ℞: radiotherapy & irridium wires if early; amputation & lymph node dissection if late.

## 64

### Advice to asymptomatic men asking for a PSA blood test (see also p534)

- Many men over 50 consider a PSA test to detect prostatic cancer. *Is this wise?*
- The test is not very accurate, and we cannot say that those having the test will live longer—even if they turn out to have prostate cancer. Most men with prostate cancer die from an unrelated cause.
- If the test is falsely positive, you may needlessly have more tests, eg prostate sampling via the back passage (causes bleeding and infection in 1-5% of men).
- Only one in three of those with a high PSA level will have cancer.
- You may be worried needlessly if later tests put you in the clear.
- If a cancer is found, there's no way to tell *for sure* if it will impinge on health. You might end up having a bad effect from treatment that wasn't needed.
- There is much uncertainty on treating those who **do** turn out to have prostate cancer: options are radical surgery to remove the prostate (this treatment may be fatal in 0.2-0.5% of patients and risks erectile dysfunction and incontinence), radiotherapy, or hormones.
- Screening via PSA has shown conflicting results. Some RCTs have shown no difference in the rate of death from prostate cancer[252]; others have found reduced mortality, eg 1 death prevented per 1055 men invited for screening (if 37 cancers detected).[253]

▶Ultimately, you must decide for yourself what you want.

### Prognostic factors in prostate cancer

A number of prognostic factors help determine if 'watchful waiting' or aggressive therapy should be advised: •Pre-treatment PSA level •Tumour stage (as measured by the TNM system; p527),[254] and •Tumour grade—as measured by its Gleason score. Gleason grading is from 1 to 5, with 5 being the highest grade, and carrying the poorest prognosis. A pathologist determines Gleason grades by analysing histology from two separate areas of tumour specimen, and adding them to get the total Gleason score for the tumour, from 2 to 10. Scores 8-10 suggest an aggressive tumour; 5-7: intermediate; 2-4: indolent.

### Benign diseases of the penis

**Balanitis** Acute inflammation of the foreskin and glans. Associated with strep and staph infections. More common in diabetics. Often seen in young children with tight foreskins R: Antibiotics, circumcision, hygiene advice.

**Phimosis** The foreskin occludes the meatus. In young boys this causes recurrent balanitis and ballooning, but time (+ trials of gentle retraction) may obviate the need for circumcision. In adulthood presents with painful intercourse, infection, ulceration and is associated with balanitis xerotica obliterans.

**Paraphimosis** Occurs when a tight foreskin is retracted and becomes irreplaceable, preventing venous return leading to oedema and even ischaemia of the glans. Can occur if the foreskin is not replaced after catheterization. ▶▶R: Ask patient to squeeze glans. Try applying a 50% glucose-soaked swab (oedema may follow osmotic gradient). Ice packs and lidocaine gel may also help. May require aspiration/dorsal slit/circumcision.

### Prostatitis

May be acute or chronic. Usually those >35yrs. *Acute prostatitis* is caused mostly by *S. faecalis* and *E. coli*, also chlamydia (and previously TB). *Features:* UTIs, retention, pain, haematospermia, swollen/boggy prostate on DRE. R: Analgesia; *levofloxacin* 500mg/24h PO for 28d. *Chronic prostatitis* may be bacterial or non-bacterial. Symptoms as above, but present for >3 months. Non-bacterial chronic prostatitis does not respond to antibiotics. Anti-inflammatory drugs, α-blockers and prostatic massage all have a place.

>90% are transitional cell carcinomas (TCCs) in the UK. What appear as benign papillomata rarely behave in a purely benign way. They are almost certainly indolent TCCs. Adenocarcinomas and squamous cell carcinomas are rare in the West (the latter may follow schistosomiasis). UK incidence ≈ 1:6000/yr. ♂:♀≈5:2. Histology is important for prognosis: **Grade 1**—differentiated; **Grade 2**—intermediate; **Grade 3**—poorly differentiated. 80% are confined to bladder mucosa, and only ~20% penetrate muscle (increasing mortality to 50% at 5yrs).

**Presentation** Painless haematuria; recurrent UTIs; voiding irritability.

**Associations** Smoking; aromatic amines (rubber industry); chronic cystitis; schistosomiasis (↑risk of squamous cell carcinoma); pelvic irradiation.

**Tests**
• Cystoscopy with biopsy is diagnostic.
• Urine: microscopy/cytology (cancers may cause sterile pyuria).
• CT urogram is both diagnostic and provides staging.
• Bimanual EUA helps assess spread.
• MRI or lymphangiography may show involved pelvic nodes.

**Staging** See TABLE.

**Treating TCC of the bladder**
• *Tis/Ta/T1:* (80% of all patients) Diathermy via transurethral cystoscopy/transurethral resection of bladder tumour (TURBT). Consider intravesical chemotherapeutic agents for multiple small tumours or high-grade tumours. A regimen of *mitomycin C, doxorubicin* and *cisplatin* as maintenence to prevent recurrence is as effective as intravesical BCG (which stimulates a non-specific immune response) and has less SEs.[255] 5yr survival ≈ 95%.
• *T2-3:* Radical cystectomy is the 'gold standard'. Radiotherapy gives worse 5yr survival rates than surgery, but preserves the bladder. 'Salvage' cystectomy can be performed if radiotherapy fails, but yields worse results than primary surgery. Post-op chemotherapy (eg M-VAC: *methotrexate, vinblastine, adriamycin,* and *cisplatin*) is toxic but effective. Neoadjuvant chemotherapy with CMV (*cisplatin, methotrexate* and *vinblastine*) has improved survival compared to cystectomy or radiotherapy alone.[256] Methods to preserve the bladder with transurethral resection or partial cystectomy + systemic chemotherapy have been tried, but long-term results are disappointing. If the bladder neck is not involved, orthotopic reconstruction rather than forming a urostoma is an option (both using ~40cm of the patient's ileum), but adequate tumour clearance must not be compromised. ►The patient should have all these options explained by a urologist and an oncologist.
• *T4:* Usually palliative chemo/radiotherapy. Chronic catheterization and urinary diversions may help to relieve pain.

**Follow-up** History, examination, and regular cystoscopy: •*High-risk tumours:* Every 3 months for 2yrs, then every 6 months; •*Low-risk tumours:* First follow-up cystoscopy after 9 months, then yearly.

**Tumour spread** Local → to pelvic structures; lymphatic → to iliac and para-aortic nodes; haematogenous → to liver and lungs.

**Survival** This depends on age at surgery. For example, the 3yr survival after cystectomy for T2 and T3 tumours is 60% if 65-75yrs old, falling to 40% if 75-82yrs old (in whom the operative mortality is 4%). With unilateral pelvic node involvement, only 6% of patients survive 5yrs. The 3yr survival with bilateral or para-aortic node involvement is nil.

**Complications** Cystectomy can result in sexual and urinary malfunction. Massive bladder haemorrhage may complicate treatment or be a feature of disease treated palliatively. Determining the cause of bleeding is key. Consider *alum* solution bladder irrigation (if no renal failure) as 1st-line treatment for intractable haematuria in advanced malignancy: it is an inpatient procedure.[257]

## TNM staging of bladder cancer

(See also p527)

| Tis | Carcinoma *in situ* | Not felt at EUA |
|-----|---------------------|-----------------|
| Ta | Tumour confined to epithelium | Not felt at EUA |
| T1 | Tumour in lamina propria | Not felt at EUA |
| T2 | Superficial muscle involved | Rubbery thickening at EUA |
| T3 | Deep muscle involved | EUA: mobile mass |
| T4 | Invasion beyond bladder | EUA: fixed mass |

EUA = examination under anaesthetic

### Is asymptomatic non-visible haematuria significant?

Dipstick tests are often done routinely for new admissions. If non-visible (previously microscopic) haematuria is found, but the patient has no related symptoms, what does this mean? Before rushing into a barrage of investigations, consider:

• One study found that incidence of urogenital disease (eg bladder cancer) was no higher in those with asymptomatic microhaematuria than in those without.[258]

• Asymptomatic non-visible haematuria is the sole presenting feature in only 4% of bladder cancers, and there is no evidence that these are less advanced than malignancies presenting with macroscopic haematuria.

• When monitoring those with treated bladder cancer for recurrence, non-visible-haematuria tests have a sensitivity of only 31% in those with superficial bladder malignancy, in whom detection would be most useful.

• Although 80% of those with flank pain due to a renal stone have microscopic haematuria, so do 50% of those with flank pain but no stone.[259]

The conclusion is not that urine dipstick testing is useless, but that results should not be interpreted in isolation. Unexplained non-visible haematuria in those >50yrs should be referred under the 2-week rule.[260] Smokers and those with +ve family history for urothelial cancer may also be investigated differently from those with no risk factors (eg ultrasound, cystoscopy ± referral), but in a young fit athlete, the diagnosis is more likely to be exercise-induced haematuria.[261] Wise doctors liaise with their patients. "Shall we let sleeping dogs lie?" is a reasonable question for some patients. Give the facts and let the patient decide, reserving to yourself the right to present the facts in certain ways, depending on your instincts, and those of a trusted colleague. Remember that medicine is for gamblers (p672), and wise gamblers assess the odds against a shifting set of circumstances.

Surgery

▶Think twice before inserting a urinary catheter.
▶Carry out rectal examination to exclude faecal impaction.
▶Is the bladder palpable after voiding (retention with overflow)?
▶Is there neurological co-morbidity: eg MS; Parkinson's disease; stroke; spinal trauma?

Anyone might 'wet themselves' on a long bus ride (we all would if it was long enough). Don't think of people as dry or incontinent, but as incontinent in some circumstances. Attending to these is as important as the physiology. Get good at treating incontinence and you will do wonders for quality of life. See p64 for symptoms.

**Incontinence in men** Enlargement of the prostate is the major cause of incontinence: urge incontinence (see below) or dribbling may result from partial retention of urine. TURP (p644) & other pelvic surgery may weaken the bladder sphincter and cause incontinence. Troublesome incontinence needs specialist assessment.

**Incontinence in women** Often under-reported with delays before seeking help.

• *Functional incontinence*, ie when physiological factors are relatively unimportant. The patient is 'caught short' and too slow in finding the toilet because of (for example) immobility, or unfamiliar surroundings.

• *Stress incontinence:* Leakage from an incompetent sphincter, eg when intra-abdominal pressure rises (eg coughing, laughing). Increasing age and obesity are risk factors. The key to diagnosis is the loss of small (but often frequent) amounts of urine when coughing etc. Examine for pelvic floor weakness/prolapse/pelvic masses.[262] Look for cough leak on standing and with full bladder. Stress incontinence is common in pregnancy and following birth. It occurs to some degree in ~50% of post-menopausal women. In elderly women, pelvic floor weakness, eg with uterine prolapse or urethrocele (OHCS p290) is a very common association.

• *Urge incontinence/overactive bladder syndrome* The urge to urinate is quickly followed by uncontrollable and sometimes complete emptying of the bladder as the detrusor muscle contracts. Urgency/leaking is precipitated by: arriving home (latchkey incontinence, a conditioned reflex); cold; the sound of running water; coffee, tea or cola; and obesity. Δ: urodynamic studies. *Cause:* detrusor overactivity, eg from central inhibitory pathway malfunction or sensitisation of peripheral afferent terminals in the bladder; or a bladder muscle problem. Check for organic brain damage (eg stroke; Parkinson's; dementia). *Other causes:* urinary infection; diabetes; diuretics; atrophic vaginitis; urethritis.

In both sexes incontinence may result from confusion or sedation. Occasionally it may be purposeful (eg preventing admission to an old people's home) or due to anger.

**Management** *Check for:* UTI; DM; diuretic use; faecal impaction; palpable bladder; GFR.

• *Stress incontinence:* Pelvic floor exercises are 1$^{st}$ line (8 contractions x3/day for 3 months). Intravaginal electrical stimulation may also be effective, but is not acceptable to many women. A ring pessary may help uterine prolapse, eg while awaiting surgical repair. *Surgical options* (eg **tension-free vaginal tape**) aim to stabilise the mid-urethra.[263] Urethral bulking is also available. If surgical options are not suitable: *Duloxetine* 40mg/12h PO may help (50% have ≥50% ↓ in incontinence episodes) SE = nausea.[264]

• *Urge incontinence:* The patient (or carer) should complete an 'incontinence' chart for 3 days to define the pattern of incontinence. Examine for spinal cord and CNS signs (including cognitive test, p70 & p85); and for vaginitis (if postmenopausal). Vaginitis can be treated with topical oestrogen therapy for a limited period. Bladder training[1] (may include pelvic floor exercises) and weight loss are important. Drugs may help reduce night-time incontinence (see BOX) but can be disappointing. Consider aids eg absorbent pad. If ♂ consider a condom catheter.

▶Do urodynamic assessment (cystometry & urine flow rate measurement) before any surgical intervention to exclude detrusor overactivity or sphincter dyssynergia.

## Managing detrusor overactivity in urge incontinence

| Agents for detrusor overactivity | Notes |
|---|---|
| Antimuscarinics: eg *tolterodine* SR 4mg/24h; SE: dry mouth, eyes/skin, drowsiness, constipation, tachycardia, abdominal pain, urinary retention, sinusitis, oedema, weight↓, glaucoma precipitation.²³¹ Up to 4mg/12 may be needed (unlicensed).²³² | Improves frequency & urgency. Alternatives: *solifenacin* 5mg/24h (max 10mg); *oxybutynin*, but more SE unless transdermal route or modified release used;◆※ *trospium* or *fesoterodine* (prefers M3 receptors).²³³ Avoid in myasthenia, and if glaucoma or UC are uncontrolled. |
| Topical oestrogens | Post-menopausal urgency, frequency + nocturia may occasionally be improved by raising the bladder's sensory threshold.◆※ Systemic therapy worsens incontinence. |
| β3 adrenergic agonist: *mirabegron* 50mg/24h; SE tachycardia; CI: severe HTN; Caution if renal/hepatic impairment. | Consider if antimuscarinics are contraindicated or clinically ineffective, or if SE unacceptable. |
| Intravesical botulinum toxin (*Botox*®) | Consider if above medications ineffective. |
| Percutaneous posterior tibial nerve stimulation (PTNS). (A typical treatment consists of x12 weekly 30 min sessions.) | Consider if drug treatment ineffective and *Botox*® not wanted. PTNS delivers neuromodulation at the S2-S4 junction of the sacral nerve plexus. |
| Neuromodulation via transcutaneous electrical stimulation²³⁴ | Sacral nerve stimulation inhibits the reflex behaviour of involuntary detrusor contractions. |
| Modulation of afferent input from bladder | Gabapentin (unlicensed).²³⁵◆※ |
| Hypnosis, psychotherapy, bladder training¹ | (These all require good motivation.) |
| Surgery (eg clam ileocystoplasty) | Reserved for troublesome or intractable symptoms. The bladder is bisected, opened like a clam, and 25cm of ileum is sewn in. |

NB: *desmopressin* nasal spray 20μg as a night-time dose has a role in ↓urine production and ∴ nocturia in overactive bladder, but is unsuitable if elderly (SE: fluid retention, heart failure, Na⁺↓).

## Not all male urinary symptoms are prostate-related!

**Detrusor over-activity** Men get this as well as women.²⁷⁰ See above. Pressure-flow studies help diagnose this (as does detrusor thickness ≥2.9mm on US).²⁷¹

**Primary bladder neck obstruction**²⁷² is a condition in which the bladder neck does not open properly during voiding. Studies in men and women with voiding dysfunction show that it is common. The cause may be muscular or neurological dysfunction or fibrosis. *Diagnosis:* Video-urodynamics, with simultaneous pressure-flow measurement, and visualization of the bladder neck during voiding. *Treatment:* Watchful waiting; α-blockers (p644); surgery.²⁷³

**Urethral stricture** This may follow trauma or infection (eg gonorrhoea)—and frequently leads to voiding symptoms, UTI, or retention. Malignancy is a rare cause. *Imaging:* Retrograde urethrogram or antegrade cystourethrogram if the patient has an existing suprapubic catheter. *Internal urethrotomy* involves incising the stricture transurethrally using endoscopic equipment—to release scar tissue. The expectation is that epithelialization ends before wound contraction still further reduces the urethral diameter.²⁷⁴ *Stents* incorporate themselves into the wall of the urethra and keep the lumen open. They work best for short strictures in the bulbar urethra (anterior urethral anatomy, from proximal to distal: prostatic urethra→posterior or membranous urethra→bulbar urethra→penile or pendulous urethra→fossa navicularis→meatus).

---

**1** Mind over bladder: •Void when you DON'T have urge; DON'T go to the bathroom when you do have urge •Gradually extend the time between voiding •Schedule your trips to toilet •Stretch your bladder to normal capacity • When urge comes, calm down and make it go using mind over bladder tricks.

Surgery

▶Testicular lump = cancer until proved otherwise.
▶Acute, tender enlargement of testis = torsion (p654) until proved otherwise.

**Diagnosing scrotal masses** (fig 2):
1 *Can you get above it?* 2 *Is it separate from the testis?* 3 *Cystic or solid?*
• Cannot get above ≈ inguinoscrotal hernia (p616) or hydrocele extending proximally
• Separate and cystic ≈ epididymal cyst
• Separate and solid ≈ epididymitis/varicocele
• Testicular and cystic ≈ hydrocele
▶Testicular and solid—tumour, haematocele, granuloma (p186), orchitis, gumma (p431). USS may help (fig 1).

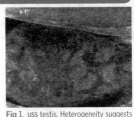

Fig 1. USS testis. Heterogeneity suggests tumour (ΔΔ: chronic inflammation).
Courtesy of Norwich Radiology Department.

**Epididymal cysts** usually develop in adulthood and contain clear or milky (spermatocele) fluid. They lie above and behind the testis. Remove if symptomatic.

**Hydroceles** (fluid within the tunica vaginalis). *Primary* (associated with a patent processus vaginalis, which typically resolves during the 1st year of life) or *secondary* to testis tumour/trauma/infection. Primary hydroceles are more common, larger, and usually in younger men. Can resolve spontaneously. *R:* aspiration (may need repeating) or surgery: plicating the tunica vaginalis (Lord's repair)/inverting the sac (Jaboulay's repair) ▶Is the testis normal after aspiration? If any doubt, do USS.

**Epididymo-orchitis** *Causes:* Chlamydia (eg if <35yrs); *E. coli*; mumps; *N. gonorrhoea*; TB. *Features:* Sudden-onset tender swelling, dysuria, sweats/fever. Take 1st catch' urine sample; look for urethral discharge. Consider STI screen. Warn of possible infertility[275] and symptoms worsening before improving. *R:* If <35yrs; *doxycycline* 100mg/12h (covers chlamydia; treat sexual partners). If gonorrhoea suspected add *ceftriaxone* 500mg IM stat. If >35yrs (mostly non-STI), associated UTI is common so try *ciprofloxacin* 500mg/12h or *ofloxacin* 200mg/12h.[276] Antibiotics should be used for 2-4 weeks. Also: analgesia, scrotal support, drainage of any abscess.

**Varicocele** Dilated veins of pampiniform plexus. Left side more commonly affected. Often visible as distended scrotal blood vessels that feel like 'a bag of worms'. Patient may complain of dull ache. Associated with subfertility, but repair (via surgery or embolization) seems to have little effect on subsequent pregnancy rates.

**Haematocele** Blood in tunica vaginalis, follows trauma, may need drainage/excision.

**Testicular tumours** The commonest malignancy in ♂ aged 15-44; 10% occur in undescended testes, even after orchidopexy. A contralateral tumour is found in 5%. Types: seminoma, 55% (30-65yrs);[277] non-seminomatous germ cell tumour, 33% (NSGCT; previously teratoma; 20-30yrs); mixed germ cell tumour, 12%; lymphoma.

*Signs:* Typically painless testis lump, found after trauma/infection ± haemospermia, secondary hydrocele, pain, dyspnoea (lung mets), abdominal mass (enlarged nodes), or effects of secreted hormones. 25% of seminomas & 50% of NSGCTs present with metastases. *Risk factors:* Undescended testis; infant hernia; infertility.

*Staging:* 1 No evidence of metastasis. 2 Infradiaphragmatic node involvement (spread via the para-aortic nodes **not** inguinal nodes). 3 Supradiaphragmatic node involvement. 4 Lung involvement (haematogenous).

*Tests:* (allow staging) CXR, CT, excision biopsy. α-FP (eg >3iu/mL)[1] and β-hCG are useful tumour markers and help monitor treatment (p535); check **before** & during R.

*R:* Radical orchidectomy (inguinal incision; occlude the spermatic cord before mobilization to ↓risk of intra-operative spread). Options are constantly updated (surgery, radiotherapy, chemotherapy). Seminomas are exquisitely radiosensitive. Stage 1 seminomas: orchidectomy + radiotherapy cures ~95%. Do close follow-up to detect relapse. Cure of NSGCT, even if metastases are present, is achieved by 3 cycles of *bleomycin* + *etoposide* + *cisplatin*. Prevention of late presentation: self-examination (see p655). 5yr survival >90% in all groups.

1 αFP is **not** ↑ in pure seminoma; may also be ↑ in: hepatitis, cirrhosis, liver cancer, open neural tube defect.

### Diagnosing groin lumps: lateral to medial thinking (see also p617)

- Psoas abscess—may present with back pain, limp and swinging pyrexia
- Neuroma of the femoral nerve
- Femoral artery aneurysm
- Saphena varix—like a hernia, it has a cough impulse
- Lymph node
- Femoral hernia
- Inguinal hernia
- Hydrocele or varicocele
- Also consider an undescended testis (cryptorchidism)

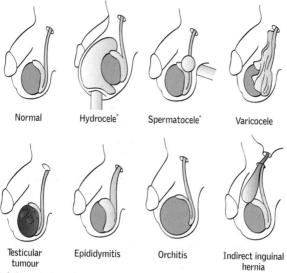

Fig 2. Diagnosis of scrotal masses. (*=transilluminates: position of pen torch shown in image)

The aim is to recognize this condition before the cardinal signs and symptoms are fully manifest, as prompt surgery saves testes. If surgery is performed in <6h the salvage rate is 90-100%; if >24h it is 0-10%.[278]

▶If in any doubt, surgery is required. If suspected refer immediately to urology.

*Symptoms:* Sudden onset of pain in one testis, which makes walking uncomfortable. Pain in the abdomen, nausea, and vomiting are common.

*Signs:* Inflammation of one testis—it is very tender, hot, and swollen. The testis may lie high and transversely. Torsion may occur at any age but is most common at 11-30yrs. With **intermittent torsion** the pain may have passed on presentation, but if it was severe, and the lie is horizontal, prophylactic fixing may be wise.[279]

*ΔΔ:* The main one is epididymo-orchitis (p652) but with this the patient tends to be older, there may be symptoms of urinary infection, and more gradual onset of pain. Also consider tumour, trauma, and an acute hydrocele. NB: **torsion of testicular or epididymal appendage** (the hydatid of Morgagni—a remnant of the Müllerian duct)—usually occurs between 7-12yrs, and causes less pain. Its tiny blue nodule may be discernible under the scrotum. It is thought to be due to the surge in gonadotrophins which signal the onset of puberty. **Idiopathic scrotal oedema** is a benign condition usually between ages 2 and 10yrs, and is differentiated from torsion by the absence of pain and tenderness.

*Tests:* Doppler USS may demonstrate lack of blood flow to testis, as may isotope scanning. Only perform if diagnosis equivocal—do not delay surgical exploration.

*Treatment:* ▶Ask consent for possible orchidectomy + **bilateral** fixation (orchidopexy)—see p570. At surgery expose and untwist the testis. If its colour looks good, return it to the scrotum and fix **both** testes to the scrotum.

## Undescended testes

**Incidence** About 3% of boys are born with at least one undescended testis (30% of premature boys) but this drops to 1% after the first year of life. Unilateral is four times more common than bilateral. (If bilateral then should have genetic testing.)
• *Cryptorchidism:* complete absence of the testicle from the scrotum (anorchism is absence of both testes).
• *Retractile testis:* the genitalia are normally developed but there is an excessive cremasteric reflex. The testicle is often found at the external inguinal ring. *R:* Reassurance (examining whilst in a warm bath, for example, may help to distinguish from maldescended/ectopic testes).
• *Maldescended testis:* may be found anywhere along the normal path of descent from abdomen to groin.
• *Ectopic testis:* most commonly found in the superior inguinal pouch (anterior to the external oblique aponeurosis) but may also be abdominal, perineal, penile and in the femoral triangle.

**Complications of maldescended and ectopic testis** Infertility; ×40 increased risk of testicular cancer (risk remains after surgery but in cryptorchidism may be ↓ if orchidopexy performed before aged 10),[280] increased risk of testicular trauma, increased risk of testicular torsion. Also associated with hernias (due to patent processus vaginalis in >90%, p615) and other urinary tract anomalies.

**Treatment of maldescended and ectopic testis** restores (potential for) spermatogenesis; the increased risk of malignancy remains but becomes easier to diagnose.

*Surgery:* Orchidopexy, usually dartos pouch procedure, is performed in infancy: testicle and cord are mobilized following a groin incision, any processus vaginalis or hernial sac is removed and the testicle is brought through a hole made in the dartos muscle into the resultant subcutaneous pouch where the muscle prevents retraction.

*Hormonal:* Hormonal therapy, most commonly human chorionic gonadotrophin (hCG), is sometimes attempted if an undescended testis is in the inguinal canal.

## 65

## Testicular self-examination: advice for patients (and male readers)

**Why?** Cancers that are detected early are the most easily treated so it makes sense to check yourself regularly. It will help you know what is normal for you and enable you to detect changes. NB: regular self-examination has not been studied enough to show if it does actually reduce the death rate from testicular cancer.[281]

**When?** Regularly; at least once a month. Ideally in the shower/bath when the muscle in the scrotum is relaxed.

**How?**

- Gently feel each testicle individually. You should feel a soft tube at the top and back of the testicle. This is the epididymis which carries and stores sperm. It may feel slightly tender. Don't confuse it with an abnormal lump. You should be able to feel the firm, smooth tube of the spermatic cord which runs up from the epididymis.
- Feel the testicle itself. It should be smooth with no lumps or swellings. It is unusual to develop cancer in both testicles at the same time, so if you are wondering whether a testicle is feeling normal or not you can compare it with the other.
- Remember—if you do notice a change in size/weight or find any abnormal lumps or swellings in your testicle, make an appointment and have it checked by your doctor as soon as possible.
- Note—most abnormalities are not cancer but collections of fluid, infection, or cysts. Cancer usually starts as a small hard painless lump. Even if it is cancer, treatment in 9 out of 10 cases, treatment can result in a complete cure. However, the earlier it is detected the easier it is to treat. More than a third of people with this cancer consult their doctor after the cancer has spread, which makes treatment more difficult. Often this is because of unfounded fears, or just hoping it will go away. Adapted from www.cancerhelp.org.uk.

Surgery

An artery with a dilatation >50% of its original diameter has an aneurysm; remember this is an ongoing process. True aneurysms are abnormal dilatations that involve all layers of the arterial wall. False aneurysms (pseudoaneurysms) involve a collection of blood in the outer layer only (adventitia) which communicates with the lumen (eg after trauma). Aneurysms may be fusiform (eg most AAAs) or sac-like (eg Berry aneurysms; fig 2 p483).

**Common sites** Aorta (infrarenal most common), iliac, femoral and popliteal arteries.

| Typical causes |
| --- |
| • Atheroma |
| • Trauma |
| • Infection, eg mycotic aneurysm in endocarditis, tertiary syphilis (esp. thoracic aneurysms) |
| • Connective tissue disorders (eg Marfan's, Ehlers-Danlos) |
| • Inflammatory, eg Takayasu's aortitis (p726) |

**Complications** Rupture; thrombosis; embolism; fistulae; pressure on other structures.

**Screening** all men at age 65yrs decreases mortality from ruptured AAA.[282] The NHS AAA screening programme is being introduced across the UK.

**Ruptured abdominal aortic aneurysm (AAA)** Death rates/year from ruptured AAAs rise with age: 125 per million in those aged 55-59; 2728 per million if over 85yrs. *Symptoms & signs:* Intermittent or continuous abdominal pain (radiates to back, iliac fossae, or groins—▶don't dismiss this as renal colic), collapse, an **expansile** abdominal mass (it expands and contracts: swellings that are pulsatile just transmit the pulse, eg nodes overlying arteries), and shock. If in doubt, assume a ruptured aneurysm.

**Unruptured AAA** *Definition:* >3cm across. *Prevalence:* 3% of those >50yrs. ♂:♀ >3:1. Less common in diabetics. *Cause:* Degeneration of elastic lamellae and smooth muscle loss.[283] There is a genetic component. *Symptoms:* Often none, they may cause abdominal/back pain, often discovered incidentally on abdominal examination (see BOX). *Monitoring:* RCTs have failed to demonstrate benefit from early endovascular repair (EVAR, see below) of aneurysms <5.5cm (where rupture rates are low).[284] Risk of rupture below this size is <1%/yr, compared to ~25%/yr for aneurysms >6cm across. ~75% of aneurysms so monitored eventually need repair and some will lose suitability for endovascular repair. Rupture is more likely if: •BP↑ •Smoker •Female •Strong family history. Modify risk factors if possible at diagnosis. *Elective surgery:* Reserve for aneurysms ≥5.5cm[283] or expanding at >1cm/yr, or symptomatic aneurysms. Operative mortality: ~5%; complications include spinal or visceral ischaemia and distal trash from dislodged thrombus debris.[285] Studies show that age >80yrs should not, in itself, preclude surgery. *Stenting (EVAR):* Major surgery can be avoided by inserting an endovascular stent via the femoral artery. EVAR has less early mortality but higher graft complications, eg failure of stent-graft to totally exclude blood flow to the aneurysm—'endoleak', & is more costly.[286] See fig 1.

## ▶▶ Thoracic aortic dissection

Blood splits the aortic media with sudden tearing chest pain (± radiation to back). As the dissection extends, branches of the aorta occlude sequentially leading to hemiplegia (carotid artery), unequal arm pulses and BP or acute limb ischaemia, paraplegia (anterior spinal artery), and anuria (renal arteries). Aortic valve incompetence, inferior MI and cardiac arrest may develop if dissection moves proximally. *Type A* (70%) dissections involve the ascending aorta, irrespective of site of the tear, whilst if the ascending aorta is not involved it is called *type B* (30%) ▶▶ All patients with type A thoracic dissection should be considered for surgery: get urgent cardiothoracic advice. Definitive treatment for type B is less clear and may be managed medically, with surgery reserved for distal dissections that are leaking, ruptured, or compromising vital organs. *Management:* •Crossmatch 10u blood; •ECG & CXR (expanded mediastinum is rare). •CT/MRI or transoesophageal echocardiography (TOE).[287] Take to ITU; hypotensives: keep systolic at ~100-110mmHg: *labetalol* (p134) or *esmolol* (p120; t½ is ultra-short) by IVI is helpful here (calcium-channel blockers may be used if β-blockers contraindicated). Acute operative mortality: <25%.

Surgery

### Emergency management of a ruptured abdominal aneurysm

Mortality—treated: 41% and improving; untreated: ~100%.[288]

▶▶ Summon a vascular surgeon and an experienced anaesthetist; warn theatre.

▶▶ Do an ECG, and take blood for amylase, Hb, crossmatch (10-40U may eventually be needed). Catheterize the bladder.

▶▶ Gain IV access with 2 large-bore cannulae. Treat shock with ORh−ve blood (if desperate), but keep systolic BP ≤100mmHg to avoid rupturing a contained leak (NB: raised BP is common early on).

▶▶ Take the patient straight to theatre. Don't waste time on x-rays: fatal delay may result, though CT can help in a stable patient with an uncertain diagnosis.

▶▶ Give prophylactic antibiotics, eg *cefuroxime* 1.5g + *metronidazole* 500mg IV.

▶▶ Surgery involves clamping the aorta above the leak, and inserting a Dacron® graft (eg 'tube graft' or, if significant iliac aneurysm also, a 'trouser graft' with each 'leg' attached to an iliac artery).

**Surgery**

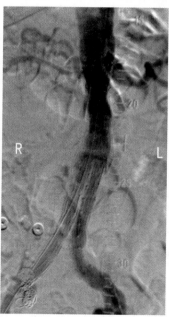

Fig 1. Stenting: not an open or closed case...this is a digital subtraction angiogram showing correct positioning of an endovascular stent at the end of the procedure. Although less invasive than open repair, some are unsuited to this method, owing to the anatomy of their aneurysm. Lifelong monitoring is needed: stents may leak and the aneurysm progress (the risk can be reduced by coiling the internal iliac arteries, as shown).[289]

Figure courtesy of Norwich Radiology Dept.

### ☼ The bomb inside you?! ♦☀

A wise doctor might reframe a patient's fear of an unexploded bomb inside them to deepen their view of his or her own health: health is not simply a question of being of sound body and mind, but entails a process of adaptation to changing environments, to growing up, to ageing, and to healing when damaged (*OHCS*, p470).

Peripheral arterial disease (PAD) occurs due to atherosclerosis causing stenosis of arteries via a multifactorial process involving modifiable and non-modifiable risk factors. 65% have co-existing clinically relevant cerebral or coronary artery disease. ▶Cardiovascular risk factors should be identified and treated aggressively. The chief feature of PAD is intermittent claudication (= *to limp*). Prevalence = 10%.

**Symptoms** Cramping pain is felt in the calf, thigh, or buttock after walking for a given distance (the **claudication distance**) and relieved by rest (calf claudication suggests femoral disease while buttock claudication suggests iliac disease). Ulceration, gangrene (p662), and foot pain **at rest**—eg burning pain at night relieved by hanging legs over side of bed—are the cardinal features of *critical ischaemia*. Buttock claudication ± impotence imply Leriche's syndrome (p718). Young, heavy smokers are at risk from Buerger's disease (thromboangiitis obliterans, p710). [291]

*Fontaine classification for peripheral arterial disease:* 1 Asymptomatic 2 Intermittent claudication 3 Ischaemic rest pain 4 Ulceration/gangrene (critical ischaemia).

**Signs** Absent femoral, popliteal or foot pulses; cold, white leg(s); atrophic skin; punched out ulcers (often painful); postural/dependent colour change; a vascular (Buerger's) angle[1] of <20° and capillary filling time >15s are found in severe ischaemia.

**Tests** Exclude DM, arteritis (ESR/CRP). FBC (anaemia, polycythaemia); U&E (renal disease); lipids (dyslipidaemia); ECG (cardiac ischaemia). Also do thrombophilia screen and serum homocysteine if <50 years. *Ankle-brachial pressure index (ABPI):* Normal = 1-1.2; Peripheral arterial disease = 0.5-0.9; Critical limb ischaemia <0.5 or ankle systolic pressure <50mmHg. Beware falsely high results from incompressible calcified vessels in severe atherosclerosis, eg DM.

**Imaging** *Colour duplex USS* is 1st line (non-invasive and readily available). If considering intervention *MR/CT angiography* (fig 2) is used to assess extent and location of stenoses and quality of distal vessels ('run-off'). It has largely replaced digital subtraction angiography.

**℞ 1** *Risk factor modification:* Quit smoking (vital). Treat hypertension and high cholesterol. Prescribe an antiplatelet agent (unless contraindicated), to prevent progression and to reduce cardiovascular risk. *Clopidogrel* is recommended as 1st-line. [292]

**2** *Management of claudication:* •*Supervised exercise programmes* reduce symptoms by improving collateral blood flow (2h per week for 3 months). Encourage patients to excercise to the point of maximal pain. •*Vasoactive drugs*, eg *naftidrofuryl oxalate*, offer modest benefit and are recommended only in those who do not wish to undergo revascularization and if exercise fails to improve symptoms.

If conservative measures have failed and PAD is severely affecting a patient's lifestyle or becoming limb threatening, intervention is required.

• *Percutaneous transluminal angioplasty (PTA)* is used for disease limited to a single arterial segment (a balloon is inflated in the narrowed segment). 5-year patency is 79% (iliac) and 55% (femoral). Stents can be used to maintain artery patency.

• *Surgical reconstruction:* If atheromatous disease is extensive but distal run-off is good (ie distal arteries filled by collateral vessels), consider arterial reconstruction with a bypass graft (fig 2). Procedures include femoral-popliteal bypass, femoral-femoral crossover and aorto-bifemoral bypass grafts. Autologous vein grafts are superior to prosthetic grafts (eg Dacron® or PTFE). [293]

*Amputation* <3% of patients with intermittent claudication require major amputation within 5 years (↑ in diabetes, p204). Amputation may relieve intractable pain and death from sepsis and gangrene. A decision to amputate must be made by the patient, usually against a background of failed alternative strategies. The knee should be preserved whenever possible as it improves mobility and rehabilitation potential (this must be balanced with the need to ensure wound healing). Rehabilitation should be started early with a view to limb fitting. *Gabapentin* (regimen on p508) can be used to treat the gruelling complication of phantom limb pain. [294]

*Future therapies:* Angiogenic gene therapy has yet to reduce amputation rates. [295]

1 Leg goes pale when raised, eg by 20° off the couch; compare sides.

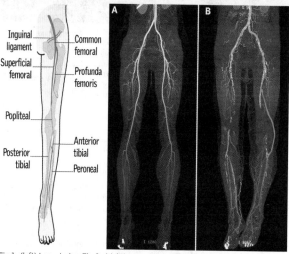

Inguinal ligament
Superficial femoral
Popliteal
Posterior tibial

Common femoral
Profunda femoris
Anterior tibial
Peroneal

**Fig 1.** (left) Leg arteries. **Fig 2.** (right) CT angiogram showing (A) normal lower limb vasculature and (B) heavily diseased arteries with previous left femoral anterior tibial bypass.

Reproduced from 'Diagnosis and management of peripheral arterial disease', G Peach, M Griffin, K G Jones, M M Thompson, R J Hinchliffe, vol 345, 2012, with permission from BMJ Publishing Group Ltd.

## Acute limb ischaemia

▶▶Surgical emergency requiring revascularization within 4–6h to save the limb. May be due to thrombosis *in situ* (~40%), emboli (38%), graft/angioplasty occlusion (15%), or trauma. Thrombosis more likely in known 'vasculopaths'; emboli are sudden, eg in those without previous vessel disease; they can affect multiple sites, and there may be a bruit. Mortality: 22%. Amputation rate: 16%.

• *Symptoms and signs:* The 6 'P's of acute ischaemia: pale, pulseless, painful, paralysed, paraesthetic, and 'perishingly cold'. Onset of fixed mottling implies irreversibility. Emboli commonly arise from the heart (AF; mural thrombus) or aneurysms. ▶In patients with **known** PAD, sudden deterioration of symptoms with deep duskiness of the limb may indicate acute arterial occlusion. This appearance is due to extensive pre-existing collaterals and must not be misdiagnosed as gout/cellulitis.

• *Management:* ▶This is an emergency and may require urgent open surgery or angioplasty. If diagnosis is in doubt, do urgent arteriography. If the occlusion is embolic, the options are surgical embolectomy (Fogarty catheter) or local thrombolysis, eg *tissue plasminogen activator* (t-PA, p339), balancing the risks of surgery with the haemorrhagic complications of thrombolysis.[298]

• Anticoagulate with *heparin* after either procedure and look for the source of emboli. ▶Be aware of possible post-op reperfusion injury and subsequent compartment syndrome.

## Carotid artery disease

Carotid artery disease accounts for 20% of strokes and TIAs. Symptomatic patients with ipsilateral stenosis ≥70% should have *carotid endarterectomy* within 2 weeks of symptom onset (see also p480). This continues to be safer than stenting.[297] *Complications:* 2–3% risk of stroke and death within 30 days; hypoglossal nerve injury. NB: there is no benefit in treating completely occluded vessels.

VVs are long, tortuous & dilated veins of the superficial venous system. **Pathology** Blood from superficial veins of the leg passes into deep veins via perforator veins (perforate deep fascia) and at the sapheno-femoral and sapheno-popliteal junctions. Valves prevent blood from passing from deep to superficial veins. If they become incompetent there is venous hypertension and dilatation of the superficial veins occurs. Risk factors: prolonged standing, obesity, pregnancy, family history, and the Pill.[298]

**Symptoms** "My legs are ugly". Pain, cramps, tingling, heaviness, and restless legs. But studies show these symptoms are only slightly commoner in those with VVs.

**Signs** Oedema; eczema; ulcers; haemosiderin; haemorrhage; phlebitis; *atrophie blanche* (white scarring at the site of a previous, healed ulcer); lipodermatosclerosis (skin hardness from subcutaneous fibrosis caused by chronic inflammation and fat necrosis). On their own varicose veins don't cause DVTs (except possibly *proximally spreading thrombophlebitis* of the long saphenous vein).

**Examination** See BOX.

**Treatment** ►NICE guidelines suggest that the criteria for specialist referral of patients with VVs should be: bleeding, pain, ulceration, superficial thrombophlebitis, or 'a severe impact on quality of life' (ie not for cosmetic reasons alone). In the UK funding for NHS treatment is usually via special funding panels.

• *Treat any underlying cause.*
• *Education:* Avoid prolonged standing and elevate leg(s) whenever possible; support stockings (compliance is a problem); lose weight; regular walks (calf muscle action aids venous return).
• *Endovascular treatment:* (less pain and earlier return to activity than surgery.)
    • *Radiofrequency ablation (VNUS closure®):* A catheter is inserted into the vein and heated to 120°C destroying the endothelium and 'closing' the vein. Results are as good as conventional surgery at 3 months.[299]
    • *Endovenous laser ablation (EVLA)* is similar but uses a laser. Outcomes are similar to surgical repair after 2yrs (in terms of quality of life and recurrence).[300]
    • *Injection sclerotherapy* Either liquid or foam can be used. Liquid sclerosant is indicated for varicosities below the knee if there is no gross saphenofemoral incompetence. It is injected at multiple sites and the vein compressed for a few weeks to avoid thrombosis (intravascular granulation tissue obliterates the lumen). Alternatively foam sclerosant is injected under ultrasound guidance at a single site and spreads rapidly throughout the veins, damaging the endothelium. Ultrasound monitoring prevents inadvertent spread of foam into the femoral vein. It achieves ~80% complete occlusion but is not more effective than liquid sclerotherapy or surgery.[301]
• *Surgery:* There are several choices, depending on vein anatomy and surgical preference, eg saphenofemoral ligation (Trendelenburg procedure); stripping from groin to upper calf (stripping to the ankle is not needed, and may damage the saphenous nerve). *Post-op:* Bandage legs tightly and elevate for 24h. Surgery is more effective than sclerotherapy in the long term.[302]
►Before surgery and after venous mapping, ensure that all varicosities are indelibly marked to either side (to avoid tattooing if the incision is made through inked skin).

**Saphena varix** Dilatation in the saphenous vein at its confluence with the femoral vein (the SFJ). It transmits a cough impulse and may be mistaken for an inguinal or femoral hernia, but on closer inspection it may have a bluish tinge.

## Examining varicose veins

**Method of examination** (Start with the patient standing.)

1 Inspect for: ulcers usually above the medial malleolus (varicose ulcers, *OHCS* p410) with deposition of haemosiderin causing brown edges, eczema, and thin skin. Inspect the legs from anterior thigh to medial calf (long saphenous vein) and the back of the calf (short saphenous vein). Palpate veins for tenderness (phlebitis) and hardness (thrombosis). If ulceration is present palpate pulses to rule out arterial disease.

2 Feel for *cough impulse* at the saphenofemoral junction (SFJ) (≈incompetence). *Percussion test:* Tap VVs distally and palpate for transmitted impulse at the SFJ (interrupted by competent valves).

3 Auscultate over varicosities for a bruit, indicating arteriovenous malformation.

4 For completion, examine the abdomen, the pelvis in females and external genitalia in males (for masses).

5 *Doppler ultrasound probes* listen for flow in incompetent valves, eg the SFJ, or the short saphenous vein behind the knee (the calf is squeezed: flow on release lasting over ½–1 second indicates significant reflux). If incompetence is not identified and treated, varicosities will return.

6 *Special tests:* Trendelenburg's test assesses if the SFJ valve is competent. Doppler USS has largely consigned this and other examination methods (eg *Tourniquet* and *Perthes' test*) to the history books.

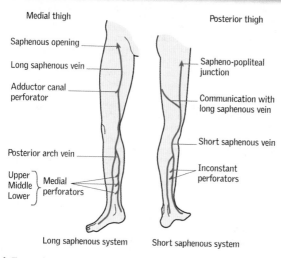

| Medial thigh | Posterior thigh |
| --- | --- |

Saphenous opening

Long saphenous vein

Adductor canal perforator

Sapheno-popliteal junction

Communication with long saphenous vein

Short saphenous vein

Posterior arch vein

Inconstant perforators

Upper
Middle — Medial perforators
Lower

Long saphenous system    Short saphenous system

Fig 1. The superficial veins of the leg.

## ☼ When do varicose veins become an illness?

Perhaps when they hurt? Or is this too simple? 'Certain illnesses are desirable: they provide a compensation for a functional disorder...' (Albert Camus); *this is known to be common with VVs.*[303] Perhaps many opt for surgery as a displacement activity to confronting deeper problems. ►We adopt the sickness role when we want sympathy. Somatization is hard to manage: here is one approach to consider:

• Give time; don't dismiss these patients as 'just the "worried well"'.
• Explore factors perpetuating illness behaviour (misinformation, social stressors).
• Agree a plan that makes sense to the patient's holistic view of themself.
• Treat any underlying depression (drugs and cognitive therapy, *OHCS* p374).

**Definitions** Gangrene is death of tissue from poor vascular supply and is a sign of critical ischaemia (see p658). Tissues are black and may slough. *Dry gangrene* is necrosis in the absence of infection. Note a line of demarcation between living and dead tissue.[1] ℞ Restoration of blood supply ± amputation. *Wet gangrene* is tissue death and infection (associated with discharge) occurring together (p205, fig 1). ℞ Analgesia; broad-spectrum IV antibiotics; surgical debridement ± amputation. *Gas gangrene* is a subset of necrotizing myositis caused by spore-forming *Clostridial species*. There is rapid onset of myonecrosis, muscle swelling, gas production, sepsis and severe pain. Risk factors include diabetes, trauma and malignancy. ℞ Remove all dead tissue (eg amputation). Give *benzylpenicillin ± clindamycin. Hyperbaric O₂* can improve survival and ↓ the number of debridements.[304]

**Necrotizing fasciitis** is a rapidly progressive infection of the deep fascia causing necrosis of subcutaneous tissue. Prompt recognition (difficult in the early stages) and aggressive treatment is required. ▸In any atypical cellulitis, get early surgical help. There is intense pain over affected skin and underlying muscle. Group A β-haemolytic streptococci is a major cause, although infection is often polymicrobial. Fournier's gangrene is necrotizing fasciitis localized to the scrotum and perineum. ℞ Radical debridement ± amputation; IV antibiotics, eg *benzylpenicillin* and *clindamycin*.

## Skin ulcers
OHCS, p604

Ulcers are abnormal breaks in an epithelial surface. Leg ulcers affect ~2% in developed countries.

**Causes** See MINIBOX—there may be multiple causes. For leg ulcers, venous disease accounts for 70%, mixed arterial and venous disease for 15% and arterial disease alone for 2%. Pressure sores: see fig 1, p477.

**History** Ask about number, pain, trauma. Go over comorbidities—eg varicose veins, peripheral arterial disease, diabetes, vasculitis. Is the history long or short? Is the patient taking steroids? Is the patient a bit odd? (remember self-induced ulcers: *dermatitis artefacta*). Has a biopsy been taken?

| Classification |
| --- |
| • Venous |
| • Arterial |
|   Large vessel |
|   Small vessel |
| • Neuropathic |
| • Diabetic |
|   Neuropathic, arterial or both |
| • Lymphoedema |
| • Vasculitic |
| • Malignant (p598) |
| • Infective |
|   TB, syphilis |
| • Traumatic (pressure) |
| • Pyoderma gangrenosum |
| • Drug induced |

**Examination** Note features such as site, number, surface area, depth, edge, base, discharge, lymphadenopathy, sensation, and healing. If in the legs, note features of venous insufficiency or arterial disease and, if possible, apply a BP cuff to perform ankle-brachial pressure index (ABPI). See BOX.

**Tests** Skin and ulcer biopsy may be necessary—eg to assess for vasculitis (will need immunohistopathology) or malignant change in an established ulcer (Marjolin's ulcer = SCC presenting in chronic wound). If ulceration is the first sign of a suspected systemic disorder then further screening tests will be required.

**Management** Managing ulcers is often difficult and expensive. Treat the cause(s) and focus on prevention. Optimize nutrition. Are there adverse risk factors (drug addiction, or risk factors for arteriopathy, eg smoking)? Get expert nursing care. Consider referral to specialist community nurse or leg ulcer/tissue viability clinic:
- 'Charing-Cross' 4-layer compression bandaging is better than standard bandages[305] (use only if arterial pulses OK: ABPI (p658) should be >0.8. Honey dressings can improve healing in mild-moderate burns, but as an adjuvant to compression bandaging for leg ulcers they do not significantly improve healing rate.[306]
- Negative pressure wound therapy (eg VAC®) helps heal diabetic ulcers.[307]
- Surgery, larval therapy and hydrogels are used to debride sloughy necrotic tissue (avoid hydrogels in diabetic ulcers due to ↑ risk of wet gangrene).
- Routine use of antibiotics does not improve healing. Only use if there is infection (not colonization).[308]

---

**1** 'The first sign of his approaching end was when one of my old aunts, while undressing him, removed a toe with one of his old socks'. Graham Greene, *A Sort of Life*, 1971, Simon & Schuster.

## Features of skin ulceration to note on examination

**Site** Above the medial malleolus ('gaiter' area) is the favourite place for *venous ulcers* (mostly related to superficial venous disease, but may reflect venous hypertension via damage to the valves of the deep venous system, eg 2° to DVT). Venous hypertension leads to the development of superficial varicosities and skin changes (*lipodermatosclerosis* = induration, pigmentation, and inflammation of the skin). Minimal trauma to the leg leads to ulceration which often takes many months to heal. Ulcers on the sacrum, greater trochanter, or heel suggest *pressure sores* (*OHCS* p605), particularly if the patient is bed-bound with suboptimal nutrition.

**Temperature** The ulcer and surrounding tissues are cold in an ischaemic ulcer. If the skin is warm and well perfused then local factors are more likely.

**Surface area** Draw a map of the area to quantify and time any healing (a wound >4 weeks old is a chronic ulcer as distinguished from an acute wound).

**Shape** Oval, circular (cigarette burns), serpiginous (*granuloma inguinale*, p416); unusual morphology can be secondary to mycobacterial infection, eg cutaneous tuberculosis or scrofuloderma (*tuberculosis colliquativa cutis*, where an infected lymph node ulcerates through to the skin).[309]

**Edge** Shelved/sloping ≈ healing; punched-out ≈ syphilis or ischaemic; rolled/everted ≈ malignant; undermined ≈ TB.

**Base** Any muscle, bone, or tendon destruction (malignancy; pressure sores; ischaemia)? There may be a grey-yellow slough, beneath which is a pale pink base. Slough is a mixture of fibrin, cell breakdown products, serous exudate, leucocytes and bacteria—it need not imply infection, and can be part of the normal wound healing process. Granulation tissue is a deep pink gel-like matrix contained within a fibrous collagen network and is evidence of a healing wound.

**Depth** If not uncomfortable for the patient (eg in neuropathic ulceration) a probe can be used to gauge how deep the ulceration extends.

**Discharge** Culture before starting any antibiotics (which usually don't work). A watery discharge is said to favour TB; bleeding can ≈ malignancy.

**Associated lymphadenopathy** suggests infection or malignancy.

**Sensation** Decreased sensation around the ulcer implies neuropathy.

**Position in phases of extension/healing** Healing is heralded by granulation, scar formation, and epithelialization. Inflamed margins ≈ extension.

Surgery

# 14 Epidemiology

## Contents

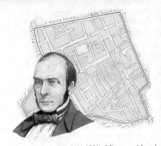

Fig 1. John Snow (1813–1858). Often considered as one of the founding figures of epidemiology, and responsible for understanding the waterborne nature of disease transmission. Most famously remembered for arranging the removal of the handle from a water pump in Broad Street in London to tackle an epidemic of cholera in the area, at that time thought to be spread by bad air or 'miasma'. However, he personally commented that the epidemic may have already been in decline, and the Council rapidly replaced the handle! He also had an interest in anaesthesia, and personally anaesthetized Queen Victoria in her last two pregnancies. Voted the "greatest doctor" of all time in 2003, pushing Hippocrates into second place.

*We thank Dr Laurie Tomlinson, our Specialist Reader, and Kit Robinson, our Junior Reader, for their contribution to this chapter.*

Epidemiology is the study of the distribution of clinical phenomena in populations. It is essential to public health research and disease prevention (p666). For example, it analyses disease outbreaks in terms of *host*, *agent*, and *environment* (the 'epidemiologist's triad')—eg starting by measuring **prevalence** and **incidence**.

**Definitions** The *period prevalence* is the number of cases during the study period, divided by the study population. If the population is unclear, then this must be specified, eg the prevalence of uterine cancer varies widely, depending on whether you specify all females, girls, or men and women. *Point prevalence* is the prevalence at a point in time. *Incidence* is the number of new cases within a specified study period, eg annual incidence. The *lifetime prevalence* of hiccups is ~100%; the (UK) incidence is millions/year—but the point prevalence may be 0 at 3AM today if no one is actually having hiccups.

**Association** Differences in disease rates between populations, eg smokers/non-smokers, point to an association between the disease and factors distinguishing the populations (eg smoking). An association is still possible with equal rates because of confounding variables (eg greater asbestos exposure in non-smokers).

*Ways of accounting for associations:* A may cause B; B cause A; a 3ʳᵈ unknown agent, X, causes A and B; or it may be a chance finding. If it looks as if A might cause B, bear in mind the **Bradford Hill 'criteria'** (he did not claim any were essential):
1 Consistent findings: the same results are got by different people and studies.
2 Temporality: the effect must occur after the cause.
3 Biological gradient: greater exposure leading to greater incidence of the effect.
4 A plausible mechanism linking cause to effect is reassuring, but not essential.[1]
5 Coherence between epidemiological and lab findings ↑ likelihood of an effect.
6 Analogy: the effect of similar factors may be considered.
7 Use of *direct experiment*. Other criteria relate to *specificity* and *strength of association*. Global scores of causation-likelihood can be calculated.[1]

**There are 2 main types of studies that explore causal connections**
*Case-control studies:* The frequency of the putative risk factor (eg smoking) is compared between two groups: those with a disease (eg lung cancer) and those without (control group). Case-control studies are retrospective in that they start after the onset of the disease (although cases may be collected prospectively).

*Cohort studies:* The study group consists of subjects exposed to the putative cause (eg smoking); and the control group comprises of unexposed subjects. The incidence of the disease is then compared between the groups over time, usually prospectively.

**Matching** An association between A and B may be due to another factor P. To eliminate this possibility, matching for X is often used in case-control studies. One powerful (but unreliable, if numbers are small) way to do this in clinical trials is for the subjects to be allocated to groups randomly. **Over-matching** If unemployment causes low income, and low income causes depression, then matching study and control groups for income would mask the genuine causal link between unemployment and depression. ►Avoid matching factors that may intervene in the causal pathway linking A and B. **Blinding** If the subject does not know which of two trial treatments she is having, the trial is single blind. To further reduce risk of bias, the experimenter should also not know (double-blind). ►In a good trial, the blind lead the blind.

---

**1** Physiology is quite often misleading: eg many deaths after MI are from arrhythmias, suppressible by anti-arrhythmics, but deaths in groups given most of these drugs are 3× *higher* than in controls.[1]

Prevention is one of the core aims of epidemiology. Although perhaps less glamorous or urgent than clever diagnosis or expensive interventions involving probes, scalpels, and imaging, preventive medicine is potentially much more powerful. The first step is to motivate your patient to take steps to benefit their own health by asking Socratic questions. "Do you want to smoke?" "What does your family think about smoking?" "Do you want your children to smoke?" "Would there be any advantages in giving up?" "Why is your health important to you?" These motivational questions with specific strategies for prevention (p87, plus when and where to turn to get help) produce more change than withering looks and lectures on lung cancer or legs dropping off.

**The law of unintended consequences** (Sod's law, p359) decrees that those whom you have to persuade the hardest to accept prevention will be those to whom a complication befalls, eg colon perforation during colonoscopy to prevent cancers in those with polyps. With this in mind, concentrate on those preventive activities that are simple, cheap, have a very low complication rate, and do not interfere (much) with how the patient runs his life.

**Individualized risk communication** Risk communication done thoughtlessly and only dwelling on positive aspects can lead to bitterness, anger, and litigation.[3] If communication is based on a person's individual risk factors for a condition (eg age, family history, smoking status, cholesterol level, eg using formulae such as that on p664), is risk communicated in ways that change behaviour? A 2003 Cochrane meta-analysis[4] suggests 'not necessarily' (although uptake of screening tests is improved). At least this technique promotes dialogue, and dialogue opens doors, minds, and possibilities for choice. *Informed participation* is the aim, not passive acceptance of advice. It does not make much difference whether information is given as an absolute risk, or as a risk score, or categorized as high, medium, or low risk. See also 'Consent' on p570.

---

### Different types of prevention

**Primary—preventing occurrence (new cases)**
- Vaccination, water fluoridation
- Advice on healthy eating, smoking cessation, safe-sex, pre-conception folate
- Screening for hypertension, hypercholesterolaemia

**Secondary—screening for early disease**
- Cervical cytology, mammography, colonoscopy
- Microalbuminuria in diabetes

**Tertiary—preventing complications**
- Aspirin/statins post MI
- Bisphosphonates in osteoporosis

**Quaternary—preventing medicalization**
- Prioritizing preventive actions
- Shielding from ruthless targets (eg easing a diabetic's BP target so he feels better or is less prone to falls).

---

### When drugs aren't the answer: the laws of quaternary prevention

1 Prevention is better than cure. (Not all prevention is good, though: see above.)
2 Don't treat symptoms without working out underlying pathologies.[5]
3 Don't treat just pathology, and go beyond the biopsychosocial straitjacket (p9).
4 Don't feel you must treat: agree with patients about what's important.
5 When you can, work *with* Nature: don't try to pull cures like rabbits out of hats.
6 Think graded *exercise* (or *bed rest*), *diet* and *hygiene* before *drugs*, *drugs*.
7 All interventions have unintended consequences. Don't be deluded about this.
8 Find something to measure to monitor disease progression and your treatment.
9 All laws have exceptions (if he's well on the wrong drug, it's the right drug).

## Screening (secondary prevention)

*Modified Wilson criteria for screening* (1-10 spells IATROGENIC[1]—to remind us that in treating healthy populations we have an especial duty to do no harm.)

1 The condition screened for should be an important one.
2 There should be an acceptable treatment for the disease.
3 Diagnostic and treatment facilities should be available.
4 A recognizable latent or early symptomatic stage is required.
5 Opinions on who to treat as patients must be agreed.
6 The test must be of *high discriminatory power* (see below), *valid* (measuring what it purports to measure, not surrogate markers which might not correlate with reality), and be *reproducible*—with safety guaranteed.
7 The examination must be acceptable to the patient.
8 The untreated natural history of the disease must be known.
9 A simple inexpensive test should be all that is required.
10 Screening must be continuous (ie not a 'one-off' affair).

*Conclusion: screening tests must be cost-effective.*

**Problems** *All screening programmes do harm; some do good as well.*[6]

1 Those most at risk do not present for screening, thus increasing the gap between the healthy and the unhealthy—the *inverse care law* (p10).
2 The 'worried well' overload services by seeking repeat screening.
3 Services for investigating those testing positive are inadequate.
4 Those who are false positives suffer stress while awaiting investigation, and remain anxious about their health despite reassurance.

►Before screening, the chances of harming a patient (by anxiety or subsequent invasive tests), as well as any benefits, must be quantified: this is *Rees' rule*.[7]

| Examples of effective screening | Unproven/ineffective screening |
|---|---|
| • Cervical smears (cervical cancer) | • Mental test score (dementia) |
| • Mammography (breast cancer) | • Urine tests (diabetes; kidney disease) |
| • Finding smokers (+ quitting advice) | • Antenatal procedures (*OHCS* p8) |
| • Looking for malignant hypertension | • PSA screening (prostate cancer, p647) |

NB: screening for cervical cancer and mammography are far from perfect: both are liable to false negatives (p674), and a negative result is interpreted as "I'm fine" (and may be seen as a licence to take risks). So signs of interval cancers (arising between screenings) may be ignored by patients who assume they are in the clear.

1 From Greek: *iatros* (physician) + genic, denoting illness caused by us doctors. You will find this word etched on all our soles, producing a malign imprint however lightly we try to tread. *Ways to reduce iatrogenic illness:* •Use EBM if possible. •Involve patients in all decisions. •Check drug labels/dosages by reading them aloud. •Be aware of drug interactions: look it up—don't assume you know. •Explain to patients how to tell if things are going wrong, and what action to take ("if ... tell me...").

*Epidemiology*

This is the conscientious and judicious use of current best evidence from research to optimize management plans and integrate them with patients' values.[8] EBM includes 6 steps: **1** Asking answerable questions. **2** Finding the best information. **3** Information appraisal for validity and relevance. **4** Dialogue to find out what the patient wants. **5** Data application to patient care. **6** Evaluation of the performance.

**The problem** More than 2,000,000 papers are published each year. Patients benefit directly from a tiny fraction of these papers. How do we find them?

**A partial solution** Journals are scanned not by experts in a specialized field, but by searchers trained to identify papers that have a direct message for clinical practice and meet predefined criteria of rigour (below). Summaries are then published, eg in *Evidence-based Medicine*.[9,10] *Questions used to evaluate papers:*
• Are the results valid? Randomized? Blinded? Were all patients accounted for who entered the trial? Was follow-up complete? Were the groups similar at the start? Was everyone treated equally, apart from the experimental intervention? NB: randomized trials are now recognized as blunt instruments: adaptive (Bayesian) designs may sometimes be a more efficient way to get to the truth (p674).[11]
• What are the results? How large (and precise) was the treatment effect?
• Will the results help my patients (cost/benefit sum)?[8]

**Problems with the solution** ► *The concept of scientific rigour is opaque.* What do we want? The science, the rigour, the truth, or what will be most useful to patients? These may overlap, but they are not the same.
• Will the best be the enemy of the good? Are useful papers rejected due to some blemish? Answer: appraise *all* evidence (often impossible).
• By insisting on *answerable* questions, EBM may subvert a patient's aims. He may only want to share his fears, not be used as a substrate for intellectual exercises.
• Is the standard the same for the evidence for *all* changes to our practice? We might avoid prescribing drug x for constipation if there is any chance that it might cause colon cancer, the choice of drugs is wide. More robust evidence is needed to persuade us to do something rather counterintuitive, eg giving heparin in DIC (p346). There is no science to tell us how robust the data need to be: we decide off the top of our head (albeit a wise head, we hope).
• What about the correspondence columns of the journals from which the winning papers are extracted? It takes years for unforeseen but fatal flaws to surface.
• There is a danger that by always asking "What is the evidence ..." we will divert resources from hard-to-prove areas (eg physiotherapy, which may be very valuable) to easy-to-prove services. The unique personal attributes of the therapist may be as important as the objective regimen.
• EBM is never 100% up-to-date, and reworking meta-analyses takes time and money, so specialists may ostensibly reject a new trial due to a tiny flaw, when the real reason is that they dread it might flip their once-perfect formulation.
• 'My increased knowledge gradually permeated or repressed the world of intuitive premonitions ...'[1]. These premonitions may be vital!
• If EBM is prescriptive, patient choice declines: not all patients are amenable to rational dialogue. Does our zeal for EBM make us arrogant and inflexible?
• The patient before us may not quite fit the type of patient who provided the research basis—and we may be tempted to ignore these small differences, which may then have major unforeseen adverse effects.

**Advantages of EBM—this is mainly that patients get better faster—also:**
• Our reading habits improve, and we can offer more rational choices to patients.
• EBM leads us to ask questions, and then to be sceptical of the answers.
• As taxpayers, we should like it (wasteful practices can be abandoned).

EBM may not have as much impact as we hope, as gaining evidence is time-consuming and expensive, and sometimes impossible. Despite these caveats, EBM is here to stay, so we may as well subscribe to its ideals—and to its journals.

**1** Carl Jung.

## Number needed to treat (NNT)

Statistical analysis is the glue that holds together the conclusions of a study. It is also the mask behind which the shortcomings of a study may hide. Having an understanding of what the statistical terms mean, and what they can be used for, will help you to decide for yourself whether a study's conclusions are valid. Some other important statistical definitions are given on p765.

If the risk of dying from an MI after 'standard treatment' is 10%, and a new treatment reduces this to 8%, the new drug can be made to look very effective by quoting the *relative risk reduction*, which is 20% ([10 – 8]/10 × 100%; ie the new drug is 20% more effective). However, the *absolute risk reduction* is 2% (10 – 8%; ie only an extra 2% of patients would derive benefit from the new treatment). In terms of the *number needed to treat*, we might say therefore that 50 patients would need treating to save one additional life ([1/absolute risk reduction] × 100). NNTs provide a useful way of quantifying benefit. In some preventive studies of mild hypertension in the young, ~800 people may need treating according to a certain regimen to prevent one stroke—when expressed like this, the treatment seems less wonderful. However, they do not take into account treatment costs or the *degree* of potential benefit.

The converse of NNT is *number needed to harm*. This is the number of people who must receive a treatment in order to produce one adverse event.

*Strengths:* NNTs are context-dependent. Thus if a new antihypertensive regimen is being compared with an old regimen where the NNT was 800 and the new regimen is only marginally better, the NNT to prevent one death or stroke *by adopting the new regimen in place of the old* may run into many thousands, as will your drugs bill if the new drug is more expensive.

*Weaknesses:* NNTs are difficult to interpret if there is a large *placebo effect*, eg in pain relief. Say the placebo response rate is 40% and that of a new analgesic is 60%, then the NNT is 5. Perhaps it is better to say to patients starting the new drug that 60% respond. *Keep your eye on the question:* NNTs can vary markedly if the question is slightly rephrased—eg from being about primary prevention to being about secondary prevention (as in the statin example above).[12] Also, one needs to be clear whether the mean or median is given as the length of follow-up. For further examples, see www.nntonline.net.

**NNT confidence intervals** Get these by taking reciprocals of the values defining the confidence interval for the absolute risk reduction (ARR). If ARR ≈ 10% with a 95% confidence interval of 5-15%, then NNT ≈ 10 (ie 100/10) and the 95% NNT-confidence interval ≈ 6.7-20 (ie 100/15 to 100/5). Non-significant treatment effects are problematic as NNTs can only be positive; here, give NNT *without* confidence intervals (Altman's rule).[13]

### Examples of NNTs

| Study | Outcome | NNT |
|---|---|---|
| Statins (p109) for primary prevention[14] | Death (MI) | 931 (78) for 5yrs |
| Statins for secondary prevention (4S) | Death (MI) | 30 (15) for 5.4yrs |
| Mild hypertension (MRC trial) | Stroke | 850 for 1yr |
| Systolic hypertension in elderly (SHEP) | Stroke | 43 for 4.5yrs |
| Aspirin in acute MI (ISIS-1) | Death | 40 |
| Streptokinase in acute MI (ISIS-2) | Death | 40 |
| ACE-i for CCF (NYHA class IV, p131) | Death | 6 for 1yr |

Epidemiology

Epidemiology

The 'gold-standard' is the double-blind, randomized trial, as they minimize bias and get at the truth as to whether this drug is any good or not. These are increasingly expensive and PROBE designs (prospective, randomized, open-label, blinded, end-point) are cheaper, easier, and may be appropriate if the outcome measure is robust (death) or can be blinded. But remember that Sod's law (p359) never sleeps, and if something can go wrong with a trial, it will—in at least 8 realms.

 1 There is no true or false answer to the question.
 2 Wrong question asked.
 3 Wrong subjects in the trial, eg all from a country where a gene conferring resistance to a treatment is prevalent. Or under-representation of the elderly.
 4 Randomization may give 2 groups that are unbalanced (the play of chance)—eg the group having the new antihypertensive may have lower BP.
 5 Blinding may be subverted if the patients can guess whether they are having the active or placebo treatment—for example by side-effects.
 6 The design may allow for rejection of the null hypothesis (that there is no difference between the two treatments)—but the null hypothesis may be irrelevant if previous studies show that the new treatment has some benefits. 73% of randomized trials made this mistake in one analysis.[15]
 7 Insufficient subjects enrolled, either by design or failure to recruit, to show a small but valuable effect. If an underpowered (the ability to detect true differences) trial *does* give 'positive' results, the size of the difference between the groups is likely to be exaggerated. (This is type I error; a type II error applies to results that indicate that there is no effect, when in fact there is.)
 8 Subgroup analysis may seem to show that a drug works in a subset of patients. But trawling of data will often produce these 'effects' if repeated often enough.

**What to do about these shortcomings?** Sometimes Bayesian probabilistic approaches will help. These ask about the probability of a range of hypotheses conditional on the data. The best dose, for example, may be found during an experiment, as a Bayesian protocol (an *adaptive design*) allows for learning during the experiment. This makes asking the wrong question less of a problem, and allows conclusions using far fewer patients (eg 50% less).[16]

In summary, no single methodology is uniquely valid and there is no coherent hierarchy of evidence. Just make do with what is available, and apply it sensibly.

**Meta-analyses** Systematic merging of similar trials *may* explain data inconsistencies. It is quicker and cheaper than doing new studies, can establish generalizability of research[17] and by trawling for unpublished trials ('grey literature') publication bias can be reduced (positive trials are more likely to be published than negative ones).[18] *Be cautious!* In one study looking at recommendations of meta-analyses where there was a later 'definitive' big trial, it turned out that meta-analyses got it wrong 30% of the time, and 20% of good meta-analyses fail to avoid bias.[19] Don't assume that all meta-analyses, even those from the cleanest stables, such as Cochrane, are free of bias owing to pharmaceutical funding.[20]

▶A big well-planned trial may be worth centuries of uncritical medical practice; but a week's experience on the wards may be more valuable than years reading journals. This is the paradox in medical education: How can we trust our own experiences knowing they are all anecdotal? How can we be open to novel ideas but avoid being merely fashionable? A stance of wary open-mindedness may serve us best.

---

**Types of study**

- Randomized trial
- Adaptive design (see above)
- Non-randomized contemporaneous trial
- Historical (retrospective) trial
- Case-control study
- N=1 trial (the patient acts as his own control—see p229)
- Other: case series, case reports, narrative: "What did it feel like on digoxin?"

## When a randomized controlled trial might not be the best method

- Generating new ideas beyond current paradigms (case reports may be better).
- Researching causes of illnesses and prognoses (cohort studies may be better).
- Evaluating diagnostic tests is best done with a cohort study and decision model.
- Where the researcher has no idea of the effective dose of a drug. A dose-ranging adaptive design where the next dose given depends on the effects of previous doses is a more efficient methodology,[11] as there can be a dynamic termination rule allowing for early discontinuation for either efficacy or futility.
- When recruiting of patients would be impossible or unethical.[21]
- If the unique gifts of the therapist might have a bigger effect than the drug used.
- When personalized medicine is the aim. For example, new cancer drugs seek to match effective treatments with patients' biomarker profiles. This may be better accomplished by adaptive designs.[22]

▶ In the end all randomized trials have to submit to the ultimate test when the statistical collides with the personal "*Will this treatment help me?*" "*Will this procedure help you?*" No randomized trial is complete until real-life decisions taken in the light of its findings are scrutinized and a narrative is compiled to suggest when results should be applied and when they should be ignored.[23] So do not ask for definitive trials: everything is provisional.

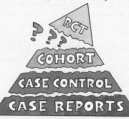

Fig 1. Hierarchy of evidence? No: think more of a network of evidence that takes into account epidemiology, lab work and experiential data.

RCT=randomized controlled trial.

Epidemiology

## Medicine and the internet and useful contacts

During the time it takes you to read this page, your better-connected patients may have checked out the latest recommendations of Guatemalan Guidelines on Gynaecomastia, or the NICE's Treatise on Toxoplasmosis. Patients have time and motivation, whereas we have little time and our motivation may be flickering. This can seem threatening to the doctor who sees himself as a dispenser of wisdom and precious remedies. It is less threatening if we consider ourselves to be in partnership with our patients. The evidence is that those who use the internet to question their therapy receive a better service. For the doctor, the role of the internet is to answer your clinical questions. Can tetanus toxoid cause purpura? Is there a connection between knee pain and constipation? Frame your questions as simply as possible. You are not asking if it is likely that this patient's purpura is due to last week's tetanus vaccine, just if it is a reported happening. Use the knowledge you are given to guide management.

*Some useful online resources:*

- **Drugs:** eMIMS (more up to date than *eBNF*, but see the *What's new* section at www.bnf.org); *eMIMS* contains many data-sheets—free and updated monthly.
- **Differential diagnoses,** eg 'what causes chest pain, knee pain, and turea?', and rare diseases—try Mentor (www.webmentorlibrary.com).
- **Research:** PubMed is free at www.ncbi.nlm.nih.gov/pubmed.
- **Meta-analyses:** (p670) eg the Cochrane Library at www.cochrane.org. Other similar resources are available through Update Software (www.update-software.com).
- **Public Health:** Central Public Health Lab: 020 8200 4400. www.hpa.org.uk. Committee on Safety of Medicines: (part of the MHRA) www.mhra.gov.uk/committees/.../MedicinesAdvisoryBodies/CommitteeonSafetyofMedicines/index.htm. Communicable Disease Surveillance Centre: 020 8200 6868. www.hpa.org.uk. Medic-Alert Foundation: 0800 581 420. www.medicalert.org.uk. Poisons information services: see p850. Transplant Service (UK) (can these organs be used?) 0845 60 60 400. Liverpool School of Tropical Medicine: 0151 705 3100. www.liv.ac.uk/lstm. London School of Hygiene and Tropical Medicine: 020 7636 8636. www.lshtm.ac.uk.

Your surgical tutor asks whether Gobble's disease is commoner in women or men. You have no idea, and make a guess. What is the chance of getting it right? Common sense decrees that it is even chances; 'Sod's law' (p359) predicts that whatever you guess, you will always be wrong. A less pessimistic view is that the balance is slightly tipped against you: according to Damon Runyon, 'all life is 6 to 5 against'.[24]

*Do new symptoms suggest a new disease or are they from an existing disease?* The answer is often counterintuitive. Suppose **s** is quite a rare symptom of Gobble's disease (seen in 5% of patients), but that it is a very common symptom of disease A (seen in 90%). If we have a man whom we already know has Gobble's disease and who goes on to develop symptom **s**, is not **s** more likely to be due to disease A, rather than Gobble's disease? The answer is usually no: *it is generally the case that **s** is due to a disease that is already known, and does not imply a new disease.*

The 'odds ratio' makes this clearer, ie the ratio of [*the probability of the symptom, given the known disease*] to [*the probability of the symptom given the new disease × the probability of developing the new disease*]. Usually this is vastly in favour of the symptom being due to the old disease, because of the prior odds of the two diseases.

**Doctors as gamblers** (fig 1). To the average mind it is distasteful to learn that doctors gamble with patients' lives. One of us (JML) has just finished consulting with 23 patients. Not too many, perhaps: it might be argued that each symptom, especially if *serious*, should be investigated until the cause is found.

Let us look at this critically. What counts as a serious symptom? One that might mean death, disfigurement, or disability. Some of these patients offered 5 symptom groups before being gently dissuaded from going on. During elucidation of these symptoms others emerged, yielding a potentially endless cycle of investigation. Certainly some of their symptoms might not seem serious ("this pain in my toe..."). But toe pain might be mortal if caused by emboli or osteomyelitis. Fingernail problems with a slight rash might mean arsenic poisoning, lethargy may mean cancer, and so on. So medicine is not for pessimists—almost anything can be made to seem fatal, so that a pessimistic doctor would never get any sleep at night for worrying about the meanings of his patients' symptoms.

Medicine is not for blind optimists either, who too easily embrace a fool's paradise of false reassurance. Rather, *medicine is for gamblers:* gamblers who are happy to use subtle clues to change their outlook from pessimism to optimism and *vice versa.* Sometimes the gambling is scientific, rational, and methodical (odds-ratio analysis): sometimes it is not, as when the gambling is based on prior knowledge (vital but ill-defined) of one's patient, or the faint apprehension of terror in this new patient's eyes that shows you that there is something wrong, and that you don't yet know what it is.

Being lucky in both types of gambling is a requisite for being a successful doctor: after all we would all rather have a lucky doctor than a wise one. In this game, especially when it gets deadly serious, the chips are not just financial (the most cost-effective next step). They betoken time (for you are spending yourself as surely as you are spending money, as you walk the wards), your reputation, and the health or otherwise of your patient. So do not worry about the fact of gambling: *gambling is your job.* If you cannot gamble you cannot cure. But try hard to assemble sufficient evidence to maximize the chances of being lucky. Professions allied to medicine often seem similar to medicine, but typically without this central role of risk-taking (midwifery is among the notable exceptions).

The foregoing explains why courage is the cardinal clinical virtue: without it we would not follow our hunches and take justified risks—and all our other clinical virtues and skills (holistic care, diagnostic acumen, and operative dexterity) would not be deployed to their full advantage, while we pass the buck.

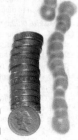

Fig 1. Her ESR is 21. Is it normal? Heads or tails? Play rouleaux-roulette to find out (p322).

### An example of the odds ratio at work

A 50-yr-old man with known carcinoma of the lung has some transient neurological symptoms and a normal CT scan. Are these symptoms due to secondaries in the brain or to transient ischaemic attacks (TIAs)?

- The chance of secondaries in the brain which cause transient neurological symptoms is 0.045 given carcinoma of the lung.
- The chance of such secondaries not showing up on a CT scan is 0.1. Therefore the chance of this cluster of symptoms is 0.0045 (ie 0.045 × 0.1).
- The chance of a normal CT + transient CNS symptoms given a TIA is 0.9.
- The chance of a 50-yr-old man developing TIA is 0.0001.
- Therefore the odds ratio is 0.0045/(0.9 × 0.0001). This equals 50.

That is, the odds ratio is ~50 to 1 in favour of secondaries in the brain.

NB: It is only very rarely that the prior odds of a new disease are so high that the new disease is more likely, eg someone presenting with anaemia already known to have breast cancer, who lives in an African community where 50% of people have hookworm-induced anaemia, is likely to have anaemia due to hookworm *as well as* breast carcinoma.

**Odds ratio and relative risk** compare the relative likelihood of an event occurring in two distinct groups. Relative risk (p671) is easier to interpret and often consistent with our intuitions. Some study designs, however, such as case-control studies, prevent the calculation of the relative risk (due to a pre-selected population). Which to use when? See childrensmercy.org/stats/journal/oddsratio.asp.

### ☼ "I did an ESR to exclude giant cell arteritis..."

William Osler wrote that 'Variability is the law of life, and as no two faces are the same, so no two bodies are alike, and no two individuals react alike and behave alike under the abnormal conditions which we know as disease. This is the fundamental difficulty of the physician, and one which he may never grasp.'[25] So whenever you hear the word 'exclude' on ward-rounds or in consulting rooms, wink at Osler—for you have discovered another one of his cases of a doctor who does not understand variability and probability. ▶*Nothing is ever excluded and everything is always provisional*—even death, for a while. (We have all been caught out by the last gasp not being the last.)

So isn't all this morass of nebulous uncertainty (fig 2) depressing? No. It's beautiful, for luckily the human brain is brilliantly constructed to solve these very problems, because life itself (off the wards, and since the beginning of time) is full of them. Medical education gets itself into a pickle when it tries to teach us too much—as if a mother would try to teach her daughter what to do on day 38 of marriage (yet this is exactly what we do with trypanosomiasis—see past editions). So, as Osler pointed out, if we give ourselves 'good methods and a proper

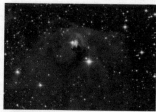

Fig 2. Like the chair you are sitting in, and your last ward round, Hind's Variable Nebula probably contains what we call a 'very young stellar object.' Learning to shine is only a matter of time.

Reproduced with permission from Panther Observatory.
www.panther-observatory.com

point of view, all other things will be added as [our] experience grows.'[25] Then, if on day 38, we find our patient is in labour, for example, we may recognize that other priorities may apply.

Epidemiology

Only rarely does a single test provide a definitive diagnosis. More often tests alter the odds of a diagnosis. When taking a history and examining patients, we make various wagers with ourselves (often barely consciously) as to how likely various diagnoses are. Further test results simply affect these odds. A test is worthwhile if it alters diagnostic odds in a clinically useful way.

**The effect of an investigation on the diagnostic odds** To work this out you need to know the *sensitivity* and *specificity* of the test. All tests have false-positive and false-negative rates, as summarized below:

| Test result | Patients with the condition | Patients without the condition |
|---|---|---|
| Result +ve for the condition | True +ve (*a*) | *False* +ve (*b*) |
| Result -ve for the condition | *False* -ve (*c*) | True -ve (*d*) |

*Specificity:* How often is the test -ve in health? $d/d+b$. *Sensitivity:* How often is the test +ve in the disease? $a/a+c$. *Positive predictive value:* How often will someone with a +ve result have the disease? $a/a+b$. *Negative predictive value:* How often will someone with a -ve result really not have the disease? $d/d+c$. Screening tests need to have a high sensitivity, to include everyone with the disease (at a cost of including some without), while diagnostic tests need a high specificity, to be certain the disease is present. For example, we know that 3-6% of chest pain patients sent home from casualty departments on the basis of a single ECG actually have myocardial infarction (MI). A single ECG is *specific* (77-100%), but not very sensitive for MI (56%). Troponin tests (p112) are very *sensitive*. So if history and ECG suggest MI, admit (treatment, p782). If story and ECG are not typical of MI, do a troponin test ≥6h after onset of chest pain—only send home if 'normal'.[1] This strategy reduces inappropriate discharge to 0.3%.[2] Note that studies showing these effects are very dependent on the local prevalence of MI. A few more MIs in the 'troponin normal' group would radically alter these results.

The *likelihood ratio* of the disease given a +ve result (LR+) is the ratio of the chance of having a +ve test if the disease is present to the chance of having a +ve test if the disease is absent: LR+=sensitivity/(1-specificity). Conversely the likelihood ratio given a -ve result, LR-, is (1-sensitivity)/specificity. Suppose we have a test of sensitivity 0.8 and specificity 0.9. LR+ will be 8:1 [ie 0.8/(1-0.9)], and LR- will be 2:9 [(1-0.8)/0.9].

**Is there any point to this test?** Work out the posterior odds assuming first a +ve and then a -ve test result—via the equation: *posterior odds = (prior odds)* × *(likelihood ratio)*. If your clinical assessment of a man with exercise-induced chest pain is that the odds of this being due to coronary artery disease (CAD) are 4:1 (80%), is it worth his doing an exercise tolerance test (sensitivity 0.72; specificity 0.8)?[26] If the test were +ve, the odds in favour of CAD would be $4 \times (0.72)/(1-0.8) = 14:1$ (93%). If -ve, they would be $4 \times (1 - 0.72)/0.8 = 1.4:1$ (58%), so the test has not in any way 'ruled out' CAD.

Experienced doctors are likely to have higher prior odds for the most likely diagnosis. The above shows that with high prior odds, a test must have high sensitivity and specificity for a negative result to bring the odds below 50%.

Another example is John, who is a 40-yr-old (not on NSAIDs, with no prior peptic ulcer) referred for '?endoscopy' because of dyspepsia. Before the result of a bedside test for *Helicobacter pylori* is known, he has a 50% chance of harbouring this organism, which, if present, is the probable cause of an ulcer.[26] The likelihood ratio for a -ve test result is 0.13[27] (sensitivity 0.88, specificity 0.91). *If the test is -ve*, the chance of John having *H. pylori* is <11%—and it may be OK to send him home with symptomatic treatment (eg ranitidine) without endoscopy—if there are no 'cancer (alarm) symptoms' (weight loss, dysphagia, etc, p242).[7] *If the test is +ve*, the probability of *H. pylori* is >90%, strongly suggesting the need for specific anti-ulcer (anti-*Helicobacter*) therapy (p242), and endoscopy if this does not cure his symptoms.

**1** Troponin T ≤0.1μg/L (or troponin I ≤0.2μg/L; labs vary); what is normal is itself a statistical issue (p652)—as is what counts as an MI.[13]
**2** Sensitivity: 97%; specificity: 93%; -ve predictive value: 99.6%; +ve predictive value: 66%; LR+: 13.9; LR-: 0.03.

### An example of epidemiology at work

Some decades ago, epidemiologists tested the hypothesis that smoking and hypertension were associated with vascular disease. Painstaking cohort studies confirmed that these were indeed *risk markers* (a term that does *not* imply causality). Over the years, as evidence accumulates, the term 'risk marker' may upgrade to *risk factor*, which *does* imply causation, and the separate idea that risk-factor modification will cause a reduction in disease. Demonstrating a dose-response relationship (with the correct time sequence) is good evidence of a causal relationship, eg showing that the greater the number of cigarettes smoked, or the higher the blood pressure, the greater the cardiovascular mortality. It is still possible that BP is a risk marker of some other phenomenon, but this is less likely if the relationship between BP and cardiovascular mortality is found to correlate *while keeping other known risk factors constant*. The work of the epidemiologist does not stop here. He or she can use actuarial statistics to weigh the relative merits and interactions of a number of risk factors, to give an overall estimate of risk for an individual. It is then possible to say things like: "If the 5yr risk of a serious cardiac event in people with no overt cardiac disease is >15%, then drug treatment of hyperlipidaemia may begin to be cost-effective—and a 10% 5yr risk may be a sufficient point to trigger antihypertensive treatment in someone with, say, a BP of 150/90". These figures are a guide only: only ~60% of those in the top 10% of the risk distribution will have an adverse event in the 5yr period. Nevertheless, this is more accurate than taking into account risk factors singly—and so we are led to our first important conclusion: *epidemiology improves and informs our dialogue with our patients.* We can give patients good evidence on which to base their choices.

*Risk equations:* Computerized records allow algorithms derived from millions of UK patients to stratify individual risk of vascular events (QRISK2) using age, sex, BMI, cholesterol/HDL, family history (1° relative <60yrs), BP, smoking and medical history (IHD, rheumatoid arthritis, AF, hypertension, renal disease), and social deprivation (via postcode).[29,30] In the UK, QRISK2 is more reliable than Framingham data even when refined for UK populations. *Accuracy:* QRISK2 classifies one in 10 UK men as high risk (10yr vascular risk ≥20% if ~30–74yrs old—the threshold recommended by NICE for statin $R_x$).[31,32] ▶Only 30% of subsequent vascular events occur in this high risk group![33] NB: ~80% of participants in QRISK had some missing data, eg cholesterol:HDL.[33]

## Contents

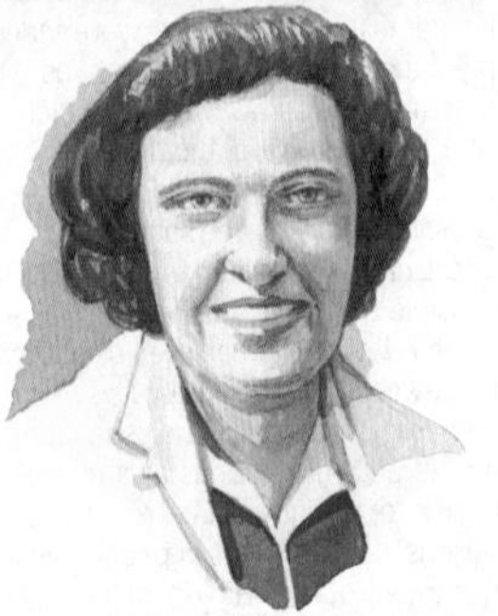

Fig 1. Rosalyn Yalow (1921-2011). Trained in nuclear physics, and made good use of this when she developed the radioimmunoassay technique to allow trace amounts of peptides to be measured in serum using antibodies. This revolutionized laboratory medicine; making reliable assays for hormones widely available; and underpinned the development of endocrinology. It was also employed to screen blood against a range of pathogens, and the technique is still commonly used today. She was awarded the Nobel prize for her work in 1977, and commenting to a group of children that: "Initially, new ideas are rejected...Later they become dogma, if you're right. And if you're really lucky you can publish your rejections as part of your Nobel presentation."

*Relevant pages elsewhere:* Reference intervals (p770); acute renal injury (p290).

## On being normal in the society of numbers

Laboratory medicine reduces our patients to a few easy-to-handle numbers: this is the discipline's great attraction—and its greatest danger. The normal range (reference interval) is usually that which includes 95% of a given population (given a normal distribution, see p764). If variation is randomly distributed, 2.5% of our results will be 'too high', and 2.5% 'too low' on an average day, when dealing with apparently normal people. This statistical definition of normality is the simplest. Other definitions may be *normative*—ie stating what an upper or lower limit *should* be. The upper end of the reference interval for plasma cholesterol may be given as 6mmol/L because this is what biochemists state to be the *desired* maximum. 40% of people in some populations will have a plasma cholesterol greater than 6mmol/L and thus may be at increased risk. The WHO definition of anaemia in pregnancy is an Hb of <110g/L, which makes 20% of mothers anaemic. This 'lax' criterion has the presumed benefit of triggering actions that result in fewer deaths from haemorrhage. So do not just ask "What is the normal range?"—also enquire about who set the range, for what population, and for what reason.

*We thank Kate McGlennan, our Junior Reader, for her contribution to this chapter.*

## General principles

- Laboratory testing may contribute to four aspects of medicine:
  - diagnosis;
  - prognosis (eg clotting in liver failure);
  - monitoring disease activity or progression (eg creatinine in chronic kidney disease);
  - screening (eg phenylketonuria in newborn babies).
- Only do a test if the result will influence management. Make sure you look at the result.
- Do not interpret laboratory results except in the light of clinical assessment (unless forced to by examiners!).
- ►Laboratory staff like to have contact with you. They are an excellent source of help and information for both requests and results.
- If a result does not fit with the clinical picture, trust clinical judgement and repeat the test. Could it be an artefact? The 'normal' range for a test (reference interval) is usually defined as the interval, symmetrical about the mean, containing 95% of results in a given population (p765). The more tests you run, the greater the probability of an 'abnormal' result of no significance (see p765).
- ►Involve the patient. Don't forget to explain to them where the test fits into their overall management plan.

## Getting the best out of the lab—a laboratory decalogue

1. Interest someone from the laboratory in your patient's problem.
2. Fill in the request form fully.
3. Give clinical details, not your preferred diagnosis.
4. Ensure that the lab knows who to contact.
5. Label specimens as well as the request form.
6. Follow the hospital labelling routine for crossmatching.
7. Find out when analysers run, especially batched assays.
8. Talk with the lab before requesting an unusual test.
9. Be thoughtful: at 16:30h the routine results are being sorted.
10. Plot results graphically: abnormalities show sooner.

## Artefacts and pitfalls in laboratory tests

- Do not take blood samples from an arm that has IV fluid running into it.
- Repeat any unexpected and inconsistent result before acting on it.
- For clotting time do not sample from a heparinized IV catheter.
- Serum K⁺ is over-estimated if the sample is old or haemolysed (this occurs if venepuncture is difficult).
- If using Vacutainers, fill *plain* tubes first—otherwise, anticoagulant contamination from previous tubes can cause errors.
- Total calcium results are affected by albumin concentration (p690).
- INR may be over-estimated if citrate bottles are under-filled.
- Drugs may cause *analytic* errors (eg prednisolone cross-reacts with cortisol). Be suspicious if results are unexpected.
- Food may affect result, eg bananas raise urinary HIAA (p278).

---

### ☼ Ford Madox Ford 1915 *'The good Soldier'*

Penguin 214, 228

► Normal values can have hidden historical, social, and political desiderata—just like the normal values novelists ascribe to their characters: *'Conventions and traditions, I suppose, work blindly but surely for the preservation of the normal type; for the extinction of proud, resolute and unusual individuals... Society must go on, I suppose, and society can only exist if the normal, if the virtuous, and the slightly deceitful flourish, and if the passionate, the headstrong, and the too-truthful are condemned to suicide and to madness. Yes, society must go on; it must breed, like rabbits. That is what we are here for ... But, at any rate, there is always Leonora to cheer you up; I don't want to sadden you. Her husband is quite an economical person of so normal a figure that he can get quite a large proportion of his clothes ready-made. That is the great desideratum of life.'*

Ca:Na⁺
K⁺

Clinical chemistry

*Dehydration:* ↑urea (disproportionate relative to smaller ↑ in creatinine),[1] ↑albumin (also useful to plot change in a patient's condition), ↑haematocrit (PCV); also ↓urine volume and ↓skin turgor.

*Abnormal kidney function:* There are two major biochemical pictures:
• *Low GFR:* ↑urea, ↑creatinine, ↑K⁺, ↑H⁺, ↑urate, ↑PO₄³⁻, ↑anion gap, ↓Ca²⁺, ↓HCO₃⁻, oliguria. Causes: early acute oliguric renal failure (p298), chronic kidney disease (p300). In chronic kidney disease also ↓Hb, ↑PTH and renal bone disease.
• *Tubular dysfunction* (damage to tubules): ↓K⁺, ↓urate, ↓PO₄³⁻, ↓HCO₃⁻, ↑H⁺, normal urea and creatinine. Other possible findings include polyuria with urinary glucose, amino acids, proteins (lysozyme, β₂-microglobulin), or phosphate. Diagnosis is made by testing renal concentrating ability (p233). *Causes:* recovery from acute renal failure, hypercalcaemia, hyperuricaemia, myeloma, pyelonephritis, hypokalaemia, Wilson's disease, galactosaemia, and heavy metal poisoning.

*Thiazide and loop diuretics:* ↓Na⁺, ↓K⁺, ↑HCO₃⁻, ↑urea.

*Bone disease:*

| | Ca²⁺ | PO₄³⁻ | Alk phos |
|---|---|---|---|
| Osteoporosis (p696) | Normal | Normal | Normal |
| Osteomalacia (p698) | ↓ | ↓ | ↑ |
| Paget's | Normal | Normal | ↑↑ |
| Myeloma | ↑ | ↑, normal | Normal |
| Bone metastases | ↑ | ↑, normal | ↑ |
| 1° Hyperparathyroidism | ↑ | ↓, normal | Normal, ↑ |
| Hypoparathyroidism | ↓ | ↑ | Normal |
| Renal failure (low GFR) | ↓ | ↑ | Normal, ↑ |

*Hepatocellular disease:* ↑bilirubin, ↑↑AST, alk phos ↑ slightly, ↓albumin. Also ↑clotting times. For details of the differences between AST and ALT, see p283.

*Cholestasis:* ↑bilirubin, ↑↑γGT, ↑alk phos, ↑AST.

*Excess alcohol intake:* Evidence of hepatocellular disease. Early evidence if ↑γGT, ↑MCV, and ethanol in blood before lunch.

*Myocardial infarction:* ↑↑troponin, ↑CK, ↑AST, ↑LDH (p112).

*Addison's disease:* ↑K⁺, ↓Na⁺ ↑urea.

*Cushing's syndrome:* May show ↓K⁺, ↑HCO₃⁻, ↑Na⁺.

*Conn's syndrome:* May show ↓K⁺, ↑HCO₃⁻. Na⁺ normal or ↑. (Also hypertension.)

*Diabetes mellitus:* ↑glucose, (↓HCO₃⁻ if acidotic).

*Diabetes insipidus:* ↑Na⁺, ↑plasma osmolality, ↓urine osmolality. (Both hypercalcaemia and hypokalaemia may cause nephrogenic diabetes insipidus.)

*Inappropriate ADH secretion (SIADH):* (see p687) ↓Na⁺ with normal or low urea and creatinine, ↓plasma osmolality. ↑urine osmolality (and > plasma osmolality), ↑urine Na⁺ (>20mmol/L).

*Some immunodeficiency states:* Normal serum albumin but *low* total protein (because immunoglobulins are missing. Also makes crossmatching difficult because expected haemagglutinins are absent; OHCS p198).

___

**1** Dehydration affects urea more than creatinine because in dehydration a greater proportion of filtered urea is reabsorbed by the kidney. Creatinine is hardly reabsorbed at all.

## Laboratory results: ▶▶when to take action NOW

- On receiving a dangerous result, first check the name and date.
- Go to the bedside. If the patient is conscious, turn off any IVI (until fluid is checked) and ask the patient how he or she is. *Any fits, faints, collapses, or unexpected symptoms?*
- Be sceptical of an unexpectedly wildly abnormal result with a well patient. Compare with previous values. Could the specimens have got muddled up? Is there an artefact? Was the sample taken from the 'drip' arm? Is a low calcium due to a low albumin (p690)? Perhaps the lab is using a new analyser with a faulty wash cycle? ▶*When in doubt, seek help and repeat the test.*

The values chosen below are somewhat arbitrary and must be taken as a guide only. Many results less extreme than those below will be just as dangerous if the patient is old, immunosuppressed, or has some other pathology such as pneumonia.

### Plasma biochemistry

▶▶ The main risks when plasma electrolytes are dangerously abnormal are of cardiac arrhythmias and CNS events such as seizures.

| Electrolyte | Lower limit | Upper limit | Relevant pages |
|---|---|---|---|
| $Na^+$ | <120mmol/L | >155mmol/L | p686 |
| $K^+$ | <2.5mmol/L | >6.5mmol/L | p688, p849 |
| Corrected $Ca^{2+}$ | <2.0mmol/L | >3.5mmol/L | p690, p692 |
| Glucose | <2.0mmol/L | >20mmol/L | p842, p844 |

### Blood gases

- $P_aO_2$ <8.0kPa = *Severe hypoxia. Give $O_2$.* See p180.
- pH <7.1 = *Dangerous acidosis. See p684 to determine the cause.*

### Haematology results

- Hb <70g/L with low mean cell volume (<75fL) or history of bleeding. This patient may need urgent transfusion (no spare capacity). See p318.
- Platelets <40×10⁹/L. May need a platelet transfusion; call a haematologist.
- *Plasmodium falciparum* seen on blood film. *Start antimalarials now.* See p396.
- ESR >30mm/h + headache. *Could there be giant cell arteritis?* See p558.

### CSF results

▶▶ Never delay treatment when bacterial meningitis is suspected.
- >1 neutrophil/mm³. *Is there meningitis: usually >1000 neutrophils?* See p832.
- Positive Gram stain. *Talk to a microbiologist; urgent blind therapy.* See p832.

**Conflicting, equivocal, or inexplicable results** ▶Get prompt help.

$Ca^{2+} Na^+$
$K^+$

Clinical chemistry

**Fluid requirement** in a normal person over 24h is roughly 2500mL. Normal daily losses are through urine (1500mL), stool (200mL), and insensible losses (800mL). This requirement is normally met through food (1000mL) and drink (1500mL).

**Intravenous fluids** are given if sufficient fluids cannot be given orally. About 2500mL fluid containing roughly 100mmol Na+ and 70mmol K+ per 24h are required. Thus, a good regimen is 2L of 5% glucose and 1L of 0.9% saline every 30h with 20mmol of K+ per litre of fluid. Alternative routes are via a central venous line or subcutaneously. However, remember that all cannulae carry a risk of MRSA infection: femoral > jugular > subclavian > peripheral, so always resume oral fluid intake as soon as possible.

▶In a sick patient, don't forget to include additional sources of fluid loss when calculating daily fluid requirements, such as drains, fevers, or diarrhoea (see BOX 2). Daily weighing helps to monitor overall fluid balance, as will fluid balance charts.

▶Examine patients regularly to assess fluid balance (see BOX 1).

### Fluid compartments and types of IV fluid

For a 70kg man *total bodily fluid* is approximately 42L (60% body weight). Of this, ⅔ is intracellular (28L) and ⅓ is extracellular (14L). Of the extracellular compartment, ⅓ is intravascular, ie blood (5L). Different types of IV fluid will equilibrate with the different fluid compartments depending on the osmotic content of the given fluid.

*5% glucose* (=dextrose) is isotonic, but contains only a small amount of glucose (50g/L) and so provides little energy (~10% daily energy per litre). The liver rapidly metabolizes all the glucose leaving only water, which rapidly equilibrates throughout all fluid compartments. It is, therefore, useless for fluid resuscitation (only 1/9 will remain in the intravascular space), but suitable for maintaining hydration. Excess 5% glucose IV may lead to water overload and hyponatraemia (p686).

*0.9% saline* ('normal saline') has about the same Na+ content as plasma (150mmol/L) and is isotonic with plasma. 0.9% saline will equilibrate rapidly throughout the extracellular compartment only, and takes longer to reach the intracellular compartment than 5% glucose. It is, therefore, appropriate for fluid resuscitation, as it will remain predominantly in the extracellular space (and thus ⅓ of the given volume in the intravascular space), as well as for maintaining hydration. Hypertonic and hypotonic saline solutions are also available, but are for specialist use only.

*Colloids* (eg Gelofusine®) have a high osmotic content similar to that of plasma and therefore remain in the intravascular space for longer than other fluids, making them appropriate for fluid resuscitation, but not for general hydration. Colloids are expensive, and may cause anaphylactic reactions. In reality, effective fluid resuscitation will use a combination of colloid and 0.9% saline.

*Hypertonic glucose (10% or 50%)* may be used in the treatment of hypoglycaemia. It is irritant to veins, so care in its use is needed. Infusion sites should be inspected regularly, and flushed with 0.9% saline after use.

*Dextrose-saline* (one-fifth 'normal saline') is isotonic, containing 0.18% saline (30mmol/L of Na+) and 4% glucose (222mmol/L). It has roughly the quantity of Na+ required for normal fluid maintenance, when given 10-hourly in adults, but is now most commonly used in a paediatric setting.

*Hartmann's solution* contains Na+ 131mmol, Cl- 111mmol, lactate 29mmol, K+ 5mmol, HCO3- 29mmol, and Ca2+ 2mmol per litre of fluid. It is an alternative to 0.9% saline, and some consider it more physiological.[1]

Ca+Na+ K+

## Assessing fluid balance

| Underfilled | Overfilled |
|---|---|
| • Tachycardia | • ↑JVP (p40) |
| • Postural drop in BP (low BP is a late sign of hypovolaemia) | • Pitting oedema of the sacrum, ankles, or even legs and abdomen |
| • ↓capillary refill time | • Tachypnoea |
| • ↓urine output | • Bibasal crepitations |
| • Cool peripheries | • Pulmonary oedema on CXR (fig 2, p293) |
| • Dry mucous membranes | See also p128 for signs of heart failure |
| • ↓skin turgor | |
| • Sunken eyes | |

The JVP is a substitute marker of central venous pressure, and when assessing fluid balance is difficult a CVP line may help to guide fluid management.

## Special cases

*Acute blood loss* Resuscitate with colloid or 0.9% saline via large-bore cannulae until blood is available.

*Children* Use dextrose-saline for fluid maintenance: 100mL/kg for the first 10kg, 50mL/kg for the next 10kg, and 20mL/kg thereafter—all per 24h.

*Elderly* More prone to fluid overload, so use IV fluids with care.

*GI losses* (diarrhoea, vomiting, NG tubes, etc) Replace lost K⁺ as well as lost fluid volume.

*Heart failure* Use IV fluids with care to avoid fluid overload (p128).

*Liver failure* Patients often have a raised total body sodium, so use salt-poor albumin or blood for resuscitation, and avoid 0.9% saline for maintenance.

*Acute pancreatitis* Aggressive fluid resuscitation is required due to large amounts of sequestered 'third space' fluid (p638).

*Poor urine output* Aim for >1 mL/kg/h; the minimum is >0.5mL/kg/h. Give a fluid challenge, eg 500mL 0.9% saline over 1h (or half this volume in heart failure or the elderly), and recheck the urine output. If not catheterized, exclude retention; if catheterized, ensure the catheter is not blocked!

*Post-operative* Check the operation notes for intraoperative losses, and ensure you chart and replace added losses from drains, etc.

*Shock* Resuscitate with colloid or 0.9% saline via large-bore cannulae. Identify the type of shock (p804).

*Transpiration losses* (fever, burns) Beware the large amounts of fluid that can be lost unseen through transpiration. Severe burns in particular may require aggressive fluid resuscitation (p858).

## Potassium in IV fluids

• Potassium ions can be given with 5% glucose or 0.9% saline, usually 20mmol/L or 40mmol/L.

• K⁺ may be retained in renal failure, so beware giving too much IV.

• Gastrointestinal fluids are rich in K⁺, so increased fluid loss from the gut (eg diarrhoea, vomiting, high-output stoma, intestinal fistula) will need increased K⁺ replacement.

▶The maximum concentration of K⁺ that is safe to infuse via a peripheral line is 40mmol/L, at a maximum rate of 20mmol/h. Fluid-restricted patients may require higher concentrations or rates in life-threatening hypokalaemia. Faster rates risk cardiac dysrhythmias and asystole, and higher concentrations thrombophlebitis, depending on the size of the vein, so give concentrated solutions >40mmol/L via a central venous catheter, and use ECG monitoring for rates over >10mmol/h. For symptoms and signs of hyper- and hypokalaemia see p688.

Clinical chemistry

**The kidney** controls the homeostasis of a number of serum electrolytes (including Na⁺, K⁺, Ca²⁺ and PO₄³⁻), helps to maintain acid-base balance, and is responsible for the excretion of many substances. It also makes erythropoietin and renin, and hydroxylates 25-hydroxyvitamin D to 1,25-dihydroxyvitamin D (see p690 for $Ca^{2+}$ and $PO_4^{3-}$ physiology). All of these functions can be affected in chronic kidney disease (p300), but it is the biochemical effects of kidney failure that are used to monitor disease progression.

**The renin-angiotensin-aldosterone system** Plasma is filtered by the glomeruli, and Na⁺, K⁺, H⁺ and water are reabsorbed from this filtrate under the control of the renin-angiotensin-aldosterone system. *Renin* is released from the juxtaglomerular apparatus (fig 1, p305) in response to low renal flow and raised sympathetic tone, and catalyses the conversion of *angiotensinogen* (a peptide made by the liver) to *angiotensin I*. This is then converted by angiotensin-converting enzyme (ACE), which is located throughout the vascular tree, to *angiotensin II*. The latter has several important actions including efferent renal arteriolar constriction (thus ↑ perfusion pressure), peripheral vasoconstriction, and stimulation of the adrenal cortex to produce *aldosterone*, which activates the Na⁺/K⁺ pump in the distal renal tubule leading to reabsorption of Na⁺ and water from the urine, in exchange for K⁺ and H⁺. Glucose spills over into the urine when the plasma concentration > renal threshold for reabsorption (≈10mmol/L, but this varies between people, and is ↓ in pregnancy).

**Control of sodium** is through the action of aldosterone on the distal convoluted tubule (DCT) and collecting duct to increase Na⁺ reabsorption from the urine. The natriuretic peptides ANP, BNP and CNP (p131) contribute to Na⁺ homeostasis by reducing Na⁺ reabsorption from the DCT and inhibiting renin. A *high GFR* (below) results in increased Na⁺ loss, and *high renal tubular flow* and haemodilution decrease Na⁺ reabsorption in the proximal tubule.

**Control of potassium** Most K⁺ is intracellular, and thus serum K⁺ levels are a poor reflection of total body potassium. The concentrations of K⁺ and H⁺ in extracellular fluid tend to vary together. This is because these ions compete with each other in the exchange with Na⁺ that occurs across most cell membranes and in the distal convoluted tubule of the kidney, where Na⁺ is reabsorbed from the urine. Thus, if the H⁺ concentration is high, less K⁺ will be excreted into the urine. Similarly K⁺ will compete with H⁺ for exchange across cell membranes and extracellular K⁺ will accumulate. Insulin and catecholamines both stimulate K⁺ uptake into cells by stimulating the Na⁺/K⁺ pump.

**Serum osmolality** is a laboratory measurement of the number of osmoles per *kilogramme* of solvent. It is approximated by *serum osmolarity* (the number of osmoles per *litre* of solution) using the equation $2(Na^+ + K^+) + Urea + Glucose$, since these are the predominant serum electrolytes. Normal serum osmolarity is 280-300mmol/L, which will always be a little less than the laboratory-measured osmolality—the *osmolar gap*. However, if the osmolar gap is greater than 10mmol/L, this indicates the presence of additional solutes: consider diabetes mellitus or high blood ethanol, methanol, mannitol, or ethylene glycol.

**Control of water** is mainly via serum Na⁺ concentration, since water intake and loss are regulated to hold the extracellular concentration of Na⁺ constant. Raised plasma osmolality (eg dehydration or ↑glucose in diabetes mellitus) causes thirst through the hypothalamic thirst centre and the release of antidiuretic hormone (ADH) from the posterior pituitary. ADH increases the passive water reabsorption from the renal collecting duct by opening water channels to allow water to flow from the hypotonic luminal fluid into the hypertonic renal interstitium. Low plasma osmolality inhibits ADH secretion, thus reducing renal water reabsorption.

**Glomerular filtration rate (GFR)** is the volume of fluid filtered by the glomeruli per minute (units mL/min), and is one of the primary measures of disease progression in chronic kidney disease. It can be estimated in a number of different ways (see BOX).

Calculating GFR is useful because it is a more sensitive indication of the degree of renal impairment than serum creatinine. Subjects with low muscle mass (eg the elderly, women) can have a 'normal' serum creatinine, despite a significant reduction in GFR. This can be important when prescribing nephrotoxic drugs, or drugs that are renally excreted, which may therefore accumulate to toxic levels in the serum.

A number of methods for estimating GFR exist, all relying on a calculation of the clearance of a substance that is renally filtered and then not reabsorbed in the renal tubule. For example, the rate of clearance of creatinine can be used as a marker for the rate of filtration of fluid and solutes in the glomerulus because it is only slightly reabsorbed from the renal tubule. The more of the filtered substance that is reabsorbed, however, the less accurate the estimate of GFR.

The **MDRD** (*Modification of Diet in Renal Disease Study Group*) equation provides an estimate of GFR from 4 simple parameters: *serum creatinine, age, gender* and *race (black/non-black)*. It is one of the best validated for monitoring patients with established moderately severe renal impairment,[2] and most labs now routinely report estimated GFR (eGFR) using the MDRD equation on all U&E reports:

$$eGFR = 32{,}788 \times serum\ creatinine^{-1.154} \times age^{-0.203} \times [1.212\ if\ black] \times [0.742\ if\ female]$$

However, a number of caveats exist, so that it is best used in monitoring declining renal function rather than labelling elderly patients with mild renal impairment:
• it is not validated for mild renal impairment, and therefore its use for screening *general* populations is questionable;
• inter-individual variations (and thus confidence intervals) are wide, although for each individual variations are small so that a decline in eGFR over a number of serum samples is always significant;
• single results may be affected by variations in serum creatinine, such as after a protein-rich meal.

The **Cockcroft-Gault equation** provides an estimate of creatinine clearance. It is an improvement on the MDRD equation because it also takes into account the patient's weight. However, 10% of creatinine is actively excreted in the tubules and therefore creatinine clearance overestimates true GFR and underestimates renal impairment.. Moreover, the equation assumes ideal body weight and is thus unreliable in the obese or oedematous. For an example of adjusting for ideal body weight, see p446. Also unreliable in unstable renal function.

$$Creat\ clearance = \frac{(140 - age) \times weight\ (kg) \times [0.85\ if\ female] \times [1.212\ if\ black]}{0.813 \times serum\ creatinine\ (\mu mol/L)}$$

Creatinine clearance can also be calculated by measuring the excreted creatinine in a **24h urine collection** and comparing it with the serum creatinine concentration. However, the accuracy of collection is vital but often poor, making this an unreliable and inconvenient method.

GFR can also be measured by injection of a radioisotope followed by sequential blood sampling ($^{51}$**Cr-EDTA**) or by an isotope scan (eg DTPA $^{99}$Tc, p190). These methods allow a more accurate estimate of GFR than creatinine clearance, since smaller proportions of these substances are reabsorbed in the tubules. They also have the advantage of being able to provide split renal function.

**Inulin clearance** (not insulin) is the gold standard for calculating GFR, because 100% of filtered inulin is retained in the luminal fluid and therefore reflects exactly the rate of filtration of water and solutes in the glomerulus. However, measuring inulin clearance again requires urine collection over several hours, and also a constant IV infusion of inulin, and is therefore inconvenient to perform.

Clinical chemistry

Arterial blood pH is closely regulated in health to 7.40 ± 0.05 by various mechanisms including bicarbonate, other plasma buffers such as deoxygenated haemoglobin, and the kidney. Acid–base disorders needlessly confuse many people, but if a few simple rules are applied, then interpretation and diagnosis are easy. The key principle is that primary changes in $HCO_3^-$ are *metabolic* and in $CO_2$ *respiratory*. See fig 1.

### A simple method

1 *Look at the pH:* is there an acidosis or alkalosis?
  • pH <7.35 is an acidosis; pH >7.45 is an alkalosis.
2 *Is the $CO_2$ abnormal?* (Normal concentration 4.7–6.0kPa)
  If so, is the change in keeping with the pH?
  • $CO_2$ is an acidic gas—is $CO_2$ raised with an acidosis, lowered with an alkalosis? If so, it is in keeping with the pH and thus caused by a *respiratory* problem. If there is no change, or an opposite one, then the change is compensatory.
3 *Is the $HCO_3^-$ abnormal?* (Normal concentration 22–28mmol/L)
  If so, is the change in keeping with the pH?
  • $HCO_3^-$ is alkaline—is $HCO_3^-$ raised with an alkalosis, lowered with an acidosis? If so, the problem is a *metabolic* one.

### An example

Your patient's blood gas shows: pH 7.05, $CO_2$ 2.0kPa, $HCO_3^-$ 8.0mmol/L. There is an *acidosis*. The $CO_2$ is low, and thus it is a compensatory change. The $HCO_3^-$ is low and is thus the primary change, ie a *metabolic* acidosis.

**The anion gap** estimates unmeasured plasma anions ('fixed' or organic acids such as phosphate, ketones, and lactate, which are hard to measure directly). It is calculated as the difference between plasma cations ($Na^+$ and $K^+$) and anions ($Cl^-$ and $HCO_3^-$). Normal range: 10–18mmol/L. It is helpful in determining the cause of a metabolic acidosis.

### Metabolic acidosis pH↓, $HCO_3^-$ ↓

*Causes of metabolic acidosis and an increased anion gap:*
Due to increased production, or reduced excretion, of fixed/organic acids. $HCO_3^-$ falls and unmeasured anions associated with the acids accumulate.
• Lactic acid (shock, infection, tissue ischaemia)
• Urate (renal failure)
• Ketones (diabetes mellitus, alcohol)
• Drugs/toxins (salicylates, biguanides, ethylene glycol, methanol)

*Causes of metabolic acidosis and a normal anion gap:*
Due to loss of bicarbonate or ingestion of $H^+$ ions ($Cl^-$ is retained).
• Renal tubular acidosis      • Addison's disease
• Diarrhoea                   • Pancreatic fistula
• Drugs (acetazolamide)       • Ammonium chloride ingestion

### Metabolic alkalosis pH↑, $HCO_3^-$↑

• Vomiting                    • Burns
• $K^+$ depletion (diuretics)  • Ingestion of base

### Respiratory acidosis pH↓, $CO_2$↑

• Type 2 respiratory failure due to any lung, neuromuscular, or physical cause (p180).
• Most commonly chronic obstructive pulmonary disease (COPD). Look at the $P_aO_2$. It will probably be low. Is oxygen therapy required? Use controlled $O_2$ (Venturi connector) if COPD is the underlying cause, as too much oxygen may make matters worse (p181).

  ►► Beware exhaustion in asthma, pneumonia and pulmonary oedema, which can present with this picture when close to respiratory arrest. These patients require urgent ITU review for ventilatory support.

### Respiratory alkalosis pH↑, $CO_2$↓

A result of hyperventilation of any cause. *CNS causes:* Stroke; subarachnoid bleed; meningitis. *Others:* Mild/moderate asthma, anxiety; altitude; $T°$↑; pregnancy; pulmonary emboli (reflex hyperventilation); drugs, eg salicylates.

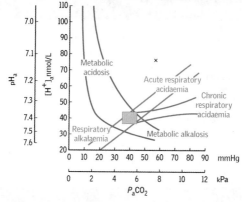

Fig 1. The shaded area represents normality. This method is very powerful. The result represented by point ×, for example, indicates that the acidosis is in part respiratory and in part metabolic. Seek a cause for each.

**Terminology** To aid understanding, we have used the terms acidosis and alkalosis, where a purist would sometimes have used acidaemia and alkalaemia.

Clinical chemistry

**Signs & symptoms** Lethargy, thirst, weakness, irritability, confusion, coma, and fits, along with signs of dehydration (p680). *Laboratory features:* ↑Na⁺, ↑PCV, ↑alb, ↑urea.

**Causes**

Usually due to water loss in excess of sodium loss:
• Fluid loss without water replacement (eg diarrhoea, vomit, burns).
• Diabetes insipidus (p232). Suspect if large urine volume. This may follow head injury, or CNS surgery, especially pituitary.
• Osmotic diuresis (for diabetic coma, see p842).
• Primary aldosteronism: rarely severe, suspect if ↑BP↑, K⁺↓, alkalosis (HCO₃⁻↑).
• Iatrogenic: incorrect IV fluid replacement (excessive saline).

**Management** Give water orally if possible. If not, give glucose 5% IV slowly (1L/6h) guided by urine output and plasma Na⁺. Use 0.9% saline IV if hypovolaemic, since this causes less marked fluid shifts and is hypotonic in a hypertonic patient. Avoid hypertonic solutions.

## Hyponatraemia

Plasma Na⁺ concentration depends on the amount of both Na⁺ and water in the plasma. Hyponatraemia therefore does not necessarily imply Na⁺ depletion. Assessing fluid status is the key to diagnosis (see fig 1).

**Signs and symptoms** Look for anorexia, nausea and malaise initially, followed by headache, irritability, confusion, weakness, ↓GCS and seizures, depending on the severity and rate of change in serum Na⁺. Cardiac failure or oedema may help to indicate the cause. Hyponatraemia also increases the risk of falls in the elderly.[3]

**Causes** See the FLOWCHART opposite. Artefactual causes include: •Blood sample was from a drip arm; •High serum lipid/protein content causing ↑serum volume, with ↓Na⁺ concentration but normal plasma osmolality; •If hyperglycaemic (≥20mmol/L) add ~4.3mmol/L to plasma Na⁺ for every 10mmol/L rise in glucose above normal.

**Iatrogenic hyponatraemia** If 5% glucose is infused continuously without adding 0.9% saline, the glucose is quickly used, rendering the fluid hypotonic and causing hyponatraemia, esp. in those on thiazide diuretics, women (especially premenopausal) and those undergoing physiological stress (eg post-operative, septic). In some patients, only marginally low plasma Na⁺ levels cause serious effects (eg ~128mmol/L)—don't attribute odd CNS signs to non-existent strokes/TIAs if Na⁺↓.

**Management**
• Correct the underlying cause; never base treatment on Na⁺ concentration alone. The presence of symptoms, the chronicity of the hyponatraemia, and state of hydration are all important. Replace Na⁺ and water at the same rate they were lost.
• *Asymptomatic chronic hyponatraemia* **fluid restriction** is often sufficient if asymptomatic, although **demeclocycline** (ADH antagonist) may be required. If hypervolaemic (cirrhosis, CCF) treat the underlying disorder first.
• *Acute or symptomatic hyponatraemia*, or if *dehydrated*, cautious rehydration with 0.9% saline may be given, but do not correct changes rapidly as *central pontine myelinolysis*[1] may result. Maximum rise in serum Na⁺ 15mmol/L per day if chronic, or 1mmol/L per hour if acute. Consider using furosemide when not hypovolaemic to avoid fluid overload.
• Vasopressor receptor antagonists ('vaptans', eg conivaptan, tolvaptan, lixivaptan and satavaptan) promote water excretion without loss of electrolytes, and appear to be effective in treating hypervolaemic and euvolaemic hyponatraemia but are expensive.[4]
▶▶*In emergency* (seizures, coma) seek expert help. Consider hypertonic saline (eg 1.8% saline) at 70mmol Na⁺/h ± furosemide. Aim for a gradual increase in plasma Na⁺ to ≈125mmol/L. Beware heart failure and central pontine myelinolysis.[1]

**1** Central pontine myelinolysis: irreversible and often fatal pontine demyelination seen in malnourished alcoholics or rapid correction of ↓Na⁺. There is subacute onset of lethargy, confusion, pseudobulbar palsy, para- or quadriparesis, 'locked-in' syndrome or coma.

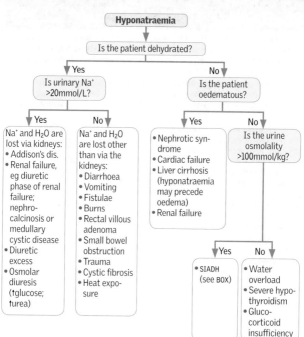

Fig 1. Hyponatraemia.

## Syndrome of inappropriate ADH secretion (SIADH)

An important, but over-diagnosed, cause of hyponatraemia. The diagnosis requires concentrated urine (Na⁺ > 20mmol/L and osmolality > 100mosmol/kg) in the presence of hyponatraemia (plasma Na⁺ < 125mmol/L) and low plasma osmolality (< 260mosmol/kg), in the absence of hypovolaemia, oedema, or diuretics.

*Causes*
• *Malignancy:* lung small-cell, pancreas, prostate, thymus, or lymphoma.
• *CNS disorders:* meningoencephalitis, abscess, stroke, subarachnoid or subdural haemorrhage, head injury, neurosurgery, Guillain-Barré, vasculitis or SLE.
• *Chest disease:* TB, pneumonia, abscess, aspergillosis, small-cell lung cancer.
• *Endocrine disease:* hypothyroidism (not true SIADH, but perhaps due to excess ADH release from carotid sinus baroreceptors triggered by ↓ cardiac output).⁵
• *Drugs:* opiates, psychotropics, SSRIs, cytotoxics.
• *Other:* acute intermittent porphyria, trauma, major abdominal or thoracic surgery, symptomatic HIV.

*Treatment* Treat the cause and restrict fluid. Consider salt ± loop diuretic if severe. Demeclocycline is used rarely. Vasopressin receptor antagonists ('vaptans', p686) are an emerging class of drug used in SIADH and other types of hyponatraemia.

Ca²⁺Na⁺
K⁺

Clinical chemistry

▶▶ A plasma potassium >6.5mmol/L is an emergency and needs urgent treatment (see p849). The worry is of myocardial hyperexcitability leading to ventricular fibrillation and cardiac arrest. First assess the patient—do they look unwell, is there an obvious cause? If not, could it be an artefactual result?

**Concerning signs and symptoms** include a fast irregular pulse, chest pain, weakness, palpitations, and light-headedness. ECG: (see ECG 9) tall tented T waves, small P waves, a wide QRS complex (eventually becoming sinusoidal), and ventricular fibrillation.

*Artefactual results:* If the patient is well, and has none of the above findings, repeat the test urgently as it may be artefactual, caused by: •haemolysis (difficult venepuncture; patient clenched fist); •contamination with potassium EDTA anticoagulant in FBC bottles (do FBCs *after* U&Es); •thrombocythaemia (K⁺ leaks out of platelets during clotting); •delayed analysis (K⁺ leaks out of RBCs; a particular problem in a primary care setting due to long transit times to the lab).⁸

**Causes**
- Oliguric renal failure
- K⁺-sparing diuretics
- Rhabdomyolysis (p307)
- Metabolic acidosis (DM)
- Excess K⁺ therapy
- Addison's disease (see p218)
- Massive blood transfusion
- Burns
- Drugs, eg ACE-i, suxamethonium
- Artefactual result (see above)

**Treatment in non-urgent cases**
- Treat the underlying cause; review medications.
- **Polystyrene sulfonate resin** (eg Calcium Resonium® 15g/8h PO) binds K⁺ in the gut, preventing absorption and bringing K⁺ levels down over a few days. If vomiting prevents PO administration, give a 30g enema, followed at 9h by colonic irrigation.
- ▶▶ If there is evidence of myocardial hyperexcitability, or K⁺ is >6.5mmol/L, get senior assistance, and treat as an emergency (see p849).

## Hypokalaemia

If K⁺ <2.5mmol/L, urgent treatment is required. Note that hypokalaemia exacerbates digoxin toxicity.

**Signs and symptoms** Muscle weakness, hypotonia, hyporeflexia, cramps, tetany, palpitations, light-headedness (arrhythmias), constipation.

**ECG** Small or inverted T waves, prominent U waves (after T wave), a long PR interval, and depressed ST segments.

**Causes**
- Diuretics
- Vomiting and diarrhoea
- Pyloric stenosis
- Rectal villous adenoma
- Intestinal fistula
- Cushing's syndrome/steroids/ACTH
- Conn's syndrome
- Alkalosis
- Purgative and liquorice abuse
- Renal tubular failure (p310 & p678)

If on diuretics, ↑HCO₃⁻ is the best indication that hypokalaemia is likely to have been long-standing. Mg²⁺ may be low, and hypokalaemia is often difficult to correct until Mg²⁺ levels are normalized. Suspect Conn's syndrome if hypertensive, hypokalaemic alkalosis in someone not taking diuretics (p220).

In *hypokalaemic periodic paralysis*, intermittent weakness lasting up to 72h appears to be caused by K⁺ shifting from extra- to intracellular fluid. See OHCS p652.

**Treatment** *If mild:* (>2.5mmol/L, no symptoms) give oral K⁺ supplement (≥80mmol/24h, eg Sando-K® 2 tabs/8h). Review K⁺ after 3 days. If taking a thiazide diuretic, and K⁺ >3.0 consider repeating and/or K⁺ sparing diuretic. *If severe:* (<2.5mmol/L, and/or dangerous symptoms) give IV potassium cautiously, not more than 20mmol/h, and not more concentrated than 40mmol/L. Do not give K⁺ if oliguric.
▶▶ **Never** give K⁺ as a fast stat bolus dose.

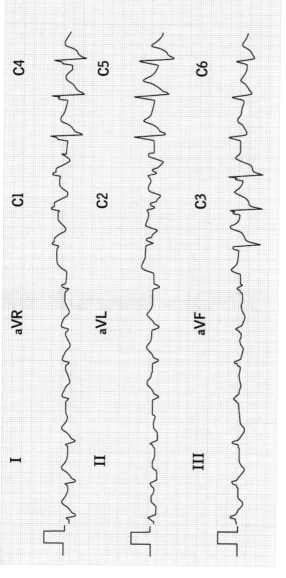

ECG 9. Hyperkalaemia—note the flattening of the P waves, prominent T waves, and widening of the QRS complex.

Ca²⁺·Na⁺
K⁺

Clinical chemistry

### Calcium and phosphate homeostasis is maintained through:

*Parathyroid hormone (PTH):* Overall effect is $\uparrow Ca^{2+}$ & $\downarrow PO_4^{3-}$. Secretion by 4 parathyroid glands is triggered by $\downarrow$serum ionized $Ca^{2+}$; controlled by -ve feedback loop. Actions are: •$\uparrow$osteoclast activity releasing $Ca^{2+}$ and $PO_4^{3-}$ from bones; •$\uparrow Ca^{2+}$ & $\downarrow PO_4^{3-}$ reabsorption in the kidney; •$\uparrow$renal production of 1,25-dihydroxy-vitamin $D_3$.

*Vitamin D and calcitonin:* Vit D is hydroxylated first in the liver to 25-hydroxy-vit D, and again in the kidney to 1,25-dihydroxy-vit D (**calcitriol**), the biologically active form, and 24,25-dihydroxy-vit D (inactive). Calcitriol production is stimulated by $\downarrow Ca^{2+}$, $\downarrow PO_4^{3-}$, and PTH. *Actions are:* •$\uparrow Ca^{2+}$ and $\uparrow PO_4^{3-}$ absorption from the gut; •inhibition of PTH release; •enhanced bone turnover; •$\uparrow Ca^{2+}$ and $\uparrow PO_4^{3-}$ reabsorption in the kidney. **Cholecalciferol** (vit $D_3$—from animal sources) and **ergocalciferol** (vit $D_2$—from vegetables) are biologically identical in their activity. Disordered regulation of calcitriol underlies familial normocalcaemic hypercalciuria, which is a major cause of calcium oxalate renal stone formation (p640).

*Calcitonin:* Made in C-cells of the thyroid, this causes $\downarrow Ca^{2+}$ and $PO_4^{3-}$, but its physiological role is unclear. It can be used as a marker of recurrence or metastasis in medullary carcinoma of the thyroid.

*Magnesium:* $\downarrow Mg^{2+}$ prevents PTH release, and may cause hypocalcaemia.

*Plasma binding:* Labs usually measure total plasma $Ca^{2+}$. ~40% is bound to albumin, and the rest is free ionized $Ca^{2+}$ which is the physiologically important amount. Therefore, **correct total $Ca^{2+}$ for albumin as follows:** add 0.1mmol/L to $Ca^{2+}$ level for every 4g/L that albumin is below 40g/L, and a similar subtraction for raised albumin. However, many other factors affect binding (eg other proteins in myeloma, cirrhosis, individual variation) so be cautious in your interpretation. If in doubt over a high $Ca^{2+}$, take blood specimens uncuffed (remove tourniquet after needle in vein, but before taking blood sample), and with the patient fasted.

## Hypercalcaemia

**Signs and symptoms** 'Bones, stones, groans, and psychic moans'. Abdominal pain; vomiting; constipation; polyuria; polydipsia; depression; anorexia; weight loss; tiredness; weakness; hypertension, confusion; pyrexia; renal stones; renal failure; ectopic calcification (of cornea—see BOX); cardiac arrest. *ECG:* QT interval$\downarrow$.

**Causes** (See fig 1) Most commonly malignancy (eg from bone metastases, myeloma, PTHrP) or primary hyperparathyroidism. Others include sarcoidosis, vit D intoxication, thyrotoxicosis, lithium, tertiary hyperparathyroidism, milk-alkali syndrome, and familial benign hypocalciuric hypercalcaemia (rare; defect in calcium-sensing receptor). HIV can cause both $\uparrow$ & $\downarrow$ $Ca^{2+}$ (perhaps from PTH-related bone remodelling).[7]

**Investigations** The main distinction is malignancy vs $1°$ hyperparathyroidism. Pointers to malignancy are $\downarrow$albumin, $\downarrow Cl^-$, alkalosis, $\downarrow K^+$, $\uparrow PO_4^{3-}$, $\uparrow$alk phos. $\uparrow$PTH indicates hyperparathyroidism. Also FBC, protein electrophoresis, CXR, isotope bone scan, 24h urinary $Ca^{2+}$ excretion (for familial hypocalciuric hypercalcaemia).

---

### Causes of metastatic (ectopic) calcification 'PARATHHORMONE'

**P**arathormone (PTH)$\uparrow$ (p214) and other causes of $Ca^{2+}\uparrow$, eg sarcoidosis;
**A**myloidosis; **R**enal failure (relates to $\uparrow PO_4^{3-}$); **A**ddison's disease (adrenal calcification)
**T**B nodes; **T**oxoplasmosis (CNS); **H**istoplasmosis (eg in lung); **O**verdose of vitamin D;
**R**aynaud's-associated diseases (eg SLE; CREST p554; dermatomyositis); **M**uscle primaries/leiomyosarcomas; **O**ssifying metastases (**o**steosarcoma) or **o**varian mets (to peritoneum); **N**ephrocalcinosis; **E**ndocrine tumours (eg gastrinoma)

$Ca^{2+}Na^+$
$K^+$

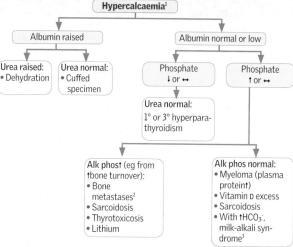

Fig 1. Hypercalcaemia.

## Treating acute hypercalcaemia

Diagnose and treat the underlying cause. If $Ca^{2+}$ >3.5mmol/L and symptomatic:

1 *Correct dehydration* if present with IV 0.9% saline.

2 *Bisphosphonates* prevent bone resorption by inhibiting osteoclast activity. A single dose of **pamidronate** lowers $Ca^{2+}$ over 2-3d; maximum effect is at 1wk. *Infuse slowly*, eg 30mg in 300mL 0.9% saline over 3h via a largish vein. Max dose 90mg (see TABLE below). *SE:* Flu symptoms, ↓$PO_4^{3-}$, bone pain, myalgia, nausea, vomiting, headache, lymphocytopenia, ↓$Mg^{2+}$, ↓$Ca^{2+}$, seizures.

3 *Further management* Chemotherapy may help in malignancy. **Steroids** are used in sarcoidosis, eg prednisolone 40-60mg/d. **Salmon calcitonin** acts similarly to bisphosphonates, and has a quicker onset of action, but is now rarely used. **NB:** The use of **furosemide** is contentious, as supporting RCT evidence is scant.[8,9] It helps to promote renal excretion of $Ca^{2+}$, but can exacerbate hypercalcaemia by worsening dehydration. Thus it should only be used once fully rehydrated, and with concomitant IV fluids (eg 0.9% saline 1L/4-6h). Avoid thiazides.

### Disodium pamidronate doses

| Calcium (mmol/L; corrected) | Single-dose pamidronate (mg) |
|---|---|
| <3 | 15-30 |
| 3-3.5 | 30-60 |
| 3.5-4 | 60-90 |
| >4 | 90 |

*Other bisphosphonates* include zoledronic acid, sodium clodronate and ibandronic acid. **Zoledronic acid** is significantly more effective in reducing serum $Ca^{2+}$ than previously used bisphosphonates.[10] Usually, a single dose of 4mg IV (diluted to 100mL, over 15min) will normalize plasma $Ca^{2+}$ within a week. *SE:* Flu symptoms, bone pain, $PO_4^{3-}$↓, confusion, thirst, taste disturbance, nausea, pulse↓, wcc↓, creatinine↑, osteonecrosis of the jaw.

1 This diagram is only a guide: use in conjunction with the clinical picture.
2 Most common primary: breast, kidney, lung, thyroid, prostate, ovary, colon.
3 Ingesting too much calcium and alkali (eg in milk) can cause hypercalcaemia with metastatic calcification and renal failure. Thyrotoxicosis causes alkalaemia because of hyperventilation.[11]

*Clinical chemistry*

▶Apparent hypocalcaemia may be an artefact of hypoalbuminaemia (p690).

**Signs and symptoms** See BOX. *Mild:* cramps, perioral numbness/paraesthesiae. Severe: carpopedal spasm (especially if brachial artery compressed, *Trousseau's sign;* see fig 1), laryngospasm, seizures. Neuromuscular excitability may also be demonstrated by tapping over parotid (facial nerve) causing facial muscles to twitch (*Chvostek's sign;* see fig 2). Cataract if chronic hypocalcaemia. *ECG:* long QT interval.

**Causes**

*With ↑ $PO_4^{3-}$*
- chronic kidney disease (p300)
- hypoparathyroidism (incl thyroid or parathyroid surgery, p214)
- pseudohypoparathyroidism (p214)
- acute rhabdomyolysis
- vitamin D deficiency
- hypomagnesaemia

*With ↔ or ↓ $PO_4^{3-}$*
- osteomalacia (↑alk phos)
- acute pancreatitis
- over-hydration
- respiratory alkalosis (total $Ca^{2+}$ is normal, but ↓ionized $Ca^{2+}$ due to ↑pH ∴ symptomatic)

**Treatment**
- *Mild symptoms:* give calcium 5mmol/6h PO, with daily plasma $Ca^{2+}$ levels.
- *In chronic kidney disease:* see p300. May require **alfacalcidol**, eg 0.5–1μg/24h PO.
- *Severe symptoms:* give 10mL of 10% **calcium gluconate** (2.25mmol) IV over 30min, and repeat as necessary. If due to respiratory alkalosis, correct the alkalosis.

---

**Features of hypocalcaemia** 'SPASMODIC'

- **S**pasms (carpopedal spasms = Trousseau's sign)
- **P**erioral paraesthesiae
- **A**nxious, irritable, irrational
- **S**eizures
- **M**uscle tone ↑ in smooth muscle—hence colic, wheeze, and dysphagia
- **O**rientation impaired (time, place and person) and confusion
- **D**ermatitis (eg atopic/exfoliative)
- **I**mpetigo herpetiformis (↓$Ca^{2+}$ and pustules in pregnancy—rare and serious)
- **C**hvostek's sign; choreoathetosis; cataract; cardiomyopathy (long QT interval on ECG)

---

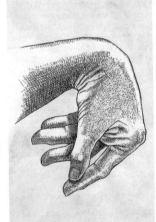

Fig 1. Trousseau's sign: on inflating the cuff, the wrist and fingers flex and draw together (carpopedal spasm).

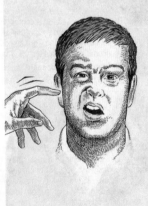

Fig 2. Chvostek's sign: the corner of the mouth twitches when the facial nerve is tapped over the parotid.

## 69

# Phosphate

**Hypophosphataemia** is common and of little significance unless severe (<0.4mmol/L). *Causes* include vitamin D deficiency, alcohol withdrawal, refeeding syndrome (p589), inadequate oral intake, severe diabetic ketoacidosis, renal tubular dysfunction and 1° hyperparathyroidism. *Signs & symptoms* include muscle weakness or rhabdomyolysis, red cell, white cell and platelet dysfunction, and cardiac arrest or arrhythmias. *Treatment* is by oral or parenteral phosphate supplementation, eg Phosphate Polyfusor® IVI (100mmol $PO_4$ in 500mL). Never give IV phosphate to a patient who is hypercalcaemic or oliguric.

**Hyperphosphataemia** is most commonly due to chronic kidney disease, when it is treated with phosphate binders, eg sevelamer 800mg/8h PO during meals. Also catabolic states such as tumour lysis syndrome (p526).

# Magnesium

Magnesium is distributed 65% in bone and 35% in cells; plasma concentration tends to follow that of $Ca^{2+}$ and $K^+$.

**Hypomagnesaemia** causes paraesthesiae, ataxia, seizures, tetany, arrhythmias. Digitalis toxicity may be exacerbated. *Causes* include diuretics, severe diarrhoea, ketoacidosis, alcohol abuse, total parenteral nutrition (monitor weekly), ↓$Ca^{2+}$, ↓$K^+$ and ↓$PO_4^{3-}$. *Treatment:* If needed, give magnesium salts, PO or IV (eg 8mmol $MgSO_4$ IV over 3min to 2h, depending on severity, with frequent $Mg^{2+}$ levels).

**Hypermagnesaemia** rarely requires treatment unless severe (>7.5mmol/L). *Causes* are renal failure or iatrogenic (eg excessive antacids). *Signs* if severe include neuromuscular depression, ↓BP, ↓pulse , hyporeflexia, CNS & respiratory depression, coma.

# Zinc

**Zinc deficiency** This may occur in parenteral nutrition or, rarely, from a poor diet (too few cereals and dairy products; anorexia nervosa; alcoholism. Rarely it is due to a genetic defect. *Symptoms:* Alopecia, dermatitis (look for red, crusted skin lesions especially around nostrils and corners of mouth), night blindness, diarrhoea. *Diagnosis:* Therapeutic trial of zinc (plasma levels are unreliable as they may be low, eg in infection or trauma, without deficiency).

# Selenium

An essential element present in cereals, nuts, and meat. Low soil levels in some parts of Europe and China cause deficiency states. Required for the antioxidant glutathione peroxidase, which ↓ harmful free radicals. Selenium is also antithrombogenic, and is required for sperm motility proteins. Deficiency may increase risk of neoplasia and atheroma, and may lead to a cardiomyopathy or arthritis. Serum levels are a poor guide. Toxic symptoms may also be found with over-energetic replacement.

**Causes of hyperuricaemia** High levels of urate in the blood (hyperuricaemia) may result from increased turnover (15%) or reduced excretion of urate (85%). Either may be drug induced.

• *Drugs:* Cytotoxics, thiazides, loop diuretics, pyrazinamide.
• *Increased cell turnover:* Lymphoma, leukaemia, psoriasis, haemolysis, muscle death (rhabdomyolysis, p307; tumour lysis syndrome, p526).
• *Reduced excretion:* Primary gout (p550), chronic kidney disease, lead nephropathy, hyperparathyroidism, pre-eclampsia (*OHCS* p48).
• *Other:* Hyperuricaemia may be associated with hypertension and hyperlipidaemia. Urate may be raised in disorders of purine synthesis such as the *Lesch-Nyhan syndrome* (*OHCS* p648).

**Hyperuricaemia and renal failure** Severe renal failure from any cause may be associated with hyperuricaemia, and rarely this may give rise to gout. Sometimes the relationship of cause and effect is reversed so that it is the hyperuricaemia that causes the renal failure. This can occur following cytotoxic treatment (tumour lysis syndrome, p526), and in muscle necrosis.

*How urate causes renal failure:* Urate is poorly soluble in water, so over-excretion can lead to crystal precipitation. Renal failure occurs most commonly because urate precipitates in the renal tubules. This may occur at plasma levels ≥1.19mmol/L. In some instances ureteric obstruction from urate crystals may occur. This responds to retrograde ureteric catheterization and lavage.

*Prevention of renal failure:* Before starting chemotherapy, ensure good hydration and initiate **allopurinol** (xanthine oxidase inhibitor) or **rasburicase** (recombinant urate oxidase), which prevent a sharp rise in urate following chemotherapy (see p526). There is a remote risk of inducing xanthine nephropathy.

*Treatment of hyperuricaemic acute renal failure:* Exclude bilateral ureteric obstruction, then give prompt **rehydration ± loop diuretic** to wash uric acid crystals out of the renal tubules, and correct electrolyte abnormalities. Once oliguria is established, **haemodialysis** is required (in preference to peritoneal dialysis). There is no evidence for either preventing (above) or treating hyperuricaemic renal failure.

**Gout** See p550.

**Urate renal stones** Urate stones (fig 1) comprise 5-10% of all renal stones and are radiolucent.

*Incidence:* ~5-10% in temperate climates (double if confirmed gout),[13] but up to 40% in hot, arid climates. ♂:♀≈4:1. But most urate stone formers have no detectable abnormalities in urate metabolism.

*Risk factors:* Acidic or strongly concentrated urine; ↑urinary excretion of urate; chronic diarrhoea; distal small bowel disease or resection (regional enteritis); ileostomy; obesity; diabetes mellitus; chemotherapy for myeloproliferative disorders; inadequate caloric or fluid intake.

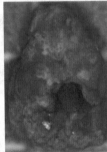

Fig 1. Urate stone.    ©Dr G Austin.

*Treatment:* **Hydration** to increase urine volume (aim > 2L/d). Unlike most other renal calculi, existing uric acid stones can often be dissolved with either systemic or topical alkalinizing agents. **Potassium citrate** or **potassium bicarbonate** at a dose titrated to alkalinize the urine to a pH of 6-7 dissolves some urate stones. If hyperuricosuria, consider dietary management ± allopurinol (xanthine oxidase inhibitor).

Clinical chemistry

Osteoporosis implies reduced bone mass. It may be 1° (age-related) or 2° to another condition or drugs. If trabecular bone is affected, crush fractures of vertebrae are common (hence the 'littleness' of little old ladies and their dowager's hump); if cortical bone is affected, long bone fractures are more likely, eg femoral neck: the big cause of death and orthopaedic expense (80% hip fractures in the UK occur in women >50yrs).

**Prevalence** (in those >50yrs): ♂6%, ♀ 18%. Women lose trabeculae with age, but in men, although there is reduced bone formation, numbers of trabeculae are stable and their lifetime risk of fracture is less.

**Risk factors** Age-independent risk factors for 1° osteoporosis: parental history, alcohol >4 units daily, rheumatoid arthritis, BMI <22, prolonged immobility, and untreated menopause. See BOX 2 for other risk factors, including for 2° osteoporosis.

**Investigations** X-ray (low sensitivity/specificity, often with hindsight after a fracture). Bone densitometry (DEXA—see BOX 1). Bloods: $Ca^{2+}$, $PO_4^{3-}$ & alk phos normal. Consider specific investigations for 2° causes if suggestive history. Biopsy is unreliable and unnecessary with non-invasive techniques available.

**Management** Loss of bone mineral density may not be entirely irreversible. Age, number of risk factors and bone mineral density (DEXA scan; see BOX) guide the pharmacological approach (eg FRAX, which is a WHO risk assessment tool for estimating 10-yr risk of osteoporotic fracture in untreated patients; see www.shef.ac.uk/frax),[14,15] although DEXA is not necessary if age >75yrs. Lifestyle measures should apply to all (including those at risk but not yet osteoporotic).

*Lifestyle measures:*
• Quit smoking and reduce alcohol consumption.
• Weight-bearing exercise may increase bone mineral density.[16]
• Balance exercises such as tai chi reduce risk of falls.
• Calcium and vitamin D-rich diet (use supplements if diet is insufficient—see below).
• Home-based fall-prevention programme, with visual assessment and a home visit. NB: hip-protectors are unreliable for preventing fractures.[17]

*Pharmacological measures:*
• Bisphosphonates: alendronate is 1ˢᵗ line (10mg/d or 70mg/wk; not if eGFR <35). Use also for prevention in long-term steroid use. If intolerant, try etidronate or risedronate. Say to swallow pills with *plenty* of water while remaining upright for >30min and wait 30min before eating or other drugs. (SE: photosensitivity; GI upset; oesophageal ulcers—stop if dysphagia or abdo pain; rarely, jaw osteonecrosis).
• Calcium and vitamin D: rarely used alone for prophylaxis, as questionable efficacy and some evidence of a small increased CV risk. Offer if evidence of deficiency, eg calcium 1g/d + vit D 800U/d. Target serum 25-hydroxy-vitamin D level ≥75nmol/L.
• Strontium ranelate helps ↓ fracture rates, and is an alternative in those intolerant of bisphosphonates. Strontium is in the same periodic group as calcium and reduces reabsorption, and may promote new bone formation.
• Hormone replacement therapy (HRT) can prevent (not treat) osteoporosis in postmenopausal women. Relative risk of breast cancer is 1.4 if used >10yrs; ↑CV risk.
• Raloxifene is a selective oestrogen receptor modulator (SERM) that acts similarly to HRT, but with ↓ breast cancer risk.
• Teriparatide (recombinant PTH) is useful in those who suffer further fractures despite treatment with other agents. There is a potential ↑ risk of renal malignancy.
• Calcitonin may reduce pain after a vertebral fracture.
• Testosterone may help in hypogonadal men by promoting trabecular connectivity.
• Denosumab, a monoclonal Ab to RANK ligand, given SC twice yearly ↓ reabsorption.

Ca²⁺Na⁺
K⁺

## DEXA bone densitometry: WHO osteoporosis criteria

Dual Energy X-ray Absorptiometry

It is better to scan the hip than the lumbar spine. Bone mineral density ($g/cm^2$) is compared with that of a young healthy adult. The 'T-score' is the number of standard deviations (SD, p765) the bone mineral density (BMD) is from the youthful average. Each decrease of 1 SD in bone mineral density ≈ 2.6-fold ↑ in risk of hip fracture.

| T-score > 0 | BMD is better than the reference. |
|---|---|
| 0 to -1 | BMD is in the top 84%: no evidence of osteoporosis. |
| -1 to -2.5 | Osteopenia. Risk of later osteoporotic fracture. Offer lifestyle advice. |
| -2.5 or worse | Osteoporosis. Offer lifestyle advice and treatment (p696). Repeat DEXA in 2yrs. |

*Some indications for DEXA:*

• NICE suggests DEXA if previous low-trauma fracture, or for women ≥ 65yrs with one or more risk factors for osteoporosis, or younger if two or more. The benefits of universal screening for osteoporosis remain unproven, but some authorities recommend this for men and women over 70—and earlier if risk factors are present.[18]
• DEXA is not needed pre-treatment for women over 75yrs if previous low-trauma fracture, or ≥ 2 present of rheumatoid arthritis, alcohol excess, or positive family history.
• Prior to giving long-term prednisolone (eg ≥3 months at >5mg/d). Steroids cause osteoporosis by promoting osteoclast bone resorption, ↓muscle mass, and ↓$Ca^{2+}$ absorption from the gut.
• Men or women with osteopenia if low-trauma non-vertebral fracture.
• Bone and bone-remodelling disorders (eg parathyroid disorders, myeloma, HIV, esp if on protease inhibitors).

## Osteoporosis risk factors 'SHATTERED'

Steroid use of >5mg/d of prednisolone; Hyperthyroidism, hyperparathyroidism, hypercalciuria; Alcohol and tobacco use†;·Thin (BMI <22); Testosterone↓ (eg antiandrogen ca prostate ℞); Early menopause; Renal or liver failure; Erosive/inflammatory bone disease (eg myeloma or rheumatoid arthritis); Dietary $Ca^{2+}$↓/malabsorption; diabetes mellitus type 1.

Clinical chemistry

In osteomalacia there is a normal amount of bone but its mineral content is low (there is excess uncalcified osteoid and cartilage). This is the reverse of osteoporosis in which mineralization is unchanged, but there is overall bone loss. Rickets is the result if this process occurs during the period of bone growth; osteomalacia is the result if it occurs after fusion of the epiphyses.

### Signs and symptoms

*Rickets:* Growth retardation, hypotonia, apathy in infants. Once walking: knock-kneed, bow-legged and deformities of the metaphyseal-epiphyseal junction (eg the rachitic rosary). Features of ↓$Ca^{2+}$—often mild (p692). Children with rickets are ill.

*Osteomalacia:* Bone pain and tenderness; fractures (esp femoral neck); proximal myopathy (waddling gait), due to ↓$PO_4^{3-}$ and vitamin D deficiency *per se*.

### Causes

- *Vitamin D deficiency:* Due to malabsorption (p280), poor diet, or lack of sunlight.
- *Renal osteodystrophy:* Renal failure leads to 1,25-dihydroxy-cholecalciferol deficiency [1,25(OH)₂-vitamin D deficiency]. See also *renal bone disease* (p302).
- *Drug-induced:* Anticonvulsants may induce liver enzymes, leading to an increased breakdown of 25-hydroxy-vitamin D.
- *Vitamin D resistance:* A number of mainly inherited conditions in which the osteomalacia responds to high doses of vitamin D (see below).
- *Liver disease:* Due to reduced hydroxylation of vitamin D to 25-hydroxy-cholecalciferol and malabsorption of vitamin D, eg in cirrhosis (p260).
- *Tumour-induced osteomalacia* (oncogenic hypophosphataemia): mediated by raised tumour production of phosphatonin fibroblast growth factor 23 (FGF-23) which causes hyperphosphaturia. ↓ serum $PO_4^{3-}$ often causes myalgia and weakness.[19]

### Investigations

*Plasma:* Mildly ↓$Ca^{2+}$ (but may be severe); ↓$PO_4^{3-}$; alk phos↑; PTH high; 25(OH)-vitamin D↓, except in vitamin D resistance. In renal failure 1,25(OH)₂-vitamin D↓ (p302).

*Biopsy:* Bone biopsy shows incomplete mineralization. Muscle biopsy (if proximal myopathy) is normal.

*x-ray:* In osteomalacia there is a loss of cortical bone; also, apparent partial fractures without displacement may be seen especially on the lateral border of the scapula, inferior femoral neck and medial femoral shaft (Looser's zones; see fig 1). Cupped, ragged metaphyseal surfaces are seen in rickets (fig 2).

### Treatment

- In dietary insufficiency, give vitamin D, eg as one Calcium D₃ Forte tablet/12h PO.
- In malabsorption or hepatic disease, give vitamin D₂ (ergocalciferol), up to 40,000U (=1mg) daily, or parenteral calcitriol, eg 7.5mg monthly.
- If due to renal disease or vitamin D resistance, give alfacalcidol (1α-hydroxy-vitamin D₃) 250ng-1μg daily, or calcitriol (1,25-dihydroxy-vitamin D₃) 250ng-1μg daily, and adjust dose according to plasma $Ca^{2+}$. ►►Alfacalcidol and calcitriol can cause dangerous hypercalcaemia.
- Monitor plasma $Ca^{2+}$, initially weekly, and if nausea/vomiting.

**Vitamin D-resistant rickets** exists in 2 forms. Type I has low renal 1α-hydroxylase activity, and type II has end-organ resistance to 1,25-dihydroxy-vitamin D₃, due to a point mutation in the receptor. Both are treated with large doses of calcitriol.

**x-linked hypophosphataemic rickets** Dominantly inherited—due to a defect in renal phosphate handling (due to mutations in the PEX or PHEX genes which encode an endopeptidase). Rickets develops in early childhood and is associated with poor growth. Plasma $PO_4^{3-}$ is low, alk phos is high, and there is phosphaturia. Treatment is with high doses of oral phosphate, and calcitriol.

Also called *osteitis deformans*, there is increased bone turnover associated with increased numbers of osteoblasts and osteoclasts with resultant remodelling, bone enlargement, deformity, and weakness. Rare in the under-40s. Incidence rises with age (3% over 55yrs old). Commoner in temperate climates, and in Anglo-Saxons.

**Clinical features** Asymptomatic in ~70%. Deep, boring pain, and bony deformity and enlargement—typically of the pelvis, lumbar spine, skull, femur, and tibia (classically a bowed sabre tibia; fig 3). *Complications* include pathological fractures, osteoarthritis, $\uparrow Ca^{2+}$, nerve compression due to bone overgrowth (eg deafness, root compression), high-output CCF (if >40% of skeleton involved) and osteosarcoma (<1% of those affected for >10yrs—suspect if sudden onset or worsening of bone pain).[20]

**Radiology x-ray** Localized enlargement of bone. Patchy cortical thickening with sclerosis, osteolysis, and deformity (eg *osteoporosis circumscripta* of the skull). Affinity for axial skeleton, long bones, and skull. **Bone scan** may reveal 'hot spots'.

**Blood chemistry** $Ca^{2+}$ and $PO_4^{3-}$ normal; alk phos markedly raised.

**Treatment** If analgesia fails, alendronate may be tried to reduce pain and/or deformity. It is more effective than etidronate or calcitonin, and as effective as IV pamidronate. Follow expert advice.

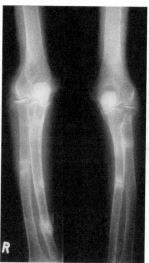

Fig 1. Osteomalacia.
Cortical bone lucency and Looser's zones are seen in both forearms of a patient with osteomalacia (fig 1). Typical ragged metaphyseal surfaces are seen in the knee and ankle joints of a child with rickets, with bowing of the long bones (fig 2). The 'sabre tibia' seen in Paget's disease, with multiple sclerotic lesions (fig 3).

Images courtesy of Dr Ian Maddison.

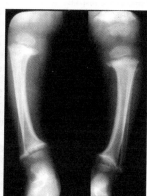

Fig 2. Rickets.

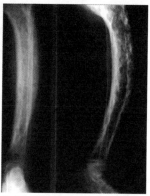

Fig 3. Paget's disease.

# Plasma proteins

The plasma contains a number of proteins including albumin, immunoglobulins, $\alpha_1$-antitrypsin, $\alpha_2$-macroglobulin, caeruloplasmin, transferrin, low-density lipoprotein (LDL), fibrinogen, complement, and factor VIII. The most abundant is albumin.

**Albumin** is synthesized in the liver; $t\frac{1}{2} \approx 20d$. It binds bilirubin, free fatty acids, $Ca^{2+}$, and some drugs. *Low albumin* results in oedema, and is caused by: • ↓*synthesis:* liver disease, acute phase response (due to ↑vascular permeability—eg sepsis, trauma, surgery), malabsorption, malnutrition, malignancy; • ↑*loss:* nephrotic syndrome, protein-losing enteropathy, burns; • *haemodilution:* late pregnancy, artefact (eg from 'drip' arm). Also posture (↑5g/L if upright) and genetic variations. *High albumin:* Dehydration; artefact (eg stasis).

**Immunoglobulins**, or antibodies, are synthesized by B cells. 5 isoforms Ig A,D,E,G,M exist in man, and IgG is the most abundant circulating form. *Specific monoclonal band* in paraproteinaemia (see p364). *Diffusely raised* in chronic infections, TB, bronchiectasis, liver cirrhosis, sarcoidosis, SLE, RA, Crohn's disease, 1° biliary cirrhosis, hepatitis, and parasitaemia. *Low* in nephrotic syndrome, malabsorption, malnutrition, and immune deficiency states (eg severe illness, renal failure, diabetes mellitus, malignancy, or congenital).

**Acute phase response** The body responds to a variety of insults with, amongst other things, the synthesis, by the liver, of a number of proteins (normally present in serum in small quantities)—eg $\alpha_1$-antitrypsin, fibrinogen, complement, haptoglobin, and CRP. A concomitant reduction in albumin level, is characteristic of conditions such as infection, malignancy (especially $\alpha_2$-fraction), trauma, surgery, and inflammatory disease.

**CRP** So-called because it binds to a polysaccharide (fraction C) in the cell wall of pneumococci. Levels help monitor inflammation/infection (normal <8mg/L). Like the ESR, it is raised in many inflammatory conditions, but changes more rapidly. It increases in hours and begins to fall within 2-3d of recovery; thus it can be used to follow disease activity (eg Crohn's disease) or the response to therapy (eg antibiotics). CRP values in mild inflammation 10-50mg/L; active bacterial infection 50-200mg/L; severe infection or trauma >200mg/L; see BOX.

# Urinary proteins

Urinary protein loss >150mg/d is pathological (p286).

**Albuminuria** is usually caused by renal disease (p286). *Microalbuminuria* is urinary protein loss between 30 and 300mg/d (so do not visible on normal dipstick) and may be seen with diabetes mellitus, ↑BP, SLE and glomerulonephritis (see p309 for role in DM).

**Bence Jones protein** consists of light chains excreted in excess by some patients with myeloma (p362). They are not detected by dipsticks and may occur with normal serum electrophoresis.

**Haemoglobinuria** is caused by intravascular haemolysis (p330).

**Myoglobinuria** is caused by rhabdomyolysis (p307).

## 70

## C-reactive protein (CRP)

*Marked elevation*
Bacterial infection
Abscess
Crohn's disease
Connective tissue diseases
  (except SLE)
Neoplasia
Trauma
Necrosis (eg MI)

*Normal-to-slight elevation*
Viral infection
Steroids/oestrogens
Ulcerative colitis
SLE
Atherosclerosis
Morbid obesity

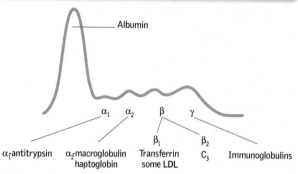

Fig 1. A normal electrophoretic scan.

Clinical chemistry

▶Reference intervals vary between laboratories. See p770 for guide normal values.

Raised levels of specific enzymes can be a useful indicator of a disease. However, remember that most can be raised for other reasons too. Levels may be raised due to cellular damage, ↑cell turnover, cellular proliferation (malignancy), enzyme induction, and ↓clearance. The major causes of *raised enzymes* are given below.

**Alkaline phosphatase** (several distinguishable isoforms exist, eg liver and bone)
• Liver disease (suggests cholestasis; also cirrhosis, abscess, hepatitis or malignancy).
• Bone disease (isoenzyme distinguishable, reflects osteoblast activity) especially Paget's, growing children, healing fractures, bone metastases, osteomalacia, osteomyelitis, chronic kidney disease and hyperparathyroidism.
• Congestive cardiac failure (moderately raised alk phos).
• Pregnancy (placenta makes its own isoenzyme).

**Alanine and aspartate aminotransferase (ALT and AST)**
• Liver disease (suggests hepatocyte damage).
• AST also ↑ in MI, skeletal muscle damage (especially crush injuries) and haemolysis.

**α-Amylase**
• Acute pancreatitis (smaller rise in chronic pancreatitis as less tissue remaining).
• *Also:* severe uraemia, diabetic ketoacidosis, severe gastroenteritis, and peptic ulcer.

**Creatine kinase (CK)** ▶A raised CK does not necessarily mean an MI.
• Myocardial infarction (p112; isoenzyme 'CK-MB'. Diagnostic if CK-MB >6% of total CK, or CK-MB mass >99 percentile of normal). CK returns to baseline within 48h (unlike troponin, which remains raised for ~10 days), ∴ useful for detecting re-infarction.
• Muscle damage (rhabdomyolysis, p307; prolonged running; haematoma; seizures; IM injection; defibrillation; bowel ischaemia; myxoedema; dermatomyositis, p554)— and *drugs* (eg statins).

**Gamma-glutamyl transferase (GGT, γGT)**
• Liver disease (particularly alcohol-induced damage, cholestasis, drugs).

**Lactate dehydrogenase (LDH)**
• Myocardial infarction (p112).
• Liver disease (suggests hepatocyte damage).
• Haemolysis (esp sickle cell crisis), pulmonary embolism, and tumour necrosis.

**Troponin**
• Subtypes troponin T and troponin I are used clinically.
• Cardiac damage or strain (MI—p112, pericarditis, myocarditis, PE, sepsis, CPR).
• Chronic kidney disease (troponin T only; elevation less marked; aetiology unknown).

Ca²⁺Na⁺
K⁺

## Enzyme inducers and inhibitors

Hepatic drug metabolism is mainly by conjugation or oxidation. The oxidative pathways are catalysed by the family of cytochrome P450 isoenzymes, the most important of which is the CYP 3A4 isoenzyme. The cytochrome P450 pathway may be either induced or inhibited by a range of commonly used drugs and foods:

| Enzyme inducers | Enzyme inhibitors | |
|---|---|---|
| Phenytoin | SSRIs | Amiodarone |
| Rifampicin | Ciprofloxacin | Diltiazem |
| Carbamazepine | Isoniazid | Verapamil |
| Alcohol | Macrolides | Omeprazole |
| St John's wort | HIV protease inhibitors | Grapefruit juice |
| Barbiturates | Imidazole and triazole antifungal agents | |

This can lead to important interactions or side-effects. For example phenytoin reduces the effectiveness of the Pill due to more rapid oestrogen metabolism, and ciprofloxacin retards the metabolism of methylxanthines (aminophylline) which leads to higher plasma levels and potentially more side-effects. The *BNF* contains a list of the major interactions between drugs.

Clinical chemistry

Clinical chemistry

Lipids travel in blood packaged with proteins as lipoproteins. There are 4 classes: chylomicrons and VLDL (mainly triglyceride), LDL (mainly cholesterol), and HDL (mainly phospholipid). The evidence that cholesterol is a major risk factor for cardiovascular disease (CVD) is now incontrovertible ('4S' STUDY,[21] WOSCOPS,[22] CARE STUDY,[23] HEART PROTECTION STUDY[24]) and indeed it may even be the 'green light' that allows other risk factors to act.[25] Half the UK population have a serum cholesterol putting them at significant risk of CVD. HDL appears to correlate inversely with CVD.

### Who to screen for hyperlipidaemia

▶NB: full screening requires a fasting lipid profile.

*Those at risk of hyperlipidaemia:* •Family history of hyperlipidaemia; •Corneal arcus <50yrs old; •Xanthomata or xanthelasmata (fig 1).

*Those at risk of CVD:* (see *risk equation*, p675) •Known CVD; •Family history of CVD <65yrs old; •DM or impaired glucose tolerance; •Hypertension; •Smoker; •↑BMI; •Low socioeconomic or Indian Asian background.

### Types of hyperlipidaemia

*Common primary hyperlipidaemia* accounts for 70% of hyperlipidaemia. ↑LDL only.

*Familial primary hyperlipidaemias* comprise multiple phenotypes (see TABLE). *Risk of CVD↑↑*, although evidence suggests protection from CVD is achieved with lower doses of statin for common primary hyperlipidaemia.[26]

*Secondary hyperlipidaemia* may be caused by Cushing's syndrome, hypothyroidism, nephrotic syndrome, or cholestasis. ↑LDL. Treat the cause first.

*Mixed hyperlipidaemia* results in ↑ both LDL and triglycerides. Caused by type 2 diabetes mellitus, metabolic syndrome, alcohol abuse, and chronic renal failure.

### Management[27,28]

- *Lifestyle advice.* Aim for BMI of 20-25. Diet with <10% of calories from saturated fats; ↑fibre, fresh fruit and vegetables, omega-3 fatty acids. ↑Exercise.
- Identify familial or 2° hyperlipidaemias. Treatment may differ—see above.
- *Treatment priorities:* using statins in primary prevention may cause side-effects and is expensive. •*Top priority:* Treat those with known CVD (there is no need to calculate their risk: ipso facto they already have high risk). •*2nd priority:* Treat all those with DM (especially if risk of cardiac event >2%/yr). •*3rd priority:* Those with a 10-year risk of CVD >20%, *irrespective of baseline lipid levels.* Current guidelines suggest a target plasma cholesterol of ≤4mmol/L.[28] There are not yet enough data to support a 4th priority of giving statins to all men over 50 and women over 65.
- *1st-line therapy:* statins, eg simvastatin (40mg PO at night), ↓cholesterol synthesis in the liver. CI: porphyria, cholestasis, pregnancy. SE: myalgia ± myositis (stop if ↑CK ≥10-fold; if any myalgia, check CK; risk is 1 per 100,000 treatment-years),[27] abdominal pain, and ↑LFTs (stop if AST ≥100U/L). Cytochrome P450 inhibitors (p702) ↑serum concentrations (eg 200mL of grapefruit juice may ↑simvastatin concentration by 300%, and atorvastatin ↑80%, but pravastatin is almost unchanged).
- *2nd-line therapy:* fibrates, eg bezafibrate (useful in mixed hyperlipidaemias), or cholesterol absorption inhibitors, eg ezetimibe (although unclear if it reduces mortality); anion exchange resins, eg colestyramine; also consider nicotinic acid (HDL↑; ·LDL↓; SE: severe flushes; aspirin 300mg ½h pre-dose helps this).
- Hypertriglyceridaemia responds best to fibrates, nicotinic acid, or fish oil.

**Xanthomata** These yellow lipid deposits may be: eruptive (itchy nodules in crops in hypertriglyceridaemia); tuberous (plaques on elbows and knees); or planar—also called palmar (orange streaks in palmar creases), 'diagnostic' of remnant hyperlipidaemia; or in tendons (p36), eyelids (xanthelasma, see fig 1), or cornea (arcus, p36).

**Abbreviations** (VLDL = (very) low-density lipoprotein; IDL = intermediate density lipoprotein; HDL = high density lipoprotein; chol = cholesterol; trig = trigylcerides.

## Primary hyperlipidaemias

Blue superscript numbers = WHO phenotype; chol/trig levels given in mmol/L.

| | | | |
|---|---|---|---|
| Familial hyperchylomicronaemia (lipoprotein lipase deficiency or apoCII deficiency)[I] | Chol <6.5 Trig 10–30 Chylomicrons ↑ | | Eruptive xanthomata; lipaemia retinalis; hepatosplenomegaly |
| Familial hypercholesterolaemia[II] (LDL receptor defects) | Chol 7.5–16 Trig <2.3 | LDL↑ | Tendon xanthoma; corneal arcus; xanthelasma |
| Familial defective apolipoprotein B-100[IIa] | Chol 7.5–16 Trig <2.3 | LDL↑ | Tendon xanthoma; arcus; xanthelasma |
| Common hypercholesterolaemia[IIa] | Chol 6.5–9 Trig <2.3 | LDL↑ | *The commonest 1° lipidaemia;* may have xanthelasma or arcus |
| Familial combined hyperlipidaemia[IIb, IV or V] | Chol 6.5–10 Trig 2.3–12 | LDL↑ VLDL↑ HDL↓ | *Next commonest 1° lipidaemia;* xanthelasma; arcus |
| Dysbetalipoproteinaemia (remnant particle disease)[III] | Chol 9–14 Trig 9–14 | IDL↑ HDL↓ LDL↓ | Palmar striae; tuberoeruptive xanthoma |
| Familial hypertriglyceridaemia[IV] | Chol 6.5–12 Trig 3.0–6.0 | VLDL↑ | |
| Type V hyperlipoproteinaemia | Trig 10–30; chylomicrons found | | Eruptive xanthomata; lipaemia retinalis; hepatosplenomegaly |

**Primary HDL abnormalities**
- Hyperalphalipoproteinaemia: ↑HDL, chol >2.
- Hypoalphalipoproteinaemia (Tangier disease): ↓HDL, chol <0.92.

**Primary LDL abnormalities**
- Abetalipoproteinaemia (ABL): trig <0.3, chol <1.3, missing LDL, VLDL and chylomicrons. Autosomal recessive disorder of fat malabsorption causing vitamin A & E deficiency, with retinitis pigmentosa, sensory neuropathy, ataxia, pes cavus and acanthocytosis.
- Hypobetalipoproteinaemia: chol <1.5, LDL↓, HDL↓. Autosomal codominant disorder of apolipoprotein B metabolism. ↑ longevity in heterozygotes. Homozygotes present with a similar clinical picture to ABL.

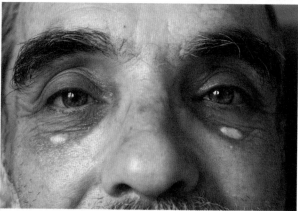

**Fig 1.** Xanthelasma. *Xanthos* is Greek for yellow, and *elasma* means plate. Xanthelasmata are lipid-laden yellow plaques, typically a few millimetres wide. They congregate around the lids, or just below the eyes, and signify hyperlipidaemia.

The porphyrias are a heterogenous group of rare diseases caused by various errors of haem biosynthesis (produced when iron is chelated into protoporphyrin IXα), which may be genetic or acquired. Depending on the stage in haem biosynthesis that is faulty, there is accumulation of either porphyrinogens, which are unstable and oxidize to porphyrins, or their precursors, porphobilinogen and δ-aminolaevulinic acid. Porphyrin precursors are neurotoxic, while porphyrins themselves induce photosensitivity and the formation of toxic free radicals.

• Alcohol, lead, and iron deficiency cause abnormal porphyrin metabolism.
• Genetic counselling (*OHCS* p154) should be offered to all patients and their families.

**Acute porphyrias** occur when the accumulation of porphyrinogen precursors predominates, and are characterized by acute neurovisceral crises, though some forms have additional photosensitive cutaneous manifestations.

*Acute intermittent porphyria* ('*the Madness of King George*') A low-penetrant autosomal dominant condition (porphobilinogen deaminase gene); 28% have no family history (*de novo mutations*). ~10% of those with the defective gene have neurovisceral symptoms. Attacks are intermittent, more common in women and those aged 18–40, and may be precipitated by drugs. Urine porphobilinogens are raised during attacks (the urine may go deep red on standing) and also, in ~50%, between attacks. Faecal porphyrin levels are normal. There is never cutaneous photosensitivity. It is the commonest form of porphyria—prevalence in UK: 1–2/100,000.

*Variegate porphyria and hereditary coproporphyria* Autosomal dominant, characterized by photosensitive blistering skin lesions and/or acute attacks. The former is prevalent in Afrikaners in South Africa. Porphobilinogen is high only during an attack, and other metabolites may be detected in faeces.

*Triggers of an acute attack* include infection, starvation (including pre-operative 'nil-by-mouth'), reproductive hormones (pregnancy, premenstrual), smoking, anaesthesia, and cytochrome P450 enzyme inducers (alcohol, and other drugs—see BOX).

*Features of an acute attack:*
• *Gastrointestinal:* abdominal pain, vomiting, constipation.
• *Neuropsychiatric:* peripheral neuropathy (weakness, hypotonia, pain, numbness), seizures (often associated with severe ↓Na⁺), psychosis (or other odd behaviour).[1]
• *Cardiovascular:* hypertension, tachycardia, shock (due to sympathetic overactivity).
• *Other:* fever, ↓Na⁺, ↓K⁺, proteinuria, urinary porphobilinogens, discoloured urine. Rare but serious complications include bulbar and respiratory paralysis.

▶▶Beware the 'acute abdomen' in acute intermittent porphyria: colic, vomiting, fever and ↑WCC—so mimicking an acute surgical abdomen. Anaesthesia could be disastrous.

*Treatment of an acute attack*
• Remove precipitants (review medications; treat intercurrent illness/infection).
• IV **fluids** to correct electrolyte imbalance.
• High **carbohydrate** intake (eg Hycal®) by NG tube, or IV if necessary.
• IV **haematin** is 1ˢᵗ-line (inhibits production of porphyrinogen precursors).
• Nausea controlled with **prochlorperazine** 12.5mg IM.
• Sedate if necessary with **chlorpromazine** 50–100mg PO/IM.
• Pain control with opiate or opioid **analgesia** (avoid oxycodone).
• Seizures can be controlled with **diazepam** (although this will prolong the attack).
• Treat tachycardia and hypertension with a β-blocker.

**Non-acute porphyrias**
*Porphyria cutanea tarda* (PCT), *erythropoietic protoporphyria*, and *congenital erythropoietic porphyria* are characterized by cutaneous photosensitivity alone, as there is no overproduction of porphyrinogen precursors, only porphyrins. PCT presents in adults with blistering skin lesions ± facial hypertrichosis and hyperpigmentation. Total plasma porphyrins and LFTs are ↑. Screen for associated disorders: hep C, HIV, iron overload, hepatocellular ca. ℞: phlebotomy, iron chelators, chloroquine, sunscreens.

## Drugs to avoid in acute intermittent porphyria

There are many, many drugs that may precipitate an acute attack ± quadriplegia, and this is by no means an exhaustive list (see *BNF/OTM*).

▶▶ For an up-to-date list of drugs considered safe in acute porphyria see www.wmic.wales.nhs.uk/porphyria_info.php.

- Diclofenac
- Alcohol
- Oral contraceptive pill & HRT
- Tricyclic antidepressants
- Benzodiazepines
- Anaesthetic agents (barbiturates, halothane)
- Metoclopramide
- ACE-inhibitors
- $Ca^{2+}$-channel blockers
- Statins
- Anticonvulsants
- Furosemide
- Sulfonylureas
- Lidocaine
- Gold salts
- Antihistamines
- Amphetamines
- Antibiotics (cephalosporins, sulfonamides, macrolides, tetracyclines, rifampicin, trimethoprim, chloramphenicol, metronidazole)

1   Be sure I looked at her eyes
    Happy and proud; at last I knew
Porphyria worshipped me; surprise
    Made my heart swell, and still it grew
While I debated what to do.
That moment she was mine, mine, fair,

    Perfectly pure and good: I found
A thing to do, and all her hair
    In one long yellow string I wound
    Three times her little throat around,
And strangled her ...

From *Porphyria's Lover* by Robert Browning.

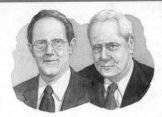

Fig 1. "No scientific discovery is named after its original discoverer", asserts Professor Stephen Stigler in 'Stigler's Law of Eponymy', and in doing so, names the sociologist RK Merton as its discoverer—deliberately making Stigler's law exemplify itself. Is the same true in medicine? At least 6 others described Alzheimer's disease before Alois Alzheimer in 1906, and Tetralogy of Fallot (named after Étienne-Louis Fallot in 1888) was first described in 1672 by Niels Stenson. Not all medical eponyms obey Stigler's law. Forty years after it was first described, the French neurologist Jean-Marie Charcot (himself associated with at least 15 medical eponyms) attributed the name 'Parkinson's Disease' to the illness outlined in James Parkinson's 1817 essay *The Shaking Palsy*. Monochromatic doctors may try to abolish eponyms by regimenting them to histologically driven disease titles. But classifications vary as facts emerge, and as a result the renaming of non-eponyms becomes essential. Eponyms, however, carry on forever, because they imply nothing about others. We like eponyms—they are our sole route to an exotic variety of obscure fame.

**Alice in Wonderland syndrome** Altered perception in size and shape of body parts or objects ± an impaired sense of passing time—as experienced by *Alice* in Lewis Caroll's novel. Seen in epilepsy, migraine and cerebral lesions.[1,2] *Alice Pleasance Liddell, 1865-∞*

**Arnold-Chiari malformation** Malformed cerebellar tonsils and medulla herniate through the foramen magnum. This may cause infantile hydrocephalus with mental retardation, optic atrophy, ocular palsies and spastic paresis of the limbs. Spina bifida, syringomyelia (p520), or focal cerebellar and brainstem signs may occur (p503). There may be bony abnormalities of the base of the skull. Often presents in early adulthood. MRI aids diagnosis.      *Julius Arnold, 1835-1915 (German pathologist); Hans Chiari, 1851-1916 (Austrian pathologist)*

**Baker's cyst** Fluid from a knee effusion escapes to form a popliteal cyst (often swollen and painful) in a sub-gastrocnemius bursa.[3] Usually secondary to degeneration. ∆∆: DVT (exclude if calf swelling); sarcoma. *Imaging:* USS; MRI. ℞: None if asymptomatic. NSAIDs/ice if painful. Spontaneous resolution may take 10-20 months. Arthroscopy + cystectomy may be needed.          *William M Baker, 1838-1896 (British surgeon)*

**Bazin's disease** (*Erythema induratum*) Localized areas of fat necrosis that produce painful, firm nodules ± ulceration and an indurated rash, characteristically on adolescent girls' calves. It is associated with TB. *Nodular vasculitis* is a variant unrelated to TB.[4]         *Pierre-Antoine-Ernest Bazin, 1807-1878 (French dermatologist)*

**Behçet's disease** A systemic inflammatory disorder of unknown cause, associated with HLA-B5. It is most common along the old Silk Road, extending from the Mediterranean to China. *Features:* Recurrent oral and genital ulceration, uveitis, skin lesions (eg erythema nodosum, papulopustular lesions); arthritis (non-erosive large joint oligoarthropathy); thrombophlebitis; vasculitis; myo/pericarditis; CNS involvement (pyramidal signs) and colitis. *Diagnosis* is mainly clinical. *Pathergy test:* needle prick leads to papule formation within 48 hours. ℞: *Colchicine* for orogenital ulceration; *Azathioprine* or *cyclophosphamide* for systemic disease. *Infliximab* has a role in ocular disease unresponsive to topical steroids.[5]      *Hulusi Behçet, 1889-1948 (Turkish dermatologist)*

**Berger's disease** (*IgA nephropathy*, p301) Ranges from microscopic haematuria to rapidly progressive glomerulonephritis. Preceded by URTI in ~45% of children, typically causing gross haematuria.[6] Biopsy shows mesangial IgA deposition. It is mostly benign, but progression to end-stage renal failure occurs in 20-40%. ℞: Corticosteroids + ACE-i/ARB if ↑BP or protienuria. Tonsillectomy can improve renal function if tonsillitis causes recurrent disease.[7]     *Jean Berger, 1930-2011 (French nephrologist)*

**Bickerstaff's brainstem encephalitis** Ophthalmoplegia, ataxia, areflexia and extensor plantars ± tetraplegia ± coma, and a **reversible brain death picture (but there is *no* structural damage).** *MRI:* hyperintense brainstem signals. GQ1b antibodies +ve.[8] Plasmapheresis may help.         *Edwin R Bickerstaff, 1920-2008 (British physician)*

## Barrett's oesophagus

Barrett's oesophagus results from prolonged exposure of normal oesophageal squamous epithelium to the refluxate of GORD (p244). This causes mucosal inflammation and erosion, leading to replacement of the mucosa with metaplastic columnar epithelium. The length affected may be a few centimetres or all the oesophagus, and can be continuous or patchy (on endoscopy). 3-5% of people with GORD develop Barrett's. ▶The most significant associated morbidity is oesophageal adenocarcinoma. Risk of progression is low: 0.6-1.6% per year in patients with low-grade dysplasia.[9] *Diagnosis:* Biopsy of endoscopically visible columnarization allows histological corroboration (using the Prague criteria). *Management:* If premalignant/high-grade dysplasia, *oesophageal resection* or *eradicative mucosectomy*[10,11] is appropriate if young and fit. Endoscopic *targeted mucosectomy*,[12] or mucosal ablation by *epithelial laser*, *radiofrequency* (HALO),[13] or *photodynamic ablation* (PD) is used in others. Annual endoscopic surveillance for low-grade dysplasia is normally recommended, but shorter endoscopic intervals are associated with ↑detection of high-grade dysplasia and adenocarcinoma[14] (no randomized trials have shown this prevents death). If no pre-malignant changes are found, surveillance endoscopy + biopsy should be performed every 1-3 years and antireflux measures used (high-dose long-term proton pump inhibitors). Those with longstanding GORD (eg >5yrs, esp. if >50yrs old) should have one-off screening endoscopy.

*Norman Rupert Barrett, 1903-1979 (British surgeon)*

## Brugada syndrome

Note right bundle branch block and the unusual morphology of the raised ST segments in $V_{1-3}$ (fig 1; there are 3 ECG variants of this pattern). This predominantly autosominal dominant condition causing faulty sodium channels predisposes to fatal arrhythmias, eg ventricular fibrillation, typically in young males (eg triggered by a fever).[15] It is preventable by implanting a defibrillator. ▶*Consider primary electrical cardiac disease in all with unexplained syncope.* Programmed electrical stimulation may be needed.[16] Relatives of those with sudden unexplained death may undergo unmasking of arrhythmias by IV ajmaline tests—but some results are false +ve.[17] Use judgement in subjecting those with ST abnormalities but no symptoms to electrophysiological tests, right ventricular myocardial biopsy, and MRI. Mutations in the SCN5A gene (encodes the cardiac voltage-gated $Na_v1.5$ channel) are found in 15-20%. Other mutations have also been described.[18]

*Pedro & Josep Brugada, described 1992 (Spanish cardiologists)*

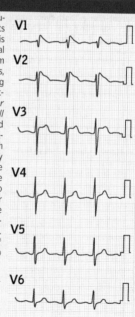

Fig 1. Note right bundle branch block and ST morphology in leads $V_{1-3}$.

Courtesy of Dr Shayashi.[19]

We thank Dr Simon Eyre, our Specialist Reader, and Kushalinii Ragubathy, our Junior Reader, for their contribution to this chapter.

See also OHCS p638-p655 concerning further unusual eponymous syndromes.

Consult the index for eponyms covered in other chapters. Biographical details: www.whonamedit.com.

ABC

**Brown-Séquard syndrome** A lesion in one half of the spinal cord (due to hemisection or unilateral cord lesion) causes: •Ipsilateral UMN weakness below the lesion (severed corticospinal tract, causing spastic paraparesis, brisk reflexes, extensor plantars) •Ipsilateral loss of proprioception and vibration (1 dorsal column severed) •Contralateral loss of pain and temperature sensation (severed spinothalamic tract which has crossed over; fig 1 also p520). *Causes:* Bullet, stab, dart, tick, tumour, disc hernia, cervical spondylosis, MS, neuroschistosomiasis, myelitis,[20] septic emboli (eg meningococcal).[21] *Imaging:* MRI. ⟶ *Charles-Édouard Brown-Séquard, 1817-1894 (Mauritian neurologist)*

**Budd-Chiari syndrome** Hepatic vein obstruction by thrombosis or tumour causes congestive ischaemia and hepatocyte damage. Abdominal pain, hepatomegaly, ascites and ↑ALT occur. Portal hypertension occurs in chronic forms. *Causes:* include hypercoagulable states (the Pill, pregnancy, malignancy, paroxysmal nocturnal haemoglobinuria, polycythaemia, thrombophilia), TB, liver, renal or adrenal tumour. *Tests:* USS + Dopplers, CT or MRI. Angioplasty, transjugular intrahepatic portosystemic shunt (TIPSS) or a surgical shunt may be needed. Anticoagulate (lifelong) unless there are varices. Consider liver transplant in fulminant hepatic necrosis or cirrhosis.[22] ⟶ *George Budd, 1808-1882 (British physician); Hans Chiari, 1851-1916 (Austrian pathologist)*

**Buerger's disease** (thromboangitis obliterans) Non-atherosclerotic smoking-related inflammation and thrombosis of veins and middle-sized arteries causing thrombophlebitis and ischaemia (→ulcers, gangrene). *Cause:* Unknown. Stopping smoking is vital. Most patients are men aged 20-45yrs (see BOX). ⟶ *Leo Buerger, 1879-1943 (US physician)*

**Caplan's syndrome** Multiple lung nodules in coal workers with RA, caused by an inflammatory reaction to anthracite (also associated with silica or asbestos exposure). CXR: bilateral peripheral nodules (0.5-5cm). ΔΔ: TB. ⟶ *Anthony Caplan, 1907-1976 (British physician)*

**Charcot-Marie-Tooth syndrome** (peroneal muscular atrophy) This inherited neuropathy starts in puberty with weak legs and foot drop + variable loss of sensation and reflexes. The peroneal muscles atrophy, leading to an inverted champagne bottle appearance. Atrophy of hand and arm muscles also occurs. The most common form, CMT1A (PMP22 myelin gene mutation on ch. 17), has AD inheritance. Quality of life is good;[23] total incapacity rare. Hand pain/paraesthesiae may respond to nerve release. ⟶ *Jean-Marie Charcot, 1825-1893; Pierre Marie, 1853-1940 (French neurologists); Howard HTooth, 1856-1926 (British physician)*

**Churg-Strauss syndrome** A triad of adult-onset asthma, eosinophilia, and vasculitis (± vasospasm ± MI ± DVT), affecting lungs, nerves, heart, and skin. A septic-shock picture/systemic inflammatory response syndrome may occur (with glomerulonephritis/renal failure, esp. if ANCA +ve). ℞: Steroids; biological agents if refractory disease, eg *rituximab*.[24] ⟶ *Jacob Churg, 1910-2005; Lotte Strauss, 1913-1985 (US pathologists)*

**Creutzfeldt-Jakob disease** (CJD) The cause is a prion (PrPSc), a misfolded form of a normal protein (PrPc), that can transform other proteins into prion proteins (hence its infectivity). ↑PrPSc leads to spongiform changes (tiny cavities ± tubulovesicular structures) in the brain.[25] Most cases are *sporadic* (incidence: 1-3/million/yr). *Variant* CJD (vCJD; ≤225 cases worldwide)[26] is transmitted via meat contaminated by CNS tissue affected by bovine spongiform encephalopathy BSE (see BOX). *Inherited forms:* (eg Gerstmann-Sträussler-Scheinker syndrome, P102L mutation in PRNP gene with ataxia ± self-mutilation), the 'normal' protein is too unstable, readily transforming to PrPSc. *Iatrogenic causes:* Contaminated surgical instruments, corneal transplants, growth hormone from human pituitaries, and blood (vCJD only).[27] Prion protein resists sterilization. *Signs:* Progressive dementia, focal CNS signs, myoclonus (present in 95%),[28] depression, eye signs (diplopia, supranuclear palsies, complex visual disturbances, homonymous field defects, hallucinations, cortical blindness). *Tests:* Tonsil/olfactory mucosa biopsy;[30] CSF gel electrophoresis; MRI. *Treatment:* None proven. Death occurs in ~6 months in sporadic and iatrogenic CJD. *Prevention:* Regulations to ↓spread of BSE and transmission to humans + ↓iatrogenic transmission.[31] ⟶ *Hans G Creutzfeldt, 1885-1964 (German pathologist); Alfons M Jakob 1884-1931 (German neurologist)*

**Crigler-Najjar syndrome** Two rare syndromes of inherited unconjugated hyperbilirubinaemia presenting in the 1st days of life with jaundice ± CNS signs. *Cause:* Mutation in UGT enzyme activity causing absent (type 1) or impaired (type 2; mild) ability to excrete bilirubin. ℞: T1: Liver transplant before irreversible kernicterus (OHCS p115) develops.[32] T2: usually no ℞ needed. ⟶ *John F Crigler b1919; Victor A Najjar b1914 (US paediatrician)*

### Signs that may distinguish variant CJD from sporadic CJD (sCJD)

- An earlier age at presentation (median 29yrs vs 60yrs in sporadic CJD).
- Longer survival and later dementia (median 14 months *vs* 4 for sporadic CJD).
- Psychiatric features are an early sign (anxiety, withdrawal, apathy, agitation, a permanent look of fear in the eyes, depression, personality change, insomnia). Hallucinations and delusions may occur—before akinetic mutism.
- Painful sensory symptoms are commoner (eg foot pain hyperaesthesia).
- More normal EEG (sporadic CJD has a characteristic spike and wave pattern).
- Mean CSF tau-pT181/tau protein ratio is 10-fold higher in vCJD than in sCJD.[33]
- Homozygosity for methionine at codon 129 of the PRP gene is typical.

### Fame and infamy in the search for lost youth

After his neurological experiments, Brown-Séquard, the most visionary of all neuroanatomists and the grandfather of HRT, proclaimed he had found the secret of perpetual youth after injecting himself with a concoction of testicular blood, semen, and testicular extracts from dogs and guinea pigs. In the 1880s over 12,000 doctors were queuing up to use his special extracts on patients, which he gave away free, provided results were reported back to him. 314 out of 405 cases of spinal syphilis improved, and his own urinary flow rate rose by 25%. Endocrinologists never forgave him for bringing their science into disrepute. To this day, no one really knows if his (literally) seminal work has given us anything of any practical value. But he might be pleased to know that testosterone is now known to have the urodynamic benefits he anticipated, at least in men with hypogonadism.[34]

Like many brilliant men, he had a cruel streak, backing clitoridectomy for preventing blindness and other imaginary complications of 'masturbatory melancholia'. Had he not been blinded by 19th-century ideas about female sexuality, could he have found a marvellous use for his concoctions, for 21st-century 'hypoactive sexual desire disorder'? Possibly, but only if he relied on placebo responses.[35,36]

### Poisoning your boss

In 1931, Buerger's disease caused gangrene in the toes of Harvey Cushing (p216)—the most cantankerous (and greatest) neurosurgeon ever. He had to be wheeled to the operating theatre to carry on his brilliant art (and to continue terrifying his assistants).[37] He had to retire partially, whereupon his colleagues presented him with a magnificent silver cigarette box, containing 2000 cigarettes (to which he was addicted)—one for each brain tumour he had removed during his long career, so verifying the truth that although we owe everything to our teachers, we must eventually kill them to move out from under their shadow.[1]

### Why bother studying rare diseases? The Liberski imperative...

For centuries, kuru was no bigger than a man's hand: a cloud barely visible on our horizon: a rare disease in cannibals beyond the Pacific. But meticulous work on kuru led to knowledge of prion diseases *before* the 1990s epidemic of vCJD. If in the 1950s, Gajdusek and Zigas had not been intrigued as to why kuru affected women and children more than men (their strange neural diet was the culprit), the discovery of vCJD would have been delayed, as no surveillance would have been in place. Neural tissue might still be in our food chain, with dreadful consequences. But further than this, the notion of 'protein-misfolding diseases'[2] would have been delayed by decades. So this is the lesson: ►*let curiosity flourish*. This is Liberski's imperative.[38] So now let's scan our horizon for other intriguing clouds.



1 *Der Vogel kämpft sich aus dem Ei. Das Ei ist die Welt. Wer geboren werden will, muss eine Welt zerstören.* The bird struggles out of the egg. The egg is the world. Whoever will be born, must first destroy a world. (Hermann Hesse. *Demian*; 1917.)

2 Cystic fibrosis (misfolded CFTR protein), Marfan's (misfolded fibrillin),[39] Fabry's (misfolded α-galactosidase), Gaucher's (misfolded β-glucocerebrosidase), retinitis pigmentosa 3 (misfolded rhodopsin); some cancers may be caused by misfolding of tumour suppressor proteins (von Hippel-Lindau protein).

**Devic's syndrome** (neuromyelitis optica; NMO) Inflammatory demyelination causes attacks of optic neuritis ± myelitis. Abnormal CSF (may mimic bacterial meningitis) and serum anti-AQP4 antibody (in 65%) help distinguish it from MS⁴⁰ (see BOX). ℞: IV steroids; plasma exchange. *Azathioprine* and *rituximab*⁴¹ help prevent relapses. *Prognosis:* Variable; complete remission may occur. *Eugène Devic, 1858-1930 (French neurologist)*

**Dressler's syndrome** This develops 2-10wks after an MI, heart surgery (or even pacemaker insertion). It is thought that myocardial injury stimulates formation of autoantibodies against heart muscle. *Symptoms:* Recurrent fever and chest pain ± pleural or pericardial rub (from serositis). Cardiac tamponade may occur, so avoid anticoagulants. ℞: Aspirin, NSAIDs or steroids. *William Dressler, 1890-1969 (US cardiologist)*

**Dubin-Johnson syndrome** Autosomal recessive There is defective hepatocyte excretion of conjugated bilirubin. Typically presents in late teens with intermittent jaundice ± hepatosplenomegaly. *Tests:* ↑bilirubin; ALT and AST are normal; bilirubinuria on dipstick; ↑ratio of urinary coproporphyrin I to III. Liver biopsy: diagnostic pigment granules.⁴² ℞: Usually none needed. *Isadore N Dubin, 1913-1981; Frank B Johnson, b1919 (US pathologists)*

**Dupuytren's contracture** (fig 1). Progressive shortening and thickening of the palmar fascia causing finger contracture and loss of extension (often 5ᵗʰ finger). *Prevalence:* ~10% of ♂ >65yrs (↑ if +ve family history). *Associations:* Smoking, alcohol use, heavy manual labour, trauma, DM, phenytoin, HIV. Peyronie's may coexist (p722). It is thought to be caused by local hypoxia. ℞: Collagenase injections.⁴³ Surgery may be needed. *Baron Guillaume Dupuytren, 1777-1835 (French surgeon, famed also for treating Napoleon's haemorrhoids)*

**Ekbom's syndrome** (Restless legs) Criteria: 1 Compelling desire to move legs 2 Worse at night 3 Relieved by movement 3 Unpleasant leg sensations (eg shootings or tinglings) worse at rest. *Mechanism:* Endogenous opioid system fault causes altered central processing of pain.☞ *Prevalence:* 1-3%. ♀:♂≈2:1. *Associations:* Iron deficiency, uraemia, pregnancy, DM, polyneuropathy, RA, COPD, persistent genital arousal disorder.⁴⁴ *Exclude:* Cramps, positional discomfort, and local leg pathology. ℞: Dopamine agonists are commonly used; also, anticonvulsants, opioids and benzodiazepines.⁴⁵ *Karl Axel Ekbom, 1907-1977 (Swedish neurologist)*

**Fabry disease** X-linked lysosomal storage disorder caused by abnormalities in the GLA gene, which leads to a deficiency in α-galactosidase A. There is accumulation of glycosphingolipids in skin (angiokeratoma ± hypohidrosis), eyes (lens opacities), heart (angina, MI, syncope, dyspnoea, LVH, arrhythmias), kidneys (renal failure), CNS (stroke) and nerves (neuropathy/acroparaesthesia) ± corneal verticillata (whorls). Most males die in the 6ᵗʰ decade due to renal failure, stroke or MI. ℞: Enzyme replacement therapy with α or β human agalsidase.⁴⁶ *Johannes Fabry, 1860-1930 (German dermatologist)*

**Fanconi anaemia** Autosomal recessive HLA-DRB1*04 Defective stem cell repair and chromosomal fragility leads to aplastic anaemia, ↑risk of AML and breast ca (BRCA2), skin pigmentation, absent radii, short stature, microcephaly, syndactyly, deafness, IQ↓, hypopituitarism, and cryptorchidism. ℞: Stem-cell transplant. *Guido Fanconi, 1892-1979 (Swiss paediatrician)*

**Felty's syndrome** A triad of rheumatoid arthritis + WCC↓ + splenomegaly (±hypersplenism, causing anaemia and ↓platelets), recurrent infections, skin ulcers and lymphadenopathy. 95% are Rh factor +ve. Splenectomy may raise the WCC. ℞: DMARDs (p549) ± *rituximab* if refractory.⁴⁷ *Augustus Roi Felty, 1895-1964 (US physician)*

**Fitz-Hugh-Curtis syndrome** Liver capsule inflammation causing RUQ pain due to transabdominal spread of chlamydial or gonococcal infection, often with PID ± 'violinstring' adhesions. ℞: Antibiotics for PID (+ treat sexual partners) ± laparoscopic division of adhesions. *Thomas Fitz-Hugh, 1894-1963 (US physician); Arthur H Curtis, 1881-1955 (US gynaecologist)*

**Foster Kennedy syndrome** Optic atrophy of one eye due to optic nerve compression (most commonly from an olfactory groove meningioma), with papilloedema of the other eye secondary to ↑ICP. There is also central scotoma and anosmia. *Robert Foster Kennedy, 1884-1952 (British neurologist)*

**Friedreich's ataxia** Autosomal recessive Expansions of the trinucleotide repeat GAA in the X25 (frataxin) gene causes degeneration of many nerve tracts: spinocerebellar tracts degenerate causing cerebellar ataxia, dysarthria, nystagmus, and dysdiadochokinesis. Loss of corticospinal tracts occurs (weakness and plantars ↑↑) with peripheral nerve damage, so tendon reflexes are paradoxically depressed (differential diagnosis p451)

## Signs distinguishing Devic's syndrome from multiple sclerosis[48]

|  | Devic's syndrome | Multiple sclerosis |
|---|---|---|
| Course | Monophasic or relapsing | Relapsing usually; see p500 |
| Attack severity | Usually severe | Often mild |
| Respiratory failure | ~30%, from cervical myelitis | Rare |
| MRI head | Usually normal | Many periventricular white-matter lesions |
| MRI cord lesions | Longitudinal, central | Multiple, small, peripheral |
| CSF oligoclonal bands | Absent | Present |
| Permanent disability | Unusual, and attack-related | In late progressive disease |
| Other autoimmunities | In ≤50% (eg Sjögren's) | Uncommon |

**Diagnostic criteria for Devic's** Optic neuritis, myelitis, and ≥2 out of 3 of: •MRI evidence of a continuous cord lesion for ≥3 segments •Brain MRI at onset non-diagnostic for MS •NMO-IgG (anti-AQP4) serum or CSF positivity (poorer prognosis).

NB: CNS involvement beyond the optic nerves and cord is compatible with NMO.

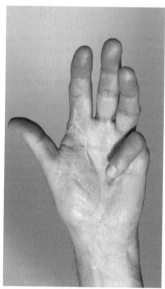

Fig 1. Dupuytren's contracture of the 5ᵗʰ finger. Note scar from previous surgery to the index finger.

There is also dorsal column degeneration, with loss of positional and vibration sense. Pes cavus and scoliosis occur. Cardiomyopathy may cause CCF. Typical age at death: ~50yrs. R: There is no cure. Treat CCF, arrhythmias and DM.

*Nikolaus Friedreich, 1825-1882 (German neurologist)*

**Froin's syndrome** ↑ CSF protein + xanthochromia with normal cell count—a sign of blockage in spinal CSF flow (eg from a spinal tumour). *Georges Froin, 1874-1932 (French physician)*

**Gardner's syndrome** Autosomal dominant A variant of familial adenomatous polyposis, caused by mutations in the APC gene (5q21). There are multiple colon polyps (which inevitably become malignant; p524),[46] benign bone osteomas, epidermal cysts, dermoid tumours, fibromas, and neurofibromas. *Fundoscopy* reveals black spots (congenital hypertrophy of retinal pigment epithelium); this helps pre-symptomatic detection. *Presentation:* Can present from 2-70yrs with colonic (eg bloody diarrhoea) or extracolonic symptoms. Prophylactic surgery (eg proctocolectomy) is the only curative treatment. Endoscopic polypectomy with long-term *sulindac* therapy has been used to postpone prophylactic colectomy.[50] *Eldon J Gardner, 1909-1989 (US physician)*

**Gélineau's syndrome** (narcolepsy) The patient, usually a young man, succumbs to irresistible attacks of inappropriate sleep ± vivid hypnogogic hallucinations, cataplexy (sudden hypotonia), and sleep paralysis (paralysis of speech and movement, while fully alert, at sleep onset or on waking). *Hypothesis:* Mutations lead to loss of hypothalamic hypocretin-containing neurons, via autoimmune destruction.[51] 95% are +ve for HLA DR2. R: Stimulants (eg methylphenidate) may cause dependence ± psychosis. Modafinil may be better. SE: anxiety, aggression, dry mouth, euphoria, insomnia, BP↑, dyskinesia, ALP↑. *Jean-Baptiste-Édouard Gélineau, 1828-1906 (French physician)*

**Gerstmann's syndrome** A constellation of symptoms suggesting a dominant parietal lesion: finger agnosia (inability to identify fingers), agraphia (inability to write), acalculia (inability to calculate) and left-right disorientation.

*Josef Gerstmann, 1887-1969 (Austrian neurologist)*

**Gilbert's syndrome** A common cause of *unconjugated* hyperbilirubinaemia due to ↓ UGT-1 activity (the enzyme that conjugates bilirubin with glucuronic acid). *Prevalence:* 1-2%; 5-15% have a family history of jaundice. It may be unnoticed for many years and usually presents in adolescence with intermittent jaundice occuring during illness, exercise or fasting. *Diagnosis:* Mild ↑ bilirubin; normal FBC and reticulocytes (ie no haemolysis). It is a benign condition. *Nicolas Augustin Gilbert, 1858-1927 (French physician)*

**Gilles de la Tourette syndrome** Tonic, clonic, dystonic, or phonic tics: jerks, blinks, sniffs, nods, spitting, stuttering, irrepressible explosive obscene verbal ejaculations (coprolalia, in 20%) or gestures (coprophilia, 6%),[52] grunts, squeaks, burps, twirlings, and nipping others ± tantrums. There may be a witty, innovatory, phantasmagoric picture, with mimicry (echopraxia), antics, impishness, extravagance, audacity, dramatizations, surreal associations, uninhibited affect, speed, 'go', vivid imagery and memory, and hunger for stimuli. *The tic paradox:* Tics are *voluntary*, but often *unwanted*: the desire to tic stems from the relief of the odd sensation that builds up prior to the tic and is relieved by it, "like scratching a mosquito bite, tics lead to more tics."[53] Tics may be controlled through the medium of dance, or when concentrating, or having sex,[54] but note: ▶"tics aren't just little annoyances now and then, they form an integral part of my existence. I tic therefore I am."[55] *Mean age of onset:* 6yrs. ♂:♀≈4:1. *Pathogenesis:* Unknown. *Molecular mimicry hypothesis:* Anti-streptococcal antibodies cross-react with basal ganglia (p136 & BOX).[56] *MRI:* Big left thalamus.[57] *Associations:* Obsessive-compulsive disorder; hyperactivity. R: (none may be wanted) Risperidone, haloperidol or pimozide.◆ Habit-reversal training.[58] Deep brain stimulation is rarely indicated, but may help—3 key structures are the medial thalamus, globus pallidus internus and internal capsule (anterior limb/nucleus accumbens).[59,60] *Marquis Georges Albert Édouard Brutus Gilles de la Tourette, 1857-1904 (French neurologist)*

**Goodpasture's disease**[1] (a pulmonary-renal syndrome). Acute glomerulonephritis + lung symptoms (haemoptysis/diffuse pulmonary haemorrhage) caused by antiglomerular basement membrane antibodies (binding kidney's basement membrane and alveolar membrane). *Tests:* CXR: infiltrates due to pulmonary haemorrhage, often in lower zones. Kidney biopsy: crescentic glomerulonephritis. R: ▶▶ Treat shock. Vigorous immunosuppressive treatment and plasmapheresis.

*Ernest William Goodpasture, 1886-1960 (US pathologist)*

## Cataplexy is highly specific for narcolepsy/Gélineau's syndrome

Daytime sleepiness has many causes, but if it occurs with cataplexy the diagnosis 'must' be narcolepsy. Cataplexy is bilateral loss of tone in antigravity muscles provoked by emotions such as laughter, startle, excitement, or anger. Associated phenomena include: falls, mouth opening, dysarthria, mutism, and phasic muscle jerking around the mouth. Most attacks are brief, but injury can occur (eg if several attacks per day). It is comparable to the atonia of rapid eye movement sleep *but without loss of awareness*. ΔΔ: bradycardia, migraine, atonic/akinetic epilepsy,[61,62] delayed sleep phase syndrome, conversion disorder, malingering, and psychosis.[63]

Don't confuse cataplexy with catalepsy—a waxy flexibility where involuntary statue-like postures are effortlessly maintained (frozen) despite looking most uncomfortable.

## The lung and its various vasculitides (eg Goodpasture's)

Lung vasculitis is most commonly seen with the primary idiopathic, small-vessel or ANCA (p555)-associated vasculitides: granulomatosis with polyangiitis (Wegener's), microscopic polyangiitis, and Churg-Strauss syndrome.[64] Medium-vessel vasculitis (classic polyarteritis nodosa), large-vessel vasculitis (Takayasu arteritis), primary immune complex-mediated vasculitis (Goodpasture's disease), and secondary vasculitis (SLE) can all affect the lung. Hepatitis C is a rare cause of lung vasculitis—usually associated with glomerulonephritis and cryoglobulinaemia.[65]

---

1 Should it be Goodpasture's **disease** or **syndrome**? The latter might refer to any pulmonary-renal vasculitis (eg caused by cryoglobulinaemia or SLE). Goodpasture's **disease** is reserved for the clinical condition characterized by lung haemorrhage, and crescentic glomerulonephritis associated with linear deposition of antibodies along the glomerular basement membrane.[66]

**Guillain-Barré syndrome** (Acute inflammatory demyelinating polyneuropathy)[67] *Incidence:* 1-2/100,000/yr. *Signs:* A few weeks after an infection a symmetrical ascending muscle weakness starts. *Triggers: Campylobacter jejuni,* CMV, mycoplasma, zoster, HIV, EBV, vaccinations. ♠☀ The trigger causes antibodies which attack nerves. In 40%, no cause is found. It may advance quickly, affecting all limbs at once, and can lead to paralysis. There is a progressive phase of up to 4 weeks, followed by recovery. Unlike other neuropathies, *proximal* muscles are more affected, eg trunk, respiratory, and cranial nerves (esp. VII). Pain is common (eg back, limb) but sensory signs may be absent. *Autonomic dysfunction:* Sweating, ↑pulse, BP changes, arrhythmias. *Nerve conduction studies:* Slow conduction. CSF: Protein↑ (eg >5.5g/L), normal CSF white cell count. Respiratory involvement (the big danger) requires transfer to ITU. Do forced vital capacity (FVC) 4 hourly. ▶*Ventilate sooner rather than later,* eg if FVC <1.5L, $P_aO_2$ <10kPa, $P_aCO_2$ >6kPa. ℞: IV immunoglobulin 0.4g/kg/24h for 5d. Plasma exchange is good too (?more SE).[68] Steroids have no role. *Prognosis:* Good; ~85% make a complete or near-complete recovery. 10% are unable to walk alone at 1yr. *Complete paralysis is compatible with complete recovery. Mortality:* 10%.

*George C Guillain, 1876–1961; Jean-Alexandre Barré, 1880–1967 (French neurologists)*

**Henoch-Schönlein purpura (HSP)** (fig 2) A small vessel vasculitis, presenting with purpura (non-blanching purple papules due to intradermal bleeding), often over buttocks and extensor surfaces, typically affecting young ♂. There may be glomerulonephritis (p300), arthritis, and abdominal pain (±intussusception), which may mimic an 'acute abdomen'. ℞: Mostly supportive.

*Eduard H Henoch, 1820–1910 (German paediatrician); Johann L Schönlein, 1793–1864 (German physician)*

**Horner's syndrome** A triad of 1 *miosis* (pupil constriction, fig 1) 2 partial *ptosis* (drooping upper eyelid) + *apparent enophthalmos* (sunken eye) 3 *anhidrosis* (ipsilateral loss of sweating). Due to interruption of the face's sympathetic supply, eg at the brainstem (demyelination, vascular disease), cord (syringomyelia), thoracic outlet (Pancoast's tumour, p722), or on the sympathetic's trip on the internal carotid artery into the skull (fig 3), and orbit. *Johann Friedrich Horner, 1831–1886 (Swiss ophthalmologist)*

**Huntington's disease** Autosomal dominant Incurable, progressive, neurodegenerative disorder presenting in middle age, often with prodromal phase of mild symptoms (irritability, depression, incoordination). Progresses to chorea, dementia ± fits and death (within ~15yrs of diagnosis). *Pathology:* Atrophy and neuronal loss of striatum and cortex. Genetic basis: Expansion of CAG repeat on Ch. 4. ℞: (p81) No treatment prevents progression. Counselling for patient and family.[69] *George Huntington, 1850–1916 (US physician)*

**Jervell and Lange-Nielsen syndrome** Autosomal recessive Congenital bilateral sensorineural deafness and long QT interval (p90, hence syncope, VT, *torsades* ± sudden death—50% by age 15 if untreated). KCNQ1 or KCNE1 gene mutation causes K⁺ channelopathy. ℞: β-blocker, pacemaker, ICD, cochlear implants.[70]

*Anton Jervell, 1901–1987; Fred Lange-Nielsen, 1919–1989 (Norwegian physicians)*

**Kaposi's sarcoma (KS)** is a spindle-cell tumour derived from capillary endothelial cells or from fibrous tissue, caused by human herpes virus (KSHV = HHV-8). It presents as purple papules (¼-1cm) or plaques on skin (fig 4) and mucosa (any organ). It metastasizes to nodes. There are 4 types: 1 Classic, especially elderly Jewish or Mediterranean ♂ (esp. in Po Valley and Sardinia, ?related to blood-sucking insects). 2 Endemic (Central Africa). In forms 1 and 2, peripheral, slow-growing skin lesions are found, visceral involvement is rare, but node involvement may cause oedema. 3 KS in immunosuppression, eg organ transplant recipients. Aggressive course with visceral involvement. Taper immunosuppressives to the lowest level that keeps the graft functional.[71] Sirolimus has a role.[72] 4 AIDS related. In HIV, KS is diagnostic of AIDS (p408) and may be life-threatening with many skin, gut and lung lesions. It affects mostly homo- or bisexual men (HIV-KS in S. Africa).[73] Prevalence is less with HAART (p414).[74] Lung KS may present in HIV +ve men and women as dyspnoea and haemoptysis.[75] Bowel KS may cause nausea, abdominal pain. *Rare sites:* CNS, larynx, eye, glands, heart, breast, wounds or biopsy sites. Δ: Biopsy. ℞: Optimize HAART;[76] ± *interferon-α*; consider topical retinoids, cryotherapy or radiotherapy for skin lesions. Chemotherapy, eg: pegylated liposomal doxorubicin ± *interleukin-12.*[77]

*Moricz Kaposi, 1837–1902 (Hungarian dermatologist)*

## Diagnostic criteria in typical Guillain-Barré polyneuritis[78]

**Features required for diagnosis:**
• Progressive weakness of all 4 limbs
• Areflexia

**Features excluding diagnosis:**

Purely sensory symptoms

Diagnosis of:  • Myasthenia
 • Botulism
 • Poliomyelitis
 • Diphtheria
 • Porphyria
 • Toxic neuropathy

**Features supporting diagnosis:**
• Progression over days, up to 4wks
• Near symmetry of symptoms
• Sensory symptoms/signs only mild
• CN involvement (eg bilateral facial weakness)
• Recovery starts ~2wks after the period of progression has finished
• Autonomic dysfunction
• Absence of fever at onset
• CSF protein ↑ with CSF WCC <10×10⁶/L
• Typical electrophysiological tests

Variants of Guillain-Barré syndrome include:

*Chronic inflammatory demyelinating polyradiculopathy (CIDP):* characterized by a slower onset and recovery.

*Miller Fisher syndrome:* Comprises of ophthalmoplegia, ataxia and areflexia. Associated with anti-GQ1b antibodies in the serum.

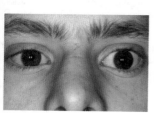

Fig 1. Right Horner's: everything reduces: pupil, eye, sweating, etc.

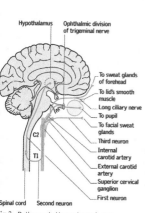

Fig 3. Pathways in Horner's syndrome.

Hypothalamus
Ophthalmic division of trigeminal nerve
To sweat glands of forehead
To lid's smooth muscle
Long ciliary nerve
To pupil
To facial sweat glands
Third neuron
Internal carotid artery
External carotid artery
Superior cervical ganglion
First neuron
C2
T1
Spinal cord  Second neuron

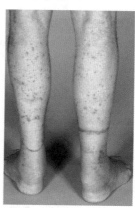

Fig 2. Henoch-Schönlein vasculitis.

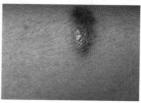

Fig 4. Kaposi's sarcoma.
Reproduced from *Oxford Handbook of Medical Dermatology*, 2010, with permission from Oxford University Press.

**Klippel-Trénaunay syndrome** A triad of port wine stain, varicose veins, and limb hypertrophy, due to vascular malformation. Usually sporadic (although AD inheritance has been reported).[79]    *Maurice Klippel, 1858-1942; Paul Trénaunay, 1875-1938 (French physicians)*

**Korsakoff's syndrome** Hypothalamic damage & cerebral atrophy due to thiamine (vitamin B₁) deficiency (eg in alcoholics). May accompany Wernicke's encephalopathy. There is ↓ability to acquire new memories, confabulation (invented memory, owing to retrograde amnesia), lack of insight & apathy. *R:* See *Wernicke's*, p728. *Donepezil* ● may have a role.[80]    *Sergei Sergeievich Korsakoff, 1853-1900 (Russian neuropsychiatrist)*

**Langerhans cell histiocytosis** (histiocytosis X) A group of disorders, either single (in 73%, eg bone) or multisystem (in 27%; at-risk organs are liver, lung, spleen, marrow) with infiltrating granulomas containing dendritic (Langerhans) cells. ♂:♀≈1.5:1. Pulmonary Langerhans cell histiocytosis presents with pneumothorax or pulmonary hypertension. CXR/CT: nodules and cysts + honeycombing in upper and middle zones. Δ: Biopsy (skin, lung). *R:* Local excision, steroids, *vinblastine ± etoposide* if severe.[81] *OHCS* p644.    *Paul Langerhans, 1847-1888 (German pathologist)*

**Leriche's syndrome** Absent femoral pulse, claudication/wasting[82] of the buttock, a pale cold leg, and erectile dysfunction (from aorto-iliac occlusive disease, eg a saddle embolus at the aortic bifurcation. Surgery may help.[83]    *René Leriche, 1879-1955 (French surgeon)*

**Löffler's eosinophilic endocarditis** Restrictive cardiomyopathy + eosinophilia (eg 120 × 10⁹/L). It may be an early stage of tropical endomyocardial fibrosis (and overlaps with hypereosinophilic syndrome, p324) but is distinct from eosinophilic leukaemia. *Signs:* Heart failure (75%) ± mitral regurgitation (49%) ± heart block. *R:* Suppress the eosinophilia (*prednisolone ± hydroxycarbamide*), and then treat with anti-heart failure medication.    *Wilhelm Löffler, 1887-1972 (Swiss physician)*

**Löffler's syndrome** (pulmonary eosinophilia) An allergic infiltration of the lungs by eosinophils. Allergens include: *Ascaris lumbricoides, Trichinella spiralis, Fasciola hepatica, Strongyloides, Ankylostoma, Toxocara, Clonorchis sinensis,*[84] sulfonamides, hydralazine, and nitrofurantoin. Often symptomless with incidental CXR (diffuse fan-shaped shadows), or cough, fever, eosinophilia (in ~20%) & larval migrans (p442). *R:* Eradicate cause. Steroids (if idiopathic).    *Wilhelm Löffler, 1887-1972 (Swiss physician)*

**Lown-Ganong-Levine syndrome** A pre-excitation syndrome, similar to Wolf-Parkinson-White (WPW, p120), characterized by a short PR interval (<0.12sec) a normal QRS complex (as opposed to the δ-waves of WPW) and risk of supraventricular tachycardia (but not AF/flutter). The cause is not completely understood, but may be due to paranodal fibres that bypass all or part of the atrioventricular node. The patient may complain of intermittent palpitations.[85]
*Bernard Lown, b1921 (US cardiologist); William F Ganong, 1924-2007 (US physiologist); Samuel A Levine, 1891-1966 (US cardiologist)*

**McArdle's glycogen storage disease (type V)** Autosomal recessive Absence of muscle phosphorylase enzyme with resulting inability to convert glycogen into glucose (eg R50X mutation of PYGM gene). Fatigue and crises of cramps ± hyperthermia. Rhabdomyolysis/myoglobinuria follow exercise. *Tests:* CK↑↑. Muscle biopsy is diagnostic (necrosis and atrophy). *R:* Moderate aerobic exercise helps (by utilizing alternative fuel substrates).[88] Avoid heavy exertion and statins. Sucrose pre-exercise improves performance, as does a carbohydrate-rich diet. Low dose creatine and *ramipril* (only if D/D ACE phenotype) may be of minimal benefit.[87]    *Brian McArdle, 1911-2002 (British paediatrician)*

**Mallory-Weiss tear** Persistent vomiting/retching *causes* haematemesis via an oesophageal mucosal tear. *George K Mallory, 1900-1986 (US pathologist); Soma Weiss, 1898-1942 (US physician)*

**Marchiafava-Bignami syndrome** Corpus callosum demyelination and necrosis, most often secondary to chronic alcoholism. Type A is characterized by coma, stupor and pyramidal tract features involving the entire corpus callosum. In type B, symptoms are mild and the corpus callosum is partially affected.[88] Δ: MRI.[89] *R:* As for Wernicke's, p728 (BOX 2).    *Ettore Marchiafava, 1847-1935; Amico Bignami, 1862-1929 (Italian pathologists)*

**Marchiafava-Micheli syndrome** (paroxysmal nocturnal haemoglobinuria, PNH) An acquired clonal expansion of a multipotent stem cell manifesting with haemolytic anaemia (from complement-mediated intravascular haemolysis), large vessel thromboses and deficient haematopoiesis (ranging from mild to pancytopenia). See BOX, fig 1 and p332.    *Ettore Marchiafava, 1847-1935 (Italian pathologist); Ferdinando Micheli, 1872-1936 (Italian physician)*

## Paroxysmal nocturnal haemoglobinuria: the darkest hour

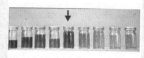
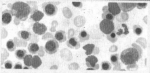

Fig 1. PNH. In this 24h urine sample, the darkest hour is before dawn.[90] Haemolysis occurs throughout the day and night, but the urine concentrated overnight produces the dramatic change in color. *Pathophysiology:* In PNH, surface proteins are missing in all blood cells due to a somatic mutation in the X-linked PIG-A gene. Cells lack the glycosyl-phosphatidylinositol (GPI) anchor that binds the surface proteins to cell membranes. This causes uncontrolled amplification of the complement system and leads to destruction of the RBC membrane and release of haemoglobin into the circulation. NB: The phenomenon of haemoglobinuria[1] is not all that reliable. A much better test even than a marrow biopsy (right-hand panel, showing a clone of PNH cells) is flow cytometric analysis of GPI-anchored proteins on peripheral blood cells. This can determine the size of the PNH clone and type of GPI deficiency (complete or partial). *R:* Most benefit from supportive measures—but allogeneic stem cell transplantation is the only cure.[91] *Eculizumab* is a monoclonal antibody that targets the C5 protein of the complement system. Blockade prevents activation of the complement distal pathway, reducing haemolysis, stabilizing haemoglobin and reducing transfusion requirements.[92]

Courtesy of Crookston Collection.

---

*Fatal effects of alcohol on the* CNS

- Inhibitions↓ (unsafe sex↑ [etc, etc])[2]
- Wernicke's encephalopathy
- Korsakoff's syndrome
- Hepatic encephalopathy
- Cerebral atrophy (dementia)
- Central pontine myelinolysis
- Cerebellar atrophy (falls [etc])
- Stroke (all varieties)
- Seizures
- Marchiafava-Bignami syndrome

1 In haemoglobinuria, urine dipstick will be positive for blood but microscopy of urine does not show RBCs (thus differentiating it from haematuria, but not myoglobinuria—where CK ± AST will be high).
2 Alcohol is frequently fatal to fetuses—in the UK *thousands* of terminations are carried out *every month* from conceptions related to binge drinking. Also, fewer inhibitions lead to more sex, and hence more deaths from cervical cancer (human papilloma virus-associated, HIV, etc).

**Marfan's syndrome** Connective tissue disorder with ↓extracellular microfibril formation and poor elastic fibres.[93] ~25% occur with no family history. *Major criteria* (diagnostic if >2): Lens dislocation (*ectopia lentis*; fig 1); aortic dissection or dilatation; dural ectasia; **skeletal features**: arachnodactyly (long spidery fingers), armspan > height, pectus deformity, scoliosis, pes planus. *Minor signs*: Mitral valve prolapse, high-arched palate, joint hypermobility. Diagnosis is clinical; MRI for dural ectasia. *R*: The danger is aortic dissection: **β**-blockers are used to slow dilatation of the aortic root. Do annual echos, with elective surgical repair when aortic diameter is >5cm. In pregnancy, the risk of dissection rises. Homocystinuria has similar skeletal deformities: *Antoine Bernard-Jean Marfan, 1858-1942 (French paediatrician)*

| *Marfan's* Autosomal dominant fibrillin gene FBN1 vs | *Homocystinuria* Cystathione β-synthetase deficiency; autosomal recessive with early vasculopathy |
|---|---|
| • Upwards lens dislocation | • Downwards lens dislocation |
| • Aortic valve incompetence | • Heart rarely affected |
| • Normal intelligence | • Mental retardation |
| • Scoliosis, flat feet, herniae | • Recurrent thromboses, osteoporosis |
| • Life expectancy is lower from cardiovascular risks | • Positive urine cyanide-nitroprusside test |
| | • Response to treatment with pyridoxine |

**Meckel's diverticulum** The distal ileum contains embryonic remnants of gastric and pancreatic tissue. There may be gastric acid secretion, causing GI pain & occult bleeding. Δ: Radionucleotide scan; laparotomy. *Johann Friedrich Meckel, 1781-1833 (German anatomist)*

**Meigs' syndrome** A triad of 1 benign ovarian tumour (fibroma) 2 pleural effusion (R>L) & 3 ascites. It resolves on tumour resection. *Joe Vincent Meigs, 1892-1963 (US gynaecologist)*

**Ménétrier's disease** Giant gastric mucosal folds up to 4cm high, in the fundus, with atrophy of the glands + ↑mucosal thickness + hypochlorhydria + protein-losing gastropathy (hence hypoalbuminaemia ± oedema). *Causes:*● CMV, streps,[94] *H. pylori*. There may be epigastric pain, vomiting ± ↓weight. It is pre-malignant. *R*: Epidermal growth factor receptor blockade with *cetuximab* is 1st-line treatment.[95] Surgery if intractable symptoms or malignant change. *Pierre Eugène Ménétrier, 1859-1935 (French pathologist)*

**Meyer-Betz syndrome** (paroxysmal myoglobinuria) This rare idiopathic condition causes necrosis of exercising muscles. There is muscle pain, weakness, and discoloured urine: pink→brown (as ↑myoglobin is excreted). Acute renal failure can result from myoglobinuria (p307). DIC is associated. *Tests:* WCC↑, LFT↑, LDH↑, CPK↑, urine myoglobin↑. *Diagnosis:* Muscle biopsy, ↑CPK and ↑serum myoglobin. Exertion should be avoided. *Friedrich Meyer-Betz, described 1910 (German physician)*

**Mikulicz's syndrome** Benign persistent swelling of lacrimal and parotid (or submandibular) glands due to lymphocytic infiltration. Exclude other causes (sarcoidosis, TB, viral infection, lymphoproliferative disorders.) It is thought to be an IgG4-related plasmacytic systemic disease.[96] *Johann Freiherr von Mikulicz-Radecki, 1850-1905 (Polish-Austrian surgeon)*

**Milroy disease** Autosomal dominant Primary congenital lymphoedema. Mutations in the VEGFR3 gene cause lymphatic malfunction with lower leg swelling from birth (fig 2) Δ: Lymphoscintigraphy; genetic testing. *R*:●Compression hosiery/bandages ●Encourage exercise ●Good skin hygiene ●Treat cellulitis actively.[97] *William Forsyth Milroy, 1855-1942 (US physician)*

**Münchausen's syndrome** Vivid liars, who are addicted to institutions, flit from hospital to hospital, feigning illness, eg hoping for a laparotomy (*laparotimophilia migrans*) or mastectomy (*mammomania non-neoplastica*), or they complain of awful bleeding (*haemorrhagica histrionica*), odd eye movements (*nystagmus confabulus*), curious fits (*neurologica diabolica*), sexual assaults (*phantasmorotica penetrans*), throat closings (*otolaryngologica prevarica*), false asthma (*bronchospasmus absurdum*) or heart attacks (*cardiopathia fantastica*). Münchausen-by-proxy entails injury to a dependent person by a carer (eg mother) to gain medical attention.

*Karl Friedrich Hieronymus, Freiherr von Münchausen, 1720-1797 (German aristocrat). Described by RAJ Asher in 1951*[98]

**Ogilvie's syndrome** (*acute colonic pseudo-obstruction*) Colonic obstruction in the absence of a mechanical cause, associated with recent severe illness or surgery. *R*: Correct U&E. Colonoscopy allows decompression, and excludes mechanical causes. Neostigmine is also effective, suggesting parasympathetic suppression is to blame.[9] Surgery is rarely needed (eg if perforation). *William Heneage Ogilvie, 1887-1971 (British surgeon)*

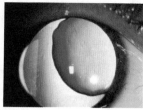

Fig 1. Lens dislocation in **Marfan's syndrome**: here the lens is dislocated superiorly and medially.

Courtesy of Prof Jonathan Trobe.

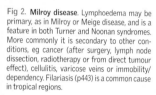

Fig 2. **Milroy disease**. Lymphoedema may be primary, as in Milroy or Meige disease, and is a feature in both Turner and Noonan syndromes. More commonly it is secondary to other conditions, eg cancer (after surgery, lymph node dissection, radiotherapy or from direct tumour effect), cellulitis, varicose veins or immobility/dependency. Filariasis (p443) is a common cause in tropical regions.

## Who was Baron Münchausen?

Baron Karl Münchausen was an 18th-century German aristocrat and fabulist, whose tall tales became first a popular book, then a byword for circular logic, and finally a medical syndrome of self-delusion. He is famous for riding cannonballs, travelling to the moon and pulling himself out of a swamp by his own hair. ▶▶In emergencies (we've all had that sinking feeling...) this method may save your life, for example in your final exams (fig 3):

*Examiner:* "What is ITP?"

*You:* "ITP is idiopathic thrombocytopenic purpura." (you have scored 50% already).

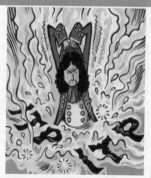

Fig 3. Münchausen during his finals.

*Examiner:* "And what is idiopathic thrombocytopenic purpura?"

*You:* "It's when a cryptogenic cause of a low platelet count leads to purpura."

You have deployed your skills with logical brilliance, without adding a single insight. For this Münchausen circularity you may be awarded 100%—unless your examiner is a philosopher, when the right answer would be "What is ITP? I don't know—and nor do you"—but don't try this too often. You see, you must never forget that medicine is marvellously scientific, and no-one is popular who dares cast doubt on this article of faith.

ABC

**Ortner's cardiovocal syndrome** Recurrent laryngeal nerve palsy from a large left atrium (eg from mitral stenosis) or aortic dissection. *Norbert Ortner, 1865-1935 (Austrian physician)*

**Osler-Weber-Rendu syndrome** (hereditary telangiectasia) Autosomal dominant Telangiectasia on the skin and mucous membranes (causing epistaxis and GI bleeds), see fig 1. It is associated with pulmonary, hepatic and cerebral arteriovenous malformations.[100]

*William Osler, 1849-1919 (Canadian); Frederick Weber, 1863-1962 (British); Henri Rendu, 1844-1902 (French)—all physicians*

**Paget's disease of the breast (PDB)** Intra-epidermal spread of an intraduct cancer, which can look just like eczema. ►Any red, scaly lesion at the nipple (see fig 2) *must* suggest PDB: do a biopsy. ℞: Breast conserving surgery + radiotherapy. Sentinal node biopsy should be performed.[101] *Sir James Paget, 1814-1899 (British surgeon)*

**Pancoast's syndrome** Apical lung ca invades the sympathetic plexus in the neck (→ipsilateral Horner's, p716) ± brachial plexus (→arm pain ± weakness) ± recurrent laryngeal nerve (→hoarse voice/bovine cough). *Henry Pancoast, 1875-1939 (US radiologist)*

**Parinaud's syndrome** (dorsal midbrain syndrome) Upward gaze palsy + pseudo-Argyll Robertson pupils (p79) ± bilateral papilloedema. *Causes:* pineal or midbrain tumours; upper brainstem stroke; MS. *Henry Parinaud, 1844-1905 (French neuro-ophthalmologist)*

**Peutz-Jeghers' syndrome** Autosomal dominant Germline mutations of tumour suppressor gene STK11 (in 66-94%) cause mucocutaneous dark freckles on lips (fig 3), oral mucosa, palms and soles + multiple GI polyps (hamartomas), causing obstruction, intussusception or bleeds. There is a 15-fold ↑ risk of developing GI cancer.∴ perform colonoscopy (from age 18yrs) and OGD (from age 25yrs) every 3yrs. NB: hamartomas are excessive focal overgrowths of normal cells in an organ composed of the same cell type. *Johannes LA Peutz, 1886-1957 (Dutch physician); Harold J Jeghers, 1904-1990 (US physician)*

**Peyronie's disease** (penile angulation) *Pathogenesis:* A poorly understood connective tissue disorder most commonly attributed to repetitive microvascular trauma during sexual intercourse, resulting in penile curvature and painful erectile dysfunction in 50%; p222). *Prevalence:* 3-9%. *Typical age:* >40. *Associations:* Dupuytren's (p712); endothelial dysfunction; atheroma; radical prostatectomy. ΔΔ: Haemangioma. *Tests:* Ultrasound/MRI. ℞: Oral potassium para-aminobenzoate (*Potaba®*), intralesional *verapamil*, *clostridial collagenase* or *interferon* α2B; topical *verapamil* 15% gel; iontophoresis with verapamil and dexamethasone. All have various success.[102] *Surgery:* (if disease stable for >3 months) tunica plication ± penile prostheses (may help penetration). Manage associated depression (seen in 48%). Penile rehabilitation can help (p222).[103] *Francois Gigot de la Peyronie, 1678-1747 (French surgeon)*

**Pott's syndrome** (spinal TB). Rare in the West, this is usually from an extra-spinal source, eg lungs. *Features:* Backache, and stiffness of *all* back movements. Fever, night sweats and weight loss occur. Progressive bone destruction leads to vertebral collapse and gibbus (sharply angled spinal curvature). Abscess formation may lead to cord compression, causing paraplegia, and bowel/bladder dysfunction (p470). *x-rays:* (fig 4) Narrow disc spaces and vertebral osteoporosis, leading to destruction with wedging of vertebrae. Lesions in the thoracic spine often lead to kyphosis. Abscess formation in the lumbar spine may track down to the psoas muscle, and erode through the skin. ℞: Anti-TB drugs (p398). *Sir Percival Pott, 1714-1788 (British surgeon)*

**Prinzmetal (variant) angina** Angina from coronary artery spasm, which may lead to MI, ventricular arrhythmias or sudden death. Severe chest pain occurs **without** physical exertion. Triggers include hyperventilation, cocaine and tobacco use. ECG: ST elevation. ℞: Establish the diagnosis. GTN treats angina. Use Ca²⁺-channel blockers (p110) and long-acting nitrates as prophylaxis. *Myron Prinzmetal, 1908-1987 (US cardiologist)*

**Raynaud's syndrome** This is peripheral digital ischaemia due to paroxysmal vasospasm, precipitated by cold or emotion. Fingers or toes ache and change colour: pale (ischaemia) →blue (deoxygenation) →red (reactive hyperaemia). It may be idiopathic (Raynaud's *disease*—prevalence: 3-20%; ♀:♂ >1:1) or have an underlying cause (Raynaud's *phenomenon*; fig 5). *Tests:* Exclude an underlying cause (see BOX). ℞: Keep warm (eg hand warmers); stop smoking. *Nifedipine* 5-20mg/8h PO helps, as may evening primrose oil, *sildenafil*, and prostacyclin (for severe attacks/digital gangrene). Relapse is common. Chemical or surgical (lumbar or digital) sympathectomy may help in those with severe disease. *AG Maurice Raynaud, 1834-1881 (French physician)*

## Prinzmetal angina and vascular hyperreactivity

Coronary spasm causes Prinzmetal angina and also contributes to coronary heart disease in general, eg acute coronary syndrome (esp. in Japan).[104] Coronary spasm can be induced by ergonovine, acetylcholine, and methacholine (the former is used diagnostically).[1] These cause vasodilatation by endothelium-derived relaxing factor when vascular endothelium is functioning normally, whereas they cause vasoconstriction if the endothelium is damaged. In the light of these facts, patients with coronary spasm are thought to have a disturbance in endothelial function as well as local hyperreactivity of the coronary arteries.

If full anti-anginal therapy does not reduce symptoms, stenting[105] or intra-coronary radiation (20Gy brachytherapy) to vasospastic segments may be tried.[106]

Prognosis is good (especially if non-smoker, no past MI, and no diabetes; progress to infarction is quite rare);[107] there is evidence that prognosis may be better with the new calcium-channel blockers such as *benidipine*.[108] β-blockers and large doses of aspirin are contraindicated.

Prinzmetal angina is associated with vascular hyperreactivity/vasospastic disorders such as Raynaud's phenomenon and migraine. It is also associated with Circle of Willis occlusion from intimal thickening (moyamoya disease).

Fig 1. Telangiectasia in Osler-Weber-Rendu syndrome.

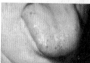

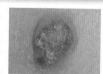

Fig 2. Paget's disease of the breast.

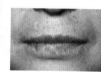

Fig 3. Perioral pigmentation, seen in Peutz-Jeghers' syndrome.

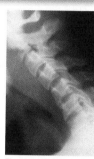

Fig 4. TB of axis: soft tissue swelling displaces the retropharyngeal air-tissue boundary forwards. There is an anterior defect in the vertebra, below the axis peg.

Figures courtesy of: Figs 1 & 3: Cox & Roper, *Clinical Skills*, 2005; Fig 4: Dr Ian Maddison, myweb.lsbu.ac.uk; Fig 5 the Crookston Collection.

## Conditions in which Raynaud's phenomenon may be exhibited[2]

*Connective tissue disorders:* Systemic sclerosis, SLE, rheumatoid arthritis, dermatomyositis/polymyositis.

*Occupational:* Using vibrating tools.

*Obstructive:* Thoracic outlet obstruction, Buerger's disease, atheroma.

*Blood:* Thrombocytosis, cold agglutinin disease, polycythaemia rubra vera (p360), monoclonal gammopathies.

*Drugs:* β-blockers.

*Others:* Hypothyroidism.

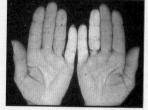

Fig 5. Raynaud's phenomenon in SLE.

ABC

1 Since Prinzmetal angina is not a 'demand-induced' symptom, but a supply (vasospastic) abnormality, exercise tolerance tests don't help. The most sensitive and specific test is IV ergonvine; 50μg at 5min intervals in a specialist lab until a +ve result or 400μg is given. When positive, the symptoms and ↑ST should be present. Nitroglycerin rapidly reverses the effects of ergonovine if refractory spasm occurs.[108]
2 Patient information on Raynaud's is available from **www.raynauds.org.uk**.

**Refsum disease** Autosomal recessive Phytanic acid accumulates in tissues and serum, due to *PHYH* or *PEX7* gene mutation. This leads to anosmia (a universal finding) and early-onset retinitis pigmentosa, with variable combinations of neuropathy, deafness, ataxia, ichthyosis and cardiomyopathy. *Tests:* Plasma phytanic acid↑. *R:* Restrict foods containing phytanic acid (animal fats, dairy products, green leafy vegetables); plasmapheresis is used for severe symptoms.[110]   *Sigvald Bernhard Refsum, 1907-1991 (Norwegian physician)*

**Romano-Ward syndrome** Autosomal dominant A mutation in a $K^+$ channel subunit causes long QT syndrome ± episodic VT, VF, *torsades* ± sudden death. (Jervell and Lange-Nielsen syn is similar, p716.)   *Cesarino Romano, 1924-2008 (Italian paediatrician); Owen C Ward, b1923 (Irish paediatrician)*

**Rotor syndrome** Autosomal recessive ⚥ A rare benign disorder of primary non-haemolytic conjugated hyperbilirubinaemia, with almost normal hepatic histology (without pigmentation, in contrast to DJS, p712).[111] Typically presents in childhood with mild jaundice. Cholescintigraphy reveals an 'absent' liver.   *Arturo Belleza Rotor, 1907-1988 (Filipino physician)*

**Sister Mary Joseph nodule** An umbilical metastatic nodule from an intra-abdominal malignancy (fig 1).   *Sister Mary Joseph Dempsey, 1856-1939 (US catholic nun & Dr William Mayo's surgical assistant)*

**Sjögren's syndrome** A chronic inflammatory autoimmune disorder, which may be primary (♀:♂≈9:1, onset 4th-5th decade) or secondary, associated with connective tissue disease (eg RA, SLE, systemic sclerosis). There is lymphocytic infiltration and fibrosis of exocrine glands, especially lacrimal and salivary glands. *Features:* ↓tear production (dry eyes, keratoconjunctivitis sicca), ↓salivation (xerostomia—dry mouth, caries), parotid swelling. Other glands are affected causing vaginal dryness, dyspareunia, dry cough and dysphagia. Systemic signs include polyarthritis/arthralgia, Raynaud's, lymphadenopathy, vasculitis, lung, liver and kidney involvement, peripheral neuropathy, myositis and fatigue. It is associated with other autoimmune diseases (eg thyroid disease, autoimmune hepatitis, PBC) and an ↑risk of non-Hodgkin's B-cell lymphoma. *Tests:* Schirmer's test measures conjunctival dryness (<5mm in 5min is +ve). Rose Bengal staining may show keratitis (use a slit-lamp). Anti-Ro (SSA; in 40%) & anti-La (SSB; in 26%) antibodies may be present (in pregnancy, these cross the placenta and cause fetal congenital heart block in 5%). ANA is usually +ve (74%); rheumatoid factor is +ve in 38%.[112] There may be hypergammaglobulinaemia. Biopsy shows focal lymphocytic aggregation. *R:* Treat sicca symptoms: eg *hypromellose* (artificial tears), frequent drinks, sugar-free pastilles/gum. NSAIDs and *hydroxychloroquine* are used for arthralgia. Immunosuppressants may be indicated in severe systemic disease.[113]   *Henrik Conrad Samuel Sjögren, 1899-1986 (Swedish ophthalmologist)*

**Stevens-Johnson syndrome** A severe form of erythema multiforme (p564), and a variant of toxic epidermal necrolysis. It is caused by a hypersensitivity reaction, usually to drugs (eg salicylates, sulfonamides, penicillin, barbiturates, carbamazepine, phenytoin), but is also seen with infections or cancer. There is ulceration of the skin and mucosal surfaces (see fig 2). Typical target lesions develop, often on the palms or soles with blistering in the centre. There may be a prodromal phase with fever, malaise, arthralgia, myalgia ± vomiting and diarrhoea. *R:* Mild disease is usually self-limiting—remove any precipitant and give supportive care (eg calamine lotion for the skin). Steroid use is controversial—trials have been variable, so ask a dermatologist and ophthalmologist. IV immunoglobulin has shown benefit. Plasmapheresis and immunosuppressive agents may have a role.[114] *Prognosis:* Mortality ~5%. May be severe for the first 10d before resolving over 30d. Damage to the eyes may persist and blindness can result.[115]   *Albert M Stevens 1884-1945; Frank C Johnson, 1894-1934 (US paediatricians)*

**Sturge-Weber syndrome (SWS)** Essential features: 1 facial cutaneous capillary malformation (port wine stain; PWS) in the ophthalmic dermatome (V1 ± V2/V3) 2 clinical signs or radiologic evidence of a leptomeningeal vascular malformation. 75% of patients with unilateral involvement develop seizures by age 1yr (95% if bilateral)—due (in part) to the increased metabolic demand of a developing brain in the setting of vascular compromise. Early management of seizures is critical to minimize brain injury. Some patients have cognitive and neurologic deficits beyond simple seizure activity. Screen early for glaucoma (50%). EEG and MRI help establish early diagnosis and treatment in patients at risk for SWS. Treat the PWS early with pulsed dye laser.   *William A Sturge, 1850-1919; Frederick P Weber, 1863-1962 (British physicians)*

## Causes of a long QT interval (eg Romano-Ward)

Many conditions and drugs (check *BNF*) cause a long QT interval. Brugada syndrome (p709) is similar, predisposing to sudden cardiac death.

*Congenital:* Romano-Ward syndrome (autosomal dominant). Jervell and Lange-Nielsen syndrome (autosomal recessive) with associated deafness (p716).

*Cardiac:* Myocardial infarction or ischaemia; mitral valve prolapse.

*HIV:* May be a direct effect of the virus or from protease inhibitors.

*Metabolic:* K⁺↓; Mg²⁺↓; Ca²⁺↓; starvation; hypothyroidism; hypothermia.

*Toxic:* Organophosphates.

*Anti-arrhythmic drugs:* Quinidine; amiodarone; procainamide; sotalol.

*Antibiotics ᵉᵗ ᵃˡ:* Erythromycin; levofloxacin; pentamidine; halofantrine.

*Antihistamines:* Terfenadine; astemizole.

*Motility drugs:* Domperidone.

*Psychoactive drugs:* Haloperidol; risperidone; tricyclics; SSRIs.

*Connective tissue diseases:* anti-RO/SSA antibodies (p554).

*Herbalism:* Ask about Chinese folk remedies (may contain unknown amounts of arsenic).[116,117] Cocaine, quinine and artemisinins (and other antimalarials) are examples of herbalism-derived products that can prolong the QT interval.

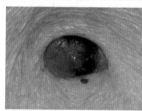

**Fig 1.** Sister Mary Joseph nodule.
Reproduced from 'Sister Joseph's Nodule', *Postgraduate Medical Journal*, J E Clague, 2002, with permission from BMJ Publishing Group Ltd.

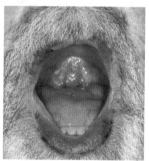

**Fig 2.** Stevens-Johnson syndrome.
Reproduced from Emberger *et al*, Stevens-Johnson syndrome associated with anti-malarial prophylaxis. *Clinical Infectious Diseases* (2003) 37:1, with permission from Oxford University Press.

ABC

**Takayasu's arteritis** (aortic arch syndrome; pulseless disease) Rare outside of Japan, this systemic vasculitis affects the aorta and its major branches. Granulomatous inflammation causes stenosis, thrombosis and aneurysms. It often affects women aged 20-40yrs. Symptoms depend on the arteries involved. The aortic arch is often affected, with cerebral, ophthalmological and upper limb symptoms, eg dizziness, visual changes, weak arm pulses. Systemic features are common—eg fever, weight loss and malaise. ↑BP is often a feature, due to renal artery stenosis. Complications include aortic valve regurgitation, aortic aneurysm and dissection; ischaemic stroke (↑BP and thrombus); and ischaemic heart disease. *Diagnosis:* ↑ESR and CRP; MRI/PET allows earlier diagnosis than standard angiography. ℞: Prednisolone (1mg/kg/d PO). Methotrexate or cyclophosphamide have been used in resistant cases. BP control is essential to ↓risk of stroke. Angioplasty ± stenting, or bypass surgery is performed for critical stenosis. *Prognosis:* ~95% survival at 15 years. *Mikito Takayasu, 1860-1938 (Japanese ophthalmologist)*

**Tietze's syndrome** (idiopathic costochondritis) Localized pain/tenderness at the costosternal junction, enhanced by motion, coughing, or sneezing. The 2nd rib is most often affected. The diagnostic key is *localized* tenderness which is marked (flinches on prodding). *Treatment:* Simple analgesia, eg NSAIDs. Its importance is that it is a benign cause of what at first seems to be alarming, eg cardiac pain. In lengthy illness, local steroid injections may be used. *Alexander Tietze, 1864-1927 (German surgeon)*

**Todd's palsy** Transient neurological deficit (paresis) after a seizure. There may be face, arm or leg weakness, aphasia or gaze palsy, lasting from ~30min-36h.[118] The aetiology is unclear. *Robert Bentley Todd, 1809-1860 (Irish-born physician)*

**Vincent's angina** (necrotizing ulcerative gingivitis) Mouth infection with ulcerative gingivitis from *Borrelia vincentii* (a spirochete) + fusiform bacilli, often affecting young ♂ smokers with poor oral hygiene. Try amoxicillin 500mg/8h and metronidazole 400mg/8h PO, + chlorhexidine mouthwash. *Jean Hyacinthe Vincent, 1862-1950 (French physician)*

**Von Hippel-Lindau syndrome** ᴬᵘᵗᵒˢᵒᵐᵃˡ ᵈᵒᵐⁱⁿᵃⁿᵗ A germline mutation of a tumour suppressor gene. It predisposes to bilateral renal cysts (with ↑risk of transformation to renal cell cancer), retinal and cerebellar haemangioblastoma, and phaeochromocytoma. See figs 1 & 2. It may present with visual impairment or cerebellar signs (eg unilateral ataxia). *Eugen von Hippel, 1867-1939 (German ophthalmologist); Arvid Lindau, 1892-1958 (Swedish pathologist)*

**Von Willebrand's disease (VWD)** Von Willebrand's factor (VWF) has 3 roles in clotting: 1 to bring platelets into contact with exposed subendothelium, 2 to make platelets bind to each other, and 3 to bind to factor VIII, protecting it from destruction in the circulation. There are >22 types of VWD; the commonest are:

*Type I:* (60-80%) ᴬᵘᵗᵒˢᵒᵐᵃˡ ᵈᵒᵐⁱⁿᵃⁿᵗ Deficiency (↓levels) of VWF. Symptoms are mild.

*Type II:* (20-30%) Abnormal VWF, with lack of high molecular weight multimers. Usually autosomal dominant inheritance. Bleeding tendency varies. There are 4 subtypes.

*Type III:* (1-5%) Undetectable VWF levels (autosomal recessive with gene deletions). VWF antigen is lacking and there is ↓factor VIII. Symptoms can be severe.

*Signs* are of a platelet-type disorder (p338): bruising, epistaxis, menorrhagia, ↑bleeding post-tooth extraction. *Tests:* APTT↑, bleeding time↑, factor VIIIC↓ (clotting activity), VWF Ag↓; INR and platelets ↔. ℞: Get expert help. Desmopressin is used in mild bleeding, VWF-containing factor VIII concentrate for surgery or major bleeds. Avoid NSAIDs. *Erik Adolf von Willebrand, 1870-1949 (Finnish physician)*

**Wallenberg's lateral medullary syndrome** This relatively common syndrome comprises lesions to multiple CNS nuclei, caused by posterior or inferior cerebellar artery occlusion leading to brainstem infarction (fig 3). *Features:* •Dysphagia, dysarthria (IX and X nuclei) •Vertigo, nausea, vomiting, nystagmus (vestibular nucleus) •Ipsilateral ataxia (inferior cerebellar peduncle) •Ipsilateral Horner's syndrome (descending sympathetic fibres) •Loss of pain and temperature sensation on the ipsilateral face (V nucleus) and contralateral limbs (spinothalamic tract). There is no limb weakness as the pyramidal tracts are unaffected.

In the rarer *medial medullary syndrome*, vertebral or anterior spinal artery occlusion causes ipsilateral tongue paralysis (XII nucleus) with contralateral limb weakness (pyramidal tract, sparing the face) and loss of position sense.

*Adolf Wallenberg, 1862-1949 (German neurologist)*

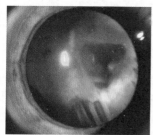

Fig 1. Von Hippel-Lindau syndrome showing retinal detachment.

Reproduced with permission from the National Eye Institute, National Institutes of Health.

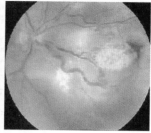

Fig 2. Von Hippel-Lindau syndrome showing a retinal tumour.

Reproduced with permission from the National Eye Institute, National Institutes of Health.

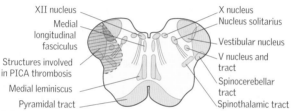

Fig 3. Cross section of the medulla showing structures involved in Wallenberg's lateral medullary syndrome (posterior inferior cerebellar artery thrombosis).

**Waterhouse-Friderichsen's (WhF) syndrome** Bilateral adrenal cortex haemorrhage, often occurring in rapidly deteriorating meningococcal sepsis, alongside widespread purpura, meningitis, coma, and DIC (fig 1). The meningococcal endotoxin acts as a potent initiator of inflammatory and coagulation cascades. Other causes include *H. influenzae*, pneumococcal, streptococcal, and staphylococcal sepsis. Adrenal failure causes shock, as normal vascular tone requires cortisol to set activity of alpha and beta adrenergic receptors, and aldosterone is needed to maintain extracellular fluid volume. *Treatment:* ►►Antibiotics, eg *ceftriaxone* (p832) and hydrocortisone 200mg/4h IV for adrenal support. ICU admission. *Rupert Waterhouse 1873-1958 (British physician); Carl Friderichsen, 1886-1979 (Danish paediatrician)*

**Weber's syndrome** (superior alternating hemiplegia) Ipsilateral oculomotor nerve palsy with contralateral hemiplegia, due to infarction of one-half of the midbrain, after occlusion of the paramedian branches of the basilar or posterior cerebral arteries. *Herman David Weber, 1823-1918 (German-born physician whose son described Sturge-Weber syndrome)*

**Wegener's\* granulomatosis** This has been renamed granulomatosis with polyangiitis (GPA), in part because of concerns over the suitability of Friedrich Wegener, a member of the Nazi party during WWII, to be the source of an eponym.[119] GPA is a multisystem disorder of unknown cause characterized by necrotizing granulomatous inflammation and vasculitis of small and medium vessels. It has a predilection for the upper respiratory tract, lungs and kidneys. *Features:* Upper airways disease is common, with nasal obstruction, ulcers, epistaxis, or destruction of the nasal septum causing a characteristic 'saddle-nose' deformity.[1] Sinusitis is often a feature. Renal disease causes rapidly progressive glomerulonephritis with crescent formation, proteinuria or haematuria. Pulmonary involvement may cause cough, haemoptysis (severe if pulmonary haemorrhage) or pleurisy. There may also be skin purpura or nodules, peripheral neuropathy, mononeuritis multiplex, arthritis/arthralgia or ocular involvement, eg keratitis, conjunctivitis, scleritis, episcleritis, uveitis. *Tests:* cANCA directed against PR3 is most specific and raised in the majority of patients (p555). Some patients express pANCA specific for MPO. ↑ESR/CRP. Urinalysis should be performed to look for proteinuria or haematuria. If these are present, consider a renal biopsy. CXR may show nodules ± fluffy infiltrates of pulmonary haemorrhage. CT may reveal diffuse alveolar haemorrhage. Atypical cells from cytology of sputum/BAL can be confused with bronchial carcinoma.[120] *Treatment:* Depends on the extent of disease. Severe disease (eg biopsy-proven renal disease) should be treated with corticosteroids and *cyclophosphamide* (or *rituximab*) to induce remission. *Azathioprine* and *methotrexate* are usually used as maintenance. Patients with severe renal disease (eg creatinine >500μmol/L) may benefit from plasma exchange in addition. *Co-trimoxazole* should be given as prophylaxis against *Pneumocystis jiroveci* and staphylococcal colonization. *Friedrich Wegener, 1907-1990 (German pathologist)*

**Wernicke's encephalopathy** Thiamine (vitamin B₁) deficiency with a classical triad of 1 confusion 2 ataxia (wide-based gait; fig 2) and 3 ophthalmoplegia (nystagmus, lateral rectus or conjugate gaze palsies). There is inadequate dietary intake, ↓ GI absorption and impaired utilization of thiamine resulting in focal areas of brain damage, including periaqueductal punctate haemorrhages (mechanism unclear). Always consider this diagnosis in alcoholics: it may also present with memory disturbance, hypotension, hypothermia, or reduced consciousness. *Recognized causes:* Chronic alcoholism, eating disorders, malnutrition, prolonged vomiting, eg with chemotherapy, GI malignancy or hyperemesis gravidarum. *Diagnosis:* Primarily clinical. Red cell transketolase activity is decreased (rarely done). *Treatment:* Urgent replacement to prevent irreversible Korsakoff's syndrome (p718). Give *thiamine* (Pabrinex®) 2 pairs of high-potency ampoules IV/IM/8h over 30min for 2d, then 1 pair OD for a further 5d. Oral supplementation (100mg OD) should continue until no longer 'at risk' (+ give other B vitamins). Anaphylaxis is rare. If there is coexisting hypoglycaemia (often the case in this group of patients), make sure thiamine is given before glucose, as Wernicke's can be precipitated by glucose administration to a thiamine-deficient patient. *Prognosis:* Untreated, death occurs in 20%, and Korsakoff's psychosis occurs in 85%—a quarter of whom will require long-term institutional care. *Karl Wernicke, 1848-1905 (German neurologist)*

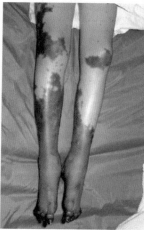

Fig 1. Meningococcal sepsis with purpura.

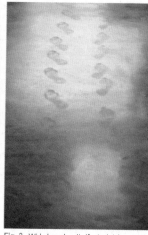

Fig 2. Wide-based gait (footprints), seen in Wernicke's encephalopathy. Before jumping to the conclusion that these footprints are those of an *OHCM* author on the way back from the pub, bear in mind that alcohol is not the only cause of Wernicke's: think of rapidly growing tumours, malabsorption, hyperemesis gravidarum, hyperthyroidism, and prolonged vomiting of any cause.[121]

**1** Common causes of a 'saddle-nose' deformity are trauma and iatrogenic (eg post-rhinoplasty). Rarer causes (popular with some finals examiners): GPA, relapsing polychondritis, syphilis, and leprosy.

**Whipple's disease**[122] A rare disease featuring GI malabsorption which usually occurs in middle-aged white males, most commonly in Europe. It is fatal if untreated and is caused by *Tropheryma whippelii*, which, combined with defective cell-mediated immunity, produces a systemic disease. *Features:* Often starts insidiously with arthralgia (chronic, migratory, seronegative arthropathy affecting mainly peripheral joints). GI symptoms commonly include colicky abdominal pain, weight loss, steatorrhea/diarrhoea, which leads to malabsorption (p280). Systemic symptoms such as chronic cough, fever, sweats, lymphadenopathy and skin hyperpigmentation also occur. Cardiac involvement may lead to endocarditis, which is typically blood culture negative. CNS features include a reversible dementia, ophthalmoplegia, and facial myoclonus (if all together, they are highly suggestive)—also hypothalamic syndrome (hyperphagia, polydipsia, insomnia). NB: CNS involvement may occur without GI involvement. *Tests:* Diagnosis requires a high level of clinical suspicion. Jejunal biopsy shows stunted villi. There is deposition of macrophages in the lamina propria-containing granules which stain positive for Periodic Acid-Schiff (PAS). Similar cells may be found in affected samples, eg CSF, cardiac valve tissue, lymph nodes, synovial fluid. The bacteria may be seen within macrophages on electron microscopy. PCR of bacterial RNA can be performed on serum or tissue. MRI may demonstrate CNS involvement. *R:* Should include antibiotics which cross the blood-brain barrier. Current recommendations: IV *ceftriaxone* (or penicillin+streptomycin) for 2wks then oral *co-trimoxazole* for some months. Shorter courses risk relapse. A rapid improvement in symptoms usually occurs. *George Hoyt Whipple, 1878-1976 (US pathologist)*

**Zellweger syndrome** (cerebrohepatorenal syndrome) Autosomal recessive A rare disorder characterized by absent peroxisomes (intracellular organelles required for many cellular activities including lipid metabolism). The syndrome has a similar molecular basis to infantile Refsum's syndrome, and although more severe, exhibits comparable biochemical abnormalities (p724). Clinical features include craniofacial abnormalities, severe hypotonia and mental retardation, glaucoma, cataracts, hepatomegaly and renal cysts. A number of causative PEX gene mutations have been identified. Life expectancy is usually a few months only. *Hans Zellweger, 1909-1990 (US paediatrician)*

**Zollinger-Ellison syndrome** This is the association of peptic ulcers with a gastrin-secreting adenoma (gastrinoma). Gastrin excites excessive gastric acid production, which may produce multiple ulcers in the duodenum and stomach. The adenoma is usually found in the pancreas, although it may arise in the stomach or duodenum. Most cases are sporadic; 20% are associated with multiple endocrine neoplasia, type 1 (MEN1, p215). 60% are malignant; metastases are found in local lymph nodes and the liver. *Symptoms:* Include abdominal pain and dyspepsia, from the ulcer(s), and chronic diarrhoea due to inactivation of pancreatic enzymes (also causes steatorrhoea) and damage to intestinal mucosa. *Incidence:* ~0.1% of patients with peptic ulcer disease. Suspect in those with multiple peptic ulcers, ulcers distal to the duodenum, or a family history of peptic ulcers (or of islet cell, pituitary, or parathyroid adenomas). *Tests:* (fig 1) ↑Fasting serum gastrin level (>1000pg/mL). Measure 3 fasting levels on different days. Hypochlorhydria (reduced acid production, eg in chronic atrophic gastritis) should be excluded as this also causes a raised gastrin level: gastric pH should be <2. The secretin stimulation test is useful in suspected cases with only mildly raised gastrin levels (100-1000pg/mL). The adenoma is often small and difficult to image; a combination of somatostatin receptor scintigraphy, endoscopic ultrasound and CT is used to localize and stage the adenoma. OGD evaluates gastric/duodenal ulceration. *R:* High-dose proton pump inhibitors (PPIs), eg *omeprazole*: start with 60mg/d and adjust according to response. Measuring intragastric pH helps determine the best dose (aim to keep pH at 2-7). All gastrinomas have malignant potential—and surgery is better sooner than later (with lymph node clearance generally recommended if >2cm in size). Surgery may be avoided in MEN1, as adenomas are often multiple, and metastatic disease is rare. If well-differentiated (G1 and G2) somatostatin analogues may be 1st-line and chemotherapy with *streptozotocin* (if available) + *doxorubicin*/5-FU is 2nd-line. In G3, *etoposide* + *cisplatin* is possible.[123] Selective embolization may be done for hepatic metastases. *Prognosis:* 5yr survival: 80% if single resectable lesion, ~20% with hepatic metastases. Screen all patients for MEN1. *Robert M Zollinger, 1903-1992; Edwin H Ellison, 1918-1970 (US surgeons)*

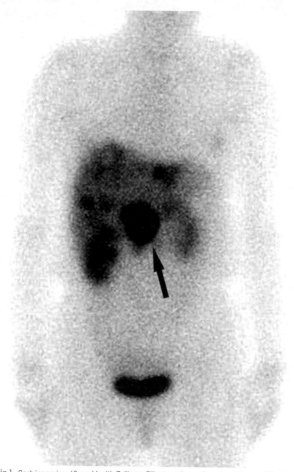

**Fig 1.** Gastrinoma in a 68-yr-old with Zollinger-Ellison syndrome. Serum gastrin was 158pg/mL (normal, 8-47pg/mL). This rather ghostly anterior $^{111}$indium pentetreotide image shows focal radiotracer uptake in the pancreatic head (arrow), the primary tumour. Note multiple liver metastases.

Courtesy of Charles Intenzo. *Scintigraphic Imaging of Body Neuroendocrine Tumors.* C Intenzo, S Jabbour, H Lin, J Miller, S Kim, D Capuzzi E Mitchell. *RadioGraphics* 2007 27 1355–1356. RSNA[124]

### Epilogue

25% of patients with rare diseases have to wait from 5-30 years for a diagnosis. 40% are misdiagnosed resulting in inappropriate drugs or psychological treatments—eg 20% of people with Ehlers-Danlos syndrome (p143) had to consult over 20 doctors before the diagnosis was made,[125] causing understandable loss of confidence in our profession. Lack of appropriate referral and rejection because of disease complexity are common problems. Let us cultivate our networks with each other and approach 'unexplained symptoms' with an open mind.

ABC

### Contents

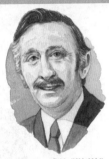

Fig 1. Godfrey Hounsfield (1919–2004). Joint winner of the 1979 Nobel Prize for Physiology or Medicine, Godfrey Hounsfield was an electrical engineer who began working on the CT scanner as a way of using x-rays to find out what was in a closed box. He constructed a computer to compile an image from multiple x-rays at different angles, creating slices that could be combined to form a 3D image. He then began testing this for potential medical applications, memorably being caught on the London tube carrying a bullock's brain for testing in an experimental whole body scanner! His name lives on in the Hounsfield scale, a measure of radiodensity used to define the images produced from CT scanners, ranging from air at -1000 Hounsfield Units, through water at 0 HU up to bone at 1000 HU.

**Other relevant pages** Chest medicine (Chapter 4); echocardiography (p106); further investigations in chest medicine (p158); cerebral artery territories (p452).

### Images in other chapters

*CXR:* Cavitating lung cancer (p155); lung metastasis (p171); idiopathic pulmonary fibrosis (p190); industrial dust diseases (p193); correct PICC line (p589); incorrect subclavian line (p589); pneumoperitoneum (p609).

*CT:* Stroke (p81 & p453); hiatus hernia (p245); liver metastases (p271); retroperitoneal fibrosis (p643); sub-arachnoid haemorrhage (p483, with 3DCT reconstruction); subdural and extradural haematomas (p487); pancreatic pseudocyst (p639); endovascular aortic stent (p657); SBO (p613); large bowel obstruction (p613); caecal cancer (p619); oesophageal cancer (p621).

*MRI:* Pituitary adenoma (p227); stroke (p475); superior sagittal sinus thrombosis (MR venogram, p485); cervical spondylosis (p512); the cauda equina (p783).

*US:* Compression US/US imaging of DVT (p579); torsion of the hydatid of Morgagni and testis cancer (p652); hydronephrosis (p645); thyroid lesion (p603).

*Nuclear medicine:* Graves' disease (p603); gastrinoma (p731).

*ERCP/MRCP:* Primary sclerosing cholangitis (p267).

*Contrast studies:* Oesophageal cancer (p241); parotid sialogram (p601).

*DSA:* Lower limb (p659).

*We thank Dr Edmund Godfrey, Dr Jennie Roberts and Professor Peter Scally, our Specialist Readers for this chapter, and Dr Tom Turmezei, who originated it. We also thank our Junior Reader, Manish Verma. Unless specified, all images are courtesy of Leeds Teaching Hospitals NHS Trust.*

## Typical effective doses

The effective dose of an examination is calculated as the weighted sum of the doses to different body tissues. The weighting factor for each tissue depends on its sensitivity. The effective dose thus provides a single dose estimate related to the total radiation risk, no matter how the radiation dose is distributed around the body. This table is certainly not to be learnt; rather it serves as a reminder of the relative exposures to radiation that we prescribe in practice. ►Remember that US and MRI involve no radiation, would they provide the answer?

| Procedure | Typical effective dose (mSv) | CXR equivalents | Approx. equivalent period of background radiation[1] |
|---|---|---|---|
| **X-ray examinations** | | | |
| Limbs and joints | <0.01 | <0.5 | <1.5 days |
| Chest (PA) | 0.02 | 1 | 3 days |
| Abdomen | 1 | 50 | 6 months |
| Lumbar spine | 1.3 | 65 | 7 months |
| CT head | 2.3 | 115 | 1 year |
| CT chest | 8 | 400 | 3.6 years |
| CT abdo/pelvis | 10 | 500 | 4.5 years |
| **Radionuclide studies** | | | |
| Lung ventilation | 0.3 | 15 | 7 weeks |
| Lung perfusion | 1 | 50 | 6 months |
| Bone | 4 | 200 | 1.8 years |
| PET head | 5 | 250 | 2.3 years |
| PET-CT | 10–20 | 500 | 4.5–9 years |

After *Making the Best Use of Department of Clinical Radiology*, 5e RCOR; with permission.

## Justifying exposure to ionizing radiation

The very nature of ionizing radiation that gives us vision into the human body also gives it lethal properties. The decision to expose patients to radiation must be made with the risks in mind, and even with strict guidelines we still have a tendency to over-exposure in medical practice. So when requesting an examination, the clinical benefits should outweigh the risks of cancer induction and genetic mutation.

The responsibility lies with us not to rely too heavily on radiology. ►Don't request examinations to comfort patients, or to replace lost images, or when the result will not affect management. To give an idea of relative doses, a CT of the abdomen and pelvis gives a typical effective dose of 500 times as much radiation as a CXR (see TABLE). This important factor also tells us about the preference of ultrasound over CT when investigating abdominal and pelvic complaints such as acute appendicitis, especially given the youthful demographics of this diagnosis. Avoid irradiating someone simply to avoid medico-legal issues.

►Unwitting exposure of the unborn fetus to radiation is inexcusable at any stage of gestation—unless the mother's life is in immediate danger—and it is the responsibility of the referring clinician to ensure that this is avoided. Discuss beforehand with the patient that you would like to do a pregnancy test, explaining why, being broad in your suppositions and tactful in your inquisitions.

One of the most nerve-wracking moments that you can encounter as a recently qualified doctor is having to request an investigation face-to-face with a seasoned consultant radiologist. Imagine that you have been asked by your team to request an ultrasound examination of the renal tract for one of your patients who has a newly raised creatinine of 300µmol/L. You aren't quite sure what to write on the request form; however, they have already moved on to the next patient. What do you write? How much do you write? Who do you ask? Put yourself on the other side. If you were a radiologist, how would you prioritize who needed what imaging and when? Keep the following in mind when requesting (never ordering!) an investigation:

1 **Patient details**
2 **Clinical details**
3 **Investigation details**

This can be broadly broken down into:

• **Who:** ▸Get the patient's name right! Include hospital number and date of birth on all requests.

• **What:** think of your clinical question, what scan do you think is required? What answer are you hoping it will give? (See MINIBOX.)

> **Radiology can help:**
> • Confirm a suspected diagnosis
> • 'Exclude' something important: remember that exclusion is never 100%
> • Define the extent of a disease
> • Monitor the progress of a disease

• **Why:** give clinical details, remember that the radiologist ultimately decides what imaging they undertake. The information you give may change the type of scan they choose, a CT chest can look at lungs, arteries, veins, soft tissues, and more. Different questions require different protocols. If you think the patient has a collection, would you like them to drain it? Always include ± intervention on the request form (eg US abdo ± drain insertion) if you think this may be required.

• **How:** it is also important to mention pertinent facts that may change the way the investigation can be carried out. For example, an agitated or confused patient may need sedation prior to an MRI of their head. A CT scan on a patient with a raised creatinine may need to be done without contrast medium. Insertion of a drain on a patient with deranged clotting may need to wait while this is corrected. Include recent creatinine, Hb and clotting on the form if appropriate. Don't forget to mention anticoagulants, eg warfarin, LMWH for intervention requests.

If in doubt, or if the investigation is very urgent, call or go down to the department in person. If you can do this for all investigations it is courteous to the radiologist, and you will learn a lot; however, they do appreciate there isn't the time to do this for every request. Radiologists appreciate being involved in the clinical decision and may be able to suggest a better way of answering your clinical question. Asking for an x-ray of the hip "fall ?#NOF" is straightforward. But "does this patient have a hepatic malignancy or is it an abscess" may require US, triple phase CT, or PET-CT.

*Pointers:*

• Know your patient well, but keep your request brief and accurate.
• Know the clinical question and how the answer will change your management.
• Look up previous imaging before you go; asking for a CT on a patient who had one yesterday makes you look foolish and will not go down well.

If your request is turned down, don't be afraid to (politely) ask why. If you or your team still feel it is warranted, look back at the request; did you miss a relevant piece of information that would change the mind of the radiologist? If you still draw a blank, try speaking to a radiologist who specializes in that particular technique. Many teams have clinical radiology meetings; think about approaching someone who appreciates why you are asking that particular question. Alternatively, go back to your team; speak to your senior, who may have a better understanding of why the investigation is needed and be able to convey this to the radiologist.

Ultimately though, remember that there is a patient at the heart of this. Don't be afraid to be their advocate. If the results of an investigation will change their management then explain this to the radiologist. Moreover, don't forget to explain it to your patient. Being whisked off to the department for investigation and intervention can be particularly terrifying if you aren't expecting it.

## Interpreting an image

You won't always be able to get a radiologist's interpretation (especially at night) so it is worth knowing broadly how to look at an image. ▶Firstly make sure the image you are looking at is of your patient. Check its date. Remembering the following points may help hone your own interpreting skills:

• **Practice makes perfect**—always look at the image before checking the report, learning how to distinguish normal from abnormal.
• **Understand how the scan is done**—makes interpretation easier and helps you appreciate which scan will give the answer you need. This also gives practical clues to the result—eg a routine CXR is performed in the postero-anterior (PA) direction (the source posterior to the patient to minimize the cardiac shadow).
• **Use a systematic approach** so that you don't miss subtleties. Don't worry, though—some things can be notoriously difficult to spot.
• **Understand your anatomy**—virtually all investigations yield a 2D image from a 3D structure (though technology keeps improving, see p745). An understanding of anatomical relationships of the area in question will help reconstruct the images in your mind.
• **Orientation**—for axial cross-sectional imaging this is as if you are looking up at the supine patient ▶from his feet. For images with non-conventional orientations (eg MRCP) look on the image for clue markings, or rely on your knowledge of anatomy—it can be tricky to visualize oblique sections!
• Remember an investigation is only one part of the clinical work-up, don't rely solely on the investigation result for your management decisions.
• Go back to see the patient after looking at the investigation and reading the radiologist's report: you might notice something that you didn't before.

## Presenting an image

Everyone has their own method for presenting, and the right way is **your own way**. As long as you cover everything systematically—because we all get 'hot-seat amnesia' at some point—the particulars will take care of themselves. Continue to polish your own method and remember a few extra tips for when an image is presented expectantly by your consultant/examiner and the floor is yours. A brief silence with a thoughtful expression as you analyse the image is fine, then...

• State the written details: name, date of birth, where and how the imaging was taken. Look for clues: weighting of an MRI, a '+ c' indicating that contrast medium has been used, the phase of the investigation (arterial/venous/portal), or even the name of the organ printed on an ultrasound.
• State the type, mode and technical quality of investigation—not always easy!

*Going through the above also gives you a bit of thinking time.* Then:

• Start with life-threatening or very obvious abnormalities. *Then be systematic:*
• Is the patient's position adequate? Any lines, leads or tubes? Note their position.
• Just like the bedside clues in a physical examination, there are clues in radiology examinations. Note oxygen masks, ECG leads, venous access, infusion apparatus, and invasive devices. Identifying what they are also helps you to look through what may otherwise appear to be a cluttered mess.
• Not everything on the image is inside the subject—some things may be on the surface/outside or not there at all, eg ring artefacts or 'stair-stepping'[1] on CT.
• Giving a differential diagnosis is good practice, as not all findings are diagnostic.
• If there is additional clinical information that would help you to make a diagnosis, don't be afraid to ask. After all, we treat patients and not images!

Remember:   •X-ray=**radiodensity** (lucency/opacity)   •CT=**attenuation**
               •US=**echogenicity**                      •MRI=**signal intensity**

---

**1** Geometry of helical CT causes periodic asymmetries and variable noise distribution, appearing as stripes (**zebra artefact**) or steps (**stair-stepping**) when surfaces are inclined relative to the table translation direction. These distort volume and diameter measurements (taking thinner slices helps).

Radiology

Images are usually taken on inspiration with the x-ray source behind the patient (postero-anterior, PA). Emergency mobile images may be antero-posterior (AP (fig 1, p741)), magnifying heart size and elevating the diaphragm. If supine, distribution of air and fluid in lungs and pleural cavities is altered.

Acclimatize yourself to the 4 cardinal elements of the chest radiograph, memorably (albeit slightly inaccurately) termed **bone, air, fat,** and 'water'/**soft tissue**. Each has its own radiographic density. ▶ *A border is only seen at an interface of 2 densities*, eg heart (soft tissue) and lung (air); this 'silhouette' is lost if air in the lung is replaced by consolidation ('water'). The silhouette sign localizes pathology (eg middle lobe pneumonia or collapse causing loss of clarity of the right heart border, fig 1). When interpreting a CXR use a systematic approach that works for you, eg from outside to inside, or inside-out. Start by assessing technical quality:

- **Rotation:** The sternal ends of the clavicles shouette overlie the transverse processes of the 4th or 5th thoracic vertebrae. A rotated film can alter the position of structures, eg rotation to the right projects the aortic arch vessels over the right upper zone, appearing as though there is a mass.
- **Inspiration:** There should be 5 to 7 ribs visible anteriorly (or 10 posteriorly). Hyperinflation can be abnormal, eg COPD. Poor inspiration can mimic cardiomegaly, as the heart is usually pulled down (hence elongated) with inspiration, and crowding of vessels at the lung bases can mimic consolidation or collapse. This is common in patients who are acutely unwell, particularly those in pain or unconscious. Take care in interpreting these images.
- **Exposure:** An under-exposed image will be too white and an over-exposed image will be too black. Both cause a loss of definition and quality. With modern software images can be adjusted, compensating for over-exposure more easily than underexposure.
- **Position:** The entire lung margins should be visible.

**Trachea** Normally central or just to the right. Deviated by collapse (towards the lesion), tension (away from the lesion), or patient rotation. Check heart position (below).

**Mediastinum** Widened by mediastinal fat; retrosternal thyroid; unfolded aorta, or aortic aneurysm; lymph node enlargement (sarcoidosis, lymphoma, metastases, TB); tumour (thymoma, teratoma); cysts (bronchogenic, pericardial); paravertebral mass (TB). There are 3 'moguls'[1] or lumps normally visible on the left border of the mediastinum that help identify pathology if abnormal. From superior to inferior they are: 1 Aortic knuckle 2 Pulmonary outflow tract 3 Left ventricle.

The mediastinum may be shifted towards a collapsed lung or away from processes that add volume (eg an effusion).

**Hila** The left hilum is higher than the right or at the same level (not lower); they should be the same size and density. May be pulled up or down by fibrosis or collapse. 1 *Enlarged hila:* Nodes; pulmonary arterial hypertension (± an enlarged 2nd mogul); bronchogenic ca. 2 *Calcification:* Sarcoid, past TB; silicosis; histoplasmosis (p440). Sarcoidosis, TB & lymphoma can give bilateral hilar + paratracheal lymphadenopathy.

**Heart** Normally less than half of the width of the thorax (cardiothoracic ratio <0.5). ⅓ should lie to the right of the vertebral column, ⅔ to the left. It may appear elongated if the chest is hyperinflated (COPD); or enlarged if the image is AP or if there is LV failure (fig 2), or a pericardial effusion. Are there calcified valves?

**Diaphragm** The right side is often slightly higher (due to the liver) *Causes of raised hemidiaphragm:* Trouble above the diaphragm—lung volume loss. Trouble with the diaphragm—stroke; phrenic nerve palsy (causes, p506; any mediastinal mass?). Trouble below the diaphragm—hepatomegaly; subphrenic abscess. NB: subpulmonic effusion (effusions having a similar contour to the diaphragm without a characteristic meniscus) and diaphragm rupture give apparent elevation. NB: bilateral palsies (polio, muscular dystrophy) cause hypoxia.

---

1 It's as if skiing down the left heart border creates these moguls or bumps of radio-opaque 'snow'.

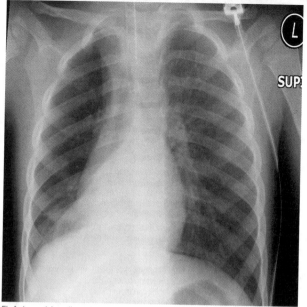

**Fig 1.** Lower lobe collapse (right lung). The right heart border is obscured and there is also volume loss in the right lower zone.

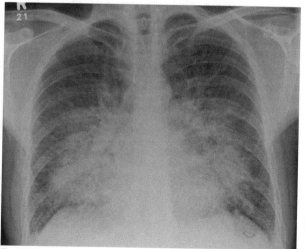

**Fig 2.** 'Bat's wing' pulmonary oedema consistent with heart failure and fluid overload (compare with fig 2, p293).

**Opacification** Lung opacities are described as nodular, reticular (network of fine lines, interstitial), or alveolar (fluffy). A single nodule may be called a SOL (space-occupying lesion).

*Nodules:*[1] (if >3cm across, the term pulmonary mass is used instead).

1 Neoplasia: metastases (often missed if small), lung cancer, hamartoma, adenoma.
2 Infections: varicella pneumonia, septic emboli, abscess (eg as an SOL), hydatid.
3 Granulomas: miliary TB, sarcoidosis, granulomatosis with polyangiitis (GPA—the new name for Wegener's granulomatosis, p728), histoplasmosis.
4 Pneumoconioses (except asbestosis), Caplan's syndrome (p710).

*Reticular opacification:* = lung parenchymal changes, can be acute (interstitial oedema, eg cardiac, atypical pneumonia, eg viral) or subacute/chronic.
 • Acute interstitial oedema
 • Infection: acute (viral, bacterial), chronic (TB, histoplasmosis)
 • Fibrosis: usual interstitial pneumonia (UIP), non-specific interstitial pneumonia (NSIP), drugs (eg methotrexate, bleomycin, crack cocaine), connective tissue disorders (rheumatoid arthritis—p548, GPA—p728, SLE, PAN, systemic sclerosis—p554, sarcoidosis), industrial lung diseases (silicosis, asbestosis)
 • Malignancy (lymphangitis carcinomatosa)

*Alveolar opacification:* = airspace opacification, can be due to any material filling the alveoli, usually divided into one or a combination of the following:
 • Pus—pneumonia
 • Blood—haemorrhage, DIC (p346)
 • Water—renal or liver failure (p294, p258), ARDS (p178), smoke inhalation (p859), drugs (heroin), $O_2$ toxicity, near drowning (OHCS p786)
 • Cells—lymphoma, bronchioloalveolar carcinoma
 • Protein—alveolar proteinosis, ARDS, fat emboli (~7 days post fracture)

*'Ring' opacities:* Either airways seen end-on (bronchitis; bronchiectasis) or cavitating lesions, eg abscess (bacterial, fungal, amoebic), tumour, or pulmonary infarct (wedge shaped with a pleural base).

*Linear opacities:* Septal lines (Kerley B lines, ie interlobular lymphatics seen with fluid, tumour, or dusts); atelectasis; pleural plaques (asbestos exposure).

*White-out* of whole hemithorax (fig 1): pneumonia, large pleural effusion, ARDS, post-pneumonectomy.

**Gas outside the lungs** Check for a pneumothorax (hard to spot if apical or in a supine image, can you see vascular markings right out to the periphery?), surgical emphysema (trauma, iatrogenic) and gas under the diaphragm (surgery, perforated viscus, trauma). *Pneumomediastinum*: air tracks along mediastinum, into the neck. Due to oesophageal or bronchial trauma (can be iatrogenic, eg from endoscope). *Pneumopericardium:* rare (usually iatrogenic).

**Bones** Check the *clavicles* for fracture, *ribs* for fractures, absence and lesions (eg metastases), *vertebral column* for degenerative disease, collapse or destruction and *shoulders* for dislocation, fracture and arthritis.

**An apparently normal CXR?** Check for tracheal compression, absent breast shadow (mastectomy), double left heart border (left lower lobe collapse, fig 2), fluid level behind the heart (hiatus hernia, achalasia), and paravertebral abscess (TB).

---

1 Remember that the apex of the lower lobe rises up to the 4th rib posteriorly, so it is difficult to ascribe the true location of a lesion on a PA image without additional information from a lateral view. It may be better to use the term 'zone' rather than lobe when localizing a lesion.

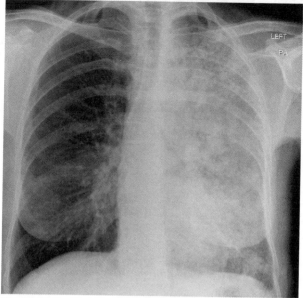

Fig 1. Opacification of the left hemithorax from consolidation.

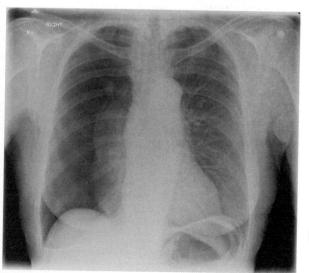

Fig 2. Large right-sided pneumothorax; note the trachea remains central, suggesting this is a simple pneumothorax, not a tension pneumothorax.

Radiology

On a night shift, one of the most frequent requests you will get as a junior doctor (after replacing cannulae and writing up fluids) is to confirm the position of various tubes, lines and leads on a CXR. This can be a daunting task, as incorrect positioning can have deadly consequences, eg an incorrectly positioned NG tube can lead to an aspiration pneumonia, a poorly positioned CVC can lead to fatal arrhythmias. However, this is a fairly straightforward task as long as you remember some basic anatomy, see figs 1 & 2:

| Line/tube/lead | Correct position for tip(s) |
|---|---|
| CVC (p788) | In the SVC or brachiocephalic vein |
| PICC | In the SVC or brachiocephalic vein |
| Tunnelled line, eg Hickmann | At the junction of the SVC and right atrium |
| Endotracheal | 5–7 cm above the carina |
| Nasogastric (p733) | 10cm beyond the gastro-oesophageal junction |
| Chest drain (p780) | In the pleural space tracking either up (for pneumothorax) or down (for effusion) |
| Cardiac pacemaker/temporary pacing wire (p790) | Atrial lead—in the right appendage  Ventricular lead—in the tip of the right ventricle |

### Normal anatomy
• The SVC begins at the right 1st anterior intercostal space
• The right atrium lies at the level of the 3rd intercostal space
• The carina should be visible at the level of T5–T7 thoracic vertebrae
• The right atrial appendage sits at the level of the 3rd intercostal space

### Common bleeps from nursing staff
**1 *Central line not aspirating***
  • Is the tip in the right place (see above) or has it gone up into the internal jugular, too far in (sitting against the tricuspid valve, does the patient have an arrhythmia?) or not far enough in (sitting against a venous valve)?
  • Is the tip kinked, suggesting it may be in a side vessel or against the vessel wall?
  • If the line looks appropriately positioned, consider flushing gently, could the line be blocked?

**2 *Patient not ventilating well***
  • Is the ET tube down the right main bronchus (causes left lung collapse, or rarely right pneumothorax)? Retract tube to correct position (above).
  • Is the ET tube blocked? Most have a secondary port allowing ventilation even if the main hole is blocked, get anaesthetic assistance!

**3 *Chest drain not bubbling/swinging***
  • Is it correctly positioned (see above)—if not in the pleural space, it cannot drain the air/fluid. Common problems include sitting in the soft tissue of the chest wall, sitting above the effusion or below the pneumothorax.
  • Is it blocked? If draining an effusion and correctly positioned, consider gently flushing with 10mL of sterile saline, then aspirating. If not successful, obtain senior advice.
  • Has the effusion/pneumothorax resolved? Pneumothoraces can rapidly resolve with a correctly positioned drain.

**4 *Unable to aspirate from NG tube***
  • Is NG tube not far enough in/coiled in oesophagus? Tip is radio-opaque and should be visible below the diaphragm, if it is coiled it may lie anywhere along the mediastinum.
  • Is NG tube passing down the trachea and into the bronchus? The oesophagus is (generally speaking) a straight vertical line, if the tube veers off to left or right before it goes below the diaphragm, assume it is in the bronchus and replace it.

The consequences of malposition can be fatal, so it is worthwhile learning this basic anatomy, and remember that if you are unsure, always ask a senior.

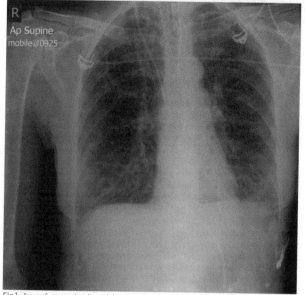

**Fig 1.** Image from ICU showing ET tube, CVC and NG tube *in situ* with ECG tracing leads placed across the chest.
Image courtesy of Dr Elen Thomson, Leeds Teaching Hospitals.

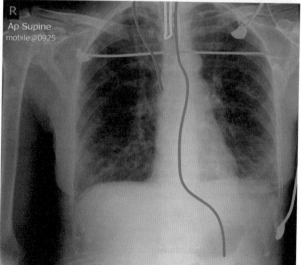

**Fig 2.** Knowing where lines and tubes should be placed is an essential skill. An ET tube (orange) should sit above the carina, this one is slightly high. The tip of the CVC (red, here a right internal jugular line) should lie in the SVC, as seen here, or just in the right atrium. The tip of the NG tube (green) must be seen below the diaphragm to ensure it is placed in the oesophagus, not the trachea. Do not confuse external leads (blue) with internal lines.

Radiology

These are rarely diagnostic and involve a radiation dose equivalent to 50 CXRs. Indications for AXR with acute abdominal symptoms are:
- Suspicion of obstruction (or intussusception, eg in paediatrics).
- Acute flare of inflammatory bowel disease to confirm/exclude megacolon.
- Renal colic with known renal stones (if first presentation, CT urogram is better).
- Ingestion of a sharp or poisonous foreign body (eg lithium battery).

Bowel gas pattern is best assessed on supine images and free intraperitoneal gas (signifying perforation) is best seen on an erect CXR (fig 1, p609).

**Gas patterns** Look for: an abnormal quantity of gas in the stomach, small intestine, or colon. Decide whether you are looking at small or large bowel (fig 1).

| Small bowel: | Large bowel: | Ileus: |
|---|---|---|
| • Smaller calibre | • Larger calibre | • Both small and large bowel visible |
| • Central; multiple loops | • Peripheral | |
| • *Valvuli conniventes:* folds that go from wall to wall, all the way across the lumen; more regular and finer than haustra | • *Semi-lunar folds:*[1] don't go all the way across the lumen, but may appear to do so if viewed from an angle | • There is no clear transition point that corresponds to an obstructing lesion |
| • Grey (contains air and fluid) | • Blacker (contains gas)[2] | |

Small bowel diameter is normally ~2.5cm, the colon ~5cm, the caecum up to 10cm. Dilated small bowel is seen in obstruction and paralytic ileus. Dilated large bowel (≥6cm) is seen in both these, and also in 'toxic dilatation', and, in the elderly, in benign hypotonicity. Grossly dilated segments of bowel (coffee bean sign) are seen in sigmoid and caecal volvulae. Loss of normal mucosal folds and bowel wall thickening are seen in inflammatory colitis (eg IBD)—fig 2. 'Thumb-printing' is protrusion of thickened mural folds into the lumen, seen in large bowel ischaemia and colitis.

**Gas outside the lumen** You must explain any gas outside the lumen of the gut. It could be: 1 Pneumoperitoneum; signs on the supine AXR include: gas on both sides of the bowel wall (Rigler's sign), a triangle of gas in the RUQ trapped beneath the falciform ligament, and a circle of gas beneath the anterior abdominal wall. 2 Gas in the urinary tract—eg in the bladder from a fistula. 3 Gas in the biliary tree (pneumobilia, see MINIBOX), or rarely 4 Intramural gas, found in bowel necrosis, after endoscopy, necrotizing enterocolitis (neonates) and rarely pneumatosis cystoides intestinalis.[3]

**Biliary tree** Any stones? ~10% visible on plain AXR. Pneumobilia (see MINIBOX).

| Pneumobilia |
|---|
| • Post-ERCP/sphincterotomy |
| • Post-surgery (eg Whipple's) |
| • Recent stone passage[4] |
| • Gallbladder-bowel fistula[3] |
| • Anaerobic cholangitis (rare) |

**Urinary tract** The kidneys normally have an equivalent length of 2½-3½ vertebral bodies and slope inferolaterally. The right is lower than the left ('pushed down' by the liver). Their outline can usually be seen as they have a surrounding layer of perinephric fat.

The ureters pass near the tips of the lumbar transverse processes, cross the sacroiliac joints, down to the ischial spines, and turn medially to join the bladder. Check the kidneys and ureteric courses for calculi (visible in 90% of cases)—this requires practice! Don't get confused by other calcifications[4]—eg phleboliths, recognized by their rounded shape and radiolucent centre, are harmless calcifications found in the perivesical veins.

**Other soft tissues** Look for size/position of: liver, spleen and bladder. A big liver will push bowel to the left side of the abdomen. An enlarged spleen displaces bowel and stomach bubble to the right. A big bladder elevates these. Liver and spleen shouldn't extend below the level of the 12th rib on a correctly aligned image.

**Medical devices** Double-J and biliary stents, nephrostomy and gastrostomy tubes, intrauterine devices, laparoscopic sterilization clips, and peritoneal dialysis (PD) catheters can all be seen on AXR.

**Bones and joints** Plain AXR is not the best image, but there may be important abnormalities. In the lumbar spine, look for scoliosis and degeneration (osteophytes, joint space narrowing).

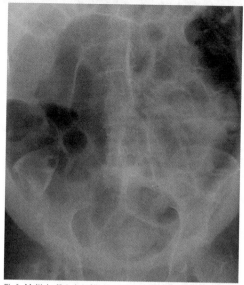

Fig 1. Multiple dilated air-filled loops of large and small bowel. This pattern is seen in ileus.
Courtesy of Norwich Radiology Department.

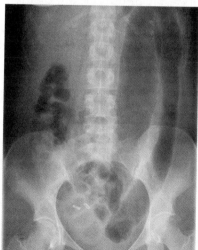

Fig 2. Abdominal film showing toxic megacolon associated with ulcerative colitis, note bowel wall thickening and loss of mucosal folds in the colon.

**1** Semi-lunar folds (plicae semilunares) lie in between adjacent haustra.

**2** The ascending colon contains liquid faeces, but the descending colon contains faecal pellets (*scyballa*).

**3** Gallstone ileus: a big stone migrates directly from an inflamed gallbladder, eg to the transverse colon. Rigler's triad (seen in 25%): 1 pneum(at)obilia 2 small bowel obstruction 3 an ectopic gallstone.

**4** The aorta may calcify, as may the pancreas (chronic pancreatitis) and gallbladder (='porcelain gallbladder') from chronic inflammation from gallstones (associates with gallbladder cancer in 22%).

Since its first use in Atkinson Morley Hospital in 1972,[5] CT has become a speedy and accurate aid to the clinician. Modern systems give whole-body images in under one breath (thanks to continuous, helical rather than sequential, axial data acquisition). Within a single slice (eg 1-5mm thick) CT records the **attenuation**[1] of different tissues to ionizing radiation and calculates a mean value for a given volume of tissue, called a **voxel**. This value is represented in greyscale as a single point, called a **pixel**, in the final 2D image. The greyscale of the image is measured on the Hounsfield scale (see fig 1) relative to the attenuation of water, which has a value of 0 Hounsfield units (HU) and ranges from less than –1000 HU (low attenuation) to more than +1000 HU (high attenuation). The human eye and the display systems have a very limited grey-scale range, so different windows are used to look at tissues of different density, eg bone or lung (fig 2).

**CT with intravenous iodinated contrast medium** gives the ability to image vascular anatomy and vascular structures (ie most organs) in arterial, venous and delayed phases after the injection of contrast medium (fig 3). It is usually given:
• IV for examining the chest, abdomen and pelvis
• IV to look for infection or neoplasia (increased blood flow to affected area)
• Orally 1 hour before examining stomach or small bowel (contrast medium = positive contrast, water = negative contrast)
• Rectally for examining colonic lumen although CT colonography or 'virtual colonoscopy' (see p757) uses insufflated air to define anatomy more clearly

CTs of the brain, spine, and musculoskeletal system are normally done without IV contrast medium. Also see *Contrast medium in imaging*, p762.

**CT as the examination of choice**
• Staging and monitoring malignant disease
• Intracranial pathology, eg stroke, trauma, ↑ICP, and space-occupying lesions
• Trauma
• Pre-operative assessment of complex masses
• Following abdominal surgery

**Streak artefact** Remember that the CT slice image is a matrix representation of the attenuation produced by rotating around the patient. High-attenuation items such as metal fillings, clips and prostheses (and even bone) can cause interference. Other CT artefacts: p735.

**Specific CT techniques**, eg 3D reconstruction (fig 4)
• *CT angiography* uses CT for imaging blood vessels.
• *CT urography* is the image of choice for the ureters.
• *Perfusion CT* maps cerebral blood flow by acquiring images after an IV bolus of contrast medium (fig 5). Although it is widely and frequently used in stroke thrombolysis,[6] there is no clear evidence base as yet. But it does have advantages of being less invasive than angiography and more available than MRI,[7] with the possibility for hub-and-spoke telenetworks to improve access to stroke thrombolysis.[8]
• *CT combined with PET* (see p752) has an increased sensitivity and specificity over each alone, although with a much higher radiation dose.

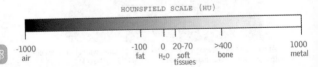

HOUNSFIELD SCALE (HU)

| –1000 air | | –100 fat | 0 H₂O | 20-70 soft tissues | >400 bone | 1000 metal |

**Fig 1.** The Hounsfield scale.

Courtesy of Dr T Turmezei

---

**1** Attenuation is loss of energy of a wave from absorption, refraction, reflection and/or divergence.

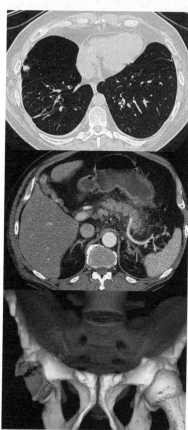

Fig 2. Axial high-resolution CT chest on a lung window algorithm; note solitary lesion in the right lung (Wegener's• granulomatosis, now known as granulomatosis with polyangiitis).
Courtesy of Norwich Radiology Dept.

Fig 3. Axial CT of the abdomen after IV contrast (arterial phase). The tortuous splenic artery is enhanced (arrow)—so is the aorta, but not the inferior vena cava.
Courtesy of Norwich Radiology Dept.

Fig 4. Surface rendered 3D CT reconstruction of the pelvis. The posterior aspect of the right acetabulum is fractured. The right femur has been removed digitally.
Courtesy of Norwich Radiology Dept.

**Radiology**

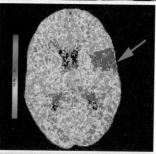

Fig 5. Head perfusion CT showing ischaemia around the Sylvian fissure (arrow).
Courtesy of Dr C Cousens.

**Too many CTs? (CT≈40% of iatrogenic radiation; ≈1.5% of all cancers)**

In one review, no substantial group of patients who were undergoing unnecessary CT could be found, but always balance benefits of CT vs other images with less or no radiation (ultrasound; MRI).[9] To get the best balance, talk to a radiologist. Risk is worst when screening healthy populations, and in children.

Radiology

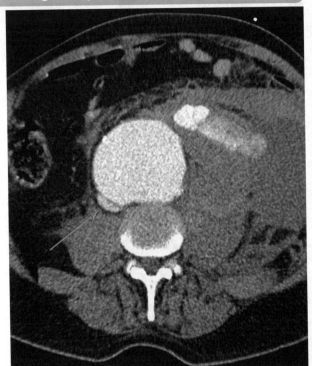

Fig 1. The history was of central abdominal pain with a non-peritonitic abdomen on examination. However, in this patient the CT shows a leaking AAA; by using CT scanning the interventional radiologists can go on to repair this using stents, inserted via arterial puncture and deployed in the aneurysm. This kind of endovascular aneurysm repair (EVAR) is increasingly used in the treatment of ruptured AAA as well as elective repair of intact but enlarging aneurysms.

**The changing role of CT in acute abdominal pain** In the days when general surgeons did their rounds towards the end of an on-call day, there would be wards of patients with undiagnosed abdominal pain having 'drip-and-suck' regimens (IVI and NGT) while awaiting improvement or the unequivocal need for surgery. On opening up, the surgeon would be confident that whatever he found he could deal with. But with the waning of the general surgeon, and the waxing of minimally invasive procedures, specialist surgical teams and highly accurate imaging, it is now best (unless immediate surgery is essential) to match the team to the condition diagnosed by imaging. CT and ultrasound are the best imaging techniques in abdominal pain. So, in this context, drip-and-suck is on the ebb, giving way to imaging, accurate diagnosis, early intervention, rapid discharge or referral to the appropriate team.

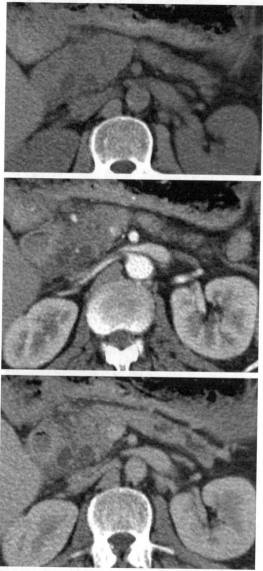

Fig 2. Triple phase CT abdomen, cropped to show the pancreas. Top panel—unenhanced image, middle panel—arterial phase of contrast medium to look for pseudocysts and parenchymal enhancement, bottom panel—portal venous phase of contrast medium to look at veins. The history here was also central abdominal pain with a non-peritonitic abdomen. Here the CT shows an enlarged pancreatic head with fat stranding around the duodenopancreatic grove, and on the portal venous phase, two small areas of fluid attenuation posteriorly consistent with small pseudocysts. The CT was diagnostic of groove pancreatitis.

1 A large proportion of the human body is fat or water (~80%).
2 Fat and water contain a large number of hydrogen nuclei (unpaired protons).
3 The spin of a positively charged hydrogen nucleus gives it magnetic polarity.

**Thus...**

• Placing the human body in a magnetic field aligns its hydrogen nuclei either with (parallel) or against (anti-parallel) the field.
• A radiofrequency (RF) pulse at the resonant frequency flips nuclei away from their original alignment by an angle depending on the amount of energy they absorb.
• When the RF pulse stops, the nuclei flip back (or **relax**) into their original alignment, emitting the energy (called an **echo**) that was absorbed from the RF field.
• Measuring and plotting the energy of the returning signal according to location (provided the nuclei haven't moved) gives a picture of fat, tissue, and water as distributed throughout the body.
• The hydrogen nuclei in flowing blood move after receiving the RF pulses. The echo is not detected, and so the vessel lumen appears black.

Rather than radiodensity or attenuation, the correct descriptive terminology for the greyscale seen in MRI is **signal intensity**: high signal appears white and low signal black (see below). **Weighting** is a quality of MRI that is dependent on the time between the RF pulses (**repetition time**, TR) and the time between an RF pulse and the echo (**echo time**, TE). MR images are most commonly T1-weighted (good for visualizing anatomy) or T2-weighted (good for visualizing disease) but can also be a mixture of both, called **proton density** (PD) weighting. FLAIR sequences produce heavily T2-weighted images. A good way to determine the weighting of an MR image is to look for water—eg in the aqueous humour of the eye, CSF, or synovial fluid (see TABLE, fig 1).

|  | T1-WEIGHTED | T2-WEIGHTED |
|---|---|---|
| TR | short (<1000ms) | long (>2000ms) |
| TE | short (<30ms) | long (>80ms) |
| LOW SIGNAL | water<br>flowing Hb<br>fresh Hb<br>haemosiderin | bone<br>flowing Hb<br>deoxyHb<br>haemosiderin<br>melanin |
| HIGH SIGNAL | bone<br>fat<br>cholesterol<br>gadolinium (p762)<br>metHb | water<br>cholesterol<br>fresh Hb<br>metHb |

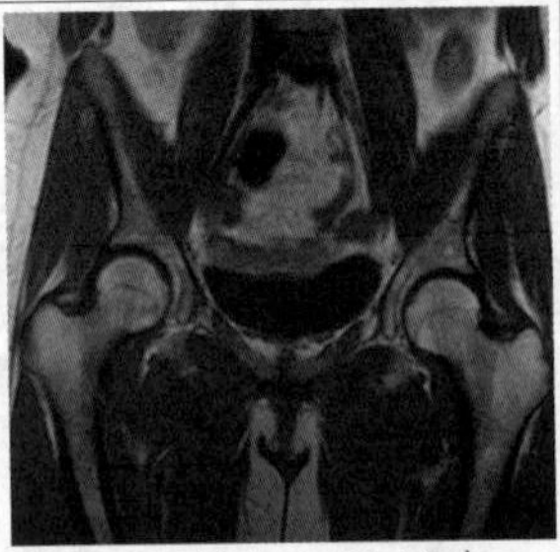

Fig 1. T1-weighted MRI of the hips.[1]

**Advantages** MRI's great bonus is that it does not involve ionizing radiation. It has no known long-term adverse effects. It is *excellent for imaging soft tissues* (water- and hence proton-dense) and is preferred over CT for many intracranial, head and neck, spinal, and musculoskeletal disorders. Multiplanar acquisition of images can provide multiple views and 3D reconstruction from one scan. MR angiography is also excellent for reconstructing vascular anatomy. This avoids the need for invasive angiography with femoral puncture or CT contrast in patients with renal impairment.

**Disadvantages** Poor imaging of lung parenchyma and GI mucosa. More claustrophobic and noisy than CT. High cost combined with limited availability.

**Contraindications** *Absolute:* •Pacemakers; other implanted electrical devices. •Metallic foreign bodies, eg intra-ocular (consider orbital x-ray to exclude), shrapnel. •Non-compatible surgical clips/coils/heart valves. *Relative:* •If unable to complete the pre-scan questionnaire. •1st trimester of pregnancy (not currently approved). •Cochlear implants. NB: orthopaedic prostheses and extracranial metallic clips are generally safe. ► If uncertain, ask a radiologist. *Contrast:* •Renal impairment (gadolinium can cause systemic fibrosis in patients with CKD[10]). •Allergy. •Pregnancy.

1 Coronal T1-weighted MRI of the hips—so normal adult bone marrow is high signal due to fatty yellow marrow, while red marrow gives a lower signal. There is also low signal from urine in the bladder.

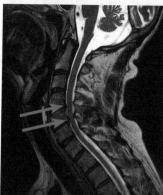

**Fig 2.** T2-weighted sagittal MRI of the cervical spine. There is impingement of the spinal cord at the C4/5 and C5/6 levels caused by degenerative disease. C2 (axis) is identifiable from the odontoid peg, which is embryologically derived from the body of C1 (atlas).

Courtesy of Norwich Radiology Department.

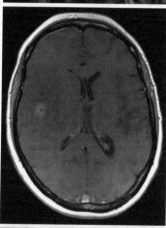

**Fig 3.** Axial T1-weighted MRI of the brain post-IV gadolinium. In the right temporo-parietal region there is a small area of high signal enhancement with a more central area of low signal, surrounded by a region of low signal (presumably vasogenic cerebral oedema) in comparison to the normal brain tissue. This is all causing mass effect with effacement of the sulci and adjacent right frontal horn of the lateral ventricle. There is very subtle midline shift.

Courtesy of Norwich Radiology Department.

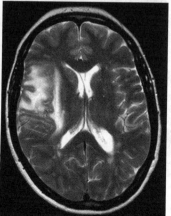

**Fig 4.** Axial T2-weighted MRI of the same patient at the same level as **fig 3**. The high signal in the temporo-parietal region shows a mass effect. The diagnosis was of a solitary metastasis. In this T2-weighted image the oedema and the cerebrospinal fluid within the ventricles and cortical sulci are of high signal due to their water content.

Courtesy of Norwich Radiology Department.

Unlike the other methods of imaging, US doesn't use electromagnetic radiation. Instead, it relies on properties of longitudinal sound waves. This has made it a popular and safe form of imaging (eg in obs & gynae, testes, gallbladders, vessels, fistulae, thyroid). High-frequency sound waves (3–15MHz) are made by a piezo-electric quartz crystal; its size, shape, and resonant frequency determine tissue penetration and image quality. NB: transducers act as transmitter and receiver due to the piezo-electric properties of quartz crystal.[1] Passage of sound waves through tissue is affected by *attenuation* and *reflection*. Attenuation disperses waves out of the receiver's range, but it is the waves reflected to the receiver that determine the image. Its quality depends on the difference in **acoustic impedance** between adjacent soft tissues.

*Processing:* with the help of software a real-time 2D image is made. During processing an average attenuation value is assumed throughout the tissue examined, so if a higher-than-average attenuation structure is in the superficial tissues, then everything deep to it will be in a low intensity (black) **acoustic shadow**. If a lower-than-average attenuation object is in the superficial tissues then everything deep to it will be high intensity (white) or **enhanced**. If a tissue interface is strongly disparate, then all the waves are reflected back, making it impossible to image beyond it. See also figs 1–4.

| Acoustic shadow |
| --- |
| • Fibrous tissue |
| • Calcification |
| • Gas |

| Acoustic enhancement |
| --- |
| • Fluid-filled and cystic structures |

**Modes** *B* (brightness) is the most common, giving 2D slices that map the different magnitudes of echo in greyscale. *M* (movement) traces the movement of structures within the line of the sound beam. It is used in imaging, eg heart valves (p106).

**Duplex ultrasonography (flow and morphology)** By combining Doppler effects (shifts in wavelength caused by movement of a source or reflecting surface) with B-mode ultrasound technology, flow characteristics of blood can be inferred (fig 1). This is extremely useful in arterial and venous studies, and echocardiography.

**Advantages** Portable; fast; non-ionizing; cheap; real-time; can be used with intervention; can enter organs, eg rectum, vagina, gut. *Endoscopic US* can be used to stage and biopsy lung and GI tract cancers, eg stomach, pancreas, [11] and also image the heart = transoesophageal echocardiogram or TOE, p106.

**Disadvantages** Operator dependent—interoperator variability high; poor quality if patient is obese; interference from bone, bowel gas, calculi, or superimposed organs can limit depth and quality of imaging.

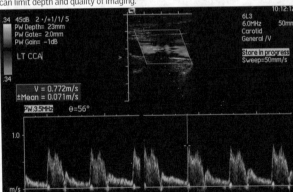

**Fig 1.** A normal Duplex US of the right common carotid artery with a flow rate=77cm/s. The Doppler trace (orange) is displayed below the main image.

**1** When a voltage is applied to a piezo-electric crystal it changes shape, emitting a sound wave when it vibrates. In reverse, when a sound wave physically alters its shape an electrical current is induced.

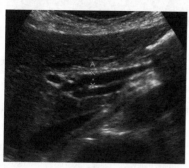

**Fig 2.** Ultrasound of the liver shows the CBD to be dilated. Distal obstruction of the CBD gives proximal dilatation of the duct. It is important to correlate the width of the CBD with the alkaline phosphatase, as the normal diameter varies with age and previous interventions.[12] Also check that the distal CBD tapers as it enters the duodenum. NB: the portal vein lies posterior to the duct (along with the hepatic artery) in the free edge of the lesser omentum. Next, ask "What is causing the obstruction?" and "Where can I get that information?"

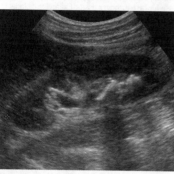

**Fig 3.** Ultrasound of the kidney. At first the image may seem normal but there is a wedge of posterior acoustic shadow cast by the object which is causing increased echogenicity in the lower pole calyces. Acoustic shadows in the kidney suggest stones—as here—or nephrocalcinosis.

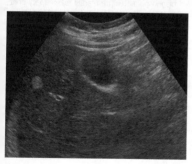

**Fig 4.** Longitudinal ultrasound of the right lobe of the liver showing a well-defined small area of echogenicity. This is the typical appearance of a liver haemangioma, a very common benign liver lesion.

All images courtesy of Norwich Radiology Department.

Radiology

The majority of imaging is concerned with passing external waves (eg radiation) through the patient to a detector, and measuring scatter, slowing or other alterations by various tissues. Nuclear medicine is the opposite; it measures emitted radiation from an internal source, introduced into the patient via injection, inhalation or ingestion. It can be diagnostic (eg PET scanning) and therapeutic (eg radio-iodine ($I^{131}$) ablation in thyrotoxicosis). When first introduced it was nicknamed 'New-Clear' medicine, but then relabelled as 'Un-Clear' medicine, as it can show where a problem is, but not usually what the problem is. Combining it with CT can overcome this.

Because molecules labelled with radioisotopes are introduced into the patient, there is exposure to ionizing radiation, though doses are usually less than those from a CT abdomen (see TABLE, p733). The selection of molecule for labelling depends on the tissue of interest, as it should be something that will be readily taken up by that tissue, eg bisphosphonates for bone, glucose for fast-turnover tissue. Examples include:

**Ventilation/perfusion (VQ) scan** Inhaled Xenon-133 ($^{133}$Xe) or technetium (Tc) plus injected $^{99m}$Tc macro-aggregates, which lodge in lung capillaries. Normal perfusion excludes PE but ventilation component requires a normal CXR for comparison (figs 1&2).

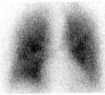
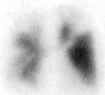
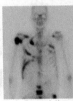

Fig 1. Ventilation scintigram.

Fig 2. Perfusion scintigram showing mismatches with fig 1.

Fig 3. Bone scintigram showing metastases.

**Bone scintigraphy** $^{99m}$Tc labelled bisphosphonates are readily taken up by bone, and concentrate in areas of pathology (tumours, metastases[1], fractures) (fig 3).

**Thyroid disease** TcO₄ is used for differentiating Graves', toxic multinodular goitre, and subacute thyroiditis (fig 1, p603) as well as identifying ectopic tissue, functioning nodules, and residual/recurrent thyroid tissue after surgery. ~15% of cold (non-functioning) nodules are malignant. Hot nodules are often toxic adenomas.

**Phaeochromocytoma** Iodine-123 ($^{123}$I) meta-iodobenzylguanidine (MIBG) is taken up by sympathetic tissues, and indicates functioning, ectopic, and metastatic adrenal medullary (+other neural crest) tumours. $^{131}$I-MIBG is also used for treatment.

**Hyperparathyroidism** $^{99m}$Tc-methoxyisobutyl isonitrile (MIBI) scans can detect parathyroid adenomas.

**Haemorrhage** Red cells are removed from the patient and labelled with $^{99m}$Tc, then re-injected to allow identification of a bleeding point. Used in both acute (3rd-line after endoscopy and CT) and chronic GI bleeding, red cell scans are more sensitive than angiography and useful in intermittent bleeding.

**Renal function** Chromium-51 ($^{51}$Cr) EDTA or DTPA ($^{99m}$Tc, p683) is used to assess GFR. $^{99m}$Tc-mercapto-acetyltriglycine (MAG3) technique assesses relative (left-right) renal function and renal transit time (eg in renovascular disease). $^{99m}$Tc-dimercaptosuccinic acid (DMSA) scanning (fig 4) is the gold standard for evaluation of renal scarring that occurs, eg in reflux nephropathy.

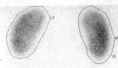

Relative kidney uptake :
Left 45 %
Right 55 %

Fig 4. DMS showing relative renal function of each kidney.

1 This is much more sensitive than x-ray, where lesions may not appear until >50% of bone matrix has been destroyed.

## Position emission tomography (PET)

This is becoming one of the key investigations in malignancy but also has a wide range of other uses. It maps glucose metabolism in the body. ¹⁸F-fluorodeoxyglucose (FDG), a short half-life (110min) glucose analogue, is taken up by metabolically active tissues. It decays rapidly to produce a positron that, after travelling a few millimetres through tissue, annihilates with an electron to produce a pair of high-energy photons (gamma rays), which PET detects. *Neoplasms* have high uptake of FDG, but so do benign inflammatory lesions. *Severely underperfused tissues*, such as those supplied by a critically stenotic coronary artery, switch from fatty acid metabolism to glycolytic metabolism, and hence take up higher levels of FDG and can also be detected by PET. This allows identification of viable (glycolytically active) tissue, eg in myocardial perfusion scanning (p754). PET can be combined with CT or MRI to provide high quality images combining anatomy with physiology, and therefore be used to guide management of malignancy and other conditions such as myocardial ischaemia.

However, PET detects all metabolically active tissue. Normal high uptake of FDG occurs in brain, liver, kidney, bladder, larynx and lymphoid tissue of pharynx and must be considered when assessing images. Inflammation or infection also increase uptake of FDG and can have a false positive result when assessing for malignancy (eg sarcoid, TB).

**Single photon emission computed tomography (SPECT)** is similar to PET but rather than using positron emission from glucose metabolism, it uses a radioisotope labelled molecule as per conventional nuclear imaging, but with two gamma cameras for detection. The images produced are of lower resolution than PET but it is more widely available as the isotopes used are longer lived and more easily available.

**Oncology** PET, PET-CT and SPECT have become some of the most widely used tools for both diagnostics and follow-up in oncology imaging. They can identify hot-spots, with high uptake of FDG, suggesting primary disease or metastases; however, because of the non-specific nature of FDG uptake, diagnosis must be confirmed with histology of suspicious lesions. They are better indicated for *staging* of many solid organ malignancies (lung, melanoma, oesophageal) as well as lymphomas, and are particularly useful for *planning* of radiotherapy and surgery for both primary disease and metastases.

### V/Q scintigram or CT pulmonary angiogram (CTPA)?

The results of the recent PIOPED II trial suggest that CTPA should be the investigation of choice for suspected pulmonary embolism. However, imaging should only be carried out where there is a moderate or high clinical suspicion of an embolism from history and examination, as well as baseline tests such as ECG and CXR.

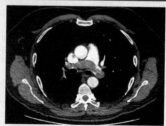
Fig 5. CT pulmonary angiogram (CTPA) with a large grey filling defect in the main pulmonary arteries, showing a saddle embolus.

- If low or moderate probability of embolism, check D-dimer; if this is negative then no further investigation is required.
- In the presence of a positive D-dimer, or where assessment gives a high probability of embolism, then CTPA should be the first choice for imaging with consideration of venous phase imaging of the pelvis and legs to assess for source of clot.
- In patients for whom contrast or high dose radiation is undesirable (CKD, young women—avoid irradiating breasts, pregnancy) consider bilateral USS Doppler legs ± V/Q as 1ˢᵗ-line.

PIOPED II suggested a positive predictive value for CTPA of 96% if there was a high clinical probability. Sensitivity was 90% and specificity 95%.

**CT**

*Cardiac CT* Recent improvements in CT technology have made routine cardiac imaging possible. 64 slice CT, because of its speed and resolution, can image coronary arteries and exclude significant disease with a negative predictive value (NPV) of 97-99%. It can also visualize CABG patency, provide coronary artery $Ca^{2+}$ scoring (a risk factor for coronary artery disease, p111), demonstrate cardiac anatomy including congenital anomalies, and estimate ventricular function.

*Vascular CT* Imaging of the vasculature has become routine in the emergency assessment room for suspected dissections, ruptured aneurysms and arterial and venous thromboses (see p753 for CTPA). CT angiography has overtaken invasive angiography in the assessment of many conditions such as stable angina and renal artery stenosis.

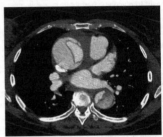

Fig 1. CT angiogram showing type A (ascending) aortic dissection with haemopericardium.

**Catheter angiography**

Wherever intervention may be required, contrast studies such as angiography are unrivalled, eg angioplasty or stenting of vessels, endovascular repair of aneurysms, clipping/coiling of aneurysms (see p760). Remember that these have a high burden of both radiation and contrast medium, so check renal function before requesting. *Complications* include those of arterial puncture (bleeding, infection, thrombosis, dissection, pseudoaneurysm formation) plus cholesterol emboli, thromboemboli and vasospasm.

**MRI**

*Cardiac MRI* has lower resolution than CT but is superior for functional assessment. This, coupled with a lack of radiation, makes it ideal for the assessment of congenital heart disease. Flow velocities can be measured and, because the flow is proportional to the pressure differences, degrees of stenosis and regurgitation across heart valves can be calculated. Myocardial infarction, perfusion and viability can also be imaged with the use of IV gadolinium contrast medium (p762). Both CT and MR use ECG-gating to acquire the imaging data and relate it to the position in the cardiac cycle, thus minimizing the movement artefact (best when the patient is in sinus rhythm).

*Vascular MRI* is used to limit radiation exposure where multiple investigations may be required over a long time period, eg follow-up of aortic root size in a young patient with Marfan's syndrome (p720) or Takayasu's arteritis (p726).

**Ultrasound**

Non-invasive with no radiation, ultrasound is excellent for assessing peripheral vessels, particularly with regard to thrombus, stenosis, malformations and vessel wall thickness. Interest has grown in the use of ultrasound as an assessment tool for cardiovascular risk. Vessel wall thickness has been suggested as a surrogate marker for atherosclerosis and there is some evidence that it may predict long-term cardiovascular outcomes.[13]

**Myocardial perfusion imaging** A non-invasive method of assessing regional myocardial blood flow and the cellular integrity of myocytes. The technique uses radionuclide tracers which cross the myocyte membrane and are trapped intracellularly. Thallium-201 ($^{201}$Tl), a K$^+$ analogue, is distributed via regional myocardial blood flow and requires cellular integrity for uptake. Newer **technetium-99** ($^{99}$Tc)-based agents are similar to $^{201}$Tl but have improved imaging characteristics, and can be used to assess myocardial perfusion and LV performance in the same study (fig 2). Myocardial territories supplied by unobstructed coronary vessels have normal perfusion whereas regions supplied by stenosed coronary vessels have poorer relative perfusion, a difference that is accentuated by exercise. For this reason, exercise tests are used in conjunction with radionuclide imaging to identify areas at risk of ischaemia/infarction. Exercise scans are compared with resting views: *reversible* (ischaemia) or *fixed defects* (infarct) can be seen and the coronary artery involved reliably predicted. Drugs (eg *adenosine*, *dobutamine* and *dipyridamole*) can also be used to induce perfusion differences between normal and underperfused tissues.

Myocardial perfusion imaging adds information in patients presenting with acute MI (to determine the amount of myocardium salvaged by thrombolysis) and in diagnosing acute chest pain in those without classical ECG changes (to define the presence of significant perfusion defects).

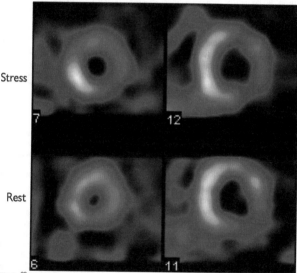

Fig 2. $^{99}$Tc perfusion study showing perfusion defect in the left ventricle anterior and lateral walls at stress which is reversible (difference between stress and rest images). This study is good for small vessel disease such as in diabetes. CT and coronary angiography do not show small vessel disease well.                    Images courtesy of Dr C Cousins.

**Multiple gated acquisition** (MUGA) scanning is a non-invasive way to measure left ventricle ejection fraction. After injection of $^{99m}$Tc labelled RBCs, a dynamic image of the left ventricle is obtained for a few hundred heartbeats by gamma camera. A widespread use for MUGA scanning has been in the pre-op assessment of patients for vascular surgery. However, one review suggested that it was an accurate predictor of long-term prognosis but not of operative risk. However, also consider that gated heart pool LVEF is more reproducible than echo. LVEF stress echocardiography and perfusion scintigraphy may have more clinical relevance in this role, particularly in monitoring of women receiving Herceptin® treatment, which can lead to cardiac dysfunction.

Radiology

### Ultrasound

US is useful for imaging gallbladder, liver, kidneys (see p758) and masses. Consider requesting when investigating abdominal pain, abnormal LFTs, jaundice, hepatomegaly, renal dysfunction and masses. Ensure the patient is 'nil by mouth' for 4 hours beforehand (aids gallbladder filling). Pelvic ultrasound needs a full bladder, consider clamping the catheter if appropriate. Ultrasound may also guide diagnostic biopsy and therapeutic aspiration of cysts or collections.

### CT

CT is widely used in the investigation of acute abdominal pain (see p744-747). It is unparalleled in the detection of free gas and intra-abdominal collections, and allows good visualization of the gut and retroperitoneal areas. Oral or IV contrast medium enhances definition (p744). The big disadvantage is the radiation dose.

*CT colonography (CTC)* Although endoscopic evaluation is still the gold standard for diagnosis of colonic neoplasia, CTC ('virtual colonoscopy' see fig 1) is increasingly used in the diagnosis of colonic abnormalities and has superceded barium enema here. CTC uses $CO_2$ insufflation, usually coupled with an oral stool tagging agent. Intravenous contrast medium is not necessarily required, but can help delineate the bowel wall. The advantage of CTC is that it can be performed in patients who are too frail to undergo the bowel purgation required for endoscopy (it requires only a low-residue diet) and if negative is a definitive test. However, if polyps or masses are seen then patients will usually go on to have a colonoscopy. It allows staging of malignancy by assessing for liver and nodal metastases at the same time as assesing the colon; this is also useful in patients with a stenosing tumour, where it can be used to assess the proximal colon when endoscopy is not possible. Disadvantages are that interpretation takes time and requires a specialist radiologist[14]. For polyps >9mm specificity is 97% but sensitivity is 85% and drops to 48% if <6mm.[15]

*Wireless capsule endoscopy* See p256.

### Magnetic resonance imaging (MRI)

MRI gives good soft tissue imaging, helping diagnose many benign and malignant lesions. Often used to image the liver, MRCP (magnetic resonance cholangiopancreatography) gives detail of the biliary system and the pancreatic duct (fig 2). MRCP has excellent sensitivity and specificity for diagnosing common bile duct stones—when these are >6mm both are 99% (although accuracy is lower for stones <6mm, see p636)—and is the imaging modality of choice.[16]

### Endoscopic retrograde cholangiopancreatography (ERCP) (fig 3)

*Indications:* No longer routinely used for diagnosis, it still has a significant therapeutic role: sphincterotomy for common bile duct stones; stenting of benign or malignant strictures and obtaining brushings to diagnose the nature of a stricture. *Method:* A catheter is advanced from a side-viewing duodenoscope via the ampulla into the common bile duct. Contrast medium is injected and x-rays taken to show lesions in the biliary tree and pancreatic ducts. *Complications:* Pancreatitis; bleeding; cholangitis; perforation. Mortality <0.2% overall; 0.4% if performing stone removal.

### Endoscopic ultrasound (EUS)

See p750. Commonly used in diagnosis of upper GI abnormalities, and is excellent for diagnosis of oesophageal, gastric and pancreatic cancers. It allows staging by assessing depth of invasion, as well as histological diagnosis by biopsy of lesions.

### Contrast studies (fig 4)

These can help in dysphagia (p240). Real-time fluoroscopic imaging studies assess swallowing function. Barium gives better contrast but iodine-based water-soluble contrast medium is used if there is a concern of perforation. *Barium enemas* are used less frequently with the increasing use of CT colonography.

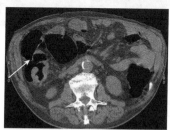

Fig 1. Axial CT colonogram: mural thickening (?ascending colon tumour).

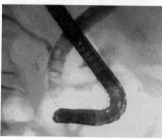

Fig 2. MRCP of the biliary system showing: left hepatic duct (yellow arrow); multiple gallstones in the gallbladder (black arrow); common bile duct (white arrow); pancreatic duct (red arrow); duodenum (green arrow).

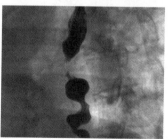

Fig 3. The ERCP shows a dilated common bile duct. The multiple filling defects are calculi within and obstructing the duct (remember the orientation of this image is flipped because the patient is prone for the procedure!).

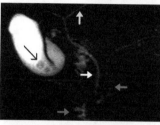

Fig 4. Barium swallow: note 'corkscrew' appearance of the oesophagus found in some motility disorders.

Figs 1–4, courtesy of Norwich Radiology Department.

Radiology

Radiology

### Ultrasound

Imaging modality of choice for genitourinary problems. Can be used to assess:

*Kidneys*
- Renal size—small in chronic kidney disease, large in renal masses, cysts, hypertrophy if other kidney missing, polycystic kidney disease (fig 1), and rarities (eg amyloidosis, p364).[17]
- Hydronephrosis, which may indicate ureteric obstruction or reflux (fig 1, p645).
- Perinephric collections (trauma, post-biopsy).
- Transplanted kidneys (collections, obstruction, perfusion).

*Lower urinary tract*
- Bladder residual volume: useful in assessment of the need to catheterize. Post-micturition residuals.
- Prostate: transrectal ultrasound enables US-guided biopsy of focal lesions. NB: prostate size does not correlate with symptoms.

*Other*
- Ovarian cysts, size, infections (pyosalpinx), uterine fibroids and other masses.
- Testicular masses, hydrocele, varicocele.

*Advantages:* Fast; cheap; independent of renal function; no IV contrast or radiation risk. *Disadvantages:* Intraluminal masses (transitional cell ca) in the upper tracts may not be seen; not a functional study; only suggests obstruction if there is dilatation of the collecting system (95% of obstructed kidneys) and so can miss obstruction from, eg, retroperitoneal fibrosis.

### CT

First-choice in renal colic. No contrast medium is used so it is safe in renal impairment; such unenhanced images miss <2% of stones,[18] and can show other pathologies (fig 2). With contrast, CT can delineate masses (cystic or solid, contrast enhancement, calcification, local/distant extension, renal vein involvement); renal trauma (presence of 2 kidneys; haemorrhage; devascularization; laceration; urine leak); and retroperitoneal lesions. CT has all but replaced intravenous urography and the radiation dose is similar.

### Plain abdominal x-ray

Can be used to look at the kidneys, the paths of the ureters, and bladder. However, in practice it is only useful for monitoring known renal calculi.

### Contrast studies

*Retrograde pyelography/ureterograms* are good at showing pelvi-calyceal, ureteric anatomy, and transitional cell carcinomas (TCCs). Contrast medium is injected via a ureteric catheter. With the advent of cystoscopy, allowing immediate intervention, these are rarely done in isolation. However, contrast medium is routinely used in cystoscopic placement of retrograde stents for obstruction.

*Percutaneous nephrostomy* Used in obstruction to decompress the renal pelvis, which is punctured under local anaesthetic with imaging guidance. Images are obtained following contrast injection (antegrade pyelogram). A nephrostomy tube is then placed to allow decompression, sometimes followed by an antegrade stent if there is no easily treatable cause of obstruction.

### Renal arteriography (fig 3)

Therapeutic indications: angioplasty; stenting; embolization (bleeding tumour, trauma, AV malformation).

### Magnetic resonance imaging (MRI)

Soft tissue resolution can help clarify equivocal CT findings. Magnetic resonance angiography (MRA) helps image renal artery anatomy/stenosis (fig 4) and is also used in the assessment of potential live donors for kidney transplant, as well as to monitor patients following embolization of tumours, arteriovenous malformations and aneurysms.

### Radionuclide imaging See p753.

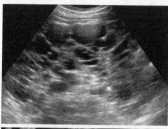

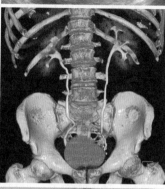

Fig 1. Ultrasound of the kidney showing multiple simple cysts.

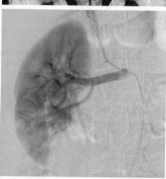

Fig 2. CT MIP (maximum intensity projection)—3D reconstruction of CT urogram showing normal appearances of both kidneys, ureters and bladder.

Fig 3. Renal artery digital subtraction angiogram (DSA; DSA is the final arbiter of renal artery stenosis). It is possible to tell that this is a DSA as no other structure has any definition or contrast in the image. There is, however, some interference from overlying bowel gas, which is not an uncommon problem. GI tract peristalsis can be diminished during the examination by using IV buscopan.

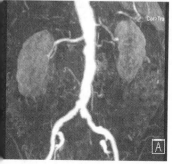

Fig 4. Coronal 3d MRA of the kidneys showing two renal arteries supplying the left kidney. This is important information pre-transplant. Anomalous renal arteries are common and, like the normal renal arteries, are end arteries, hence the consequence of infarction if tied at surgery.

Radiology

### CT

CT is the imaging modality of choice for patients presenting with acute neurological symptoms suggestive of a stroke. It is better than MRI at showing *acute haemorrhage* and *fractures*, and is much easier to do in ill or anaesthetized patients, and so is good in emergencies. The attenuation of biological soft tissues is in a narrow range from about +80 for blood and muscle, to 0 for CSF, and down to -100 for fat (Hounsfield units, p744). IV contrast medium initially gives an angiographic effect, whitening the vessels. Later, if there is a defect in the blood-brain barrier (eg tumours or infection) contrast medium will opacify a lesion's margins, giving enhancing white areas.

- Some CNS areas, eg pituitary gland, choroid plexus, have no blood-brain barrier and enhance normally.
- Fresh blood is of higher attenuation (ie whiter) than brain tissue.
- In old haematomas Hb breaks down and loses attenuation, so a subacute subdural haematoma at 2wks may be of the same attenuation as adjacent brain.
- A chronic subdural haematoma will be of relatively low attenuation.

CT is often used in *acute stroke* to exclude haemorrhage (eg pre-anticoagulation) and now to detect clot in a major artery, such as the middle cerebral or basilar, as part of management decisions regarding thrombolysis. The actual area of infarction/ischaemia will not show up for a day or so, and will be low-attenuation cytotoxic oedema (affecting white and grey matter—look for loss of grey matter definition).

*Tumours and abscesses* appear similar, eg a ring enhancing mass, surrounding vasogenic oedema, and mass effect. Vasogenic oedema (from leaky capillaries) is extracellular and spreads through the white matter (grey matter spared). Mass effect causes compression of the sulci and ipsilateral ventricle, and may also cause herniation (subfalcine, transtentorial, or tonsillar). ▶See p487 (and also fig 2).

Another indication for CT is acute, *severe headache*, eg suggestive of subarachnoid haemorrhage. An unenhanced CT may show acute blood, but if not will demonstrate if there is hydrocephalus or any other abnormality that might make lumbar puncture unsafe.

*Cranial CT perfusion* assesses cerebral blood flow without the need for invasive catheter angiography (fig 5, p745). 3D CT angiography gives excellent mapping of the cerebral circulation (fig 3), and can be done directly after unenhanced CT, looking for an aneurysm if the unenhanced CT shows subarachnoid haemorrhage.

### Magnetic resonance imaging (MRI)

See p748. Example of MRI in stroke: p475. The chief image sequences are:

- *T1-weighted images:* Give good anatomical detail to which the T2 image can be compared. Fat is brightest (signal intensity ↑); other tissues are darker to varying degrees. Flowing blood is low signal. Gadolinium-DTPA contrast medium (p762) usually results in an increase in signal intensity.
- *T2-weighted images:* These provide the best detection of most lesions as they usually contain some oedema or fluid and therefore appear white (eg fig 4, p749). Fat and fluid appear brightest. Flowing blood is again low signal.

*Magnetic resonance angiography* maps carotid, vertebrobasilar and cerebral arterial circulations (and sinuses, veins). Functional MRI can image local blood flow.

### Catheter angiography

Fig 4 is less commonly used since the advent of MRA and CT angiography and perfusion techniques, though it has the advantage of allowing immediate therapy—eg co embolization of saccular aneurysms.

### Radionuclide imaging

See p752. PET is mostly used as a research tool in dementia, but perfusion scintigraphy scan be used in the assessment of Alzheimer's disease, other dementias, and localizing epileptogenic foci. Dopamine scintigraphy can be used to assess local cerebral uptake in Parkinson's disease.

Radiology

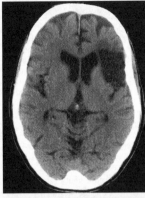

**Fig 1.** Unenhanced axial CT head: note the old infarct in the left middle cerebral artery territory.

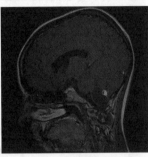

**Fig 2.** T1-weighted MRI of the brain showing a haemangioblastoma in a patient with Von Hippel-Lindau syndrome (p726). Note enhancement with contrast medium.

Courtesy of Dr Edmund Godfrey.

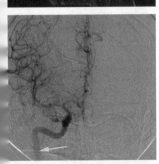

**Fig 3.** Digital subtraction angiogram (DSA). The right internal carotid artery (yellow arrow), anterior cerebral artery (green arrow) and middle cerebral artery (red arrow) are shown.

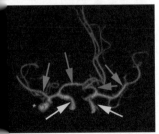

**Fig 4.** A 3D reconstruction of a CT angiogram of the paired internal carotid arteries (yellow arrows) and their branches (anterior cerebral arteries—green arrows, middle cerebral arteries—red arrows), seen from the front and slightly to the right. There is an aneurysm of the right middle cerebral artery (*).

Figs 1, 3 & 4 courtesy of Norwich Radiology Department.

*Radiology*

The use of x-irradiation in imaging relies on the principle that tissues of different electron densities produce different degrees of attenuation. Two adjacent tissues of a similar electron density are indistinguishable on plain x-ray. Increasing electron density increases attenuation and makes tissues appear more radio-opaque. Although this can occur pathophysiologically (eg calcification in chronic pancreatitis or malignancy) it can be induced artificially by the use of a contrast medium and thus create a visible interface. Contrast medium is usually administered by the following routes:

- *PO:* barium- or iodine-based agents for swallow, meal, or follow-through.
- *Inhaled:* technetium or xenon used in ventilation scintigraphy.
- *IV:* iodine- or gadolinium- (see below) based contrast agents.
- *PR:* $CO_2$ can be introduced to the colon for CT colonography, iodinated contrast medium is used for water-soluble enemas.

IV contrast medium has the most widespread clinical application.

**Iodine-based contrast agents** Iodine is used because of its relatively high electron density and good physiological tolerance. When used with CT, the examination is said to be contrast enhanced—look for '+ c' amongst the scan details. Caution should be exercised in patients with the following because of the increased risk of adverse reactions (have latest renal function to hand): renal or cardiac impairment; myeloma; diabetes; sickle cell disease; the elderly and infants; a history of allergy to contrast medium or iodine. Minor reactions include nausea, vomiting and a sensation of warmth. More severe reactions include urticaria, bronchospasm, angioedema and low BP (1:250); theoretical risk of death for 1:150,000 ►Metformin must be withheld for 48h after IV contrast administration because of the risk of lactic acidosis[19]. ►Avoid iodine-based agents in patients with active hyperthyroidism. Contrast induced acute kidney injury is problematic in acutely unwell patients—see p307.

**Barium sulfate** is the most common contrast medium used in examination of the GI tract. Water-insoluble particles of 0.6–1.4μm diameter are mixed with large organic molecules such as pectin and gum to promote good flow, mucosal adherence and high density in thin layers. *Complications:* chemical pneumonitis or peritonitis. Never administer if you suspect perforated viscus.

**Water-soluble iodine-based contrast agents** are used instead of barium where there is a risk of peritoneal contamination (eg fistula, megacolon, ulceration, diverticulitis, bowel anastomosis, acute intestinal haemorrhage), but gastrograffin should never be used where there is a risk of aspiration as it can cause pulmonary oedema; discuss alternatives with your radiologist. ►Contains iodine so establish allergy history and thyroid status.

**Air** In CT colonography air (or $CO_2$) is insufflated as a negative contrast medium after barium administration to enhance mucosal definition. Water can also be used PR to outline the lumen of the colon.

**Gadolinium** is a lanthanide series element with paramagnetic qualities that is administered intravenously as gadolinium-DTPA) to enhance the contrast of certain structures in MRI. It works by reducing the time to relaxation (TR) of hydrogen nuclei in its proximity and appears as high signal on T1-weighted scans. It does not cross the blood-brain barrier so is useful in enhancing isointense extra-axial tumours such as meningiomas. It can also highlight areas where the blood-brain barrier has broken down secondary to inflammatory or neoplastic processes. It is renally excreted: ►check eGFR: if reduced, gadolinium is contraindicated, as up to 30% may develop *progressive nephrogenic systemic fibrosis/nephrogenic fibrosing dermopathy* which causes generalized fibrosis which impairs movement and breathing—and which may be fatal. Aberrations in calcium-phosphate metabolism and erythropoietin treatment seem to increase risk.[20]

Other adverse reactions include headache, nausea and local irritation at the site of injection, with idiosyncratic reaction reported in less than 1%.

Asking yourself *"Does this investigation need to be done right now?"* will often yield the answer *"No!"*, yet there are a few occasions when early imaging can provide vital diagnostic information and influence the prognosis for a patient:
• Acute cauda equina syndrome (p470): ▶▶MRI lumbar spine.
• Suspected thoracic aorta dissection (p656): ▶▶CT thorax + IV contrast, MRI or transoesophageal echo (TOE). The mediastinum is rarely widened on CXR.
• Acute kidney injury (p290 & p848): ▶▶US of renal tract to exclude obstruction.
• Acute pulmonary oedema: ▶▶Portable CXR: don't delay to get an ideal film.
• Acute abdomen with signs of peritonism: ▶▶Erect CXR to find intraperitoneal free gas (fig 1, p609; ≈ GI perforation). Remember: post-op there will be detectable gas (air/$CO_2$) in the abdomen for ~10 days.[21] Early CT (<6h after onset of symptoms) in addition to plain films appears not to give added diagnostic information in peptic perforation.[22]
• Any patient with post-traumatic midline cervical spine tenderness—not just for the emergency department: ▶▶Hard collar and backboard immobilization followed by a CT. All the vertebrae down to the top of T1 must be visualized and cleared before it is safe to take the collar off.
• Sudden onset focal neurology, worst-ever headache, deteriorating GCS: ▶▶CT head, then LP if no evidence of ↑ICP.

Remember that imaging—or re-imaging for a poor quality film—should never delay the definitive treatment of an emergency condition, eg:
• Tension pneumothorax (p824 and fig 1): ▶▶decompression not CXR.
• Intra-abdominal haemorrhage or viscus rupture (p608): ▶▶laparotomy.
• High clinical suspicion of torsion of testis (p654): ▶▶surgery not Doppler US.
Prior to the advent of interventional radiology, a collapsed, shocked patient with an acute abdomen would have skipped CT and gone straight for a laparotomy. However, you should bear in mind that ruptured aneurysms are increasingly being managed by endovascular repair under CT guidance (p656) so this is one area where rapid imaging may be preferable to immediate intervention.

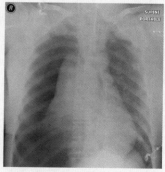

Fig 1. This is a great educational image from ICU. The inexperienced doctor could be distracted by the poor quality image, missing the lung bases: technicians do their best under difficult conditions. To ask for a new CXR here would be a mistake ▶▶note the large right-sided tension pneumothorax needing immediate decompression!

*Lungs:* The right lung field is too black compared to the left, the right hemidiaphragm is also depressed and the right lung is seen collapsed against the mediastinum.

*Pleura:* The pleural recess is seen at the right base. *Mediastinum:* Left-shifted, obstructing venous return—so cardiac output↓, and a threat to life. Is it being pushed or pulled? Check hila, bones and soft tissues. Is the ET tube down the right main bronchus, inflating the right lung and collapsing the left? No. Is the right lung collapsed? Yes. ▶▶Right tension pneumothorax. Needle thoracocentesis decompression and a chest drain are needed now. Once this has been done it is evident that, although the ET tube and internal jugular line are appropriately placed, the tip of the NG tube (trace the wire—see p741) is too high and needs repositioning before use (see p741) or there is risk of feed/medications entering the lungs.

**Contents**

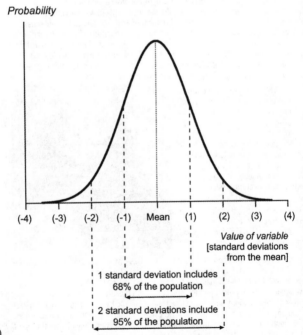

 Fig 1.
Reproduced with permission from *Concepts of Epidemiology*, Bhopal R, Oxford University Press 2008

Once upon a time, in a famous hospital named R— in the middle of England, there lived a crusty old surgeon and a brilliant young house officer. The surgeon issued infallible and peremptory edicts such as "All my patients with a haemoglobin less than 100 must be transfused." Everyone did as the surgeon said (this was a long time ago) except for the wily house officer who understood statistics, sampling error, and the play of chance. One day she was rung up by the haematologist who asked her "Why have you requested 3 blood counts on Mrs Wells today? One is enough. You are wasting our resources!" "Not so," said the house officer. "The first Hb was 98, the second was 97 and the third was 101g/L. I knew if I was persistent, I stood a good chance of preventing an unnecessary transfusion. She is a patient of Mr X." The two conspirators smiled at each other down the telephone, and no more was said. Of course the right way of dealing with this problem is through clinical governance and dialogue with the surgeon. But the point remains: numbers are elastic, despite, on occasion, being given to 3 decimal places. Don't believe in them as absolute entities, and don't believe that the normal range is anything other than arbitrary; think before you act: think statistically. *Think like Gauss.*

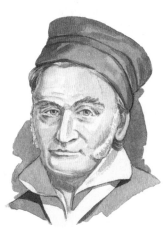

Fig 2. Carl Friedrich Gauss (1777-1855). His Gaussian ('Normal') distribution bell-shaped graph is the theoretical basis of reference intervals (normal values—see below). In some ways Gauss would have made an ideal handbook author: he left behind him a tiny notebook of just 19 pages which solved 146 problems in mathematics including non-Euclidean geometry—his motto being *pauca sed matura* (few but ripe). His messages were brief and perhaps *too* much to the point (not surprisingly, since he invented the first telegraph in 1833)—on being disturbed during deep thought to be told that his wife was dying it is reported that he replied "Tell her to wait a moment until I'm through..."[1]

Image courtesy of Axel Wittman.

### Some definitions

- *Range:* The lowest and highest value of all observations in the set being studied.
- *Arithmetic mean:* The sum of all observations ÷ by the number of observations.
- *Median:* The median is the middle value (eg 9 data points are higher and 9 are lower). If their distribution is Normal, then the median coincides with the mean.
- *Standard deviation (SD):* The square root of the variance (the average of the square of the distance of each data point from the mean). When the distribution of the observations is Normal, 95% of observations are located in the interval 'mean ± 1.96 SD'. This is the basis of the reference interval.
- *Standard error of the mean:* This gives an estimate of the reliability of the mean of a sample representing the mean of the population from which the sample was taken, and is the SD of the sample ÷ by the square root of the number of observations in the sample. Thus the larger the sample size, the smaller the standard error of the mean. Sample means are always Normally distributed, even if the underlying population they are taken from is not, thus you would expect 95% of those sample means to fall within the range '*population mean ± 1.96 × population* SD'.

Reference intervals, etc.

▶ Ranges should only be used as a guide to treatment. A drug in an apparently too low concentration may still be clinically useful.² Some patients require (and tolerate) levels in the 'toxic' range.

▶ The time since the last dose should be specified on the request form.

*Amikacin* Peak (1h post IV dose): 20-30mg/L. Trough: <10mg/L.

*Carbamazepine* Optimal concentration: 20-50μmol/L (4-12mg/L).

*†Digoxin* (6-12h post dose) 1-2.6nmol/L (0.8-2μg/L). <1.3nmol/L may be toxic if there is hypokalaemia. *Signs of toxicity*—CVS: arrhythmias, heart block. CNS: confusion, insomnia, agitation, seeing too much yellow (xanthopsia), delirium. GI: nausea. *NB*: in those over 65yrs, 0.5-0.9ng/mL may be sufficient and if the indication is CCF.²

*†Gentamicin* (p381) and *tobramycin* The potential for oto- and nephrotoxicity is high if aminoglycosides are used inappropriately, so use local expert advice/guidelines. *Signs of toxicity*: tinnitus, deafness, nystagmus, vertigo, renal failure. Although historically given two or three times daily, many now favour **once-daily dosing**, such as the Hartford protocol (fig 1),³ with fewer SEs, and better bactericidal activity. They are suitable only for short therapeutic courses, and are contraindicated in severe renal or liver failure, ascites, burns, high cardiac output states (eg anaemia, Paget's disease), children, and pregnancy. In endocarditis, dosing 8-hourly increases the synergistic bactericidal effect of prescribing gentamicin with other agents. **Divided daily dosing** in such cases may be calculated as 1mg/kg/8h (or 12-hourly in renal failure), or more accurately using a nomogram such as that shown in fig 2. Peak (1h post-dose) and trough (just before dose) levels should be monitored daily—*peak*: 5-10mg/L (3-5mg/L in IE); *trough*: <2mg/L (<1mg/L in IE). Adjust the dose if peak level is out of range, and dose **interval** if trough level is out of range.

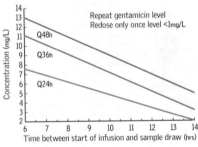

Fig 1. Hartford protocol for 7mg/kg once-daily gentamicin dosing IVI over 15min. Adjust the dosing interval depending on the zone into which the level falls. Q48h means give every 48h; Q24h means give once daily. Above the blue line repeat the gentamicin level and redose only once level <1mg/L. Use lean body weight (p446).

*Antimicrobial Agents and Chemotherapy*, 1995, Vol 39, pages 650-655, with permission from American Society for Microbiology.

†*Lithium* (12h post dose). Guidelines vary: 0.4-0.8mmol/L is reasonable. *Early* signs of toxicity (Li⁺ >1.5mmol/L): tremor. *Intermediate*: lethargy. *Late*: (Li⁺ >2mmol/L) spasms, coma, fits, arrhythmias, renal failure (haemodialysis may be needed). See *OHCS* p354.

*Phenobarbital* Trough: 60-180μmol/L (15-40mg/L).

*†Phenytoin* Trough: 40-80μmol/L (10-20mg/L). Beware if ↑↓ albumin, as the assay is for bound phenytoin, while it is free phenytoin that is pharmacologically important. *Signs of toxicity*: ataxia, diplopia, nystagmus, sedation, dysarthria.

*Theophylline* 10-20mg/mL (55-110μmol/L). (▶see p821) Take sample 4-6h after starting an infusion (which should be stopped for ~15min just before the specimen is taken). *Signs of toxicity*: arrhythmias, anxiety, tremor, convulsions.

*Vancomycin* Trough: 5-10 mg/L (10-15mg/L in SBE/IE and less-sensitive MRSA infections). Start monitoring 48h after 1st dose.

---

* Trough levels should be taken just before the next dose.
† Drugs for which *routine* monitoring is indicated.

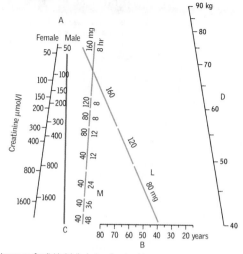

**Fig 2.** Nomogram for divided daily dosing of gentamicin.

1 Join with a straight line the serum creatinine concentration appropriate to the sex on scale A and the age on scale B. Mark the point at which this line cuts line C.

2 Join with a line the mark on line C and the body weight on line D. Mark the points at which this line cuts lines L and M, to get loading and maintenance doses, respectively.

3 Confirm the appropriateness of this regimen at an early stage by measuring serum levels, especially in severe illness and renal impairment.

4 Adjust dose if peak concentration (1h after IM dose; ½h after IV dose) is outside the range 5–10mg/L. A trough concentration (just before dose) above 2mg/L indicates the need for a longer dosage interval.

Note: '↑' means the effect of the drug in italics is increased (eg through inhibition of metabolism or renal clearance). '↓' means that its effect is decreased (eg through enzyme induction). See p702 for a list of cytochrome P450 inducers and inhibitors.

*Adenosine* ↓ by: aminophylline. ↑ by: dipyridamole.

*Aminoglycosides* ↑ by: loop diuretics.

*Antidiabetic drugs* (all) ↑ by: alcohol, β-blockers, bezafibrate, monoamine oxidase inhibitors. ↓ by: contraceptive steroids, corticosteroids, diazoxide, diuretics, (possibly also lithium).

　*Metformin* ↑ by: cimetidine. With alcohol: lactic acidosis risk.

　*Sulfonylureas* ↑ by: azapropazone, chloramphenicol, bezafibrate, co-trimoxazole, miconazole, sulfinpyrazone. ↓ by: rifampicin (nifedipine occasionally).

*Antiretroviral agents (HIV):* See p414.

*Angiotensin-converting enzyme (ACE) inhibitors* ↓ by: NSAIDs, oestrogens.

*Antihistamines* Avoid anything that ↑concentrations and risk of arrhythmias, eg anti-arrhythmics, antifungals, antipsychotics, β-blockers, diuretics, halofantrine, macrolide antibiotics (erythromycin, azithromycin, etc), protease inhibitors (p414), SSRIs (p454), tricyclics.

*Azathioprine* ↑ by: allopurinol.

*β-blockers* Avoid verapamil. ↓ by: NSAIDs. Lipophilic β-blockers (eg propranolol) are metabolized by the liver, and concentrations are ↑ by cimetidine. This does not happen with hydrophilic β-blockers (eg atenolol).

*Carbamazepine* ↑ by: erythromycin, isoniazid, verapamil.

*Ciclosporin* ↑ by: erythromycin, grapefruit juice, nifedipine. ↓ by: phenytoin.

*Cimetidine* ↑ the effect of: amitriptyline, lidocaine, metronidazole, pethidine, phenytoin, propranolol, quinine, theophylline, warfarin.

*Contraceptive steroids* ↓ by: antibiotics, barbiturates, carbamazepine, phenytoin, rifampicin.

*Digoxin* ↑ by: amiodarone, carbenoxolone and diuretics (due to ↓ K⁺), quinine, verapamil.

*Diuretics* ↓ by: NSAIDs—particularly indometacin.

*Ergotamine* ↑ by: erythromycin (ergotism may occur).

*Fluconazole:* Avoid concurrent astemizole.

*Lithium* ↑ by: thiazide diuretics.

*Methotrexate* ↑ by: aspirin, NSAIDs. Many antibiotics (check *BNF*).

*Phenytoin* ↑ by: chloramphenicol, cimetidine, disulfiram, isoniazid, sulfonamides. ↓ by: carbamazepine.

*Potassium-sparing diuretics with ACE-inhibitors:* Hyperkalaemia.

*Theophyllines* ↑ by: cimetidine, ciprofloxacin, erythromycin, contraceptive steroids, propranolol. ↓ by: barbiturates, carbamazepine, phenytoin, rifampicin. See p821.

*Valproate* ↓by: carbamazepine, phenobarbital, phenytoin.

*Warfarin* and *nicoumalone* (=acenocoumarol) ↑ by: alcohol, allopurinol, amiodarone, aspirin, chloramphenicol, cimetidine, ciprofloxacin, co-trimoxazole, danazol, dipyridamole, disulfiram, erythromycin (and broad-spectrum antibiotics), gemfibrozil, glucagon, ketoconazole, metronidazole, miconazole, nalidixic acid, neomycin, NSAIDs, phenytoin, quinidine, simvastatin (but not pravastatin), sulfinpyrazone, sulfonamides, tetracyclines, levothyroxine.

*Warfarin* and *nicoumalone* ↓ by: aminoglutethimide, barbiturates, carbamazepine, contraceptive steroids, dichloralphenazone, griseofulvin, rifampicin, phenytoin, vitamin K.

*Zidovudine (AZT)* ↑ by: paracetamol (increased marrow toxicity).

**IVI solutions to avoid**

*Dextrose:* Avoid furosemide, ampicillin, hydralazine, insulin, melphalan, phenytoin, and quinine.

*0.9% saline:* Avoid amphotericin, lidocaine, nitroprusside.

(For $B_{12}$, folate, Fe, and TIBC, see p770-1)

| Measurement | Reference interval | Your hospital |
|---|---|---|
| White cell count (WCC) | 4.0-11.0 × $10^9$/L | |
| Red cell count | ♂ 4.5-6.5 × $10^{12}$/L | |
| | ♀ 3.9-5.6 × $10^{12}$/L | |
| Haemoglobin | ♂ 130-180g/L | |
| | ♀ 115-160g/L | |
| Packed red cell volume (PCV) or haematocrit | ♂ 0.4-0.54L/L | |
| | ♀ 0.37-0.47L/L | |
| Mean cell volume (MCV) | 76-96fL | |
| Mean cell haemoglobin (MCH) | 27-32pg | |
| Mean cell haemoglobin concentration (MCHC) | 300-360g/L | |
| Red cell distribution width (RCDW, RDW) | 11.6-14.6% (p319) | |
| Neutrophils | 2.0-7.5 × $10^9$/L; 40-75% WCC | |
| Lymphocytes | 1.3-3.5 × $10^9$/L; 20-45% WCC | |
| Eosinophils | 0.04-0.44 × $10^9$/L; 1-6% WCC | |
| Basophils | 0.0-0.10 × $10^9$/L; 0-1% WCC | |
| Monocytes | 0.2-0.8 × $10^9$/L; 2-10% WCC | |
| Platelet count | 150-400 × $10^9$/L | |
| Reticulocyte count | 0.8-2.0%[1] 25-100 × $10^9$/L | |
| Erythrocyte sedimentation rate | Depends on age (p366) | |
| Prothrombin time (citrated bottle) (factors I, II, VII, X) | 10-14s | |
| Activated partial thrombo-plastin time (VIII, IX, XI, XII) | 35-45s | |
| D-dimer (citrated bottle, as for INR)[2] | <0.5mg/L | |

*Proposed therapeutic ranges for prothrombin time: see p345.*

1 Only use percentages as reference interval if red cell count is normal; otherwise, use the absolute value.
2 D-dimer assay is useful for *excluding* thromboembolic disease if the assay is normal. The D-dimer is so non-specific, however, that a raised level is unhelpful, thus the assay should only be requested if the probability of thromboembolic disease is low (eg Wells score; see p581). It needs to get to the lab quickly.

Reference intervals, etc.

*See p676 for the philosophy of the normal range; see OHCS p222 for children.*

Drugs (and other substances) may interfere with any chemical method; as these effects may be method dependent, it is difficult for the clinician to be aware of all the possibilities. If in doubt, discuss with the lab.

| Substance | Specimen | Reference interval *(labs vary, so a guide only)* | Your hospital |
|---|---|---|---|
| Adrenocorticotrophic hormone | P | <80ng/L | |
| Alanine aminotransferase (ALT) | P | 5–35u/L | |
| Albumin[1] | P | 35–50g/L | |
| Aldosterone[2] | P | 100–500pmol/L | |
| Alkaline phosphatase | P | 30–150u/L (adults) | |
| α-amylase | P | 0–180 Somogyi u/dL | |
| α-fetoprotein | S | <10ku/L | |
| Angiotensin II[2] | P | 5–35pmol/L | |
| Antidiuretic hormone (ADH) | P | 0.9–4.6pmol/L | |
| Aspartate transaminase | P | 5–35u/L | |
| Bicarbonate[1] | P | 24–30mmol/L | |
| Bilirubin | P | 3–17µmol/L | |
| BNP (see p689) | P | <50ng/L | |
| Calcitonin | P | <0.1µg/L | |
| Calcium (ionized) | P | 1.0–1.25mmol/L | |
| Calcium[1] (total) | P | 2.12–2.65mmol/L | |
| See p690 to correct for albumin | | | |
| Chloride | P | 95–105mmol/L | |
| Cholesterol[3] (see p704) | P | <5.0mmol/L | |
|   VLDL (see p704) | P | 0.128–0.645mmol/L | |
|   LDL | P | <2.0mmol/L | |
|   HDL | P | 0.9–1.93mmol/L | |
| Cortisol | P | AM 450–700nmol/L midnight 80–280nmol/L | |
| Creatine kinase (CK) | P | ♂ 25–195u/L ♀ 25–170u/L | |
| Creatinine[1] (∝ to lean body mass) | P | 70–150µmol/L | |
| Ferritin | P | 12–200µg/L | |
| Folate | S | 2.1µg/L | |
| Follicle-stimulating hormone (FSH) | P/S | 2–8u/L in ♀ (luteal); >25u/L in menopause | |
| Gamma-glutamyl transpeptidase | P | ♂ 11–51u/L ♀ 7–33u/L | |
| Glucose (fasting) | P | 3.5–5.5mmol/L | |
| Growth hormone | P | <20mu/L | |
| HbA1c = glycosylated Hb (DCCT) | B | 4–6%. 7% ≈ good DM control | |
| HbA1c IFCC (more specific than DCCT) | B | 20–42mmol/mol; 53 ≈ good DM control | |
| Iron | S | ♂ 14–31µmol/L ♀ 11–30µmol/L | |
| Lactate | P | Venous 0.6–2.4mmol/L | |
| | ABG | Arterial 0.6–1.8mmol/L | |
| Lactate dehydrogenase (LDH) | P | 70–250u/L | |
| Lead | B | <1.8mmol/L | |
| Luteinizing hormone (LH) (premenopausal) | P | 3–16u/L (luteal) | |

1 See *OHCS* p15 for reference intervals in pregnancy.
2 The sample requires special handling: contact the laboratory.
3 Desired upper limit of cholesterol would be <6mmol/L. In some populations, 7.8mmol/L is the top end of the distribution.

| | | |
|---|---|---|
| Magnesium | P | 0.75–1.05mmol/L |
| Osmolality | P | 278–305mosmol/kg |
| Parathyroid hormone (PTH) | P | <0.8–8.5pmol/L |
| Potassium | P | 3.5–5.0mmol/L |
| Prolactin | P | ♂ <450u/L |
| | | ♀ <600u/L |
| Prostate specific antigen (PSA) | P | 0–4μg/mL, age specific, see p538 |
| Protein (total) | P | 60–80g/L |
| Red cell folate | B | 0.36–1.44μmol/L (160–640μg/L) |
| Renin² (erect/recumbent) | P | 2.8–4.5/ 1.1–2.7pmol/mL/h |
| Sodium¹ | P | 135–145mmol/L |
| Thyroid-binding globulin (TBG) | P | 7–17mg/L |
| Thyroid-stimulating hormone (TSH) | P | 0.5–5.7mu/L widens with age, p208 assays vary; 4–5 is a grey area |
| Thyroxine (T₄) | P | 70–140nmol/L |
| Thyroxine (free) | P | 9–22pmol/L |
| Total iron-binding capacity | S | 54–75μmol/L |
| Triglyceride | P | 0.55–1.90mmol/L |
| Triiodothyronine (T₃) | P | 1.2–3.0nmol/L |
| Troponin T (see p112) | P | <0.1μg/L |
| Urate¹ | P | ♂ 210–480μmol/L |
| | | ♀ 150–390μmol/L |
| Urea¹ | P | 2.5–6.7mmol/L |
| Vitamin B₁₂ | S | 0.13–0.68nmol/L (>150ng/L) |
| Vitamin D | S | 60–105nmol/L |

### Arterial blood gases reference intervals

pH: 7.35–7.45
$P_aO_2$: >10.6kPa

$P_aCO_2$: 4.7–6.0kPa
Base excess: ±2mmol/L

Note: 7.6mmHg = 1kPa (atmospheric pressure ≈ 100kPa)

| Urine reference intervals | Reference interval | Your hospital |
|---|---|---|
| Cortisol (free) | <280nmol/24h | |
| Hydroxyindole acetic acid | 16–73μmol/24h | |
| Hydroxymethylmandelic acid (HMMA, VMA) | 16–48μmol/24h | |
| Metanephrines | 0.03–0.69μmol/mmol creatinine (or <5.5μmol/day) | |
| Osmolality | 350–1000mosmol/kg | |
| 17-oxogenic steroids | ♂ 28–30μmol/24h | |
| | ♀ 21–66μmol/24h | |
| 17-oxosteroids (neutral) | ♂ 17–76μmol/24h | |
| | ♀ 14–59μmol/24h | |
| Phosphate (inorganic) | 15–50mmol/24h | |
| Potassium | 14–120mmol/24h | |
| Protein | <150mg/24h | |
| Protein | creatinine ratio <3mg/mmol | |
| Sodium | 100–250mmol/24h | |

P=plasma (eg citrate bottle); S=serum (clotted; no anticoagulant); B=whole blood (edetic acid EDTA bottle). ABG = arterial blood gas.

## Contents

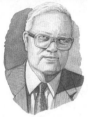

Fig 1. Ivan Seldinger (1921-1998). Swedish radiologist who pioneered a technique to access both vessels and hollow organs throughout the body, by means of threading a catheter over a flexible guide wire. He published this technique in 1953 as a new method of percutaneous angiography, but it is now widely used for all forms of access from central line insertion, pacemakers, angiography and angioplasty, and drainage of fluid (infected collections, pleural effusions, pneumothorax, ascites). He received many awards for his work, which has revolutionised practical procedures by allowing percutaneous rather than open approaches, minimising infection and reducing recovery times.

▶With the new focus on practical skills training in Foundation and Core training programmes, there is much more emphasis on ensuring junior doctors are confident in carrying out procedures, and the old adage of 'see one, do one, teach one' is no longer relevant. 'Just having a go' when you aren't confident can have devastating consequences for the patient, but also for you and your future. Seek out opportunities to learn practical procedures, in an elective setting, so that your first attempt isn't a life-or-death emergency attempt. For example, time in theatres or intensive care units can hone skills in NG tube insertion, IV cannulation, urethral catheterization, central venous access, arterial line insertion, airway management, lumbar punctures, ascitic drains and chest drain insertion. Many seniors will be happy to make time to teach if you contact them in advance—speak to anaesthetists, respiratory physicians, surgeons, ED and ICU staff. Let them know you are interested and leave your bleep, you'll find your experiential learning increases significantly!

▶Even in an emergency setting, it is often wiser to obtain help rather than carrying out an urgent procedure for the first time (fig 1)—but some procedures must occasionally be performed at once—see EMERGENCY BOX, p775.

▶NHS Never Events have come to the fore in recent years, and several relate to practical procedures. A Never Event is a serious, largely preventable patient safety incident that should *never* occur if the available preventative measures have been implemented. Examples include misplacement of NG tube, misidentification of patient, and overdose of midazolam during conscious sedation, such as for insertion of central venous access. A Never Event can have serious consequences for the Trust and for you. Patient safety should come first in your mind, but your own safety and future should not be far behind.[1]

**Relevant pages in other chapters:** Arrhythmias (p118); bone marrow biopsy (p358); cardiogenic shock (p814); consent, (p570); intravenous fluid therapy (p680); liver failure (p258); local anaesthetics (TABLE, p575); meningitis (p832); pleural effusion (p184); pneumothorax (p182, p824); renal biopsy (p300); subarachnoid haemorrhage (p482); tension pneumothorax (p824); the venous system of the thoracic inlet (BOX, p589).

*We thank our Specialist Reader, Dr Andrew Johnston, and our Junior Reader, Timothy Crocker-Buqué for their contribution to this chapter.*

## Nasogastric tubes

These tubes are passed into the stomach via the nose—orogastric if via the mouth—and drain externally. Large (eg 16 Fr) are good for drainage but can be uncomfortable for patients. Small (eg 10 Fr) are more comfortable for feeding but can be difficult to aspirate and are poor for drainage.

- To decompress the stomach/gastrointestinal tract especially when there is obstruction, eg gastric outflow obstruction, ileus, intestinal obstruction.
- For gastric lavage.
- To administer feed/drugs, especially in critically ill patients or those with dysphagia, eg motor neuron disease, post CVA.

**Passing the tube** Nurses are experts and will ask you (who may never have passed one) to do so only when they fail—so the first question to ask is: "Have you asked the charge-nurse from the ward next door?"

- Wear non-sterile gloves and an apron to protect both you and the patient.
- Explain the procedure. Take a new, cool (hence less flexible) tube. Have a cup of water to hand. Lubricate well with aqueous gel.
- Use the tube, by holding it against the patient's head, to estimate the length required to get from the nostril to the back of the throat.
- Place lubricated tube in nostril with its natural curve promoting passage down, rather than up. The right nostril is often easier than the left but, if feasible, ask the patient for their preference. Advance directly backwards (not upwards).
- When the tip is estimated to be entering the throat, rotate the tube by ~180° to discourage passage into the mouth.
- Ask the patient to swallow a sip of water, and advance as they do, timing each push with a swallow. **If this fails:** Try the other nostril, then oral insertion.
- The tube has distance markings along it: the stomach is at ~35-40cm in adults, so advance > this distance, preferably 10-20cm beyond. Tape securely to the nose.

**Confirming position:** This is vital prior to commencing any treatment through the tube. Misplaced naso- or orogastric tubes have led to a number of preventable deaths, and a misplaced tube is an NHS Never Event (see opposite).

- Use pH paper (pH gradations of 0.5 and a pH range of 0-6 or 1-11) to test that you are in the stomach: aspirated gastric contents are acid (pH ≤5.5) although antacids or PPIs may increase the pH. Small tubes can be difficult to aspirate, try withdrawing or advancing a few centimetres or turning the patient on the left side to help dip the tube in gastric contents. Aspirates should be >0.5mL and tested directly on unhandled pH paper. Allow 10s for the colour change to occur.
- If the pH is >5.5 and the NGT is needed for drug or feed administration then the position must be checked radiologically. Request a CXR/abdo X-ray (tell the radiologist why you need it). Look for the radio-opaque line/tip (this can be hard to see, look below the diaphragm, but if in doubt, ask for help from the radiologist).
- The 'whoosh' test is NOT an accepted method of testing for tube position.
- Either spigot the tube, or allow to drain into a dependent catheter bag secured to clothing (zinc oxide tape around tube to form a flap, safety pin through flap).

▶Do not pass a tube nasally if there is any suspicion of a facial fracture.

▶Get senior help if the patient has recently had upper GI surgery—it is not good practice to push the tube through a fresh anastomosis!

**Complications** •Pain, or, rarely: •Loss of electrolytes •Oesophagitis •Tracheal or duodenal intubation •Necrosis: retro- or nasopharyngeal •Stomach perforation.

**Weaning** When planning removal of an NGT *in situ* for decompression or relief of obstruction, it is wise to wean it so that the patient manages well without it. Drainage should be <750mL/24 hours for successful weaning.

- First it should be on free drainage with, eg, 4hrly aspirations;
- Then spigot with 4hrly aspirations;
- Then spigot only. If this is tolerated along with oral intake then it is probably safe to remove the tube; if not, then take a step backwards.

►Much of what we do is not evidence based; however, in more recent years, particularly in intensive care units, the rise of hospital acquired infections and multidrug resistant organisms has prompted a review of standard practice and a series of evidence based interventions put together as a 'care bundle' to reduce hospital acquired infections. The technique for placing a cannula is best shown by the bedside by an expert, but keeping these simple rules in mind means the risk of infection from the cannula is significantly reduced.[2]

**Preparation is key, remember the following before you start:**

1 **Equipment:** set up a tray with cleaning swabs, gauze, cannulae (swallow your pride and take at least three of different sizes), dressings, 0.9% saline, 10mL syringe, needle-free adaptor (eg octopus with bionector), blood tubes if required, portable sharps bin → needlestick injuries do happen.

2 **Patient:** have them lying down, explain procedure, obtain verbal consent, place tourniquet around arm, rest the arm below the heart to aid venous filling.

3 **Site:** look for the best vein—it should be palpable, some of the best veins are not easily visible, some of the most visible collapse on insertion. Tapping gently helps. ►**Never cannulate:** AV fisulae arms, limbs with lymphoedema. ►**Avoid** sites crossing a joint (if possible), the cephalic vein in a renal patient.

4 **Consider:** *EMLA®* cream, cold spray or 1% lidocaine for children or those with needle phobia. *EMLA®* takes 45min to work, but can save you hassle later.[3]

**Insertion care bundle**

1 Aseptic technique 2 Hand hygiene 3 Apron + non-sterile gloves 4 Skin preparation—2% chorhexidine in 70% isopropyl alcohol (allow to dry for 30 seconds). Do not repalpate vein after cleaning unless wearing sterile gloves 5 Dressing—sterile and transparent so that insertion site can be observed.

**After insertion**

1 Take blood with syringe or adaptor 2 Remove tourniquet 3 Attach needle-free device (if appropriate) and flush with 10mL 0.9% saline 4 Apply dressing 5 Let nursing staff know that cannula is in place and ready for use 6 Document insertion according to local policy 7 Write up appropriate fluids or parenteral medication.

When seeing your patient on the daily ward round, and to avoid being called to review or replace cannulae at 6pm, do a RAID assessment:[4] consider if the drip is:

**R**equired—can the patient manage with oral medication/fluids?

**A**ppropriate—should you consider a PICC, central line, long-term line, etc?

**I**nfected—any signs of inflammation or infection? Remove if yes. Peripheral cannulae should be replaced every 72-96 hours

**D**ressed properly—many drips are replaced early because they have 'fallen out', or are kinked from poor dressings

Tissued or infected cannulae need replacing, either with another peripheral cannula, or with a longer-term access device, such as a PICC line.

**If you fail after 3 attempts** ►Shocked patients need fluid quickly: if you are having trouble putting in a drip, call your senior. The advice below assumes that the drip is not immediately life-saving. ►►If it is, see EMERGENCY BOX.

• Ask for help—from colleagues or seniors—do not be ashamed, everyone has to learn and even senior doctors have bad days; a fresh pair of eyes can be all it takes. As a house officer, one of us was asked to place a drip when a very shame-faced consultant had 'had a go' to prove he still could, and found out that he couldn't!

• Help yourself—try putting the hand in warm water, using a small amount of GTN paste over the hand, or using ultrasound if available to help you identify the vein.

• If there is no one else to help, take a break and come back in half an hour. Veins come and go, and coming back with fresh eyes can make all the difference.

## Intravenous cannulae sizes and UK colour conventions

| Gauge | Colour | Diameter (mm) | Length (mm) | Flow rate (mL/min°) |
|-------|--------|---------------|-------------|---------------------|
| 14G | | 2.0 | 45 | 250 |
| 16G | | 1.7 | 42 | 170 |
| 18G | | 1.2 | 40 | 90 |
| 20G | | 1.0 | 32 | 55 |
| 22G | | 0.28 | 25 | 25 |
| 24G | | 0.07 | 19 | 24 |

V=Maximum flow rate under gravity.

According to Poiseuille's law[1] the flow rate ($Q$) of a fluid through a tubular structure is inversely proportional to viscosity (h) and length (l) and proportional to the pressure difference across it ($P_i - P_o$) and the radius *to the power of 4($r^4$)*. Hence:

$$Q \propto \frac{(P_i - P_o) \, r^4}{h \, l}$$

## A last throw of the dice

Just once it may come down to you. For some, this is one of the challenges and thrills in medicine. There may be no one else available to help when there is an absolute and urgent indication for IV drugs/fluids/blood—and all of the above measures have been tried, and have failed. Think of lonesome night shifts, over-run emergency departments, a disaster scene, war, or medicine in the field. The following measures are not recommended for non-life-threatening scenarios:

▶▶ Don't worry. Have a good look again. Feet (avoid in diabetics)? Inside of the forearm? Upper arm?

▶▶ Have you really exhausted all of your options for help from a colleague? Maybe the anaesthetist or ICU registrar is approachable—they do have remarkable skills.

▶▶ Is the patient familiar with his/her own veins (eg previous IV drug abuser)?

▶▶ If there is only a small amount of IV medication required and a small, short vein, you may be able to gain access with a carefully placed butterfly needle that is taped down. Some drugs cannot be passed this way (eg **amiodarone**, K⁺).

▶▶ The external jugular vein may become prominent when the patient is head down (Trendelenburg) by 5–10° (▶not in situations of fluid overload, LVF, ↑ICP). Only attempt cannulation of this vein if you are not going to jeopardize future central line insertion, and if you can clearly determine the surrounding anatomy.

▶▶ In an arrest situation, the 2010 Advanced Life Support Guidelines recommend the intraosseous route in both adults and children if venous access is not possible.

*Only do the following if you have had the appropriate training/experience:*

▶▶ In children, consider cannulating a scalp vein.

▶▶ Central venous catheterization (p789). This may be just as hard in a profoundly hypovolaemic arrest patient, and a good knowledge of local anatomy and of the procedure (± ultrasound guidance) will be invaluable.

NB: A cut down to the long saphenous vein may (must!) be attempted, *in extremis*,[s] even if you have no prior experience (at this site you won't kill by being ham-fisted). ▶▶ Make a transverse incision 1-2cm anterior and superior to the medial malleolus ▶▶ Free the vein with forceps ▶▶ Cannulate it under direct vision. ▶ Here, 'first do no harm' is trumped by 'nothing ventured, nothing gained'.

Hopefully, it shouldn't ever have to come to these measures, but one day...

---

**1** Poiseuille's law is a neat piece of physiology and worth remembering—it is applicable in some form to almost every system in the body. Note that it is a 4th-power law: a small change in the radius makes a huge difference to flow.

Practical procedures

Urinary tract infections are the second commonest healthcare associated infection, and urinary catheters are frequently to blame. Think, does the patient really need a catheter? If so, use the smallest you can and take out as soon as possible.

*Size:* (in French gauge): 12=small; 16=large; 20=very large (eg 3-way). *Material:* Latex is soft (►ask about allergy). A silastic (silicone) catheter may be used long term, but costs more. Silver alloy coating reduces infections.[6] *Shape:* Foley is typical (fig 1); coudé (elbow) catheters have an angled tip to ease around prostates but are more risky; 3-way catheters are used in clot or debris retention and have an extra lumen for irrigation fluid, attached to the irrigation set via an extra port on the distal end (fig 2). Get urology advice before starting irrigation. Condom catheters are often preferred by patients (less discomfort) even though they may leak and fall off.[7]

**Catheter problems:** • *Infection* ~5% develop bacteraemia (most will have bacterial colonization, antibiotics may not be required unless systemically unwell—discuss with microbiology). A stat dose of, eg, *gentamicin 80mg,* is sometimes given pre-insertion despite a lack of evidence for benefit.[8] Check your local policy. • *Bladder spasm* may be painful—try reducing the water in the balloon or an anticholinergic drug, eg *oxybutinin.*

| Checklist |
| --- |
| • Gloves |
| • Catheter |
| • *Lidocaine* jelly |
| • 10mL water |
| • Cleaning solution |
| • Drape |
| • Kidney dish |
| • Gauze swabs |
| • Forceps (optional) |
| • Drainage bag |
| • Specimen container |

**Catheterize as per the recommended care bundle!**

**1 Per urethram:** Aseptic technique required.

*Indications* • Relieve urinary retention, • Monitor urine output in critically ill patients, • Collect uncontaminated urine for diagnosis. ► It is contraindicated in urethral injury (eg pelvic fracture) and acute prostatitis.

• Explain the procedure, and obtain verbal consent. Prepare a catheterization pack (if not pre-packed, see MINIBOX).

• Lie the patient supine: women with knees flexed and hips abducted with heels together. Use a gloved hand to clean urethral meatus in a pubis-to-anus direction, holding the labia apart with the other hand. With uncircumcised men (check with the patient!), retract the foreskin to clean the glans; use a gloved hand to hold the penis still. The hand used to hold the penis or labia should not touch the catheter. Place a sterile drape with a hole in the middle to help you maintain asepsis. Remember: left hand dirty, right hand clean.

• Put sterile lidocaine 1-2% gel on the catheter tip and ≤10mL into the urethra (≤5mL if ♀). In men, lift and gently stretch the penis upwards to eliminate any urethral folds that may lead to false passage formation.

• Use steady gentle pressure to advance the catheter, rotating slightly can help it slide in. ►Never force the catheter. Tilting the penis up towards the umbilicus while inserting may help negotiate the prostate. Insert to the hilt; wait until urine emerges before inflating the balloon. Remember to check the balloon's capacity before inflation (written on the outer end). Collect a sterile specimen and attach a drainage bag. Pull the catheter back so that the balloon comes to rest at the bladder neck.

• If you are having trouble getting past the prostate try: more lubrication; a gentle twisting motion; a larger catheter; or call the urologists, who may use a guide-wire.

►Remember to reposition the foreskin in uncircumcised men after the catheter is inserted to prevent oedema of the glans and paraphimos.

*Documentation:* in the notes be sure to document the indication for catheterization, size of catheter, whether insertion was difficult or straightforward, any complications, residual volume and colour of urine. It is good practice to document that the foreskin has been replaced. Sign with your name, date and designation.

**2 Suprapubic catheterization:** Sterile technique required ►Absolutely contraindicated unless there is a large bladder palpable or visible on ultrasound, because of the risk of bowel perforation. Be wary, particularly if there is a history of abdominal or pelvic surgery. Suprapubic catheter insertion is high risk and you should be trained before attempting it, speak to the urologists first!

## Self-catheterization

This is a good, safe way of managing chronic retention from a neuropathic bladder (eg in multiple sclerosis, diabetic neuropathy, spinal tumour or trauma). Never consider a patient in difficulties from a big residual volume to be too old, young, or disabled to learn. 5-yr-old children can learn the technique, and can have their lives transformed—so motivation may be excellent. There may be fewer UTIs as there is no residual urine—and less reflux obstructive uropathy. Assessing suitability entails testing sacral dermatomes: a 'numb bum' implies ↓ sensation of a full bladder; higher sensory loss may mean catheterization will be painless. Get help from your continence adviser who will be in a position to teach the patient or carer that catheterizations must be gentle (the catheter is of a much smaller calibre), particularly if sensation is lacking, and must number >4/d ('always keep your catheter with you; don't wait for an urge before catheterizing'). See fig 3.

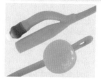 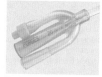 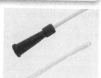

**Fig 1.** A size 14F latex Foley catheter with the balloon inflated via the topmost port of the outer end (green).[1] Images © Dr Tom Turmezei (they are not to scale).

**Fig 2.** The external end of a size 20F 3-way catheter. The lowest port is for the bladder irrigation fluid and the uppermost port (yellow) is for balloon inflation.

**Fig 3.** A size 10F catheter for self-catheterization. They are usually smaller than indwelling catheters, eg 10F compared to 14F. Note that this catheter also has no balloon.

## "The catheter is not draining..."

You will be asked to check catheters that are not draining. Check the fluid chart and the patient:

- *Previously good output, now anuric* = blocked catheter until proven otherwise. Was the urine clear previously or bloodstained? Consider flushing the catheter: with aseptic technique flush and withdraw 20mL of sterile 0.9% saline with a bladder syringe. This may get the flow going again. A 3-way catheter may be needed if there is clot or debris retention. If it blocks again, replace it. Repeated flushes lead to infection.
- *Slow decline in urine output over several hours:* in a dehydrated/post-op patient a fluid challenge of 250mL Gelofusine® STAT (slowly if renal/cardiac comorbidity) may help, come back and check the response in 30min. Check all other parameters (eg pulse, BP, CVP) and increase rate of IV fluids if appropriate.
- ►► Acute kidney injury (the new name for acute renal failure, p848): if urine output has tailed off and now stopped, the cause is often renal hypoperfusion (ie pre-renal failure), but consider other factors, eg nephrotoxic drugs.
- *Catheter is bypassing:* a condom catheter may be more appropriate.
- *Catheter has dislodged* into the proximal (prostatic♂) urethra, possible even if the balloon is fully inflated. Consider this if a flush enters but cannot be withdrawn. If the patient still needs a catheter then replace it, consider a larger size.
- ►► The catheter has perforated the lower urinary tract on insertion and is not lying in the bladder or urethra. If suspected, call the urologists immediately.

**Remember:** urine output should be >400mL in 24h or >0.5mL/kg/h (see p578).

## Trial without catheter (TWOC)

When it is time to remove a catheter, the possibility of urinary retention must be considered. If very likely, arrange for a urology outpatient TWOC in 2 weeks, or start an α-blocker first; otherwise remove the catheter first thing one morning. If retention does occur, insert a long-term catheter (eg silicone) and arrange urology clinic follow-up.

1 We would like to thank Addenbrooke's Hospital Urology Department for supplying the catheters.

For patients with refractory or recurrent ascites that is symptomatic, it is possible to drain the ascites using a long pig-tail catheter. Paracentesis in such patients even in the presence of spontaneous bacterial peritonitis may be safe.[9] Learn at the bedside from an expert.

*Contraindications (these are relative, not absolute):* End-stage cirrhosis; co-agulopathy; hyponatraemia (≤126mmol/L); sepsis. The main complication of the procedure is severe hypovolaemia secondary to reaccumulation of the ascites, so intravascular replenishment with a plasma expander is required. For smaller volumes, eg less than 5L, 500mL of 5% human albumin or gelofusine would be sufficient. For volumes over 5L, reasonable replacement would be 100mL 20% *human albumin* IV for each 1-3 litres of ascites drained[10] (check your local policy). You may need to call the haematology lab to request this in advance.

**Procedure** Requires sterile technique.
• Ensure you have good IV access—eg 18G cannula in the antecubital fossa.
• Explain the procedure including the risks of infection, bleeding, hyponatraemia, renal impairment and damage to surrounding structures (such as liver, spleen and bowel), and obtain consent from the patient. Serious complications occur in less than 1 in 1000 patients.[11] Ask the patient to empty their bladder.
• Examine the abdomen carefully, evaluating the ascites and checking for orga-nomegaly. Mark where you are going to enter. If in doubt, ask the radiology de-partment to ultrasound the abdomen and mark a spot for drainage. Approach from the left side unless previous local surgery/stoma prevents this—call a senior for support and advice if this is the case.
• Prepare a tray with 2% chlorhexidine solution, sterile drapes, 1% lidocaine, sy-ringes, needles, sample bottles and your drain. Clean the abdomen thoroughly and place sterile drapes, ensure you maintain sterile technique throughout. Infil-trate the local anaesthetic.
• Perform an ascitic tap (see p779) first so that you know you are in the correct place, remove 20mL fluid for MC&S.
• Away from the patient, carefully thread the catheter over the (large and long) needle using the guide so that the pig-tail has been straightened out. Remove the guide.
• With the left hand hold the needle ~1 inch from the tip—this will stop it from advancing too far (and from performing an aortic biopsy!). With the right hand, hold the other end.
• Gently insert the needle perpendicular to the skin at the site of the ascitic tap up to your hold with your left hand—ascites should now drain easily. If necessary advance the needle and catheter a short distance until good flow is achieved.
• Advance the catheter over the needle with your left hand, keeping the needle in exactly the same place with your right hand. ►Do not re-advance the needle be-cause it will go through the curled pig-tail and do not withdraw it because you won't be able to thread in the catheter.
• When fully inserted, remove the needle, connect the catheter to a drainage bag (keep it below the level of the abdomen) and tape it down securely to the skin.
• The patient should stay in bed as the ascites drains.
• Document clearly in the notes the indication for the procedure, that consent was obtained, clotting and U&Es checked pre-procedure, how much lidocaine was re-quired, how much fluid was removed for investigations, and whether there were any complications to the procedure.
• Replenish intravascular volume with human albumin (see above).
• Ask the nursing staff to remove the catheter after 6h or after a pre-determined volume has been drained (up to 20L can come off in 6 hours!) and document this clearly in the medical notes. Drains are normally removed after 4-6 hours to prevent infection.
• Check U&E after the procedure and re-examine the patient.

## Diagnostic taps

If you are unsure whether a drain is needed, a diagnostic tap can be helpful. Whatever fluid you are sampling, a green needle carries far less risk than a formal drain. It also allows you to decide whether a drain is required.

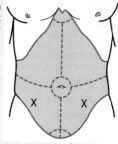

Ascites may be sampled to give a cytological or bacterial diagnosis, eg to exclude spontaneous bacterial peritonitis (SBP; p260). Before starting, know the patient's platelets + clotting times. If they are abnormal, seek help before proceeding.

- Place the patient flat and tap out the ascites, marking a point where fluid has been identified, avoiding vessels, stomas and scars (adhesions to the anterior abdominal wall). The left side may be safer—less chance of nicking liver.

Fig 1. Always tap out the ascites, but aim approximately for 5cm medial to and superior to the anterior superior iliac spine. If in doubt, ask for an ultrasound to mark the spot.

- Clean the skin. Infiltrate some local anaesthetic, eg 1% *lidocaine* (see p575).
- Insert a 21G needle on a 20mL syringe into the skin and advance while aspirating until fluid is withdrawn, try to obtain 60mL of fluid.
- Remove the needle, apply a sterile dressing.
- Send fluid to microbiology (15mL) for *microscopy and culture*, *biochemistry* (5mL for protein, see p184), and *cytology* (40mL). Call microbiology to forewarn them if urgent analysis of the specimen is required.

## Diagnostic aspiration of a pleural effusion

- If not yet done, a CXR may help evaluate the side and size of the effusion.
- Percuss the upper border of the pleural effusion and choose a site 1 or 2 intercostal spaces below it (usually posteriorly or laterally). If there is any doubt about the size or site of the effusion, ask for an ultrasound to mark a spot.
- Clean the area around the marked spot with 2% chlorhexidine solution.
- Infiltrate down to the pleura with 5-10mL of 1% lidocaine.
- Attach a 21G needle to a syringe and insert it just above the upper border of the rib below the mark to avoid the neurovascular bundle (see BOX above). Aspirate whilst advancing the needle. Draw off 10-30mL of pleural fluid. Send fluid to the lab for *chemistry* (protein, glucose, pH, LDH, amylase); *bacteriology* (microscopy and culture, auramine stain, TB culture); *cytology* and, if indicated, *immunology* (rheumatoid factor, antinuclear antibodies, complement).
▶▶If you cannot obtain fluid with a 21G needle, seek help.
- If any cause for concern, arrange a repeat CXR.

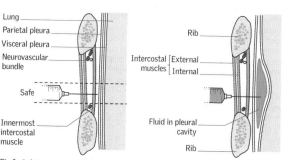

Lung
Parietal pleura
Visceral pleura
Neurovascular bundle

Safe

Innermost intercostal muscle

Rib
Intercostal { External
muscles { Internal

Fluid in pleural cavity

Rib

Fig 2. Safe approach to entering the pleura by the intercostal route.

Practical procedures

### Indications
- Pneumothorax: ventilated; tension; persistent/recurrent despite aspiration (eg <24h after $1^{st}$ aspiration); large $2^{nd}$ spontaneous pneumothorax if >50yrs old
- Malignant pleural effusion, empyema or complicated parapneumonic effusion
- Pleural effusion compromising ventilation, eg in ICU patients
- Traumatic haemopneumothorax
- Post-operatively: eg thoracotomy; oesophagectomy; cardiothoracic surgery.

►Most effusions are now drained using ultrasound guidance and a Seldinger technique. The Seldinger technique is also used for pneumathoraces except in traumatic or post-operative situations and for this reason is detailed below.

### Sterile procedure[12]
- Identify the point for drainage. In effusions this should be done with ultrasound, ideally under direct guidance or with a marked spot (make sure the patient doesn't move!). For pneumothoraces check the drainage point from CXR/CT/examination.
- Preparation: Trolley with dressing pack; 2% chlorhexidine; needles; 10mL syringes; 1% lidocaine; scalpel; suture; Seldinger chest drain kit; underwater drainage bottle; connection tubes; sterile $H_2O$; dressings. Incontinence pad under patient.
- Choose insertion site: $4^{th}-6^{th}$ intercostal space, anterior- to mid-axillary line—the 'safe triangle' (see BOX and fig 1). A more posterior approach, eg the $7^{th}$ space posteriorly, may be required to drain a loculated effusion (under direct US visualization!) and occasionally the $2^{nd}$ intercostal space in the mid-clavicular line may be used for apical pneumothoraces—however, both approaches tend to be less comfortable.
- Maintain sterile technique—clean and place sterile drapes. Scrub for insertion.
- Prepare your underwater drain by filling the bottle to the marked line with sterile water. Ensure this is kept sterile until you need it.
- Infiltrate down to pleura with 10mL of 1% lidocaine and a 21G needle. Check that air/fluid can be aspirated from the proposed insertion site; if not do not proceed.
- Attach the Seldinger needle to the syringe containing 1-2mL of sterile saline. The needle is bevelled and will direct the guidewire, in general advance bevel up for pneumothoraces, bevel down for effusions.
- Insert the needle gently, aspirating constantly. When fluid/air is obtained in the syringe, stop, note insertion depth from the markings on the Seldinger needle. Remove syringe, thread the guidewire through the needle. Remove the needle and clamp the guidewire to the sterile drapes to ensure it does not move. Using the markings on the Seldinger needle, move the rubber stops on the dilators to the depth noted earlier, to prevent the dilator slipping in further than intended.
- Make a nick in the skin where the wire enters, and slide the dilators over the wire sequentially from smallest to largest to enlarge the hole, keep gauze on hand. Slide the Seldinger drain over the wire into the pleural cavity. Remove the wire and attach a three-way tap to the drain, then connect to the underwater drainage bottle.
- Suture the drain in place using a drain stitch—make a stitch in the skin close to the drain site, tie this fairly loosely with a double knot. Then tie the suture to the drain. It is usually best to be shown this before attempting it for yourself. Dress the drain, and ensure it is well taped down.
- Check that the drain is swinging (effusion) or bubbling (pneumothorax) and ensure the water bottle remains below the level of the patient at all times. If the drain needs to be lifted above the patient, clamp it briefly. ►You should never clamp chest drains inserted for pneumothoraces. Clamping for pleural effusions can control the rate of drainage and prevent expansion pulmonary oedema.
- Request a CXR to check the position of the drain.

**Removal** *in pneumothorax* Consider when drain is no longer bubbling and CXR shows re-inflation. Give analgesia beforehand, eg morphine.[13] Smartly withdraw during expiration or Valsalva. There is no need to clamp the drain beforehand as reinsertion is unlikely.[14] *In effusions* generally the drain can be removed when drainage is <200mL/24h, but for cirrhotic hydrothoraces the chest drain is treated similarly to the ascitic drain (see p778) with HAS supplementation and removal at 4-6 hours.

## The 'safe triangle' for insertion of a chest drain

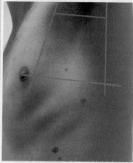

Fig 1. The safe 'triangle' is not really a triangle, as the axilla cuts off the point of the triangle. Draw a line along the lateral border of pectoralis major, a line along the anterior border of latissimus dorsi, and a line superior to the horizontal level of the nipple. The apex of the triangle is the axilla.

Often chest drains are inserted directly under ultrasound guidance, or with a pre-marked spot; however, in an emergency or for aspiration, the landmarks of the safe triangle are important to know.

### Complications
• Thoracic or abdominal organ injury •Lymphatic damage ∴ chylothorax
• Damage to long thoracic nerve of Bell ∴ wing scapula •Rarely, arrhythmia.[15]

### Watch out for
• Retrograde flow back into the chest
• Persistent bubbling—there may be a continual leak from the lung
• Blockage of the tube from clots or kinking—no swinging or bubbling
• Malposition—check position with CXR.

## Relieving a tension pneumothorax

**Symptoms** Acute respiratory distress, chest pain, ▶▶respiratory arrest.

**Signs** Hypotension; distended neck veins; asymmetrical lung expansion; trachea and apex deviated away from side of reduced air entry and hyperresonance to percussion. ▶▶There is no time for a CXR (but see fig 1, p763).

**Aim** To release air from the pleural space. In a tension pneumothorax air is drawn into the intrapleural space with each breath, but cannot escape due to a valve-like effect of the tiny flap in the parietal pleura. The increasing pressure progressively embarrasses the heart and the other lung.

▶▶**100% oxygen.**

▶▶**Insert a large-bore IV cannula** (eg Venflon®) usually through the 2nd intercostal space in the midclavicular line or the 'safe triangle' for chest drain insertion (see BOX). Remove the stylet, allowing the trapped air to escape, usually with an audible hiss. This converts the tension pneumothorax to an open pneumothorax. Tape securely. ▶Don't recover the cannula as tensioning will recur.

▶▶Proceed to formal chest drain insertion (see p780).

## Aspiration of a pneumothorax

▶p825

Identify the 2nd intercostal space in the midclavicular line (or 4-6th intercostal space in the midaxillary line) and infiltrate with 1% *lidocaine* down to the pleura overlying the pneumothorax.
• Insert a 16G cannula into the pleural space. Remove the needle and connect the cannula to a 3-way tap and a 50mL syringe. Aspirate up to 2.5L of air (50mL×50). Stop if resistance is felt, or if the patient coughs excessively.
• Request a CXR to confirm resolution of the pneumothorax. If successful, consider discharging the patient and repeating the CXR after 24h to exclude recurrence, and again after 7-10d. Advise to avoid air travel for 6 weeks after a normal CXR. Diving should be permanently avoided.
• If aspiration is unsuccessful (in a significant, symptomatic pneumothorax), insert an intercostal drain (see p780).

**Contraindications** •Bleeding diathesis; •Cardiorespiratory compromise; •Infection at site of needle insertion. Most importantly: ▶▶ ↑Intracranial pressure (suspect if very severe headache, ↓level of consciousness with falling pulse, rising BP, vomiting, focal neurology, or papilloedema)—LP in these patients will cause coning, so unless it is a routine procedure, eg for known idiopathic intracranial hypertension, obtain a CT prior to LP. CT is not infallible, so be sure your indication for LP is strong.

**Method** Explain to the patient what sampling CSF entails, why it is needed, that co-operation is vital, and that they can communicate with you at all stages.

• Place the patient on his or her left side, with the back on the edge of the bed, fully flexed (knees to chin). A pillow under the head and another between the knees may keep them more stable.
• Landmarks: plane of iliac crests through the level of L3/4 (see fig 1). In adults, the spinal cord ends at the L1/2 disc (fig 2). Mark L3/4 intervertebral space (or one space below, L4/5), eg by a gentle indentation of a needle cap on the overlying skin (better than a ballpoint pen mark, which might be erased by the sterilizing fluid).
• Use aseptic technique (hat, mask, gloves, gown) and 2% chlorhexidine in 70% alcohol to clean the skin, allow to dry and then place sterile drapes.
• Open the spinal pack. Assemble the manometer and 3-way tap. Have 3 plain sterile tubes and 1 fluoride tube (for glucose) ready.
• Using a 25G (orange) needle, raise a bleb of local anaesthetic, then use a 21G (green) needle to infiltrate deeper.
• Wait 1min, then insert spinal needle (22G, stilette in place) perpendicular to the body, aiming slightly up towards umbilicus. Feel resistance of spinal ligaments, and then the dura, then a 'give' as the needle enters the subarachnoid space. NB: keep the bevel of the needle facing up, parallel with dural fibres.
• Withdraw stilette. Check CSF fills needle and attach manometer (3-way tap turned off towards you) to measure 'opening' pressure.
• Catch fluid in three sequentially numbered bottles (10 drops per tube).
• Reinsert stilette,[16] then remove needle and apply dressing. Document the procedure clearly in the notes including CSF appearance and opening pressure.
• Send CSF promptly for *microscopy, culture, protein, lactate and glucose* (do plasma glucose too)—call the lab to let them know. If applicable, also send for: cytology, fungal studies, TB culture, virology (± herpes and other PCR), syphilis serology, oligoclonal bands (+serum sample for comparison) if multiple sclerosis suspected. Is there xanthochromia (p482)?
• There is no evidence that lying flat post procedure prevents headache,[17] check CNS observations and BP regularly if you have concerns. Post-LP headache is partly preventable by reinserting the stilette before needle withdrawal,[16] and reducing CSF leakage by using finer needles shaped to part the dura rather than cut it: see BOX.
• If you fail: ask for help—try with the patient sitting or with radiology guidance.

**CSF composition** *Normal values:* Lymphocytes <5/mm³; no polymorphs; protein <0.4g/L; glucose >2.2mmol/L (or ≥50% plasma level); pressure <200mm CSF. *In meningitis:* See p833. *In multiple sclerosis:* See p500.

*Bloody tap:* This is an artefact due to piercing a blood vessel, which is indicated (unreliably) by fewer red cells in successive bottles, and no yellowing of CSF (xanthochromia). To estimate how many white cells ($W$) were in the CSF before the blood was added, use the following:

$$W = CSF\ WCC - [(blood\ WCC \times CSF\ RBC) \div blood\ RBC].$$

If the blood count is normal, the rule of thumb is to subtract from the total CSF WCC (per µL) one white cell for every 1000 RBCs. To estimate the true protein level, subtract 10mg/L for every 1000 RBCs/mm³ (be sure to do the count and protein estimation on the same bottle). NB: high protein levels in CSF make it appear yellow. *Subarachnoid haemorrhage:* Xanthochromia (yellow supernatant on spun CSF). Red cells in equal numbers in all bottles (unreliable). RBCs will excite an inflammatory response (eg CSF WCC raised), most marked after 48h. *Raised protein:* Meningitis; MS; Guillain-Barré syndrome. *Very raised CSF protein:* Spinal block; TB; or severe bacterial meningitis.

## Complications

• Post-dural puncture headache • Infection • Bleeding • Cerebral herniation (rare, check for signs of ↑ICP before proceeding) • Minor/transient neurological symptoms, eg paraesthesia, radiculopathy.

Any change in lower body neurology after an LP (pain, weakness, sensory changes, bladder/bowel disturbance) should be treated as cauda equina compression (haematoma/abscess) until proven otherwise. Obtain an urgent MRI spine.

**NB**: post-LP brain MRI scans often show diffuse meningeal enhancement with gadolinium. This is thought to be a reflection of increased blood flow secondary to intracranial hypotension. Interpret these scans with caution and in the context of the patient's clinical situation. Ensure the reason for the scan and current neurological examination are discussed with the radiologist pre procedure.

## Post-LP headache

**Risk** 10–30%, typically occurring within 24h of LP, resolution over hours to 2wks (mean: 3–4d). Patients describe a constant, dull ache, more frontal than occipital. The most characteristic symptom is of **positional exacerbation**—worse when upright. There may be mild meningism or nausea. The pathology is thought to be continued leakage of CSF from the puncture site and intracranial hypotension, though there may be other mechanisms involved.[18]

**Prevention** Use the smallest spinal needle that is practical (22G) and keep the bevel aligned as described on p782. Blunt needles (more expensive!) can reduce risk and are recommended (ask an anaesthetist about supply, headache following spinal anaesthesia occurs in only ~1%, partly due to this and partly due to the smaller needles used);[19] however, collection of CSF takes too long (>6min) if needles smaller than 22G are used.[20] Before withdrawing the needle, reinsert the stilette.[16]

**Treatment** Despite years of anecdotal advice to the contrary, none of the following has ever been shown to be a risk factor: position during or after the procedure; hydration status before, during, or after; amount of CSF removed; immediate activity or rest post-LP.[21] Time is a consistent healer. For severe or prolonged headaches, ask an anaesthetist about a **blood patch**.[22] This is a careful injection of 20mL of autologous venous blood into the adjacent epidural space (said to 'clog up the hole'). Immediate relief occurs in 95%.

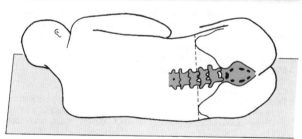

**Fig 1.** Defining the 3rd–4th lumbar vertebral interspace.
Adapted with permission from Vakil; Diagnosis & Management of Medical Emergencies, OUP.

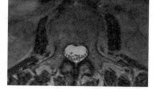

**Fig 2.** Axial T2-weighted MRI of the lumbar spine. The conus ends at the L1/L2 level with continuation of the cauda equina. Lumbar puncture below the L2 level will not damage the cauda equina as the nerve roots will part around an LP needle.

Image courtesy of Norwich Radiology Dept.

Practical procedures

▶Do not wait for a crisis before familiarizing yourself with the defibrillator, as there are several types. All hospitals should include this information in your induction but check how the machine on your ward works.

**Indications** To restore sinus rhythm if VF/VT; AF, flutter, or supraventricular tachycardias if other treatments (p120) have failed, or there is haemodynamic compromise (p124 & p818). This may be done as an emergency, eg VF/VT, or electively, eg AF.

**Aim** To completely depolarize the heart using a direct current.

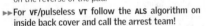

## Procedure

- Unless critically unwell, conscious patients require a general anaesthetic or monitored heavy sedation.[1]
- If elective cardioversion of AF ensure adequate anticoagulation beforehand.
- Almost all defibrillators are now paddle-free and use 'hands-free' pads instead (less chance of skin arc than jelly). Place the pads (eg Littmann™ Defib Pads) on chest, 1 over apex (p37) and 1 below right clavicle. The positions are often given by a diagram on the reverse of the pad.

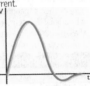

Fig 1. The dampened sine monophasic waveform.

▶▶For VF/pulseless VT follow the ALS algorithm on inside back cover and call the arrest team!

*Cardioversion:* Synchronize the shock with the rhythm by pressing the 'SYNC' button on the machine. This ensures the shock does not initiate a ventricular arrhythmia. However, this only works for cardioversion; **if the sync mode is engaged in VF, the defibrillator will not discharge!**

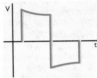

Fig 2. Rectilinear biphasic waveform with truncated exponential decay. Most new external defibrillators use this waveform.

- *Monophasic defibrillators* (fig 1): Set the energy level at 360J for VF/VT (ARREST SITUATION); 200J for AF; 50J for atrial flutter.[23,24]
- *Biphasic defibrillators* (fig 2): Impedance is less with a biphasic shock and 120-200J is used for shocks for VF/VT. They use less energy and are just as effective as monophasic defibs in cardioversion. 120-200J will cardiovert most arrhythmias.
- *Automatic external defibrillators* (AED): Can be used by anyone who can turn them on and apply the pads. Follow the instructions given by the AED.

## Shocking

1 Consider anticoagulation in AF.[2]
2 Clearly state that you are charging the defibrillator.
3 Make sure no one else is touching the patient, the bed, or anything is in turn touching these.
4 Clearly state that you are about to shock the patient.
5 Press the button(s) on the electrode(s) to give the shock. If there is a change in rhythm before you shock and the shock is no longer required, turn the dial to 'discharge'. Do not allow anyone to approach until the reading has dropped to 0J.
6 After a shock: watch ECG; repeat the shock. Up to 3 are usual for AF/flutter.
7 Get an up-to-date 12-lead ECG.

▶In children, use 2J/kg, then 4J/kg in VF/VT; if monophasic, and if >10kg, use adult paddles; *OHCS* p239.

1 Remember that overdose of midazolam for sedation in a conscious patient is an NHS 'Never Event', so make sure you know what you are doing and have the support of an anaesthetist or someone else who is trained in sedation and airway management, eg intensivist, or emergency department physician.
2 The risk of emboli is increased if the patient presents >48 hours after onset of AF; if in doubt, anticoagulate or, if patient less stable, request a TOE to check for thrombi.

## 78

## Taking arterial blood gas (ABG) samples

The reaction of a patient to ABG sampling is often very different to when they are subjected to venepuncture, so try to explain that the blood sample you are about to take is going to feel different and is for a different purpose (p156 for indications and analysis). The usual site is the radial artery at the wrist. ▶Check with the patient that they do not have an arteriovenous fistula for haemodialysis. Never, ever sample from a fistula!

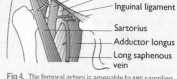

Fig 3. The ideal position for the wrist, slightly hyperextended, resting on an unopened litre bag of fluid or a bandage is ideal. In an unconscious patient or for arterial line insertion, taping the thumb to the bed can hold the wrist in the perfect position if you do not have an assistant.

*Procedure:*
• Get kit ready; include: portable sharps bin; pre-heparinized syringe; needle (blue size (23G) is good, although many syringes now come pre-made with needle); gloves; 2% chlorhexidine/70% alcohol swab; gauze; tape.
• Feel thoroughly for the best site. Look at both sides.
• Wipe with cleaning swab. Let the area dry. Get yourself comfortable.
• If the patient is drowsy or unconscious, ask an assistant to hold the hand and arm with the wrist slightly extended (fig 3).
• Before sampling, expel any excess heparin in the syringe. Infiltration over the artery with a small amount of 1% *lidocaine* (p575) through a 25G (orange) needle makes the procedure painless.
• Hold the syringe like a pen, with the needle bevel up. Let the patient know you are about to take the sample. Feel for the pulse with your other hand and enter at 45°, aiming beneath the finger you are feeling with.
• In most syringes, the plunger will move up on its own in a pulsatile manner if you are in the artery; rarely, entry into a vein next to the artery will give a similar result. Colour of the blood is little guide to its source!
• Allow the syringe to fill with 1-2mL, then remove the needle and apply firm pressure for 5 minutes (10 if anticoagulated).
• Expel any air from the syringe as this will alter the oxygenation of the blood. Cap and label the sample, check the patient's temperature and $FiO_2$ (0.21 if on air!). Take the sample to the nearest analysis machine or send it by express delivery to the lab (which may

Fig 4. The femoral artery is amenable to ABG sampling.

- Femoral nerve
- Femoral artery
- Femoral vein
- Inguinal ligament
- Sartorius
- Adductor longus
- Long saphenous vein

be by your own feet, get someone else to apply pressure) as it should be analysed within 15 minutes of sampling.
• Syringes and analysis machines differ, so get familiar with the local nuances.

The other site that is amenable to ABG sampling is the femoral artery. Surprisingly this may be less uncomfortable as it is a relatively less sensitive area and because, when supine, the patient cannot see the needle and thus may feel less apprehensive. The brachial artery can also be used, but be aware that the median nerve sits closely on its medial side and it is an end-artery. Normal values: p771.

**Cricothyroidotomy** = an emergency procedure to overcome airway obstruction above the level of the larynx. It should only be done in absolute "can't intubate, can't ventilate" situations, ie where ventilation is impossible with a bag and mask (± airway adjuncts) and where there is an immediate threat to life. If not, call anaesthetics or ENT for immediate help.

**Indications** Upper airway obstruction when endotracheal intubation not possible, eg irretrievable foreign body; facial oedema (burns, angio-oedema); maxillofacial trauma; infection (epiglottitis).

**Procedure** Lie the patient supine with neck extended (eg pillow under shoulders) unless there is suspected cervical-spine instability. Run your index finger down the neck anteriorly in the midline to find the notch in the upper border of the thyroid cartilage (the Adam's apple): just below this, between the thyroid and cricoid cartilages, is a depression—the cricothyroid membrane (see fig 1). If you cannot feel the depression and it is an emergency, you can access the trachea directly approximately halfway between the cricoid cartilage and the suprasternal notch.

Ideally use a purpose-designed kit (eg QuickTrach, MiniTrach), all hospitals will stock one version. If no kit is available then a cannula (needle cricothyroidotomy) can buy time, and in out-of-hospital situations a blade and empty biro case have saved lives!

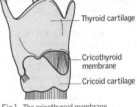

- Thyroid cartilage
- Cricothyroid membrane
- Cricoid cartilage

Fig 1. The cricothyroid membrane.

**1** *Needle cricothyroidotomy:* Pierce the membrane perpendicular to the skin with large-bore cannula (14G) attached to syringe: withdrawal of air confirms position; lidocaine may or may not be required. Slide cannula over needle at 45° to the skin superiorly in the sagittal plane (see fig 3). Use a Y-connector or improvise connection to $O_2$ supply at 15L/min: use thumb on Y-connector to allow $O_2$ in over 1s and $CO_2$ out over 4s ('transtracheal jet insufflation'). This is the preferred method in children <12yrs. This will only sustain life for 30–45min before $CO_2$ builds up. However, if the patient has a completely obstructed airway then they will not be able to exhale through this, and it will lead to cardiovascular compromise and pneumothoraces.

**2** *Cricothyroidotomy kit:* Most contain a guarded blade, and a large (4–6mm) shaped cannula (cuffed or uncuffed depending on brand) over an introducer, plus a connector and binding tape. The patient will have to be ventilated via a bag, as the resistance is too high to breathe spontaneously. This will sustain for 30–45min.

**3** *Surgical cricothyroidotomy:* Smallest tube for prolonged ventilation is 6mm. Introduce high-volume low-pressure cuff tracheostomy tube through a horizontal incision in membrane. Take care not to cut the thyroid or cricoid cartilages.

**Complications** Local haemorrhage ± aspiration; posterior perforation of trachea ± oesophagus; subglottic stenosis; laryngeal stenosis if membrane over-incised in childhood; tube blockage; subcutaneous tunnelling; vocal cord paralysis or hoarseness (the recurrent laryngeal nerve runs superiorly in the tracheo-oesophageal groove).

▶NB: needle and kit cricothyroidotomies are temporary measures pending formal tracheostomy.

### Emergency needle pericardiocentesis[1] (fig 2)

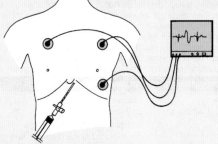

Fig 2. Emergency needle pericardiocentesis.

- Get your senior's help (for whom this page may serve as an *aide-mémoire*).
- Equipment: 20mL syringe, long 18G cannula, 3-way tap, ECG monitor, skin cleanser. Use echo guidance if time allows.
- If time allows, use full aseptic technique, at a minimum clean skin with 2% chlorhexidine in 70% alcohol (eg ChloraPrep®) and wear sterile gloves, and, if conscious, use local anaesthesia and sedation, eg with slow IV *midazolam*: titrate up to 3.5-5mg—start with 2mg over 1min, 0.5-1mg in elderly (in whom the maximum dose is 3.5mg; inject at the rate of ≤2mg/min)—antidote: *flumazenil* 0.2mg IV over 15s, then 0.1mg every 60s, up to 1mg in total.
  ▶Ensure you have IV access and full resuscitation equipment to hand.
- Introduce needle at 45° to skin just below and to left of xiphisternum, aiming for tip of left scapula. Aspirate continuously and watch ECG. Frequent ventricular ectopics or an injury pattern (ST segment↓) on ECG imply that the myocardium has been breached—withdraw slightly. As soon as fluid is obtained through the needle, slide the cannula into place.
- Evacuate pericardial contents through the syringe and 3-way tap. Removal of only a small amount of fluid (eg 20mL) can produce marked clinical improvement. If you are not sure whether the fluid you are aspirating is pure blood (eg on entering a ventricle), see if it clots (heavily bloodstained pericardial fluid does not clot), or measure its PCV (though this may be difficult in the acute setting but some blood gas analysers may give this).
- You can leave the cannula *in situ* temporarily, for repeated aspiration. If there is reaccumulation, insert a drain but pericardiectomy may be needed.
- Send fluid for microscopy and culture, as needed, including tests for TB.

*Complications:* Laceration of ventricle or coronary artery (± subsequent haemopericardium); aspiration of ventricular blood; arrhythmias (ventricular fibrillation); pneumothorax; puncture of aorta, oesophagus (± mediastinitis), or peritoneum (± peritonitis).

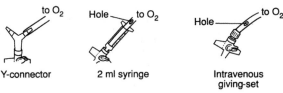

Fig 3. Methods of providing oxygen.

1 Procedures used by cardiologists for elective pericardiocentesis may differ, involving the use of guide-wires, screening, and catheters.

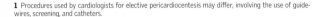

Central venous cannulae may be inserted to measure central venous pressure (CVP), to administer certain drugs (eg amiodarone, chemotherapy), or for intravenous access (fluid, parenteral nutrition). In an emergency, the procedure can be done using the landmark method (see opposite), though NICE recommends that all routine internal jugular catheters should be placed with US guidance.[25] Even if the line is not placed under direct ultrasound visualization, a look to check vessel size, position in relation to artery, and patency (no thrombus or stenosis) is extremely useful.

### Contraindications to central venous cannulation

| Absolute | Relative |
|---|---|
| Infection at insertion site | Coagulopathy |
| | Ipsilateral carotid endarterectomy |
| | Newly inserted cardiac pacemaker leads |
| | Thrombus within the vein |
| | Venous stenosis |
| | Ipsilateral abnormal anatomy |

**Sites of insertion** include the internal jugular vein (see below and BOX, p41), subclavian vein, and the femoral vein (often used in an emergency see BOX, p785). The choice depends largely on operator experience, but evidence suggests that the femoral approach is associated with a higher rate of line infection and thrombosis.[26] Overall, the internal jugular approach (with ultrasound guidance) is most commonly used and risks fewer complications than the subclavian. If possible, get written consent (p570). Check clotting + platelets. The technique for internal jugular (routine) and femoral (emergency) is given below.

**Complications** (~20%). Insertion is not without hazard, so decide whether the patient requires a line first, and then ask for help if you are inexperienced.
▶Bleeding; arterial puncture/cannulation; AV fistula formation.
• Air embolism.
• Pneumothorax; haemothorax; chylothorax (lymph).
• Phrenic nerve palsy.[1] The right phrenic nerve passes over the brachiocephalic artery, posterior to the subclavian vein. Hiccups may be a sign of injury.[27]
• Phlebitis; thrombus formation on tip or in vein. If high risk for thromboembolism (eg malignancy), consider anticoagulation (eg low molecular weight heparin).
• Bacterial colonization; cellulitis; sepsis. This can be reduced by adherence to a strict aseptic technique, and use of antibiotic- or heparin-coated catheters.[28]

▶If taking blood cultures in a febrile patient with a central venous line, remember to take samples from the central line and from a new peripheral site (ie not a pre-existing cannula).

**Peripherally inserted central cannulas (PICC lines)** are a good alternative to central lines, as they can stay *in situ* for up to 6 months, and provide access for blood sampling, fluids, antibiotics (allowing home IV therapy). They are placed using a Seldinger technique, puncturing the brachial or basilic vein then threading the line into the subclavian or superior vena cava. Because of the insertion site there is a much lower risk of pneumo- or haemothorax, but they are tricky to insert in an emergency.

**Removing central lines** Should be done carefully with aseptic technique. Put the patient slightly head down, remove dressings, clean and drape the area, remove sutures. Ask the patient to inhale and hold their breath, then breath out smoothly while you are pulling the line out. This helps to prevent air emboli. Apply pressure for 5 minutes (longer if coagulopathic).

---

**1** Think of phrenic nerve palsy whenever there is orthopnoea (CXR: raised hemidiaphragm). Other causes: lung ca; myeloma; thymoma; neck trauma; cervical spondylosis; thoracic surgery; C3-5 zoster; HIV; Lyme dis.; TB; paraneoplastic syndrome; muscular dystrophy; big left atrium; phrenic nucleus lesion (eg MS).[29]

**Internal jugular** should be the approach of choice in a non-emergency situation. Ideally the right side as it offers a direct route to the heart and there is less chance of misplacement of the line compared to the left. The subclavian approach is trickier and best taught by an expert. Use ultrasound guidance if at all possible, ideally to insert the line under direct vision, but at least to define the anatomy. If possible, have the patient attached to a cardiac monitor in case of arrhythmias.

- Position the patient slightly head down to avoid air embolism and fill the veins to improve your chances of success. NB: ►this can compromise cardiac function and precipitate acute LVF so check if your patient has a cardiac history. Minimize the time the patient is head down; if they are unable to lie flat, consider a femoral approach. Turn their head slightly to the left.
- This should be a sterile procedure so use full aseptic technique (hat, mask, gloves, gown) and clean with 2% chlorhexidine in 70% isopropyl alcohol before draping. Ensure your equipment is prepared, flush the catheter lumens with saline.
- If ultrasound is not available, the *landmark procedure* can be used to identify insertion point—approximately at the junction of the two heads of sternocleidomastoid at about the level of the thyroid cartilage (fig 1). Feel gently for the carotid pulse, then infiltrate with 1% lidocaine just lateral to this. The vein is usually superficial (fig 2).

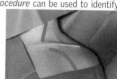

**Fig 1.** Position of internal jugular and subclavian veins (red) compared to the clavicle (yellow).

- Insert the introducer needle with a 5mL syringe attached, advance gently at a 45 degree angle, aiming for the ipsilateral nipple and aspirating continuously. If you are using ultrasound, watch the needle tip enter the vein, if the landmark approach keep your fingers on the carotid pulse.
- As soon as blood is aspirated, lay down the ultrasound and hold the introducer needle in position, remove the syringe and thread the guidewire through the needle. It should pass easily, if there is resistance try lowering the angle of the needle and gently advancing the wire. If the wire will not pass do not remove it alone, the tip can shear off and embolize, remove the needle with the wire, apply pressure and attempt a second puncture.

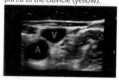

**Fig 2.** Vessels seen on ultrasound. The compressible vein is above the artery.

- If the wire threads easily, insert to 30cm (see markings on the wire), remove the needle keeping hold of the wire at all times. Make a nick in the skin with a scalpel at the insertion point, and gently thread the dilator over the wire. You do not need to insert the dilator far, only as far as the vein (you often feel a loss of resistance as the dilator enters the vein, so insert gently, the authors have seen several pneumothoraces from enthusiastic dilating).
- Remove the dilator, keeping hold of the wire, thread the flushed catheter over the wire, then remove the wire. The line should sit at about 13cm on the right side (17cm on the left). Check you can aspirate blood from each lumen, then flush them.
- Suture the catheter in place (many have little 'wings' for suturing) and dress. Request a CXR to confirm position and exclude pneumothorax. The tip of the catheter should sit vertically in the SVC.

**Femoral vein** In an emergency situation where ultrasound is not easily accessible, if the patient is unable to lie flat, or where speed is of the essence, the femoral approach is often the safest, as there is no risk of pneumothorax, haemothorax and a much reduced risk of arrhythmia. The technique is similar to internal jugular, except the insertion point is just medial to the femoral artery at the groin crease.

**Subclavian vein** Should be taught by an expert and should ideally be carried out under ultrasound guidance. Many experienced physicians prefer this approach, but even in experienced hands there is a higher risk of complications compared to ultrasound guided internal jugular lines.[30]

Often it is wiser to liaise with a specialist pacing centre to arrange prompt, definitive pacing than to try temporary transvenous pacing, which often has complications (see below) which may delay a definitive procedure.

### Possible indications in the acute phase of myocardial infarction

- *Complete AV block:*
  - With inferior MI (right coronary artery occlusion) pacing may only be needed if symptomatic; spontaneous recovery may occur.
  - With anterior MI (representing massive septal infarction).
- *Second-degree block:*
  - Wenckebach (p119; implies decremental AV node conduction; may respond to atropine in an inferior MI; pace if anterior MI).
  - Mobitz type 2 block is usually associated with distal fascicular disease and carries high risk of complete heart block, so pace in both types of MI.
- *First-degree block:* Observe carefully: 40% develop higher degrees of block.
- *Bundle branch block:* Pace prophylactically if evidence of trifascicular disease (p94) or non-adjacent bifascicular disease.
- *Sino-atrial disease + serious symptoms:* Pace unless responds to atropine.

### Other indications where temporary pacing may be needed

- Pre-op: if surgery is required in patients with type 2 or complete heart block (whether or not MI has occurred); do 24h ECG; liaise with the anaesthetist.
- Drug poisoning, eg with β-blockers, digoxin, or verapamil.
- Symptomatic bradycardia, uncontrolled by atropine or isoprenaline.
- Suppression of drug-resistant VT and SVT (overdrive pacing; do on ICU).
- Asystolic cardiac arrest with P-wave activity (ventricular standstill).
- During or after cardiac surgery—eg around the AV node or bundle of His.

### Technique for temporary transvenous pacing Learn from an expert.

- *Preparation:* Monitor ECG; have a defibrillator to hand, ensure the patient has peripheral access; check that a radiographer with screening equipment is present.[1] If you are screening, wear leads. Ensure you use full aseptic technique throughout.
- *Insertion:* Place the introducer into the (ideally right) internal jugular vein (p789) or subclavian. If this is difficult, access to the right atrium can be achieved via the femoral vein. Pass the pacing wire through the introducer into the right atrium, ideally under radiological screening. It will either pass easily through the tricuspid valve or loop within the atrium. If the latter occurs, it is usually possible to flip the wire across the valve with a combined twisting and withdrawing movement (fig 1). Advance the wire slightly. At this stage the wire may try to exit the ventricle through the pulmonary outflow tract. A further withdrawing and rotation of the wire will aim the tip at the apex of the right ventricle. Advance slightly again to place the wire in contact with the endocardium. Remove any slack to ↓risk of subsequent displacement.
- *Checking the threshold:* Connect the wire to the pacing box and set the 'demand' rate slightly higher than the patient's own heart rate and the output to 3V. A paced rhythm should be seen. Find the pacing threshold by slowly reducing the voltage until the pacemaker fails to stimulate the tissue (pacing spikes are no longer followed by paced beats). The threshold should be less than 1V, but a slightly higher value may be acceptable if it is stable—eg after a large infarction.
- *Setting the pacemaker:* Set the output to 3V or over 3 times the threshold value (whichever is higher) in 'demand' mode. Set the rate as required. Suture the wire to the skin, and fix with a sterile dressing.
- Check the position of the wire (and exclude pneumothorax) with a CXR.
- Recurrent checks of the pacing threshold are required over the next few days. The formation of endocardial oedema can raise the threshold by a factor of 2-3.

**Complications** Pneumothorax; sepsis; cardiac perforation; pacing failure: from loss of capture, loss of electrical continuity in pacing circuit, or electrode displacement.

---

1 Balloon-flotation techniques do not need radiographic guidance and have been shown to be quicker and easier to insert, with fewer complications compared to placement of semi-rigid electrode wires.[31]

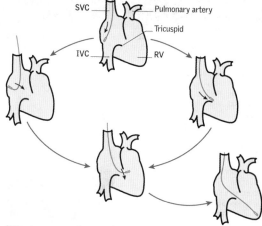

## 79

**Fig 1.** Siting a temporary cardiac pacemaker.

### Non-invasive transcutaneous cardiac pacing

This method (performed through a defibrillator with external pacing facility) has the advantages of being quicker, less risky than the transvenous route, and easier to perform. Its main disadvantage is the pain caused by skeletal muscle contraction in the non-sedated patient. Indications for pacing via the transcutaneous route are as OPPOSITE, **plus** if transvenous pacing (or someone able to perform it) is unavailable or will be delayed in an emergency situation.

►► Give sedation and analgesia, eg *midazolam + morphine* IV titrated to effect.

►► Clipping chest hair may help improve electrical contact; ►don't shave the skin, as nicks can predispose to electrical burns. Ensure the skin is dry.

►► Almost all modern transcutaneous devices can function through defibrillation 'hands free' pads, and so these can be applied as for defibrillation (see p784). If necessary, the pads can be placed in an AP position: anteriorly over the $V_2$–$V_3$ electrode position and posteriorly at the same level, just below the scapula.

►► Select 'demand' mode, (which synchronizes the stimulus with the R wave, so avoiding pacing on the T wave—which can provoke VF or VT) and adjust the ECG gain so that QRS complexes can be seen.

►► Select an appropriate pacing rate: eg 60-90bpm in an adult.

►► Set the pacing current at the lowest setting and turn on the pacemaker.

►► Increase the pacing current until electrical capture occurs (normally from 50-100mA), which can be confirmed by seeing a wide QRS complex and a T wave on the trace (ventricular electrical capture). This does not necessarily mean that there has been mechanical capture—one clinical trial has described using emergency cardiac ultrasound to assess for this.[32]

►► There will be some interference from skeletal muscle contraction on the ECG trace, as well as possible artefact, which could be mistaken for a QRS complex. The absence of a T wave is an important discriminator between the two.

►► CPR can continue with the pads in place, though only when the pacing unit is **off**.

►► Once adequate cardiac output has been maintained, seek expert help and arrange transvenous pacing.

Many diseases can present as emergencies, but if you know about the following, you will be very unlucky to lose a patient from a disease not listed here, on a general medical take, provided you remember to ask for help.

## Emergency presentations

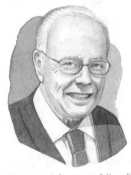

Fig 1. Dr James K. Styner was piloting a light aircraft in 1976 when weather conditions caused a crash that killed his wife and seriously injured three of his four children. With his eldest son he stabilised the other children and transferred all three to a local hospital, where he was appalled that the local doctors were unprepared for treating multiple trauma cases. He famously said "When I can provide better care in the field with limited resources than my children and I received at the primary facility, there is something wrong with the system and the system has to be changed." Following this incident he collaborated with several colleagues and in 1978 began offering an Advanced Trauma and Life Support course, now available in over 40 countries worldwide and considered the gold standard for initial management of trauma cases. He still practises today as an orthopaedic surgeon in California.

*Emergencies covered in other chapters* See inside front cover.
In OHCS—*Paediatrics:* Life support and cardiac arrest (OHCS p238–p239); is he seriously ill? (OHCS p103); epiglottitis (OHCS p158). *Adults:* The major disaster (OHCS p806); trauma (OHCS chapter 11); drowning (OHCS p724); ectopic pregnancy (OHCS p262); eclampsia (OHCS p48); amniotic fluid embolus (OHCS p89); obstetric shock (OHCS p55); glaucoma (OHCS p430); pre-hospital care/first aid (OHCS p790–p814).

⚠ Sources include: *BMJ; NEJM; Oxford Handbook of Acute Medicine;* and the MOD clinical guidelines for operations.[1]

## Introduction to emergencies

Some doctors enjoy the adrenaline rush of seeing an emergency case and pulling someone back from the edge of death. Some fear the emergency take, worried as to what they will miss, how many will die. There is no right approach; the emergency room needs both thought and practicality to manage patients. A patient who comes in flat and can be resuscitated gives the whole team a boost, as right there in front of us is the proof that we can make a difference. However, a patient who comes in well and collapses, dying before we can even decide what is wrong, can bring the whole team down. There are nights where we save life after life, and nights where we can't, sometimes a death is inevitable, despite our best efforts. You are a doctor, but you are a human being as well, and losing a patient can feel like a personal failure. However, remember that when we lose a patient it is the disease that has killed them, not us. Try to take a few minutes and reflect on what happened; ask if you could have done anything differently. Should you have sought help sooner? Discussing with a senior can be helpful, as can writing down your reflection, not in a portfolio for discussion at your appraisal, but in anonymous format for your own education. Watch the team at an arrest, the best doctors are the ones who have learned to stand back, assess the whole situation, and take enough time to see where the critical intervention is needed. There is no substitute for experience, nobody becomes a Consultant overnight, but watch the best clinicians at work and you will learn both practical and life skills.

Most important in an emergency situation is communication. Wherever you can, involve the relatives and the whole team in discussions, but remember that at the heart of this is a patient. What do they want? Never be afraid to ask the patient directly, they may hold very strong views. However, it is up to us as physicians to be honest with them about their prognosis, do not offer a treatment you know is not in the best interests of the patient, and this includes resuscitation. When faced with death, many patients are afraid, our role is to try to relieve that fear, whether by intervening to delay death, or by easing their passing. But we cannot ever prevent death, we simply delay it. As Shakespeare says in *Julius Caesar*:

"Of all the wonders that I have yet heard, it seems to me most strange that men should fear, seeing that death, a necessary end, will come when it will come."

## ABCDE preliminary assessment (primary survey)[2 NICE]

| | |
|---|---|
| Airway | Protect cervical spine, if injury possible.<br>*Assessment:* any signs of obstruction? Ascertain patency.<br>*Management:* establish a patent airway. |
| Breathing | *Assessment:* determine respiratory rate, check bilateral chest movement, percuss and auscultate.<br>*Management:* if no respiratory effort, treat as arrest[2] (see inside back cover), intubate and ventilate. If breathing compromised, give high-concentration $O_2$, manage according to findings, eg relieve tension pneumothorax. |
| Circulation | *Assessment:* check pulse and BP; check if peripherally shut down; check capillary refill; look for evidence of haemorrhage.<br>*Management:* if shocked, treat as on p804.<br>If no cardiac output, treat as arrest (see inside back cover). |
| Disability | Assess 'level of consciousness' with AVPU score (alert? responds to voice? to pain? unresponsive?); check pupils: size, equality, reactions. *Glasgow coma scale*, if time allows. |
| Exposure | Undress patient, but cover to avoid hypothermia. |

Quick history from relatives assists diagnosis: *Events* surrounding onset of illness, evidence of overdose/suicide attempt, any suggestion of trauma? *Past medical history:* Especially diabetes, asthma, COPD, alcohol, opiate or street drug abuse, epilepsy or recent head injury; recent travel. *Medication:* Current drugs. *Allergies*.

Once ventilation and circulation are adequate, proceed to carry out history, examination, investigations, and management in the usual way.

We thank Dr Andrew Johnston and Bernard Ho, our Junior Reader, for their contribution.

The vast majority of headaches are benign, but when taking a history do not forget to ask about the following (early diagnosis can save lives):

**Worrying features or 'red flags'**[1]
• First and worst headache—*subarachnoid haemorrhage*
• Thunderclap headache—*subarachnoid haemorrhage* (p484 for other causes)
• Unilateral headache and eye pain—*cluster headache, acute glaucoma*
• Unilateral headache and ipsilateral symptoms—*migraine, tumour, vascular*
• Cough-initiated headache—*raised ICP/venous thrombosis*
• Worse in the morning or bending forward—*raised ICP/venous thrombosis*
• Persisting headache ± scalp tenderness in over-50s—*giant cell arteritis*
• Headache with fever or neck stiffness—*meningitis*
• Change in the pattern of 'usual headaches'
• Decreased level of consciousness

*Two other vital questions:*
• Where have you been? (malaria)
• Might you be pregnant? (pre-eclampsia; especially if proteinuria and BP↑)

Always examine a patient presenting with a severe headache, if nothing about history or examination is concerning, both you and the patient will be reassured, but subtle abnormalities are important not to miss.

**No signs on examination**
• Tension headache
• Migraine
• Cluster headache
• Post-traumatic
• Drugs (nitrates, calcium-channel antagonists)
• Carbon monoxide poisoning or anoxia
• Subarachnoid haemorrhage

**Signs of meningism?**
• Meningitis (may not have fever or rash)
• Subarachnoid haemorrhage (examination may be normal)

**Decreased conscious level or localizing signs?**
• Stroke
• Encephalitis/meningitis
• Cerebral abscess
• Subarachnoid haemorrhage (see p482-3, figs 2 & 3)
• Venous sinus occlusion (focal neurological deficits)
• Tumour
• Subdural haematoma
• TB meningitis

**Papilloedema?**
• Tumour
• Venous sinus occlusion (focal neurological deficits)
• Malignant (accelerated phase) hypertension
• Idiopathic intracranial hypertension
• Any CNS infection, if prolonged (eg >2wks)—eg TB meningitis

**Others**
• Giant cell arteritis (ESR↑ and tender scalp over temporal arteries)
• Acute glaucoma (painful red eye—get pressures checked urgently)
• Vertebral artery dissection (neck pain and cerebellar/medullary signs)
• Cervical spondylosis
• Sinusitis
• Paget's disease (alk phos ↑↑)
• Altitude sickness

1 Adapted from C Hawkes 2002 *Hosp Med* 63 732-42.

There may not be time to ask or the patient may not be able to give you a history in acute breathlessness, this in itself can be a helpful sign (inability to complete sentences in one breath = severe breathlessness, inability to speak/impaired conscious level = life threatening). Collateral history of known respiratory disease, anaphylaxis or other history can be extremely helpful but do not delay. Assess the patient for the following:

**Wheezing?**
- Asthma (p820)
- COPD (p822)
- Heart failure (p812)
- Anaphylaxis (p806)

**Stridor?** (Upper airway obstruction)
- Foreign body or tumour
- Acute epiglottitis (younger patients)
- Anaphylaxis
- Trauma, eg laryngeal fracture

**Crepitations?**
- Heart failure
- Pneumonia
- Bronchiectasis
- Fibrosis

**Chest clear?**
- Pulmonary embolism (p828)
- Hyperventilation
- Metabolic acidosis, eg diabetic ketoacidosis (DKA)
- Anaemia
- Drugs, eg salicylates
- Shock (may cause 'air hunger', p804)
- Pneumocystis jirovecii pneumonia
- CNS causes

**Others**
- Pneumothorax—pain, increased resonance, tracheal deviation (if tension pneumothorax)
- Pleural effusion—'stony dullness'

**Key investigations**
- Baseline observations—$O_2$ sats, pulse, temperature, peak flow
- ABG if saturations <94% or concern about acidosis/drugs/sepsis
- ECG (signs of PE, LVH, MI?)
- CXR
- Baseline bloods: glucose, FBC, U&E, consider drug screen

First exclude any potentially life-threatening causes, by virtue of history, brief examination, and limited investigations. Then consider other potential causes. For the full assessment of cardiac pain, see p88 & p112.

**Life-threatening**
• Acute myocardial infarction
• Angina/acute coronary syndrome
• Aortic dissection
• Tension pneumothorax
• Pulmonary embolism
• Oesophageal rupture

**Others**
• Pneumonia
• Chest wall pain:
    • Muscular
    • Rib fractures
    • Bony metastases
    • Costochondritis
• Gastro-oesophageal reflux
• Pleurisy
• Empyema
• Pericarditis
• Oesophageal spasm
• Herpes zoster
• Cervical spondylosis
• Intra-abdominal:
    • Cholecystitis
    • Peptic ulceration
    • Pancreatitis
• Sickle-cell crisis

Before discharging patients with undiagnosed chest pain, be sure in your own mind that the pain is not cardiac (this pain is usually dull, may radiate to jaw, arm, or epigastrium, and is usually associated with exertion). Carry out key investigations and discuss options with a colleague, and the patient. *Safety-net*, telling the patient to return or seek advice if they develop worrying features (specify these) or the pain does not settle.

**Key investigations**
• CXR
• ECG
• FBC, U&E, and troponin (p112). Consider D-dimer

▶Just because the patient's chest wall is tender to palpation, this doesn't mean the cause of the chest pain is musculoskeletal. Even if palpation reproduces the same type of pain, ensure that you exclude all potential life-threatening causes. Although chest wall tenderness has discriminatory value against cardiac pain, it may be a feature of a pulmonary embolism.

**Definition** *Unrousable unresponsiveness.* Quantify using the *Glasgow coma scale.*

**Causes of impaired conscious level/coma**

*Metabolic:* Drugs, poisoning, eg carbon monoxide, alcohol, tricyclics

Hypoglycaemia, hyperglycaemia (ketoacidotic, or HONK, p844)

Hypoxia, $CO_2$ narcosis (COPD)

Septicaemia

Hypothermia

Myxoedema, Addisonian crisis

Hepatic/uraemic encephalopathy

*Neurological:* Trauma

Infection: meningitis (p832); encephalitis, eg herpes simplex—give IV aciclovir if the slightest suspicion (p400), *tropical*: malaria (▶▶p394; do thick films), typhoid, typhus, rabies, trypanosomiasis

Tumour: 1° or 2°

Vascular: stroke, subdural/subarachnoid, hypertensive encephalopathy

Epilepsy: non-convulsive status (p489) or post-ictal state

**Immediate management** see fig 1 (and coma CNS exam, p802)

- Assess **A**irway, **B**reathing, and **C**irculation. Consider intubation if GCS <8 (p802). Support the circulation if required (ie IV fluids). Give $O_2$ and treat any seizures. Protect the cervical spine unless trauma is known not to be the cause.
- Check blood glucose; give 50mL 20% glucose IV stat if hypoglycaemia possible.
- IV thiamine if any suggestion of Wernicke's encephalopathy; see below.
- IV naloxone (0.4-2mg IV) for opiate intoxication (may also be given IM or via ET tube); IV flumazenil (p854) for benzodiazepine intoxication only if airway compromised as risk of seizures especially if concomitant tricyclic intoxication.

**Examination** ▶ *Vital signs are vital—obtain full set, including temperature.*

- Signs of trauma—haematoma, laceration, bruising, CSF/blood in nose or ears, fracture 'step' deformity of skull, subcutaneous emphysema, 'panda eyes'.
- Stigmata of other illnesses: liver disease, alcoholism, diabetes, myxoedema.
- Skin for needle marks, cyanosis, pallor, rash (meningitis; typhus), poor turgor.
- Smell the breath (alcohol, hepatic fetor, ketosis, uraemia).
- Opisthotonus (fig 1, p425) ≈meningitis or tetanus. Decerebrate/decorticate? p802.
- Meningism (p460, p832) ▶but do *not* move neck unless cervical spine is cleared.
- Pupils (p803) size, reactivity, gaze.
- Heart/lung exam for BP, murmurs, rubs, wheeze, consolidation, collapse.
- Abdomen/rectal for organomegaly, ascites, bruising, peritonism, melaena.
- Are there any foci of infection (abscesses, bites, middle ear infection)?
- Any features of meningitis: neck stiffness, rash, focal neurology?
- Note the *absence* of signs, eg *no* pin-point pupils in a known heroin addict.

**Quick history** from family, ambulance staff, bystanders: Abrupt or gradual onset? How found—suicide note, seizure? If injured, suspect cervical spinal injury and do not move spine (*OHCS* p766). Recent complaints—headache, fever, vertigo, depression? Recent medical history—sinusitis, otitis, neurosurgery, ENT procedure? Past medical history—diabetes, asthma, ↑BP, cancer, epilepsy, psychiatric illness? Drug or toxin exposure (especially alcohol or other recreational drugs)? Any travel?

*If the diagnosis is unclear*

- Treat the treatable: Pabrinex® IV for Wernicke's encephalopathy, p728; $O_2$; naloxone as above; glucose (50mL of 50% IV); septic specifics: cefotaxime 2g/12h IV (meningitis, p832), artemether/quinine (malaria, p396), aciclovir (encephalitis, p834).
- Do routine biochemistry, haematology, thick films, blood cultures, blood ethanol, drug screen, etc.
- Arrange urgent CT head, if normal, and no CI, proceed to LP.

The diagnosis should now be clear, eg hyperglycaemia; alcohol excess; poisoning; uraemia; pneumonia; subarachnoid (p482); hypertensive/hepatic encephalopathy.

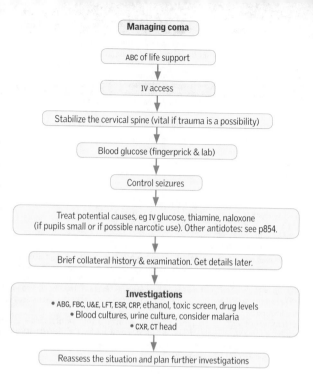

Fig 1. Managing coma. NB: check pupils every few minutes during the early stages, particularly if trauma is the likely cause. Doing so is the quickest way to find a localizing sign (so helpful in diagnosis, but remember that false localizing signs do occur)—and observing changes in pupil behaviour (eg becoming fixed and dilated) is the quickest way of finding out just how bad things are.

Emergencies

This gives a reliable, objective way of recording the conscious state of a person. It can be used by medical and nursing staff for initial and continuing assessment. It has value in predicting ultimate outcome. 3 types of response are assessed, note in each case the best response (or best of any limb) which should be recorded.

| Best motor response | Best verbal response | Eye opening |
|---|---|---|
| 6 Obeying commands | 5 Oriented (time, place, person) | 4 Spontaneous |
| 5 Localizing to pain | 4 Confused conversation | 3 In response to speech |
| 4 Withdrawing to pain | 3 Inappropriate speech | 2 In response to pain |
| 3 Flexor response to pain | 2 Incomprehensible sounds | 1 None |
| 2 Extensor response to pain | 1 None | |
| 1 No response to pain | | |

An overall score is made by summing the score in the 3 areas assessed.
- No response to pain + no verbalization + no eye opening = 3
- Severe injury, GCS ≤8—consider airway protection
- Moderate injury, GCS 9-12
- Minor injury, GCS 13-15.

Causing pain is not a pleasant thing, there are acceptable and unacceptable methods. Try fingernail bed pressure with a pen/pencil, supraorbital pressure or sternal pressure (not a rub). Abnormal responses to pain can help to localize the damage:
- *Flexion* = decorticate posture (arms bent inwards on chest, thumbs tucked in a clenched fist, legs extended) implies damage above the level of the red nucleus in the midbrain.[1]
- *Extension* = decerebrate posture (adduction and internal rotation of shoulder, pronation of forearm) indicates midbrain damage below the level of the red nucleus.

NB: an abbreviated coma scale, AVPU, is sometimes used in the initial assessment ('primary survey') of the critically ill:

A = alert

V = responds to vocal stimuli

P = responds to pain

U = unresponsive

NB: the GCS scoring is different in young children; see *OHCS* p201.

---

1 Red nucleus output reinforces upper limb antigravity flexion. When its output is damaged, the unregulated reticulospinal and vestibulospinal tracts reinforce extension tone of upper and lower limbs.[4]

## The neurological examination in coma

This is aimed at locating the pathology in 1 of 2 places. Altered level of consciousness implies either:

1 A diffuse, bilateral, cortical dysfunction (usually producing loss of awareness with normal arousal), or

2 Damage to the ascending reticular activating system (ARAS) located throughout the brainstem from the medulla to the thalami (usually producing loss of arousal with unassessable awareness). The brainstem can be affected directly (eg pontine haemorrhage) or indirectly (eg compression from trans-tentorial or cerebellar herniation secondary to a mass or oedema).

### Systematic examination

- Level of consciousness; describe using *objective* words/AVPU.
- Respiratory pattern (p53) - Cheyne-Stokes (brainstem lesions or compression) hyperventilation (acidosis, hypoxia, or, rarely, neurogenic), ataxic or apneustic (breath-holding) breathing (brainstem damage with grave prognosis).
- Eyes—almost all patients with ARAS pathology will have eye findings.

  1 *Visual fields* In light coma, test fields with visual threat. No blink in one field suggests hemianopia and contralateral hemisphere lesion.

  2 *Pupils Normal direct and consensual reflexes present* = intact midbrain. *Mid-position (3-5mm) non-reactive ± irregular* = midbrain lesion. *Unilateral dilated and unreactive* ('fixed') = 3$^{rd}$ nerve compression. *Small, reactive* = pontine lesion ('pin-point pontine pupils') or drugs. *Horner's syndrome* (p716, fig 1) = ipsilateral lateral medulla or hypothalamus lesion, may precede uncal herniation. Beware patients with false eyes or who use eye drops for glaucoma.

  3 *Extraocular movements (EOMS)*—observe resting position and spontaneous movement; then test the vestibulo-ocular reflex (VOR) with either the *doll's-head manoeuvre* (normal if the eyes keep looking at the same point in space when the head is quickly moved laterally or vertically) or *ice water calorics* (normal if eyes deviate towards the cold ear with nystagmus to the other side). If present, the VOR exonerates most of the brainstem from the VII$^{th}$ nerve nucleus (medulla) to the III$^{rd}$ (midbrain). *Don't move the head unless the cervical spine is cleared.*

  4 *Fundi*—papilloedema, subhyaloid haemorrhage, hypertensive retinopathy, signs of other disease (eg diabetic retinopathy).

- Examine for CNS asymmetry (tone, spontaneous movements, reflexes). One way to test for hemiplegia in coma is to raise both arms together and compare how they fall under gravity. If one descends fast, like a lead weight, but the other descends more gracefully, you have found a valuable focal sign. The same applies to the legs.

**Essence** Circulatory failure resulting in inadequate organ perfusion. Often defined by low BP—(SBP) systolic <90mmHg—or mean arterial pressure (MAP) <65mmHg—with evidence of tissue hypoperfusion, eg mottled skin, urine output (UO) of <0.5mL/kg for 1 hour, serum lactate >2mmol/L. *Signs:* Low GCS/agitation, pallor, cool peripheries, tachycardia, slow capillary refill, tachypnoea, oliguria.

**MAP = cardiac output (CO)** × systemic vascular resistance (**SVR**). CO = stroke volume × heart rate. So shock can result from inadequate CO or a loss of SVR, or both.

### Inadequate cardiac output
- *Hypovolaemia:*
  - Bleeding: trauma, ruptured aortic aneurysm, GI bleed.
  - Fluid loss: vomiting, burns, 'third space' losses, eg pancreatitis, heat exhaustion.
- *Pump failure:*
  - Cardiogenic shock, eg ACS, arrhythmias, aortic dissection, acute valve failure.
  - Secondary causes, eg pulmonary embolism, tension pneumothorax, cardiac tamponade.

### Peripheral circulatory failure (loss of SVR)
- *Sepsis:* Infection with any organism can cause acute vasodilation from inflammatory cytokines. Gram -ves can produce endotoxin, causing sudden and severe shock but without signs of infection (fever, raised WCC). Classically patients with sepsis are warm & vasodilated, but may be cold & shut down. Other diseases, eg pancreatitis, can give a similar picture associated with the inflammatory cascade.
- *Anaphylaxis:* p806.
- *Neurogenic:* Eg spinal cord injury, epidural or spinal anaesthesia.
- *Endocrine failure:* Addison's disease, p846 or hypothyroidism; see p844.
- *Other:* Drugs, eg anaesthetics, antihypertensives. Inability to use oxygen, eg cyanide poisoning.

**Assessment** ▶▶ABCDE (p793) With shock we are dealing primarily with 'C' so get large-bore IV access × 2 and check ECG for rate, rhythm (very fast or very slow will compromise cardiac output), and signs of ischaemia.

*General review:* Cold and clammy suggests cardiogenic shock or fluid loss. Look for signs of anaemia or dehydration, eg skin turgor, postural hypotension? Warm and well perfused, with bounding pulse points to septic shock. Any features suggestive of anaphylaxis—history, urticaria, angio-oedema, wheeze?

*CVS:* usually tachycardic (unless on β-blocker, or in spinal shock—*OHCS* p772) and hypotensive. But in the young and fit, or pregnant women, the systolic BP may remain normal, although the pulse pressure will narrow, with up to 30% blood volume depletion. Difference between arms (>20mmHg)—aortic dissection?

*JVP or central venous pressure:* If raised, cardiogenic shock likely.

*Check abdomen:* Any signs of trauma, or aneurysm? Any evidence of GI bleed?

**Management** ▶If BP unrecordable, call the cardiac arrest team.
- *Septic shock:*
  - Ideally take cultures before antibiotics (2 × peripheral blood culture plus, eg. urine, sputum, CSF) but do not delay starting treatment!
  - Give antibiotics within first hour, choice depends on local policy and suspected source. Empirical $R$ if no clear source, eg Tazocin® (4.5g tds) + gentamicin (eg 5mg/kg od; see p766) + vancomycin (1g/12h IVI) if MRSA. Adjust doses in CKD.
  - After fluid bolus of 20mL/kg crystalloid (or 7mL/kg colloid) repeat BP and ABG. If SBP remains <90 or lactate >4mmol/L then consider referral to ICU for early goal-directed therapy[5]—aim CVP 8-12, MAP >65mmHg, UO >0.5mL/kg/h.
  - Low-dose steroids may improve BP but do not improve mortality, recombinant activated protein C does not improve outcome and has been withdrawn from the market.
- *Anaphylaxis:* See p806.
- *Cardiogenic shock:* See p814.

- *Hypovolaemic shock:* Identify and treat underlying cause. Raise the legs.
  - Give fluid bolus 10–15mL/kg crystalloid or 3–5mL/kg colloid, if shock improves, repeat, titrate to HR (aim <100), BP (aim SBP >90) and UO (aim >0.5mL/kg/h)
  - If no improvement after 2 boluses, consider referral to ICU.
- *Haemorrhagic shock:* Stop bleeding if possible. See TABLE for grading.
  - If still shocked despite 2L crystalloid or present with class III/IV shock (see table) then crossmatch blood (request O Rh-ve in an emergency, see p342)
  - Give FFP alongside packed red cells (1:1 ratio) and aim for platelets >100 and fibrinogen >1. Discuss with haematology early.
- *Heat exposure (heat exhaustion):*
  - Tepid sponging + fanning; avoid ice and immersion. Resuscitate with high-sodium IVI, such as 0.9% saline ± hydrocortisone 100mg IV. Dantrolene seems ineffective. Chlorpromazine 25mg IM may be used to stop shivering. Stop cooling when core temperature <39°C.

| Class of shock | 1 | 2 | 3 | 4 |
|---|---|---|---|---|
| Blood loss (estimated mL or % of circulating vol) | <750mL or <15% | 750–1500mL 15–30% | 1500–2000mL 30–40% | >2000mL >40% |
| Heart rate (HR) | <100bpm | >100bpm | 120–140bpm | >140bpm |
| Systolic BP | Normal | Normal | Low | Unrecordable |
| Pulse pressure | Normal | Narrow | Narrow | V narrow/absent |
| Capillary refill | Normal | >2 seconds | >2 seconds | Absent |
| Respiratory rate | 14–20/min | 20–30/min | >30/min | >35/min |
| Urine output | >30mL/h | 20–30mL/h | 5–20mL/h | Negligible |
| Cerebral function | Normal/anxious | Anxious/hostile | Anxious/confused | Confused/unresponsive |

NB: remember that higher flow rates can be achieved through peripheral lines than through 'standard' gauge central lines. If cause unclear: $R$ as hypovolaemia—the most common cause, and reversible.

## SIRS, sepsis, and related syndromes

The pathogenesis of sepsis and septic shock is becoming increasingly understood. The 'systemic inflammatory response syndrome' (SIRS) is thought to be a central component, involving cytokine cascades, free-radical production, and the release of vasoactive mediators. SIRS is defined as the presence of 2 or more of the following features:[6]
- Temperature >38°C or <36°C
- Tachycardia >90bpm
- Respiratory rate >20 breaths/min or $P_aCO_2$ <4.3kPa
- WBC >12×10⁹/L or <4×10⁹/L, or >10% immature (band) forms

Related syndromes include:

*Sepsis:* SIRS occurring in the presence of infection.

*Severe sepsis:* Sepsis with evidence of organ hypoperfusion, eg hypoxaemia, oliguria, lactic acidosis, or altered cerebral function.

*Septic shock:* Severe sepsis with hypotension (systolic BP <90mmHg or MAP ≤ 60) despite adequate fluid resuscitation, or the requirement for vasopressors/inotropes to maintain blood pressure.

*Septicaemia* was used to denote the presence of multiplying bacteria in the circulation, but has been replaced with the definitions above.

Type-I IgE-mediated hypersensitivity reaction. Release of histamine and other agents causes: capillary leak; wheeze; cyanosis; oedema (larynx, lids, tongue, lips); urticaria. More common in atopic individuals. An *anaphylactoid reaction* results from direct release of mediators from inflammatory cells, without involving antibodies, usually in response to a drug, eg acetylcysteine.

### Examples of precipitants
• Drugs, eg penicillin, and contrast media in radiology
• Latex
• Stings, eggs, fish, peanuts, strawberries, semen (rare)

### Signs and symptoms
• Itching, sweating, diarrhoea and vomiting, erythema, urticaria, oedema
• Wheeze, laryngeal obstruction, cyanosis
• Tachycardia, hypotension

### Mimics of anaphylaxis
- Carcinoid (p278–279)
- Phaeochromocytoma (p220, p847)
- Systemic mastocytosis
- Hereditary angioedema

## Management of anaphylaxis

Secure the airway—give 100% O₂
Intubate if respiratory obstruction imminent

↓

Remove the cause; raising the feet
may help restore the circulation

↓

Give adrenaline IM *0.5mg* (ie *0.5mL of 1:1000*)
Repeat every 5min, if needed as guided by BP, pulse,
and respiratory function, until better

↓

Secure IV access

↓

Chlorphenamine 10mg IV and
hydrocortisone 200mg IV

↓

IVI (0.9% saline, eg 500mL over ¼h; up to 2L may be needed)
Titrate against blood pressure

↓

If wheeze, treat for asthma (p820)
May require ventilatory support

↓

If still hypotensive, admission to ICU and an IVI of adrenaline may be needed ± aminophylline (p821) and nebulized
salbutamol (p821): get expert help.

↓

### Further management
• Admit to ward. Monitor ECG.
• Measure mast cell tryptase 1-6h after suspected anaphylaxis.
• Continue chlorphenamine 4mg/6h PO if itching.
• Suggest a 'MedicAlert' bracelet naming the culprit allergen.
• Teach about self-injected adrenaline (eg 0.3mg, Epipen®) to
prevent a fatal attack.
• Skin-prick tests showing specific IgE help identify allergens
to avoid.

Fig 1. Management of anaphylaxis.

▶▶Adrenaline (=epinephrine) is given IM and NOT IV unless the patient is severely
ill, or has no pulse. The IV dose is **different**: 100μg/min—titrating with the response.
This is 0.5mL of 1:10,000 solution per minute. Stop as soon as a response has been
obtained.

If on a β-blocker, consider salbutamol IV in place of adrenaline.

Acute coronary syndrome (ACS) includes unstable angina, STEMI (what most of us mean by acute MI), and NSTEMI (see p810). STEMI is a common medical emergency, and prompt appropriate treatment saves lives. If in doubt, seek immediate help.

**Initial treatment** Take brief history, do a quick physical examination and take a 12-lead ECG. Blood tests on admission: U&E, troponin, glucose, cholesterol, FBC, CXR.

- *Aspirin* 300mg PO (if not already given); consider prasugrel (60mg PO if no history of stroke/TIA and <75yrs) or ticagrelor (180mg PO) as newer alternatives to clopidogrel (300mg PO) as they have been shown to be superior in outcome studies.[10, 11, 12]
- *Morphine* 5–10mg IV (repeat after 5min if necessary). Give anti-emetic with the 1st dose of morphine: metoclopramide 10mg IV (1st line) or cyclizine 50mg IV (2nd line).
- *GTN* routine use now not recommended in the acute setting unless patient is hypertensive or in acute LVF. Useful as anti-anginal in chronic/stable patients.
- *Oxygen* is recommended if patients have SaO$_2$ <95%, are breathless or in acute LVF.
- *Restore coronary perfusion* Either primary PCI (if available) or thrombolysis.
  - *Primary PCI* ▶▶should be offered to all patients who present with an acute STEMI who either are at or can be transferred to a primary PCI centre within 120 minutes of first medical contact. If this is not possible, patients should receive fibrinolysis and be transferred to a primary PCI centre after the infusion for either rescue PCI (if fibrinolysis unsuccessful) or angiography if successful.
  - *Fibrinolysis* ▶▶ benefit reduces steadily from onset of chest pain, target time is <30min from admission, and is contraindicated >24h from onset of symptoms. ▶Do not thrombolyse ST depression alone, T-wave inversion alone or normal ECG.
- *Anticoagulation* an injectable anticoagulant must be used in primary PCI. Bivalirudin is preferred, if not available use enoxaparin ± a GP IIb/IIIa blocker.

**Complications**
- Recurrent ischaemia or failure to reperfuse is not uncommon (usually detected as persisting pain and ST-segment elevation immediately after thrombolysis) so all patients should be transferred to a primary PCI centre for ongoing management.
- Stroke.
- Pericarditis: analgesics, try to avoid NSAIDs.
- Cardiogenic shock: see p814, and heart failure: see p812.

**Right ventricular infarction** Confirm by demonstrating ST elevation in rV$_{3/4}$ and/or echo. NB: rV$_4$ means that V$_4$ is placed in the right 5th intercostal space in the midclavicular line. Treat hypotension and oliguria with fluids (avoid nitrates and diuretics). Monitor BP carefully, and assess early signs of pulmonary oedema. Intensive monitoring and inotropes may be useful in some patients.

### Thrombolysis

**ECG criteria for thrombolysis**
- ST elevation >1mm in 2 or more limb leads or >2mm in 2 or more chest leads.
- LBBB (unless known to have LBBB previously).
- Posterior changes: Deep ST depression and tall R waves in leads V$_1$ to V$_3$.

*Contraindications*

| | |
|---|---|
| • Previous intracranial haemorrhage | • GI bleeding (<1 month) |
| • Ischaemic stroke <6months | • Known bleeding disorder |
| • Cerebral malignancy or AVM | • Aortic dissection |
| • Recent major trauma/surgery/head injury (<3wks) | • Non-compressible punctures <24h eg liver biopsy, lumbar puncture |

*Relative CI:* TIA <6months, oral anticoagulant therapy, pregnancy/<1wk post partum, refractory hypertension (>180mmHg/110mmHg), advanced liver disease, infective endocarditis, active peptic ulcer, prolonged/traumatic resuscitation.

Choice of agent: tissue plasminogen activators are preferred 1st line. *Alteplase, reteplase or tenecteplase* are all associated with fewer deaths than streptokinase, although a slight increase in stroke risk. Alteplase should be followed with an unfractionated heparin infusion. Tenecteplase is preferred in the out-of-hospital setting as it is a single bolus.

▶Patients with STEMI who do not receive reperfusion should be treated with *fondaparinux*,[14] or enoxaparin/unfractionated heparin if not available.

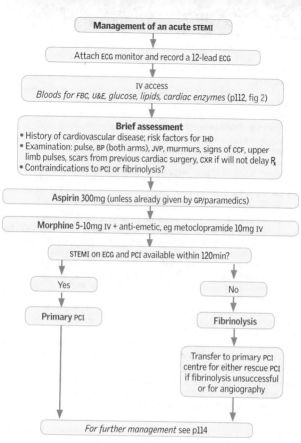

**Management of an acute STEMI**

Attach ECG monitor and record a 12-lead ECG

IV access
*Bloods for FBC, U&E, glucose, lipids, cardiac enzymes (p112, fig 2)*

**Brief assessment**
• History of cardiovascular disease; risk factors for IHD
• Examination: pulse, BP (both arms), JVP, murmurs, signs of CCF, upper limb pulses, scars from previous cardiac surgery, CXR if will not delay Rx
• Contraindications to PCI or fibrinolysis?

Aspirin 300mg (unless already given by GP/paramedics)

Morphine 5-10mg IV + anti-emetic, eg metoclopramide 10mg IV

STEMI on ECG and PCI available within 120min?

Yes

No

**Primary PCI**

**Fibrinolysis**

Transfer to primary PCI centre for either rescue PCI if fibrinolysis unsuccessful or for angiography

*For further management see p114*

Fig 1. Management of an acute STEMI.

Emergencies

Patients should be managed medically until symptoms settle, unless high risk. They are then investigated by angiography with a view to possible percutaneous coronary intervention or surgery (CABG).

### Assessment

*Brief history:* (p34) previous angina, relief with rest/nitrates, history of cardiovascular disease, risk factors for IHD.

*Examination:* (p36) pulse, BP, JVP, cardiac murmurs, signs of heart failure, peripheral pulses, scars from previous cardiac surgery.

**Investigations** ECG: ST depression; flat or inverted T waves; or normal.
U&E, troponin, glucose, random cholesterol, FBC, CXR (later on CCU if no recent CXR). Measurement of cardiac troponins helps to predict which patients are at risk of a cardiac event, and who can be safely discharged early.[14] Note that 2 different forms of troponin are measured: troponin T and troponin I: they have different reference intervals (consult your lab).

**Management** ►See fig 1 for acute management, but p808 if ST elevation.

The aim of therapy is to optimize anti-ischaemic and antiplatelet therapy.

*Oral antiplatelet therapy: Aspirin* 300mg initially, followed by 75mg/d **and either** *clopidogrel* (300mg initially then 75mg/d PO), ticagrelor (180mg then 90mg/12h PO) or prasugrel (50–60mg then 10mg/d PO) should be given to the following groups of patients and continued for 12 months: •↑troponin •ACS already on aspirin •↓ST on resting ECG •ACS after recent MI •Patients being transferred for angioplasty •Aspirin intolerant. Clopidogrel should not be used routinely for patients with suspected cardiac pain in the absence of ECG changes or raised troponin.

*Anticoagulation:* ideally fondaparinux (Factor Xa inhibitor) 2.5mg daily; if not available, use low molecular weight heparin (LMWH, eg enoxaparin 1mg/kg/12h) or unfractionated heparin (aim APTT 50–70s) until discharge.

*Glycoprotein IIb/IIIa inhibitors:* (see FLOWCHART). Consider in patients with recurrent or persistent chest pain and ECG changes despite standard treatment.

*Nitrates* (PO or IV) for recurrent chest pain.

*Beta-blockers:* if tachycardic or hypertensive and no signs of heart failure, unless contraindicated (consider diltiazem as alternative). Continue if previously on Rx.

*ACE-i* should be given to all patients unless there are CI (monitor renal function).

*Lipid management:* as for STEMI (p114).

**Prognosis** Overall risk of death ~1–2%, but ~15% for refractory angina despite medical therapy. Risk stratification can help predict those most at risk and allow intervention to be targeted at those individuals. The following are associated with an increased risk:
• History of unstable angina
• ST depression or widespread T-wave inversion
• Raised troponin (except patients with ST elevation MI)
• Age >70 years
• General comorbidity, previous MI, poor LV function or DM.

►High-risk patients should be considered for inpatient coronary angiography.

### Further measures and preparing for discharge
• Wean off *glyceryl trinitrate* (GTN) infusion when stabilized on oral drugs.
• Continue fondaparinux (or LMWH or heparin) until discharge.
• Check serial ECGs, and troponin >12h after pain.
• Address modifiable risk factors: smoking, hypertension, hyperlipidaemia, diabetes.
• Gentle mobilization.
• Ensure patient on dual antiplatelet therapy, β-blocker if depressed LV function, ACE inhibitor and statin.

►*If symptoms recur, refer to cardiologist for urgent angiography & PCI or CABG.*

## Acute management of ACS without ST-segment elevation

Admit to CCU and monitor closely

If SaO₂ <90% or breathless, low flow O₂

Analgesia: eg morphine 5-10mg IV + metoclopramide 10mg IV

Nitrates: GTN spray or sublingual tablets as required

Aspirin: 300mg PO and second antiplatelet agent (clopidogrel, ticagrelor, prasugrel) unless contraindicated

Oral β-blocker: eg metoprolol 50mg/12h if hypertensive/ tachycardic/LV function <40%

If β-blocker contradicted (asthma, COPD, LVF, bradycardia, coronary spasm), give rate-limiting calcium antagonist (eg verapamil¹ 80-120mg/8h PO, or diltiazem 60-120mg/8h PO)

Fondaparinux 2.5mg OD SC or LMWH 1mg/kg/12h SC

IV nitrate if pain continues (eg GTN 50mg in 50mL 0.9% saline at 2-10mL/h) titrate to pain, and maintain systolic BP >100mmHg

Record ECG while in pain

### Invasive strategy (high-risk pt)
* *Rise in troponin*
* *Dynamic ST or T wave changes*
* *Secondary criteria—diabetes, CKD, LVEF <40%, early angina post MI, recent PCI, prior CABG, intermediate to high-risk GRACE score²*

Infusion of a GPIIb/IIIa antagonist (eg tirofiban) and refer for angiography as inpatient (<72h after onset)

1 Urgent (<120min after presentation) if ongoing angina despite R̲ and evolving ST changes, signs of cardiogenic shock or life-threatening arrhythmias
2 Early (<24h) if GRACE score >140 and high-risk patient
3 Within 72h if lower risk patient

### Conservative strategy (low-risk pt)
* *No recurrence of chest pain*
* *No signs of heart failure*
* *Normal ECG*
* *Negative baseline + 6-9-hour troponin³*
* *No inducible ischaemia*

May be discharged if a repeat troponin is negative. Treat medically and arrange further investigation, eg stress test, angiogram

Fig 1. Acute management of ACS without ST-segment elevation. ¹⁵

1 Do not use verapamil and a β-blocker together (can cause asystole).

2 GRACE = Global Registry of Acute Coronary Events. Risk is scored based on age, heart rate, BP, renal function, Killip class of heart failure, and other events, eg raised troponin. Very complicated to calculate so recommendation by European Society of Cardiology is to use an online calculator, eg http://www.outcomes-umassmed.org/grace/.

3 Many labs are changing from traditional 12-hour troponins, check your local policy.

### Causes
- Cardiovascular, usually left ventricular failure (post-MI or ischaemic heart disease). Also valvular heart disease, arrhythmias, and malignant hypertension.
- ARDS (p178) from any cause, eg trauma, malaria, drugs. Then look for predisposing factors, eg trauma, post-op, sepsis. *Is aspirin overdose or glue-sniffing/drug abuse likely*? Ask friends/relatives.
- Fluid overload.
- Neurogenic, eg head injury.

**Differential diagnosis** Asthma/COPD, pneumonia, and pulmonary oedema are often hard to distinguish, especially in the elderly, where they may co-exist. If the patient is extremely unwell and you are not sure, consider treating all three (eg with salbutamol nebulizer, furosemide IV, diamorphine, amoxicillin—p378).

**Symptoms** Dyspnoea, orthopnoea (eg paroxysmal), pink frothy sputum. NB: note drugs recently given and other illnesses (recent MI/COPD or pneumonia).

**Signs** Distressed, pale, sweaty, pulse↑, tachypnoea, pink frothy sputum, pulsus alternans, JVP↑, fine lung crackles, triple/gallop rhythm (p42), wheeze (cardiac asthma). Usually sitting up and leaning forward. Quickly examine for possible causes.

### Investigations
- CXR (p129, p737-741): cardiomegaly, signs of pulmonary oedema: look for shadowing (usually bilateral), small effusions at costophrenic angles, fluid in the lung fissures, and Kerley B lines (linear opacities).
- ECG: signs of MI, dysrhythmias.
- U&E, troponin, ABG.
- Consider echo.
- Plasma BNP (p131) may be helpful if diagnosis in question (high negative predictive value).[16]

### Management
▶▶Begin treatment before investigations. See fig 1.

*Monitoring progress:* BP; pulse; cyanosis; respiratory rate; JVP; urine output; ABG.

*Once stable and improving:*
- Daily weights, aim reduction of 0.5kg/day, check obs at least QDS.
- Repeat CXR.
- Change to oral furosemide or bumetanide.
- If on large doses of loop diuretic, consider the addition of a thiazide (eg bendroflumethiazide or metolazone 2.5-5mg daily PO).
- ACE-i if LVEF <40%. If ACE-i contraindicated, consider hydralazine and nitrate (may also be more effective in African-Caribbeans).[17]
- Also consider β-blocker and spironolactone (if LVEF <35%).
- Is the patient suitable for biventricular pacing or cardiac transplantation?
- Consider digoxin ± warfarin, especially if AF.

Nesiritide, recombinant human brain natriuretic peptide, is not recommended for use in acute heart failure as the largest RCT showed only borderline improvement in dyspnoea with no improvement in mortality or rehospitalization, and a significant increase in hypotension.[18]

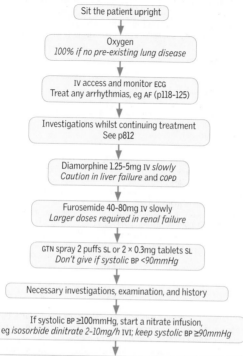

**Management of acute heart failure**

Sit the patient upright

Oxygen
*100% if no pre-existing lung disease*

IV access and monitor ECG
Treat any arrhythmias, eg AF (p118-125)

Investigations whilst continuing treatment
See p812

Diamorphine 1.25-5mg IV *slowly*
*Caution in liver failure* and COPD

Furosemide 40-80mg IV slowly
*Larger doses required in renal failure*

GTN spray 2 puffs SL or 2 × 0.3mg tablets SL
*Don't give if systolic BP <90mmHg*

Necessary investigations, examination, and history

If systolic BP ≥100mmHg, start a nitrate infusion,
eg *isosorbide dinitrate 2-10mg/h* IVI; keep systolic BP ≥90mmHg

If the patient is worsening:
• Further dose of furosemide 40-80mg
• Consider CPAP—improves ventilation by recruiting more alveoli, driving fluid out
  of alveolar spaces and into vasculature (get help before initiating!)
• Increase nitrate infusion if able to do so without dropping systolic BP <100

If systolic BP <100mmHg, treat as cardiogenic shock (p814) and refer to ICU

**Fig 1.** Management of heart failure.
Notes:[19,20]
• If failure to improve, reassess and consider alternative diagnoses, eg hypertensive
  heart failure, aortic dissection, pulmonary embolism, pneumonia.
• CPAP (5-10cmH$_2$O) in dyspnoeic patients (if no ↓BP or emergent need for intubation)
  can reduce the need for intubation, and possibly in-hospital mortality.
• Consider IV nitrate therapy for patients with dyspnoea.

Emergencies

This has a high mortality and is very difficult to treat. ▸Ask a senior physician's help both in formulating an *exact* diagnosis and in guiding treatment.

Cardiogenic shock is a state of inadequate tissue perfusion primarily due to cardiac dysfunction. It may occur suddenly, or after progressively worsening heart failure.

## Causes
- Myocardial infarction
- Arrhythmias
- Pulmonary embolism
- Tension pneumothorax
- Cardiac tamponade
- Myocarditis; myocardial depression (drugs, hypoxia, acidosis, sepsis)
- Valve destruction (endocarditis)
- Aortic dissection

## Management

If the cause is myocardial infarction prompt revascularization (acute angioplasty or fibrinolysis) is vital[1]; ▸▸see p808 for indications and contraindications.
- Manage in Coronary Care Unit, or ICU.
- Investigation and treatment may need to be done concurrently.
- See fig 1 for details of management.
- *Investigations:* ECG, U&E, troponins/cardiac enzymes, ABG, CXR, echocardiogram. If indicated, CT thorax (aortic dissection/PE) or V/Q scan.
- *Monitor* CVP, BP, ABG, ECG, urine output. Do a 12-lead ECG every hour until the diagnosis is made. Consider a CVP line and an arterial line to monitor pressure, if these are *in situ* consider using PICCO, LIDCO[2] or other measures of cardiac output and volume status. Catheterize for accurate urine output.

## Cardiac tamponade

*Essence:* Pericardial fluid collects → intrapericardial pressure rises → heart cannot fill → pumping stops.

*Causes:* Trauma, lung/breast cancer, pericarditis, myocardial infarct, bacteria, eg TB. *Rarely:* Urea↑, radiation, myxoedema, dissecting aorta, SLE. Also coronary artery dissection (secondary to PCI) and/or ruptured ventricle.

*Signs:* Falling BP, a rising JVP, and muffled heart sounds (Beck's triad); JVP↑ on inspiration (Kussmaul's sign); pulsus paradoxus (pulse fades on inspiration). Echocardiography may be diagnostic. CXR: globular heart; left heart border convex or straight; right cardiophrenic angle <90°. ECG: electrical alternans (p148).

*Management:* This can be very difficult. Everything is against you: time, physiology, and your own confidence, as the patient may be too ill to give a history, and signs may be equivocal—but bitter experience has taught us not to equivocate for long.

▸▸Request the presence of your senior at the bedside (do not make do with telephone advice). With luck, prompt pericardiocentesis (p787) brings swift relief. While awaiting this, give O₂, monitor ECG, and set up IVI. Take blood for group and save. NB: there may be a role for cardiothoracic surgery (eg CABG, ventricular repair, or pericardial window) as a definitive solution to some causes.

---

**1** SHOCK trial 2003 V Menon *Congest Heart Fail* 9 35. NNT for acute angioplasty = 5.
**2** Pulse contour cardiac output and lithium dilution cardiac output. Both use injection (PICCO = cold water, LIDCO = lithium) to estimate filling pressure, extravascular water (ie pulmonary oedema) and cardiac output. The time from injection via a central vein to detection via an arterial line, plus dilution, gives estimates of cardiac output and volume status and can guide fluid and inotrope therapy.

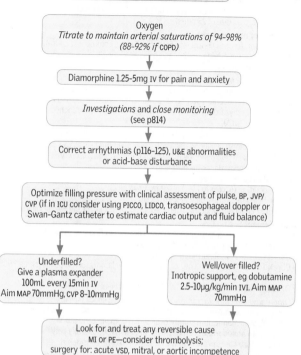

**Fig 1.** Management of cardiogenic shock. MAP = Mean arterial pressure

ECG shows rate of >100bpm and QRS complexes >120ms (>3 small squares on ECGs done at the standard UK rate of 25mm/s).

### Principles of management
1 If in doubt, treat as ventricular tachycardia (the commonest cause).
2 Identify the underlying rhythm and treat accordingly.

### Differential diagnosis
- *Ventricular tachycardia (VT) including torsade de pointes.* Single ventricular ectopics should not cause confusion; if >3 together at a rate >100, this is VT.
- SVT with aberrant conduction, eg AF, atrial flutter with bundle branch block.
- Pre-excited tachycardias, eg AF, atrial flutter, or AV re-entry tachycardia with underlying WPW (p120).

**Identifying the underlying rhythm** may be hard; get help. Diagnosis is based on the history (if IHD/MI likelihood of a ventricular arrhythmia is >95%), 12-lead ECG, and lack of response to IV adenosine (p120). *ECG findings in favour of VT:*
- Positive QRS concordance in chest leads
- Marked left axis deviation
- AV dissociation (occurs in 25%) or 2:1 or 3:1 AV block
- Fusion beats or capture beats (ECG p123, fig 1)
- Also bear in mind Brugada's criteria, eg RSR complex in V1 (and +ve QRS in V1): p123.

### Management See fig 1.
- Connect patient to a cardiac monitor and have a defibrillator to hand.
- Monitor $O_2$ sats and if <90% give supplemental oxygen.
- Correct electrolyte abnormalities, esp $K^+$ and $Mg^{2+}$.
- Check for adverse signs. Low cardiac output (clammy, consciousness↓, BP <90); oliguria; angina; pulmonary oedema.
- Obtain 12-lead ECG (request CXR) and obtain IV access.

*If haemodynamically unstable:* ►► Synchronized DC shock (see inside back cover).
- Correct any hypokalaemia and hypomagnesaemia: up to 60mmol KCl at 30mmol/h, and 4mL 50% magnesium sulfate over 30min both via central line.
- Follow with amiodarone 300mg IV over 10–20min (peripherally only in emergency).
- For refractory cases procainamide or sotalol may be considered.

*If haemodynamically stable:* Correct hypokalaemia and hypomagnesaemia: as above.
- Amiodarone 300mg IV over 20–60min (avoid if long QT) via central line.
- If this fails, use synchronized DC shock.

*After correction of VT:* Establish the cause (via the history and tests above).
- Maintenance anti-arrhythmic therapy may be required. If VT occurs after MI, give IV amiodarone infusion for 12–24h; if 24h after MI, also start oral anti-arrhythmic: sotalol (if good LV function) or amiodarone (if poor LV function).
- Prevention of recurrent VT: surgical isolation of the arrhythmogenic area or an implantable cardioverter defibrillator (ICD) may help.

*Ventricular fibrillation:* (ECG p123, fig 3) Use non-synchronized DC shock (there is no R wave to trigger defibrillation, p784): see inside back cover.

*Ventricular extrasystoles (ectopics):* These are the commonest post-MI arrhythmia but they are also seen in healthy people (often >10/h). Patients with frequent ectopics post-MI have a worse prognosis, but there is no evidence that antidysrhythmic drugs improve outcome, indeed they may increase mortality.

*Torsade de pointes:* A form of VT, with a constantly varying axis, often in the setting of long-QT syndromes (ECG p123, fig 4). Causes (p725): congenital or from drugs (eg some antidysrhythmics, tricyclics, antimalarials, antipsychotics). Torsade in the setting of congenital long-QT syndromes can be treated with high doses of β-blockers.

In acquired long-QT syndromes (p725), stop all predisposing drugs, correct hypokalaemia, and give magnesium sulfate (2g IV over 10min). Alternatives include: overdrive pacing (pace at a faster rate, then slow reduce) or isoprenaline IVI to increase heart rate.

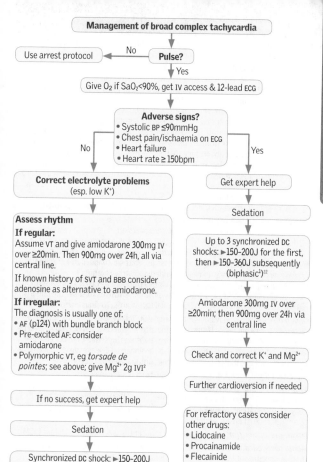

Fig 1. Management of broad complex tachycardia.

1 If monophasic shock used, start at 200J, subsequent shocks at 360.
2 Magnesium sulfate—give 4mL of 50% magnesium sulfate (which is 8mmol or 2g) over 10 minutes.

Emergencies

ECG shows rate of >100bpm and QRS complex duration of <120ms (<3 small squares on ECGs done at the standard UK rate of 25mm/s).

**Differential diagnosis**
- *Sinus tachycardia:* Normal P wave followed by normal QRS—not an arrhythmia! Do not attempt to cardiovert; if necessary (ie not a physiological response to fever/hypovolaemia) rate control with β-blockers.
- *Atrial tachyarrhythmias:* Rhythm arises in atria, AV node is a bystander.
  - Atrial fibrillation (AF): absent P wave, irregular QRS complexes.
  - Atrial flutter: atrial rate ~260-340bpm. Sawtooth baseline, due to a re-entrant circuit usually in the right atrium. Ventricular rate often 150bpm (2:1 block).
  - Atrial tachycardia: abnormally shaped P waves, may outnumber QRS.
  - Multifocal atrial tachycardia: ≥3 P wave morphologies, irregular QRS complexes.
- *Junctional tachycardia:* AV node is part of the pathway. P wave either buried in QRS complex or occurring after QRS complex.
  - AV nodal re-entry tachycardia.
  - AV re-entry tachycardia, includes an accessory pathway, eg WPW (p120).

**Principles of management** See fig 1.
▶▶If the patient is compromised, use DC cardioversion.
- Otherwise, identify the underlying rhythm and treat accordingly. The most important thing is to decide whether the rhythm is regular or not (irregular is likely AF).
- Vagal manoeuvres (carotid sinus massage, Valsalva manoeuvre) transiently increase AV block, and may unmask an underlying atrial rhythm.
- If unsuccessful, give **adenosine**, which causes transient AV block. It has a short half-life (10-15s) and works by: **1** transiently slowing ventricles to show the underlying atrial rhythm; **2** cardioverting a junctional tachycardia to sinus rhythm.

*Giving adenosine:*[1] 6mg IV bolus into a large vein, followed by 0.9% saline flush, while recording a rhythm strip. If unsuccessful, after 2 min give 12mg, then one further 12mg bolus. Warn about SE: transient chest tightness, dyspnoea, headache, flushing. *Relative CI:* Asthma, 2nd/3rd-degree AV block or sinoatrial disease (unless pacemaker). *Interactions:* Potentiated by dipyridamole; antagonized by theophylline.

**Specifics** *Sinus tachycardia:* Identify and treat underlying cause.

*Supraventricular tachycardia:* If adenosine fails, use **verapamil** ~5mg IV over 2-3min. NB: NOT if on a β-blocker. If no response, a further 5mg IV over 3min (if age <60yrs). Alternatives: **atenolol** 2.5mg IV repeated at 5min intervals until 10mg given; or **amiodarone**. If unsuccessful, use DC cardioversion.

*Atrial fibrillation/flutter:* Manage with rate control; seek help if resistant (p124).

*Atrial tachycardia:* Rare; may be due to digoxin toxicity: withdraw digoxin, consider digoxin-specific antibody fragments. Maintain $K^+$ at 4-5mmol/L.

*Multifocal atrial tachycardia:* Most commonly occurs in COPD. Correct hypoxia and hypercapnia. Consider **verapamil** if rate remains >110bpm.

*Junctional tachycardia:* Where anterograde conduction through the AV node occurs, vagal manoeuvres are worth trying. **Adenosine** will usually cardiovert a junctional rhythm to sinus rhythm. If it fails or recurs, β-blockers (or verapamil—*not* with β-blockers, digoxin, or class I agents such as quinidine). If this does not control symptoms, consider radiofrequency ablation.

▶Seek specialist advice if resistant junction tachycardia, or accessory pathway.

**Wolff-Parkinson-White (WPW) syndrome** *(ECG p125)* Caused by congenital accessory conduction pathway between atria and ventricles. Resting ECG shows short PR interval and widened QRS complex due to slurred upstroke or 'delta wave'. 2 types: WPW type A (+ve δ wave in $V_1$), WPW type B (-ve δ wave in $V_1$). Present with SVT which may be due to an AVRT (p120), pre-excited AF, or pre-excited atrial flutter. Risk of degeneration to VF and sudden death. $R_x$: **Flecainide, propafenone, sotalol**, or **amiodarone**. Refer to cardiologist for electrophysiology and ablation of the accessory pathway.

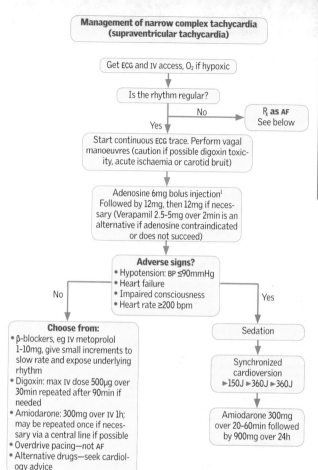

Fig 1. Management of narrow complex tachycardia (supraventricular tachycardia).

## Irregular narrow complex tachycardia

- Treat as AF—by far the most likely diagnosis.
- Control rate with either β-blocker or digoxin.
- If onset <48h consider cardioversion with either amiodarone, 300mg IVI over 20-60min, then 900mg over 24h; or DC shock, see p784.
- Consider anticoagulation with heparin and/or warfarin to reduce the risk of stroke.

1 Consult *BNF* if on dipyridamole or has had a heart transplant.
See Resuscitation Council (UK) guidance for more details (www.resus.org.uk).

▶The severity of an attack is easily underestimated.

▶An atmosphere of calm helps.

**Presentation** Acute breathlessness and wheeze.

**History** (p48) Ask about usual and recent treatment; previous acute episodes and their severity and best peak expiratory flow rate (PEF). Have they been admitted to ICU?

**Differential diagnosis** Acute infective exacerbation of COPD, pulmonary oedema, upper respiratory tract obstruction, pulmonary embolus, anaphylaxis.

**Investigations** PEF—but may be too ill; arterial blood gases if saturations <92%; CXR (if suspicion of pneumothorax, infection or life-threatening attack); FBC; U&E.

**Assessing the severity of an acute asthmatic attack**

*Severe attack:*
• Unable to complete sentences
• Respiratory rate >25/min
• Pulse rate >110 beats/min
• Peak expiratory flow 33–50% of predicted or best

*Life-threatening attack:*
• Peak expiratory flow <33% of predicted or best
• Silent chest, cyanosis, feeble respiratory effort
• Bradycardia or hypotension
• Exhaustion, confusion, or coma
• Arterial blood gases:
    •normal/high $P_aCO_2$ >4.6kPa (32mmHg)
    •$P_aO_2$ <8kPa (60mmHg), or $S_aO_2$ <92%
    •low pH, eg <7.35

**Treatment** ▶Life-threatening or severe asthma, see fig 1.
• Salbutamol 5mg nebulized with oxygen and give prednisolone 30mg PO.
• If PEF remains <75%, repeat salbutamol.
• Monitor oxygen saturation, heart rate, and respiratory rate.

**Discharge** Patients, before discharge, must have:
• Been stable on discharge medication for 24h.
• Had inhaler technique checked.
• Peak flow rate >75% predicted or best with diurnal variability <25%.
• Steroid (inhaled *and* oral) and bronchodilator therapy.
• their own PEF meter and have management plan.
• GP appointment within 1wk.
• Respiratory clinic appointment within 4wks.

**Drugs used in acute asthma**

*Salbutamol* (β₂-agonist) SE: tachycardia, arrhythmias, tremor, K⁺↓.

*Hydrocortisone* and *prednisolone* (steroid; reduces inflammation).

*Aminophylline* is used much less frequently and is not routinely recommended in current BTS guidelines, but may be initiated by respiratory team or ICU. It inhibits phosphodiesterase; ↑[cAMP]. SE: pulse↑, arrhythmias, nausea, seizures. The amount of IVI aminophylline may need altering according to the individual patient: always check the BNF. Monitor ECG.
• *Factors that may necessitate reduction of dose:* Cardiac or liver failure, drugs that increase the half-life of aminophylline, eg cimetidine, ciprofloxacin, erythromycin, contraceptive steroids.
• *Factors that may require* ↑ *dose:* Smoking, drugs that shorten the half-life, eg phenytoin, carbamazepine, barbiturates, rifampicin.

▶Aim for plasma concentration of 10–20μg/mL (55–110μmol/L). Serious toxicity (BP↓ arrhythmias, cardiac arrest) can occur at concentrations ≥25μg/mL. Measure plasma K⁺: theophyllines may cause K⁺↓. Don't load patients already on oral preparations. Stick with one brand (bioavailability varies).

## Management of acute severe asthma

**Assess severity of attack**
PEF, ability to speak, RR, pulse rate, $O_2$ sats
Warn ICU if severe or life-threatening attack

**Immediate treatment**[1]
Salbutamol 5mg (or terbutaline 10mg) nebulized with $O_2$
Hydrocortisone 100mg IV or prednisolone 40-50mg PO or both if very ill
Start $O_2$ if saturations <92% (also check ABG), aim sats 94-98%

**If life-threatening features present:**
- Inform ICU and seniors
- Give salbutamol nebulizers every 15min, or 10mg continuously per hour. Monitor ECG; watch for arrhythmias
- Add in ipratropium 0.5mg to nebulizers
- Give single dose of magnesium sulfate ($MgSO_4$) 1.2-2g IV over 20min

**▶▶If not improving:**
Refer to ICU for consideration of ventilatory support and intensification of medical therapy, eg aminophylline, IV salbutamol if any of the following signs are present:
- Deteriorating PEF
- Persistent/worsening hypoxia
- Hypercapnia
- ABG showing low pH or high H⁺
- Exhaustion, feeble respiration
- Drowsiness, confusion, altered conscious level
- Respiratory arrest

**If improving within 15-30 minutes:**
- Nebulized salbutamol every 4 hours
- Prednisolone 40-50mg PO OD for 5-7 days
- Monitor peak flow and $O_2$ sats, aim 94-98% with supplemental if needed

Fig 1. Management of acute severe asthma.

1 NB: The routine use of antibiotics is not recommended in exacerbations of asthma.

Emergencies

A common medical emergency especially in winter. May be triggered by viral or bacterial infections.

**Presentation** Increasing cough, breathlessness, or wheeze. Decreased exercise capacity.

**History** (p48) Ask about usual/recent treatments (especially home oxygen), smoking status, and exercise capacity (may influence a decision to ventilate the patient).

**Differential diagnosis** Asthma, pulmonary oedema, upper respiratory tract obstruction, pulmonary embolus, anaphylaxis.

**Investigations**
• Arterial blood gases (p785).
• CXR to exclude pneumothorax and infection.
• FBC; U&E; CRP. Theophylline level if patient on therapy at home.
• ECG.
• Send sputum for culture if purulent.
• Blood cultures if pyrexial.

**Management**
• Look for a cause, eg infection, pneumothorax.
• See fig 1 for acute management.
• Prior to discharge, liaise with GP regarding steroid reduction, domiciliary oxygen (p176), smoking cessation, and pneumococcal and flu vaccinations (p160).

*Treatment of stable COPD and more advanced disease:* See p176, p177.

*Considering the ceiling of care:*

In the acute setting it is very easy for us to intervene, there are many things we can do, but it is often important to consider what we *should* do and what is in the best interests of the patient. Invasive ventilation for exacerbations of COPD can be a minefield, as it can be difficult to wean patients off ventilatory support, and brings with it the risk of ventilator-associated pneumonias and pneumothoraces from ruptured bullae. If possible, speak to the patient early, before deterioration, try to ascertain their wishes. Patients who have previously been ventilated may not wish to repeat the experience. Consider age, FEV₁, comorbidities, functional status, whether the patient requires home oxygen, and whether the patient has previously been admitted to ICU (and if so, whether they were easily weaned from invasive ventilation). Involve the patient, the family, your seniors and ICU early in making a decision about the ceiling of care for an individual patient.

---

### Oxygen therapy

• The greatest danger is hypoxia, which probably accounts for more deaths than hypercapnia. *Don't leave patients severely hypoxic.*
• However, in some patients, who rely on their hypoxic drive to breathe, too much oxygen may lead to a reduced respiratory rate and hypercapnia, with a consequent fall in conscious level. Always prescribe $O_2$ as if it were a drug.
• Care is always required with $O_2$, especially if there is evidence of $CO_2$ retention. Start with 24–28% $O_2$ in such patients.

►► Whenever you initiate or change oxygen therapy, do an ABG within the next hour or sooner if the patient is deteriorating.

• Monitor the patient carefully. Aim to raise the $P_aO_2$ above 8.0kPa with a rise in $P_aCO_2$ <1.5kPa.
• In patients without evidence of retention at baseline use 28–40% $O_2$, but still monitor and repeat ABG.

## Management of acute COPD

**Nebulized bronchodilators**
Salbutamol 5mg/4h and ipratropium 500µg/6h
**Investigate:** CXR, ABG

**Controlled oxygen therapy if $S_aO_2$ <88% or $P_aO_2$ <7 kPa**
Start at 24-28%, aim sats 88-92% (94-98% if no hypercapnia on ABG)
Adjust according to ABG, aim $P_aO_2$ >8.0kPa with a rise in $P_aCO_2$ <1.5kPa[25]

**Steroids**
IV hydrocortisone 200mg and oral prednisolone
30mg OD (continue for 7-14d)

**Antibiotics**
Use if evidence of infection, eg amoxicillin 500mg/8h PO,
alternatively clarithromycin or doxycycline (p381)

Physiotherapy to aid sputum expectoration

**If no response to nebulizers and steroids:**
Consider IV aminophylline[1]

**If no response**
1 Consider non-invasive positive pressure ventilation[2] (NIPPV) if
respiratory rate >30 or pH <7.35, or $P_aCO_2$ rising despite best
medical treatment

2 Consider intubation and ventilation if pH <7.26 and $P_aCO_2$ is
rising despite non-invasive ventilation

3 Consider a respiratory stimulant drug, eg doxapram 1.5-4mg/
min IV. *SE: agitation, confusion, tachycardia, nausea.* In
patients who are not suitable for mechanical ventilation. It is
a short-term measure, used only if NIV is not available

Fig 1. Management of acute COPD.

Aminophylline: Do not give a loading dose to patients on maintenance methylxanthines
(theophyllines/aminophylline; see p820). Load with 250mg over 20min, then infuse at a rate of ~500µg/
kg/h (300µg/kg/h if elderly), where kg is ideal body weight, p446. Check plasma levels if given for >24h.
ECG monitoring is required.

1 This may alone serve as a rescue therapy, be an intermittent step before ventilation, or be considered
as a 'ceiling of therapy' for those deemed not suitable for mechanical ventilation.

▶▶**Tension pneumothorax** requires immediate relief (see below). Do not delay management by obtaining a CXR.

### Causes
• *Spontaneous* (especially in young thin men) due to rupture of a subpleural bulla
• *Chronic lung disease*: asthma; COPD; cystic fibrosis; lung fibrosis; sarcoidosis
• *Infection*: TB; pneumonia; lung abscess
• *Traumatic*: including iatrogenic (CVP line insertion, pleural aspiration or biopsy, percutaneous liver biopsy, positive pressure ventilation).
• *Carcinoma*
• *Connective tissue disorders*: Marfan's syndrome, Ehlers-Danlos syndrome

### Clinical features
*Symptoms:* Can be asymptomatic (especially in fit young people with small pneumothoraces) or sudden onset of dyspnoea and/or pleuritic chest pain. Patients with asthma or COPD may present with a sudden deterioration. Mechanically ventilated patients can suddenly develop hypoxia or an increase in ventilation pressures.

*Signs:* Reduced expansion, hyper-resonance to percussion and diminished breath sounds on the affected side. *With a tension pneumothorax, the trachea will be deviated away from the affected side and the patient will be very unwell.*

**Tests** ▶*A CXR should not be performed if a tension pneumothorax is suspected, as it will delay immediate necessary treatment.* Otherwise, request an expiratory film, and look for an area devoid of lung markings, peripheral to the edge of the collapsed lung (see p739). Ensure the suspected *pneumothorax is not a large emphysematous bulla.* Check ABG in dyspnoeic/hypoxic patients and those with chronic lung disease.

**Management** Depends on whether it is a primary or secondary (underlying lung disease) pneumothorax, size and symptoms—see fig 1.
• Pneumothorax due to trauma or mechanical ventilation requires a chest drain.
• Aspiration of a pneumothorax, see p781.
• Insertion and management of a chest drain, see p780.

*Surgical advice:* Arrange if: bilateral pneumothoraces; lung fails to expand after intercostal drain insertion; 2 or more previous pneumothoraces on the same side; or history of pneumothorax on the opposite side.

## ▶▶Tension pneumothorax                    (see p763)

▶▶This is a medical emergency.

**Essence** Air drawn into the pleural space with each inspiration has no route of escape during expiration. The mediastinum is pushed over into the contralateral hemithorax, kinking and compressing the great veins. Unless the air is rapidly removed, cardiorespiratory arrest will occur.

**Signs** Respiratory distress, tachycardia, hypotension, distended neck veins, trachea deviated away from side of pneumothorax. Increased percussion note, reduced air entry/breath sounds on the affected side.

### Treatment
To remove the air, insert a large-bore (14-16G) needle with a syringe, partially filled with 0.9% saline, into the 2$^{nd}$ intercostal interspace in the midclavicular line on the side of the suspected pneumothorax. Remove plunger to allow the trapped air to bubble through the syringe (with saline as a water seal) until a chest tube can be placed. Alternatively, insert a large-bore Venflon in the same location.

▶▶Do this *before* requesting a CXR.
▶▶Then insert a chest drain. See p780.

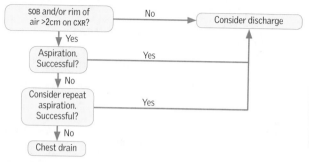

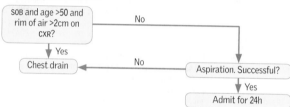

Fig 1. Acute management of pneumothorax.

*Aspiration of a pneumothorax:* ►►see p781.

*Intercostal tube drainage:* For insertion, see p780.

• Use a small tube (10-14F) unless blood/pus is also present.
• Never clamp a bubbling tube.
• Tubes may be removed 24h after the lung has re-expanded and air leak has stopped (ie the tube stops bubbling). This is done during expiration or a Valsalva manoeuvre.
• If the lung fails to re-expand within 48h, or if there is a persistent air leak, specialist advice should be obtained, as suction or surgical intervention may be required.
• If suction is required, high-volume, low-pressure (-10 to -20cmH$_2$O) systems are required.

An infection of the lung parenchyma. Incidence of community-acquired pneumonia is 5–11 per 1000 adults. Of these, 1–3 per 1000 will require hospitalization, and mortality in those hospitalized is up to 14%.

**Common organisms**
- *Streptococcus pneumoniae* is the commonest cause (60–75%).
- *Haemophilus influenzae*.
- *Mycoplasma pneumoniae*.
- *Staphylococcus aureus* found more commonly in ICU patients.
- *Legionella* species and *Chlamydia psittaci*.
- Gram-negative bacilli, often hospital-acquired or immunocompromised, eg *Pseudomonas*, especially in those with COPD.
- Viruses including influenza account for up to 15%.

**Symptoms**
- Fever, rigors, malaise, anorexia, dyspnoea, cough, purulent sputum (classically 'rusty' with pneumococcus), haemoptysis, and pleuritic chest pain.

**Signs**
- Fever, cyanosis, herpes labialis (pneumococcus), confusion, tachypnoea, tachycardia, hypotension, signs of consolidation (diminished expansion, dull percussion note, increased tactile vocal fremitus/vocal resonance, bronchial breathing), and a pleural rub.

**Investigations**
- CXR (X-ray images, fig 1 on p739).
- Oxygen saturation and arterial blood gases if $S_aO_2$ <92% or severe pneumonia.
- FBC, U&E, LFT, CRP, atypical serology (remember to put date of onset on form).
- Urine pneumococcal (and legionella) antigen.
- Viral throat swabs if appropriate.
- Blood cultures if pyrexial.
- Pleural fluid may be aspirated for culture.
- Bronchoscopy and bronchoalveolar lavage if the patient is immunocompromised or on ICU.

**Severity**

Calculate the core adverse features 'CURB-65' score
- Confusion (abbreviated mental test ≤8)
- Urea >7mmol/L
- Respiratory rate ≥30/min
- BP <90/60mmHg
- Age ≥65

*Score:*
>      0–1 home treatment if possible
>      2 hospital therapy
>      ≥3 indicates severe pneumonia and should consider ICU referral

Other features increasing the risk of death are: co-existing disease; bilateral/multilobar involvement; $P_aO_2$ <8kPa or $S_aO_2$ <92%.

**Management** See fig 1.

**Complications** (of infection or treatment)

Pleural effusion, empyema, lung abscess, respiratory failure, septicaemia, pericarditis, myocarditis, cholestatic jaundice, acute kidney injury.

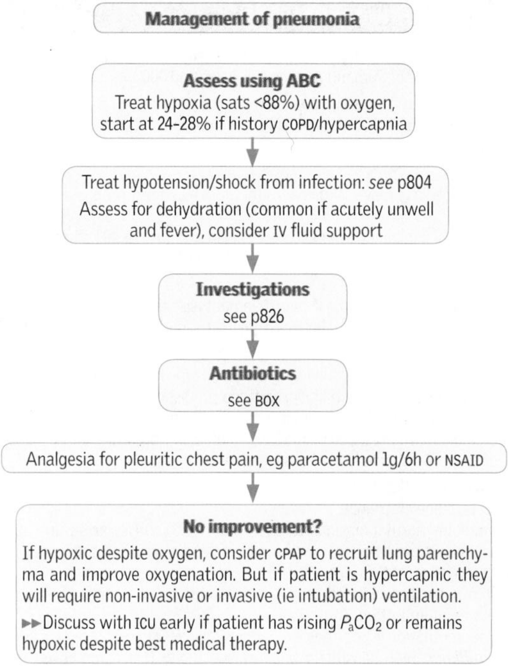

| **Management of pneumonia** |

**Assess using ABC**
Treat hypoxia (sats <88%) with oxygen,
start at 24-28% if history COPD/hypercapnia

Treat hypotension/shock from infection: *see* p804
Assess for dehydration (common if acutely unwell
and fever), consider IV fluid support

**Investigations**
see p826

**Antibiotics**
see BOX

Analgesia for pleuritic chest pain, eg paracetamol 1g/6h or NSAID

**No improvement?**
If hypoxic despite oxygen, consider CPAP to recruit lung parenchyma and improve oxygenation. But if patient is hypercapnic they will require non-invasive or invasive (ie intubation) ventilation.
►► Discuss with ICU early if patient has rising $P_aCO_2$ or remains hypoxic despite best medical therapy.

Fig 1. Management of pneumonia.

---

**Empirical treatment of severe pneumonia (CURB 3-5)**

► Regimens vary, so consult local guidelines—the following are British Thoracic Society suggestions. For fuller advice see p161.
Co-amoxiclav 1.2g/8h IV AND clarithromycin 500mg/12h IVI.
If penicillin allergic use cephalosporin instead of co-amoxiclav. Ciprofloxacin is an alternative to clarithromycin.
*If atypical suspected* Legionella pneumophilia add levofloxacin + rifampicin, *Chlamydophila* species (p162) add tetracycline, *Pneumocystis jiroveci* add high-dose co-trimoxazole (p411).
*If hospital acquired or neutropenic consider* aminoglycoside IV (eg gentamicin, p766) + antipseudomonal penicillin (eg ticarcillin, p378).

Emergencies

▶Always suspect pulmonary embolism (PE) in sudden collapse 1–2wks after surgery. Mortality rate in England and Wales: 30,000–40,000/yr.

**Mechanism** Venous thrombi, usually from DVT, pass into the pulmonary circulation and block blood flow to lungs. The source is often occult.

**Risk factors**
• Malignancy.
• Surgery—especially pelvic and lower limb (much lower if prophylaxis used).
• Immobility.
• Combined oral contraceptive pill (there is also a slight risk attached to HRT).
• Previous thromboembolism and inherited thrombophilia, see p368.

**Signs and symptoms**
• Acute dyspnoea, pleuritic chest pain, haemoptysis, and syncope.
• Hypotension, tachycardia, gallop rhythm, JVP↑, loud $P_2$, right ventricular heave, pleural rub, tachypnoea, cyanosis, AF.

With thromboprophylaxis PE following surgery is far less common, but PE may occur after any period of immobility, or with no predisposing factors. Breathlessness may be the only sign. Multiple small emboli may present less dramatically with pleuritic pain, haemoptysis, and gradually increasing breathlessness. ▶Look for a source of emboli—especially DVT (is a leg swollen?).

**Investigations** ▶p182
• U&E, FBC, baseline clotting.
• *ECG:* commonly normal or sinus tachycardia; right ventricular strain pattern $V_{1-3}$ (p94), right axis deviation, RBBB, AF, may be deep S waves in I, Q waves in III, inverted T waves in III ('$S_I Q_{III} T_{III}$').
• *CXR:* often normal; decreased vascular markings, small pleural effusion. Wedge-shaped area of infarction. Atelectasis.
• *ABG:* hyperventilation + poor gas exchange: $P_aO_2$↓, $P_aCO_2$↓, pH often ↑, p156.
• *Serum D-dimer:* high sensitivity but low specificity (↑ if thrombosis, inflammation, post-op, infection, malignancy) ∴ excludes PE if normal D-dimer.
• *CT pulmonary angiography* (CTPA) is sensitive and specific in determining if emboli are in pulmonary arteries. If unavailable, a *ventilation-perfusion (V/Q) scan* can aid diagnosis. If V/Q scan is equivocal, pulmonary angiography or bilateral venograms may help (MRI venography or plethysmography are alternatives).

**Management** See fig 1 for immediate management.
• Try to prevent further thrombosis with compression stockings.
• Low molecular weight heparin (LMWH) concurrently with warfarin until INR >2.
• If obvious remedial cause, 6 weeks of warfarin (p345) may be enough; otherwise, continue for ≥3–6 months (long term if recurrent emboli, or underlying malignancy).
• Is there an underlying cause, eg thrombophilic tendency (p368), malignancy (especially prostate, breast, or pelvic cancer), SLE, or polycythaemia?
▶If good story and signs, make the diagnosis. Start treatment (FLOWCHART) before definitive investigations: most PE deaths occur within 1h.

**Prevention** Early post-op mobilization is the simplest method; also consider:
• Antithromboembolic (TED) stockings.
• Low molecular weight heparin prophylaxis SC.
• Avoid contraceptive pill if at risk, eg major or orthopaedic surgery.
• Recurrent PEs may be prevented by anticoagulation. Vena caval filters are of limited use unless patients cannot be anticoagulated.

Don't just think of prophylactic low molecular weight heparin (LMWH, p580) for post-op patients. Many acutely ill medical patients are equally at risk (5–15% have DVTs, and >50% of all thromboembolic events are in these patients; prevalence of PE: 0.3–1.5%).[29] Do proper risk analysis—especially in those with MI, pneumonia, malignancy, inflammatory bowel disease, prolonged immobility/on ICU, and stroke (there is no ↑ risk of CNS bleeds if LMWH is used).[30]

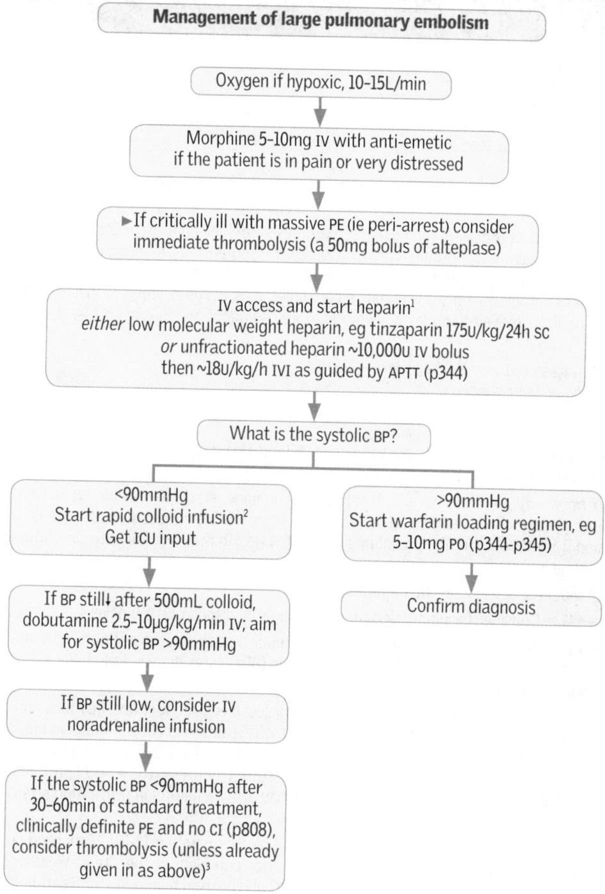

## Management of large pulmonary embolism

Oxygen if hypoxic, 10-15L/min

Morphine 5-10mg IV with anti-emetic
if the patient is in pain or very distressed

►If critically ill with massive PE (ie peri-arrest) consider
immediate thrombolysis (a 50mg bolus of alteplase)

IV access and start heparin[1]
*either* low molecular weight heparin, eg tinzaparin 175u/kg/24h SC
*or* unfractionated heparin ~10,000u IV bolus
then ~18u/kg/h IVI as guided by APTT (p344)

What is the systolic BP?

**<90mmHg**
Start rapid colloid infusion[2]
Get ICU input

**>90mmHg**
Start warfarin loading regimen, eg
5-10mg PO (p344-p345)

If BP still↓ after 500mL colloid,
dobutamine 2.5-10μg/kg/min IV; aim
for systolic BP >90mmHg

Confirm diagnosis

If BP still low, consider IV
noradrenaline infusion

If the systolic BP <90mmHg after
30-60min of standard treatment,
clinically definite PE and no CI (p808),
consider thrombolysis (unless already
given in as above)[3]

Fig 1. Management of large pulmonary embolism.

**1** A bolus of unfractionated heparin may be preferred in massive PE for its faster onset, and unfractionated heparin may also be useful where there may be a need for rapid reversal of anticoagulation.
**2** Controversial, but some authorities say it is best to infuse plasma-expanding fluids even if CVP↑, to maintain BP and organ perfusion, see *Concise OTM* (OUP, 2000) p151—but see Task Force on PE, European Society Cardiology *Eur Heart J* 2000 21 1301.
**3** A standard regimen is: alteplase 50mg bolus IV over 1-2min. See also formulary.

## Causes
- Peptic ulcer disease (PUD) 35-50%.
- Gastroduodenal erosions 8-15%.
- Oesophagitis 5-15%.
- Mallory-Weiss tear 15%.
- Varices 5-10%.
- Other: upper GI malignancy, vascular malformations. Consider also facial trauma, nose bleed, or haemoptysis as causes of *swallowed* blood.

**Signs and symptoms** (p56-63) Haematemesis, or melaena, dizziness (especially postural), fainting, abdominal pain, dysphagia? Hypotension (in young may be postural only), tachycardia (not if on β-blocker), ↓JVP, ↓urine output, cool and clammy, signs of chronic liver disease (p260), eg telangiectasia, purpura, jaundice (biliary colic + jaundice + melaena suggests haemobilia). NB: ask about previous GI problems, drug use, alcohol.

**Management** (see Rockall score, p253)[32]
*Is the patient shocked?*
- Cool and clammy to touch (especially nose, toes, fingers) ↓capillary refill.
- Pulse >100bpm, JVP not visible
- Systolic BP <100mmHg or postural drop (>20mmHg on standing).
- Urine output <30mL/h.

*If haemodynamically stable:* Insert 2 big cannulae; start slow saline IVI to keep lines patent; check bloods and monitor vital signs + urine output. Consider transfusion if loss >30% circulating volume (see p805) NB: Hb may not fall until circulating volume is restored.
*If shocked:* See fig 1 for management.
*CVP line:* Consider for high-risk patients, eg ↑age, CV disease, on β-blockers.
*Acute drug therapy:* Following successful endoscopic therapy in patients with major ulcer bleeding, omeprazole or pantoprazole (80mg stat IV over 5min followed by 8mg/h for 72h) is recommended.
*Variceal bleeding:* (p254) Resuscitate then proceed to urgent endoscopy for banding or sclerotherapy. Give terlipressin 2mg SC qds (caution in PUD). If massive bleed or bleeding continues, pass a Sengstaken-Blakemore tube (p255, see BOX). A bleed is the equivalent of a large protein meal so start treatment to avoid hepatic encephalopathy (p258). Omeprazole 40mg PO may also be helpful in preventing stress ulceration.
*Endoscopy:* Within 4h if you suspect variceal bleeding; within 12-24h if shocked on admission or significant comorbidity. Endoscopy can identify the site of bleeding, estimate the risk of rebleeding (see FLOWCHART) and be used to administer treatment.
*No site of bleeding identified:* Bleeding site missed on endoscopy; bleeding site has healed (Mallory-Weiss tear or Dieulafoy's lesion); nose bleed (swallowed blood); site distal to 3rd part of the duodenum (Meckel's diverticulum, colonic site).
*Helicobacter pylori:* Check status in all patients; eradicate if positive (p243).

**Rebleeds** Serious event: 40% of patients who rebleed will die. If 'at risk' maintain a high index of suspicion. If a rebleed occurs, check vital signs every 15min and call senior cover for repeat endoscopy and/or surgical intervention.

*Signs of a rebleed:*
- Rising pulse rate.
- Falling JVP ± decreasing hourly urine output.
- Haematemesis or melaena.
- Fall in BP (a late and sinister finding) and decreased conscious level.

## Immediate management if shocked

Protect airway and keep NBM
Insert two large-bore cannulae (14-16G)

↓

Urgent bloods: FBC, U&E, LFT, glucose, clotting
screen, crossmatch 6 units

↓

Rapid IV crystalloid infusion up to 1L

↓

If signs of grade III or IV shock (p805) give blood
Group specific or O Rh-ve until crossmatch done

↓

Otherwise slow crystalloid infusion[1]
to keep lines open

↓

Transfuse as dictated by haemodynamics

↓

Correct clotting abnormalities
Vitamin K, FFP, platelet concentrate

↓

Consider referral to ICU or HDU, and consider CVP
line to guide fluid replacement. Aim for >5cmH₂O
CVP may mislead if there is ascites or CCF

↓

Catheterize and monitor urine output. Aim for >30mL/h

↓

Monitor vital signs every 15min until stable, then hourly

↓

Notify surgeons of all severe bleeds

↓

Urgent endoscopy for diagnosis ± control of bleeding
• Within 4 hours if variceal bleeding
• Within 12-24 hours if patient unstable on admission

Fig 1. Immediate management if shocked.

### Rockall scoring system for prognosis in acute GI bleeding

| Variable | Score 0 | 1 | 2 | 3 |
|---|---|---|---|---|
| Age | <60 | 60-79 | >80 | |
| Shocked? | No | SBP >100 | SBP <100 | |
| | | Pulse >100 | Pulse >100 | |
| Comorbidity? | None | | CCF, IHD, any major | Renal/liver failure or malignancy |
| Diagnosis | Mallory-Weiss or normal | All other diagnoses | Malignancy | |
| Bleeding visible? | None/spot | | Visible blood/clot spurting vessel | |

Score <3 means an excellent prognosis; >8 means a high risk of death

1 Avoid saline in patients with decompensated liver disease (ascites, peripheral oedema) as it worsens ascites and, despite a low serum sodium, patients have a high body sodium. Use whole blood or salt-poor albumin for resuscitation, and 5% dextrose for maintenance.

▶**When to act now** Headache, pyrexia, neck stiffness, altered mental state: if any 2 co-exist and not yet in hospital, give benzylpenicillin 1.2g IM/IV before admitting.[33]

**Organisms** Meningococcus or pneumococcus. Less commonly *Haemophilus influenzae*; *Listeria monocytogenes*. CMV, cryptococcus (p411), or TB (p399) if immunocompromised, eg HIV +ve, organ transplant, malignancy.

**Differential** Malaria, encephalitis, septicaemia, subarachnoid, dengue, tetanus.

### Features[34]

*Early*: Headache, leg pains, cold hands and feet, abnormal skin colour.

*Later:*
- Meningism: neck stiffness, photophobia, Kernig's sign (pain + resistance on passive knee extension with hip fully flexed).
- Conscious level ↓, coma.
- Seizures (~20%) ± focal CNS signs (~20%) ± opisthotonus (p425, fig 1).
- Petechial rash (non-blanching—fig 1; may only be 1 or 2 spots, or none).

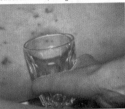
Fig 1. Glass test for petechiae.
Courtesy of Meningitis Research Foundation

Signs of galloping sepsis: slow capillary refill; DIC; BP↓. T° and pulse: ↑ or normal.

### Management[35]

- ▶ Start antibiotics (below) immediately; see fig 1 for acute management.
- *Signs of disease causing meningitis:* zoster; cold sore/genital vesicles (HSV); HIV signs (lymphadenopathy, dermatitis, candidiasis, uveitis); bleeding ± red eye (leptospirosis); parotid swelling (mumps); sore throat ± jaundice ± nodes (glandular fever, p401); splenectomy scar (∴ immunodeficient).
- *If ICP raised,* summon help immediately and inform neurosurgeons.
- *Prophylaxis:* (discuss with public health/ID) • Household contacts in droplet range. • Those who have kissed the patient's mouth. Give **rifampicin** (600mg/12h PO for 2d; children >1yr 10mg/kg/12h; <1yr 5mg/kg/12h) or **ciprofloxacin** (500mg PO, 1 dose child 5-12yrs: 250mg stat): neither is guaranteed in pregnancy, but are recommended.

---

**Antibiotic therapy for meningitis**

▶Local policies vary. If in doubt, ask. The following are suggestions only, where the organism is unknown:
- <55yrs: **cefotaxime** 2g/6h slow IV.
- >55yrs: **cefotaxime** as above + **ampicillin** 2g IV/4h (for *Listeria*).
- **Aciclovir** (p834) if viral encephalitis suspected.
- Once organism isolated, seek urgent microbiological advice.

---

### Investigations

- U&E, FBC (WBC↓≈immunocompromise: get help), LFT, glucose, coagulation screen.
- Blood culture, throat swabs (1 for bacteria, 1 for virology), rectal swab for viruses. Serology, eg EBV (p401); HIV (p412; contact lab).
- Lumbar puncture (p782) is usually done after CT but if GCS 15, no symptoms of raised ICP and no focal neurology can be done without. CI: suspected intracranial mass lesion, focal signs, papilloedema, trauma, middle ear pathology, major coagulopathy. Measure opening pressure:
  - 7-18cm CSF is normal
  - In meningitis may be >40; typically 14-30
- Send CSF for MC&S, Gram stain, protein, glucose, virology/PCR, and lactate (see FLOW-CHART for interpretation and normal values).
- In aseptic meningitis (usually self-limiting) do CSF PCR: 46% are from enteroviruses (eg Coxsackie A & B; echoviruses); 31% herpes simplex type 2 (HSV2); 4% HSV1. HSV meningitis is self-limiting if immunocompetent, unlike HSV encephalitis (a different entity).[36] For mumps, etc, see OHCS p142.
- CXR (signs of TB? If so, consider TB meningitis, p399).

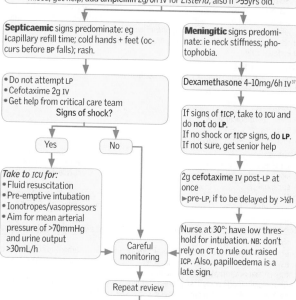

**Management of suspected bacterial meningitis**[33]

**ABCs:** IVI + fluid resus. Ask a nurse to draw up cefotaxime 2g. If immunocompromised, get help; add **ampicillin** 2g/6h IV for *Listeria*, also if >55yrs old.

**Septicaemic** signs predominate: eg ↓capillary refill time; cold hands + feet (occurs before BP falls); rash.

**Meningitic** signs predominate: ie neck stiffness; photophobia.

- Do not attempt LP
- Cefotaxime 2g IV
- Get help from critical care team

Signs of shock?

Yes / No

*Take to ICU for:*
- Fluid resuscitation
- Pre-emptive intubation
- Ionotropes/vasopressors
- Aim for mean arterial pressure of >70mmHg and urine output >30mL/h

Dexamethasone 4-10mg/6h IV[37]

If signs of ↑ICP, take to ICU and do **not** do **LP**.
If no shock or ↑ICP signs, do **LP**.
If not sure, get senior help

2g cefotaxime IV post-LP at once
► pre-LP, if to be delayed by >½h

Nurse at 30°; have low threshold for intubation. NB: don't rely on CT to rule out raised ICP. Also, papilloedema is a late sign.

Careful monitoring

Repeat review

**Subsequent therapy:** Discuss antibiotic therapy with microbiology and adjust based on organism and local sensitivities. Maintain normovolaemia with IVI if needed. Isolate for 1st 24h. If response to the above is poor consider pre-emptive intubation and ventilation ± inotropic/vasopressor support (p804). Inform Public Health, p373.

*Fig 1.* Management of suspected bacterial meningitis.

## Lumbar puncture in meningitis

| CSF in meningitis | Pyogenic | Tuberculous (p399) | Viral ('aseptic') |
|---|---|---|---|
| Appearance | Often turbid | Often fibrin web | Usually clear |
| Predominant cell | Polymorphs | Mononuclear | Mononuclear* |
| Cell count/mm³ | Eg 90-1000 or more | 10-1000 | 50-1000 |
| Glucose | <⅔ plasma | <⅔ plasma | >⅔ plasma |
| Protein (g/L) | >1.5 | 1-5 | <1 |
| Bacteria | In smear & culture | Often none in smear | None seen or cultured |

**Normal values:** ≤5 lymphocytes/mm³ may be normal, so long as there are no neutrophils. Protein: 0.15–0.45g/L. CSF glucose: 2.8-4.2mmol/L: *Causes of ↓CSF glucose:* sepsis; parasitic meningitis, eg from eating snails (do CSF eosinophil count); also herpes encephalitis, hypoglycaemia, sarcoid, CNS vasculitis. A CSF lactate level of ≥3.5mmol/L (31.5mg/dL) predicts bacterial meningitis quite well.[38]

\* Predominant cell type may also be lymphocytes in TB, listerial, and cryptococcal meningitis.

Emergencies

▶Suspect encephalitis whenever odd behaviour, ↓consciousness, focal neurology or seizure is preceded by an infectious prodrome (T°↑, rash, lymphadenopathy, cold sores, conjunctivitis, meningeal signs). It is often wise to treat (see below) before the exact cause is known—usually viral, and often never identified. Without the infectious prodrome consider *encephalopathy*: hypoglycaemia, hepatic encephalopathy, diabetic ketoacidosis, drugs, hypoxic brain injury, uraemia, SLE, beri-beri (give vit B₁ if in doubt p728).

### Signs and symptoms
- Bizarre encephalopathic behaviour or confusion
- ↓GCS or coma
- Fever
- Headache
- Focal neurological signs
- Seizures
- History of travel or animal bite.

### Causes
- *Viral:* HSV-1 & 2, arboviruses, CMV, EBV, VZV (varicella-zoster virus), HIV (seroconversion), measles, mumps, rabies, Japanese B encephalitis, West Nile virus, tick-borne encephalitis.
- *Non-viral:* any bacterial meningitis, TB, malaria, listeria, Lyme disease, legionella, leptospirosis, aspergillosis, cryptococcus, schistosomiasis, typhus (fig 3, p389).

### Investigations
- *Bloods:* blood cultures; serum for viral PCR (also throat swab and MSU); toxoplasma IgM titre; malaria film.
- *Contrast-enhanced CT:* focal bilateral temporal lobe involvement is suggestive of HSV encephalitis. Meningeal enhancement suggests meningoencephalitis. Do before LP. MRI is alternative if allergic to contrast.
- *LP:* typically moderately ↑CSF protein and lymphocytes, and ↓glucose (p833). Send CSF for viral PCR including HSV (CSF PCR is 95% specific for HSV-1).
- *EEG:* urgent EEG showing diffuse abnormalities may help confirm a diagnosis of encephalitis, but does not indicate a cause.

### Management
▶Mortality in untreated viral encephalitis is ~70%. ▶▶Aim to start aciclovir within 30min[30] of the patient arriving (10mg/kg/8h IV over 1h) for 14 days as empirical treatment for HSV (21 days if immunosuppressed). Adjust aciclovir dose according to eGFR: use every 12h if eGFR 25–50; every 24h if eGFR 10–25. Consult product literature if eGFR <10. Specific therapies also exist for CMV and toxoplasmosis (p404).
- Supportive therapy, in high-dependency unit or ICU environment if necessary.
- Symptomatic treatment: eg phenytoin for seizures (p836).

# Cerebral abscess

Suspect this in any patient with ↑ICP, especially if there is fever or ↑WCC. It may follow ear, sinus, dental, or periodontal infection; skull fracture; congenital heart disease; endocarditis; bronchiectasis. It may also occur in the absence of systemic signs of inflammation.

**Signs** Seizures, fever, localizing signs, or signs of ↑ICP. Coma. Signs of sepsis elsewhere (eg teeth, ears, lungs, endocarditis).

**Investigations** CT/MRI p760 (eg 'ring-enhancing' lesion); ↑WCC, ↑ESR; biopsy.

**Treatment** Urgent neurosurgical referral; treat ↑ICP (p840). If frontal sinuses or teeth are the source, the likely organism will be *Strep. milleri* (microaerophilic), or oropharyngeal anaerobes. In ear abscesses, *B. fragilis* or other anaerobes are most common. Bacterial abscesses are often peripheral; toxoplasma lesions (p404) are deeper (eg basal ganglia). NB: ask yourself: is the patient immunocompromised? Discuss with infectious diseases/microbiology.

Emergencies

This means seizures lasting for >30min, or repeated seizures without intervening consciousness. Mortality and the risk of permanent brain damage increase with the length of attack. Aim to terminate seizures lasting more than a few minutes as soon as possible (<20min).

Status usually occurs in patients with known epilepsy. If it is the 1st presentation, the chance of a structural brain lesion is high (>50%). Diagnosis of tonic-clonic status is usually clear. Non-convulsive status (eg absence status or continuous partial seizures with preservation of consciousness) may be more difficult: look for subtle eye or lid movement. For other signs, see p489, p494-497. An EEG can be very helpful. ▶*Could the patient be pregnant* (any pelvic mass)? If so, eclampsia (*OHCS* p48) is the likely diagnosis, check the urine and BP: call a senior obstetrician—immediate delivery may be needed.

### Investigations
• Bedside glucose, the following tests can be done once $R$ has started: lab glucose, ABG, U&E, $Ca^{2+}$, FBC, ECG.
• Consider anticonvulsant levels, toxicology screen, LP, culture blood and urine, EEG, CT, carbon monoxide level.
• Pulse oximetry, cardiac monitor.

**Treatment** See fig 1. Basic life support—and these agents:
1 *Lorazepam:* 0.1mg/kg (usually 4mg) as a slow bolus into a large vein. If no response within 10min give a second dose. Beware respiratory arrest during the last part of the injection. Have full resuscitation facilities to hand for all IV benzodiazepine use. The rectal route is an alternative for diazepam if IV access is difficult.[1] *Buccal midazolam* is an easier to use oral alternative; dose for those 10yrs old and older 10mg; if 1-5yrs 5mg, if 5-10yrs 7.5mg; squirt half the volume between the lower gum and the cheek on each side. While waiting for this to work, prepare other drugs. If fits continue ...
2 *Phenytoin infusion:* 15-20mg/kg IVI (roughly 1g if 60kg, and 1.5g if 80kg; max 2g), at a rate of ≤50mg/min (don't put diazepam in same line: they don't mix). Beware BP↓ and do not use if bradycardic or heart block. Requires BP and ECG monitoring. 100mg/6-8h is a maintenance dose (check levels). If fits continue ...
3 *Diazepam infusion:* eg 100mg in 500mL of 5% dextrose; infuse at about 40mL/h (max 3mg/kg/24h) until seizures respond. Close monitoring, especially respiratory function, is vital. It is most unusual for seizures to remain unresponsive following this. If they do, allow the idea to pass through your mind that they could be pseudoseizures (p720), particularly if there are odd features (pelvic thrusts; resisting attempts to open lids and your attempts to do passive movements; arms and legs flailing around).
4 *Dexamethasone:* 10mg IV if vasculitis/cerebral oedema (tumour) possible.
5 *General anaesthesia:* ▶For refractory status: get anaesthetist/ICU involved early.

As soon as seizures are controlled, start oral drugs (p496). Ask what the cause was, eg hypoglycaemia, pregnancy, alcohol, drugs, CNS lesion or infection, hypertensive encephalopathy, inadequate anticonvulsant dose (p494).

⚠️ 1 Diazepam Rectubes®: give 0.5mg/kg stat dose—eg ~2-3 10mg tubes PR (respiratory problems at this dose are *very* rare: all survived). If your back is still against the wall with no response after 10min, try 1 last 10mg tube. Halve dose if elderly. *For children's Stesolid® regimen* (it is different), see *OHCS* p206.

**Management of status epilepticus**

Open and maintain the airway, lay in recovery position
Remove false teeth if poorly fitting, insert oral/nasal airway,
intubate if necessary

↓

Oxygen, 100% + suction (as required)

↓

IV access and take blood:
U&E, LFT, FBC, glucose, Ca²⁺
Toxicology screen if indicated
Anticonvulsant levels

↓

**Slow IV bolus phase**—to stop seizures: eg lorazepam
2-4mg. Give 2ⁿᵈ dose of lorazepam if no response within 10min.

↓

Thiamine 250mg IV over 30min if alcoholism or
malnourishment suspected.
Glucose 50mL 50% IV, unless glucose known to be normal
Treat acidosis if severe (contact ICU)

↓

Correct hypotension with fluids

↓

**IV infusion phase:** If seizures continue, start phenytoin,
15-20mg/kg IVI, at a rate of ≤50mg/min. Monitor ECG and BP.
100mg/6-8h is a maintenance dose (check levels).
**Alternative:** diazepam infusion: 100mg in 500mL
of 5% glucose; infuse at ~40mL/h as opposite

↓

**General anaesthesia phase:** Continuing seizures require expert help
with paralysis and ventilation with continuous EEG monitoring in ICU

Fig 1. Management of status epilepticus.
NB: ▶**never** spend longer than 20min on someone with status epilepticus without
having help at the bedside from an anaesthetist.

▶If the pupils are unequal, diagnose rising intracranial pressure (ICP), eg from extradural haemorrhage, and summon urgent neurosurgical help (p486). Retinal vein pulsation at fundoscopy helps exclude ↑ICP.

**Initial management** (See fig 1) Write full notes. Record times.
- Involve neurosurgeons at an early stage, especially with comatose patients, or if raised ICP suspected.
- Examine the CNS. Chart pulse, BP, T°, respirations + pupils every 15min.
- Assess anterograde amnesia (loss from the time of injury, ie post-traumatic) and retrograde amnesia—its extent correlates with the severity of the injury, and it never occurs without anterograde amnesia.
- Nurse semi-prone if no spinal injury; meticulous care to bladder and airway.

*Who needs a CT head?*
If any of the following are present, a CT is required immediately:
- GCS <13 at any time, or GCS 13 or 14 at 2h following injury
- Focal neurological deficit
- Suspected open or depressed skull fracture, or signs of basal skull fracture (haemotympanum, 'panda' eyes, CSF leak through nose/ears, Battle's sign)
- Post-traumatic seizure
- Vomiting >once
- Loss of consciousness AND any of the following:
  - Age ≥65
  - Coagulopathy
  - 'Dangerous mechanism of injury', eg car crash or fall from great height
  - Anterograde amnesia of >30min

*When to ventilate immediately:*
- Coma ≤8 on Glasgow coma scale (GCS; p802)
- $P_aO_2$ <9kPa in air (<13kPa in $O_2$) or $P_aCO_2$ >6kPa
- Spontaneous hyperventilation ($P_aCO_2$ <3.5kPa)
- Respiratory irregularity (p53)

*Ventilate before neurosurgical transfer if:*
- Deteriorating level of consciousness
- Bilateral fractured mandible
- Bleeding into mouth, eg skull base fracture
- Seizures

**Risk of intracranial haematoma in adults**
- Fully conscious, no skull fracture = <1:1000
- Confused, no skull fracture = 1:100
- Fully conscious, skull fracture = 1:30
- Confused, skull fracture = 1:4

**Criteria for admission**
- Difficult to assess (child; post-ictal; alcohol intoxication)
- CNS signs; severe headache or vomiting; fracture
- Brief loss of consciousness does **not** require admission if well and a responsible adult is in attendance

*Drowsy trauma patients (GCS <15 to >8) smelling of alcohol:* Alcohol is an unlikely cause of coma if plasma alcohol <44mmol/L. If unavailable, estimate blood alcohol level from the osmolar gap (p682). If blood alcohol ≈ 40mmol/L, osmolar gap ≈ 40mmol/L. Never assume signs are just from alcohol.

**Complications** *Early:* Extradural/subdural haemorrhage, seizures. *Late:* Subdural (p486), seizures, diabetes insipidus, parkinsonism, dementia.

**Indicators of a bad prognosis** Old age, decerebrate rigidity, extensor spasms, prolonged coma, ↑BP, $P_aO_2$↓ (on blood gases), T° >39°C. 60% of those with loss of consciousness of >1 month will survive 3–25yrs, but may need daily nursing care.

For *Spinal cord injury & Persistent vegetative states*, see OHCS (p766-774 & p776).

## Immediate management plan for head injury

ABC

⬇

Oxygen if saturations <92% or hypoxic on ABG
Intubate and hyperventilate if necessary
Immobilize neck until injury to cervical spine excluded

⬇

Stop blood loss and support circulation
Treat for shock if required (p804)

⬇

Treat seizures with lorazepam ± phenytoin (p836)

⬇

**Assess level of consciousness (GCS)**
Anterograde and retrograde amnesia

⬇

Rapid examination survey

⬇

**Investigations:**
U&Es, glucose, FBC, blood alcohol,
toxicology screen, ABG and clotting

⬇

Neurological examination

⬇

**Brief history**
When? Where? How? Had a fit? Lucid interval? Alcohol?

⬇

**Evaluate lacerations of face or scalp**
Palpate deep wounds with sterile glove to check for
step deformity. Note obvious skull/facial fractures[1]

⬇

**Check for CSF leak, from nose (rhinorrhoea) or ear (otorrhoea)**
Any blood behind the ear drum?
If either is present, suspect basilar skull fracture: do CT
Give tetanus toxoid, and refer at once to neurosurgeons

⬇

**Palpate the neck posteriorly for tenderness and deformity**
If detected, or if the patient has obvious head injury, or injury above the
clavicle with loss of consciousness, immobilize the neck and get cervical
spine X-ray or CT neck ± chest/abdo/pelvis (trauma series)

⬇

**Radiology**
As indicated: CT of head/trauma CT series (see p744)

Fig 1. Immediate management plan for head injury.

1 Periorbital ('panda' eyes/racoon sign) or postauricular (Battle sign) ecchymoses.

**Emergencies**

The volume inside the cranium is fixed, so any increase in the contents can lead to raised ICP. This can be mass effect, oedema or obstruction to fluid outflow. Normal ICP in adults is <15mmHg.

## Causes
• Primary or metastatic tumours.
• Head injury.
• Haemorrhage (subdural, extradural, subarachnoid, intracerebral, intraventricular).
• Infection: meningitis, encephalitis, brain abscess.
• Hydrocephalus.
• Cerebral oedema.
• Status epilepticus.

## Signs and symptoms
• Headache (worse on coughing, leaning forwards), vomiting.
• Altered GCS: drowsiness; listlessness, irritability, coma.
• History of trauma.
• Falling pulse and rising BP (Cushing's response); Cheyne–Stokes respiration.
• Pupil changes (constriction at first, later dilatation—do not mask these signs by using agents such as tropicamide to dilate the pupil to aid fundoscopy).
• ↓visual acuity; peripheral visual field loss.
• Papilloedema is an unreliable sign, but venous pulsation at the disc may be absent (absent in ~50% of normal people, but *loss* of it is a useful sign).

## Investigations
• U&E, FBC, LFT, glucose, serum osmolality, clotting, blood culture.
• Consider toxicology screen.
• CXR—any source of infection that might indicate abscess?
• CT head.
• Then consider lumbar puncture if safe. Measure the opening pressure!

## Treatment
The goal is to ↓ICP and avert secondary injury. Urgent neurosurgery is required for the definitive treatment of ↑ICP from focal causes (eg haematomas). This is achieved via a craniotomy or burr hole. Also, an ICP monitor (or bolt) may be placed to monitor pressure. Surgery is generally *not* helpful following ischaemic or anoxic injury.

*Holding measures* are listed in fig 1.

## Herniation syndromes
*Uncal herniation* is caused by a lateral supratentorial mass, which pushes the ipsilateral inferomedial temporal lobe (uncus) through the temporal incisura and against the midbrain. The III$^{rd}$ nerve, travelling in this space, gets compressed, causing a dilated ipsilateral pupil, then ophthalmoplegia (a fixed pupil localizes a lesion poorly but is 'ipsi-lateralizing'). This may be followed (quickly) by contralateral hemiparesis (pressure on the cerebral peduncle) and coma from pressure on the ascending reticular activating system (ARAS) in the midbrain.

*Cerebellar tonsil herniation* is caused by ↑pressure in the posterior fossa forcing the cerebellar tonsils through the foramen magnum. Ataxia, VI$^{th}$ nerve palsies, and upgoing plantar reflexes occur first, then loss of consciousness, irregular breathing, and apnoea. This syndrome may proceed very rapidly given the small size of, and poor compliance in, the posterior fossa.

*Subfalcian (cingulate) herniation* is caused by a frontal mass. The cingulate gyrus (medial frontal lobe) is forced under the rigid falx cerebri. It may be silent unless the anterior cerebral artery is compressed and causes a stroke—eg contralateral leg weakness ± abulia (lack of decision-making).

⚠

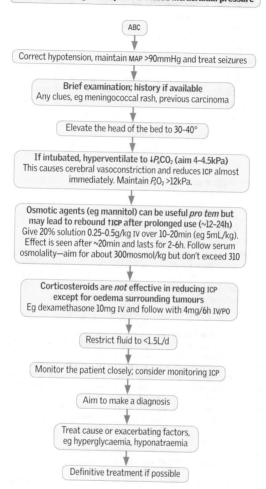

**Immediate management plan for raised intracranial pressure**

ABC

Correct hypotension, maintain MAP >90mmHg and treat seizures

**Brief examination; history if available**
Any clues, eg meningococcal rash, previous carcinoma

Elevate the head of the bed to 30-40°

**If intubated, hyperventilate to $\downarrow P_aCO_2$ (aim 4-4.5kPa)**
This causes cerebral vasoconstriction and reduces ICP almost
immediately. Maintain $P_aO_2$ >12kPa.

Osmotic agents (eg mannitol) can be useful *pro tem* but
may lead to rebound $\uparrow$ICP after prolonged use (~12-24h)
Give 20% solution 0.25-0.5g/kg IV over 10-20min (eg 5mL/kg).
Effect is seen after ~20min and lasts for 2-6h. Follow serum
osmolality—aim for about 300mosmol/kg but don't exceed 310

Corticosteroids are *not* effective in reducing ICP
except for oedema surrounding tumours
Eg dexamethasone 10mg IV and follow with 4mg/6h IV/PO

Restrict fluid to <1.5L/d

Monitor the patient closely; consider monitoring ICP

Aim to make a diagnosis

Treat cause or exacerbating factors,
eg hyperglycaemia, hyponatraemia

Definitive treatment if possible

Fig 1. Immediate management plan for raised intracranial pressure.

**Mechanism** Normally the body metabolizes carbohydrates, leading to efficient energy production. Ketoacidosis is an alternative metabolic pathway, normally used in starvation states, it is far less efficient, and produces acetone as a by product (hence the fruity breath of patients in ketosis). In acute diabetic ketoacidosis, there is excessive glucose, but because of the lack of insulin, this cannot be taken up into cells to be metabolized, so pushing the body into a starvation-like state where ketoacidosis is the only mechanism of energy production. The combination of severe acidosis and hyperglycaemia can be deadly, so early recognition and treatment is important.

**Typical picture** Gradual drowsiness, vomiting and dehydration in type 1 diabetic (very rarely type 2) ►Do glucose in *all* those with unexplained vomiting, abdo pain, polyuria, polydipsia, lethargy, anorexia, ketotic breath, dehydration, coma, or deep breathing (sighing 'Kussmaul' hyperventilation). *Triggers:* Infection, eg UTI; surgery; MI; pancreatitis; chemotherapy; antipsychotics;[43] wrong insulin dose/non-compliance.

### Diagnosis
1 Acidaemia (blood pH <7.3)
2 Hyperglycaemia
3 Ketonaemia

*Tests:* ECG, CXR. *Urine:* Dipstick and MSU. *Blood:* Capillary and lab glucose, ketones, U&E, $HCO_3^-$, amylase, osmolality, ABG/VBG (p843), FBC, blood culture.
Plasma osmolarity = 2[$Na^+$]+[urea]+[glucose] mmol/L. Anion gap: p684.

**Severe DKA** If one or more of the following features is present on admission, consider transfer to HDU/ICU for monitoring and central venous access. Get senior help!

- Blood ketones >6mmol/L
- Venous bicarbonate <5mmol/L
- Venous/arterial pH <7.1
- K <3.5mmol/L on admission
- GCS <12
- $O_2$ sats <92% on air (assuming no respiratory disease)
- Systolic BP <90mmHg
- Pulse >100 or <60 bpm
- Anion gap above 16

### Pitfalls in diabetic ketoacidosis
- *Plasma glucose* is usually high, but not always, especially if insulin continued.
- *High WCC* may be seen in the absence of infection.
- *Infection:* often there is no fever. Do MSU, blood cultures, and CXR. Start broad-spectrum antibiotics (eg co-amoxiclav, p378) early if infection is suspected.
- *Creatinine:* some assays for creatinine cross-react with ketone bodies, so plasma creatinine may not reflect true renal function.
- *Hyponatraemia* is common, due to osmolar compensation for the hyperglycaemia. ↑ or ↔ [$Na^+$] indicates severe water loss. As treatment commences $Na^+$ rises as water enters cells. $Na^+$ is also low due to an artefact; corrected plasma [$Na^+$] = $Na^+$ + 2.4[(glucose −5.5)/5.5].
- *Ketonuria* does not equate with ketoacidosis. Anyone may have up to ++ketonuria after an overnight fast. Not all ketones are due to diabetes—consider alcohol if glucose normal. Always check venous blood ketones.
- *Recurrent ketoacidosis:* blood glucose may return to normal long before ketones are removed from the blood, and a rapid reduction in the amount of insulin administered may lead to lack of clearance and return to DKA. This may be avoided by maintaining a constant rate of insulin, eg 4–5u/h IVI, and co-infusing glucose 10–20% to keep plasma glucose at 6–10mmol/L—the extended insulin regimen.
- *Acidosis* but without gross elevation of glucose may occur, but consider overdose (eg aspirin) and lactic acidosis (in elderly diabetics).
- *Serum amylase* is often raised (up to ×10) and non-specific abdominal pain is common, even in the absence of pancreatitis.

**Complications** ►Cerebral oedema (get help if sudden CNS decline), aspiration pneumonia, hypokalaemia, hypomagnesaemia, hypophosphataemia, thromboembolism.
►Talk with the patient: ensure there are no further preventable episodes.

## Management plan for diabetic ketoacidosis

**ABC approach, 2 large-bore cannulae**
If SBP <90mmHg give 500mL bolus saline, if no response give a second bolus and get ICU advice. If SBP >90 or response to first bolus, start fluids as below.

↓

*Tests:* As per p842, venous blood gas (VBG) for pH, bicarbonate and lab glucose, ketones, U&Es (for K⁺ and Na⁺) as minimum

↓

*Insulin* add 50u actrapid to 50mL 0.9% saline. Infuse continuously at 0.1u/kg/h. Only give a stat dose if there is a delay in starting the infusion. Continue the patient's long-acting insulin.
Aim for a fall in blood ketones of 0.5mmol/L/h, or a rise in venous bicarbonate of 3mmol/L/h with a fall in glucose of 3mmol/L/h. If not achieving this, increase insulin infusion by 1u/h until target rates achieved.

↓

Check VBG for pH, bicarb, glucose and K⁺ at 1h, 2h and 2hrly thereafter

↓

Assess need for K⁺ replacement (see below)

↓

Consider catheter if not passed urine by 1h, aim for urine output 0.5ml/kg/h. Consider NG tube if vomiting or drowsy.
Start all patients on low molecular weight heparin

↓

Avoid hypoglycaemia! When glucose <14mmol/L start 10% glucose at 125mL/h to run alongside saline and prevent hypoglycaemia

↓

Continue fixed-rate insulin until ketones <0.3mmol/L, venous pH >7.3 and venous bicarb >18mmol/L. Do not rely on urinary ketones to indicate resolution—they stay positive after DKA resolved.
Find and treat infection/cause for DKA.

Fig 1. Management plan for diabetic ketoacidosis.

### Fluid replacement
- 0.9% saline is the replacement fluid of choice.
- Typical fluid deficit is 100mL/kg, so for an average 70kg man = 7 litres.
- In this example, give 1L in 1st hour, 1L over 2 hours, 1L over 2 hours, 1L over 4 hours, 1L over 4 hours, 1L over 6 hours. Always reassess at 12 hours.
- Be more cautious with fluids if young adult, elderly, pregnant, comorbidities.
- Bicarbonate may increase risk of cerebral oedema and is not recommended.

### Potassium replacement
- Typical deficit = 3–5mmol/kg, plasma K⁺ falls with treatment as K⁺ enters cells.
- Don't add K⁺ to the 1st bag. Monitor UO hourly; start adding K⁺ when >30mL/h.
- Check U&E hourly initially, and replace as required:

| Serum K⁺ (mmol/L) | Amount of KCl to add per litre of IV fluid |
|---|---|
| >5.5 | Nil |
| 3.5–5.5 | 40mmol |
| <3.5 | Seek help from HDU/ICU re higher doses |

Less will be needed in renal failure or oliguria.

*Other emergencies:* Hyperosmolar non-ketotic coma and hypoglycaemia: p844.

**Hypoglycaemic coma** Usually *rapid* onset; may be preceded by odd behaviour (eg aggression), sweating, pulse↑, seizures. *Management:* ►►Give 20–30g glucose IV, eg 200–300mL of 10% dextrose. This is preferable to 50–100mL 50% glucose which harms veins. Expect prompt recovery. Glucagon 1mg IV/IM is nearly as rapid as dextrose but will not work in drunk patients. Dextrose IVI may be needed for severe prolonged hypoglycaemia. Once conscious, give sugary drinks and a meal.

**Hyperglycaemic hyperosmolar non-ketotic (HONK) coma** Typically those with type 2 DM are at risk of this.[44] The history is longer (eg 1wk), with marked dehydration and glucose >35mmol/L. Acidosis is absent as there is no switch to ketone metabolism. Osmolality (p842) is >340mosmol/kg. ►*Occlusive events are a danger* (focal CNS signs, chorea, DIC, leg ischaemia/rhabdomyolysis[45]) DVT—give LMWH prophylaxis to all unless contraindication (p344).[46,47] Rehydrate slowly with 0.9% saline IVI over 48h, typical deficits are 110–220mL/kg, ie 8–15L for a 70kg adult. Replace $K^+$ when urine starts to flow (see DKA BOX, p843). Only use insulin if blood glucose not falling by 5mmol/L/h with rehydration or if ketonaemia—start slowly 0.05u/kg/h. Keep blood glucose at least 10–15mmol/L for first 24 hours to avoid cerebral oedema.[48] Look for the cause, eg MI, drugs, or bowel infarct.

**Lactic acidosis** is a rare but serious complication of DM with metformin use or septicaemia. Blood lactate: >5mmol/L. Seek expert help. Treat sepsis vigorously, maintain blood pressure and hence tissue perfusion. Stop metformin.

## Thyroid emergencies

**Myxoedema coma** The ultimate hypothyroid state before death.

*Signs and symptoms:* Looks hypothyroid (p212, p213, fig 1); often >65yrs; hypothermia; hyporeflexia; glucose↓; bradycardia; coma; seizures. May have had radioidine, thyroidectomy, or pituitary surgery (signs of hypopituitarism, p224). Patient may have seemed psychotic (myxoedema madness)[49] just before the coma (eg precipitated by infection, MI, stroke, or trauma).

*Examination:* Goitre; cyanosis; BP↓ (cardiogenic); heart failure; signs of precipitants.

*Treatment:* Preferably on ICU.
• Blood for: T3, T4, TSH, FBC, U&E (Na⁺ often↓), cultures, cortisol, glucose.
• ABG for $P_aO_2$. High-flow $O_2$ if cyanosed. Ventilation may be needed.
• Correct any hypoglycaemia.
• Give T3 (liothyronine) 5–20µg/12h IV slowly. Be cautious: you may precipitate manifestations of ischaemic heart disease. Alternative regimens involve levothyroxine.[50]
• Give hydrocortisone 100mg/8h IV—vital if pituitary hypothyroidism is suspected (ie no goitre, no previous radioidine, and no previous thyroid surgery).
• If infection suspected, give antibiotic, eg cefuroxime 1.5g/8h IVI.
• Caution with fluid, rehydrate as needed but watch for cardiac dysfunction, BP may not respond to fluid and inotropes may be needed.[51]
• Active warming (blankets, fluids) may be needed for *hypothermia.* Beware complications (hypoglycaemia, pancreatitis, arrhythmias). See p860.

*Further R:* T3 5–20µg/4–12h IV until sustained improvement (~2-3d) then levothyroxine 50µg/24h PO. Hydrocortisone + IV fluids as needed (hyponatraemia is dilutional).

**Hyperthyroid crisis (thyrotoxic storm)** *Sign and symptoms:* ♀:♂≈4:1. Severe hyperthyroidism also see p210: T°↑, agitation, confusion, coma, tachycardia, AF, D&V, goitre, thyroid bruit, acute abdomen (exclude surgical causes), heart failure, cardiovascular collapse.[52]

*Precipitants:* Recent thyroid surgery or radioidine; infection; MI; trauma.

*Diagnosis:* Do not wait for test results if urgent treatment is needed. Do TSH, free T4 and free T3. Confirm with technetium uptake if possible.

*Treatment:* Ask an endocrinologist. **Grand strategy:** 1 Counteract peripheral effects of thyroid hormones. 2 Inhibit thyroid hormone synthesis. 3 Treat systemic complications. See fig 1 for how to put this into effect.[53] If you are not making headway in 24h, consider thyroidectomy if you can find a good anaesthetist and surgeon.[54,55]

## Management plan for thyrotoxic storm

IV access, fluids if dehydrated. NG tube if vomiting.

↓

Take blood for: T3, T4, TSH, cultures (if infection suspected).

↓

Sedate if necessary (eg chlorpromazine 50mg PO/IM). Monitor BP.

↓

If no contraindication, and cardiac output OK, give propranolol 40mg/8h PO; max IV dose: 1mg over 1min; may need repeating. In asthma/poor cardiac output, propranolol has caused cardiac arrest in thyroid storm, so ultra-short-acting β-blockers have a role, eg IV esmolol. Consider diltiazem if β-blockers contraindicated. ►Get help.

↓

High-dose digoxin may be needed to slow the heart, but ensure adequately β blocked, give with cardiac monitoring.

↓

Antithyroid drugs: carbimazole 15–25mg/6h PO (or via NGT); after 4h give Lugol's solution (aqueous iodine oral solution) 0.3mL/8h PO well diluted in water for 7–10 days to block thyroid.

↓

Hydrocortisone 100mg/6h IV or dexamethasone 4mg/8h PO to prevent peripheral conversion T4 to T3.

↓

Treat suspected infection, eg with co-amoxiclav 1.2g/8h IVI.

↓

Adjust IV fluids as necessary; cool with tepid sponging ± paracetamol.

↓

*Continuing treatment:* After 5d reduce carbimazole to 15mg/8h PO. After 10d stop propranolol and iodine. Adjust carbimazole (p210).

Fig 1. Management plan for thyrotoxic storm.

**Signs and symptoms** Patients may present in shock (pulse↑; vasoconstriction; postural hypotension; oliguria; weak; confused; comatose)—often (but not always!) in a patient with known Addison's (eg when oral steroid has not been increased to cover stress such as pneumonia), or someone on long-term steroids who has forgotten their tablets. Remember bilateral adrenal haemorrhage (eg meningococcaemia) as a cause. An alternative presentation is with hypoglycaemia.

**Precipitating factors** Infection, trauma, surgery, missed medication.

**Management** If suspected, treat before biochemical results.
• Bloods for cortisol and ACTH (this needs to go straight to laboratory, call ahead!), U&Es—can have high K⁺ (check ECG and give calcium gluconate if needed, see p849) and low Na⁺ (salt depletion, should resolve with rehydration and steroids).
• Hydrocortisone 100mg IV stat.
• IV fluid bolus, crystalloid or colloid to support BP.
• Monitor blood glucose: the danger is hypoglycaemia.
• Blood, urine, sputum for culture, then antibiotics if concern about infection.

**Continuing treatment**
• Glucose IV may be needed if hypoglycaemic.
• Give IV fluids as guided by clinical state and to correct U&E imbalance.
• Continue hydrocortisone, eg 100mg/8h IV or IM.
• Change to oral steroids after 72h if patient's condition good. The tetracosactrin (=tetracosactide) test is impossible while on hydrocortisone.
• Fludrocortisone may well be needed if the cause is adrenal disease: ask an expert.
• Search for (and vigorously treat) the underlying cause. Get endocrinological help.

## Hypopituitary coma

Think of decompensated chronic hypophyseal failure whenever hypothermia, refractory hypotension ± septic signs *without* fever occur with short stature or loss of axillary/pubic hair ± gonadal atrophy.[56] ▶Waiting for lab confirmation may be fatal. It *usually* develops gradually in a person with known hypopituitarism. If rapid onset due to pituitary infarction (eg postpartum Sheehan's, p224), subarachnoid haemorrhage is often misdiagnosed as symptoms include headache and meningism.

**Presentation** Headache; ophthalmoplegia; consciousness↓; hypotension; hypothermia; hypoglycaemia; signs of hypopituitarism (p224).

**Tests** Cortisol; T4; TSH; ACTH; glucose. Pituitary fossa CT/MRI.

**Treatment** ▶Hydrocortisone, eg 100mg IV/6h.
• Only after hydrocortisone begun: liothyronine (L-tri-iodothyronine sodium), eg 10µg/12h PO or by slow IV: 5–20µg/12h (4-hourly may be needed).
• Prompt surgery is needed if the cause is pituitary apoplexy (p226).

Patients with phaeochromocytoma may have had undiagnosed symptoms for some time, but stress, abdominal palpation, parturition, general anaesthetic, or contrast media used in imaging[1] can cause acute *hypertensive crises*.

**Signs and symptoms** Pallor, pulsating headache, hypertension, feels 'about to die', pyrexial. *ECG*: signs of LVF, ↑ST segment, VT and cardiogenic shock.[57]

**Treatment** ▸Get help. Take to ICU.

Principle is combined α and β blockade, but α must be started first, as unopposed β blockade can worsen hypertension.

- Start with short-acting, IV α-blocker, eg **phentolamine** 2–5mg IV.[58] Repeat to maintain safe BP.
- When BP controlled, give long-acting α-blocker, eg **phenoxybenzamine** 10mg/24h PO (increase by 10mg/d as needed, up to 30mg/12h PO); SE: postural hypotension; dizziness; tachycardia; nasal congestion; miosis; idiosyncratic marked BP drop after 1st dose. The idea is to ↑ the dose until BP is controlled and there is no significant postural hypotension. Alternative α1-selective blockers, eg doxazosin, are preferred in some centres, particularly if surgery is not an option, eg metastatic tumour.
- A β1-blocker may also be given at this stage to control any tachycardia or myocardial ischaemia/dysrhythmias (p108).
- **Surgery** is usually done electively after 4–6wks to allow full α-blockade and volume expansion. When admitted for surgery the phenoxybenzamine dose is increased until significant postural hypotension.

---

1 NB: low-osmolarity IV contrast may be OK.[58]

▶Seek expert help promptly.

Acute kidney injury is a common problem in emergency admissions, and anyone arriving with sepsis, acute fluid losses or dehydration, hypotension or oliguria is at risk. See p290-293 for comprehensive assessment and management, this emergency information covers the first few hours of admission.

**Symptoms and signs** May be none, or fatigue, malaise, rash, joint pains, nausea/vomiting, chest pain, palpitations, shortness of breath, fluid overload, abdominal pain, oliguria, hypo- or hypertension.

**Investigations**
- Urgent ABG/VBG for $K^+$
- *ECG* for hyperkalaemic changes (see ECG, p 689)
- *Bloods:* U&Es, $Ca^{2+}$, $PO_4^{3-}$, FBC, ESR, CRP, clotting, LFTs, CK in all. Consider 'renal screen': protein electrophoresis, hepatitis serology, autoantibodies (ANCA, ANA, anti-GBM), complement, ASOT, rheumatoid factor, cryoglobulins.
- *Urine:* dipstick, send for microscopy, culture, albumin/creatinine ratio
- USS
- CXR

**Causes**
- *Pre-renal:* hypotension of any cause, eg sepsis, hypovolaemia, cardiac dysfunction
- *Renal:* drugs, glomerulonephritis, vasculitis (p558)
- *Post-renal:* obstruction (p642), eg prostatic, stones (usually very painful)

**Principles of treatment**
*See fig 1*
- Treat life-threatening hyperkalaemia
- Treat hypotension, sepsis or other pre-renal cause
- Catheterize to try to treat any post-renal component
- Treat pulmonary oedema with IV diuretics
- Contact renal team early if no urine output following catheterization and correction of hypotension, particularly if hyperkalaemia, pulmonary oedema or signs of uraemic pericarditis (extremely rare) (p148)
- Urgent USS to rule out obstruction above the level of the bladder (ie not corrected with catheterization)
- Consider whether patient needs transfer to ICU (especially if more than one organ dysfunction, eg AKI in association with sepsis from pneumonia—may need ventilatory and inotropic support as well as renal support)

**Contact renal team for urgent dialysis if:**
▶▶Hyperkalaemia unresponsive to medical treatment or in an oliguric patient

▶▶Pulmonary oedema unresponsive to medical treatment

▶▶Uraemic complications such as pericarditis, encephalopathy

▶▶Severe metabolic acidosis (pH <7.2 or base excess below -10)

### Management of AKI

Urgent ABG/VBG to check K⁺
ECG for signs of hyperkalaemia (see below)

Treat hyperkalaemia:
1 Stabilize cardiac membrane with 10mL 10% calcium gluconate
2 Drive K⁺ into cells with 10units actrapid in 50mL 20% glucose
NB: remember this is a **temporary treatment** only—speak to renal team!

Assess intravascular volume: BP (inc postural), JVP, skin turgor, fluid
balance sheet, weight, attach to cardiac monitor

Catheterize to assess hourly urine output, and establish fluid charts

If dehydrated, give fluid challenge.
250–500mL of saline over 30min

#### Reassess
Repeat fluid challenge if still dehydrated (give fluids until JVP visible and
systolic BP >100mmHg. Caution in patients with cardiac dysfunction)

Once fluid replete, continue fluids at 20mL
+ previous hour's urine output per hour

If volume overloaded, consider urgent dialysis.
If patient is passing urine then consider driving diuresis as per treatment of
pulmonary oedema (p812) with furosemide, diamorphine to vasodilate and
nitrate infusion

If clinical suspicion of sepsis, take cultures, then treat vigorously.
**Do not leave possible sources of sepsis (eg IV lines) *in situ* if not needed**

Refer to renal team for opinion early, particularly if poor response to initial
treatment or oliguria with hyperkalaemia

Fig 1. Management of AKI.

---

#### Hyperkalaemia

The danger is ventricular fibrillation. K⁺ >7.0mmol/L requires urgent treatment, as
does K⁺ >6mmol/L or potentially lower values if there are ECG changes:
• Tall 'tented' T waves ± flat P waves ± increased PR interval (p. 688, ECG p. 689).
• Widening of the QRS complex—leading eventually, and dangerously, to a sinusoidal pattern and VF/VT.

Emergencies

**Diagnosis** Mainly from the history. The patient may not tell the truth about what has been taken. If there are any tablets with the patient, use *MIMS Colour Index*, *eMIMS* images, *BNF* descriptions, or the computerized system 'TICTAC' (ask pharmacy) to identify tablets and plan specific treatment.

**TOXBASE** is the best resource for managing acute poisoning: **www.toxbase.org**— check with your Emergency Department about log-in details for your hospital.[71]

Clues may become apparent from examination:
• *Fast or irregular pulse:* Salbutamol, antimuscarinics, tricyclics, quinine, or phenothiazine poisoning.
• *Respiratory depression:* Opiate (p854) or benzodiazepine (p855) toxicity.
• *Hypothermia:* Phenothiazines (p855), barbiturates.
• *Hyperthermia:* Amphetamines, MAOIs, cocaine, or ecstasy (p855).
• *Coma:* Benzodiazepines, alcohol, opiates, tricyclics, or barbiturates.
• *Seizures:* Recreational drugs, hypoglycaemic agents, tricyclics, phenothiazines, or theophyllines.
• *Constricted pupils:* Opiates (p854) or insecticides (organophosphates, p855).
• *Dilated pupils:* Amphetamines, cocaine, quinine, or tricyclics.
• *Hyperglycaemia:* Organophosphates, theophyllines, or MAOIs.
• *Hypoglycaemia:* (p844) Insulin, oral hypoglycaemics, alcohol, or salicylates.
• *Renal impairment:* Salicylate (p 856), paracetamol (p856), or ethylene glycol.
• *Metabolic acidosis:* Alcohol, ethylene glycol, methanol, paracetamol, or carbon monoxide poisoning—p854.
• ↑*Osmolality:* Alcohols (ethyl or methyl); ethylene glycol. See p682.

**Management** See fig 1 for a general guide to management.
• *Take blood* as appropriate (p852). Always check paracetamol and salicylate levels.
• *Empty stomach* if appropriate (p852).
• *Consider specific antidote* (p854) or oral activated charcoal (p852).
• *If you are not familiar with the poison* get more information. *Toxbase* (www. toxbase.org) should be your first thought. If no information here or in doubt how best to act, phone the Poisons Information Service: in the UK phone 0844 892 0111.

**Continuing care** Measure temperature, pulse, BP, and blood glucose regularly. Keep on cardiac monitor. If unconscious, nurse semi-prone, turn regularly. Catherize if the bladder is distended, or acute kidney injury (p848) is suspected, or forced diuresis undertaken. Consider ICU, eg if respiration↓.

**Psychiatric assessment** Be sympathetic despite the hour! Interview relatives and friends if possible. Aim to establish:
• *Intentions at time:* Was this a suicide attempt, if so was the act planned? What precautions against being found? Did the patient seek help afterwards? Does the patient think the method was dangerous? Was there a final act (eg suicide note)?
• *Present intentions.* Do they still feel suicidal? Do they wish it had worked?
• *What problems* led to the act: do they still exist?
• Is there a *psychiatric disorder* (depression, alcoholism, personality disorder, schizophrenia, dementia)?
• What are the patient's *resources* (friends, family, work, personality)?

*The assessment of suicide risk:* The following increase the chance of future suicide: original intention was to die; present intention is to die; presence of psychiatric disorder; poor resources; previous suicide attempts; socially isolated; unemployed; male; >50yrs old. See *OHCS* p338. There is an increased risk of death in the first year following initial presentation.

*Referral to psychiatrist:* This depends partly on local resources. Refer all with presence of psychiatric disorder or high suicide risk. Consider discussing all presentations with deliberate self-poisoning.

*Mental Capacity Act or the Mental Health Act:* (in England and Wales) may provide for the detention of the patient against his or her will: see *OHCS* p400.

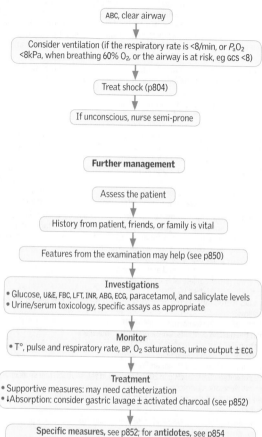

**Fig 1.** Emergency care in acute poisoning.

Emergencies

**Plasma toxicology** For all unconscious patients, paracetamol and aspirin levels and blood glucose are required. The necessity of other assays depends on the drug taken and the index of suspicion. Be guided by the Poisons Information Service. More common assays include: digoxin; methanol; lithium; iron; theophylline. Toxicological screening of urine, especially for recreational drugs, may be of use in some cases (although not always, see BOX p853).

**GI decontamination:** recommended for many drugs. The treatment of choice is now activated charcoal rather than gastric lavage. If in doubt, consult Toxbase or Poisons Information Service.

**Activated charcoal** reduces the absorption of many drugs from the gut when given as a single dose of 50g with water, eg salicylates, paracetamol. It is given in repeated doses (50g/4h) to increase elimination of some drugs from the blood, eg carbamazepine, dapsone, theophyllines, quinine, phenobarbital, and paraquat. Lower doses are used in children. Do not use with petroleum products, corrosives, alcohols, clofenotane, malathion or metal salts (eg iron, lithium).

**Gastric lavage** Rarely used. Lavage after 30–60min may make matters worse. ▶*Do not empty stomach* if petroleum products or corrosives such as acids, alkalis, bleach, descalers have been ingested (*exception:* paraquat), or if the patient is unconscious or unable to protect their airway (unless intubated). ▶Never induce vomiting.

**Gastric emptying and lavage** NB: we do not recommend gastric lavage is attempted unless specifically suggested by toxbase or poisons information service. If comatose, or no gag reflex, ask for an anaesthetist to protect airway with cuffed endotracheal tube. If conscious, get verbal consent.
• Monitor $O_2$ by pulse oximetry. See p156.
• Have suction apparatus to hand and working.
• Position the patient in left lateral position.
• Raise the foot of the bed by 20cm.
• Pass a lubricated tube (14mm external diameter) via the mouth, asking the patient to swallow.
• Confirm position in stomach (see page 773).
• Siphon the gastric contents. Check pH with litmus paper.
• Perform gastric lavage using 300–600mL tepid water at a time. Massage the left hypochondrium then siphon fluid.
• Repeat until no tablets in siphoned fluid.
• Leave activated charcoal (50g in 200mL water) in the stomach unless alcohol, iron, $Li^+$, or ethylene glycol ingested.
• When pulling out tube, occlude its end (prevents aspiration of fluid remaining in the tube).

**Haemodialysis** This may be needed for poisoning from ethylene glycol, lithium, methanol, phenobarbital, salicylates, and sodium valpoate.

⚠ Help on the web: healthcare providers in the UK can register for free toxological advice at **www.toxbase.org** or call 0844 892 0111 for Poisons Information Service.

## Legal highs

Increasingly 'designer' drugs, which can be legal to buy, are leading to acute poisoning and complications requiring admission. These drugs pose a difficult problem for the admitting physician, as the chemical make-up and mechanisms of action are often unclear. Although many are legal, they can be as deadly as many well-known recreational drugs, leading to deaths[60,61] and life-threatening complications such as rhabdomyolysis.[62] Be aware that these drugs are out there, and ask specifically about legal highs when taking a history, as there are often no screening tools for these drugs.

**Benzodiazepines** Flumazenil (for respiratory arrest) 200µg over 15s; then 100µg at 60s intervals if needed. Usual dose range: 300–600µg IV over 3–6min (up to 1mg; 2mg if on ICU). May provoke fits. Use only after expert advice.

**β-blockers** Severe bradycardia or hypotension. Try atropine up to 3mg IV. Give glucagon 2–10mg IV bolus + 5% glucose if atropine fails then infusion of 50µg/kg/h. Also consider including phosphodiesterase inhibitor infusions (eg enoximone 5–20µg/kg/min). If unresponsive, consider pacing.

**Cyanide** This fast-killing poison has affinity for $Fe^{3+}$, and inhibits the cytochrome system, ↓aerobic respiration (therefore patients are acidotic with raised lactate). Depending on degree of poisoning presentation can be:
• *Mild* Dizziness, anxiety, tachycardia, nausea, drowsiness/confusion
• *Moderate* Vomiting, reduced consciousness, convulsions, cyanosis
• *Severe* Deep coma, fixed unreactive pupils, cardiorespiratory failure, arrhythmias, pulmonary oedema
*Treatment:* ▸▸100% $O_2$, GI decontamination. If mild, supportive care is usually sufficient. If moderate/severe then specific treatment to bind cyanide is required. Give sodium nitrite/sodium thiosulfate, or dicobalt edetate 300mg IV over 1min, then 50mL 50% glucose IV (repeat once if no response after a minute); or hydroxocobalamin (Cyanokit®) 5g over 15min repeated once if required. *Get expert help.* See p859.

**Carbon monoxide** Despite hypoxaemia skin is pink (or pale), not blue, as carboxyhaemoglobin (COHb) displaces $O_2$ from Hb binding sites. For the same reasons $SpO_2$ from a pulse oximeter may be normal. Check ABG in a co-oximeter (ie ensure it measures haemoglobin, $SaO_2$, Meth-Hb and COHb) which will show low $SaO_2$ and high CoHb (normal <5%). *Symptoms:* Headache, vomiting, pulse↑, tachypnoea, and, if COHb >50%, fits, coma, and cardiac arrest.
*Treatment* ▸▸Remove the source. Give 100% $O_2$ until COHb <10%. Metabolic acidosis usually responds to correction of hypoxia. If severe, anticipate cerebral oedema and give mannitol IVI (p841). Confirm diagnosis with an ABG quickly as levels may soon return to normal. Monitor ECG. If COHb >20%, patient has neurological or psychological features, or cardiovascular impairment, fails to respond to treatment, or is pregnant consider hyperbaric $O_2$: discuss with the poisons service.

**Digoxin** *Symptoms:* Cognition↓, yellow-green visual halos, arrhythmias, nausea, and anorexia. If serious arrhythmias are present, correct hypokalaemia, and inactivate with digoxin-specific antibody fragments (DigiFab®). If load or level is unknown, give 20 vials (800mg)—adult or child >20kg. Consult Compendium/SPC (p850). If the amount of digoxin ingested is known, the SPC will tell you how much DigiFab® to give.

**Heavy metals** Enlist expert help.

**Iron** Desferrioxamine 15mg/kg/h IVI; max 80mg/kg/d. NB: gastric lavage if iron ingestion in last hour; consider whole bowel irrigation.

**Oral anticoagulants** If major bleed, treat with vitamin K, 5mg slow IV; give prothrombin complex concentrate 50U/kg IV (or if unavailable, fresh frozen plasma 15mL/kg IVI). For abnormal INR with no (or minimal) bleeding, see BNF. If it is vital that anticoagulation continues, enlist expert help. Discuss with haematology. NB: coagulation defects may be delayed for 2–3d following ingestion.

**Opiates** (Many analgesics contain opiates.) Give naloxone, eg 0.4–2mg IV; repeat every 2min until breathing is adequate (it has a short *t*½, so it may need to be given often or IM; max ~10mg). Naloxone may precipitate features of opiate withdrawal—diarrhoea and cramps, which will normally respond to diphenoxylate and atropine (Lomotil®—eg 2 tablets/6h PO). Sedate as needed (see p11). High-dose opiate misusers may need methadone (eg 10–30mg/12h PO) to combat withdrawal. Register opiate addiction (*OHCS* p362), and refer for help.

**Phenothiazine poisoning** (eg chlorpromazine) No specific antidote. *Dystonia (torticollis, retrocollis, glossopharyngeal dystonia, opisthotonus):* try procyclidine, eg 5-10mg IM or IV. Treat shock by raising the legs (± plasma expander IVI, or inotropes if desperate). Restore body temperature. *Monitor ECG.* Avoid lidocaine in dysrhythmias. Use lorazepam IV for prolonged fits in the usual way (p836). *Neuroleptic malignant syndrome* consists of: hyperthermia, rigidity, extrapyramidal signs, autonomic dysfunction (labile BP, pulse↑, sweating, urinary incontinence), mutism, confusion, coma, WCC↑, CK↑; it may be treated with cooling. Dantrolene 1-2.5mg/kg IV (p574) (max 10mg/kg/day) can help, bromocriptine and amantadine are alternatives.

**Carbon tetrachloride poisoning** This solvent, used in many industrial processes, causes vomiting, abdominal pain, diarrhoea, seizures, coma, renal failure, and tender hepatomegaly with jaundice and liver failure. IV N-acetylcysteine may improve prognosis. Seek expert help.

**Organophosphate insecticides** inactivate cholinesterase—the resulting increase in acetylcholine causes the SLUD response: salivation, lacrimation, urination, and diarrhoea. Also look for sweating, small pupils, muscle fasciculation, coma, respiratory distress, and bradycardia. *Treatment:* Wear gloves; remove soiled clothes. Wash skin. Take blood (FBC and serum cholinesterase activity). Give atropine IV 2mg every 10min till full atropinization (skin dry, pulse >70, pupils dilated). Up to 3 days' treatment may be needed. Also give pralidoxime 30mg/kg IVI over 20min, then 8mg/kg/h, max 12g in 24h. See Toxbase.[1] Even if fits are not occurring, diazepam 5-10mg IV slowly seems to help.

**Paraquat poisoning** (Found in weed-killers.) This causes D&V, painful oral ulcers, alveolitis, and renal failure. Diagnose by urine test. Give activated charcoal at once (100g followed by a laxative, then 50g/3-4h). ▶Get expert help. Avoid O₂ early on (promotes lung damage).

**Ecstasy poisoning** Ecstasy is a semi-synthetic, hallucinogenic substance (MDMA, 3,4-methylenedioxymethamphetamine). Its effects range from nausea, muscle pain, blurred vision, amnesia, fever, confusion, and ataxia to tachyarrhythmias, hyperthermia, hyper/hypotension, water intoxication, DIC, K⁺↑, acute kidney injury (AKI), hepatocellular and muscle necrosis, cardiovascular collapse, and ARDS. There is no antidote and treatment is supportive. Management depends on clinical and lab findings, but may include:
• Administration of activated charcoal and monitoring of BP, ECG, and temperature for at least 12h (rapid cooling may be needed).
• Monitor urine output and U&E (AKI 292, p848-849), LFT, CK, FBC, and coagulation (DIC p346). Metabolic acidosis may benefit from treatment with bicarbonate.
• Anxiety: diazepam 0.1-0.3mg/kg PO. IV dose: p836.
• Narrow complex tachycardias (p818) in adults: consider metoprolol 5mg IV.
• Hypertension can be treated with nifedipine 5-10mg PO or phentolamine 2-5mg IV. Treat hypotension conventionally (p804).
• Hyperthermia: attempt to cool, if rectal T° >39°C consider dantrolene 1mg/kg IV (may need repeating: discuss with your senior and a poisons unit, below). Hyperthermia with ecstasy is akin to serotonin syndrome, and propranolol, muscle relaxation and ventilation may be needed.

**Snakes (adders)** *Anaphylaxis* p806. *Signs of envenoming:* BP↓ (vasodilatation, viper cardiotoxicity); D&V; swelling spreading proximally within 4h of bite; bleeding gums or venepuncture sites; anaphylaxis; ptosis; trismus; rhabdomyolysis; pulmonary oedema. *Tests:* WCC↑; clotting↓; platelets↓; U&E; urine RBC↑; CK↑; P_aO₂↓, ECG. *Management:* Avoid active movement of affected limb (so use splints/slings). *Avoid incisions and tourniquets.* ▶Get help from local/national poisons service. Is antivenom indicated (IgG from venom-immunized sheep)?—eg 10mL IV over 15min (adults *and* children) of European Viper Antiserum (from Monviato) for adder bites (see BNF); —20mL if severe envenoming have adrenaline to hand—p806. Monitor ECG. For foreign snakes, see BNF.

---

Help on the web: healthcare providers in the UK can register for free toxological advice at **www.toxbase.org** or call 0844 892 0111 for Poisons Information Service.

Aspirin is a weak acid with poor water solubility. It is present in many over-the-counter preparations. Uncoupling of oxidative phosphorylation leads to anaerobic metabolism and the production of lactate and heat. Effects are dose-related and potentially fatal: •150mg/kg: mild toxicity •250mg/kg: moderate •>500mg/kg: severe toxicity. Levels over 700mg/L are potentially fatal.

**Signs and symptoms** Unlike paracetamol, there are many early features:
• Vomiting, dehydration, hyperventilation, tinnitus, vertigo, sweating.
• Rarely ↓GCS, seizures, ↓BP and heart block, pulmonary oedema, hyperthermia.
Patients present initially with respiratory alkalosis due to a direct stimulation of the central respiratory centres and then develop a metabolic acidosis. Hyper- or hypoglycaemia may occur.

**Management** _General:_ p850-p851. Correct dehydration. Keep patient on ECG monitor. Give activated charcoal to all presenting ≤1h—consider even if delayed presentation, slow release formations or bezoar formation (can delay absorption): at least one dose of 1g/kg (max 50g). Consider repeat doses (2 further doses of 50g, 4h apart).

1 _Bloods:_ Paracetamol and salicylate level, glucose, U&E, LFT, INR, ABG, HCO₃⁻, FBC. Salicylate level may need to be repeated after 2h, due to continuing absorption if a potentially toxic dose has been taken. Monitor blood glucose 1-2hrly, beware hypoglycaemia, if severe poisoning, monitor salicylate levels, serum pH and U&E.

2 _Urine:_ Check pH, consider catheterization to monitor output and pH.

3 _Correct acidosis:_ If plasma salicylate level >500mg/L (3.6mmol/L) or severe metabolic acidosis, consider alkalinization of the urine, eg with 1.5L 1.26% sodium bicarbonate IV over 3h. Aim for urine pH 7.5-8. NB: monitor serum K⁺ as hypokalaemia may occur, and should be treated (caution if acute kidney injury—AKI).

4 _Dialysis_ may well be needed if salicylate level >700mg/L, and if AKI or heart failure, pulmonary or cerebral oedema, confusion or seizures, severe acidosis despite best medical therapy, or persistently ↑plasma salicylate. Contact nephrology early.

5 Discuss any serious cases with the local toxicological service or national poisons information service.

## Paracetamol poisoning

150mg/kg,[1] or 12g in adults may be fatal (75mg/kg if malnourished). However, prompt treatment can prevent liver failure and death. ►1 tablet of paracetamol = 500mg.

**Signs and symptoms** None initially, or vomiting ± RUQ pain. Later: jaundice and encephalopathy from liver damage (the main danger) ± acute kidney injury.

**Management** _General measures_ p850, GI decontamination is recommended in those presenting <4h after OD. Activated charcoal 1g/kg (max 50g) is the treatment of choice, reducing serum levels more than gastric lavage[63] and limiting liver injury.[64]
• Glucose, U&E, LFT, INR, ABG, FBC, HCO₃⁻; blood paracetamol level at 4h post-ingestion.
• If <10-12h since overdose, not vomiting, and plasma paracetamol is above the line on the graph (see fig 1), start N-acetylcysteine.
• If >8-24h and suspicion of large overdose (>7.5g) err on the side of caution and start N-acetylcysteine, stopping it if level below treatment line and INR/ALT normal. _N-acetylcysteine_ is given by IVI: +ve 150mg/kg in 5% dextrose over 15min 1 hour.[2] Then 50mg/kg in 500mL of 5% dextrose over 4h. Then 100mg/kg/16h in 1L of 5% dextrose. Rash is a common SE: treat with chlorphenamine + observe; do not stop unless anaphylatoid reaction with shock, vomiting, and wheeze (occur <10%). An alternative (if acetylcysteine unavailable) is methionine 2.5g/4h PO for 16h (total: 10g), but absorption is unreliable if vomiting.
• If ingestion time is unknown, or it is staggered, or presentation is >15h from ingestion, treatment _may_ help. ►Get advice.
• The graph may mislead if HIV +ve (hepatic glutathione↓), or if long-acting paracetamol has been taken, or if pre-existing liver disease or induction of liver enzymes has occurred. ►Beware ↓glucose—do BM hourly; INR/12h.

## Ongoing management:
- Next day do INR, U&E, LFT. If INR rising, continue N-acetylcysteine until <1.4.
- If continued deterioration, discuss with the liver team. Don't hesitate to get help

### Criteria for referral to specialist liver unit

In 1989 King's College Hospital in London proposed criteria for liver transplantation for fulminant liver failure. These have since been modified,[65] and these modified criteria probably still have the best predictive value of fulminant hepatic failure in paracetamol overdose. Discuss early with liver unit if:
- Lactate >3.5mg/dL (0.39mmol/L) 4h after early fluid resuscitation
- pH <7.3 or lactate >3mg/dL (0.33mmol/L) after full fluid resuscitation at 12h
- INR >2.0 at 24h, >4 at 48h, >6 at 72h (peak elevation 72-96h)
- Creatinine >300µmol/L (3.4mg/dL) at any point
- Grade 3 or 4 hepatic encephalopathy
- Phosphate >1.2mmol/L (3.75mg/dL) at 48h

Refer all with signs of CNS oedema: BP >160/90 (or brief SBP rises >200mmHg), bradycardia, decerebrate posture, extensor spasms, poor pupil responses.

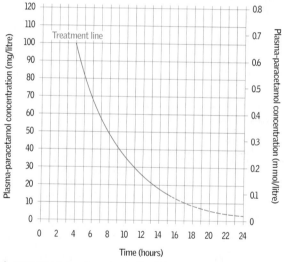

Fig 1. Plasma concentration of paracetamol vs time. If the patient's plasma paracetamol concentration is above the treatment line, overdose occurred <10-12 hours ago and there is no vomiting, give N-acetylcysteine by IV infusion. If there is doubt about the timing of the overdose, or ingestion has been 'staggered' over more that 1 hour, give acetylcysteine without waiting for levels. Treatment can be stopped if levels are low.

Reproduced from Drug Safety Update September 2012, vol 6, issue 2: A1 © Crown Copyright 2013.

1 If the patient weighs >110kg, use a body weight of 110kg to avoid underestimating toxicity.
2 The volume of glucose to give is 3mL/kg (of 5% solution).

Emergencies

Resuscitate and arrange transfer for all major burns (>25% partial thickness in adults and >20% in children). Assess site, size, and depth of burn (fig 1, to help calculate fluid requirements). Referral is still warranted in cases of full thickness burns >5%, partial thickness burns >10% in adults or >5% in children or the elderly, burns of special sites, chemical and electrical burns and burns with inhalational injury.

**Assessment** *Burn size* is important to assess (see fig 1, BOX 2) as it influences the size of the inflammatory response (vasodilatation, increased vascular permeability) and thus fluid shift from the intravascular volume. Ignore erythema. *Burn depth* determines healing time/scarring; assessing this can be hard, even for the experienced. The big distinction is whether the burn is partial thickness (painful, red, and blistered) or full thickness (insensate/painless; grey-white). NB: burns can evolve, particularly over the first 48h.

**Resuscitation**
- *Airway:* Beware of upper airway obstruction developing if hot gases inhaled. Suspect if history of fire in enclosed space, soot in oral/nasal cavity, singed nasal hairs or hoarse voice. A flexible laryngo/bronchoscopy is useful. Involve anaesthetists early and consider early intubation. Obstruction can develop in the first 24h.
- *Breathing:* Exclude life-threatening chest injuries (eg tension pneumothorax) and constricting burns—consider escharotomy if chest burns are impairing thorax excursion (*OHCS* p733). Give 100% $O_2$. Suspect carbon monoxide poisoning (p.854) from history, cherry-red skin and carboxyhaemoglobin level (COHb). With 100% $O_2$ $t\frac{1}{2}$ of COHb falls from 250min to 40min (consider hyperbaric $O_2$ if: pregnant; CNS signs; >20% COHb). $SpO_2$ (oximetry) is unreliable in CO poisoning.
- *Circulation:* Partial thickness burns >10% in a child and >15% in adults require IV fluid resuscitation. Put up 2 large-bore (14G or 16G) IV lines. Do not worry if you have to put these through burned skin, intraosseous access is valuable in infants and can be used in adults (see p236). Secure them well: they are literally lifelines.

Use a *burns calculator* flow chart or a formula, eg: *Parkland formula* (popular): 4 × weight (kg) × % burn = mL Hartmann's solution in 24h, half given in 1$^{st}$ 8h. Replace fluid from the time of burn, not from the time first seen in hospital. *Formulae are only guides:* adjust IVI according to clinical response and urine output; aim for 0.5mL/kg/h (1mL/kg/h in children), ~50% more in electrical burns and inhalation injury. Monitor T° (core and surface); catheterize the bladder. Beware of over-resuscitation ('fluid creep') which can lead to complications such as abdominal compartment syndrome.

**Treatment** 'Cool the burn, warm the patient'. Do *not* apply cold water to extensive burns for long periods: this may intensify shock. Take care with circumferential full thickness burns of the limbs as compartment syndrome may develop rapidly particularly after fluid resuscitation. Decompress (escharotomy and fasciotomy) as needed. If transferring to a burns unit, do not burst blisters or apply any special creams as this can hinder assessment. Simple saline gauze or paraffin gauze is suitable; cling film is useful as a temporary measure and relieves pain. Titrate morphine IV for good analgesia. Ensure tetanus immunity. Antibiotic prophylaxis is not routinely used.

**Definitive dressings** There are many dressings for partial thickness burns, eg biological (pigskin, cadaveric skin), synthetic (Mepitel®, Duoderm®) and silver sulfadiazine cream alone (Flamazine®) or with cerium nitrate as Flammacerium®; it forms a leathery eschar which resists infection.[66] Major full thickness burns benefit from early tangential excision and split-skin grafts as the burn is a major source of inflammatory cytokines causing SIRS (systemic inflammatory response syndrome—see p804 for management) and forms a rich medium for bacterial growth.

## Smoke inhalation

Consider if:
- History of exposure to fire and smoke in an enclosed space
- Hoarseness or change in voice
- Harsh cough
- Stridor
- Burns to face
- Singed nasal hairs
- Soot in saliva or sputum
- Inflamed oropharynx

Initially laryngospasm leads to hypoxia and straining (leading to petechiae), then hypoxic cord relaxation leads to true inhalation injury. Free radicals, cyanide compounds, and carbon monoxide (CO) accompany thermal injury. Cyanide (p.854) compounds (generated, eg, from burning plastics) stop oxidative phosphorylation, causing dizziness, headaches, and seizures. Tachycardia + dyspnoea soon give way to bradycardia + apnoea. CO is generated later in the fire as oxygen is depleted. NB: COHb levels do not correlate well with the severity of poisoning and partly reflect smoking status and urban life. Use nomograms to extrapolate peak levels.

▶▶100% O₂ is given to elute both cyanide and CO.

▶▶Involve ICU/anaesthetists early if any signs of airway obstruction or respiratory failure: early intubation and ventilation may be useful.

▶▶Enlist expert help in cyanide poisoning—see p854.

**Emergencies**

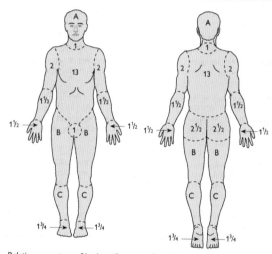

Relative percentage of body surface area affected by growth

| Area | Age | 0 | 1 | 5 | 10 | 15 | Adult |
|---|---|---|---|---|---|---|---|
| A: half of head | | 9½ | 8½ | 6½ | 5½ | 4½ | 3½ |
| B: half of thigh | | 2¾ | 3¼ | 4 | 4¼ | 4½ | 4¾ |
| C: half of leg | | 2½ | 2½ | 2¾ | 3 | 3¼ | 3½ |

Fig 1. Lund and Browder charts.[1]

**1** Accurate but time-consuming compared with the 'rule of nines': arm: 9%; front of trunk 18%; head and neck 9%; leg 18%; back of trunk 18%; perineum 1%. The rule of nines generally over-estimates burn area (better than under-estimating).[67] A **modified rule of nines for children:** from birth up to 1yr, surface area of head and neck is 18% and each leg is 14%. For each year after, the head loses 1% and each leg gains 0.5%—so adult proportions are reached by age 10yrs.

*We thank Professor Tor Chiu for help in preparing this topic.*

Emergencies

▶*Have a high index of suspicion and a low-reading thermometer.* Most patients are elderly and do not complain, or feel, cold—so they have not tried to warm up. In the young, hypothermia is usually from cold exposure (eg near-drowning), or is secondary to impaired consciousness (eg following excess alcohol or drug overdose).

**Definition** Hypothermia implies a core (rectal) temperature <35°C.

**Causes** In the elderly, hypothermia is often caused by a combination of factors:
• Impaired homeostatic mechanisms: usually age-related
• Low room temperature: poverty, poor housing
• Impaired thermoregulation: pneumonia, MI, heart failure
• Reduced metabolism: immobility, hypothyroidism, diabetes mellitus
• Autonomic neuropathy (p509); eg diabetes mellitus, Parkinson's
• Excess heat loss: psoriasis and any other widespread dermatological diseases (i.e. TEN/erythrodermic eczema)
• Cold awareness↓: dementia, confusion
• Increased exposure to cold: falls, especially at night when cold
• Drugs: major tranquillizers, antidepressants, diuretics, alcohol

**The patient**
• If the patient is shivering then the hypothermia is mild, if they are not shivering despite temp <35°C then the hypothermia is severe
• Symptoms and signs include confusion, agitation, reduced GCS, coma, bradycardia, hypotension and arrhythmias (AF, VT, VF), esp if temp <30°C

There are many stories of people 'returning to life' when warmed despite absence of vital signs, see BOX. It is essential to rewarm (see below) and re-examine.

**Diagnosis** Check oral or axillary T°. If ordinary thermometer shows <36.5°C, use a low-reading one PR. Is the rectal temperature <35°C? Infra-red ear thermometers can accurately reflect core temperature.

**Tests** Urgent U&E, plasma glucose, and amylase. Thyroid function tests; FBC; blood cultures. Consider blood gases. The ECG may show J-waves (fig 1).

**Treatment** Use ABCDE approach (p793)—but don't expose to cold.
• All patients should receive warm, humidified O₂, ventilate if comatose or respiratory insufficiency.
• Remove wet clothing, *slowly rewarm*, aiming for rise of ½°C/h (check rectal temperature, BP, pulse, and respiratory rate every 30min) using blankets or active external warming (hot air duvets). If temp rising too quickly stop and allow to cool slightly. Rapid rewarming causes peripheral vasodilatation and shock. A falling BP can be a sign of too rapid warming.
• Warm IVI.
• Cardiac monitor is essential (AF, VF and VT can occur at any time during rewarming or on stimulation).
• Consider antibiotics for the prevention of pneumonia (p160). Give these routinely in patients over 65yrs with a temperature <32°C.
• Consider urinary catheter (to monitor renal function).

NB: in sudden hypothermia from immersion or profound hypothermia with cardiovascular instability/cardiac arrest, the temperature needs to be raised rapidly. Options include warmed fluid lavage (intravesical, nasogastric, intrapleural, intraperitoneal) and intravascular warming (cardiopulmonary bypass, dialysis). In the event of cardiac arrest, defibrillation is usually unsuccessful if the temperature is <30°C (consider amiodarone, bretylium). Resuscitation must continue until the core temp is above 33°C (*OHCS* p786.)

**Complications** Arrhythmias (if there is a cardiac arrest continue resuscitating until T° >33°C, as cold brains are less damaged by hypoxia); pneumonia; pancreatitis; acute kidney injury; disseminated intravascular coagulation. *Prognosis:* Depends on age and degree of hypothermia. If age >70yrs and T° <32°C then mortality >50%.

**Before hospital discharge** Anticipate problems. Will it happen again? What is their network of support? Review medication (could you stop tranquillizers?)? How is progress to be monitored? Liaise with GP/social worker.

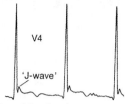

**Fig 1.** J-wave in hypothermia.
Courtesy of Dr R Luke and Dr E McLachlan.

### ☼ "I did not die but nothing of life remained..."

Remember that death is a process not an event, and that in hypothermia, *all* processes are suspended, as this chilling quotation from Dante shows. In the last round of the 9th circle of *Hell*, Dante tells how those betraying their benefactors are encased in ice (*canto xxxiv*) 'Com'io divenni allor ge-lato e fioco...Io non morì e non rimasi vivo—How frozen I then became: I did not die but nothing of life remained'.

**Human records:** Mitsuaka Uchikoshi appears to have 'hibernated'◢ for 24 days on Mount Rokko (core T°≈22°C). Erica Nordy came to life in 2 hours after her heart stopped (core T°: 16°).

**Planning** All hospitals have a detailed *Major Incident Plan*, but additionally the tasks of key personnel can be distributed on individual *Action Cards*.

**At the scene** Call the police to notify them of the Major Incident and ask them to take command. They will set up a central command centre to assess and manage the incident, depending on casualty numbers they will inform multiple hospitals of the need to prepare for the imminent arrival of casualties.

*Safety* is paramount—your own and others. Be visible (luminous monogrammed jacket) and wear protective clothing where appropriate (safety helmet; waterproofs; boots; respirator in chemical environment).

*Triage:* See *OHCS* p797. There are several commercial systems available to label patients so emergency personnel can see at a glance the scale of the incident. The key is to divide patients by the urgency of care/transfer to hospital:

1 Emergency (label RED = will die in a few minutes if no treatment)
2 Urgent (label YELLOW = will die in ~2h if no treatment)
3 Non-urgent (label GREEN = walking wounded/those who are stable and can wait)
4 Deceased (label BLUE/WHITE).

*Communications* are essential; each emergency service will dispatch a control vehicle and will have a designated incident officer for liaison. Support medical staff from hospital report to the medical incident officer (MIO)—he or she is usually the first doctor on the scene. Their job is to assess then communicate to the receiving hospital the number + severity of casualties, to organize resupply of equipment and to replace fatigued staff. The MIO must resist temptation to treat casualties as this compromises their role.

*Equipment:* Must be portable and include: intubation and cricothyrotomy set; intravenous fluids (colloid); bandages and dressings; chest drain (+flutter valve); amputation kit (when used, ideally 2 doctors should concur); drugs—*analgesic:* morphine; *anaesthetic:* ketamine 2mg/kg IV over >60s (0.5mg/kg is a powerful analgesic without respiratory depression); limb splints (may be inflatable); defibrillator/monitor ± pulse oximeter.

*Evacuation:* Remember that with immediate treatment on scene, the priority for evacuation may be reduced (eg a tension pneumothorax—RED—once relieved can wait for evacuation and becomes YELLOW), but those who may suffer by delay at the scene must go first. Send any severed limbs to the same hospital as the patient, ideally chilled—but not frozen.

**At the hospital** a 'major incident' is declared. The *first receiving* hospital will take most of the casualties; the *support* hospital(s) will cope with overflow and may provide mobile teams so that staff are not depleted from the first hospital. A control room is established and the medical coordinator ensures staff have been summoned and informed of their roles, nominates a triage officer, and supervises the best use of inpatient beds and ICU/theatre resources.

These may be caused by domestic (eg gas explosion) or industrial (eg mining) accidents, or by terrorist bombs. Death may occur without any obvious external injury. Injury occurs in a number of ways:

1 *Blast wave:* A transient (milliseconds) wave of overpressure expands rapidly producing cellular disruption, shearing forces along tissue planes (submucosal/subserosal haemorrhage) and re-expansion of compressed trapped gas—bowel perforation, fatal air embolism.

2 *Blast wind:* This can totally disrupt a body or cause avulsive amputations. Bodies can be thrown and sustain injuries on landing.

3 *Missiles:* Penetration or laceration from missiles are by far the commonest injuries. Missiles arise from the bomb or are secondary, eg glass.

4 *Flash burns:* These are usually superficial and occur on exposed skin.

5 *Crush injuries:* Beware sudden death or acute kidney injury from rhabdomyolysis after release.

6 *Contamination:* There is increasing concern about the use of biological or radioactive material in terrorist bombs. Even domestic or industrial blasts can scatter chemicals widely and cause both superficial and penetrating contamination. Consider the location and mechanism of the blast, and seek advice.

7 *Psychological injury:* Eg post-traumatic stress disorder (*OHCS* p347).

**Treatment** Approach the same as any major trauma (*OHCS* p724). Rest and observe any suspected of exposure to significant blast but without other injury. Gun-shot injury: see *OHCS* p722. Major blast injuries, whatever the cause, should be reported to the police for investigation, particularly if multiple casualties are involved.

Emergencies

*Abbreviations:* F indexes a notable figure or image; dis = disease; syn = syndrome.

We thank Shahzad Arain, Timothy Crocker-Buqué, William Hunt, Amelia Lloyd, Konstantinos Kritikos, Eleanor Zimmermann and Ayoma Ratnappuli for their help with the index.

All indexes can be improved: let us know how at ohcm.index@oup.com

▶These pages outline typical adult doses, and the commoner side-effects, of medications that a new house officer will be called upon to prescribe. If in any doubt, consult a drug fomulary (eg British National Formulary, *BNF*, www.bnf.org) esp if eGFR↓.

| Drug | Dose and frequency | Notes |
|---|---|---|
| *Analgesics* | (see p454 for more details on analgesia) | |
| Aspirin | 300-900mg/4-6h PO, max 4g/24h | SE of NSAIDs: gastritis; bronchospasm; hypersensitivity. CI: GI ulcer/bleeding; NSAID-induced asthma; coagulopathy. Avoid aspirin in child (risks Reye's syndrome). |
| Diclofenac | 50mg/8h PO/PR | |
| Ibuprofen | 400mg/6h PO, max 2.4g/24h | |
| Paracetamol | 0.5-1g/4-6h PO, max. 4g/24h | Avoid if hepatic impairment. Patients with chronic pain (eg malignancy) may require higher doses. SE of opioids: nausea and vomiting; constipation; drowsiness; hypotension; respiratory depression, dependence. CI: Acute respiratory depression, acute alcoholism. Use carefully in head injury, as may hinder neurological assessment. |
| Codeine phosphate | 30-60mg/4h PO/IM, max 240mg/24h | |
| Dihydrocodeine tartrate | 30mg/4-6h PO, OR 50mg/4-6h IM/SC | |
| Meptazinol | 200mg/3-6h PO, OR 50-100mg/2-4h IM/IV | |
| Oxycodone | 5mg/6h PO | |
| Pethidine | 50-100mg/4h PO/IM/SC | |
| Tramadol | 50-100mg/4h PO/IM/IV | |
| Morphine | 5-10mg/4h PO/IM/SC | |
| *Antibiotics* | (see p366-374) | |
| *Anti-emetics* | | |
| Cyclizine | 50mg/8h PO/IM/IV | Use 25mg/8h in elderly |
| Metoclopramide | 10mg/8h PO/IM/IV | May cause extrapyramidal SE, especially in young adults. |
| Ondansetron | 8mg/8h PO, or 4mg IM/IV | |
| *Antihistamines* | | |
| Chlorphenamine | 10-20mg IM/IV, max 40mg/24h OR 4mg/6h PO | SE of antihistamines: Drowsiness; urinary retention; dry mouth; blurred vision; GI disturbance; arrhythmias. Drowsiness is less common with newer drugs, eg cetirizine, fexofenadine. |
| Cetirizine | 5-10mg/24h PO | |
| Levocetirizine | 5mg/24h PO | |
| Fexofenadine | 120-180mg/24h PO | |
| Loratadine | 10mg/24h PO | |
| Desloratadine | 5mg/24h PO | |
| *Gastric acid-reducing drugs* | | |
| Cimetidine | 400mg/12h PO | SE of H$_2$-blockers: GI disturbance; ↑LFT. |
| Ranitidine | 150mg/12h PO | |
| Omeprazole | 20-40mg/24h PO | SE of PPIs: GI disturbance; hypersensitivity. ▶Acid-reducing drugs may mask symptoms of gastric cancer; use with care in middle-aged patients. |
| Esomeprazole | 20-40mg/24h PO | |
| Lansoprazole | 15-30mg/24h PO | |
| Pantoprazole | 20-40mg/24h PO/IV | |

| Drug | Dose and frequency | Notes |
|---|---|---|
| *Heparins* | (see p334 for more details on anticoagulation) | |
| Unfractionated heparin | *DVT prophylaxis:* 5000u/12h SC | SE of heparins: bleeding; thrombocytopenia; hypersensitivity; hyperkalaemia; osteoporosis after prolonged use. CI: coagulopathy; peptic ulcer; recent cerebral bleed; recent trauma or surgery; active bleeding. |
| Enoxaparin (Clexane®) | *DVT prophylaxis:* 20–40mg/24h SC. *DVT/PE treatment:* 1.5mg/kg/24h SC until warfarinized. Unstable angina: use fondaparinux, see p810 | |
| Tinzaparin | *DVT prophylaxis:* 3500u/24h SC (eg starting 2h pre-op). *DVT/PE treatment:* 175u/kg per 24h SC till warfarinized. | |
| Dalteparin (Fragmin®) | *DVT prophylaxis:* Start 2h pre-op 2500–5000u/24h SC. *DVT/PE treatment:* 150u/kg/d SC (18,000u/24h max). MI/STEMI, see p811. | |
| *Hypnotics* | | |
| Temazepam | 10–20mg PO at night | SE: Drowsiness; dependence. Zopiclone also causes bitter taste and GI disturbances. CI: Respiratory depression; myasthenia. |
| Zopiclone | 3.75–7.5mg PO at night | |
| *Tranquillizers* | | |
| Haloperidol | 0.5–1mg IM/IV initially in elderly (2–5mg younger patients), then every 4–8h till response, max 18mg in total. | SE: Extrapyramidal effects, sedation, hypotension, anti-muscarinic effects, neuroleptic malignant syndrome. Monitor BP. |
| *Others* | | |
| Naloxone | *In opiate overdose:* 0.4–2mg IV repeated every 2–3min to a maximum of 10mg if respiratory function does not improve. *To reverse opiate-induced respiratory depression:* 100–200µg IV every 2min. | SE: Tachycardia; fibrillation. Can precipitate opiate withdrawl. |
| Flumazenil | *To reverse benzodiazepines:* 200µg IV over 15s, then 100µg every 60s if required, up to 1mg max. | SE: Convulsions (esp. in epileptics); nausea and vomiting; flushing. Avoid if patient has a life-threatening illness controlled by benzodiazepines (eg status epilepticus). |

**See also:** laxatives (p248), inhalers (p175), digoxin (p116), insulin sliding scales (p591), fluids (p680), oxygen prescribing (p181).

## ▶▶Cardiorespiratory arrest

Ensure safety of patient and yourself. Confirm diagnosis (unconscious, apnoeic, absent carotid pulse). Call for help.

**Causes** MI; PE; trauma; tension pneumothorax, electrocution; shock; hypoxia; hypercapnia; hypothermia; U&E imbalance; drugs, eg digoxin.

**Basic life support** Shout for help. Ask someone to call the arrest team and bring the defibrillator. Note the time. Begin CPR as follows (ABC):

*Airway:* Head tilt (if no spine injury) + chin lift/jaw thrust. Clear the mouth.

*Breathing:* Check breathing then give 2 breaths after 1$^{st}$ set of compressions, each inflation ~1s long. Use specialized bag and mask system (eg Ambu® system) if available and 2 resuscitators present. Otherwise, mouth-to-mouth with valved pocket mask.

*Chest compressions:* Give 30 compressions to 2 breaths (30 : 2). CPR should not be interrupted except to give shocks or to intubate. Use the heel of hand with straight elbows. Centre over the lower ⅓ of the sternum; aim for 4cm compression at 100/min.

**Advanced life support** For algorithm and details, see over. Notes:
Place defibrillator paddles on chest as soon as possible and set monitor to read through the paddles if delay in attaching leads. Assess rhythm: is this VF/pulseless VT?
• In **VF/pulseless VT**, defibrillate without delay: 360J monophasic, 150–360J biphasic.
• **Asystole and electromechanical dissociation** (synonymous with pulseless electrical activity) are rhythms with a poorer prognosis than VF/VT, but potentially remediable (see BOX next page). Treatment may be life-saving.
• Obtain IV access and intubation if skilled person present, otherwise secure airway.
• Look for reversible causes of cardiac arrest, and treat accordingly.
• Check for pulse if ECG rhythm compatible with a cardiac output.
• **Reassess ECG rhythm.** Repeat defibrillation if still VF/VT. All shocks now at 360J.
• Send someone to find the patient's notes and the patient's usual doctor. These may give clues as to the cause of the arrest.
• If IV access fails, the intraosseous route (IO) is recommended for adults as well as children. Endotracheal delivery and intracardiac injection are not recommended.

**When to stop attempts at resuscitation** No general rule, as survival is influenced by the rhythm and the cause of the arrest. In patients without myocardial disease, do not stop until core temperature is >33°C and pH and potassium are normal. Consider stopping resuscitation attempts after 20min if there is refractory asystole or electromechanical dissociation.

**After successful resuscitation:**
• 12-lead ECG; CXR, U&Es, glucose, FBC, CK/troponin. ABG.
• Titrate oxygen to saturations of 94–98%, hyperoxaemia can worsen prognosis.[1]
• Transfer to ICU for consideration of therapeutic hypothermia.
• Monitor vital signs.
• Whatever the outcome, explain to relatives what has happened.

**When '*do not attempt resuscitate*' may be a valid decision** (UK DOH guidelines)
  if a patient's condition is such that resuscitation is unlikely to succeed.
  a mentally competent patient has consistently stated or recorded the fact that or she does not want to be resuscitated.
  the patient has signed an advanced directive forbidding resuscitation.
  resuscitation is not in a patient's interest as it would lead to a poor quality of life (often a great imponderable!). ▶*Ideally, involve patients and relatives in the decision before the emergency.* When in doubt, try to resuscitate.

**1** Association between arterial hyperoxia following resuscitation from cardiac arrest and in-hospital mortality. Kilgannon JH, Jones AE, Shapiro NI, *et al JAMA* 2010;303(21):2165-2171.

## UK Adult Basic Life-Support Algorithm 2010

The algorithm assumes that only one rescuer is present, with no equipment. (If a defibrillator is to hand, get a rhythm readout, and defibrillate, as opposite, as soon as possible.)

### Adult Basic Life Support

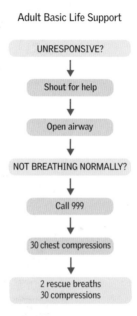

Algorithm reproduced with the permission of the Resuscitation Council (UK), © 2010.

Send or go for help as soon as possible, according to guidelines.

| **Managing the airway** | **Chest compressions** |
|---|---|
| You open the airway by tilting the head and lifting the chin—but only do this if there is no question of spinal trauma.<br><br>Use a close-fitting mask if available, held in place by thumbs pressing downwards either side of the mouth-piece, palms against cheeks. The mask should have a one-way valve to protect you. | Cardiopulmonary resuscitation (CPR) involves compressive force over the lower sternum, with the heels of the hands placed one on top of the other, directing the weight of your body through your vertical, straight arms.<br><br>Depth of compression:  4cm<br>Rate of compressions:  100/min |

Remember that these are guidelines only, and that the exact circumstances of the cardiorespiratory arrest will partly determine best practice. The guidelines are also more consensus based than evidence based (p644), and are likely to be adapted from time to time.